DVD AVAILABLE FROM THE
LIBRARY OFFICE

THE SHOULDER

THE SHOULDER

VOLUME TWO

EDITORS

Charles A. Rockwood, Jr., M.D.
Professor and Chairman Emeritus
Department of Orthopaedics
The University of Texas Health Science Center at San Antonio
San Antonio, Texas

Frederick A. Matsen III, M.D.
Professor and Chairman
Department of Orthopaedics and Sports Medicine
University of Washington School of Medicine
Seattle, Washington

Michael A. Wirth, M.D.
Professor, Department of Orthopaedics
The University of Texas Health Science Center at San Antonio
San Antonio, Texas

Steven B. Lippitt, M.D.
Northeast Ohio Orthopaedic Associates
Associate Professor of Orthopaedic Surgery
Northeastern Ohio Universities College of Medicine
Akron General Medical Center
Akron, Ohio

3rd EDITION

SAUNDERS
An Imprint of Elsevier

SAUNDERS
An Imprint of Elsevier

The Curtis Center
Independence Square West
Philadelphia, Pennsylvania 19106

THE SHOULDER   ISBN 0-7216-0148-0
Copyright © 2004, Elsevier. All rights reserved.

Notice

Orthopaedics is an ever-changing field. Standard safety precautions must be followed but as new research and clinical experience broaden our knowledge, changes in treatment and drug therapy may become necessary or appropriate. Readers are advised to check the most current product information provided by the manufacturer of each drug to be administered to verify the recommended dose, the method and duration of administration, and contraindications. It is the responsibility of the treating physician, relying on experience and knowledge of the patient, to determine dosages and the best treatment for each individual patient. Neither the publisher nor the author assumes any liability for any injury and/or damage to persons or property arising from this publication.

The Publisher

Library of Congress Cataloging-in-Publication Data

The shoulder / editors, Charles A. Rockwood, Jr. . . . [et al.].—3rd ed.
      p. ; cm.
         Includes bibliographical references and index.
         ISBN 0-7216-0148-0
         1. Shoulder—Diseases.   2. Shoulder—Surgery.   I. Rockwood, Charles A., Jr.
      [DNLM: 1. Shoulder.   2. Shoulder Joint. WE 810 S55861 2004]
RC939.S484 2004
617.5'72—dc22   2003057379

Publishing Director, Surgery: Richard Lampert
Developmental Editor: Arlene Chappelle
Publishing Services Manager: Tina Rebane

Printed in the United States of America.

Last digit is the print number: 9   8   7   6   5   4   3   2   1

We dedicate these volumes to our families, who have given us their fullest support and encouragement during our careers as shoulder surgeons. We also dedicate our work to the millions of individuals who experience shoulder problems, with the hope that our efforts will enable them to receive the best possible management leading to a prompt return to comfort and function. Finally, we dedicate our book to all those who are captivated by the shoulder and who pursue greater insights into its function, its malfunction, and the effective treatment of its clinical disorders.

CAR

FAM

MAW

SBL

CONTRIBUTORS

David. W. Altchek, M.D.
Associate Professor of Orthopaedics, Weill Medical
College of Cornell University, Hospital for Special
Surgery, New York, New York
Shoulder Arthroscopy

Laurie B. Amundsen, M.D.
Assistant Professor, Department of Anesthesiology,
University of Washington School of Medicine, Seattle,
Washington
Anesthesia for Shoulder Procedures

Kai-Nan An, Ph.D.
Professor and Chair, Division of Orthopedic Research,
Mayo Clinic, Rochester, Minnesota
Biomechanics of the Shoulder

Arash Araghi, D.O.
Shoulder Fellow, Department of Orthopaedic Surgery,
NYU–Hospital for Joint Diseases, New York, New York
Occupational Shoulder Disorders

Michel A. Arcand, M.D.
Memorial Orthopaedic Specialists, Memorial Hospital of
Rhode Island, Pawtucket, Rhode Island
The Biceps Tendon

Carl J. Basamania, M.D.
Assistant Professor of Surgery, Duke University Medical
Center, Durham, North Carolina
Fractures of the Clavicle

Louis U. Bigliani, M.D.
Frank E. Stinchfield Professor and Chairman, Center for
Shoulder, Elbow and Sports Medicine, Department of
Orthopaedic Surgery, Columbia-Presbyterian Medical
Center, Columbia University, New York, New York
Fractures of the Proximal Humerus

Theodore A. Blaine, M.D.
Assistant Director and Assistant Professor, Center for
Shoulder, Elbow and Sports Medicine, Department of
Orthopaedic Surgery, Columbia-Presbyterian Medical
Center, Columbia University, New York, New York
Fractures of the Proximal Humerus

Desmond J. Bokor, M.B.B.S., F.R.A.C.S.
Consultant Orthopaedic Surgeon, Western Sydney
Orthopaedic Associates, and Honorary Orthopaedic
Surgeon, University of Sydney and Westmead Hospital,
Sydney, Australia
Clinical Evaluation of Shoulder Problems

Jonathan Botts, B.A.
Research Assistant, Hospital for Special Surgery, New
York, New York
*Developmental Anatomy of the Shoulder and Anatomy of the
Glenohumeral Joint*

Ernest M. Burgess, M.D.[†]
Formerly Clinical Professor, Department of
Orthopaedics, University of Washington; Endowed
Chair of Orthopaedic Research, University of
Washington School of Medicine; Senior Scientist,
Prosthetics Research Study, Seattle, Washington
Amputations and Prosthetic Replacement

Wayne Z. Burkhead, Jr., M.D.
Clinical Associate Professor, University of Texas
Southwestern Medical Center; Attending Physician,
W. B. Carrell Memorial Clinic, Dallas, Texas
The Biceps Tendon

Mary Beth Cermak, M.D.
Medical Director, Hamot Surgery Center, and
Orthopaedic Surgeon, Shriners' Hospital for Children,
Erie, Pennsylvania
*Fractures, Dislocations, and Acquired Problems of the Shoulder
in Children*

Michael J. Coen, M.D.
Assistant Professor, Department of Orthopaedic
Surgery, Loma Linda University School of Medicine,
Loma Linda University Medical Center, Loma Linda,
California
Gross Anatomy of the Shoulder

Ernest U. Conrad III, M.D.
Professor of Orthopaedics, University of Washington
School of Medicine; Director of Sarcoma Service,
Director of Division of Orthopaedics, and Director of
Bone Tumor Clinic, Children's Hospital, University of
Washington, Children's Hospital and Medical Center,
Seattle, Washington
Tumors and Related Conditions

Edward V. Craig, M.D.
Professor of Clinical Surgery, Cornell University Medical
College; Attending Surgeon, Hospital for Special
Surgery, New York, New York
Fractures of the Clavicle

[†]Deceased

Joanna M. Davies, M.B.B.S.
Assistant Professor, University of Washington, Seattle, Washington
Anesthesia for Shoulder Procedures

Anthony F. DePalma, M.D.
Formerly Chairman, Department of Orthopaedic Surgery, Thomas Jefferson University Hospital, Philadelphia, Pennsylvania
Congenital Anomalies and Variational Anatomy of the Shoulder

Geoffrey F. Dervin, M.D., M.Sc., F.R.C.S.C.
Professor, Department of Orthopaedics, University of Ottawa, Ottawa Hospital, General Campus, Ottawa, Ontario, Canada
Calcifying Tendinitis

Mark Drakos, M.D.
Resident, Hospital for Special Surgery, New York, New York
Developmental Anatomy of the Shoulder and Anatomy of the Glenohumeral Joint

Stephen Fealy, M.D.
Assistant Attending, Orthopedic Surgery, Hospital for Special Surgery, Cornell University Medical Center, New York, New York
Developmental Anatomy of the Shoulder and Anatomy of the Glenohumeral Joint

John M. Fenlin, Jr., M.D.
Director of Shoulder Service, Jefferson University Hospital, and Clinical Professor of Orthopedic Surgery, Jefferson Medical College, The Rothman Institute, Philadelphia, Pennsylvania
Congenital Anomalies and Variational Anatomy of the Shoulder

Charles L. Getz, M.D.
Fellow of Shoulder and Elbow Surgery, University of Pennsylvania Medical School, Presbyterian Hospital, Philadelphia, Pennsylvania
Congenital Anomalies and Variational Anatomy of the Shoulder

Thomas P. Goss, M.D.
Professor of Orthopaedic Surgery, Department of Orthopaedics, and Chief of Shoulder Surgery and Attending Orthopaedic Surgeon, University of Massachusetts Memorial Medical Center, Worcester, Massachusetts
Fractures of the Scapula

Peter Habermeyer, M.D.
Professor, ATOS Praxisklinik, Heidelberg, Germany
The Biceps Tendon

Manny Halpern, Ph.D.
Senior Manager of Ergonomic Services, Occupational and Industrial Orthopaedic Center (OIOC), Hospital for Joint Diseases Orthopaedic Institute, Program of Ergonomics and Biomechanics, New York University, New York, New York
Occupational Shoulder Disorders

Douglas T. Harryman II, M.D.[†]
Formerly Assistant Professor, Department of Orthopaedic Surgery, University of Washington School of Medicine, Seattle, Washington
The Stiff Shoulder

Richard J. Hawkins, M.D.
Clinical Professor, University of Colorado, Denver, Colorado; Clinical Professor, University of Texas Southwestern Medical School, Dallas, Texas; Consultant, Vail Valley Medical Center and Steadman Hawkins Clinic, Vail, Colorado
Clinical Evaluation of Shoulder Problems

Eiji Itoi, M.D., Ph.D.
Professor and Chairman, Department of Orthopedic Surgery, Akita University School of Medicine, Akita, Japan
Biomechanics of the Shoulder

Kirk L. Jensen, M.D.
Assistant Clinical Professor, Department of Orthopaedic Surgery, University of California, San Francisco; Staff, San Francisco General Hospital, San Francisco; Staff, Orthopaedic Surgery, Summit Medical Center, Oakland, California
X-Ray Evaluation of Shoulder Problems

Christopher M. Jobe, M.D.
Professor, Orthopaedic Surgery, Department of Orthopaedic Surgery, Loma Linda University School of Medicine, Loma Linda University Medical Center; Consulting Staff, Jerry L. Pettis Memorial Veterans Administration Hospital, Loma Linda, California
Gross Anatomy of the Shoulder; The Shoulder in Sports

Frank W. Jobe, M.D.
Clinical Professor, Department of Orthopaedics, University of Southern California, Keck School of Medicine; Orthopaedic Consultant, Los Angeles Dodgers; Orthopaedic Consultant, PGA Tour and Senior PGA Tour; Associate, Kerlan-Jobe Orthopaedic Clinic, Los Angeles, California
The Shoulder in Sports

Sumant G. Krishnan, M.D.
Clinical Assistant Professor, Department of Orthopaedic Surgery, University of Texas Southwestern Medical Center; Attending Physician, Shoulder and Elbow Service, W. B. Carrell Memorial Clinic, Dallas, Texas
Clinical Evaluation of Shoulder Problems

Mark D. Lazarus, M.D.
Associate Professor, Department of Orthopaedic Surgery, The Rothman Institute, Thomas Jefferson University School of Medicine, Philadelphia, Pennsylvania
The Stiff Shoulder

[†]Deceased

William N. Levine, M.D.
Director of Sports Medicine, and Associate Director, Center for Shoulder, Elbow and Sports Medicine, Department of Orthopaedic Surgery, Columbia-Presbyterian Medical Center, Columbia University, New York, New York
Fractures of the Proximal Humerus

Steven B. Lippitt, M.D.
Associate Professor of Orthopaedic Surgery, Northeastern Ohio Universities College of Medicine, Akron General Medical Center, Akron, Ohio
Glenohumeral Instability; Rotator Cuff; Glenohumeral Arthritis and Its Management

Joachim F. Loehr, M.D.
Professor, Department of Orthopaedics, University of Luebeck, Germany
Calcifying Tendinitis

Frederick A. Matsen III, M.D.
Professor and Chairman, Department of Orthopaedics and Sports Medicine, University of Washington School of Medicine, Seattle, Washington
Glenohumeral Instability; Rotator Cuff; Glenohumeral Arthritis and Its Management; Effectiveness Evaluation and the Shoulder

Bernard F. Morrey, M.D.
Professor of Orthopedic Surgery, Mayo Medical School; Emeritus Chairman, Department of Orthopedics, Mayo Clinic, Rochester, Minnesota
Biomechanics of the Shoulder

Stephen J. O'Brien, M.D.
Associate Professor of Orthopaedic Surgery, Hospital for Special Surgery, Cornell University Medical College; Assistant Scientist, Associate Attending Orthopaedic Surgeon, New York Hospital, New York, New York
Developmental Anatomy of the Shoulder and Anatomy of the Glenohumeral Joint

Ira M. (Moby) Parsons, M.D.
Seacoast Orthopaedics and Sports Medicine, Somersworth, New Hampshire
Glenohumeral Arthritis and Its Management; Effectiveness Evaluation and the Shoulder

Marilyn M. Pink, Ph.D., P.T.
Director of Biomechanic Laboratory, Centinela Hospital Medical Center, Inglewood, California
The Shoulder in Sports

Robin R. Richards, M.D., F.R.C.S.C.
Professor of Surgery, University of Toronto; Surgeon-in-Chief, Sunnybrook and Women's College Health Sciences Centre, Toronto, Ontario, Canada
Sepsis of the Shoulder: Molecular Mechanisms and Pathogenesis

Charles A. Rockwood, Jr., M.D.
Professor and Chairman Emeritus, Department of Orthopaedics, The University of Texas Health Science Center at San Antonio, San Antonio, Texas
X-Ray Evaluation of Shoulder Problems; Fractures of the Clavicle; Disorders of the Acromioclavicular Joint; Disorders of the Sternoclavicular Joint; Glenohumeral Instability; Rotator Cuff; Glenohumeral Arthritis and Its Management

Robert L. Romano, M.D.
Clinical Professor, Department of Orthopaedics, University of Washington School of Medicine; Staff Physician, Providence Medical Center, Seattle, Washington
Amputations and Prosthetic Replacement

James O. Sanders, M.D.
Chief of Staff, Shriners Hospitals for Children, Erie, Pennsylvania
Fractures, Dislocations, and Acquired Problems of the Shoulder in Children

Peter T. Simonian, M.D.
Clinical Professor, Department of Orthopaedic Surgery, University of Washington School of Medicine, Seattle, Washington; Medical Director, Simonian Sports Medicine Clinic, Fresno, California
Muscle Ruptures Affecting the Shoulder Girdle

Douglas G. Smith, M.D.
Associate Professor, Department of Orthopaedic Surgery, University of Washington School of Medicine, Harborview Medical Center, Seattle, Washington
Amputations and Prosthetic Replacement

Kevin L. Smith, M.D.
Associate Professor, Department of Orthopaedics and Sports Medicine, University of Washington, and Shoulder and Elbow Service, Bone and Joint Center, University of Washington Medical Center, Seattle, Washington
Effectiveness Evaluation and the Shoulder

Robert J. Spinner, M.D.
Assistant Professor of Neurologic Surgery, Orthopedics and Anatomy, Department of Neurologic Surgery, Mayo Medical School, Mayo Clinic, Rochester, Minnesota
Nerve Problems About the Shoulder

Scott P. Steinmann, M.D.
Assistant Professor of Orthopedic Surgery, Mayo Medical School, Mayo Clinic, Rochester, Minnesota
Nerve Problems About the Shoulder

James E. Tibone, M.D.
Moss Foundation Professor, The Moss Foundation Professorship in Sports Medicine in memory of Dr. Robert K. Kerlan, and Clinical Professor, Department of Orthopaedics, University of California, Keck School of Medicine; Associate, Kerlan-Jobe Orthopaedic Clinic, Los Angeles, California
The Shoulder in Sports

Robert M. Titelman, M.D.
Resurgeons Orthopaedics, Atlanta, Georgia
Glenohumeral Instability; Rotator Cuff

Hans K. Uhthoff, M.D.
Professor Emeritus, University of Ottawa; Attending
Physician, Ottawa Hospital, General Campus, Ottawa,
Ontario, Canada
Calcifying Tendinitis

Todd W. Ulmer, M.D.
Acting Director, Sports Medicine, University of
Washington, Department of Orthopaedics and Sports
Medicine, Seattle, Washington
Muscle Ruptures Affecting the Shoulder Girdle

Christopher J. Wahl, M.D.
Center for Orthopaedics, New Haven, Connecticut
Shoulder Arthroscopy

Gilles Walch, M.D.
Clinique St. Anne-Lumiere, Lyon, France
The Biceps Tendon

Russell F. Warren, M.D.
Professor of Orthopaedics, Weill Medical College of
Cornell University; Surgeon-in-Chief, Hospital for
Special Surgery, New York, New York
Shoulder Arthroscopy

Gerald R. Williams Jr., M.D.
Associate Professor, Department of Orthopaedic
Surgery, University of Pennsylvania Health System;
Chief, Shoulder and Elbow Service, and Chief of
Orthopaedic Surgery, Presbyterian Medical Center,
Philadelphia, Pennsylvania
Disorders of the Acromioclavicular Joint

Michael A. Wirth, M.D.
Professor, Department of Orthopaedics, The University
of Texas Health Science Center at San Antonio, San
Antonio, Texas
*Disorders of the Sternoclavicular Joint; Glenohumeral
Instability; Rotator Cuff; Glenohumeral Arthritis and Its
Management*

D. Christopher Young, M.D.
Associate Clinical Professor, Orthopaedic Surgery,
Medical College of Virginia; Orthopaedic Surgeon, West
End Orthopaedic Clinic, Richmond, Virginia
Disorders of the Acromioclavicular Joint

Craig Zeman, M.D.
Orthopaedic Surgeon, Ventura Orthopaedic and Sports
Medical Group, Oxnard, California
The Biceps Tendon

Joseph D. Zuckerman, M.D.
Department of Orthopaedic Surgery, NYU—Hospital for
Joint Diseases, New York, New York
Occupational Shoulder Disorders

FOREWORD
to the Third Edition

Publishing companies do not re-issue books that are inaccurate, unused, or unpopular. So, there is a good reason to be excited about the third edition of *The Shoulder*, edited by Drs. Rockwood, Matsen, Wirth, and Lippitt. Not too long ago, as history is measured, we considered ourselves to be in the early stages of learning about the shoulder joint—its functional anatomy, its injury patterns, and, very importantly, its optimal treatment.

Since the first edition of this book, our technical capabilities in imaging, instrumentation, and pain control have improved tremendously. Chapters dealing with these aspects of shoulder care reflect this heightened scrutiny. Continuing interest in and understanding of both developmental and functional anatomy allow us to comprehend the biomechanics of not only the pathologic shoulder, but also the normal shoulder. Without a clear picture of normal shoulder function, our devising and refinement of correctional procedures would lack a clear direction.

The editors have succeeded in assembling a panel of chapter authors with acknowledged skills in shoulder diagnosis and management. Perhaps more importantly, the contributing authors also demonstrate a commitment to the pursuit of better understanding and more effective treatments, rather than just relying on traditional methods. And, even more importantly, these authors are also discriminating about incorporating some of these newer techniques that may represent a triumph of technology over reason.

Finally, some of you know, and most of you can imagine, how much work it is to write and assemble a quality text such as this. It is our considerable good fortune to have these editors at the forefront of our profession, willing and able to undertake this arduous task, and producing a work of such outstanding breadth and quality.

FRANK W. JOBE, M.D.
Kerlan-Jobe Orthopaedic Clinic
Centinela Hospital Medical Center
Inglewood, California
January, 2004

FOREWORD
to the First Edition

It is a privilege to write the Foreword for *The Shoulder* by Drs. Charles A. Rockwood, Jr., and Frederick A. Matsen III. Their objective when they began this work was an all-inclusive text on the shoulder that would also include all references on the subject in the English literature. Forty-six authors have contributed to this text.

The editors of *The Shoulder* are two of the leading shoulder surgeons in the United States. Dr. Rockwood was the fourth President of the American Shoulder and Elbow Surgeons, has organized the Instructional Course Lectures on the Shoulder for the Annual Meeting of the American Academy of Orthopaedic Surgeons for many years, and is a most experienced and dedicated teacher. Dr. Matsen is President-Elect of the American Shoulder and Elbow Surgeons and is an unusually talented teacher and leader. These two men, with their academic know-how and the help of their contributing authors, have organized a monumental text for surgeons in training and in practice, as well as one that can serve as an extensive reference source. They are to be commended for this superior book.

CHARLES S. NEER II, M.D.
Professor Emeritus, Orthopaedic Surgery,
Columbia University; Chief, Shoulder Service,
Columbia-Presbyterian Medical Center, New York

PREFACE

Dear Readers,

Thank you for joining us in our interest in the body's most fascinating joint: the shoulder.

Where else are we challenged by complex anatomy, huge functional demands, and clinical problems ranging from congenital disorders to fractures, arthritis, instability, stiffness, tendon disorders, and tumors? To help patients with these problems we have powerful diagnostic and therapeutic tools that we must understand how to use effectively: clinical examination, radiographs, ultrasound, MRI, arthroscopy, and open surgery. We are now learning that the value of these tools must be considered in terms of their effectiveness in improving the comfort and function of the shoulder as assessed by the patient.

The two of us have been partners in the shoulder for over two decades. While we have never practiced together, it became evident early on that the San Antonio and the Seattle schools of thought were more often congruent than divergent—whether the topic was the rotator cuff, instability, or glenohumeral arthritis. We have also gained a great respect for those with other ideas, be they in other parts of the United States or abroad. Our courses and travels have put us in contact with creative thinkers and innovators from around the world. To capture the extant diversity of thought regarding the shoulder is a formidable challenge. In this task we have enlisted the help of Steven Lippitt and Michael Wirth as editors as well as a great group of chapter contributors. In this the third edition of *The Shoulder*, we have expanded the horizon while still honing in on the methods preferred by the authors selected for each of the chapters.

We encourage you to be aggressive in your pursuit of new shoulder knowledge and conservative in your adoption of the many new approaches being proposed for the evaluation and management of the shoulder. We hope this book will give you a basis for considering what might be in the best interest of your patients. We hope you enjoy reading this book as much as we enjoyed editing it.

Best wishes to each of you—happy shouldering!

CHARLES A. ROCKWOOD, JR.
FREDERICK A. MATSEN III
January, 2004

CONTENTS

VOLUME TWO

CHAPTER 14

Glenohumeral Instability

Frederick A. Matsen III, M.D.,   Robert M. Titelman, M.D.,   Steven B. Lippitt, M.D.,
Charles A. Rockwood, Jr., M.D.,   and Michael A. Wirth, M.D.

• • • •

It deserves to be known how a shoulder which is subject to frequent dislocations should be treated. For many persons owing to this accident have been obliged to abandon gymnastic exercises, though otherwise well qualified for them; and from the same misfortune have become inept in warlike practices, and have thus perished. And this subject deserves to be noticed, because I have never known any physician [to] treat the case properly; some abandon the attempt altogether, and others hold opinions and practice the very reverse of what is proper.

- Hippocrates 2400 years ago

In every case the anterior margin of the glenoid cavity will be found to be smooth, rounded, and free of any attachments, and a blunt instrument can be passed freely inwards over the bare bone on the front of the neck of the scapula.

- Perthes 1906

. . . the only rational treatment is to reattach the glenoid ligament (or the capsule) to the bone from which it has been torn.

- Bankart 1939[34]

HISTORICAL REVIEW

Early Descriptions

The first report of a shoulder dislocation is found in humankind's oldest book, the Edwin Smith Papyrus (3000-2500 BC).[793] Hussein[305] reported that in 1200 BC in the tomb of Upuy, an artist and sculptor to Ramses II, there was a drawing of a scene that was strikingly similar to Kocher's method of reduction (Fig. 14–1).

The most detailed early description of anterior dislocations came from the father of medicine, Hippocrates, who was born in 460 BC on the island of Cos.[1] Hippocrates described the anatomy of the shoulder, the types of dislocations, and the first surgical procedure. In one of his classic procedures for reduction, he stressed the need for suitably sized, leather-covered balls to be placed into the axilla, for without them the heel could not reach the head of the humerus in his reduction maneuver. Other Hippocratic techniques are described by Brockbank and Griffiths (Fig. 14–2).[73]

Hippocrates criticized his contemporaries for improper burning of the shoulder, a treatment popular at the time. In this first description of a surgical procedure for recurrent dislocation of the shoulder, he described how physicians had burned the top, anterior, and poste-

rior aspects of the shoulder, which only caused scarring in those areas and promoted downward dislocation. He advocated the use of cautery in which an oblong, red-hot iron was inserted through the axilla to make eschars, but only in the lower part of the joint. Hippocrates displayed considerable knowledge of the anatomy of the shoulder, and he warned the surgeon to not let the iron come in contact with the major vessels and nerves because it would cause great harm. Following the burnings, he bound the arm to the side, day and night for a long time, "for thus more especially will cicatrization take place, and the wide space into which the humerus used to escape will become contracted."

Interested readers are referred to the text by H. F. Moseley,[490] which has a particularly good section on the historical aspects of management of shoulder instability.

Humeral Head Defect

In 1861, Flower[190] described the anatomic and pathologic changes found in 41 traumatically dislocated shoulders from specimens in London museums. He wrote that "where the head of the humerus rests upon the edge of the glenoid fossa absorption occurs, and a groove is evacuated, usually between the articular head and the greater tuberosity." In 1880, Eve[170] reported an autopsy of a

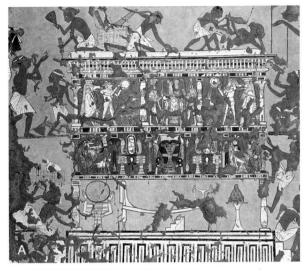

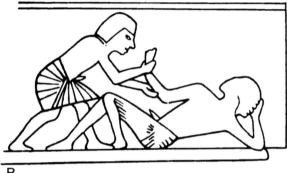

■ Figure 14–1
The Kocher technique is 3000 years old. **A,** Drawing from the tomb of Upuy in the year 1200 BC. (All rights reserved, The Metropolitan Museum of Art. Egyptian Expedition of the Metropolitan Museum of Art, Rogers Fund, 1930. Photograph—1978 The Metropolitan Museum of Art.) **B,** Schematic drawing of the picture in the upper right corner of the tomb painting depicting a patient on the ground while a man—possibly a physician—is manipulating a dislocated shoulder in the technique of Kocher. *(From Hussein MK: Kocher's method is 3,000 years old. J Bone Joint Surg Br 50:669-671, 1968.)*

patient who died 12 hours after an acute anterior dislocation in which he found a deep groove in the posterolateral aspect of the head. Joessel[334] also observed the defect. According to Hill and Sachs,[283] beginning in 1882, publications by Kuster,[373] Cramer,[119] Löbker,[416] Schüller,[637] Staffel,[671] and Francke[192] described the finding of a posterolateral defect in humeral heads resected for relief of chronic or recurrent dislocation.

In 1887, Caird[81] of Edinburgh concluded that a true subcoracoid dislocation must have an indentation fracture of the humeral head that is produced by the dense, hard anterior lip of the glenoid fossa. In cadaver experiments, he was able to produce the head defect. He said that the hard, dense glenoid lip would cut into the soft cancellous bone like a knife (Fig. 14–3).

Roentgen's discovery of x-rays in 1895 ushered in new evaluations and studies of the anatomy of the anterior glenoid and humeral head defects. The first description of the radiographic changes in the humeral head associated with recurrent instability is attributed to Francke[192] in

1898, only 3 years after Roentgen's discovery.[278] Hermodsson demonstrated that the posterolateral humeral head defect is the result of a compression fracture caused by the anterior glenoid rim following the exit of the humeral head from the glenoid fossa.[278] He also observed that (1) the defect is seen in the majority of cases; (2) the longer the head is dislocated, the larger the defect will be; (3) the defects are generally larger in anteroinferior dislocations than in anterior dislocations; and (4) the defect is usually larger in recurrent anterior dislocations of the shoulder.

In 1925, Pilz[566] reported the first detailed radiographic examination of recurrent dislocation of the shoulder and stated that routine radiographs were of little help. He stressed the need for an angled-beam projection to observe the defect. In 1940, Hill and Sachs[283] published a very clear and concise review of the available information on the humeral head compression fracture defect that now carries their names.

Anterior Capsule and Muscle Defects

According to the Hunterian Lecture given by Reeves in 1967, Roger of Palermo in the 13th century taught that the lesion in an acute dislocation was a capsular rupture. Bankart,[32] following the concepts of Broca and Hartmann,[72] Perthes,[564] Flower,[190] and Caird,[81] claimed that the essential lesion was detachment of the labrum and capsule from the anterior glenoid as a result of forward translation of the humeral head (referred to by subsequent authors as the Bankart lesion) (see Fig. 14–3). Later experimental and clinical work by Reeves[582] and Townley[704] suggested that other lesions may be responsible for recurrent dislocation, such as failure of the initial injury to incite a healing response, detachment of the subscapularis tendon, and variance in attachment of the inferior glenohumeral ligament.

Moseley and Overgaard[493] found laxity in 25 consecutive cases, and DePalma and associates[140] reported subscapularis laxity, rupture, and decreased muscle tone in 38 consecutive cases. Several of their cases and some from Hauser[258] revealed a definite defect along the anterior or inferior aspect of the subscapularis tendon, as though it had been partially torn from its bone attachment, along with separation of the muscle fibers that insert into the humerus directly below the lesser tuberosity. McLaughlin,[456] DePalma and associates,[140] Jens,[323] and Reeves[584] have noted at the time of surgery before arthrotomy that with abduction and external rotation, the humeral head would dislocate under the lower edge of the subscapularis tendon. Symeonides[685] took biopsy samples of the subscapularis muscle tendon unit at the time of surgery and found microscopic evidence of "healed post-traumatic lesions." He stated that instability results because traumatic lengthening of the subscapularis muscle leads to loss of the power necessary to stabilize the shoulder.

Rotator Cuff Injuries

In 1880, Joessel[334] reported on his careful postmortem studies of four cases of known recurrent dislocation of the

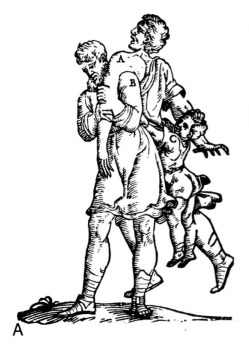

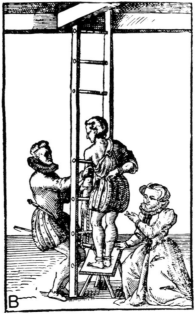

■ **Figure 14–2**
Modified techniques of Hippocrates to reduce dislocations of the shoulder. **A,** Reduction over the operator's shoulder. (From the Venice edition of Galen in 1625.) **B,** Reduction over the rung of a ladder. When the stepstool on which the patient is standing is withdrawn, the weight of the patient's body produces a reduction of the dislocation. (From deCruce in 1607.) **C,** Use of the rack to reduce a shoulder dislocation (Vidius). **D,** Reduction of a dislocation by a medieval type of screw traction (From Scultetus in 1693). *(From Brockbank W and Griffiths DL: Orthopaedic surgery in the 16th and 17th centuries. J Bone Joint Surg Br 30:365–375, 1948.)*

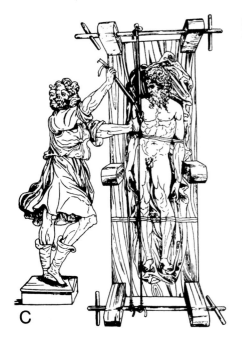

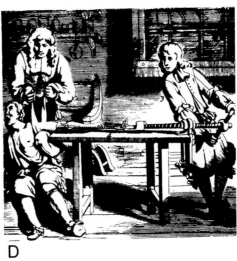

shoulder. In all cases he found a rupture of the postero-lateral portion of the rotator cuff from the greater tuberosity and a greatly increased shoulder joint capsule volume (Figs. 14–4 and 14–5). He also noted fractures of the humeral head and the anterior glenoid rim (Fig. 14–6). Joessel concluded that cuff disruptions that did not heal predisposed to recurrence of the problem, that recurrences were facilitated by the enlarged capsule, and that fractures of the glenoid or the head of the humerus resulted in a smaller articular surface, which may tend to produce recurrent dislocation. However, his four patients were elderly and may have had the degenerative cuff changes so common in older people.

Treatment of Acute Traumatic Dislocations

Hippocrates[287] discussed in detail at least six different techniques to reduce a dislocated shoulder. From century to century the literature has included woodcuts, drawings, and redrawings illustrating modifications of Hippocrates' teachings by such investigators as Paré, de Cruce, Vidius, and Scultetus. Hippocrates' original technique[1] is still used on occasion. The stockinged foot of the physician is used as countertraction. The heel should not go into the axilla (i.e., between the anterior and posterior axillary folds) but should extend across the folds and against the chest wall. Traction should be slow and gentle; as with all

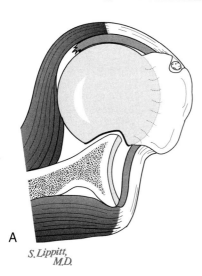

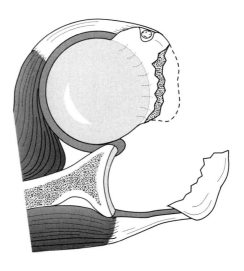

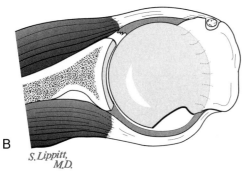

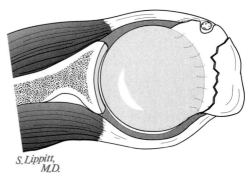

■ **Figure 14–3**
A, Anterior dislocation shown in an axillary projection with a posterior lateral humeral head defect (Hill-Sachs defect) and a tear of the anterior capsule and labrum from the glenoid lip (Bankart lesion). **B,** The dislocation is reduced, but the humeral head and capsular lesions remain.

■ **Figure 14–5**
This anterior dislocation is shown in the axillary projection with a displaced fracture of the greater tuberosity.

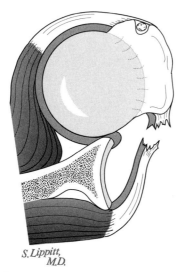

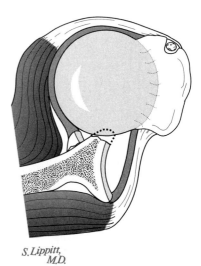

■ **Figure 14–4**
An anterior dislocation shown in an axillary projection with a tear in the posterior rotator cuff.

■ **Figure 14–6**
This anterior dislocation is shown in the axillary projection with a displaced fracture of the anterior glenoid rim.

traction techniques, the arm may be gently rotated internally and externally to disengage the head.

In 1870, Theodore Kocher,[363] a Nobel Prize winner for medicine in 1909, gave a somewhat confusing report of his technique for levering in an anteriorly dislocated shoulder. Had Kocher not been so famous as a thyroid surgeon, his article might have received only scant attention.

In 1938 Milch[472] described a technique for reduction in the supine position whereby the arm is abducted and externally rotated and the thumb is used to gently push the head of the humerus back in place. Lacey[374] modified the technique by performing the maneuver with the patient prone on an examining table. Russell and associates[623] reported on the ease and success of this technique.

In the Kocher technique, the humeral head is levered on the anterior glenoid and the shaft is levered against the anterior thoracic wall until the reduction is completed. DePalma[137] warned that undue forces used in rotation leverage can damage the soft tissues of the shoulder joint, the vessels, and the brachial plexus. Beattie and coworkers[43] reported a fracture of the humeral neck during a Kocher procedure. Other authors have described spiral fractures of the upper shaft of the humerus and further damage to the anterior capsular mechanism when the Kocher leverage technique of reduction was used. McMurray[463] reported that of 64 dislocations reduced by the Kocher method, 40% became recurrent, whereas of 112 dislocations reduced by gently lifting the head in place, only 12% became recurrent.

Since 1975, numerous articles have described simple techniques to reduce a dislocated shoulder: the forward elevation maneuver,[320,731] the external rotation method,[405,478] scapular manipulation,[9] the modified gravity method,[408] the crutch and chair technique,[552] the chair and pillow technique,[756] and others.[105,434]

Operative Reconstructions for Anterior Instability

Most of the published literature on shoulder dislocations is concerned with the problem of recurrent anterior dislocations. As mentioned previously, Hippocrates[287] described the use of a white-hot poker to scar the anteroinferior part of the capsule. Since then, hundreds of operative procedures have been described for the management of recurrent anterior dislocations. Readers who have a yearning for the detailed history should read the classic texts by Moseley[490] and Hermodsson.[278]

Various operative techniques have been based on the posterolateral defect and soft tissue disruptions on the front of the shoulder. Bardenheuer[36] in 1886 and Thomas[692,693] from 1909 to 1921 discussed capsular plication or shrinking; in 1888, Albert[7] performed arthrodesis; and in 1901, Hildebrand[282] deepened the glenoid socket.

In 1906, Perthes[564] wrote a classic paper on the operative treatment of recurrent dislocations. He stated that the operation should be directed at repairing the underlying lesion (i.e., repair of the capsule, the glenoid labrum detachment from the anterior bony rim, and the rotator cuff tear). He repaired the capsule with suture to the anterior glenoid rim through drill holes and, in several cases, used staples to repair the anterior capsular structures. This report gave the first description of repair of the anterior labrum and capsule to the anterior glenoid rim. Two patients were monitored for 17 years, one for 12 years, two for 3 years, and one for 1 year and 9 months. All had excellent function with no recurrence.

The muscle sling myoplasty operation was used in 1913 by Clairmont and Ehrlich.[100] The posterior third of the deltoid, with its innervation left intact, was removed from its insertion on the humerus, passed through the quadrilateral space, and sutured to the coracoid process. When the arm was abducted, the deltoid contracted, which held up the humeral head. Finsterer,[185] in a similar but reversed procedure, used the coracobrachialis and the short head of the biceps from the coracoid and transferred them posteriorly. Both operations failed because of high recurrence rates.

In 1923, Bankart[32] first published his operative technique and noted that only two classes of operations were used at that time for recurrent dislocation of the shoulder: (1) those designed to diminish the size of the capsule by plication or pleating[692,693] and (2) those designed to give inferior support to the capsule.[100,103] Bankart condemned both in preference to his procedure. He stated that the essential lesion was detachment or rupture of the capsule from the glenoid ligament. He recommended repair with interrupted sutures of silkworm gut passed between the free edge of the capsule and the glenoid ligament. At that time he did not repair the lateral capsule to the bone of the anterior glenoid rim. In his 1939 article, Bankart[34] described the essential lesion as "detachment of the glenoid ligament from the anterior margin of the glenoid cavity" and stated that "the only rational treatment is to reattach the glenoid ligament (or the capsule) to the bone from which it has been torn." He further wrote that "the glenoid ligament may be found lying loose either on the head of the humerus or the margin of the glenoid cavity." He recommended repair of the lateral capsule down to the raw bone of the anterior glenoid and that it be held in place with suture through drill holes made in the anterior glenoid rim with sharp, pointed forceps. Although no references were listed in either article, Bankart must have been greatly influenced by the previously published work of Broca and Hartmann[72] and particularly that of Perthes,[564] which described virtually identical pathology and repair.

Beginning in 1929, Nicola[512-516] published a series of articles on management of recurrent dislocation of the shoulder. He used the long head of the biceps tendon and the coracohumeral ligament as a suspension checkrein to the front of the shoulder. Henderson[273,274] described another checkrein operation that looped half the peroneus longus tendon through drill holes in the acromion and the greater tuberosity. In 1927, Gallie and LeMesurier[197] described the use of autogenous fascia lata suture in the treatment of recurrent dislocation of the shoulder. This procedure has been modified by Bateman.[41]

Posterior Glenohumeral Instability

In 1839 in a Guy's Hospital report,[113] Sir Astley Cooper described in detail a dislocation of the os humeri on the dorsum scapulae. This report is a classic, for Cooper presented most of the characteristics associated with posterior dislocations: the dislocation occurred during an epileptic seizure; the pain was greater than with the usual anterior dislocation; external rotation of the arm was entirely impeded, and the patient could not elevate his arm from his side; the shoulder had an anterior void or flatness and a posterior fullness; and the patient was "unable to use or move his arm to any extent." In this report of a case in which Cooper had acted as a consultant, reduction could not be accomplished and the patient never recovered the use of his shoulder. Postmortem examination of the shoulder, performed 7 years later, revealed that the subscapularis tendon was detached and the infraspinatus muscles were stretched posteriorly about the head of the humerus. The report suggested that the detached subscapularis was "the cause of the symptoms." Cooper further described resorption of the anterior aspect of the humeral head where it was in contact with the posterior glenoid—probably the first description of the so-called reversed Hill-Sachs lesion.

Another classic article on the subject was published in 1855 by Malgaigne,[433] who reported on 37 cases of posterior dislocation of the shoulder. Three cases were his own and 34 were reviewed from the literature. This series of cases was collected 40 years before the discovery of x-rays, and it points out that with adequate physical examination of the patient, the correct diagnosis can be made.

RELEVANT ANATOMY

The Skin

Shoulder stabilization surgery can usually be accomplished through cosmetically acceptable incisions in the lines of the skin (see also Chapter 2). Anteriorly, the surgeon can identify and mark the prominent anterior

axillary crease by adducting the shoulder. An incision placed in the lower part of this crease provides excellent access to the shoulder for anterior repair and yet heals nicely with subcuticular closure (Figs. 14–7 and 14–8). When cosmesis is a concern, the incision can be made more into the axilla as described by Leslie and Ryan.[396]

Posteriorly, an analogous vertical incision in line with the extended posterior axillary crease (best visualized by extending the shoulder backward) also heals well (Fig. 14–9). Fortuitously, these creases lie directly over the joint to which the surgeon needs access.

The First Muscle Layer

The shoulder is covered by the deltoid muscle arising from the clavicle, acromion, and scapular spine. The anterior deltoid extends to a line running approximately from the midclavicle to the midlateral portion of the humerus. This line passes over the cephalic vein, the anterior venous drainage of the deltoid, and the coracoid process. The deltoid is innervated by the axillary nerve, whose branches swoop upward as they extend anteriorly (Fig. 14–10). The commonly described "safe zone" 5 cm distal to the acromion does not take into account these anterior branches, which may come as close as 2 cm to the acromion. At the deltopectoral groove, the deltoid meets the clavicular head of the pectoralis major, which assists the anterior deltoid in forward flexion. The medial and lateral pectoral nerves are not in the surgical field of shoulder stabilization. Splitting the deltopectoral interval just medial to the cephalic vein preserves the deltoid's

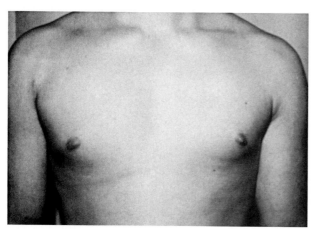

■ **Figure 14–7**

A cosmetic anterior approach on the patient's right shoulder. The incision is made in the axillary skin crease.

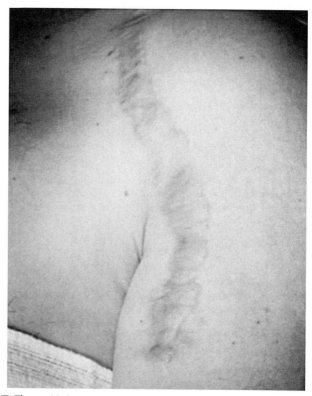

■ **Figure 14–8**

A noncosmetic approach across the front of the shoulder.

venous drainage and takes the surgeon to the next layer. It is important to note that extension of the shoulder tightens the pectoralis major and the anterior deltoid, as well as the coracoid muscles, and thus compromises the exposure. Accordingly, surgical assistants must be reminded to hold the shoulder in slight flexion to relax these muscles and facilitate access to the joint.

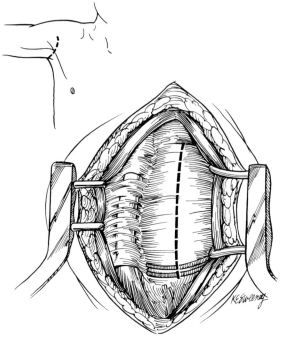

■ Figure 14–9
A posterior approach for treatment of posterior glenohumeral instability. The incision is centered over the posterior glenoid rim *(inset)*. Note the deltoid-splitting approach to minimize the amount of deltoid origin that must be released. Also note the incision in the infraspinatus and teres minor tendons. *(From Matsen FA and Thomas SC: Glenohumeral instability. In Evarts CM [ed]: Surgery of the Musculoskeletal System, 2nd ed. New York: Churchill Livingstone, 1989.)*

Posteriorly, the medial edge of the deltoid is too medial to provide useful access to the glenohumeral joint. Access must be achieved by splitting the deltoid, which is most conveniently done at the junction of its middle and posterior thirds. This junction is marked by the posterior corner of the acromion. The site is favorable for a split because it overlies the joint and also because the axillary nerve exiting the quadrangular space divides into two trunks (its anterior and posterior branches) near the inferior aspect of the split.

The Coracoacromial Arch and Clavipectoral Fascia

The coracoid process is the "lighthouse" of the anterior aspect of the shoulder in that it provides a palpable guide to the deltopectoral groove, a locator for the coracoacromial arch, and an anchor for the coracoid muscles (the coracobrachialis and short head of the biceps) that separate the lateral "safe side" from the medial "suicide" where the brachial plexus and major vessels lie. The surgeon comes to full appreciation of the value of such a lighthouse when it is lacking—for example, when re-exploring a shoulder for complications of a coracoid transfer procedure. The clavipectoral fascia covers the floor of the deltopectoral groove. Rotating the humerus enables the surgeon to identify the subscapularis moving beneath this fascial layer. Incising the fascia up to but not through the coracoacromial ligament preserves the stabilizing function of the coracoacromial arch.

The Humeroscapular Motion Interface

The humeroscapular motion interface (Fig. 14–11) separates the structures that do not move on humeral rotation (the deltoid, coracoid muscles, acromion, and coracoacromial ligament) from those that do (the rotator cuff,

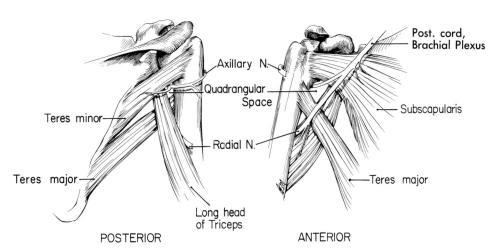

■ Figure 14–10
Relationships of the axillary nerve to the subscapularis muscle, the quadrangular space, and the neck of the humerus. With anterior dislocations, the subscapularis is displaced forward, which creates a traction injury in the axillary nerve. The nerve cannot move out of the way because it is held above by the brachial plexus and below where it wraps around behind the neck of the humerus. *(From Rockwood CA and Green DP [eds]: Fractures, 3 vols, 2nd ed. Philadelphia: JB Lippincott, 1984.)*

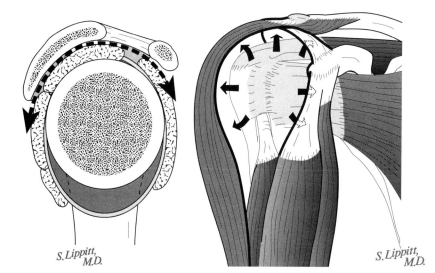

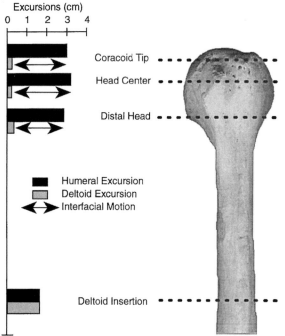

■ **Figures 14-11**

The humeroscapular motion interface is an important location of motion between the humerus and the scapula. The deltoid, acromion, coracoacromial ligament, coracoid process, and tendons attaching to the coracoid lie on the superficial side of this interface, whereas the proximal end of the humerus, rotator cuff, and biceps tendon sheath lie on the deep side. *(Modified from Matsen FA III, Lippitt SE, Sidles JA, and Harryman DT II: Practical Evaluation and Management of the Shoulder. Philadelphia: WB Saunders, 1994.)*

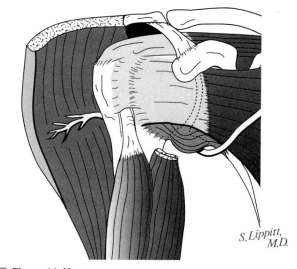

■ **Figure 14–13**

The axillary nerve in the humeroscapular motion interface between the cuff and the humerus on the inside and the coracoid muscles and the deltoid on the outside. *(From Matsen FA III, Lippitt SB, Sidles JA, and Harryman DT II: Practical Evaluation and Management of the Shoulder. Philadelphia: WB Saunders, 1994.)*

■ **Figure 14–12**

Mean humeroscapular interface motion recorded in vivo from five normal subjects with the use of magnetic resonance imaging. The humerus at the right shows the levels at which the motions were measured. The excursion (in centimeters) of the humerus *(black)* and the deltoid *(gray)* from maximal internal to maximal external rotation is indicated by the *horizontal bars.* The magnitudes of motion at the interface between the deltoid and the humerus are indicated by the *double-headed arrows.* The mean excursion at the humerothoracic motion interface was approximately 3 cm proximally and 0 cm at the deltoid insertion. *(From Matsen FA III, Lippitt SB, Sidles JA, and Harryman DT II: Practical Evaluation and Management of the Shoulder. Philadelphia: WB Saunders, 1994.)*

long head of the biceps tendon, and humeral tuberosities). During shoulder motion, substantial gliding takes place at this interface (Fig. 14–12). The humeroscapular motion interface provides a convenient plane for medial and lateral retractors and is also the plane in which the principal nerves lie.

The axillary nerve runs in the humeroscapular motion interface, superficial to the humerus and cuff and deep to the deltoid and coracoid muscles (Fig. 14–13; see also Fig. 14–10). Sweeping a finger in a superior-to-inferior direction along the anterior aspect of the subscapularis muscle catches the axillary nerve, which hangs like a watch chain across the muscle belly. Tracing this nerve proximally and medially leads the finger to the bulk of the brachial plexus. Tracing it laterally and posteriorly leads the finger beneath the shoulder capsule toward the quadrangular space. From a posterior vantage, the axillary nerve is seen to exit the quadrangular space beneath the teres minor and extend laterally, where it is applied to the deep surface of the deltoid muscle. By virtue of its prominent location in close proximity to the shoulder joint anteriorly, inferiorly, and posteriorly, the axillary nerve is the most frequently injured structure in shoulder surgery.

The musculocutaneous nerve lies on the deep surface of the coracoid muscles and penetrates the coracobrachialis with one or more branches lying a variable distance distal to the coracoid. (The often-described 5-cm "safe zone" for the nerve beneath the process refers only to the average position of the main trunk and not to an area that can be entered recklessly.) The musculocutaneous nerve is vulnerable to injury from retractors placed under the coracoid muscles and to traction injury during coracoid transfer. Knowledge of the position of these nerves can make the shoulder surgeon both more comfortable and more effective.

The Rotator Cuff

The next layer of the shoulder is the rotator cuff. The tendons of these muscles blend in with the capsule as they insert into the humeral tuberosities.[101] Thus, in reconstructions that require splitting of these muscles from the capsule, such splitting is more easily accomplished medially, before the blending becomes complete. The nerves to these muscles run on their deep surfaces: the upper and lower subscapular to the subscapularis and the suprascapular to the supraspinatus and infraspinatus. Medial dissection on the deep surface of these muscles may jeopardize their nerve supply.[788] The superior portion of the subscapularis tendon has been found to have significantly higher stiffness and ultimate load than its inferior portion has.[243]

The capsule is relatively thin between the supraspinatus and the subscapularis (the "rotator interval"). This thinness allows the cuff to slide back and forth around the coracoid process as the arm is elevated and lowered. Splitting this interval toward the base of the coracoid may be helpful when mobilization of the subscapularis is needed.

The tendon of the long head of the biceps originates from the supraglenoid tubercle (Figs. 14–14 and 14–15). It runs beneath the cuff in the area of the rotator interval and exits the shoulder beneath the transverse humeral ligament and between the greater and lesser tuberosities. It is subject to injury when incising the upper subscapularis from the lesser tuberosity. In the bicipital groove of the humerus, this tendon is endangered by procedures that involve lateral transfer of the subscapularis tendon across the groove (see also Chapters 1 and 2).

The Scapulohumeral Ligaments

Though often suggested as the "primary stabilizers" of the glenohumeral joint, the scapulohumeral ligaments are now recognized to play a role primarily in positions near the extremes of the allowed range of motion. The thickness of the capsule decreases as it nears the humerus. The capsule is found to be thickest in the inferior pouch at 2.8 mm, whereas it is 2.4 mm in its anterior portion and 2.2 mm in the posterior portion. The thickness ranges from 1.3 to 4.5 mm in cadaveric specimens.[99] The glenohumeral joint capsule is normally large, loose, and redundant, which allows for full and free range of motion of the shoulder. By virtue of their mandatory redundancy, the capsule and its ligaments are lax throughout most of

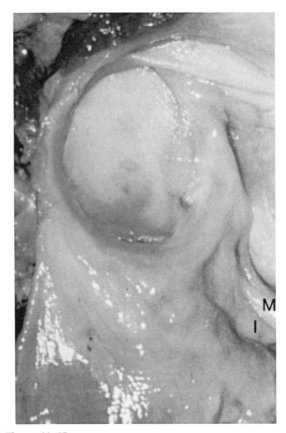

■ Figure 14–15
Cadaver dissection of the glenoid, biceps tendon insertion, and associated glenohumeral ligaments. This dissection demonstrates the anterior glenohumeral ligaments. Note the relationship of the anterior inferior (I) and the anterior middle (M) glenohumeral ligaments to the anterior rim of the glenoid.

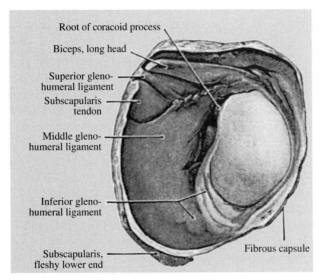

■ Figure 14–14
Anterior glenohumeral ligaments. This drawing shows the anterosuperior, anterior middle, and anteroinferior glenohumeral ligaments. The middle and inferior anterior glenohumeral ligaments are often avulsed from the glenoid or the glenoid labrum in traumatic anterior instability. *(From Grant's Atlas of Anatomy, 4th ed. Baltimore: Williams & Wilkins, 1956.)*

A　　　　　　　　B

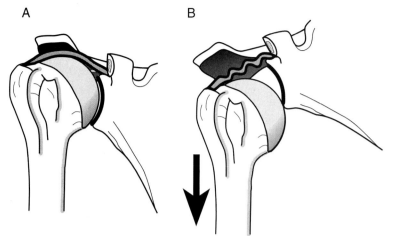

■ **Figure 14–16**

Scapular dumping. With the scapula in a normal position (A), the superior capsular mechanism is tight and supporting the head in the glenoid concavity. Drooping of the lateral aspect of the scapula (B) relaxes the superior capsular structures and rotates the glenoid concavity so that it does not support the head of the humerus. *(From Matsen FA III, Lippitt SB, Sidles JA, and Harryman DT II: Practical Evaluation and Management of the Shoulder. Philadelphia: WB Saunders, 1994.)*

the range of joint motion. Thus, they can exert major stabilizing effects only when they come under tension as the joint approaches the limits of its range of motion. In the midrange of shoulder motion, the center of the humeral head remains within 2.2 mm of the center of the glenoid on magnetic resonance imaging (MRI).[635] This limited stabilizing effect shows the importance of mechanisms of glenohumeral stability other than the capsule and its ligaments. The capsular structures are also believed to contribute to stability through their proprioceptive functions.[498]

The three anterior glenohumeral ligaments were first described by Schlemm.[636] Since then, many observers have described their anatomy and role in limiting glenohumeral rotation and translation (see Figs. 14–14 and 14–15).*

Codman[106] and others pointed out the variability of the ligaments (see Fig. 14–15).[133,137,183,493,525,760] These authors also demonstrated great variation in the size and number of synovial recesses that form in the anterior capsule above, below, and between the glenohumeral ligaments. They observed that if the capsule arises at the labrum, few if any synovial recesses are present (in this situation, because of generalized blending of all three ligaments, no room is left for synovial recesses or weaknesses, and hence the anterior glenohumeral capsule is stronger). However, the more medially the capsule arises from the glenoid (i.e., from the anterior scapular neck), the larger and more numerous the synovial recesses are. The end result is a thin, weak anterior capsule. In an embryologic study involving 52 specimens, Uhthoff and Piscopo[712] demonstrated that the anterior capsule inserted into the glenoid labrum in 77% and into the medial neck of the scapula in 23%. This variation in anatomy was later classified into two different types, I and II. A type I attachment occurs when the fibers primarily originate from the labrum, with some fibers attaching to the glenoid, and it is seen 80% of the time. A type II origin of the capsuloligamentous structures occurs solely from the glenoid neck and is seen in 20% of cadaveric specimens.[155]

The superior glenohumeral ligament (SGHL) is identified as the most consistent capsular ligament.[139] It crosses the rotator interval capsule and lies between the supraspinatus and subscapularis tendons. Another interval capsular structure, the coracohumeral ligament, originates at the base of the coracoid, blends into the cuff tendons, and inserts into the greater and lesser tuberosities.[102,254,327,370,541,675]

Harryman and colleagues pointed out that these two ligaments and the rotator interval capsule come under tension with glenohumeral flexion, extension, external rotation, and adduction.[254] When they are under tension, these structures resist posterior and inferior displacement of the humeral head. Clinical and experimental data have shown that releasing or surgically tightening the rotator interval capsule increases or decreases the allowed posterior and inferior translational laxity, respectively.[38,254,505,520,735]

It is these ligaments and capsule, as well as the inferior glenoid lip, that provide static restraint against inferior translation.[38] It is of anatomic interest and clinical significance that when the lateral aspect of the scapula is allowed to droop inferiorly, the resulting passive abduction of the humerus relaxes the rotator interval capsule and the superior ligaments; as a result, the humeral head can be "dumped" out of the glenoid fossa (Fig. 14–16).[441] Drooping of the lateral part of the scapula is normally prevented by the postural action of the scapular stabilizers, particularly the trapezius and serratus. Elevation of the lateral aspect of the scapula with the arm at the side enhances inferior stability in two ways: the resulting glenohumeral adduction tightens the superior capsule and ligaments, and the scapular rotation places more of the inferior glenoid lip beneath the humeral head.[314,735]

Whereas the SGHL and coracohumeral ligament come under tension with external rotation in adduction, the middle glenohumeral ligament (MGHL) is tensioned by external rotation when the humerus is abducted to 45 degrees.[685,688,708] The MGHL originates anterosuperiorly on the glenoid and inserts midway along the anterior humeral articular surface adjacent to the lesser tuberosity. In over a third of shoulders, the MGHL is absent or poorly defined, a situation that may place the shoulder at greater risk for anterior glenohumeral instability.[487]

With greater degrees of shoulder abduction, for example, in the "apprehension" position, the inferior

---

*See references 133, 136, 183, 184, 456, 493, 527, 583, 708, 753.

glenohumeral ligament (IGHL) and the inferior capsular sling come into play.[688,708] The IGHL originates below the sigmoid notch and courses obliquely between the anteroinferior glenoid and its humeral capsular insertion.[525] O'Brien and coworkers have described an anterior thickening of the IGHL, the anterior superior band.[525] The anterior and posterior aspects of the IGHL are said to function as a cruciate construct in which they alternately tighten in external and internal rotation.[525,735,741] These ligaments can be stretched out with repeated use. The dominant shoulders of handball athletes were placed in 90 degrees of abduction and external rotation and then brought into extension while being observed in a computed tomographic (CT) scanner. The dominant shoulders were seen to have more external rotation of the humeral head and more of a shift from the posterior aspect of the glenoid to its center than noted in normal shoulders when brought into the late cocking position.[27]

When the humerus is elevated anteriorly in the sagittal plane (flexion), the posterior inferior capsular pouch along with the rotator interval capsule comes into tension.[253,254,525,588,735] If the humerus is internally rotated while elevated in the sagittal plane, the interval capsule slackens but the posterior inferior pouch tightens. Posteroinferior capsular tension also limits flexion, internal rotation, and horizontal adduction.[253,254,588] Excessive tightness of this portion of the capsule is a well-recognized clinical entity (see Chapter 15 on the rotator cuff).

Coracoacromial Ligament

Resection of the coracoacromial ligament in cadaveric shoulders was found to result in significantly greater anterior translation of the humeral head with the shoulder in 0 and 30 degrees of abduction. At 0 degrees of abduction, significantly greater inferior translation occurred after resection of the coracoacromial ligament.[48] This observation should encourage caution with needless resection of the ligament.

Glenoid Labrum

The glenoid labrum is a fibrous rim that serves to deepen the glenoid fossa and allow attachment of the glenohumeral ligaments and the biceps tendon to the glenoid (see Figs. 14–14, 14–15, and 14–17). Anatomically, it is the interconnection of the periosteum of the glenoid, the glenoid bone, the glenoid articular cartilage, the synovium, and the capsule. Although microscopic studies have shown that a small amount of fibrocartilage is located at the junction of the hyaline cartilage of the glenoid and the fibrous capsule, the vast majority of the labrum consists of dense fibrous tissue with a few elastic fibers (Fig. 14–18).[201,493,704] The posterosuperior portion of the labrum is continuous with the tendon of the long head of the biceps. Anteriorly, it is continuous with the IGHL (see Fig. 14–15).[227,489,492,706] Hertz and colleagues[280] detailed the microanatomy of the labrum, whereas Prodromos and associates,[573] DePalma,[137] and Olsson[534] described changes in the glenoid labrum with age.

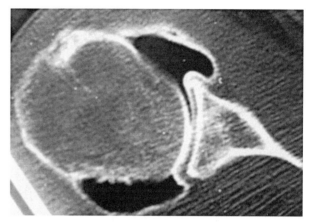

■ Figure 14–17
Computed tomographic arthrogram of the glenohumeral joint. The depth of the bony glenoid is enhanced by contributions of the articular cartilage and the glenoid labrum, which further increases the stability of the glenohumeral joint. Note that in this position, the anterior and posterior capsuloligamentous structures are relaxed and cannot contribute to stability.

In cadavers, isolated labral lesions are not usually sufficient to allow glenohumeral dislocation.[546,582,584,704] Cadaveric studies have shown diminished stability with labral lesions. Resection of the labrum was found to decrease the stability ratio of cadaveric shoulders with an average age of 76.7 years by 9.6%, thus indicating that the labrum plays a significant role even in this age group.[245] Clinical studies reveal a high incidence of labral deficiency in patients with recurrent traumatic instability.[34,126,135,442,612,713]

The reader is referred to a review of the gross anatomy of the glenohumeral joint surfaces, ligaments, labrum, and capsule by Warner (Chapter 1).[440] Fehringer and colleagues have recently added to our understanding of the role of the labrum by showing that a simple incision in its attachment to the glenoid uncenters the humeral head.[180]

MECHANICS OF GLENOHUMERAL STABILITY

The most remarkable feature of the glenohumeral joint is its ability to precisely stabilize the humeral head in the center of the glenoid on one hand and to allow a vast range of motion on the other. This balance of stability and mobility is achieved by a combination of mechanisms particular to this articulation.

● In contrast to the hip joint, the glenohumeral joint does not offer a deep stabilizing socket. An acetabular-like socket would limit motion by contact of the anatomic neck of the humerus with its rim. Instead, the small arc of the glenoid captures relatively little of the humeral articular surface, so neck-rim contact is avoided for a wide range of positions (Fig. 14–19).[129,432,441,626,708]

● In contrast to hinge-like joints with shallow sockets, such as the knee, interphalangeal joints, elbow, and ankle, the glenohumeral joint does not offer isometric articular ligaments that provide stability as the joint is flexed around a defined anatomic axis. Instead, the

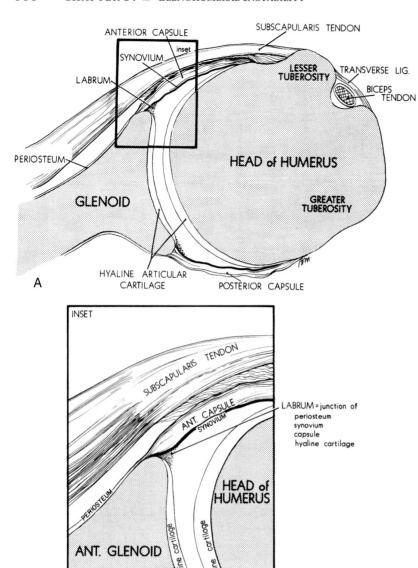

■ **Figure 14–18**
Normal shoulder anatomy. **A,** Horizontal section through the middle of the glenohumeral joint demonstrating normal anatomic relationships. Note the close relationship of the subscapularis tendon to the anterior capsule. **B,** Close-up view in the area of the labrum. The labrum consists of tissues from the nearby hyaline cartilage, capsule, synovium, and periosteum. *(From Rockwood CA and Green DP [eds]: Fractures, 3 vols, 2nd ed. Philadelphia: JB Lippincott, 1984.)*

glenohumeral ligaments play important stabilizing roles only at the extremes of motion; they are lax and relatively ineffectual in most functional positions of the joint (Fig. 14–20).[441,735]

In spite of its lack of a deep socket or isometric ligaments, the normal shoulder precisely constrains the humeral head to the center of the glenoid cavity throughout most of the arc of movement.[299,300,569,570] It is remarkable that this seemingly unconstrained joint is able to provide such precise centering, resist the gravitational pull on the arm hanging at the side for long periods, remain located during sleep, allow for the lifting of large loads, permit throwing a baseball at speeds approaching 100 miles an hour, and maintain stability during the application of an almost infinite variety of forces of differing magnitude, direction, duration, and abruptness.

The mechanics of glenohumeral stability can be most easily understood in terms of the relationship between the net force acting on the humeral head and the shape of the glenoid fossa. A working familiarity with the mechanics

of glenohumeral stability will greatly enhance one's understanding of the workings of the normal joint, laboratory models of instability, clinical problems of instability, and clinical strategies for managing glenohumeral instability.

The basic laws of glenohumeral stability can be stated as follows:

1. The glenohumeral joint will not dislocate as long as the net humeral joint reaction force* (Fig. 14–21) is directed within the effective glenoid arc† (Figs. 14–22 and 14–23).
2. The humeral head will remain centered in the glenoid fossa if the glenoid and humeral joint surfaces are con-

---

*The "net humeral joint reaction force" is the resultant of all muscular, ligamentous, inertial, gravitational, and other external forces applied to the head of the humerus (other than the force applied by the glenoid).
†Because the rim of the glenoid is deformable under load, the "effective glenoid arc" is the arc of the glenoid available to support the humeral head under the specified loading conditions.

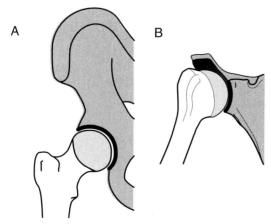

■ **Figure 14–19**

In contrast to the hip (**A**), the shallow glenoid captures relatively little of the articulating ball (**B**). *(From Matsen FA III, Lippitt SB, Sidles JA, and Harryman DT II: Practical Evaluation and Management of the Shoulder. Philadelphia: WB Saunders, 1994.)*

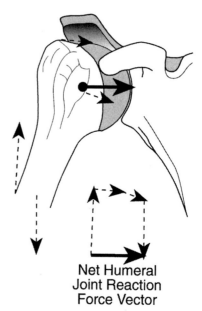

Net Humeral Joint Reaction Force Vector

■ **Figure 14–21**

The net humeral joint reaction force is the vector sum of all forces acting on the head of the humerus relative to the glenoid fossa. *(From Matsen FA III, Lippitt SB, Sidles JA, and Harryman DT II: Practical Evaluation and Management of the Shoulder. Philadelphia: WB Saunders, 1994.)*

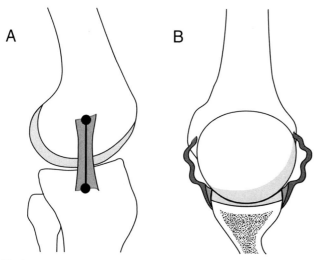

■ **Figure 14–20**

In contrast to the knee, where the ligaments remain isometric during joint motion (**A**), the glenohumeral ligaments must be slack in most of the joint's positions (**B**). *(Modified from Matsen FA III, Lippitt SB, Sidles JA, and Harryman DT II: Practical Evaluation and Management of the Shoulder. Philadelphia: WB Saunders, 1994.)*

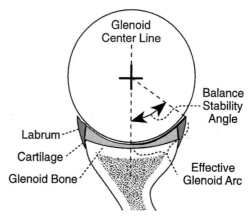

■ **Figure 14–22**

The effective glenoid arc is the arc of the glenoid able to support the net humeral joint reaction force. The balance stability angle is the maximal angle that the net humeral joint reaction force can make with the glenoid center line (see Fig. 14–26) before dislocation occurs. The shape of the bone, cartilage, and labrum all contribute to the effective glenoid arc and the balance stability angle.

gruent and if the net humeral joint reaction force is directed within the effective glenoid arc.

The effective shape of the glenoid is revealed by the *glenoidogram*, which rather than showing how the glenoid *looks*, shows how it *works* (Figs. 14–24 and 14–25).[387,442] The glenoidogram is the path taken by the center of the humeral head as it is translated away from the center of the glenoid fossa in a specified direction under defined loads. The shape of the glenoidogram indicates the extent of the effective glenoid arc in that direction. If the net humeral joint reaction force passes outside the effective glenoid arc, the joint becomes unstable. The glenoidogram is oriented with respect to the *glenoid center line*, a reference line perpendicular to the center of the glenoid fossa (Figs. 14–26 and 14–27). The maximal angle that the net humeral joint reaction force can make with the glenoid

center line in a given direction is the *balance stability angle* (see Figs. 14–22 and 14–28). Balance stability angles vary for different directions around the glenoid. The requisite for a stable glenohumeral joint is that the net humeral joint reaction force be maintained within the balance stability angles.

The Net Humeral Joint Reaction Force

The direction of the net humeral joint reaction force is controlled actively by elements of the rotator cuff and

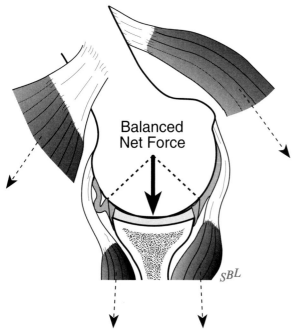

■ Figure 14–23
The deltoid and cuff muscle forces *(dotted arrows)* maintain the net humeral joint reaction force *(solid arrow)* within the balance stability angles *(dotted lines)*. *(Modified from Matsen FA III, Lippitt SB, Sidles JA, and Harryman DT II: Practical Evaluation and Management of the Shoulder. Philadelphia: WB Saunders, 1994.)*

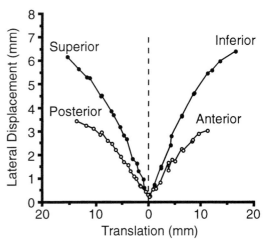

■ Figure 14–25
Measured glenoidograms for four different directions of translation in a young cadaver shoulder. The *dotted vertical line* represents the glenoid center line (see Fig. 14–26) . The effective glenoid depth in this shoulder was 3.4 mm for translation in the posterior direction, 3.2 mm in the anterior direction, 6.2 mm in the superior direction, and 6.4 mm in the inferior direction. Note the high degree of symmetry about the glenoid center line and the deep valley when the head is exactly centered in the glenoid socket. *(From Matsen FA III, Lippitt SB, Sidles JA, and Harryman DT II: Practical Evaluation and Management of the Shoulder. Philadelphia: WB Saunders, 1994.)*

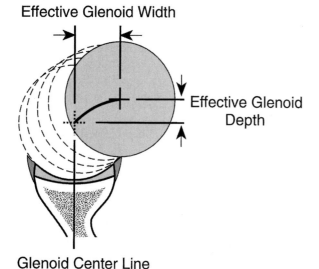

■ Figure 14–24
A glenoidogram is the path of the humeral head as it translates in a specified direction across the face of the glenoid away from the glenoid center line under defined loads. A glenoidogram shows the effective glenoid depth and width for the specified direction of translation and loading conditions. *(Modified from Matsen FA III, Lippitt SB, Sidles JA, and Harryman DT II: Practical Evaluation and Management of the Shoulder. Philadelphia: WB Saunders, 1994.)*

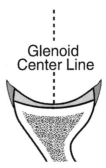

■ Figure 14–26
The glenoid center line is a line perpendicular to the surface of the glenoid fossa at its midpoint. *(Modified from Matsen FA III, Lippitt SB, Sidles JA, and Harryman DT II: Practical Evaluation and Management of the Shoulder. Philadelphia: WB Saunders, 1994.)*

other shoulder muscles. Each active muscle generates a force whose direction is determined by the effective origin and insertion of that muscle (Fig. 14–29). Neural control of the magnitude of these muscle forces provides the mechanism by which the direction of the net humeral

joint reaction force is controlled. For example, by increasing the force of contraction of a muscle whose force direction is close to the glenoid center line, the direction of the net humeral joint reaction force can be aligned more closely with the glenoid fossa (Fig. 14–30). The elements of the rotator cuff are well positioned to contribute to this muscle balance.*

In addition to the compression provided by the rotator cuff musculature, the deltoid assists in this capacity as well. The middle and posterior portions of the deltoid have been shown to be more important than the anterior portion in producing concavity compression.[390] The lateral portion of the deltoid was found to be important

---

*See references 39, 40, 55, 80, 252, 311, 316, 348, 546, 563, 602, 630, 717, 718, 721, 779.

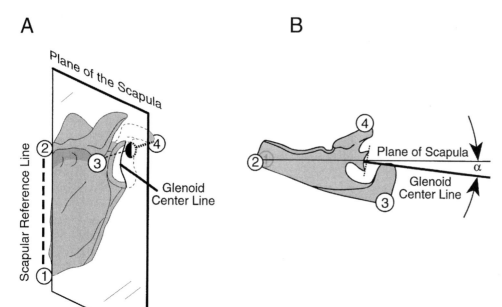

A

Plane of the Scapula

Scapular Reference Line

Glenoid Center Line

B

Plane of Scapula

Glenoid Center Line

α

■ **Figure 14–27**
The glenoid center line can be related to scapular coordinates and the plane of the scapula. The following reference points are all easily palpated: (1) the inferior pole of the scapula, (2) the medial end of the spine of the scapula, (3) the posterior angle of the acromion, and (4) the coracoid tip. The scapular reference line connects reference points 1 and 2. The plane of the scapula passes through points 1 and 2 and halfway between points 3 and 4. The glenoid center line usually makes a slightly posterior angle (α) with the plane of the scapula. *(Modified from Matsen FA III, Lippitt SB, Sidles JA, and Harryman DT II: Practical Evaluation and Management of the Shoulder. Philadelphia: WB Saunders, 1994.)*

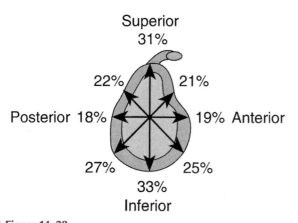

Superior
31%

22%   21%

Posterior 18%   19% Anterior

27%   25%

33%
Inferior

■ **Figure 14–28**
The balance stability angle varies around the face of the glenoid. For a normal glenoid, the superior and inferior balance stability angles are greater than the anterior and posterior balance stability angles. This figure shows the balance stability angles measured in eight directions around the face of the glenoid. Values are means for 10 cadaver shoulders with a compressive load of 50 N. *(Modified from Matsen FA III, Lippitt SB, Sidles JA, and Harryman DT II: Practical Evaluation and Management of the Shoulder. Philadelphia: WB Saunders, 1994.)*

Effective Point of Application

F

R

F_D

SBL

F_C

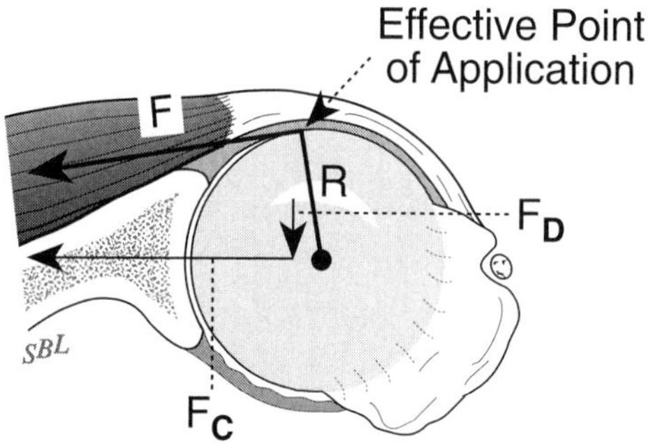

■ **Figure 14–29**
Each active muscle generates a force (F) whose direction is determined by the effective origin and insertion of that muscle. Note that the rotator cuff tendons wrap around the head of the humerus, so their effective point of attachment is on the humeral articular surface. Note also that each muscle force has a compressive (F_c) and a displacing (F_d) component. The product of the force multiplied by the radius (R) is the torque (F × R). *(Modified from Matsen FA III, Lippitt SB, Sidles JA, and Harryman DT II: Practical Evaluation and Management of the Shoulder. Philadelphia, WB Saunders, 1994.)*

in resisting inferior subluxation, with 8.2 mm of superior translation of the humeral head produced in a cadaveric study. The posterior portion of the deltoid produced 7.7 mm of superior translation.[244] The long head of the biceps muscle may contribute to shoulder stability as well. Shoulders with anterior instability in 90 degrees of abduction and 120 degrees of external rotation had significantly more electromyographic activity in the long head of the biceps than did stable shoulders in the same position.[357]

Strengthening and neuromuscular training help optimize neuromuscular control of the net humeral joint reaction force. Conversely, the net humeral joint reaction force is difficult to optimize when muscle control is impaired by injury, disuse, contracture, paralysis, loss of coordination, or tendon defects (Fig. 14–31). Neuromuscular training may be guided by proprioceptors in the labrum and ligaments.[235,256,324,720] Blasier and coworkers[54] and Kronberg and colleagues[368] showed that individuals with generalized joint laxity have less acute proprioception and altered muscle activation. Zuckerman and associates demonstrated that motion and position sense are compromised in the presence of traumatic anterior instability and are restored 1 year after surgical reconstruction.[796]

The reader is referred to reviews of neuromuscular stabilization of the shoulder by Lieber and Friden[440] (Chapter 4) and by Speer and Garrett[440] (Chapter 8). In the same

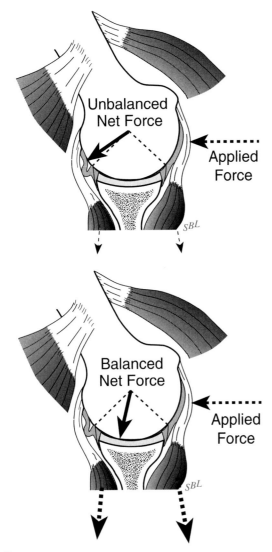

■ **Figure 14–30**
Stabilizing the glenohumeral joint against an applied translational force. Strong contraction of the cuff muscles provides an increased compression force into the glenoid concavity. As a result, the net humeral force is balanced within the glenoid concavity.

reference are found reviews of the role of capsular feedback and pattern generators in shoulder kinematics by Grigg[440] (Chapter 9) and the role of muscle optimization by Flanders[440] (Chapter 39).

The Balance Stability Angle and the Stability Ratio

The balance stability angle is the maximal angle that the net humeral joint reaction force can make with the glenoid center line before glenohumeral dislocation occurs. The tangent of this balance stability angle is the ratio between its displacing component (perpendicular to the glenoid center line) and its compressive component (parallel to the glenoid center line), which is known as the *stability ratio*. The stability ratio is the maximal displacing force in a given direction that can be stabilized by a specified compressive load, assuming frictional effects to be

minimal.* The effective glenoid arc, the balance stability angle, and stability ratios vary around the perimeter of the glenoid (see Fig. 14–28). It is handy to note that for small angles, the stability ratio can be estimated by dividing the balance stability angle by 57 degrees.†

The stability ratio is frequently used in the laboratory because it is relatively easy to measure: a compressive load is applied, and the displacing force is progressively increased until dislocation occurs. For example, Lippitt and colleagues[413] found that a compressive load of 50 N resisted displacing loads of up to 30 N and that the effectiveness of this stabilization mechanism varied with the depth of the glenoid (Fig. 14–32). Investigation of these parameters provides important information on stability mechanics; for example, resection of the labrum has been shown to reduce the stability ratio by 20%.[413] Furthermore, a 3-mm anterior glenoid defect has been shown to reduce the balance stability angle over 25% from 18 to 13 degrees.[441] Fractures of the anterior glenoid rim were noted to produce significantly more instability when they involve 21% or more of the glenoid, an average of 6.8 mm in width.[312]

Clinically, the stability ratio can be sensed by using the "load and shift" test wherein the examiner applies a compressive load pressing the humeral head into the glenoid while noting the amount of translating force necessary to move the humeral head from its centered position.[652] This test gives the examiner an indication of the adequacy of the glenoid concavity and is one of the most practical ways to detect deficiencies of the glenoid rim.

The Effective Glenoid Arc

The glenoid concavity is formed by a combination of the shape of the underlying bone and the overlying cartilage and labrum (see Figs. 14–22 and 14–24).[299,664] The effective glenoid arc may be compromised by congenital deficiency (glenoid hypoplasia), excessive compliance, traumatic lesions (rim fractures or Bankart defects), or wear (Fig. 14–33).‡ The effective arc may be augmented by anatomic repair of fractures or Bankart lesions (Fig. 14–34), by rim augmentation, by congruent glenoid bone grafting, and by glenoid osteotomy.[387]

The effective shape of the glenoid is revealed by the glenoidogram. As the humeral head is translated from

---

* Measured stability ratios may be influenced by the friction of the joint surfaces and by other stabilizing mechanisms such as adhesion/cohesion and the glenoid suction cup (which will be discussed later). These effects tend to increase the displacing force necessary to dislocate the humeral head for a given compressive load. It is essential to control for these effects in the laboratory. Specifically, the under-lubricated, aged cadaver joints available to the laboratory may have substantially greater coefficients of friction in vitro than the exquisitely lubricated and smooth joint of a young person in vivo.

† At small angles, the tangent of an angle is approximately equal to the angle expressed in radians. Thus, the stability ratio (tangent of the balance stability angle) is approximately the balance stability angle divided by 57 degrees per radian.

‡ See references 8, 30, 33, 115, 125, 299, 334, 387, 413, 441–443, 503, 550, 612, 691.

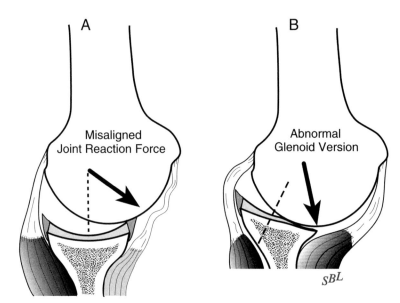

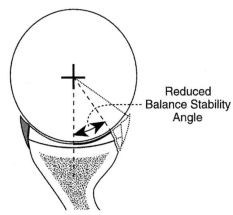

■ **Figure 14–31**
A, Stability is compromised by muscle imbalance. In this example, the humerus is aligned with the glenoid center line, but the net humeral joint reaction force is misaligned because of weakness of the posterior cuff musculature. **B,** Balance stability is compromised with abnormal glenoid version. In this example, the humerus is aligned with the plane of the scapula, but severe glenoid retroversion results in a posteriorly directed glenoid center line that is divergent from the net humeral joint reaction force. *(Modified from Matsen FA III, Lippitt SB, Sidles JA, and Harryman DT II: Practical Evaluation and Management of the Shoulder. Philadelphia, WB Saunders, 1994.)*

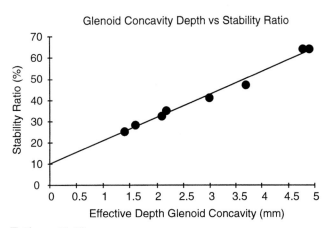

■ **Figure 14–32**

A nearly linear relationship exists between the effective depth of the glenoid concavity and the stability ratio with a 50-N compressive load. These data include points representing superior, inferior, anterior, and posterior translation before and after excision of the glenoid labrum. *(From Matsen FA III, Lippitt SB, Sidles JA, and Harryman DT II: Practical Evaluation and Management of the Shoulder. WB Saunders, Philadelphia, 1994.)*

■ **Figure 14–33**

The balance stability angle and the effective glenoid arc are reduced by a fracture of the glenoid rim. *(Modified from Matsen FA III, Lippitt SB, Sidles JA, and Harryman DT II: Practical Evaluation and Management of the Shoulder. Philadelphia: WB Saunders, 1994.)*

the center of the glenoid to the rim in a given direction, the center of the humeral head traces the glenoidogram, which has a characteristic "gullwing" shape. The glenoidogram is different for different directions of translation (see Fig. 14–25, which presents data recorded for the superior, inferior, anterior, and posterior directions in a typical shoulder). The shape of the glenoidogram can be predicted from the humeral radius of curvature, the glenoid radius of curvature, and the balance stability angle.*

Predicted glenoidograms are qualitatively similar to glenoidograms measured experimentally (compare Figs. 14–35 and 14–25). The glenoidogram also reveals another important aspect of shoulder stability: the slope of the glenoidogram at any point is equal to the tangent of the balance stability angle (which equals the stability ratio) at that point. For most glenoidograms it can be seen that the

slope is steepest when the humeral head is centered in the glenoid (Fig. 14–35). Thus, the joint has the highly desirable property of being most stable when the head is centered. As the humeral head is moved away from the center, the slope of the glenoidogram and the stability ratio become less. Accordingly, as the head is displaced from the glenoid center, it becomes progressively more unstable.

---

*Glenoidograms can be predicted given the radius of curvature of the humeral head (R_h), the radius of curvature of the glenoid fossa (R_g), the effective glenoid width (W), the effective glenoid depth (D), and the balance stability angle (BSA) in radians. For each value of x (the distance away from the glenoid center line), the perpendicular distance of the center of the humeral head away from the glenoid bottom, y, is given by $D - R_h + (R_h \cdot R_h - [W - x] \cdot [W - x])^{1/2}$. The sample spreadsheet displays the case in which $R_g = R_h = 25$ mm and the BSA = 30 degrees = 0.5236 radians. In this case, the effective glenoid width (W) = $Rg \cdot \sin(BSA)$, and the effective glenoid depth (D) = $Rg \cdot (1 - \cos[BSA])$. The results of this prediction are shown in Table 14-1 and in Figure 14–35.

TABLE 14-1.   Predicted Coordinates of the Glenoidogram

Effective Glenoid Width (W) $R_g \cdot \sin(\text{BSA})$	Effective Glenoid Depth (D) $R_g \cdot (1 - \cos[\text{BSA}])$	X	Y $D - R_b + (R_b \cdot R_b - [W - X] \cdot [W - X])^{1/2}$
12.5	3.35	0	0
12.5	3.35	0.1	0.057428086
12.5	3.35	0.2	0.114245197
12.5	3.35	0.3	0.170456105
12.5	3.35	0.4	0.226065482
12.5	3.35	0.5	0.281077905
12.5	3.35	0.6	0.335497855
12.5	3.35	0.7	0.38932972
12.5	3.35	0.8	0.442577799
12.5	3.35	0.9	0.495246303
12.5	3.35	1.0	0.547339357

BSA, balance stability angle.

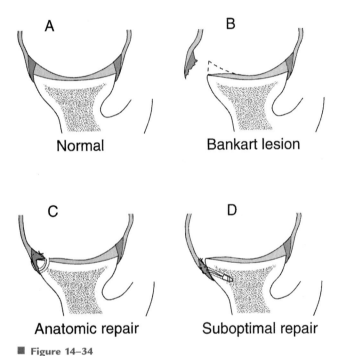

■ **Figure 14–34**

Normally, the capsule and labrum deepen the effective glenoid fossa (**A**). This effect is lost in the presence of a Bankart lesion, particularly if the articular cartilage is worn away (**B**). Anatomic repair of the detached glenoid labrum and glenohumeral ligaments to the glenoid rim helps restore the effective glenoid arc (**C**). By contrast, when the labrum and capsule heal to the neck, the effective glenoid arc is not restored (**D**). *(Modified from Matsen FA III, Lippitt SB, Sidles JA, and Harryman DT II: Practical Evaluation and Management of the Shoulder. Philadelphia: WB Saunders, 1994.)*

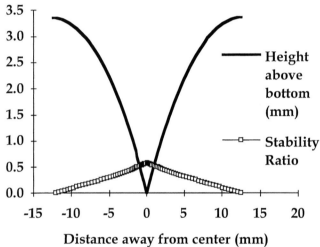

■ **Figure 14–35**

The glenoidogram predicted for a shoulder with glenoid and humeral radii (R_g and R_h) of 25 mm and a balance stability angle (A) of 30 degrees. For a position *x* millimeters from the center, the effective glenoid depth (*y*) was calculated from the formula $y = R_g \cdot (1 - \cos A) - R_h + (R_h^2 - [R_g \cdot (\sin A) - x]^2)^{1/2}$. Also shown are the local stability ratios (equal to the slope of the glenoidogram) for the different humeral positions along the glenoidogram. Note that the stability ratio is maximal when the humeral head is centered in the glenoid.

Once enough force is applied to displace the head from the center, that same amount of force would easily displace the humeral head over the glenoid lip. Note also that when the humeral head is translated to the lip of the glenoid, the stability ratio is, as expected, zero. These observations relate to the "jerk" tests described for anterior[394] and posterior[441] instability; in these tests, there is no translation of the humeral head until the point at which sudden and substantial translation occurs.[387,413]

Glenoid Version

Glenoid version is the angle that the glenoid center line makes with the plane of the scapula (see Fig. 14–27). The glenoid center line usually points a few degrees posterior to the plane of the scapula (see Fig. 14–27). Changing the version of the glenoid articular surface imposes a corresponding change in the humeroscapular positions in which the net humeral joint reaction force will be contained by the effective glenoid arc. Glenoid version may be altered by glenoid dysplasia (Fig. 14–36),[770] fractures, glenoid osteotomy,[770] and glenoid arthroplasty. Abnormal glenoid version positions the glenoid fossa in an abnormal relationship to the forces generated by the scapulohumeral muscles. Normalization of abnormal glenoid version is often a critical step in glenohumeral reconstruction.

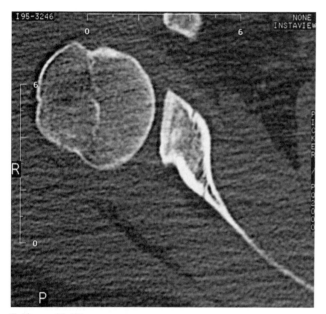

■ Figure 14–36

A computed tomographic scan of a shoulder with glenoid dysplasia manifested as absence of the posterior glenoid lip and glenoid retroversion.

Apparent changes in glenoid version can arise from loss of part of the glenoid rim (see Figs. 14–31 and 14–33).[70,304,580] Dias and colleagues did not find any difference in apparent glenoid version between normal subjects and recurrent anterior dislocators.[144] Dowdy and O'Driscoll[151] found only minor variance in radiographic glenoid version among patients with and without recurrence after stabilization surgery. However, Hirschfelder and Kirsten[289] detected increased glenoid retroversion in both the symptomatic and asymptomatic shoulders of individuals with posterior instability, and Grasshoff and coworkers[229] found increased anteversion in shoulders

with recurrent anterior instability. It has been shown that the dominant shoulder of throwing athletes has an average of 17 degrees of retroversion of the humeral head and 3 degrees of retroversion of the glenoid.[122] It was demonstrated in a cadaveric study by Churchill and colleagues that black men and women have less glenoid retroversion than white men and women do, 0.2 and 2.65 degrees respectively.[97] No significant difference was found between men and women.

Changes in version may be difficult to quantitate on axillary radiographs unless the view is carefully standardized (Fig. 14–37). Even with optimal radiographic technique, the important contributions of cartilage and labrum to the depth and orientation of the fossa[299,664] cannot be seen on plain radiographs or CT scans. When it is important to know the orientation of the cartilaginous joint surface in relation to the scapular body, a double-contrast CT scan is necessary (see Fig. 14–17).

Patients with posterior instability were found to be more likely to have glenoid rim deficiency than were those with normal or anteriorly unstable shoulders.[751]

Scapular Positioning

A special feature of the glenohumeral joint is that the glenoid can be positioned on the thorax (in contrast to the fixed acetabulum of the hip). This scapular alignment greatly increases the range of positions in which the criteria for glenohumeral stability can be met (Fig. 14–38). Consider the arm to be elevated 90 degrees in the sagittal thoracic plane. This position can be achieved with the scapula protracted or retracted. If the scapula is protracted, the humerus is closely aligned with the glenoid center line. When the humerus is in this position, most of the humeroscapular muscles are oriented to compress the humeral head into the glenoid fossa. Alternatively, if the scapula is maximally retracted, the humerus is almost at

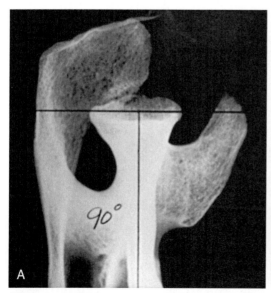
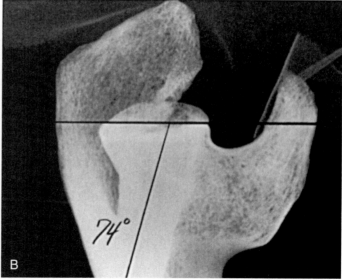

■ Figure 14–37

Two radiographs of the same cadaver scapula showing the variation in apparent glenoid retroversion, depending on the radiographic projection.

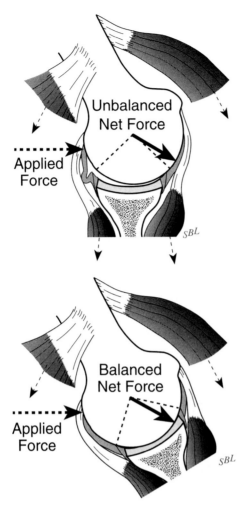

■ Figure 14–38
Stabilization against an applied translational force by repositioning the glenoid concavity to support the net humeral force.

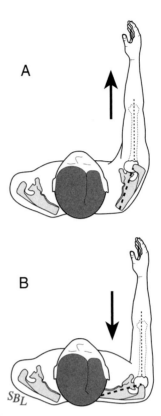

■ Figure 14–39
Essentially identical humerothoracic positions can be achieved with different humeroscapular positions, which in turn have different implications for balancing the net humeral force. **A,** The humerus is elevated so that it is closely aligned with the glenoid center line. This position should be the most stable. **B,** The same humerothoracic position can be achieved with the humerus almost perpendicular to the glenoid center line, but this orientation challenges the ability of the joint to balance the net humeral force. *(From Matsen FA III, Lippitt SB, Sidles JA, and Harryman DT II: Practical Evaluation and Management of the Shoulder. Philadelphia: WB Saunders, 1994.)*

right angles to the glenoid center line (Fig. 14–39). In this position, the net humeral joint reaction force is directed posteriorly and may not be contained within the balance stability angle.[66,219,310,543,570,737]

Which humeroscapular position is used to achieve a given humerothoracic position is a question of habit and training. Coordination of scapular position and glenohumeral muscle balance is an important element of the neuromuscular control of glenohumeral stability.

Atwater[25] has documented that in most throwing and striking skills, the shoulder abduction angle is usually 100 degrees. Higher and lower release points are achieved by tilting the trunk rather than by increasing or decreasing the shoulder abduction angle relative to the trunk.

Ligaments

Properties of Ligaments

Each glenohumeral ligament has clinically important properties that can be characterized by the relationship of the distance between its origin and insertion and its tension.[191] These properties include the following:

1. Its resting length (how far its origin and insertion can be separated with minimal force)
2. Its elastic deformability (how much additional separation of the origin and insertion can be achieved by the application of larger forces without permanently changing the ligament's properties)
3. Its plastic deformability (beyond the ligament's elastic limit, how much additional separation between the origin and insertion can be achieved by the application of larger forces that permanently deform the ligament up to the point where the ligament fails).

These properties can be demonstrated as a plot of the ligament's tension versus the distance between the ligament's origin and insertion. The same relationship pertains whether the ligament's origin and insertion are separated by translation of the humeral head or by rotation (Fig. 14–40).

At point "A," the origin and insertion of the ligament are closely approximated. At point "B," the origin and insertion have been separated enough to initiate tension in the ligament. Thus, the resting length of the ligament is shown as A-B. Stefko and coworkers[673] measured the length of the anterior band of the IGHL to be 37 mm.

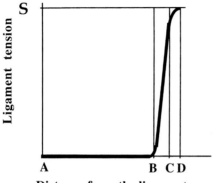

Distance from the ligament
origin to the ligament insertion
or
Angle from position A
where the ligament origin and
insertion are approximated

■ **Figure 14–40**
The distance from the ligament origin to the ligament insertion or the angle from position A, where the ligament origin and insertion are approximated.

Additional separation of the origin and insertion causes increasing ligament tension. Up to point "C," this separation is elastic (i.e., it does not result in permanent change in the ligament). Further separation of the origin and insertion plastically deforms the ligament up to point "D," where the ligament fails at a tension of "S." The midsubstance strain to failure has been measured as being from 7% to 11%.[673]

Such graphs are helpful in describing the properties of ligaments:

The *strength* of a ligament is the amount of tension that it can take before failure (S).

The *laxity* of a ligament is the amount of translation (Fig. 14–41) or rotation (Fig. 14–42) that it allows from a specified starting position when a small load is applied. Ligaments with long A-B distances demonstrate substan-

tial laxity if the starting point for laxity testing is close to "A." Laxity is diminished when the joint is positioned near the extremes of motion (Fig. 14–43), that is, when the starting point for the laxity measurement is close to "B" (see Fig. 14–40). Ligaments with small A-B distances are short or contracted. *Translational laxity and rotational laxity are equivalent*: they both reflect the ability to separate the attachment points of the ligament.

A typical relationship between humeroscapular position and torque (capsular tension × humeral head radius) is shown in (Fig. 14–44).[441] Note that the greatest part of glenohumeral motion and function takes place in the area where no tension is being placed on the capsule (corresponding to zone A-B in Fig. 14–40). Also note that at the limits of motion (corresponding to zone B-C), the torque increases rapidly with changes in position as suggested by the rapid increase in tension shown in Figure 14–40.

These diagrams help distinguish laxity from instability. Normally stable shoulders may demonstrate substantial laxity; consider the very lax, but very stable glenohumeral joints of gymnasts. In a most important study, Emery and Mullaji[163] found that of 150 asymptomatic shoulders in schoolchildren, 50% demonstrated positive signs of "increased laxity."

Some investigators have measured increased laxity in patients with glenohumeral instability.[108,325,326,344,436] However, recent evidence indicates that these differences are not always significant.[255,409,441] Starting in a neutral position, the translational laxity of eight normal living subjects was found to be 8 ± 4, 8 ± 6, and 11 ± 4 mm in the anterior, posterior, and inferior directions, respectively. Interestingly, virtually identical laxity was measured in 16 patients who required surgery for symptomatic recurrent instability (Fig. 14–45), thus indicating that in these subjects, the measured laxity was not the determinant of glenohumeral stability.[409,441] Sperber and Wredmark[670] found no differences in joint volume or capsular elasticity between healthy and unstable shoulders. These results indicate that the amount of laxity cannot be used to distinguish clinically stable shoulders from those that are unstable.

■ **Figure 14–41**
Glenohumeral translation is movement of the center of the humeral head with respect to the face of the glenoid. The amount of translation allowed is determined by both the initial position of the joint and the length of the ligament that becomes tight.

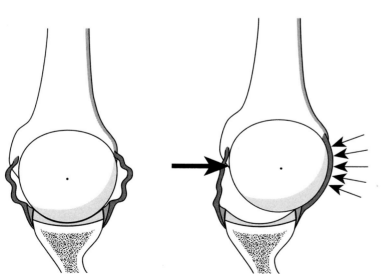

SBL

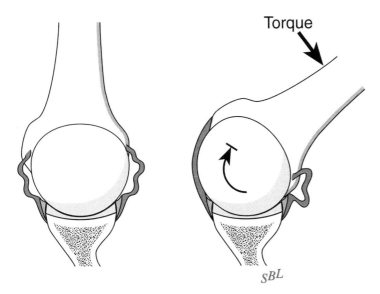

Torque

■ **Figure 14–42**
Glenohumeral rotation is movement of the humerus around the center of the humeral head, which remains centered in the glenoid fossa. The amount of rotation allowed is determined by both the initial position of the joint and the length of the ligament that becomes tight.

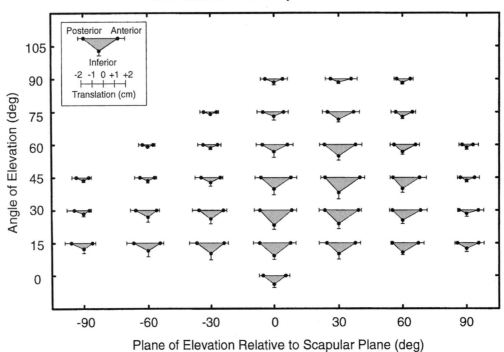

■ **Figure 14–43**
Mean translational laxity as measured in eight cadaveric shoulders. The applied translational force was 30 N (approximately 6 lb), and it was applied along each of the following axes: anterior, posterior, and inferior. The planes of elevation are measured relative to the plane of the scapula (see Fig. 14–27), not the thoracic plane. The angles of elevation are measured relative to the scapular reference line (see Fig. 14–27). Standard deviations are shown at the vertex of each triangle. *(From Matsen FA III, Lippitt SB, Sidles JA, and Harryman DT II: Practical Evaluation and Management of the Shoulder. Philadelphia: WB Saunders, 1994.)*

The *stretchiness* of a ligament is its elasticity. Ligaments with long B-C distances (Fig. 14-40) are stretchy and have "soft" end points on clinical laxity tests. Ligaments with short B-C distances are stiff and have "firm" end points on clinical laxity tests.

Biochemical composition (as in Ehlers-Danlos syndrome), anatomic variation (anomalies of attachment), use (or disuse), age, disease (e.g., diabetes, frozen shoulder), injury, and surgery (e.g., capsulorrhaphy) can affect the strength, laxity, and stretchiness of glenohumeral ligaments.

The reader is referred to reviews of the material properties of the IGHL by Mow and colleagues[440] (Chapter 2) and the role of ligaments in glenohumeral stability by Lew and associates[440] (Chapter 3).

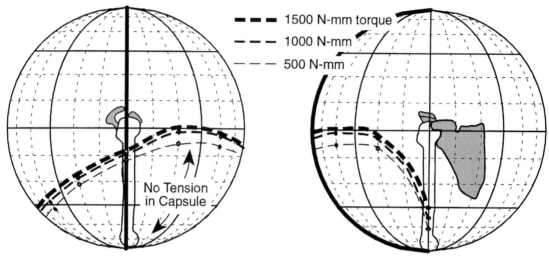

■ **Figure 14–44**

The range of humeroscapular elevation with no capsular tension. This global diagram represents data from a cadaver experiment in which the humerus was elevated in various scapular planes with free axial rotation. Elevation was performed until the torque reached 500, 1000, and 1500 N-mm. The positions associated with these torque levels are indicated by the isobars. The area within the inner isobars indicates the range of positions in which no tension is placed on the capsuloligamentous structures. *(From Matsen FA III, Lippitt SB, Sidles JA, and Harryman DT II: Practical Evaluation and Management of the Shoulder. Philadelphia: WB Saunders, 1994.)*

Ligamentous Stabilization

The glenohumeral ligaments exert two stabilizing effects:

1. They serve as *checkreins* in which the range of joint positions is restricted to those that can be stabilized by muscle balance. This function is important because at extreme glenohumeral positions, the net humeral joint reaction force becomes increasingly difficult to balance within the glenoid (Fig. 14–46). For example, excessive abduction, extension, and external rotation of the shoulder may allow the net humeral joint reaction force vector to point beyond the anterior-inferior balance stability angle. Similarly, excessive posterior capsular laxity allows the net humeral joint reaction force to achieve large angles with the glenoid center line; these angles may exceed the posterior balance stability angle. Furthermore, at the extremes of motion, the muscles tend to be near their maximal extension, a position in which their force-generating capacity is diminished.[404]

The patient can modify the checkrein function by altering the position of the scapula (see Fig. 14–16). Surgeons can likewise modify the checkrein function: capsular tightening moves points B, C, and D closer to point A, thereby reducing laxity (see Fig. 14–41). The checkrein function is inoperant when the ligament is not under tension (i.e., when the humeroscapular position is within the tension-free zone (A-B in Fig. 14–40; see also Fig. 14–44).

2. When torque is applied to the humerus so that a ligament comes under tension, this ligament applies a force to the proximal end of the humerus. Because of the attachments of the ligament, this *countervailing force* both compresses the humeral head into the glenoid fossa and resists displacement in the direction of the tight ligament (Fig. 14–47).

An analysis of ligament function* demonstrates the limits of the stability provided by ligaments acting alone. For example, such an analysis suggests that if the torque resulting from a modest 10-lb force applied to the arm at a distance of 40 inches from the center of a humeral head with a 1-inch radius were resisted only by the tension in the IGHL, the IGHL would need to be able to withstand a tension of 400 lb (Fig. 14–48).

If tension in the ligament exceeds the strength of the ligament (S), the ligament breaks. A few investigations

---

*The magnitude of the countervailing force is determined by the applied torque and limited by the strength of the ligament. The direction of this force is tangent to the humeral head at the point of its contact with the glenoid rim.

The countervailing force mechanism operates in the arc B-C, where the ligament is elastically deformed. If the ligament behaves perfectly elastically, the tension in the ligament provides a stabilizing force (T) in which

T = (Angular position − Angle B) · Diameter of humeral head · $\pi/360°$ · Spring constant of the ligament

This relationship predicts the following:

- Until angle B is reached, no force is generated by the ligament.
- The larger the angle past position B, the more force that is generated (up to the elastic limit).
- Stiffer ligaments generate more force for a given angular displacement.
- Larger humeral heads generate more force for each degree of angular displacement.

Ligament tension results from applied torque. When an externally applied force B acts at a distance E from the center of the humeral head, it creates a torque (Q) that is the product of B and E (Fig. 14–48). If this torque is resisted by a ligament closely applied to the humeral head (i.e., the effective moment arm equals the head radius [R]), the tension in the ligament (T) is

$$T = Q/R = B \cdot E/R$$

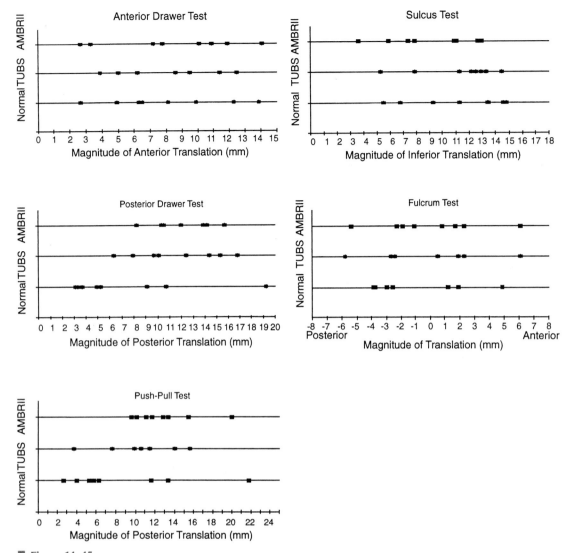

■ **Figure 14–45**
The magnitude of translation on laxity tests for three groups of shoulders in vivo: eight normal shoulders, eight shoulders with symptomatic atraumatic instability (AMBRII), and eight shoulders with symptomatic traumatic instability (TUBS). Each shoulder is represented by a mark on the *horizontal lines*. Note that for each of these laxity tests, the range of translations for the normal subjects is essentially the same as the range of translations for subjects with symptomatic instability requiring surgical repair. *(From Matsen FA III, Lippitt SB, Sidles JA, and Harryman DT II: Practical Evaluation and Management of the Shoulder. Philadelphia: WB Saunders, 1994.)*

have attempted to measure the strength of the glenohumeral capsular ligaments. Kaltsas[346] has studied some of the material properties of the shoulder capsule and found it to be more elastic and stronger than the capsule of the elbow. He noted that the entire glenohumeral capsule ruptured at 2000 N of distraction (450 lb). Stefko and colleagues[673] found the average load to failure of the entire IGHL to be 713 N, or 160 lb. Bigliani and coworkers[52] noted in 16 cadaver shoulders that the IGHL could be divided into three anatomic regions: a superior band, an anterior axillary pouch, and a posterior axillary pouch, the thickest of which was the superior band (2.8 mm). With relatively low strain rates, the stress at failure was found to be nearly identical for the three regions of the ligament, an average of 5.5 MPa, which is 5.5 N (1.2 lb) per square millimeter. Therefore, to function as the primary stabilizer for a load of 300 lb as in the aforementioned

example, the IGHLs of these cadavers would need to be 250 mm² in cross section. Thus, no experimental measurements have demonstrated that the IGHL alone is sufficiently strong to balance the torque resulting from a load of 10 lb applied to the arm at a distance of 30 inches from the center of the humeral head.

Excessive ligament tension can produce obligate translation of the humeral head. Harryman and colleagues[253] demonstrated that certain passive motions of the glenohumeral joint forced translation of the humeral head away from the center of the joint. This obligate translation occurs when the displacing force generated by ligament tension (quantity "P" in Fig. 14–47) overwhelms the concavity compression stability mechanism (Fig. 14–49). In Harryman's study, anterior humeral translation occurred at the extremes of flexion and cross-body adduction, whereas posterior humeral translation occurred at

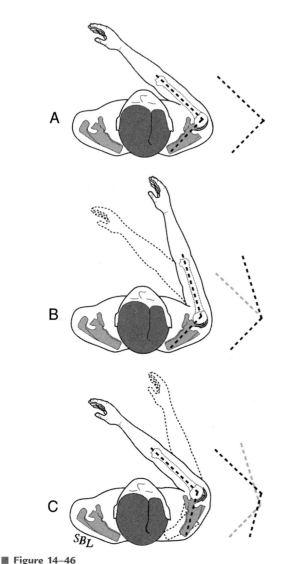

the extremes of extension and external rotation. Operative tightening of the posterior portion of the capsule increased anterior translation on flexion and cross-body adduction and caused it to occur earlier in the arc of motion than in an intact joint. Operative tightening of the posterior part of the capsule also resulted in significant superior translation with flexion of the glenohumeral joint. These data indicate that glenohumeral translation may occur in sports when the joint is forced to the extremes of its motion, such as at the transition between late cocking and early acceleration. Such obligate translation may account for the posterior labral tears and calcifications seen at the posterior glenoid in throwers. In addition, these results point to the hazard of overtightening the glenohumeral capsule, which may result in a form of secondary osteoarthritis known as capsulorrhaphy arthropathy. Hawkins and Angelo[261] pointed to these complications of obligate translation in overtightened capsular repairs.

■ **Figure 14–46**

A, Excessive posterior capsular laxity allows an excessively small angle between the humerus and the plane of the scapula; as a result, posterior stability is challenged. **B,** Normal tightness appropriately limits the allowed angular position to the range that can be stabilized. **C,** Cross-body adduction is achieved by scapular protraction, as well as by humeroscapular angulation.

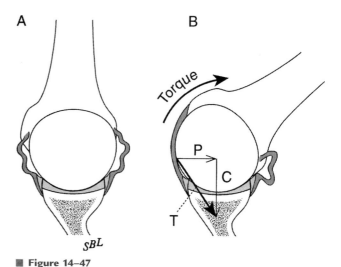

■ **Figure 14–47**

A, When the glenohumeral ligaments are slack, they exert no force. **B,** When torque is applied, the ligaments come under tension (T). This ligament tension exerts a compressive force (C) directed into the glenoid and a displacing force (P) pushing the humeral head away from the tight ligament.

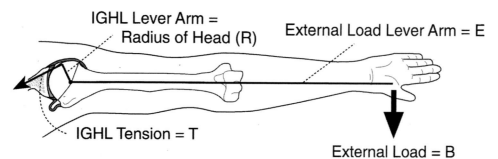

■ **Figure 14–48**

Torque balance. In the absence of other forces, the product of ligament tension (T) and the humeral head radius (R) must equal the product of the external load (B) and its lever arm (E). If the point of application of the external force is 40 inches away from the center of the head and if the radius of the head is 1 inch, the tension in the ligament must be 40 times the external force. IGHL, inferior glenohumeral ligament. *(Modified from Matsen FA III, Lippitt SB, Sidles JA, and Harryman DT II: Practical Evaluation and Management of the Shoulder. Philadelphia: WB Saunders, 1994.)*

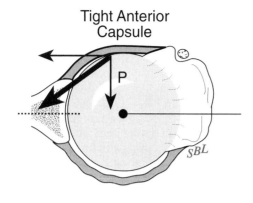

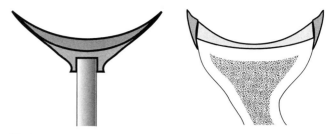

■ **Figure 14–50**

In cross section, the glenoid looks much like a rubber suction cup with respect to its feathered, compliant edges and more rigid center. *(Modified from Matsen FA III, Lippitt SB, Sidles JA, and Harryman DT II: Practical Evaluation and Management of the Shoulder. Philadelphia: WB Saunders, 1994.)*

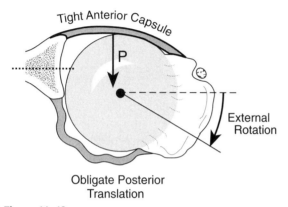

■ **Figure 14–49**

If the humerus is rotated beyond the point at which the ligaments become tight, the displacing force (P) can push the humeral head out of the glenoid center—a phenomenon known as obligate translation. *(Modified from Matsen FA III, Lippitt SB, Sidles JA, and Harryman DT II: Practical Evaluation and Management of the Shoulder. Philadelphia: WB Saunders, 1994.)*

Adhesion/Cohesion

Adhesion/cohesion is a stabilizing mechanism by which joint surfaces wet with joint fluid are held together by the molecular attraction of the fluid to itself and to the joint surfaces. Fluids such as water and joint fluid demonstrate the property of cohesion; that is, they tend to stick together. Some surfaces, such as clean glass or articular cartilage, can be wet with water or synovial fluid, which means that the fluid adheres to them. When two surfaces with adherent fluid are brought into contact, the adhesion of the fluid to the surfaces and the cohesion of the fluids tend to hold the two surfaces together (like two wetted microscope slides). The amount of stability generated by adhesion/cohesion is related to the adhesive and cohesive properties of the joint fluid, the "wetability" of the joint surfaces, and the area of contact between the glenoid socket and the humerus. Joint fluid has the highly desirable properties of (1) high tensile strength (difficult to pull apart) and (2) low shear strength (allows easy sliding of the two joint surfaces on each other with low resistance).[653]

The adhesion/cohesion effect is reduced by any factor that lowers the cohesion of joint fluid (such as in inflammatory joint disease), reduces wetability of the joint surfaces (as may occur in degenerative joint disease), or diminishes the glenohumeral contact area (such as in a displaced articular surface fracture or a congenitally small glenoid). It is also noteworthy that adhesion/cohesion forces do not stabilize a prosthetic shoulder replacement because metal and polyethylene are insufficiently compliant to provide the necessary nearly perfect congruence and because water does not adhere to their surfaces.

The Glenohumeral "Suction Cup"

This mechanism provides stability by virtue of the seal of the labrum and capsule to the humeral head (Fig. 14–50). A suction cup adheres to a smooth surface by expressing the interposed air or fluid and then forming a seal with the surface. A rubber suction cup is noncompliant in the center but becomes more flexible toward its periphery. In a similar manner, the center of the glenoid is covered with a relatively thin layer of articular cartilage. At greater distances from the center, the articular cartilage becomes thicker and thus provides greater flexibility. More peripherally, the glenoid labrum and, finally, the capsule provide even more flexibility. This graduated flexibility permits the socket to conform and seal to the smooth humeral articular surface. Compression of the head into the glenoid fossa expels any intervening fluid so that a "suction" is produced that resists distraction.

The glenoid suction cup stabilization mechanism was demonstrated by Harryman and associates.[252] In elderly cadaver shoulders without degenerative changes, the suction cup resisted an average of 20 ± 3 N of lateral traction (about 4 lb). Creating a defect in the labrum completely eliminated the suction cup effect. No suction cup effect could be demonstrated in the two shoulders with mild degenerative change of the joint surface. It is likely that this effect would be even stronger in younger living shoulders in which the articular cartilage, glenoid labrum, and joint capsule are larger, more hydrated, and more compliant. Like stabilization from adhesion/cohesion, the glenoid suction cup centers the head of the humerus in the glenoid without muscle action and is effective in midrange positions in which the capsule and ligaments are not under tension.

Limited Joint Volume

Limited joint volume is a stabilizing mechanism in which the humeral head is held to the glenoid by the relative vacuum created when they are distracted (Figs. 14–51 and 14–52). Although it is common to speak of the gleno-humeral joint space, there is essentially no space and minimal free fluid within the confines of the articular surfaces and the joint capsule of a normal glenohumeral joint. The scarcity of fluid within the joint can be confirmed on MRI scans of normal joints, on inspection of normal joints, and on attempts to aspirate fluid from normal joints. The appearance of the *potential* joint volume can only be demonstrated after instilling fluids such as air, saline, or contrast material into the joint. Osmotic action by the synovium removes free fluid, thus keeping slightly negative pressure within a normal joint.[398,495,653] This negative intra-articular pressure holds the joint together with a force proportional to the joint surface area and the magnitude of the negative intra-articular pressure. For example, if the colloid osmotic pressure of normal synovial fluid is 10 mm Hg and the colloid osmotic pressure of the synovial interstitium is 14 mm Hg, the equilibrium pressure in the joint fluid will be −4 mm Hg.[653] This negative intra-articular pressure adds a small amount of resistance to distraction (about 1 oz/inch²) to the limited joint volume effect. Because a normal joint is sealed, attempted distraction of the joint surfaces lowers the intra-articular pressure even more, thereby progressively adding substantial resistance to greater displacement.[252,313]

The limited joint volume effect is reduced if the joint is vented (opened to the atmosphere) or the capsular boundaries of the joint are very compliant. In the latter circumstance, attempted distraction draws the flexible capsule into the joint and produces a "sulcus" (Figs. 14–51 and 14–52). The decreased stability from venting the joint was initially described by Humphry in 1858[303] and subsequently by others.* Gibb and colleagues[215,441] found that simply venting the capsule with an 18-gauge needle reduced the force necessary to translate the head of the humerus halfway to the edge of the glenoid by an average of 50%. Wulker and coworkers[780] found that venting the joint increased displacement of the joint with an applied load of 50 N by 50% in all directions.

From these results it is expected that glenohumeral stability from limited joint volume is compromised by arthrography, arthroscopy, articular effusions, hemarthrosis, and other situations in which free fluid is allowed to enter the glenohumeral joint. In a very interesting study, Habermeyer and associates[240,241] found that the mean stabilizing force obtained by atmospheric pressure was 146 N (32 lb). In 15 stable living shoulders, traction on the arm caused negative intra-articular pressure proportionate to the amount of force exerted. In contrast, unstable shoulder joints with a Bankart lesion did not exhibit this phenomenon.

These stabilizing mechanisms may be overwhelmed by the application of traction, as in cracking of the

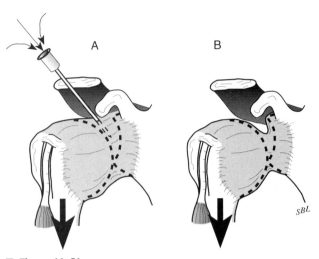

■ Figure 14–51

Normally, the glenohumeral capsule establishes a limited joint volume, so distraction of the humeral head produces a relative vacuum within the capsule that resists further displacement. **A,** Venting of the capsule eliminates the limited joint volume effect. **B,** The limited joint volume effect is reduced if the capsule is excessively compliant and can be displaced into the joint. *(From Matsen FA III, Lippitt SB, Sidles JA, and Harryman DT II: Practical Evaluation and Management of the Shoulder. Philadelphia: WB Saunders, 1994.)*

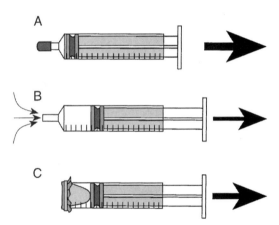

■ Figure 14–52

Limited joint volume effect demonstrated with a syringe model. Substantial force is required to pull the plunger from a plugged syringe **(A)**. This stabilizing effect is lost if the syringe is uncapped **(B)** or if the end of the syringe is covered with compliant material **(C)**. *(From Matsen FA III, Lippitt SB, Sidles JA, and Harryman DT II: Practical Evaluation and Management of the Shoulder. Philadelphia: WB Saunders, 1994.)*

metacarpophalangeal joint. A "crack" is produced as the joint cavitates: subatmospheric pressure within the joint releases gas (>80% carbon dioxide) from solution in the joint fluid. This release of gas is accompanied by a sudden increase in separation of the joint surfaces. Once a joint has cracked, it cannot be cracked again until about 20 minutes later when all the gas has been reabsorbed.[608,714]

Stability at Rest

It is apparent that a relaxed glenohumeral joint is held together without either active muscle contraction or

---

*See references 117, 175, 372, 502, 541, 542, 651, 694, 695, 779.

ligament tension. The intact shoulder of a fresh anatomic specimen,[372] the anesthetized and paralyzed shoulder of a patient in the operating room, and the arm relaxed at the side[38] all maintain the normal relationships of the glenoid and humeral joint surfaces. This resting stability is due to a group of mechanisms, including adhesion/cohesion, the glenoid suction cup, and limited joint volume. These mechanisms save energy, as pointed out by Humphry in 1858[303]: "We have only to remember that this power is in continual operation to appreciate the amount of animal force that is economized."

Superior Stability: The Same Plus a Unique Addition

Superior stability benefits from all the same mechanisms as anterior, posterior, and inferior stability: glenoid orientation, muscle balance, glenoid shape, ligamentous effects, adhesion/cohesion, the suction cup, and limited joint volume. Compression of the humeral head into the glenoid concavity is an important mechanism by which the head of the humerus is centered and stabilized in the

glenoid fossa to resist superiorly directed loads (Fig. 14–53). Even when a substantial supraspinatus defect is present, compression from the subscapularis and infraspinatus can hold the humeral head centered in the glenoid (Fig. 14–54). More severe cases of chronic rotator cuff deficiency, however, may be associated with superior subluxation of the head of the humerus and wear on the superior lip of the glenoid fossa (Fig. 14–55). This erosive wear flattens the superior glenoid concavity and thereby reduces the effective glenoid depth in that direction. Once the effective superior glenoid depth is lost, repair of the rotator cuff tendons or complex capsular reconstructions cannot completely restore the glenohumeral stability previously provided by concavity compression (Fig. 14–55).

In addition to mechanisms that stabilize the shoulder in other directions, superior stability has a unique aspect: a ceiling effect provided by the superior cuff tendon interposed between the humeral head and the coracoacromial arch. As every shoulder surgeon has observed, in a normal shoulder in a resting position, no gap is present between the humeral head, the superior cuff tendon, and the coracoacromial arch. As a result, the slightest amount of superior translation compresses the cuff tendon between the humeral head and the arch. Thus, when the humeral head is pressed upward (for example, when pushing up from an armchair or with isometric contraction of the deltoid), further superior displacement is opposed by a downward force exerted by the coracoacromial arch through the cuff tendon to the humeral head. Ziegler and coworkers[791] confirmed this stabilizing effect in cadavers by demonstrating

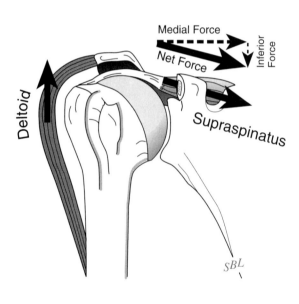

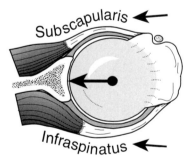

■ **Figure 14–53**
The supraspinatus muscle compresses the humeral head into the glenoid and thereby provides stability against displacement by the force of the deltoid. It is not optimally oriented to depress the head of the humerus because the inferiorly directed component of its force is small. *(From Matsen FA III, Lippitt SB, Sidles JA, and Harryman DT II: Practical Evaluation and Management of the Shoulder. Philadelphia: WB Saunders, 1994.)*

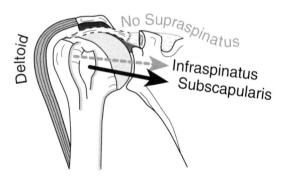

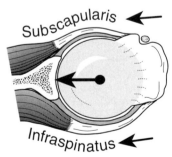

■ **Figure 14–54**
Compressive force from the infraspinatus and subscapularis can stabilize the humeral head in the absence of a supraspinatus, provided that the glenoid concavity is intact. *(Modified from Matsen FA III, Lippitt SB, Sidles JA, and Harryman DT II: Practical Evaluation and Management of the Shoulder. Philadelphia: WB Saunders, 1994.)*

acromial deformation when the neutrally positioned humerus was loaded in a superior direction. By attaching strain gauges percutaneously to the acromion they were able to measure its deformation under load. The acromion thus became an in situ load transducer. By applying known loads to the acromion, they were able to derive calibration load-deformation curves that were

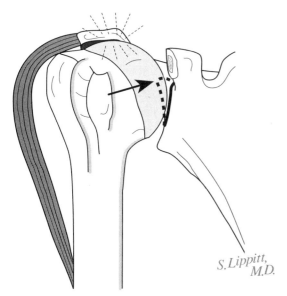

■ **Figure 14–55**
Erosion of the superior glenoid concavity compromises the concavity compression stability mechanism and allows upward translation. *(Modified from Matsen FA III, Lippitt SB, Sidles JA, and Harryman DT II: Practical Evaluation and Management of the Shoulder. Philadelphia: WB Saunders, 1994.)*

essentially linear. Superiorly directed loads applied to the humerus were then correlated with the resulting acromial loads and with superior humeral displacement. In 10 fresh cadaver specimens with the superior cuff tendon intact but not under tension, superiorly directed loads of 80 N produced only 1.7 mm of superior displacement of the humeral head relative to the acromion. When the cuff tendon was excised, a similar load produced superior displacement of 5.4 mm (*P* < .0001). In specimens in which the cuff tendon was intact, an upward load of 20 N gave rise to an estimated acromial load of 8 N. Greater humeral loads up to 80 N were associated with a linear increase in acromial load of up to 55 N when an upward load of 80 N was applied (Fig. 14–56). In a single in vivo experiment in which the acromion was instrumented and calibrated as in the cadavers, very similar relationships between upward humeral load and acromial load were noted (Fig. 14–56). These acromial loads must have been transmitted through the intact cuff tendon. When the tendon was excised, the humeral head rose until it contacted and again loaded the acromial undersurface (Fig. 14–57).

Flatow and colleagues[189] used a cadaver model to explore the active and passive restraints to superior humeral translation. Whereas Ziegler's study was conducted with the arm in neutral position with axial loads, Flatow's involved abducting the humerus with simulated deltoid and cuff muscle forces. Both groups noted that the presence of the supraspinatus tendon limited superior translation of the humeral head, even with no tension from simulated muscle action.

Both Ziegler and Flatow cautioned that the effectiveness of the cuff tendon as a superior stabilizing mechanism is dependent on an intact coracoacromial arch. Sacrifice of the ceiling of the joint, the coracoacromial

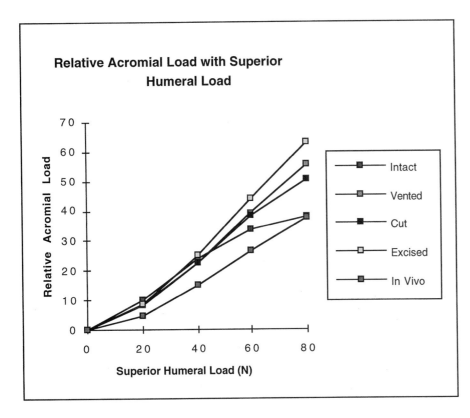

Relative Acromial Load with Superior Humeral Load

- ■ Intact
- ■ Vented
- ■ Cut
- □ Excised
- ■ In Vivo

■ **Figure 14–56**
Relative acromial load as a function of a superiorly directed humeral load. The chart compares loads for (1) intact specimens, (2) after venting of the joint to air, (3) after cutting (but not excising) the cuff tendon, and (4) after excising the superior cuff tendon. Also included are the data from (5) a single in vivo experiment performed with the identical instrumentation. Note that the difference in these acromial load–humeral load relationships is minimal, even when the cuff tendon has been excised. In the latter case, the humeral head loaded the acromion directly rather than through the interposed cuff tendon.

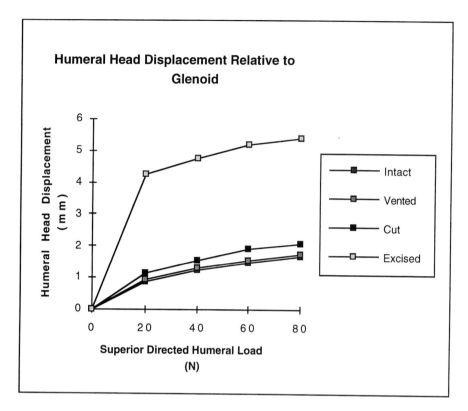

Humeral Head Displacement Relative to Glenoid

■ **Figure 14–57**
Mean superior humeral displacement (relative to the scapula) as a function of the superior humeral load. The chart compares displacements for (1) intact specimens, (2) after venting of the joint to air, (3) after cutting (but not excising) the cuff tendon, and (4) after excising the superior cuff tendon.

ligament, or the undersurface of the acromion can be expected to compromise the resistance to superior displacement of the humeral head.

The reader is referred to Soslowsky and colleagues' review[440] of stabilization of the glenohumeral joint surfaces by articular contact and by contact in the subacromial space (Chapter 5).

TYPES OF GLENOHUMERAL INSTABILITY

Glenohumeral instability is an inability to maintain the humeral head centered in the glenoid fossa.[440,441] Clinical cases of instability can be characterized according to the circumstances under which they occur, the degree of instability, and the direction of instability.

Circumstances of Instability

Congenital instability may result from local anomalies such as glenoid dysplasia[767] or from systemic conditions such as Ehlers-Danlos syndrome. Instability is acute if seen within the first days after its onset; otherwise it is *chronic*. A dislocation is *locked* (or *fixed*) if the humeral head has been impaled on the edge of the glenoid, thus making reduction of the dislocation difficult. If a glenohumeral joint has been unstable on multiple occasions, the instability is *recurrent*. Recurrent instability may consist of repeated glenohumeral dislocations, subluxations, or both.

Instability may arise from a *traumatic* episode in which an injury occurs to the bone, rotator cuff, labrum, capsule, and/or a combination of ligaments. Recurrent traumatic

instability typically produces symptoms when the arm is placed in a position near that of the original injury. Conversely, instability may arise from *atraumatic* decompensation of the stabilizing mechanisms. The degree to which the shoulder was "torn loose" as opposed to "'born loose" or just "got loose" is critical in determining the best management strategy.

We have found that most patients with recurrent instability fall into one of two groups. On one hand, patients with a *traumatic* etiology usually have *unidirectional* instability, often have obvious pathology such as a *Bankart* lesion, and frequently require *surgery* when the instability is recurrent—thus the acronym *TUBS*. On the other hand, patients with *atraumatic* instability often have *multidirectional* laxity that is frequently *bilateral* and usually responds to a *rehabilitation* program. However, should surgery be performed, the surgeon must pay particular attention to performing an *inferior* capsular shift and closing the rotator *interval*—thus the acronym *AMBRII*. Rowe[609] carefully analyzed 500 dislocations of the glenohumeral joint and determined that 96% were traumatic (caused by a major injury) and the remaining 4% were atraumatic. DePalma,[138] Rockwood,[596] and Collins and Wilde[110] also recognized the importance of distinguishing between traumatic and atraumatic instability of the shoulder.

Patients with atraumatic instability may have generalized joint laxity. Imazato[308] and Hirakawa[288] demonstrated that patients with "loose" shoulders have relatively immature, more soluble, and less cross-linked collagen fibers in their capsule, muscles, and skin than controls do; presumably, tissues such as the glenoid labrum would contain immature collagen as well, thus making them more deformable under load. Further evidence of constitutional factors is gained from a number of reports of positive family histories and bilateral involvement in individuals with shoulder dislocations (Fig. 14–58). O'Driscoll and Evans[532] and Dowdy and O'Driscoll[150] found a family history of shoulder instability in 24% of patients who required surgery for anterior glenohumeral instability. Morrey and Janes[488] reported a positive family history in approximately 15% of patients who were operated on for recurrent anterior shoulder instability. A positive family history was also noted twice as frequently in patients whose postoperative course was complicated by recurrent instability as in those with successful surgery. Rowe and colleagues[612] reported a positive family history in 27% of 55 patients with anterior shoulder instability

who were treated with a Bankart procedure. Bilateral instability was noted in 50% of patients with a positive family history versus 26% of those with a negative family history, which suggests the possibility of genetic predisposition.

When instability develops with no or minimal injury,[204,574,616] the initial reason for the loss of stability is often unclear. However, it appears that once lost, the factors maintaining stability may be difficult to regain. Certain phenomena may be self-perpetuating: when the humeral head rides up on the glenoid rim, the rim becomes flattened and less effective and allows easier translation. Furthermore, when normal neuromuscular control is compromised, the feedback systems that maintain head centering fail to provide effective input. Thus, the joint becomes launched on a cycle of instability leading to loss of the effective glenoid concavity and loss of neuromuscular control leading to more instability.

If a patient intentionally subluxates or dislocates the shoulder, the instability is described as *voluntary*. If the instability occurs unintentionally, it is *involuntary*. Voluntary and involuntary instability may coexist. Voluntary anterior dislocation may occur with the arm at the side or in abduction/external rotation. Voluntary posterior dislocation may occur with the arm in flexion, adduction, and internal rotation or with the arm at the side. The association of voluntary dislocation of the shoulder with emotional instability and psychiatric problems has been noted by several authors (Figs. 14–59 and 14–60).[84,613] The desire to voluntarily dislocate the shoulder cannot be treated surgically. However, the fact that patients can voluntarily demonstrate their instability does not necessarily mean that they are emotionally impaired.

Neuromuscular causes of shoulder instability have been reported as well. Percy[561] described a woman in whom

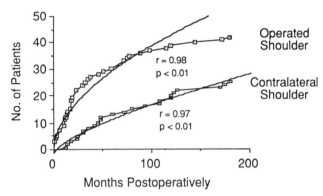

■ **Figure 14–58**
Incidence of contralateral shoulder instability from the data of O'Driscoll and Evans. In 13% of the patients with normal contralateral shoulders at the time of surgery, contralateral instability developed within the next 15 years. *(From O'Driscoll SW and Evans DC: The DuToit staple capsulorrhaphy for recurrent anterior dislocation of the shoulder: Twenty years of experience in six Toronto hospitals. Paper presented at the American Shoulder and Elbow Surgeons 4th Open Meeting, 1988, Atlanta.)*

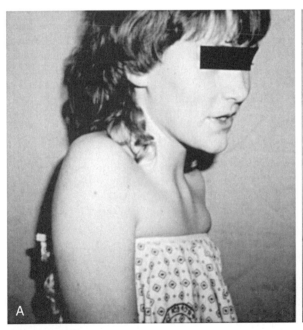
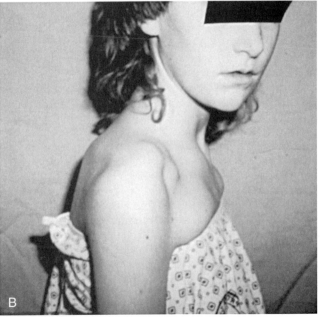

■ **Figure 14–59**
Voluntary instability. This patient had no significant history of injury but could voluntarily dislocate her shoulder with minimal discomfort. She is shown with the right shoulder reduced (**A**) and posteriorly dislocated (**B**).

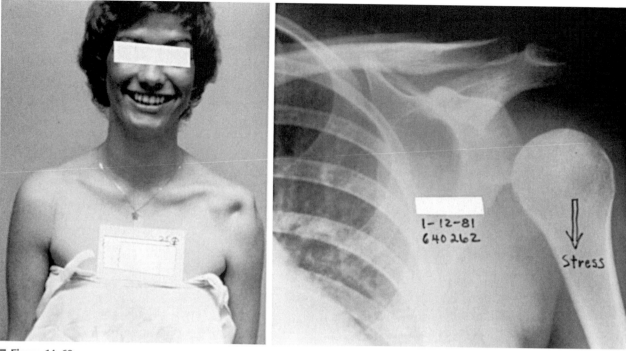

■ **Figure 14–60**
A patient with voluntary inferior instability. She performed this maneuver without discomfort. *(From Rockwood CA and Green DP [eds]: Fractures, 3 vols, 2nd ed. Philadelphia: JB Lippincott, 1984.)*

posterior dislocation developed after an episode of encephalitis. Kretzler and Blue[366] discussed the management of posterior dislocation of the shoulder in children with cerebral palsy. Sever,[644] Fairbank,[174] L'Episcopo,[393] Zachary,[790] and Wickstrom[757] reported techniques for the management of neurologic dislocation of the shoulder as a result of upper brachial plexus birth injuries. Stroke is another important neurologic cause of instability.[795]

Degree of Instability

Recurrent instability may be characterized as dislocation, subluxation, or apprehension. *Dislocation* of the glenohumeral joint is complete separation of the articular surfaces; immediate, spontaneous relocation may not occur. Glenohumeral *subluxation* is defined as symptomatic translation of the humeral head on the glenoid without complete separation of the articular surfaces. Subluxation of the glenohumeral joint is usually transient: the humeral head returns spontaneously to its normal position in the glenoid fossa. In a series of patients with anterior shoulder subluxation reported by Rowe and Zarins,[616] 87% of cases were traumatic, and over 50% of patients were not aware that their shoulders were unstable. Like dislocations, subluxations may be traumatic or atraumatic; anterior, posterior, or inferior; or acute or recurrent; or they may occur after previous surgical repairs that did not achieve complete shoulder stability. Recurrent subluxations may coexist with or be initiated by glenohumeral dislocation. Rowe and Zarins[609,617] reported seeing a Hill-Sachs compression fracture in 40% of patients in their series on subluxation of the shoulder, an observation indicating that at some time these shoulders had been

completely dislocated. *Apprehension* refers to the fear that the shoulder will subluxate or dislocate. This fear may prevent the individual from participating fully in work or sports.

Traumatic Instability

Traumatic instability may have consequences beyond recurrent dislocation of the shoulder. Nine percent of rugby players who stopped playing did so because of dislocation of the shoulder.[389] This figure was higher than the rate in players who ceased because of concussion, 4%. The likelihood of glenohumeral arthrosis developing has been shown to be 10 to 20 times higher in patients who have had a shoulder dislocation.[439]

Direction of Instability

Dislocations of the shoulder account for approximately 45% of all dislocations.[351] Of these, almost 85% are anterior glenohumeral dislocations.[92]

Anterior Dislocations

Subcoracoid dislocation is the most common type of anterior dislocation. The usual mechanism of injury that causes a subcoracoid dislocation is a combination of shoulder abduction, extension, and external rotation producing forces that challenge the anterior capsule and ligaments, the glenoid rim, and the rotator cuff mechanism. The head of the humerus is displaced anteriorly with respect to the glenoid and is inferior to the coracoid

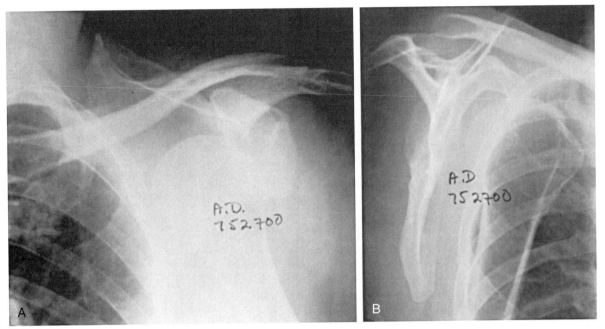

■ **Figure 14–61**
Subcoracoid dislocation. **A,** This anteroposterior view reveals that the head is medially displaced away from the glenoid fossa. With this view it is difficult to be sure whether the head is dislocated anteriorly or posteriorly. **B,** On a true scapular lateral view, the humeral head is completely anterior to the glenoid fossa. *(From Rockwood CA and Green DP [eds]: Fractures, 3 vols, 2nd ed. Philadelphia: JB Lippincott, 1984.)*

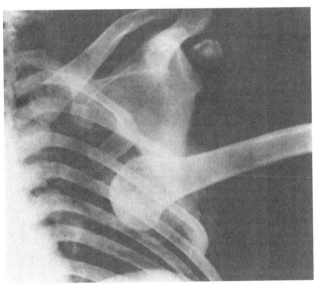

■ **Figure 14–62**
Intrathoracic anterior dislocation of the left shoulder. Note the wide interspace laterally between the third and fourth ribs and the avulsion fracture of the greater tuberosity, which remained in the vicinity of the glenoid fossa. *(From Rockwood CA Jr, Green DP, and Bucholz RW [eds]: Fractures in Adults. Philadelphia: JB Lippincott, 1991.)*

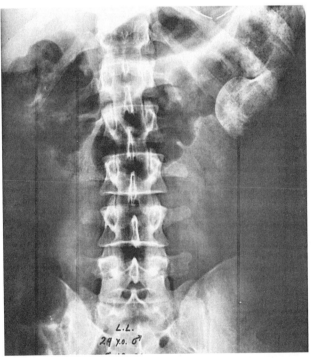

■ **Figure 14–63**
Abdominal radiograph revealing the proximal end of the humerus in the left upper quadrant.

process (Fig. 14-61). Other types of anterior dislocation include subglenoid (the head of the humerus lies anterior to and below the glenoid fossa), subclavicular (the head of the humerus lies medial to the coracoid process, just inferior to the lower border of the clavicle), intrathoracic (the head of the humerus lies between the ribs and the thoracic cavity) (Fig. 14-62),[217,491,558,633,754] and retroperitoneal (Figs. 14-63 and 14-64).[766] These rarer types of dislocation are usually associated with severe trauma and have a high incidence of fracture of the greater tuberosity of the humerus and rotator cuff avulsion. Neurologic, pulmonary, and vascular complications can occur, as can subcutaneous emphysema. West[754] reported a case of intrathoracic dislocation in which on reduction, the humerus was felt to slip out of the chest cavity with a sensation similar to that of slipping a large cork from a bottle. His patient, who had an avulsion fracture of the greater tuberosity and no neurologic deficit, regained functional range of motion and returned to his job as a carpenter.

Posterior Dislocations

Posterior dislocations may leave the humeral head in a subacromial (head behind the glenoid and beneath the acromion), subglenoid (head behind and beneath the

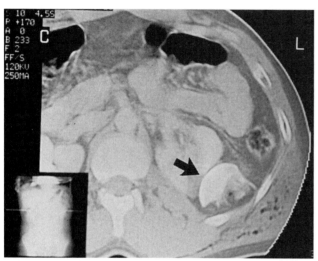

■ **Figure 14–64**
Enhanced computed tomographic scan of the abdomen. Note the retroperitoneal location of the humeral head posterior to the left kidney (arrow).

glenoid), or subspinous (head medial to the acromion and beneath the spine of the scapula) location. Subacromial dislocation is the most common by far (Fig. 14-65). Posterior dislocations are frequently locked. Hawkins and coworkers[265] reviewed 41 such cases related to motor vehicle accidents, surgery, and electroshock therapy.

The incidence of posterior dislocations is estimated at 2% but is difficult to ascertain because of the frequency with which this diagnosis is missed. Thomas[690] reported seeing only four cases of posterior shoulder dislocation in 6000 x-ray examinations. The literature reflects that the diagnosis of posterior dislocation of the shoulder is missed in over 60% of cases.[166,269,467,559,724] A 1982 article by Rowe and Zarins[617] indicated that the diagnosis was missed in 79% of cases! McLaughlin[454] stated that posterior shoulder dislocations are sufficiently uncommon that their occurrence creates a "diagnostic trap."

One of the largest series of posterior dislocations of the shoulder (37 cases) was recorded by Malgaigne[433] in 1855, 40 years before the discovery of x-rays. He and his colleagues made the diagnosis by performing a proper physical examination! Cooper[113] stated that the physical findings are so classic that he called it "an accident which cannot be mistaken."

Posterior dislocation may result from axial loading of an adducted, internally rotated arm,[481] from violent muscle contraction, or from electrical shock or convulsive seizures (see references 5, 84, 186, 260, 407, 448, 474, 535, 574, 642). In the case of involuntary muscle contraction, the combined strength of the internal rotators (latissimus dorsi, pectoralis major, and subscapularis muscles) simply overwhelms the external rotators (infraspinatus and teres minor muscles) (Fig. 14-66). Heller and coworkers proposed a classification of posterior shoulder dislocations.[271]

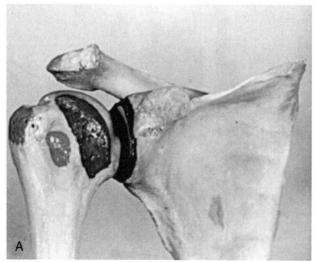
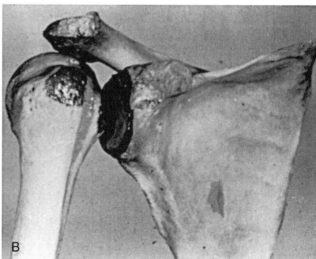

■ **Figure 14–65**
A subacromial posterior dislocation can appear deceptively normal on radiographs. **A,** Normal position of the humeral head in the glenoid fossa. **B,** In the subacromial type of posterior shoulder dislocation, the arm is in full internal rotation and the articular surface of the head is completely posterior, with only the lesser tuberosity left in the glenoid fossa. This positioning explains why abduction—and particularly external rotation—is blocked in posterior dislocations of the shoulder. *(From Rockwood CA and Green DP [eds]: Fractures, 3 vols, 2nd ed. Philadelphia: JB Lippincott, 1984.)*

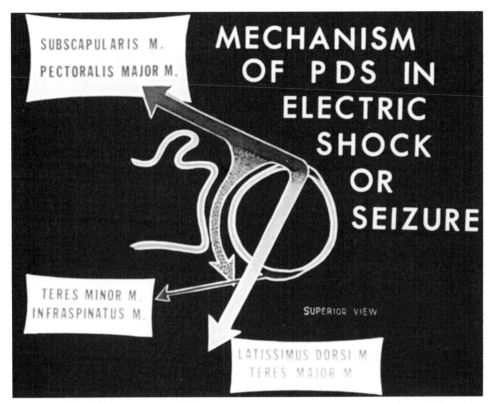

■ **Figure 14–66**
Mechanism of posterior dislocation of the shoulder (PDS) caused by an accidental electrical shock or a convulsive seizure. The strong internal rotators simply overpower the weak external rotators.

Inferior Dislocations

Inferior dislocation of the glenohumeral joint was first described by Middeldorpf and Scharm[471] in 1859. Lynn[423] in 1921 carefully reviewed 34 cases, and Roca and Ramos-Vertiz[595] in 1962 reviewed 50 cases from the world literature. Laskin and Sedlin[381] reported a case in an infant. Three bilateral cases have been described by Murrard,[497] Langfritz,[380] and Peiro and coworkers.[560] Nobel[519] reported a case of subglenoid dislocation in which the acromion-olecranon distance was shortened by 1.5 inches.

Inferior dislocation may be produced by a hyperabduction force that causes abutment of the neck of the humerus against the acromion process and subsequent leverage of the head out of the glenoid inferiorly (see Figs. 14-67 through 14-70). The humerus is then locked with the head below the glenoid fossa and the humeral shaft pointing overhead, a condition called luxatio erecta (Figs. 14-67 and 14-71). The clinical picture of a patient with luxatio erecta is so clear that it can hardly be mistaken for any other condition. The humerus is locked in a position somewhere between 110 and 160 degrees of adduction (Figs. 14-68 and 14-69). Severe soft tissue injury or fractures about the proximal end of the humerus occur with this dislocation (Figs. 14-68 and 14-71). At the time of surgery or autopsy, various authors have found avulsion of the supraspinatus, pectoralis major, or teres minor muscles and fractures of the greater tuberosity.[369,381,423,471,497,595] Neurovascular involvement is common.[200,397,423,465] Lev-El and Rubinstein[397] reported a patient with an injury to the axillary artery in whom a thrombus subsequently developed that required resection and a vein graft. Gardham and Scott[200] reported a case in 1980 in which the axillary artery was damaged in its third

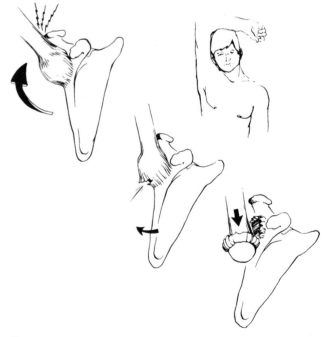

■ **Figure 14–67**
Mechanism of luxatio erecta. With hyperabduction of the humerus, the shaft abuts the acromion process, which stresses and then tears the capsule inferiorly and levers the head out inferiorly. The head and neck may be buttonholed through a rent in the inferior capsule, or the entire capsule may be separated. The rotator cuff muscles are always detached, and an associated fracture of the greater tuberosity may be present. *(From Rockwood CA Jr, Green DP, and Bucholz RW [eds]: Fractures in Adults. Philadelphia: JB Lippincott, 1991.)*

part and was managed with a bypass graft using the saphenous vein. Rockwood and Wirth found that in 19 patients with this condition, all 19 had a brachial plexus injury and some vascular compromise before reduction. The force may be so great that it forces the head out through the soft tissues and skin. Lucas and Peterson[420] reported the case of a 16-year-old boy who caught his arm in the power takeoff of a tractor and suffered an open luxatio erecta injury. Reduction of an inferior dislocation can often be accomplished by traction and countertraction maneuvers (Fig. 14–72). When closed reduction

cannot be achieved, the buttonhole rent in the inferior capsule must be surgically enlarged before reduction can occur.

Superior Dislocations

Speed[665] reported that Langier, in 1834, was the first to record a case of superior dislocation of the glenohumeral joint; Stimson[679] reviewed 14 cases that had been reported in the literature before 1912. In the current literature, little is mentioned about this type of dislocation, but undoubtedly occasional cases do occur. The usual cause is an extreme forward and upward force on an adducted arm. With displacement of the humerus upward, fractures may occur in the acromion, acromioclavicular joint, clavicle, coracoid process, or humeral tuberosities (Fig. 14–73). Extreme soft tissue damage occurs to the capsule rotator cuff, biceps tendon, and surrounding muscles. Clinically, the head rides above the level of the acromion. The arm is short and adducted to the side. Shoulder movement is restricted and quite painful, and neurovascular complications are usually present.

Bilateral Dislocations

Mynter[499] first described this condition in 1902; according to Honner,[290] only 20 cases were reported before 1969. Bilateral dislocations have been reported by McFie,[448] Yadav,[781] Onabowale and Jaja,[535] Segal and colleagues,[642] and Carew-McColl.[84] Most of these cases were the result of convulsions or violent trauma. Peiro and coworkers[560] reported bilateral erect dislocation of the shoulders in a man caught in a cement mixer. Bilateral dislocation of the shoulder secondary to accidental electrical shock has been described by Carew-McColl[84] and by Fipp.[186] Nicola and coworkers[511] reported cases of bilateral posterior fracture-dislocation after a convulsive seizure. Ahlgren and associates[5] reported three cases of bilateral posterior

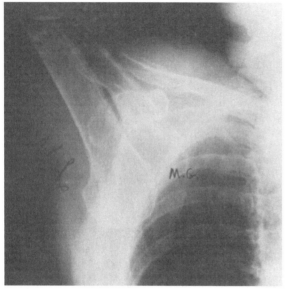

■ **Figure 14–68**
An anteroposterior x-ray film of an inferior dislocation reveals that the entire humeral head and surgical neck of the humerus are inferior to the glenoid fossa. *(From Rockwood CA Jr, Green DP, and Bucholz RW [eds]: Fractures in Adults. Philadelphia: JB Lippincott, 1991.)*

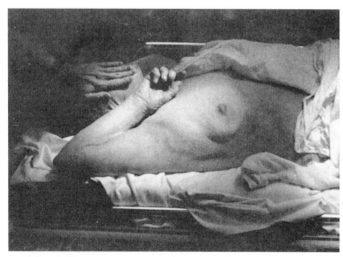
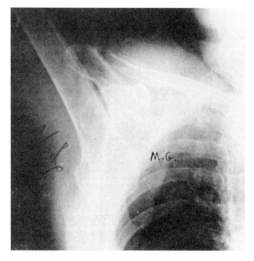

■ **Figure 14–69**
Inferior dislocation (luxatio erecta) of the right shoulder of a 75-year-old woman. Note that the arm is directed upward in relation to the trunk *(left)*. The hand of the flexed elbow is lying on the anterior of the chest. An anteroposterior x-ray film of the inferior dislocation reveals that the entire humeral head and surgical neck of the humerus are inferior to the glenoid fossa *(right)*. *(From Rockwood CA Jr, Green DP, and Bucholz RW [eds]: Fractures in Adults. Philadelphia: JB Lippincott, 1991.)*

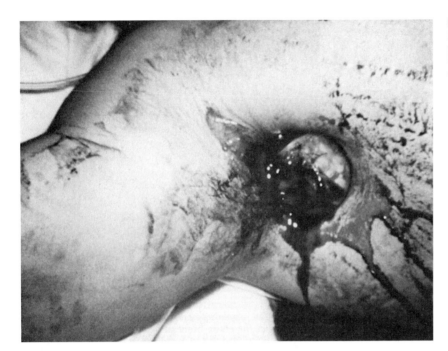

■ **Figure 14–70**
Photograph of the right shoulder and axilla of a patient who had an open inferior dislocation of the humeral head out through the axilla. *(Courtesy of George Armstrong.)*

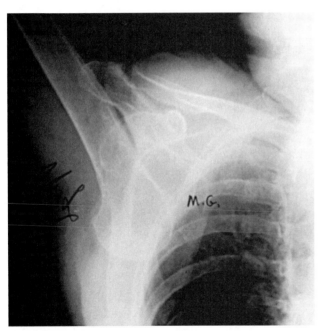

■ **Figure 14–71**
This anteroposterior radiograph of an inferior dislocation reveals that the entire humeral head and surgical neck of the humerus are inferior to the glenoid fossa.

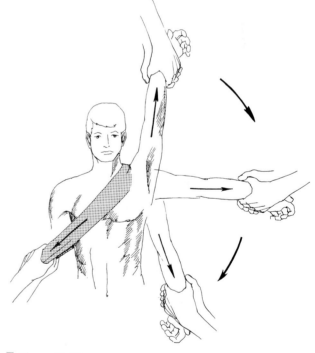

■ **Figure 14–72**
Technique of reduction of an inferior dislocation (luxatio erecta) of the glenohumeral joint. Countertraction is applied by an assistant using a folded sheet across the superior aspect of the shoulder and neck. Traction on the arm is first applied upward, and then gradually the arm is brought into less abduction and finally placed at the patient's side as demonstrated. *(From Rockwood CA Jr, Green DP, and Bucholz RW [eds]: Fractures in Adults. Philadelphia: JB Lippincott, 1991.)*

fracture-dislocation associated with a convulsion. Lindholm and Elmstedt[407] presented a case of bilateral posterior fracture-dislocation after an epileptic seizure, which was treated by open reduction and internal fixation with screws. Parrish and Skiendzielewski[553] reported a patient with bilateral posterior fracture-dislocation after status epilepticus. The diagnosis was missed for over 12 hours. Pagden and associates[545] reported two cases of posterior shoulder dislocation after seizures related to regional anesthesia. Costigan and coworkers[116] reported a case of undiagnosed bilateral anterior dislocation of the shoulder in a 74-year-old patient admitted to the hospital for an unrelated problem. The patient had no complaints related to the shoulders and was able to place both hands on her head and behind her back.

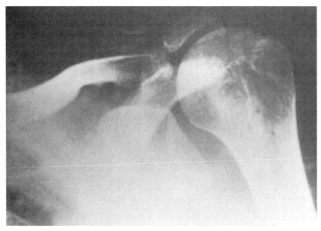

■ **Figure 14–73**
Superior dislocation of the left shoulder. Note that the head of the humerus is displaced superiorly from the glenoid fossa and that the fracture of the acromion process has also been displaced upward. *(From Rockwood CA Jr, Green DP, and Bucholz RW [eds]: Fractures in Adults. Philadelphia: JB Lippincott, 1991.)*

CLINICAL FINDINGS

Dislocation

History

The history should define the mechanism of the injury, including the position of the arm, the amount of force applied, and the point of force application.[574,616,617] Injury with the arm in extension, abduction, and external rotation favors anterior dislocation. Electroshock, seizures, or a fall on the flexed and adducted arm are commonly associated with posterior dislocation. If the instability is recurrent, the history defines the initial injury, the position or action that results in instability, how long the shoulder stays "out," whether radiographs are available with the shoulder out of joint, and what means have been necessary to reduce the shoulder. The history also solicits evidence of neurologic or rotator cuff problems after previous episodes of shoulder instability. Previous treatment of the recurrent instability, as well as the effectiveness of this treatment, should be documented.

Physical Examination of a Dislocated Shoulder

Anterior Dislocation

An acutely dislocated shoulder is usually very painful, and muscles are in spasm in an attempt to stabilize the joint. The humeral head may be palpable anteriorly. The posterior of the shoulder shows a hollow beneath the acromion. The arm is held in slight abduction and external rotation; internal rotation and adduction are usually limited. Because of the frequent association of nerve injuries[132] and, to a lesser extent, vascular injuries,[57] an essential part of the physical examination of an anteriorly dislocated shoulder is assessment of the neurovascular status of the upper extremity and charting of the findings before reduction.

Posterior Dislocation

Recognition of a posterior dislocation may be impaired by the lack of a striking deformity of the shoulder and by the fact that the shoulder is held in the traditional sling position of adduction and internal rotation. However, a directed physical examination will reveal the diagnosis. The classic features of a posterior dislocation include the following:

1. Limited external rotation of the shoulder (often to less than 0 degrees)
2. Limited elevation of the arm (often to less than 90 degrees)
3. Posterior prominence and rounding of the shoulder in comparison to the normal side
4. Flattening of the anterior aspect of the shoulder
5. Prominence of the coracoid process on the dislocated side

Asymmetry of the shoulder contours can often best be visualized by viewing the shoulders from above while standing behind the patient (Fig. 14–74).

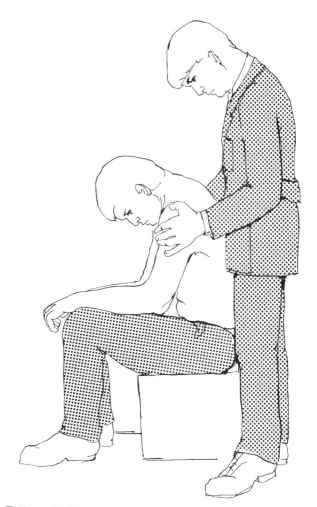

■ **Figure 14–74**
Inspection of the anterior and posterior aspects of the shoulders can best be accomplished by having the patient sit on a low stool with the examiner standing behind him. The injured shoulder can then be easily compared with the uninjured one. *(From Rockwood CA and Green DP [eds]: Fractures, 3 vols, 2nd ed. Philadelphia: JB Lippincott, 1984.)*

Motion is limited because the head of the humerus is fixed on the posterior glenoid rim by muscle forces, or the head may actually be impaled on the glenoid rim. With the passage of time, the posterior rim of the glenoid may further impact the fracture of the humeral head and produce a deep hatchet-like defect or a V-shaped compression fracture, which engages the head even more securely. Patients with old, unreduced posterior dislocations of the shoulder may have 30 to 40 degrees of glenohumeral abduction and some humeral rotation as a result of enlargement of the groove. With long-standing disuse of the muscles about the shoulder, atrophy will be present; such atrophy accentuates the flattening of the anterior portion of the shoulder, the prominence of the coracoid, and the fullness of the posterior portion of the shoulder.

Proper physical examination is essential. Rowe and Zarins[617] reported 23 cases of unreduced dislocation of the shoulder, 14 of which were posterior. Hill and McLaughlin[285] reported that in their series the average time from injury to diagnosis was 8 months. In the interval before the diagnosis of posterior dislocation of the shoulder is made, the injury may be misdiagnosed as a "frozen shoulder"[285,457] for which vigorous therapy may be mistakenly instituted in an attempt to restore range of motion.

Radiographic Evaluation

When a shoulder is dislocated, radiographs need to demonstrate (1) the direction of the dislocation, (2) the existence of associated fractures (displaced or not), and (3) possible barriers to relocation. The glenohumeral joint is most reliably imaged with three standardized views referred to the plane of the scapula: an anteroposterior view in the plane of the scapula (Fig. 14–75), a scapular lateral view (Fig. 14–76), and an axillary view (Fig. 14–77). The complete series of three views oriented to the scapula provides much more information than does the commonly obtained view in the plane of the body (Fig. 14–78). McLaughlin has said that reliance on anteroposterior radiographs will lead an unwary orthopaedist into a "diagnostic trap."[454] Dorgan[149] reported that in addition to obesity, technical factors may prevent accurate identification of the glenohumeral joint in the transthoracic lateral view.

Anteroposterior View in the Plane of the Scapula

In 1923, Grashey[228] recognized that to take a true anteroposterior radiograph of the shoulder joint, the direction of the x-ray beam must be perpendicular to the plane of the scapula. This view is most easily accomplished by placing the scapula flat on the cassette (a position that the patient can help achieve) and passing the x-ray beam at right angles to this plane and centering it on the coracoid process (Figs. 14–75 and 14–79). This view can be taken with the arm in a sling and the body rotated to the desired position (Figs. 14–80 and 14–81). In a normal shoulder this view reveals clear separation of the humeral subchondral bone from that of the glenoid (see Fig. 14–75).

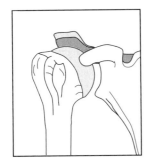

■ **Figure 14–75**
The anteroposterior view in the plane of the scapula is obtained by orienting the beam perpendicular to the plane of the scapula (see Fig. 14–27) and centering it on the coracoid tip while the film is parallel to the plane of the scapula. *(From Typischer Rontgenfilder, 1923.)*

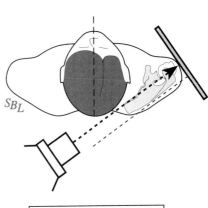
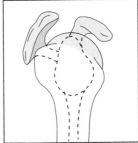

■ **Figure 14–76**
A lateral view in the plane of the scapula is obtained by orienting the beam parallel to the plane of the scapula and centering it on the glenoid while the film is perpendicular to the plane of the scapula.

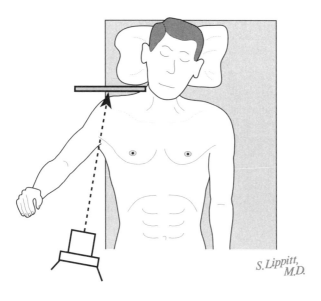

S.Lippitt, M.D.

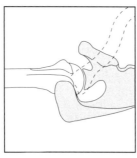

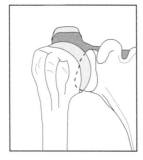

■ **Figure 14–77**
The axillary view is obtained by orienting the beam parallel to the scapula and centering it between the coracoid tip and the posterior angle of the acromion.

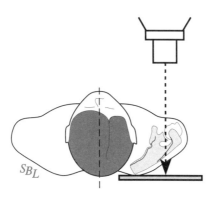

SBL

■ **Figure 14–78**
The anteroposterior view in the plane of the body presents an overlapping and often confusing view of the glenohumeral joint.

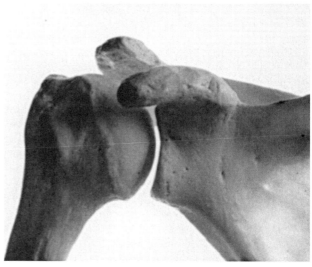

■ **Figure 14–79**
A simulated x-ray view of a scapular anteroposterior view using backlighted skeletal models. This view reveals the radiographic glenohumeral joint space and provides a good opportunity to detect fractures of the humerus or glenoid lip.

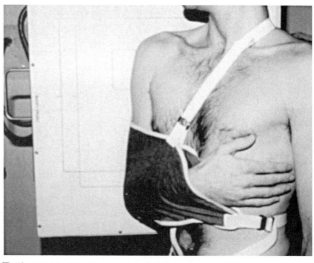

■ **Figure 14–80**
Positioning of the patient in a sling for an anteroposterior radiograph in the plane of the scapula. The scapula is placed flat on the cassette. The x-ray beam is positioned at right angles to the cassette and centered on the coracoid process.

Lateral View in the Plane of the Scapula

This view is taken at right angles to the anteroposterior view in the plane of the scapula (Figs. 14–76, 14–82, and 14–83).[454,457,458,501,597] Like the anteroposterior view, it can be obtained by positioning the body without moving the dislocated shoulder. The radiographic beam is passed in a medial-to-lateral direction parallel to the body of the scapula while the cassette is held perpendicular to the beam at the anterolateral aspect of the shoulder (Figs. 14–76 and 14–83).[597] In this view, the contour of the scapula projects as the letter "Y."[620] The downward stem of the Y is projected by the body of the scapula; the upper

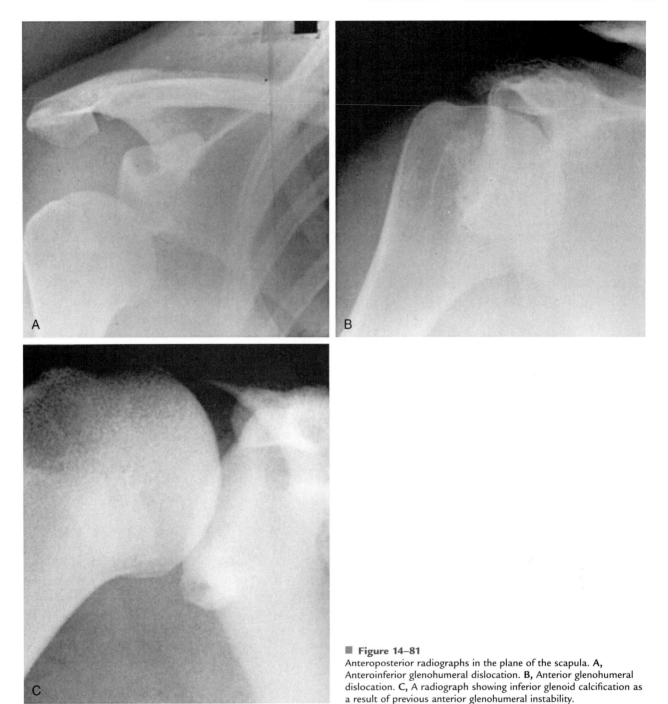

■ **Figure 14–81**
Anteroposterior radiographs in the plane of the scapula. **A,**
Anteroinferior glenohumeral dislocation. **B,** Anterior glenohumeral
dislocation. **C,** A radiograph showing inferior glenoid calcification as
a result of previous anterior glenohumeral instability.

forks are projected by the coracoid process anteriorly and
by the spine and acromion posteriorly (Figs. 14–84 and
14–85). The glenoid is located at the junction of the stem
and the two arms of the Y. In a normal shoulder, the
humeral head is at the center of the arms of the Y, that is,
in the glenoid fossa. In posterior dislocations, the head is
seen posterior to the glenoid (see Fig. 14–85); in anterior
dislocations, the head is anterior to it (see Fig. 14–84).

Axillary View

In this view, first described by Lawrence in 1915,[385,466] the
cassette is placed on the superior aspect of the shoulder.

This view requires that the humerus be abducted sufficiently to allow the radiographic beam to pass between it
and the thorax. Fortunately, sufficient abduction can be
achieved by gentle positioning of the dislocated shoulder
or by modifications of the technique (Figs. 14–77 and
14–86 to 14–89). The axillary radiograph is critical in
evaluation of a dislocated shoulder: it unambiguously
reveals not only the direction and magnitude of head displacement relative to the glenoid but also the presence
and size of head compression fractures, fractures of the
glenoid, and fractures of the humeral tuberosities (Figs.
14–90 to 14–94). The axillary view may also be helpful in
judging the bony competence and version of the glenoid

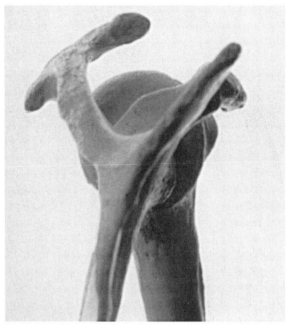

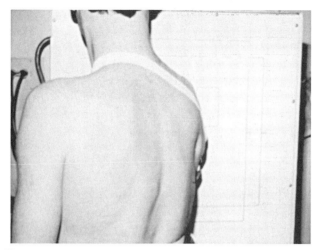

■ Figure 14–83
Position of the patient in a sling for a scapular lateral radiograph. The scapula is positioned perpendicular to the cassette. The beam should be placed parallel to the spine of the scapula and perpendicular to the cassette.

■ Figure 14–82
Simulated scapular lateral x-ray view with backlighted skeletal models. The x-ray beam is passed parallel to the plane of the scapula and is centered on the scapular spine. The view reveals the anteroposterior relationship of the head of the humerus in the glenoid fossa. The glenoid fossa is identified as the intersection of the spine of the scapula, the coracoid process, and the body of the scapula.

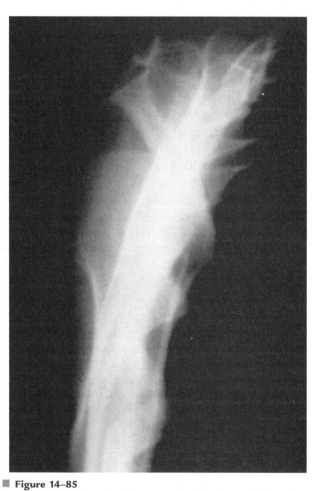

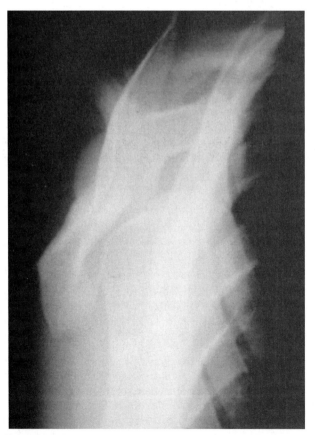

■ Figure 14–85
A scapular lateral view showing a posterior glenohumeral dislocation. The head of the humerus is dislocated posterior to the glenoid fossa and in this view appears to be sitting directly below the spine of the scapula.

■ Figure 14–84
Scapular lateral view showing an anterior glenohumeral dislocation. Note that the humerus is no longer centered at the base of the Y.

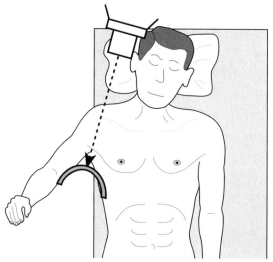

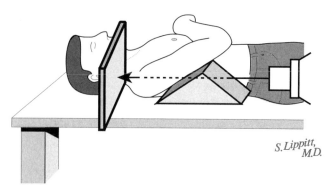

■ Figure 14–88
A trauma axillary lateral radiograph. This arm is flexed on a foam wedge. *(Modified from Tietge RA and Ciullo JV: The CAM axillary x-ray. Orthop Trans 6:451, 1982.)*

■ Figure 14–86
The axillary view with a curved cassette, a method that is useful if the arm cannot be adequately abducted for a routine axillary view.

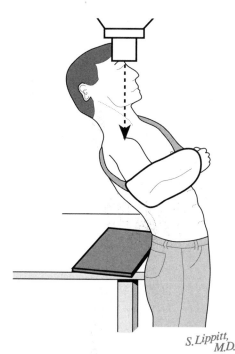

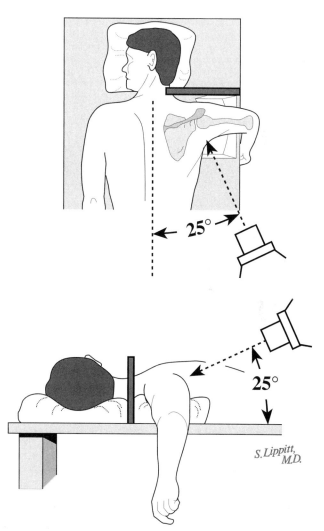

■ Figure 14–87
The Velpeau axillary lateral x-ray technique. With the arm in a sling, the patient leans backward until the shoulder is over the cassette. *(Modified from Bloom MH and Obata WG: Diagnosis of posterior dislocation of the shoulder with use of the Velpeau axillary and angle-up roentgenographic views. J Bone Joint Surg Am 49:943-949, 1967.)*

■ Figure 14–89
The West Point axillary lateral view. The patient is prone with the beam inclined 25 degrees down and 25 degrees medially. *(Modified from Rokous JR, Feagin JA, and Abbott HG: Modified axillary roentgenogram. Clin Orthop 82:84-86, 1972.)*

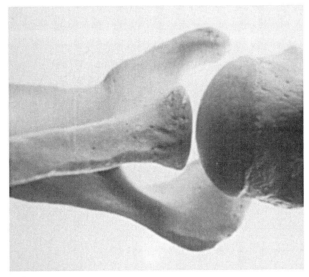

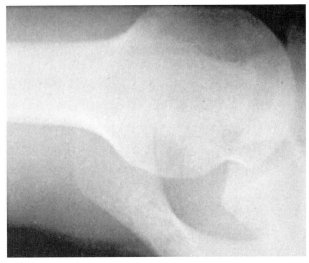

■ **Figure 14–90**
Simulated axillary view using a backlighted skeletal model. An x-ray beam is passed up the axilla to project the glenoid fossa between the coracoid process anteriorly and the scapular spine posteriorly. This projection reveals the radiographic glenohumeral joint space, the anteroposterior position of the head of the humerus relative to the glenoid, and a view of fractures of the glenoid lip and humerus.

■ **Figure 14–91**
Axillary view. Note the posterior humeral head defect (Hill-Sachs lesion) secondary to a previous anterior glenohumeral dislocation.

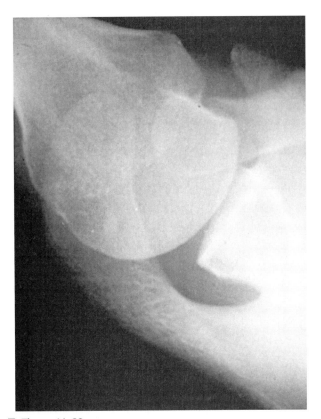

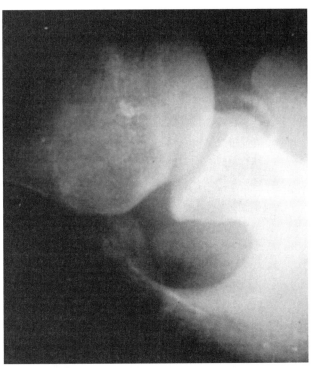

■ **Figure 14–93**
Axillary view showing an anterior glenoid defect and calcification as a result of an anterior glenohumeral dislocation. A posterior lateral humeral head defect is also seen.

■ **Figure 14–92**
Axillary view. This patient has an anterior humeral head defect that occurred as a result of a posterior glenohumeral dislocation.

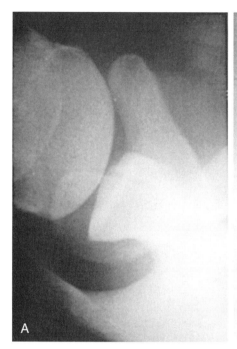
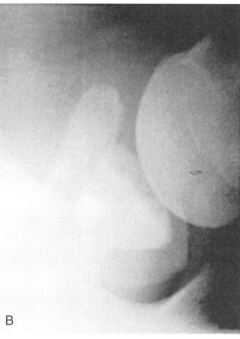

■ **Figure 14–94**
Bilateral axillary views. **A,** Rounding of the anterior glenoid rim as a result of recurrent anterior glenohumeral dislocation is evident on this axillary view. **B,** The normal side is shown for comparison.

fossa, but the projection must be standardized to avoid misinterpretation (see Fig. 14–37).

In his text on radiographic positioning, Jordan demonstrated the various techniques for obtaining axillary lateral views.[343] Cleaves[104,466] and Teitge and Ciullo[572] have described variations on this view (see Fig. 14–88). Rockwood has pointed out that in a situation in which the patient cannot abduct the arm sufficiently, a curved cassette or a rolled cardboard cassette can be placed in the axilla and the radiographic beam passed from a superior position (see Fig. 14–86). Bloom and Obata[58] modified the axillary technique so that the arm does not have to be abducted (see Fig. 14–87). They called this modification the Velpeau axillary lateral view. While wearing a sling or Velpeau dressing, the patient leans backward 30 degrees over the cassette on the table. The x-ray tube is placed above the shoulder and the beam is projected vertically down through the shoulder onto the cassette.

In summary, in the evaluation of a possibly dislocated shoulder or a fractured-dislocated shoulder, we recommend the three orthogonal projections of the shoulder (anteroposterior and lateral in the plane of the scapula and axillary views), which provide a sensitive assessment of shoulder dislocation. The use of fewer views or other less interpretable projections may obscure significant pathologic processes. If the three views cannot be taken, if a question has arisen regarding the diagnosis, or if the anatomy needs to be defined in greater detail, a CT scan may be of great assistance (Figs. 14–18 and 14–95 to 14–98).[359,589,650] By using modern methods of three-dimensional reconstruction, anterior inferior glenoid lesions and posterior lateral humeral head lesions can be shown in striking detail (Figs. 14–99 and 14–100). It is of note that the patient whose shoulder is shown in these figures obtained an excellent result after nonoperative treatment

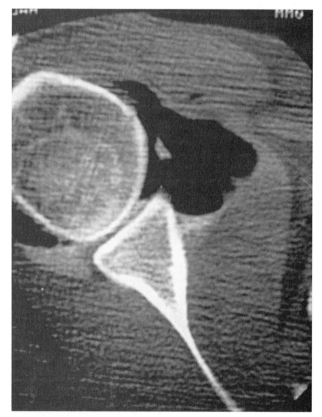

■ **Figure 14–95**
Computed tomographic scan of the glenohumeral joint with air contrast. This study demonstrates a bony avulsion from the anterior glenoid rim.

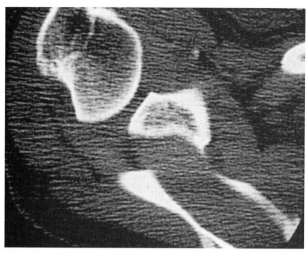

■ **Figure 14–96**
Computed tomographic scan of the glenohumeral joint. The posterior humeral head defect and the anterior glenoid defect are well demonstrated.

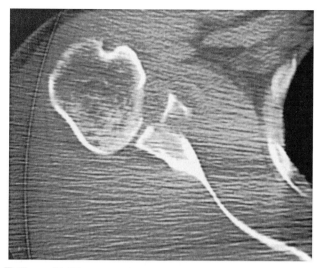

■ **Figure 14–97**
Computed tomographic scan of the glenohumeral joint showing a fracture of the anterior glenoid rim secondary to anterior glenohumeral dislocation.

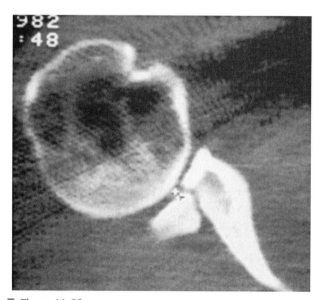

■ **Figure 14–98**
Computed tomographic scan of the glenohumeral joint demonstrating a fracture of the posterior glenoid rim as a result of posterior dislocation of the glenohumeral joint.

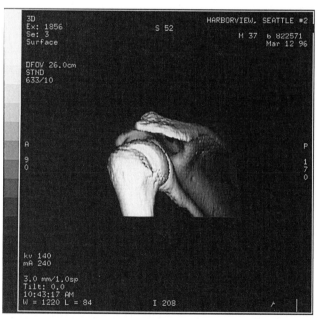

■ **Figure 14–99**
Three-dimensional computed tomographic reconstruction after reduction of a first-time dislocation showing a posterior lateral humeral head defect.

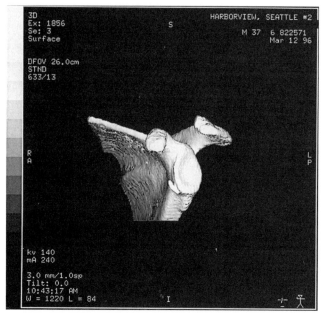

■ **Figure 14–100**
Three-dimensional computed tomographic reconstruction after reduction of a first-time dislocation showing anterior glenoid avulsion.

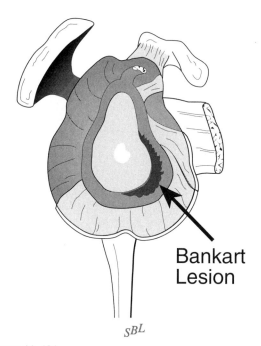

Bankart Lesion

SBL

■ **Figure 14–101**
The capsulolabral detachment typical of traumatic instability. *(Modified from Matsen FA III, Lippitt SB, Sidles JA, and Harryman DT II: Practical Evaluation and Management of the Shoulder. Philadelphia: WB Saunders, 1994.)*

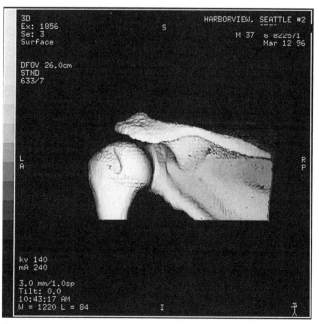

■ **Figure 14–102**
Three-dimensional computed tomographic reconstruction of the left shoulder of a 37-year-old man 3 days after his first traumatic glenohumeral dislocation. The patient recovered normal shoulder function with nonoperative management.

in spite of the damage shown on the radiographic reconstructions.

INJURIES ASSOCIATED WITH ANTERIOR DISLOCATIONS

Ligaments and Capsule

A common feature of traumatic anterior dislocations is avulsion of the anteroinferior glenohumeral ligaments and capsule from the glenoid lip, especially in younger individuals (Figs. 14–3, 14–101, 14–102). Nonhealing of this avulsion is a major factor in recurrent traumatic instability. Occasionally, the capsule may be avulsed from the anteroinferior portion of the humerus, sometimes with a fleck of bone.

Fractures

Fractures of the glenoid (Figs. 14–6, 14–98, 14–103), humeral head (Figs. 14–91 and 14–92), and tuberosities (Figs. 14–5 and 14–104 to 14–106) may accompany traumatic dislocations. A CT scan may be helpful in determining the degree of posterior displacement of fractures (Figs. 14–96 to 14–98, 14–107, and 14–108).

It is important to seek evidence of a nondisplaced humeral neck fracture on the prereduction radiographs lest this fracture be displaced during attempted closed reduction (see Fig. 14–106).[181]

Other fractures, such as those of the coracoid process, may be associated with glenohumeral dislocations.[45,777]

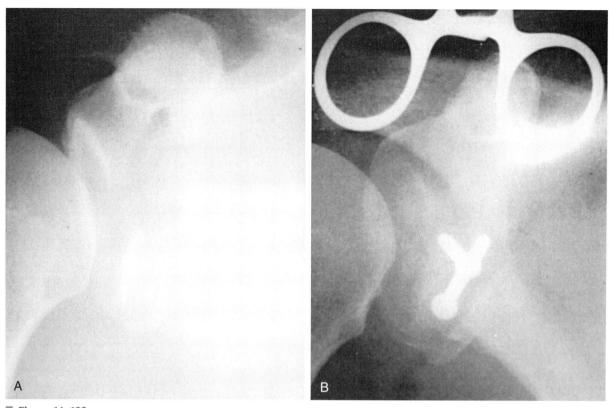

■ **Figure 14–103**
Anterior glenoid rim fracture. **A,** An anteroposterior radiograph demonstrates an anterior glenoid rim fracture secondary to traumatic anterior dislocation. **B,** An intraoperative anteroposterior radiograph shows reduction and screw fixation of an anterior glenoid rim fracture.

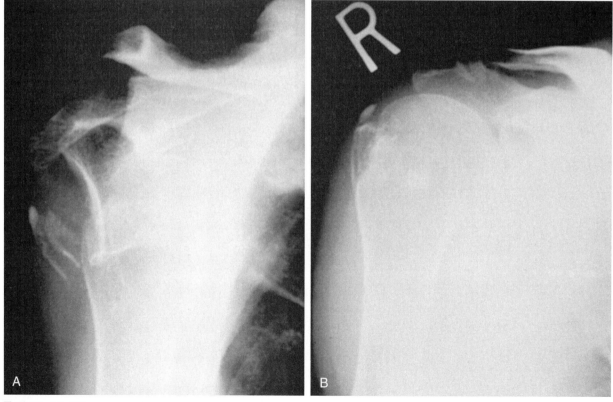

■ **Figure 14–104**
Greater tuberosity fracture. **A,** An anteroposterior radiograph before reduction shows a fracture of the greater tuberosity.
B, Postreduction anteroposterior radiograph of a greater tuberosity fracture.

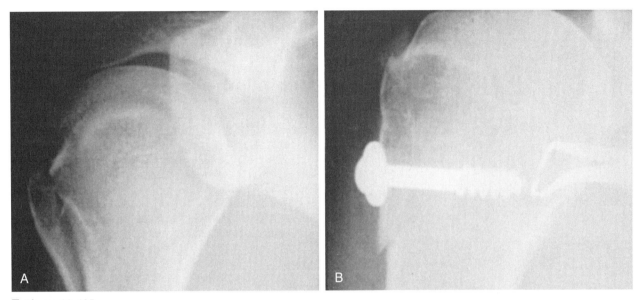

■ **Figure 14–105**

A, Radiograph showing a displaced greater tuberosity fracture. **B,** Intraoperative radiograph showing screw fixation of a greater tuberosity fracture.

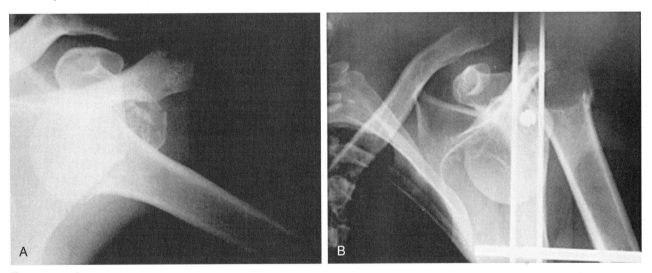

■ **Figure 14–106**

A, Anteroposterior view showing an anteroinferior dislocation with an associated greater tuberosity fracture. **B,** Anteroposterior view after a reduction attempt showing displacement of a humeral neck fracture.

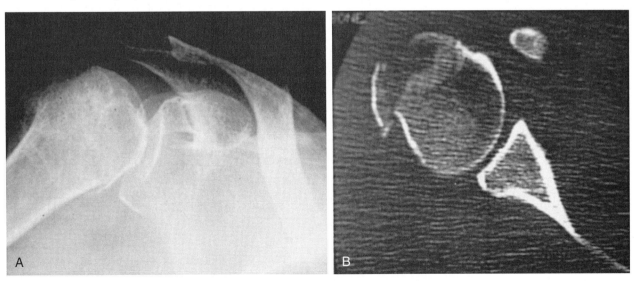

■ **Figure 14–107**

Minimally displaced greater tuberosity fracture. **A,** An anteroposterior radiograph shows a minimally displaced greater tuberosity fracture. **B,** A computed tomographic scan shows the position of the greater tuberosity.

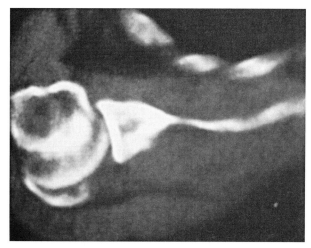

■ Figure 14–108
Computed tomographic scan of a significantly displaced greater tuberosity fracture.

Cuff Tears

Rotator cuff tears may accompany anterior and inferior glenohumeral dislocations (see Fig. 14-4). The frequency of this complication increases with age: in patients older than 40 years, the incidence exceeds 30%; in those older than 60 years, it exceeds 80%.[318,556,565,584,663,685,701]

Rotator cuff tears may be manifested as pain or weakness on external rotation and abduction.[262,507,565,582,756] Sonnabend reported a series of primary shoulder dislocations in patients older than 40 years.[663] Of the 13 patients who had complaints of weakness or pain after 3 weeks, 11 had rotator cuff tears. However, the presence of a rotator cuff tear may be masked by a coexisting axillary nerve palsy.[223,336]

Shoulder ultrasonography,[426] arthrography, or MRI is considered for evaluation of the possibility of an associated cuff tear (1) when shoulder dislocations occur in patients older than 40 years, (2) when initial displacement of the humeral head has been substantial (such as in a subglenoid dislocation), and (3) when pain or loss of rotator cuff strength has persisted for 3 weeks after a glenohumeral dislocation. Toolanen found sonographic evidence of rotator cuff lesions in 24 of 63 patients older than 40 years at the time of anterior glenohumeral dislocation.[702]

Prompt operative repair of these acute cuff tears is usually indicated. Itoi and Tabata[318] reported 16 rotator cuff tears in 109 shoulders with a traumatic anterior dislocation. The cuff was surgically repaired in 11 shoulders, and the results were graded as satisfactory in 73% of cases.

Neviaser and coauthors[508] reported on 37 patients older than 40 years in whom the diagnosis of cuff rupture was initially missed after an anterior dislocation of the shoulder. The weakness from the cuff rupture was often erroneously attributed to axillary neuropathy. Recurrent anterior instability caused by rupture of the subscapularis and anterior capsule from the lesser tuberosity developed in 11 of these patients. None of these shoulders had a Bankart lesion. Repair of the capsule and subscapularis restored stability in all of the patients.

Vascular Injuries

Several reports of arterial and neurologic injury with shoulder dislocation reinforce the importance of a thorough neurovascular evaluation.[272,438,536]

Vascular damage most frequently occurs in elderly patients with stiffer, more fragile vessels. The injury may be to the axillary artery or vein or to branches of the axillary artery—the thoracoacromial, subscapular, circumflex, and rarely, the long thoracic. Sometimes these injuries can be combined, as pointed out by Kirker, who described a case of rupture of the axillary artery and axillary vein along with a brachial plexus palsy.[360] Injury may occur at the time of either dislocation or reduction.[14,124,236,321]

Anatomy

The axillary artery is divided into three parts that lie medial to, behind, and lateral to the pectoralis minor muscle (Fig. 14–109). Injuries most commonly involve the second part, where the thoracoacromial trunk may be avulsed, and the third part, where the subscapular and circumflex branches may be avulsed or the axillary artery may be totally ruptured.

Mechanism of Injury

Damage to the axillary artery can take the form of a complete transection, a linear tear of the artery caused by avulsion of one of its branches, or an intravascular thrombus, perhaps related to an initial tear. The artery is relatively fixed at the lateral margin of the pectoralis minor muscle. With abduction and external rotation, the artery is taut; when the head dislocates, it forces the axillary artery forward, and the pectoralis minor acts as a fulcrum over which the artery is deformed and ruptured.[75,321,475]

Watson-Jones[744] reported the case of a man who had multiple anterior dislocations that he reduced himself. Finally, when the man was older, the axillary artery ruptured during one of the dislocations and he died. Vascular injuries may occur either at the time of dislocation or

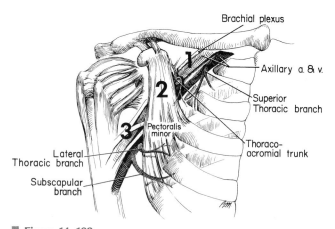

■ Figure 14–109
The axillary artery is divided into three parts by the pectoralis minor muscle; the second part is behind it, and the third part is lateral to it. (From Rockwood CA and Green DP [eds]: Fractures, 3 vols, 2nd ed. Philadelphia: JB Lippincott, 1984.)

during attempted reduction. Sometimes it is unclear which is the case.[360,510,676]

Injury at the Time of Dislocation

Vascular injuries are commonly associated with inferior dislocation.[200,397,423,465] Gardham and Scott[200] reported occlusion of the axillary artery with an erect dislocation of the shoulder in a 40-year-old patient who had fallen headfirst down an escalator. Although vascular injuries are most common in older individuals, they can occur at any age.[49,152,188,395,629,674] Banatta and coworkers[35] reported the case of a 13-year-old boy who ruptured his axillary artery after a subcoracoid dislocation sustained while wrestling.

Injury at the Time of Reduction

Vascular damage at the time of reduction occurs primarily in the elderly, particularly when a chronic old anterior dislocation is mistaken for an acute injury and closed reduction is attempted. The largest series of vascular complications associated with closed reduction of the shoulder has been reported by Calvet and coworkers,[83] who in 1941 collected 90 cases. This paper, which revealed the tragic end results, must have accomplished its purpose because very few reports have appeared in the literature since then dealing with the complications that occur during reduction. In their series, in which 64 of 91 reductions were performed many weeks after the initial dislocation, the mortality rate was 50%. The other patients either lost the arm or function of the arm. Besides the long delay from dislocation to reduction, these injuries may also be due to the use of excessive force. Delpeche observed a case in which the force of 10 men was used to accomplish the shoulder reduction; such force damaged the axillary vessel.[237]

Signs and Symptoms

Vascular damage may be obvious or subtle. Findings may include pain, expanding hematoma, pulse deficit, peripheral cyanosis, peripheral coolness and pallor, neurologic dysfunction, and shock. Doppler or an arteriogram should confirm the diagnosis and locate the site of injury.

Treatment and Prognosis

Patients suspected of having major arterial injury are managed as a surgical emergency, with establishment of a major intravenous line and obtaining blood for transfusion. Jardon and coworkers[321] pointed out that bleeding can be temporarily controlled by digital pressure on the axillary artery over the first rib. These authors also recommend that the axillary artery be explored through the subclavicular operative approach, as described by Steenburg and Ravitch.[672]

The treatment of choice for a damaged axillary artery is either direct repair or a bypass graft after resection of the injury. Excellent results have been reported with

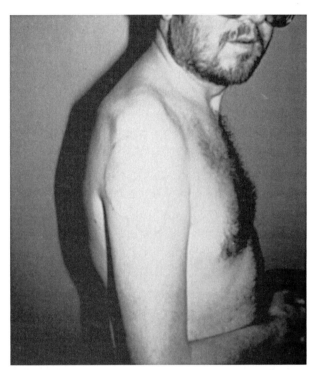

■ **Figure 14–110**
This patient sustained an axillary nerve palsy secondary to glenohumeral dislocation. Note the area of decreased sensation diagrammed on the lateral aspect of the proximal end of the humerus. Also note the presence of significant wasting.

prompt management of these vascular injuries.* The results of simple ligation of the vessels in elderly patients have been disappointing, probably because of poor collateral circulation and the presence of arteriosclerotic vascular disease in these typically older individuals.[341,360,719] Even when ligation has been performed in younger patients with good collateral circulation, approximately two thirds of these patients have lost function of the upper extremity, for example, because of the development of upper extremity claudication.

Nerve Injuries

The brachial plexus and the axillary artery lie immediately anterior, inferior, and medial to the glenohumeral joint.[227] It is not surprising, therefore, that neurovascular injuries frequently accompany traumatic anterior glenohumeral dislocations (Fig. 14–110).

Anatomy

The axillary nerve originates off the posterior cord of the brachial plexus. It crosses the anterior surface of the subscapularis muscle and angulates sharply posteriorly to travel along the inferior shoulder joint capsule. It then leaves the axilla to exit through the quadrangular space below the lower border of the teres minor muscle, where

---

*See references 75, 121, 148, 200, 216, 277, 321, 397, 451, 594, 677.

it hooks around the posterior and lateral aspect of the humerus on the deep surface of the deltoid muscle.

Mechanism of Injury

The dislocated humeral head displaces the subscapularis and the overlying axillary nerve anteroinferiorly and creates traction and direct pressure on the nerve.[475,476,677] The injury to the nerve may be a neurapraxia (no structural damage, recovery in approximately 6 weeks), an axonotmesis (disruption of the axons, preservation of the nerve sheath, axonal regrowth at 1 inch per month), or a neurotmesis (complete nerve disruption, guarded prognosis for recovery).

Incidence

The reported incidence of nerve injuries in series of acute dislocations is substantial, often as high as 33%.* If careful electrodiagnostic studies are carried out prospectively, the incidence of nerve injury may be as high as 45%.[132]

The axillary nerve is most commonly involved; up to a third of first-time anterior dislocations are associated with axillary nerve involvement.[57,236,391,557,610] The likelihood of an axillary nerve injury increases with the age of the patient, the duration of the dislocation, and the amount of trauma that initiated the dislocation.[57,556] Other nerves injured are the radial, musculocutaneous, median, ulnar, and the entire brachial plexus.

Diagnosis

The diagnosis of nerve injury is considered in any patient with neurologic symptoms or signs such as weakness or numbness after a dislocation. A nerve injury may also be manifested as delayed recovery of active shoulder motion after glenohumeral dislocation. Blom and Dahlback[57] demonstrated that axillary neuropathy may exist without numbness in the usual sensory distribution of the axillary nerve. Electromyography provides objective evaluation of neurologic function, provided that 3 or 4 weeks has intervened between the injury and the evaluation.[57]

Treatment and Prognosis

Most axillary nerve injuries resulting from anterior dislocation are traction neurapraxias and will recover completely. However, if recovery has not occurred in 3 months, the prognosis is not as good.[23,57,76,132]

Recurrence of Instability after Anterior Dislocations

Effect of Age

The age of the patient at the time of the initial dislocation has a major influence on the incidence of redislocation.[609,614] Several authors have reported that individuals younger than 20 years at the time of the initial dislocation have up to a 90% chance of having recurrent instability.† In patients older than 40 years, the incidence drops sharply to 10% to 15%.[460,614] Hovelius and colleagues[294] reported a careful prospective study with a somewhat lower incidence of recurrence in each age group: 33% in those younger than 20, 25% between 20 and 30, and 10% between 30 and 40 years of age. The majority of all recurrences occur within the first 2 years after the first traumatic dislocation.‡

Effect of Trauma, Sports, Gender, and Dominance

Rowe[609,614] has pointed out that the recurrence rate varies inversely with the severity of the original trauma; in other words, the more easily the dislocation occurred initially, the more easily it recurs. The recurrence rate in athletes may be higher than in nonathletes[654] and higher in men than women.[490] Dominance of the affected shoulder does not seem to have a major effect on the recurrence rate.[614]

Effect of Postdislocation Treatment

In many reports, the incidence of recurrence appears to be relatively insensitive to the type (sling versus plaster Velpeau) and duration of immobilization (0 versus 4 weeks) of the shoulder after the initial dislocation.[158,293,459,614]

By contrast, others have reported that longer periods of immobilization (over 3 weeks) are associated with a reduced incidence of recurrence.[351,680]

In a definitive 10-year prospective study, Hovelius and coworkers studied the effect of immobilization on the incidence of recurrence.[294] After reduction, 247 primary anterior dislocations were partially randomized to either a 3- to 4-week period of immobilization or to a sling to be discarded after comfort was achieved. The authors concluded that the immobilization did not affect the rate of recurrence. The results provide useful "rules of thumb": overall, half of these shoulders had recurrent dislocations, half the recurrences were treated surgically, and half of the recurrences treated nonoperatively were stable without surgery at 10 years. One of six patients had dislocation of the opposite shoulder. Eleven percent of the shoulders had at least mild evidence of secondary degenerative joint disease. Interestingly, this secondary disease was observed in both surgical and nonsurgical cases.

Aronen and Regan[21] reported a 3-year average follow-up study of 20 primary dislocations in Navy midshipmen treated with a 3-month aggressive postdislocation program. The program consisted of 3 weeks of sling immobilization followed by progressive strengthening. The patients were not allowed to return to activity until they had no evidence of weakness or atrophy and no apprehension on abduction and external rotation. In this series, no recurrent dislocations and two recurrent subluxations occurred. Similarly, Yoneda[783] reported good

---

*See references 76, 137, 202, 460, 496, 554, 557, 609, 709, 725, 742.

†See references 19, 276, 292, 296, 361, 459, 460, 490, 609, 654, 755.
‡See references 3, 34, 137, 171, 459, 489, 491, 609, 610, 704.

results in 83% of patients in a program emphasizing postimmobilization exercises.

Effect of Fractures

The incidence of recurrence is lower when a first-time shoulder dislocation is associated with a greater tuberosity fracture.[134,292,294,460,608,609,613] Hovelius[292] reported that these fractures were three times as common in patients older than 30 years: 23% versus 8% in patients younger than 30 years.

Other fractures, such as substantial posterior lateral humeral head lesions and fractures of the glenoid lip, are likely to be associated with an increased incidence of recurrent instability.

In conclusion, it appears that the injuries sustained by young patients in association with traumatic dislocations are relatively unlikely to heal in a manner yielding a stable shoulder. Probably the most important of these unhealing injuries are (1) avulsion of the glenohumeral capsular ligaments from the anterior glenoid lip and (2) posterolateral humeral head defects. Older patients may tend to stretch the capsule or fracture the greater tuberosity, either of which is likely to heal and result in a stable shoulder. In atraumatic instability, there is no traumatic lesion and thus a high chance of recurrence. The degree of trauma and the age of the patient seem to be the most important factors in determining the recurrence rate.

INJURIES ASSOCIATED WITH POSTERIOR DISLOCATIONS

Fractures

Fractures of the posterior glenoid rim and proximal part of the humerus (upper shaft, tuberosities, and head) are quite common in traumatic posterior dislocations of the shoulder.[528,529,6903,761] The commonly associated compression fracture of the anteromedial portion of the humeral

head is produced by the posterior cortical rim of the glenoid. It is best seen on an axillary view or a CT scan (Figs. 14–92 and 14–111).

This lesion, sometimes called a "reversed Hill-Sachs lesion," often occurs at the time of the original posterior dislocation. It becomes larger with multiple posterior dislocations of the shoulder. Large humeral head defects are also seen in old unreduced posterior dislocations.

The posterior rim of the glenoid may be fractured and displaced in posterior dislocations (see Fig. 14–98). Such injury occurs not only with direct forces from an anterior direction that push the humeral head out posteriorly but also with indirect types of dislocations such as occur during seizures or accidental electrical shock.

Fracture of the lesser tuberosity of the humerus may accompany posterior dislocations. The subscapularis muscle comes under considerable tension in this dislocation and may avulse the lesser tuberosity onto which it inserts. Although the fracture may be seen on anteroposterior and lateral radiographs of the glenohumeral joint, it is best seen on the axillary view and on CT scan.

Posterior dislocations of the humerus may be overlooked in the presence of a comminuted fracture of the proximal end of the humerus or humeral shaft fractures. In the series of 16 cases of posterior dislocation of the shoulder reported by O'Conner and Jacknow,[529] 12 had comminuted fractures of the proximal part of the humerus. In 8 of the 12 cases of fracture, the diagnosis of posterior dislocation was initially missed.

Other Associated Injuries

Injuries to the rotator cuff and neurovascular structures are less common with posterior than with anterior dislocations. However, they do occur. Moeller[481] reported a patient who had an open acute posterior dislocation of the left shoulder. The shoulder was totally unstable after reduction because of tears of the rotator cuff, biceps tendon, and subscapularis tendons. The patient had associated injury to the axillary and suprascapular nerves.

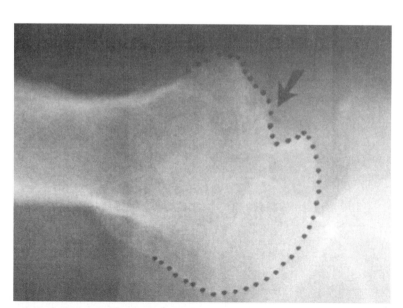

■ **Figure 14–111**

Axillary lateral x-ray film demonstrating an anteromedial compression fracture of the humeral head ("reverse Hill-Sachs lesion") after a traumatic posterior shoulder dislocation. *(From Rockwood CA Jr, Green DP, and Bucholz RW [eds]: Fractures in Adults. Philadelphia: JB Lippincott, 1991.)*

TREATMENT

Acute Traumatic Anterior Dislocations

Timing of Reduction and Analgesia

Acute dislocations of the glenohumeral joint should be reduced as gently and expeditiously as possible, ideally after a complete set of radiographs is obtained to rule out associated bony injuries. Early relocation promptly eliminates the stretch and compression of neurovascular structures, minimizes the amount of muscle spasm that must be overcome to effect reduction, and prevents progressive enlargement of the humeral head defect in locked dislocations. The extent of anesthesia required to accomplish a gentle reduction depends on many factors, including the amount of trauma that produced the dislocation, the duration of the dislocation, the number of previous dislocations, whether the dislocation is locked, and to what extent the patient can voluntarily relax the shoulder musculature. When seen acutely, some dislocations can be reduced without the use of medication. At the other extreme, reduction of a long-standing, locked dislocation may require a brachial plexus block or general anesthesia with muscle relaxation. Many practitioners use narcotics and muscle relaxants to aid in the reduction of shoulder dislocations. A potential trap exists: the dosages required to produce muscle relaxation while the shoulder is dislocated may be sufficient to produce respiratory depression once the shoulder is reduced. Our recommendation is that if these medications are to be used, they should be administered through an established intravenous line. Such practice produces a more rapid onset, a short duration of action, and the opportunity to adjust the required dose more appropriately. Furthermore, resuscitation (if necessary) is facilitated by the prospective presence of such a route of access. Airway management tools should be readily available.

Lippitt and colleagues[411,412] compared two methods of analgesia for the reduction of anterior dislocations: (1) intravenous analgesia and muscle relaxation and (2) intra-articular lidocaine. With respect to the first, they found a 75% success rate and a 37% complication rate in a retrospective series of 52 reductions in which intravenous narcotics (morphine, 3 to 24 mg, or meperidine, 12.5 to 100 mg, with or without diazepam, 1.5 to 15 mg, or midazolam, 1 to 10 mg) were used for analgesia. They remarked on the difficulty of determining the appropriate intravenous dose of narcotics. The level of pain, age, smoking history, alcohol consumption, cardiac disease, and regional perfusion are just a few of the factors that may influence the narcotic requirement.[28] Older patients and intoxicated patients are more sensitive to the respiratory depressant effects of narcotics. Because pain counteracts the respiratory depressant effect, patients sedated by narcotics are at increased risk of respiratory depression after removal of the painful stimulus when the shoulder is reduced. Complications from intravenous analgesia included respiratory depression, hypotension, hyperemesis, and oversedation. With respect to the second method, the use of 20 mL of 1% plain intra-articular lidocaine,

Lippitt and associates found a 100% success rate in the reduction of 40 dislocations with no complications. One patient inadvertently received 400 instead of 200 mg of lidocaine, and transient tinnitus, perioral numbness, and mild dysarthria developed. A survey revealed that both patients and physicians were satisfied with this method. The authors speculated that the success of intra-articular injection may be due to a combination of pain relief allowing reduction, relief from muscle spasm, and venting of the joint. Intra-articular lidocaine has been shown to be effective in the reduction of dislocations in other studies as well.[143,538] This technique may be particularly useful in patients with complicating factors such as medical problems or facial trauma and in whom respiratory depression with intravenous analgesia is not desired.

Method of Reduction

Once the shoulder is relaxed, a variety of gentle methods can be used to achieve reduction. Gentle traction on the arm is common to most (Figs. 14–112 and 14–113). One such method is known as the Stimson technique. Though named for Lewis A. Stimson[678,679] of New York City, Stimson credited Dr. Cole, a house staff physician of the

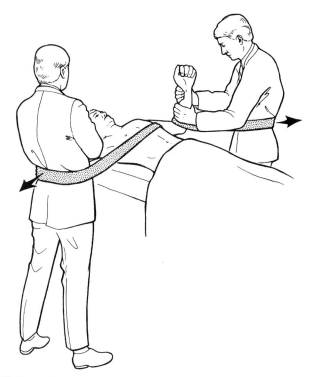

■ **Figure 14–112**

Reduction technique for an anterior glenohumeral dislocation. The patient lies supine with a sheet placed around the thorax and then around the assistant's waist to provide countertraction. The surgeon stands on the side of the dislocated shoulder near the patient's waist with the elbow of the dislocated shoulder flexed to 90 degrees. A second sheet is tied loosely around the waist of the surgeon and looped over the patient's forearm, thus providing traction while the surgeon leans back against the sheet and grasps the forearm. Steady traction along the axis of the arm will usually achieve reduction. The surgeon's hands are free to gently rock the humerus from internal to external rotation or provide gentle outward pressure on the proximal part of the humerus from the axilla.

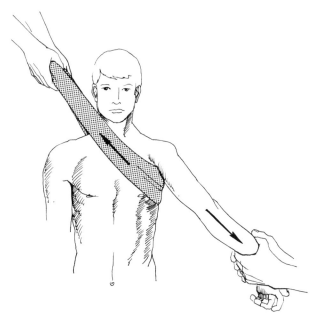

■ **Figure 14–113**
Closed reduction of the left shoulder with traction against countertraction. *(From Rockwood CA and Green DP [eds]: Fractures, 3 vols, 2nd ed. Philadelphia: JB Lippincott, 1984.)*

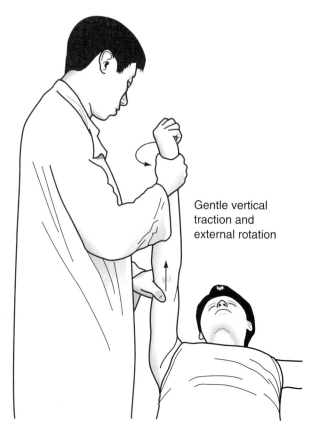

Gentle vertical traction and external rotation

■ **Figure 14–114**
The Spaso technique for reduction of anterior glenohumeral dislocations.

Chambers Street Hospital. In the Stimson method, the patient is placed prone on the edge of the examining table while downward traction is gently applied.[678] The traction force may be applied by the weight of the arm, by weights taped to the wrist, or by the surgeon. It may take several minutes for the traction to produce muscle relaxation. It is important that patients not be left unattended in this position, particularly if narcotics and muscle relaxants have been administered.

A new method of reducing shoulder dislocations has been described as the Spaso technique. This method places the patient in the supine position with the arm at the side. Longitudinal traction is applied as the arm is brought into forward flexion to produce an external rotational moment (Figure 14–114).[787]

■ AUTHORS' PREFERRED METHOD OF ANTERIOR REDUCTION

ANALGESIA

Although analgesia may not be necessary to achieve reduction, we are impressed with the safety and effectiveness of intra-articular lidocaine as described by Lippitt and coworkers (Fig. 14–115).[411,412] In this method, a maximum of 20 mL of 1% plain lidocaine is injected with an 18-gauge needle placed 2 cm below the lateral edge of the acromion just posterior to the dislocated humeral head and directed toward the glenoid fossa. The amount of lidocaine is limited to 200 mg.[631] Placement of the needle in the joint is confirmed by a combination of (1) feeling the needle penetrate the glenohumeral capsule, (2) aspirating joint fluid/hemarthrosis and ensuring that the injection is not

intravascular, (3) gently palpating the glenoid fossa with the needle, and (4) verifying easy flow on injection and return of the injected lidocaine solution. Fifteen minutes is allowed to maximize the analgesic effect of the lidocaine before manipulation.

MANEUVER

Reduction of either anterior or posterior glenohumeral dislocations can usually be effected by traction on the abducted and flexed arm with countertraction on the body (Figs. 14–112 and 14–113). The patient is placed supine with a sheet around the thorax and the loose ends on the side opposite the shoulder dislocation, where they are held by an assistant. The surgeon stands on the side of the dislocated shoulder near the waist of the patient. The elbow of the dislocated shoulder is flexed to 90 degrees (to relax the neurovascular structures), and traction is applied through a sheet looped over the patient's forearm, or traction can be applied directly. Steady traction along the axis of the arm will usually effect reduction. To this basic maneuver, one may add gentle rocking of the humerus from internal to external rotation or outward pressure on the proximal end of the humerus from the axilla. These additions are particularly useful if prereduction axillary roentgenograms show the humeral head to be impaled on the glenoid rim. Postreduction roentgenograms are used to confirm reduction and detect fractures. A postreduction neurovascular examination is routine.

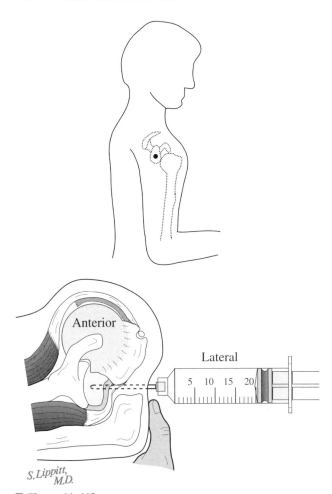

■ **Figure 14–115**
Intra-articular lidocaine injection for anesthesia during reduction of an anterior dislocation. The needle is inserted just posterior to the dislocated humeral head.

Chronic Anterior Traumatic Dislocations

Reduction and Analgesia

A glenohumeral joint that has been dislocated for several days is a chronic dislocation. The principles and methods for reducing a chronic dislocation are similar to those relating to an acute dislocation, except for the fact that the patient and the shoulder are usually more fragile and the relocation is more difficult. As the chronicity of the dislocation increases, so do the difficulties and complications of reduction. When one encounters an elderly patient with pain in the shoulder whose radiographs reveal an anterior dislocation, a very careful history is needed to determine whether the initial injury occurred recently or quite a while earlier.

Chronic dislocations are seen most commonly in elderly people and in those whose general health or mental status may prevent them from seeking help for the injury. The event causing the injury may be relatively trivial.[47,478] Old age, chronicity of dislocation, and soft bone make closed reduction difficult and dangerous.[452] If closed reduction is to be performed, it should be done with minimal traction, without leverage, and with total muscle relaxation under controlled general anesthesia. If the dislocation is over a week old, the humeral head is likely to be firmly impaled on the anterior glenoid with such soft tissue contraction that gentle closed reduction is impossible.

Open Reduction

If a gentle attempt at closed reduction fails, open reduction is considered. Open reduction can be a complex procedure because of the altered position of the axillary artery and branches of the brachial plexus and because the structures are tight and scarred. When the risks of attempting reduction appear to outweigh the advantages, the dislocated position may be accepted. Sometimes the symptoms of chronic dislocation are surprisingly minimal.[199]

To perform an open reduction, the subscapularis and anterior portion of the capsule are incised near their insertion onto the lesser tuberosity to allow substantial external rotation of the dislocated shoulder. External rotation and lateral traction will usually disimpact the humerus from the glenoid. While lateral traction is maintained, the humerus is gently internally rotated under direct vision to ensure that the articular surface of the humerus passes safely by the anterior glenoid lip and into the glenoid fossa. Leverage is avoided because the head is usually very soft. If the posterolateral head defect is greater than 40% or if the head collapses during reduction, a humeral head prosthesis may be necessary to restore a functional joint surface. The subscapularis and capsule are then repaired. The shoulder is carefully inspected for evidence of cuff tear or vascular damage.

Results of Treatment of Chronic Dislocations

Schulz and associates[638] reported a series of 17 posterior and 44 anterior chronic dislocations. These dislocations occurred primarily in elderly people, and more than half the dislocations were associated with fracture of the tuberosities, humeral head, humeral neck, glenoid, or coracoid process. More than a third involved neurologic deficits. Closed reduction was attempted in 40 shoulders and was successful in 20. Of the 20 shoulders successfully reduced (3 posterior and 17 anterior), the duration of dislocation exceeded 4 weeks in only one instance. Open reduction was performed in 20 and humeral head excision in 6. Eight patients were not treated, and five shoulders were irreducible.

Perniceni and Augereau[562] described reinforcement of the anterior shoulder complex in three patients after reduction of neglected anterior dislocations of the shoulder. They used the Gosset[224] technique, which places a rib graft between the coracoid and the glenoid rim. Rowe and Zarins[617] reported on 24 patients with unreduced dislocations of the shoulder and operated on 14 of them.

Management after Reduction of an Anterior Dislocation

Evaluation

After reducing the dislocation, anteroposterior and lateral x-ray views are obtained in the plane of the scapula to verify the adequacy of the reduction and provide an additional opportunity to detect fractures of the glenoid and proximal end of the humerus. The patient's neurologic status is again checked, including the sensory and motor function of all five major nerves in the upper extremity. The strength of the pulse is verified, and evidence of bruits or an expanding hematoma is sought.[236] The integrity of the rotator cuff is initially evaluated by observing the strength of isometric external rotation and abduction.

Trimmings[707] demonstrated that aspiration of hemarthrosis from the shoulder can be an effective means of reducing discomfort after the shoulder is reduced.

Protection

Because recurrent glenohumeral instability is the most common complication of a glenohumeral dislocation, postreduction treatment focuses on optimizing shoulder stability. Thus, two potentially important elements in postreduction treatment are protection and muscle rehabilitation. Reeves demonstrated that after repair of the subscapularis in primates, 3 months was necessary before normal capsular patterns of collagen bundles were observed, 5 months before the tendon was histologically normal, and 4 to 5 months before tensile strength was regained.[583] It is unknown whether labral tears or ligamentous avulsions from the glenoid heal or how long it might take. In any event, it is apparent that the shoulder cannot be immobilized for the full length of time required for complete healing. Immobilization in external rotation rather than the standard internally rotated position is suggested by Itoi and colleagues, who used MRI to examine shoulders after dislocation and found the anterior labrum to have 1.9 mm of separation from the glenoid while the shoulder is in internal rotation but only 0.1 mm when the arm is externally rotated.[317] No clinical follow-up information was given. (The reader is referred to the previous section "Recurrence of Instability after Anterior Dislocations," "Effect of Postdislocation Treatment" for a review of some of the literature on the effectiveness of different postreduction management programs.)

The authors treat first-time dislocations in a manner similar to the postoperative management of dislocation repairs. Thus, younger patients are placed on the "90-0 program," in which flexion is limited to 90 degrees and external rotation is limited to 0 degrees for the first 3 weeks while strength is maintained with cuff and deltoid isometrics. The elbow is fully extended at least several times a day to prevent "sling soreness." Because stiffness of the shoulder, elbow, and hand is more likely to develop in persons older than 30 years, the duration of immobilization is progressively reduced for individuals of increasing age.[361,459,460,609,783] Patients are checked 3 weeks after relocation and examined for stiffness; if external rotation to 0 degrees is difficult, formal stretching exercises are started. Otherwise, the patient is allowed to increase use of the shoulder as comfort permits.

Strengthening

At 3 weeks, the patient institutes more vigorous rotator cuff–strengthening exercises with rubber tubing or weights. The patient is informed that strong subscapularis and infraspinatus muscles are ideally situated to increase glenohumeral stability.[626]

Burkhead and Rockwood,[78] Glousman and coworkers,[219] and Tibone and Bradley[697] emphasized the importance of strengthening not only the rotator cuff but also the scapular stabilizing muscles because of their vital importance in providing a stable platform for shoulder function. Even in the case of recurrent instability, Burkhead and Rockwood[78] found that a complete exercise program was effective in the management of 12% of patients with traumatic subluxation, 80% with anterior atraumatic subluxation, and 90% with posterior instability.

Swimming is recommended at 6 weeks to enhance endurance and coordination. By 3 months after the dislocation, most patients should have almost full flexion and rotation of the shoulder. Patients are not allowed to use the injured arm in sports or for over-the-head labor until they have achieved (1) normal rotator strength, (2) comfortable and nearly full forward elevation, and (3) confidence in their shoulder with it in the necessary positions. Any deviation from the expected course of recovery requires careful re-evaluation for occult fractures, loose bodies, rotator cuff tears, peripheral nerve injuries, and glenohumeral arthritis.

Indications for Early Surgery in Shoulders Dislocated Anteriorly

Soft Tissue Interposition

Tietjen[700] reported a case in which surgery was required to retrieve the avulsed supraspinatus, infraspinatus, and teres minor from their interposition between the humeral head and the glenoid.

Bridle and Ferris[71] reported a case of apparent successful closed reduction of an anterior shoulder dislocation that appeared to be confirmed on an anteroposterior radiograph. However, the patient continued to experience severe pain, and a subsequent axillary lateral view demonstrated persistent anterior subluxation of the glenohumeral joint. At the time of open reduction the ruptured muscle belly of the subscapularis was found interposed between the humeral head and glenoid. Inao and associates[309] reported a case of an acute anterior shoulder dislocation that was irreducible by closed treatment because of interposition of the posteriorly displaced tendon of the long head of the biceps.

Displaced Fracture of the Greater Tuberosity

Although fractures of the greater tuberosity are not uncommonly associated with anterior shoulder dislocation, the tuberosity usually reduces into an acceptable position when the shoulder is reduced (Figs. 14–5 and 14–104). Occasionally, the greater tuberosity fragment displaces up under the acromion process or is pulled posteriorly by the cuff muscles. If the greater tuberosity remains displaced after reduction of the shoulder joint (Fig. 14–108), consideration should be given to anatomic reduction and internal fixation of the fragment and repair of the attendant split in the tendons of the rotator cuff (Fig. 14–105). It is relatively easy to determine the amount of superior displacement of the tuberosity fragment on an anteroposterior radiograph in the plane of the scapula. Posterior displacement can be more difficult to discern. It is important to look for the "vacant tuberosity" sign, wherein the normal contour of the greater tuberosity is lacking. If one is concerned about the anteroposterior position of the tuberosity on plain films, a CT scan should be considered. If the tuberosity is allowed to heal with posterior displacement, it may produce the functional equivalent of both a rotator cuff tear and a bony block to external rotation.

Glenoid Rim Fracture

Aston and Gregory[24] reported three cases in which a large anterior fracture of the glenoid occurred as a result of a fall on the lateral aspect of the abducted shoulder. A fracture of the glenoid lip may require open reduction and internal fixation if an intra-articular incongruity or an inadequate effective glenoid arc is present (see Fig. 14–98).

Special Problems

Occasionally, it may be a consideration to perform early surgical reconstruction in a patient who requires absolute and complete shoulder stability before being able to return to work or sports. Hertz and coauthors[279] reported a 2.4-year follow-up of 31 patients with an initial dislocation treated by primary repair of an arthroscopically demonstrated Bankart lesion: none had recurrent instability. Arciero and colleagues[18,19] initiated a study at West Point in which the Bankart lesion was repaired arthroscopically after the initial dislocation. Their initial data indicated a decrease in recurrent instability from 80% with nonoperative management to 14% with early repair.[17-19]

Posterior Dislocations

Reduction

Reduction of acute, traumatic posterior dislocations may be much more difficult than reduction of acute, traumatic anterior dislocations. Hawkins and coworkers[265] reviewed 41 cases of locked posterior shoulder dislocations. The average interval between injury and diagnosis was 1 year! In seven shoulders the deformity was accepted. Closed reduction was successful in only 6 of the 12 cases in which it was attempted.

Intravenous narcotics combined with muscle relaxants or tranquilizers may provide insufficient analgesia and muscle relaxation; general anesthesia with muscle paralysis may be required. Atraumatic closed reduction can usually be accomplished once the muscle spasm has been eliminated. With the patient in the supine position, longitudinal and lateral traction is applied to the arm while it is gently rocked in internal and external rotation. Once the head is disimpacted, it is lifted anteriorly back into the glenoid fossa. In locked posterior dislocations, it may be necessary to gently stretch out the posterior cuff and

capsule by maximally internally rotating the humerus before reduction is attempted. Care should be taken to not force the arm into external rotation before reduction is achieved; if the head is locked posteriorly on the glenoid rim, forced external rotation could produce a fracture of the head or shaft of the humerus.

If gentle closed reduction of a locked posterior glenohumeral dislocation is not possible, open reduction may be accomplished through an anterior deltopectoral approach.[147,265,335,371,375,458,604,633] Because local anatomy is significantly distorted, the tendon of the long head of the biceps is used as a guide to the lesser tuberosity. The subscapularis is released either by osteotomy of the lesser tuberosity or by direct incision. With the glenoid thus exposed, open reduction is carried out by gently pulling the humeral head laterally and then lifting its articular surface up on the face of the glenoid.

Postreduction Care

If after closed reduction the shoulder is stable in the sling position, this type of postreduction management is most convenient for the patient. However, if recurrent instability is a concern, the shoulder is immobilized in a shoulder spica or brace with the amount of external rotation necessary to provide stability.[90,91] Scougall[641] has shown experimentally in monkeys that a surgically detached posterior glenoid labrum and capsule heal soundly without repair. He concluded that the best position of immobilization, to allow healing of all the posterior structures, was in abduction, external rotation, and extension and that the position should be maintained for 4 weeks.

Although some have recommended pin fixation for 3 weeks after reduction,[761] this method carries a risk of pin breakage and infection.

Early Surgery in Acute Traumatic Posterior Dislocation

Indications for surgery include a displaced lesser tuberosity fracture, a significant posterior glenoid fracture, an irreducible dislocation, an open dislocation, or an unstable reduction.

A major cause of recurrent instability after reduction of a posterior dislocation is the presence of a large anteromedial humeral head defect. If at the time of reduction stability cannot be obtained because of such a defect, it may be rendered extra-articular by filling it with the subscapularis tendon as described by McLaughlin[397,453-455,458] or the lesser tuberosity as described by Neer.[516,597] If the humeral head defect involves over 30% of the articular surface, prosthetic replacement may be indicated; otherwise, instability may recur with internal rotation. Hawkins and coworkers demonstrated the use of each of these techniques in a series of locked posterior dislocations.[265]

After surgery, the arm may be immobilized in a sling and swathe for 2 weeks as recommended by McLaughlin, the arm may be positioned at the side posterior to the coronal plane with a strip of tape or canvas restraint as recommended by Rowe and Zarins,[617] or a modified spica in neutral rotation may be used for 6 weeks, followed by an additional 3 to 6 months of rehabilitative exercises as recommended by Rockwood.[597]

Keppler and colleagues suggested using rotational osteotomy of the humerus for the postreduction management of locked posterior dislocations.[353]

Chronic Posterior Dislocation

If a patient, especially an older patient, has had a chronic posterior dislocation for months or years with minimal pain and a functional range of motion, surgery may not be indicated. However, if disability exists and the glenohumeral joint has good bone stock, open reduction with a subscapularis or lesser tuberosity transfer or shoulder arthroplasty can be considered.[617]

■ AUTHORS' PREFERRED METHOD OF TREATMENT

Our management of acute traumatic posterior dislocations begins with a definition of the extent and chronicity of the injury. A complete radiographic evaluation that includes anteroposterior and lateral views in the plane of the scapula and an axillary view is necessary. Careful note is made of associated fractures, including the extent of the impression fracture of the anteromedial humeral head. Under anesthesia and muscle relaxation, gentle closed reduction is attempted with the application of axial traction on the arm. If the head is locked on the glenoid rim, gentle internal rotation may stretch out the posterior capsule to facilitate reduction. Lateral traction on the proximal part of the humerus may unlock the humeral

head. Once it is unlocked, the humerus is gently externally rotated. After reduction is achieved and confirmed by postreduction radiographs, the reduction is maintained for 3 weeks in a cummerbund "handshake" cast (Fig. 14–116) or orthotic (Fig. 14–117) in neutral rotation and slight extension. External rotation and deltoid isometrics are carried out during this period of immobilization. After removal of the cast, a vigorous internal and external rotator-*strengthening* program is initiated. Range of motion is allowed to return with active use, beginning with elevation in the plane of the scapula. Vigorous physical activities are not resumed until the shoulder is strong and 3 months has elapsed since reduction. Swimming is encouraged to develop endurance and muscle coordination.

When a humeral head defect involves 20% to 40% of the humeral head, a subscapularis transfer into the defect to prevent recurrent instability is considered. When the humeral head defect is greater than 40%, a proximal humeral prosthesis to replace the lost articular surface is considered. When the dislocation is obviously chronic, consideration can be given to accepting the dislocation and focusing on enhancing the patient's ability to carry out activities of daily living.

RECURRENT INSTABILITY: EVALUATION

After an initial dislocation, the shoulder may return to functional stability, or it may fall victim to recurrent glenohumeral instability. Although intermediate forms of recurrent instability do occur, the great majority of recurrently unstable shoulder may be thought of as being either atraumatic or traumatic in origin.

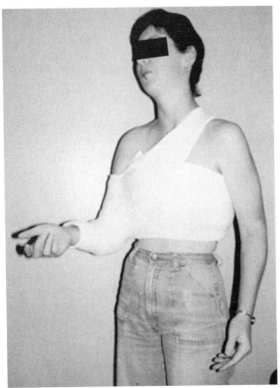

■ Figure 14–116
A handshake cast. After closed reduction of an acute traumatic posterior dislocation is confirmed by radiographs, a cast is applied in neutral rotation and slight extension for 3 weeks.

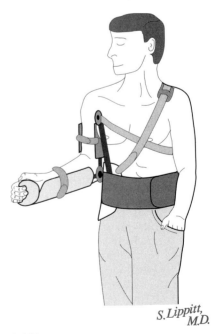

■ Figure 14–117
An orthosis is used to immobilize the arm after reduction of a posterior dislocation or a global capsular repair. (*Modified from Matsen FA III, Lippitt SB, Sidles JA, and Harryman DT II: Practical Evaluation and Management of the Shoulder. Philadelphia: WB Saunders, 1994.*)

Recurrent Atraumatic Instability

Atraumatic instability is instability that arises without the type of trauma necessary to tear the stabilizing soft tissues or create a humeral head defect, tuberosity fracture, or glenoid lip fracture. Certain shoulders may be more susceptible to atraumatic instability. A small or functionally flat glenoid fossa may jeopardize the concavity compression, adhesion/cohesion, and glenoid suction cup stability mechanisms. Thin, excessively compliant capsular tissue may invaginate into the joint when traction is applied and thus limit the effectiveness of stabilization from limited joint volume. A large, potentially capacious capsule may allow humeroscapular positions outside the range of balance stability. Weak rotator cuff muscles may provide insufficient compression for the concavity compression stabilizing mechanism. Poor neuromuscular control may fail to position the scapula to balance the net humeral joint reaction force. Voluntary or inadvertent malpositioning of the humerus in excessive anterior or posterior scapular planes may cause the net humeral joint reaction force to lie outside the balance stability angles. Once initiated, the instability may be perpetuated by compression of the glenoid rim as a result of chronically poor humeral head centering. Excessive labral compliance may predispose to this loss of effective glenoid depth.

Any of these factors, individually or in combination, could contribute to instability of the glenohumeral joint. For example, posterior glenohumeral subluxation may be caused by the combination of a relatively flat posterior glenoid and the tendency to retract the scapula during anterior elevation of the arm; such a combination results in use of the elevated humerus in excessively anterior scapular planes. Excessively compliant capsular tissue in conjunction with relatively weak rotator cuff muscles could contribute to inferior subluxation on attempted lifting of objects with the arm at the side. If the lateral aspect of the scapula is allowed to droop (whether voluntarily or involuntarily), the superior capsular structures are relaxed and permit inferior translation of the humerus with respect to the glenoid (see Fig. 14–16).[315]

Because it usually results from loss of midrange stability, atraumatic instability is more likely to be multidirectional. Pathogenic factors such as a flat glenoid, weak muscles, and a compliant capsule may produce instability anteriorly, inferiorly, posteriorly, or in a combination of directions. Although the onset of atraumatic instability may be provoked by a period of disuse or a minor injury, many of the underlying contributing factors may be developmental. As a result, the tendency for atraumatic instability is likely to be bilateral and familial as well.

It is apparent that atraumatic instability is not a simple diagnosis, but rather a syndrome that may arise from a multiplicity of factors. To help recall the various aspects of this syndrome, we use the acronym AMBRII. The instability is **A**traumatic, usually associated with **M**ultidirectional laxity and with **B**ilateral findings. Treatment is predominantly by **R**ehabilitation directed at restoring optimal neuromuscular control. If surgery is necessary, it may need to include reconstruction of the rotator **I**nterval capsule-coracohumeral ligament mechanism and tightening of the **I**nferior capsule. The diagnosis and management of this condition have been presented in detail.[107,410,441,530]

The History

Most patients with AMBRII are younger than 30 years (Fig. 14–118). Because the instability occurs in the midrange positions of the shoulder, atraumatic instability typically causes discomfort and dysfunction in ordinary activities of daily living. Commonly, such patients have the greatest difficulty sleeping, lifting overhead, and throwing (Table 14–2 and Fig. 14–119). Their general health status as revealed by the SF 36 is not as good on average as that of a comparable group of patients with traumatic instability (Fig. 14–120).

The onset is usually insidious, but it may occur after a minor injury or period of disuse. The unwanted translations may range from a sensation of a minor "slip" in the joint to complete dislocation of the humeral head from the glenoid. The displacement characteristically reduces spontaneously, after which the patient is usually able to return to previous activities without much pain or problem. As the condition progresses, the patient notices that the shoulder has become looser and may feel it slip out and clunk back in with increasing ease and in an increasing number of activities. The shoulder may become uncomfortable, even with the arm at rest. Patients may volunteer that they can make the shoulder "pop out" and that at times the shoulder feels as though it "needs to be popped out" on purpose.

It is important to document from the history the circumstances surrounding the onset of the problem, as well as each and every position of the shoulder in which the patient experiences instability. It is also important to note whether the opposite shoulder is symptomatic as well. A family history may reveal other kindred similarly affected, in addition to conditions known to predispose to atraumatic instability, such as Ehlers-Danlos syndrome.

Many patients admit that they had a habit of dislocating the joint but that they can now no longer control the stability of the joint. The surgeon must determine whether habitual dislocation remains a feature of the

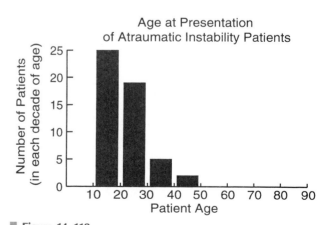

■ **Figure 14–118**

Age distribution of 51 patients with atraumatic instability. *(From Matsen FA III, Lippitt SB, Sidles JA, and Harryman DT II: Practical Evaluation and Management of the Shoulder. Philadelphia: WB Saunders, 1994.)*

TABLE 14–2. Characteristics of Patients with Traumatic Instability (TUBS), Atraumatic Instability (AMBRII), and Failed Instability Repairs

	TUBS	AMBRII	Failed Repairs
No. of Patients	101	70	76
% Female	26%	38%	28%
% Right side	55%	68%	51%
Age	29 ± 11	27 ± 10	31 ± 8
% Able to Perform Function	*TUBS (101)*	*AMBRII (70)*	*Failed Repairs (76)*
Sleep on side	43	19	11
Comfort by side	87	71	56
Wash opposite shoulder	69	64	39
Hand behind head	77	75	48
Tuck in shirt	89	81	54
Place 8 lb on shelf	53	35	28
Place 1 lb on shelf	91	75	65
Place coin on shelf	93	77	73
Toss overhand	31	35	15
Do usual work	69	46	42
Toss underhand	83	70	44
Carry 20 lb	73	61	46
Health Status	*TUBS (101)*	*AMBRII (70)*	*Failed Repairs (76)*
Physical role	52	35	28
Comfort	60	43	43
Physical function	85	78	71
Emotional role	86	72	70
Social function	84	73	66
Vitality	67	58	55
Mental health	78	74	68
General health	81	78	68

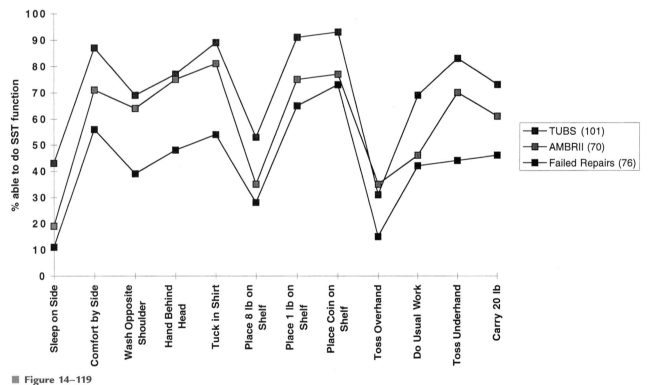

■ Figure 14–119

Comparison of responses to the 12 questions of the Simple Shoulder Test for groups of patients with traumatic instability (TUBS), atraumatic instability (AMBRII), and failed instability repairs.

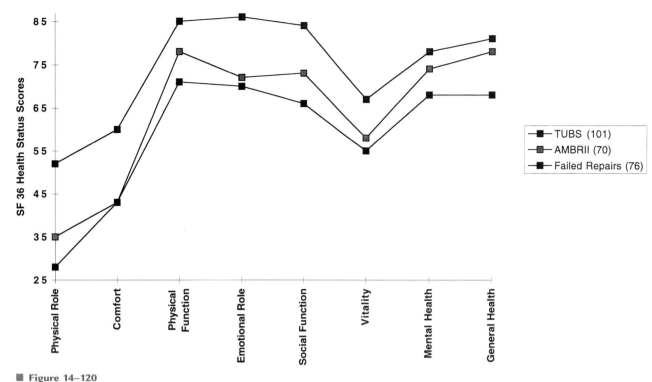

■ **Figure 14–120**

Comparison of scores on the SF 36 General Health Status Questionnaire for groups of patients with traumatic instability (TUBS), atraumatic instability (AMBRII), and failed instability repairs.

patient's problem. It is obvious that it is difficult for surgery to cure habitual instability.

Finally, it is important to document the patient's expectations of the shoulder to ensure that the goals are within reach before treatment is started.

The Physical Examination

Demonstration of Instability

Patients are routinely asked whether they can dislocate the shoulder at will (Figs. 14–59, 14–60, and 14–121). Such voluntary instability enables the surgeon to see the different positions of concern and directions of translation. By palpating the scapula, the surgeon can estimate the relative position of the humerus and scapula when the shoulder is translated and reduced. Three common demonstrations of instability may be noted:

1. The patient may demonstrate a spontaneous "jerk" test by bringing the internally rotated arm horizontally across the chest; this action causes the humeral head to subluxate posteriorly. Then, by returning the elevated humerus to the coronal plane, the shoulder produces a "clunk" on reduction of the glenohumeral joint (much like the Ortolani and Barlow signs of the hip).
2. The patient may demonstrate that the shoulder subluxates inferiorly when attempting to lift an object or tie a shoe.
3. The patient may demonstrate that the shoulder translates when the arm is elevated in the posterior humerothoracic planes, with spontaneous reduction on return to the coronal plane.

Laxity Tests

Laxity tests examine the amount of translation allowed by the shoulder starting from positions in which the ligaments are normally loose. The amount of translation on laxity testing is determined by the length of the capsule and ligaments, as well as by the starting position (i.e., more anterior laxity will be noted if the arm is examined in internal rotation, which relaxes the anterior structures, than if it is examined in external rotation, which tightens the anterior structures).

When interpreting the significance of the degree of translation on laxity tests, it is important to use the contralateral shoulder as an example of what is "normal" for the patient. Not infrequently, the laxity on the symptomatic side will be similar to that on the asymptomatic side. Investigations of clinical laxity tests have shown that the range of translation for shoulders with atraumatic instability was similar to that of normal shoulders or shoulders with traumatic instability (see Fig. 14–45).[253] However, a distinguishing feature of many shoulders with atraumatic instability is that resistance to translation is diminished when the humeral head is pressed into the glenoid fossa, thus suggesting that the effective glenoid concavity is diminished. It is helpful if the patient recognizes one or more of the directions of translation as being responsible for the clinical symptoms. Finally, it is important to point out that these are tests of *laxity,* not tests of *instability;* many normally stable shoulders, such as those of gymnasts, will demonstrate substantial translation on these laxity tests even though they are asymptomatic.

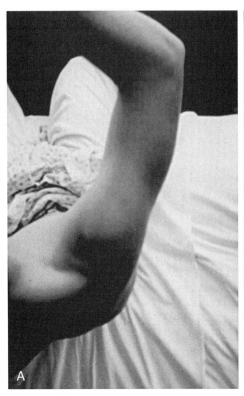
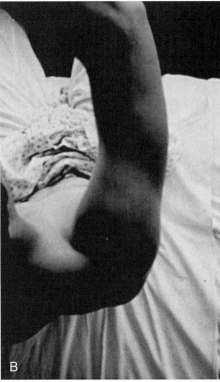

■ **Figure 14–121**

The voluntary jerk test. **A,** Normal appearance of the shoulder before the patient performs a jerk test. **B,** With movement of the arm horizontally across the body, the humeral head slides off the back of the glenoid with a jerk of dislocation and a prominence in the posterior aspect of the patient's shoulder. When the arm is moved back to the position shown in **A,** a jerk of reduction occurs.

Drawer Test (Fig. 14–122)

The patient is seated with the forearm resting on the lap and the shoulder relaxed. The examiner stands behind the patient. One of the examiner's hands stabilizes the shoulder girdle (scapula and clavicle) while the other grasps the proximal end of the humerus. These tests are performed with (1) a minimal compressive load (just enough to center the head in the glenoid) and (2) a substantial compressive load (to gain a feeling for the effectiveness of the glenoid concavity). Starting from the centered position with a minimal compressive load, the humerus is first pushed forward to determine the amount of anterior displacement relative to the scapula. The anterior translation of a normal shoulder reaches a firm end point with no clunking, no pain, and no apprehension. A clunk or snap on anterior subluxation or reduction may suggest a labral tear or Bankart lesion. The test is then repeated with a substantial compressive load applied before translation is attempted to gain an appreciation of the competency of the anterior glenoid lip. The humerus is returned to the neutral position and the posterior drawer test is performed with light and again with substantial compressive loads to judge the amount of translation and the effectiveness of the posterior glenoid lip, respectively.[652]

Sulcus Test (Figs. 14–123 and 14–124)

The patient sits with the arm relaxed at the side. The examiner centers the head with a mild compressive load and then pulls the arm downward. Inferior laxity is demonstrated if a sulcus or hollow appears inferior to the acromion. Competency of the inferior glenoid lip is demonstrated by pressing the humeral head into the glenoid while inferior traction is applied.

Push-Pull Test (Fig. 14–125)

The patient lies supine with the shoulder off the edge of the table. The arm is in 90 degrees of abduction and 30 degrees of flexion. Standing next to the patient's hip, the examiner pulls up on the wrist with one hand while pushing down on the proximal part of the humerus with the other. The shoulders of normal, relaxed patients will often allow 50% posterior translation on this test.

Stability Tests

Stability tests examine the ability of the shoulder to resist challenges to stability in positions in which the ligaments are normally under tension.

Fulcrum Test (Fig. 14–126)

The patient lies supine at the edge of the examination table with the arm abducted to 90 degrees. The examiner places one hand on the table under the glenohumeral joint to act as a fulcrum. The patient's arm is gently and progressively extended and externally rotated over this fulcrum. Maintaining gentle passive external rotation for a minute fatigues the subscapularis and thereby challenges the capsular contribution to anterior stability of the shoulder. A patient with anterior instability will usually become apprehensive as this maneuver is carried out (watch the eyebrows for a clue that the shoulder is getting ready to dislocate). In this test, normally no translation occurs because it is performed in a position in which the anterior ligaments are placed under tension.

Crank or Apprehension Test (Fig. 14–127)

The patient sits with the back toward the examiner. The arm is held in 90 degrees of abduction and external

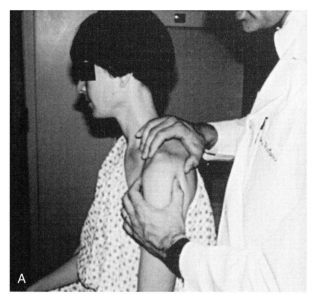
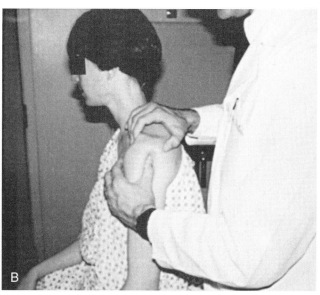

■ **Figure 14–122**

Drawer test. **A,** With the patient seated and the forearm resting in the lap, the examiner stands behind the patient and stabilizes the shoulder girdle with one hand while grasping the proximal end of the humerus with the other and pressing the humeral head gently toward the scapula to center it in the glenoid. **B,** The head is then pushed forward to determine the amount of anterior displacement relative to the scapula. It can then be returned to the neutral position, and a posterior force is applied to determine the amount of posterior translation relative to the scapula.

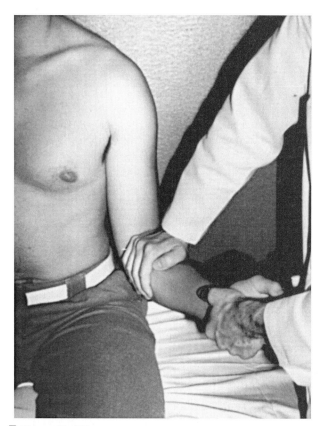

■ **Figure 14–123**

The sulcus test. The patient is seated with the arm relaxed and at the side. The examiner pulls downward on the arm. Inferior instability is demonstrated if a sulcus (or hollow) appears inferior to the acromion. The result of the sulcus test in this patient is negative.

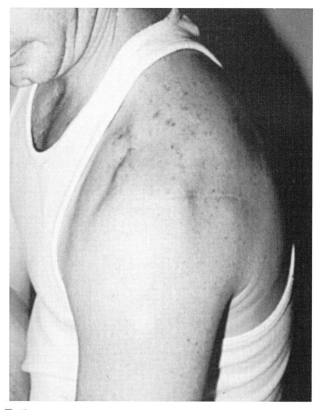

■ **Figure 14–124**

The sulcus sign. This patient had a posterior repair for glenohumeral instability. However, he continues to have inferior instability and demonstrates the sulcus (or hollow) just inferior to the anterior acromion during this sulcus test.

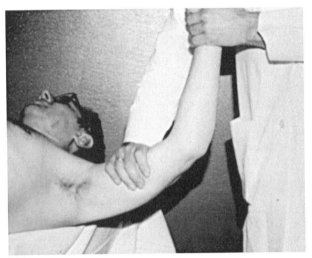

■ Figure 14–125
The push-pull test. The patient lies supine and relaxed with the shoulder at the edge of the examination table. The examiner pulls up on the wrist with one hand while pushing down on the proximal part of the humerus with the other. Approximately 50% posterior translation of the humerus on the glenoid is normal in relaxed patients.

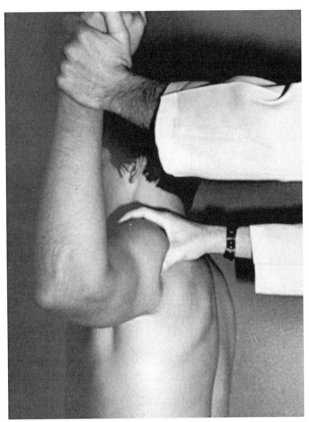

■ Figure 14–127
The crank test. The arm is held in 90 degrees of abduction and external rotation. The examiner's left hand is pulling back on the patient's wrist while the right hand stabilizes the back of the shoulder. A patient with anterior instability becomes apprehensive with this maneuver.

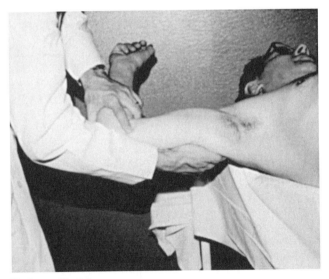

■ Figure 14–126
The fulcrum test. With the patient supine and the shoulder at the edge of the examination table, the arm is abducted to 90 degrees. The examiner's right hand is used as a fulcrum while the arm is gently and progressively extended and externally rotated. In the presence of anterior instability, the patient becomes apprehensive or the shoulder translates with this maneuver.

rotation. The examiner pulls back on the patient's wrist with one hand while stabilizing the back of the shoulder with the other. A patient with anterior instability will usually become apprehensive with this maneuver. As with the fulcrum test, no translation is expected in a normal shoulder because this test is performed in a position in which the anterior ligaments are placed under tension.

Jerk Test (Figs. 14–121 and 14–128)

The patient sits with the arm internally rotated and flexed forward to 90 degrees. The examiner grasps the elbow and

axially loads the humerus in a proximal direction. While axial loading of the humerus is maintained, the arm is moved horizontally across the body. A positive test is indicated by a sudden jerk as the humeral head slides off the back of the glenoid. When the arm is returned to the original position of 90-degree abduction, a second jerk may be observed, that of the humeral head returning to the glenoid.

Strength Tests

The strength of abduction and rotation are tested to gauge the power of the muscles contributing to stability through concavity compression. The strength of the scapular protractors and elevators is also tested to determine their ability to position the scapula securely.

Radiographs

In atraumatic instability, shoulder radiographs characteristically show no bony pathology, specifically, no postero-lateral humeral head defect, no glenoid rim fracture or new bone formation, and no evidence of tuberosity fracture. Because these patients typically demonstrate midrange instability, radiographs may show translation of the humeral head with respect to the glenoid; for example, the axillary view may show posterior subluxation. Occasionally, radiographs may suggest factors underlying

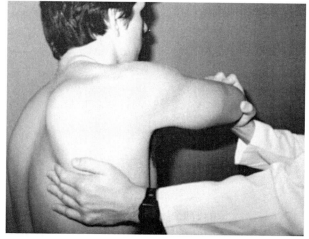

■ **Figure 14–128**
The jerk test. The patient's arm is abducted to 90 degrees and internally rotated. The examiner axially loads the humerus while the arm is moved horizontally across the body. The left hand stabilizes the scapula. A patient with a recurrent posterior instability may demonstrate a sudden jerk as the humeral head slides off the back of the glenoid or when it is reduced by moving the arm back to the starting position.

the atraumatic instability, such as a relatively small or hypoplastic glenoid or a posteriorly inclined or otherwise dysplastic glenoid. The bony glenoid fossa may appear quite flat; however, it is difficult to relate the apparent depth of the bony socket to the effective depth of the fossa formed by cartilage and labrum covering the bone.

Arthroscopy

Using arthroscopy, Burkhart and colleagues have shown the bare spot of the glenoid to be a consistent reference point for the center of the glenoid.[77] Adequacy of the glenoid may be assessed by determining the amount of glenoid surrounding the bare area. The presence of a drive-through sign has been used as an indicator of laxity. In a study of 339 patients undergoing shoulder arthroscopy for any reason, the drive-through sign was found to have a sensitivity of 92% for the diagnosis of instability but only 37.6% sensitivity. The positive and negative predictive values were 29.9% and 94.2%, respectively.[447]

We do not use stress radiography, arthrography, MRI, or arthroscopy routinely in the diagnosis of atraumatic instability.

Recurrent Traumatic Instability

Traumatic instability is instability that arises from an injury of sufficient magnitude to tear the glenohumeral capsule, ligaments, labrum, or rotator cuff or produce a fracture of the humerus or glenoid. A typical patient is a 17-year-old skier whose recurrent anterior instability began with a fall on an abducted, externally rotated arm (although the condition has been reported in individuals as young as 3 years).[164] To injure these strong structures, substantial force must be applied to them. The most common pathology associated with traumatic instability

is avulsion of the anteroinferior capsule and ligaments from the glenoid rim. Considerable force is required to produce this avulsion in a healthy shoulder. Although this load may be applied directly (for example, by having the proximal end of the humerus hit from behind), an indirect loading mechanism is more common. Indirect loading is most easily understood in terms of a simple model of the torques involved. When the upper extremity is abducted and externally rotated by a force applied to the hand, the following equation for torque equilibrium is a useful approximation, *if* we attribute the major stabilizing role to the ligament (see Fig. 14–48):

$$T = B \cdot E/R$$

where T is the tension in the inferior glenohumeral ligament, R is the radius of the humeral head, B is the abduction external rotation load applied to the hand, and E is the distance from the center of the humeral head to the hand. If the radius of the humeral head is 2.5 cm and the distance from the center of the head to the hand is 1 m, this formula suggests that the inferior glenohumeral ligament would experience a load 40 times greater than that applied to the hand. From this example we can see that a relatively small load is required to produce the characteristic lesion of traumatic instability if this load is applied indirectly through the lever arm of the upper extremity.

Avulsion of the anterior glenohumeral ligament mechanism (see Fig. 14–34) deprives the joint of stability in positions in which this structure is a checkrein, such as in maximal external rotation and extension of the arm elevated near the coronal plane. Thus, it is evident that in recurrent traumatic instability, problems are most likely to occur when the arm is placed in a position approximating that in which the original injury occurred (see Figs. 14–126 and 14–127). Midrange instability may also result from a traumatic injury because the glenoid concavity may be compromised by avulsion of the labrum or fracture of the bony lip of the glenoid (see Fig. 14–33). Lessening of the effective glenoid arc compromises the effectiveness of concavity compression, reduces the balance stability angles, decreases the surface available for adhesion/cohesion, and compromises the ability of the glenoid suction cup to conform to the head of the humerus.

The corner of the glenoid abuts against the insertion of the cuff to the tuberosity when the humerus is extended, abducted, and externally rotated (Fig. 14–129).[414,441,483,607,729,730] Thus, the same forces that challenge the inferior glenohumeral ligament are also applied to the greater tuberosity–cuff insertion area. It is not surprising, therefore, that posterolateral humeral head defects, tuberosity fractures, and cuff injuries may be a part of the clinical picture of traumatic instability. The exact location and type of traumatic injury depend on the age of the patient and the magnitude, rate, and direction of force applied. Avulsions of the glenoid labrum, glenoid rim fractures, and posterolateral humeral head defects are more commonly seen in young individuals. In patients older than 35 years, traumatic instability tends to be associated with fractures of the greater tuberosity and rotator cuff tears. This tendency increases with increasing age at

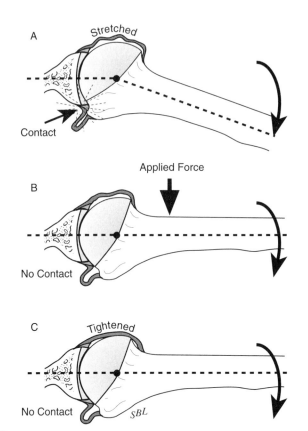

■ **Figure 14–129**

Posterior contact between the glenoid lip and the insertion of the cuff onto the tuberosity occurs in the apprehension, or fulcrum, position, especially if the anteroinferior aspect of the capsule has been stretched and is allowing the humerus to extend to an unusually posterior scapular plane. This contact can challenge the integrity of the posterior cuff insertion and the tuberosity (**A**). Application of a posteriorly directed force on the front of the shoulder may change the humeroscapular position enough to relieve this posterior abutment. This maneuver is similar to that described as the relocation test; however, this diagram suggests that the mechanism for relief of discomfort is avoidance of posterior abutment rather than elimination of subluxation (**B**). A similar protection from posterior abutment may be achieved by tightening the anterior part of the capsule, thus preventing extension of the humerus to a substantially posterior scapular plane (**C**). *(From Matsen FA III, Lippitt SB, Sidles JA, and Harryman DT II: Practical Evaluation and Management of the Shoulder. Philadelphia: WB Saunders, 1994.)*

the time of the initial traumatic dislocation. Thus, as a rule, younger patients require management of anterior lesions and older patients require management of posterior lesions.

Posterior lateral humeral head defects are common features of traumatic instability. These lesions are often noted after the first traumatic dislocation and tend to increase in size with recurrent episodes. This impaction injury usually occurs when the anterior corner of the glenoid is driven into the posterior lateral humeral articular surface. It is evident that this injury is close to the cuff insertion. Large head defects compromise stability by diminishing the articular congruity of the humerus.

To help recall the common aspects of traumatic instability, we use the acronym TUBS. The instability arises from a significant episode of **T**rauma, characteristically from abduction and extension of the arm elevated in the coronal plane. The resulting instability is usually

Unidirectional in the anteroinferior direction. The pathology is generally an avulsion of the labrum and capsuloligamentous complex from the anterior inferior lip of the glenoid, commonly referred to as a **B**ankart lesion. With functionally significant recurrent traumatic instability, **S**urgical reconstruction of this labral and ligament avulsion is frequently required to restore stability.

The reader is referred to a review of the pathology and pathogenesis of traumatic instability by Wirth and Rockwood.[768]

The History

Most patients with TUBS are between the ages of 14 and 34 (Fig. 14–130). These patients characteristically have difficulty throwing overhand, but many patients also have problems sleeping, putting their hand behind their head, and lifting a gallon to head level (see Table 14–2 and Fig. 14–119). Their general health status as revealed by the SF 36 self-assessment questionnaire is better on average than that of a comparable group of patients with atraumatic instability (Fig. 14–120).

The Initial Dislocation

The most important element in the history is a definition of the original injury. As is evident to anyone who has attempted to re-create these lesions in a cadaver, substantial force is required to produce a traumatic dislocation—in most cadaver specimens, it is impossible to duplicate the Bankart injury mechanism because the humerus fractures first! In characteristic anterior traumatic instability, the structure that is avulsed is the strongest part of the shoulder's capsular mechanism: the anterior inferior glenohumeral ligament. To tear this ligament, substantial force must be applied to the shoulder when the arm is in a position to tighten this ligament. Thus, the usual mechanism of injury involves the application of a large extension–external rotation force to the arm elevated near the coronal plane. Such a mechanism may occur in a fall while snow skiing, while executing a high-speed cut in water skiing, in an arm tackle during football, with a block of a volleyball or basketball shot, or in relatively violent

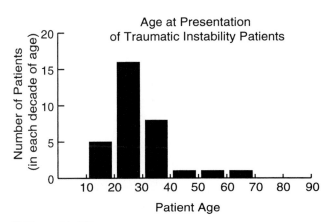

■ **Figure 14–130**

Age distribution of 32 patients with traumatic instability. *(From Matsen FA III, Lippitt SB, Sidles JA, and Harryman DT II: Practical Evaluation and Management of the Shoulder. Philadelphia: WB Saunders, 1994.)*

industrial accidents in which a posteriorly directed force is applied to the hand while the arm is abducted and externally rotated. Awkward lifting on the job and rear-end automobile accidents would not be expected to provide the conditions or mechanism needed for this injury. Direct questioning and persistence are often necessary to elicit a full description of the mechanism of the initial injury, including the position of the shoulder and the direction and magnitude of the applied force. Yet this information is critical to establishing the diagnosis.

An initial traumatic dislocation often requires assistance in reduction rather than reducing spontaneously as is usually the case in atraumatic instability. Radiographs from previous emergency room visits may be available to show the shoulder in its dislocated position. Axillary or other neuropathy may have accompanied the glenohumeral dislocation. Any of these findings individually or in combination support the diagnosis of traumatic as opposed to atraumatic instability.

Traumatic instability may occur without a complete dislocation. In this situation, the injury produces a traumatic lesion, but the lesion is insufficient to allow the humeral head to completely escape from the glenoid. The shoulder may be unstable because as a result of the injury, it manifests apprehension or subluxation when the arm is placed near the position of injury. Such patients have no history of the need for reduction nor radiographs with the shoulder in the dislocated position. Thus, the diagnosis rests to an even greater extent on a careful history that focuses on the position and forces involved in the initial episode.

Subsequent Episodes of Instability

Characteristically, a shoulder with traumatic instability is comfortable when troublesome positions are avoided. However, the apprehension or fear of instability may prevent the individual from returning to work or sports. Recurrent subluxation or dislocation may occur when the shoulder is unexpectedly forced into the abducted, externally rotated position or during sleep when the patient's active guard is less effective. The patient may have a history of increasing ease of dislocation as the remaining stabilizing factors are progressively compromised.

The Physical Examination

The goal of physical examination is largely to confirm the impression obtained from the history: that a certain combination of arm position and application of force produces the actual or threatened glenohumeral instability that is of functional concern to the patient. If the diagnosis has been rigorously established from the history, for example, by documented recurrent anterior dislocations, it is not necessary to risk redislocation on the physical examination. If such rigorous documentation is not available, however, the examiner must challenge the ligamentous stability of the shoulder in the suspected position of vulnerability and be prepared to reduce the shoulder should a dislocation result.

The most common direction of recurrent traumatic instability is anteroinferior. Stability in this position is challenged by externally rotating and extending the arm elevated to various degrees in the coronal plane (see Figs. 14-126 and 14-127). It may be necessary to hold the arm in the challenging position for 1 to 2 minutes to fatigue the stabilizing musculature. When the muscle stabilizers tire, the capsuloligamentous mechanism is all that is holding the humeral head in the glenoid. At this moment a patient with traumatic anterior instability becomes apprehensive because of recognition that the shoulder is about to come out of joint. This recognition is strongly supportive of the diagnosis of traumatic anterior instability.

The magnitude of translation on standard tests of glenohumeral laxity (see Figs. 14-122 to 14-125) does not necessarily distinguish stable from unstable shoulders (see Fig. 14-45). However, an experienced examiner may detect diminished resistance to anterior translation on the drawer test when the humeral head is compressed into the glenoid fossa; the diminished resistance in this case is indicative of loss of the anterior glenoid lip. This maneuver may also elicit grinding as the humeral head slides over the bony edge of the glenoid from which the labrum has been avulsed or elicit catching as the head passes over a torn glenoid labrum.

Pain on abduction, external rotation, and extension is not specific for instability. Such pain may relate to shoulder stiffness or alternatively to abutment of the glenoid against the cuff insertion to the head posteriorly.[441,607,729,730] Relief of this pain by anterior pressure on the humeral head may result from diminished stretch on the anterior capsule or from relief of the abutment posteriorly (Fig. 14-129).

In all patients with traumatic instability, particularly those older than 35 years, the strength of internal and external rotation must be examined to explore the possibility of cuff weakness or tear. Finally, a neurologic examination is performed to determine the integrity of the axillary nerve and other branches of the brachial plexus.

Radiographs and Other Tests

Radiographs frequently help provide confirmation of traumatic glenohumeral instability.

Humeral Head Changes

One of the most common findings is indentation or impaction in the posterior aspect of the humeral head from contact with the anteroinferior corner of the glenoid when the joint was dislocated (Figs. 14-3, 14-92, and 14-131). In their classic article,[283] Hill and Sachs evaluated the relationship of humeral head defects to shoulder instability. They concluded that more than two thirds of anterior shoulder dislocations are complicated by a bony injury of the humerus or scapula. We quote:

Compression fractures as a result of impingement of the weakest portion of the humeral head, that is, the posterior lateral aspect of the articular surface against the anterior rim of the glenoid fossa, are found so frequently in cases of habitual dislocation that they have been described as a typical defect. These defects are sustained at the time of the original dislocation. A special sign is the sharp, vertical, dense medial border of the groove known as the line of

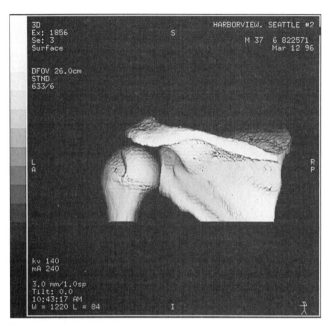

■ **Figure 14–131**
Three-dimensional computed tomographic reconstruction of the left shoulder of a 37-year-old man 3 days after his first traumatic glenohumeral dislocation. The bony defect in the posterior lateral aspect of the humeral head is clearly shown. The patient recovered normal shoulder function with nonoperative management.

condensation, the length of which is correlated with the size of the defect.

They reported the defect in only 27% of 119 acute anterior dislocations but in 74% of 15 recurrent anterior dislocations. However, they stated that the incidence of the groove defect was low, undoubtedly because it was only in the last 6 months of their 10-year study (1930 to 1940) that they used special radiographic views. The size of the defect varied in length (cephalocaudal) from 5 mm to 3 cm, in width from 3 mm to 2 cm, and in depth from 10 mm to 22 mm.[284]

A number of special projections have been used to enhance visualization of the Hill-Sachs defect.[4,146,246,278,283,490,537,559,685] Two of these views bear special mention.

The Stryker Notch View

The patient is supine on the table with the cassette placed under the shoulder.[246] The palm of the hand of the affected shoulder is placed on top of the head, with the fingers directed toward the back of the head. The elbow of the affected shoulder should point straight upward. The x-ray beam tilts 10 degrees toward the head and is centered over the coracoid process (Fig. 14–132). This technique was developed by William S. Stryker and reported by Hall and coworkers.[246] They stated that they could demonstrate the humeral head defect in 90% of 20 patients with a history of recurring anterior dislocation of the shoulder.

The Apical Oblique View

Garth and coworkers[204,205] described the apical oblique projection of the shoulder (Fig. 14–133). In this technique

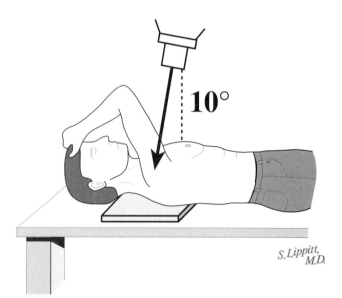

■ **Figure 14–132**
Stryker notch view. *(Modified from Hall RH, Isaac F, and Booth CR: Dislocations of the shoulder with special reference to accompanying small fractures. J Bone Joint Surg Am 41:489-494, 1959.)*

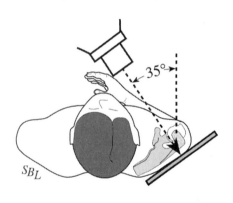

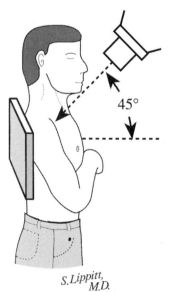

■ **Figure 14–133**
Apical oblique radiograph: a true anteroposterior view of the glenohumeral joint with a 45-degree caudal tilt of the x-ray beam. *(Modified from Garth WP Jr, Slappey CE, and Ochs CW: Roentgenographic demonstration of instability of the shoulder: The apical oblique projection. A technical note. J Bone Joint Surg Am 66:1450-1453, 1984.)*

the patient sits with the scapula flat against the cassette (as for the anteroposterior view in the plane of the scapula). The arm may be in a sling. The x-ray beam is centered on the coracoid and directed perpendicular to the cassette (45 degrees to the coronal plane), except that it is angled 45 degrees caudally. The beam passes tangential to the articular surface of the glenohumeral joint and the posterolateral aspect of the humeral head. This view is likely to reveal both anterior glenoid lip defects and posterior lateral impression fractures of the humeral head.

The incidence of the Hill-Sachs defect reported depends on both the radiographic technique and the patient population. Symeonides[685] reported the humeral head defect in 23 of 45 patients who had recurrent anterior dislocations of the shoulder. However, at the time of surgery he could confirm only 18 of 45.

Eyre-Brook[173] reported a 64% incidence of the Hill-Sachs defect in 17 recurrent anterior dislocations, and Brav[69] recorded a rate of 67% in 69 recurrent dislocations. Rowe and colleagues[611] noted the defect in 38% of 125 acute dislocations and in 57% of 63 recurrent dislocations. Adams[3] reported that the defect was found at the time of surgery in 82% of 68 patients. Palmer and Widen[548] found the defect at surgery in all of 60 patients.

Calandra and coworkers[82] used diagnostic arthroscopy to prospectively study the incidence of Hills-Sach lesions. In a young population of 32 patients with a mean age of 28 years, the frequency of this lesion was 47% for initial anterior shoulder dislocations.

Danzig and colleagues[127] reported that in cadaveric and clinical studies, no single view will always reveal the humeral head compression fracture. Pavlov and coworkers[559] and Rozing and associates[619] found that the Stryker notch view taken in internal rotation best revealed the posterolateral humeral head defect (Fig. 14–132).

The demonstration of a posterior lateral humeral head defect strongly indicates that the shoulder has been subject to a traumatic anterior dislocation. When these factors are already known—for example, in a 17-year-old whose recurrent anterior dislocations began with a well-documented abduction–external rotation injury in football—it is not necessary to spend a great deal of effort demonstrating the humeral head defect because (1) it is very likely to be present even if not seen on radiographs and (2) the existence of such a lesion does not in itself alter our management of the patient.

Glenoid Changes

Standard radiographs may reveal a periosteal reaction to the ligamentous avulsion at the glenoid lip or a fracture (see Figs. 14–6 and 14–97), erosion (see Fig. 14–94), or new bone formation (see Figs. 14–81 and 14–93) at the glenoid rim. Modifications of the axillary view may help in the identification of glenoid rim changes. Rokous and colleagues[603] described what has become known as the "West Point" axillary view.[597] In this technique, the patient is placed prone on the x-ray table with the involved shoulder on a pad raised 7.5 cm from the top of the table. The head and neck are turned away from the involved side. With the cassette held against the superior aspect of the

shoulder, the x-ray beam is centered on the axilla, 25 degrees downward from the horizontal and 25 degrees medial. The resulting radiograph is a tangential view of the anteroinferior rim of the glenoid (see Fig. 14–89). Using this view, Rokous and associates demonstrated bony abnormalities of the anterior glenoid rim in 53 of 63 patients whose histories indicated traumatic instability of the shoulder. Cyprien and coworkers[125] demonstrated lessening of the glenoid diameter and shortening of the anterior glenoid rim in shoulders with recurrent anterior dislocation. Blazina and Satzman[56] also reported anteroinferior glenoid rim fractures seen on the axillary view in nine of their cases.

Special Radiographic Techniques

Although pathology can be seen with additional radiographic views,[231,479,552,582] CT arthrography,* fluoroscopy,[522] or MRI, these additional tests are rarely cost-effective in the clinical evaluation and management of shoulders with characteristic traumatic instability.[165,415] Although CT evidence of labral or capsular pathology is unlikely to change management of the shoulder, contrast CT scans may help document flattening of the antero-inferior glenoid concavity caused by loss of articular cartilage (see Fig. 14–95). CT scans may also be useful in defining the magnitude of bone loss when sizable humeral head or glenoid defects are suggested on plain radiographs (see Figs. 14–96 and 14–97).[225,643] When previous glenoid bone blocks have been carried out or hardware inserted, CT scans are useful for examining the possibility of their encroachment on the humeral head.[119,120,128]

Although many articles have been written on the use of MRI for imaging an unstable shoulder (Fig. 14–134) (e.g., see references 94, 233, 307, 354, 470, 506, 548, 590, 621, 723), the clinical usefulness of this examination awaits definition. Iannotti and colleagues[307] reported that the sensitivity and specificity of MRI in the diagnosis of labral tears associated with glenohumeral instability were 88% and 93%, respectively (Fig. 14–135). However, in a blinded study, Garneau and associates[203] found that it was insensitive and nonspecific for labral pathology. Even if MRI reliably yielded this information, it is unclear how it would be cost-effective in management because patients with refractory instability would be considered for surgery with or without such data.

MRI after postoperative recurrence of instability is less accurate than on unoperated shoulders. For imaging of recurrent labral lesions, MR arthrography has a higher sensitivity for detecting recurrent labral lesions than MRI does, 100% versus 71%, respectively.[727] The specificity of MR arthrography in this study was 60% versus 80% for standard MRI. Indirect MR arthrography in this study had 100% sensitivity and specificity in six shoulders, two of which had recurrent labral tears.

Rotator Cuff Imaging

Patients whose onset of traumatic instability occurred after the age of 35 may have evidence of rotator cuff

---

*See references 68, 120, 159, 352, 362, 449, 462, 577, 578, 649.

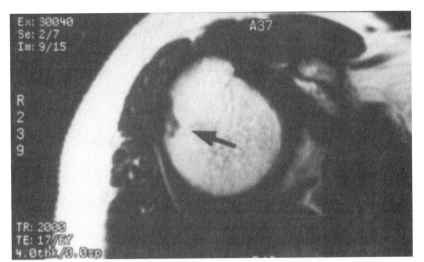

■ **Figure 14–134**

Magnetic resonance imaging demonstrating a focal abnormality in the anterolateral aspect of the humeral head that is consistent with a recent episode of anterior glenohumeral instability. The plain x-ray films were interpreted as normal. *(From Rockwood CA Jr, Green DP, and Bucholz RW [eds]: Fractures in Adults. Philadelphia: JB Lippincott, 1991.)*

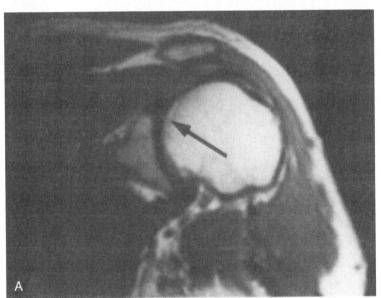

■ **Figure 14–135**

A-C, Lesion of the long head of the biceps tendon origin and superior glenoid labrum as seen on magnetic resonance imaging and arthroscopic examination. *(From Rockwood CA Jr, Green DP, and Bucholz RW [eds]: Fractures in Adults. Philadelphia: JB Lippincott, 1991.)*

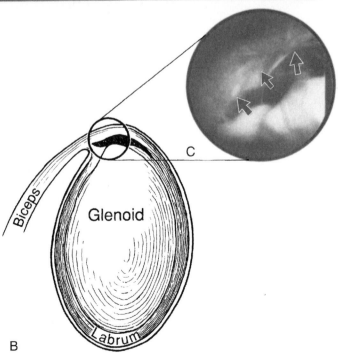

pathology on the history and physical examination. Particular concern arises if weakness of external rotation or elevation persists longer than a week or so. In these situations, preoperative imaging of cuff integrity may play an important role in surgical planning; for example, the approach for rotator cuff repair is quite different from the approach for repair of an anteroinferior capsular lesion. Arthrography, ultrasound, or MRI may be useful in this situation.

Electromyography

Electromyography may be helpful in the evaluation of a patient with recurrent traumatic instability if the history and physical examination suggest residual brachial plexus lesions.

Arthroscopy

Diagnostic arthroscopy is not a necessary prelude to open surgical repair of documented recurrent traumatic instability. Although it rarely changes the surgical approach, shoulder arthroscopy has helped define some of the pathology associated with recurrent instability. Such lesions include labral tears, capsular rents, humeral head defects, and rotator cuff defects (Fig. 14–135).*

A classification of anterior labral "Bankart" lesions was proposed by Green and Christensen.[232] In 37 cases, they described the arthroscopic appearance common to five separate groups. Type I is the normal intact labrum, type II is a simple detachment of the labrum from the glenoid, type III is an intrasubstance tear of the glenoid labrum, type IV is a detachment of the labrum with significant fraying or degeneration, and type V is complete degeneration or absence of the glenoid labrum.

Neviaser found that occasionally, the anterior labroligamentous periosteal sleeve is avulsed from the glenoid.[509] This injury has become known as the ALPSA lesion. The posterior labral periosteal sleeve avulsion (POLPSA lesion) recently described by Simons and colleagues has been shown to be associated with posterior instability,[655] tends to occur in younger patients, and is similar to the anterior version, the ALPSA lesion. The labrum is intact, but separated from the glenoid by an avulsion of its periosteum. The POLPSA lesion has been seen on MRI evaluation.[786]

Gleyze and Habermeyer noted that shoulders with more than five recurrent dislocations were found to have erosion of the anterior articular cartilage.[218] Harryman detected labral damage in all patients treated for recurrent anterior traumatic instability (Fig. 14–136) and in 20% of patients treated for significant articular erosion to subchondral bone (Fig. 14–137).[250]

Other lesions may be associated with Bankart lesions. Snyder and associates[661] and Warner and coworkers[739] found an association of superior labral detachment and Bankart lesions.

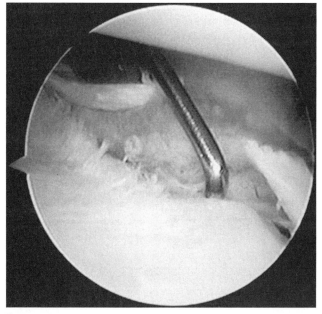

■ Figure 14–136

A Bankart lesion in a patient with recurrent anteroinferior instability. Note the traumatic disruption of the glenoid labrum, fraying of articular cartilage at the glenoid rim, and anterior capsular scarring with synovitis along the inferior glenohumeral ligament. *(Courtesy of Douglas T. Harryman II, MD, Department of Orthopaedics, University of Washington.)*

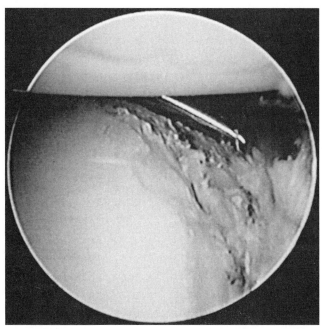

■ Figure 14–137

Chronic anteroinferior instability with evidence of erosion of articular cartilage to subchondral bone and degenerative erosion of the labrum. *(Courtesy of Douglas T. Harryman II, MD, Department of Orthopaedics, University of Washington.)*

---

*See references 12, 84, 195, 204, 242, 286, 338, 406, 462, 480, 533, 551, 758, 759, 794.

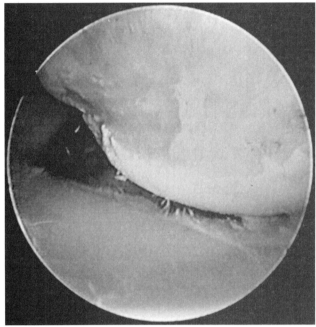

■ **Figure 14–138**
Visualizing the anterior rim of the glenoid and the posterior edge of the humeral articular surface adjacent to a large Hill-Sachs defect with the humerus in abduction–external rotation (same shoulder as seen in Fig. 14–136). *(Courtesy of Douglas T. Harryman II, MD, Department of Orthopaedics, University of Washington.)*

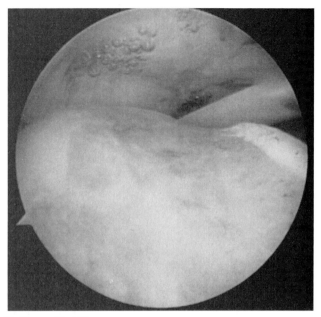

■ **Figure 14–140**
An extensive Hill-Sachs defect that crosses the superior humeral articular surface. Even with this degree of articular surface loss, an arthroscopic Bankart repair was performed with use of the Seattle Bankart guide and has been entirely successful. *(Courtesy of Douglas T. Harryman II, MD, Department of Orthopaedics, University of Washington.)*

Wolf and colleagues reported that 6 of 64 patients with anterior instability had avulsion of the glenohumeral ligaments from the humerus, whereas 47 had true Bankart lesions (73.5%).[775]

Arthroscopy has revealed defects in the articular cartilage of the posterior lateral humeral head that would not be detected on radiographs (Figs. 14–138 to 14–140).

RECURRENT INSTABILITY: TREATMENT

Nonoperative Management

As has been emphasized in the section "Mechanisms of Glenohumeral Stability," coordinated, strong muscle contraction is a key element in stabilization of the humeral head in the glenoid. Patients with traumatic instability were found to have statistically significant humeral translation toward their direction of instability in abduction and external rotation. Patients with atraumatic instability also had decentralization of the humeral head, but in nonuniform directions. Those with traumatic instability were able to recenter the head with muscular action, whereas atraumatic patients were not.[726] This inability suggests that patients with atraumatic instability may have an insufficient glenoid concavity. Under these conditions, optimal neuromuscular control is required of the rotator cuff muscles, deltoid and pectoralis major, and the scapular musculature. These dynamic stabilizing mechanisms require muscle strength, coordination, and training. Such a program is likely to be of particular benefit in patients with atraumatic (AMBRII) instability[304,502] because optimizing neuromuscular control can help

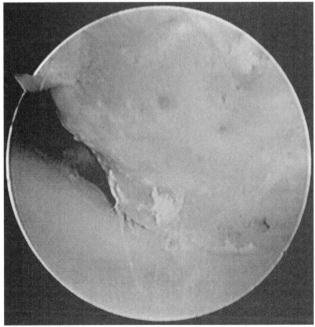

■ **Figure 14–139**
External rotation is increased until the humeral head suddenly dislocates over the edge of the anterior glenoid rim. After repair, external rotation of the glenohumeral joint must be checked adequately to maintain articular contact. *(Courtesy of Douglas T. Harryman II, MD, Department of Orthopaedics, University of Washington.)*

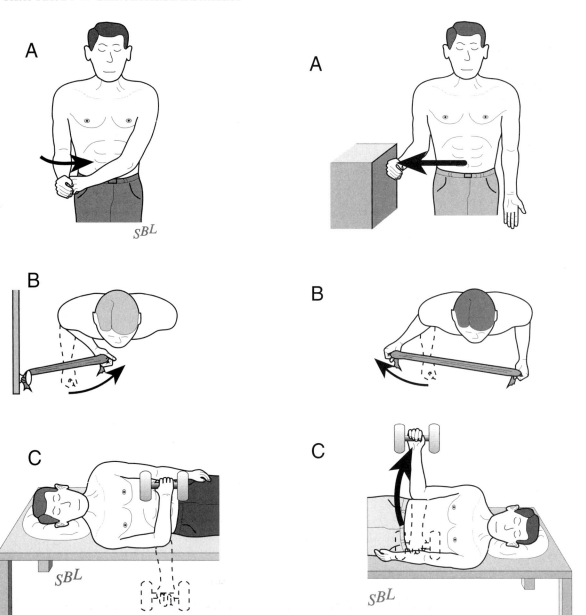

■ **Figure 14–141**
Internal rotation can be strengthened with isometrics (**A**), rubber tubing (**B**), or free weights (**C**). *(From Matsen FA III, Lippitt SB, Sidles JA, and Harryman DT II: Practical Evaluation and Management of the Shoulder. Philadelphia: WB Saunders, 1994.)*

■ **Figure 14–142**
External rotation strengthening with isometrics (**A**), rubber tubing (**B**), or free weights (**C**). *(From Matsen FA III, Lippitt SB, Sidles JA, and Harryman DT II: Practical Evaluation and Management of the Shoulder. Philadelphia: WB Saunders, 1994.)*

balance the humeral head in the glenoid. Nonoperative management is also an especially attractive option for children, for patients with voluntary instability,[502] for those with posterior glenohumeral instability, and for those requiring a supranormal range of motion (such as baseball pitchers and gymnasts, in whom surgical management often does not permit return to a competitive level of function).[262,301,613,625]

Strengthening of the rotator cuff, deltoid, and scapular motors can be accomplished with a simple series of exercises (Figs. 14–141 to 14–144). During the early phases of the program, the patient is taught to use the shoulder only in the most stable positions, that is, those in which the humerus is elevated in the plane of the scapula (avoiding, for example, elevation in the sagittal plane with the arm in internal rotation if the patient has a tendency to posterior instability). As coordination and confidence improve, progressively less intrinsically stable positions are attempted. Taping may provide a useful reminder to avoid unstable positions (Fig. 14–145). The shoulder is then progressed to smooth repetitive activities such as swimming or rowing, which can play an essential role in retraining the neuromuscular patterns required for stability.

Finally, it is important to avoid all activities and habits that promote glenohumeral subluxation or dislocation;

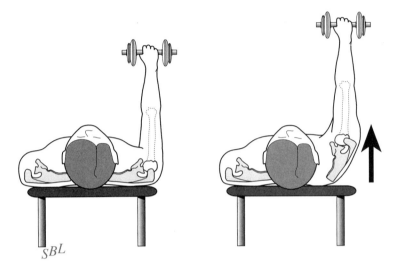

■ Figure 14–143
In the press plus, the arm is pushed upward until the shoulder blade is lifted off the table or bed. (From Matsen FA III, Lippitt SB, Sidles JA, and Harryman DT II: Practical Evaluation and Management of the Shoulder. Philadelphia: WB Saunders, 1994.)

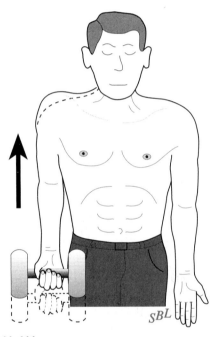

■ Figure 14–144
The shoulder shrug exercise is performed by lifting the tip of the shoulder toward the ear while holding the elbow straight. (From Matsen FA III, Lippitt SB, Sidles JA, and Harryman DT II: Practical Evaluation and Management of the Shoulder. Philadelphia: WB Saunders, 1994.)

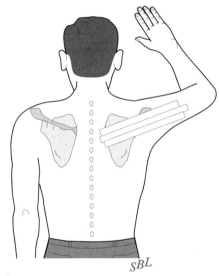

■ Figure 14–145
Training tape is applied across the back of the shoulder as a reminder to avoid unbalanced positions. (Modified from Matsen FA III, Lippitt SB, Sidles JA, and Harryman DT II: Practical Evaluation and Management of the Shoulder. Philadelphia: WB Saunders, 1994.)

patients are taught that each time that their shoulder goes out, it gets easier for it to go out the next time.

Rockwood and colleagues[600] and Burkhead and Rockwood[78] found that 16% of patients with traumatic subluxation, 80% of those with anterior atraumatic subluxation, and 90% of those with posterior instability responded to a rehabilitation program (Fig. 14–146). Brostrom and associates[74] found that exercises improved all but 5 of 33 unstable shoulders, including traumatic and atraumatic types. Anderson and colleagues demonstrated the effectiveness of an exercise program that used rubber bands to improve internal rotator strength.[11] Wirth and coworkers demonstrated that nonoperative

management can be successful even in patients with a congenital factor in their instability. They reported 16 patients with hypoplasia of the glenoid.[767] A subset of this group consisted of five patients with bilateral glenoid hypoplasia and multidirectional instability as indicated by symptomatic increased translation of the humeral head during anterior, inferior, and posterior drawer testing. In addition, generalized ligamentous laxity of the metacarpophalangeal joints, elbows, or knees was noted in all five patients. Four of the patients had been involved in occupational or recreational activities, or both, that had placed heavy demands on the shoulders. Four of these patients had considerable improvement in ratings for pain and the ability to carry out work and sports activities at an average of 3 months after they had begun a strengthening program designed by Rockwood. None of the patients needed vocational rehabilitation despite the

Shoulder Strengthening Exercises

Shoulder Service - Department of Orthopaedics
University of Texas Health Science Center
at San Antonio

Do each exercise _____ times. Hold each
time for _____ counts. Do exercise program
_____ times per day.

Begin with _____ Theraband for _____ weeks.
Then use _____ Theraband for _____ weeks.
Then use _____ Theraband for _____ weeks.

EXERCISE 3

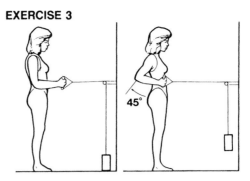

EXERCISE 1

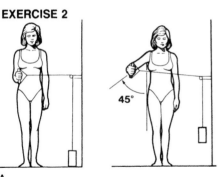

EXERCISE 4

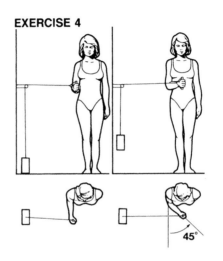

EXERCISE 2

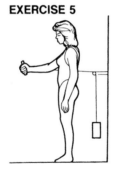

EXERCISE 5

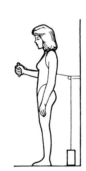

A

■ **Figure 14–146**
A, Shoulder-strengthening exercises. Initially, the patient is given rubber TheraBands to strengthen the rotator cuff muscles and the three parts of the deltoid. After achieving proficiency in rubber resistance with exercises 1 to 5, the patient is given an exercise kit that consists of a pulley, hook, rope, and handle. The pulley is attached to the hook, which is fixed to the wall, and the five exercises are performed. Initially, the patient is instructed to use 5 or 10 lb of weight; the weight is gradually increased over a period of several months to as much as 25 lb. The purpose of the five exercises is to strengthen the three parts of the deltoid muscles, the internal rotators, and the external rotators.

heavy demands on their shoulders associated with their occupational or recreational activities.

These results again support the concept of concavity compression and point out that when the concavity is compromised, stability can often be restored by optimizing balance of the compression mechanism.

Open Operative Management of Traumatic Anterior Instability

Surgical stabilization of the glenohumeral joint is considered for patients with traumatic instability if the condition repeatedly compromises shoulder comfort or function in spite of a reasonable trial of internal and external rotator strengthening and coordination exercises.

When contemplating a surgical approach to anterior traumatic glenohumeral instability, it is essential to preoperatively identify any factors that may compromise the surgical result, such as a tendency for voluntary dislocation, generalized ligamentous laxity, multidirectional instability, or significant bony defects of the humeral head or glenoid. If these conditions exist, it is necessary to modify the management approach. It is noteworthy that these factors can and should be identified preoperatively.

In the past, many surgical procedures have been described for the treatment of recurrent anterior glenohumeral instability. Tightening and to some degree realigning the subscapularis tendon and partially eliminating external rotation were the goals of the Magnuson-Stack and the Putti-Platt procedures. The Putti-Platt operation also tightened and reinforced the anterior

Shoulder Strengthening and Stretching Exercises

■ **Figure 14–146**
Continued B, In addition, the patient is instructed in exercises to strengthen the scapular stabilizer muscles. To strengthen the serratus anterior and the rhomboids, the patient is instructed to first do wall pushups, then gradually do knee pushups, and later do regular pushups. The shoulder shrug exercise is used to strengthen the trapezius and levator scapulae muscles.

Wall Push-Up

30°

Do each exercise _____ times.
Do exercise program _____ times a day.

Knee Push-Up

Regular Push-Up

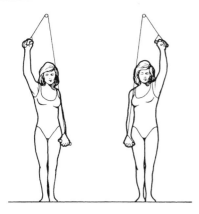

Do each exercise _____ times.
Hold each time for _____ counts.
Do exercise program _____ times a day.

Shoulder Shrug

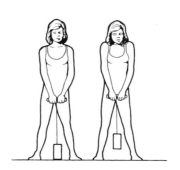

Do each exercise _____ times.
Hold each time for _____ counts.
Use _____ pounds of weight.
Do exercise program _____ times a day.

B

capsule. Reattachment of the capsule and glenoid labrum to the glenoid lip was the goal of the DuToit staple capsulorrhaphy and the Eyre-Brook capsulorrhaphy.[171,172] The Bristow procedure transferred the tip of the coracoid process with its muscle attachments to create a musculotendinous sling across the anteroinferior glenohumeral joint. An anterior glenoid bone buttress was the objective of the Oudard and Trillat procedures. Augmentation of the bony anterior glenoid lip was the goal of anterior bone block procedures such as the Eden-Hybinette procedure. Haaker and coworkers[239] added an autogenous bone graft to the glenoid rim for recurrent instability. In their series of recurrent instabilities in 24 young soldiers, they used screws to fix an anterior iliac crest graft to the anterior glenoid rim. At the conclusion of graft placement, the glenoid labrum is replaced over the graft.

Large posterolateral humeral head defects have been approached by limiting external rotation, by filling the defect with the infraspinatus tendon, or by performing a rotational osteotomy of the humerus.[90,91,681,746]

As will be seen later, most of the reported series on the various types of reconstruction have yielded "excellent" results. However, it is very difficult to determine how each author graded the results. For example, if the patient has no recurrence after repair but has loss of 45 degrees of external rotation and cannot throw, is that a fair, good, or excellent result? The simple fact that the shoulder no longer dislocates cannot be equated with an excellent result. Although the older literature suggested that the goal of surgery for anterior dislocation of the shoulder was to limit external rotation, more modern literature suggests that a reconstruction can both prevent recurrent dislocation and allow nearly normal range of motion and comfortable function.

Capsulolabral Reconstruction

The objective of anatomic repair for traumatic instability is reconstruction of the avulsed capsule and labrum at the glenoid lip, often referred to as a Bankart repair. This type of repair was apparently first performed by Perthes[564] in 1906, who recommended repair of the anterior capsule to the anterior glenoid rim. He was not in doubt about the pathology of traumatic instability: "In every case the anterior margin of the glenoid cavity will be found to be smooth, rounded, and free of any attachments, and a blunt instrument can be passed freely inwards over the bare bone on the front of the neck of the scapula." He reattached the capsule to the glenoid rim by placing drill holes through the bone. Credit for this type of repair should go to Perthes, but the popularity of the technique is due to the work of Bankart,[32,34] who first performed the operation in 1923 on one of his former house surgeons. The procedure commonly used today is based on Bankart's 1939 article in which he discusses repair of the capsule to the bone of the anterior glenoid through the use of drill holes and suture. The subscapularis muscle, which is carefully divided to expose the capsule, is reapproximated without any overlap or shortening. Bankart reported 27 consecutive cases with "full movements of the joint and in no case has there been any recurrence of the dislocation."[56,603,610,616]

It is important to emphasize several significant differences between Bankart's original method and the capsulolabral reconstruction currently recommended. Today we do not osteotomize the coracoid, we do not shave off bone from the anterior glenoid, and finally, we strive to reattach the capsule and any residual labrum up on the surface of the glenoid lip rather than on the anterior aspect of the glenoid as shown by Bankart.

Hovelius and coworkers[297] found a 2% redislocation rate after the Bankart procedure versus a 19% rate after the Putti-Platt procedure. Over one third of the patients younger than 25 years were dissatisfied with the results of the Putti-Platt procedure. Rowe and Zarins[616] reported a series of 50 subluxating shoulders in which good or excellent results were achieved in 94% after a Bankart repair. A Bankart lesion was found in 64% of these shoulders. Rowe and coworkers[611] reported on 51 shoulders with a fracture of the anterior rim of the glenoid. Eighteen shoulders had a fracture involving one sixth or less of the glenoid, 26 involved one fourth of the glenoid, and 7 had one third of the anterior glenoid fractured off. In this group of patients who were treated with a Bankart repair without particular attention paid to the fracture, the overall incidence of failure was 2%. Prozorovskii and colleagues[575] reported no recurrences in the long-term follow-up of 41 Bankart repairs. Martin and coworkers[437] reported excellent results and minimal degenerative change in a 10-year follow-up of 53 patients managed with a Bankart repair.

Although many variations on the method of attaching the capsule to the glenoid have been described, no method has been demonstrated to be safer or more secure than suture passed through drill holes in the lip of the glenoid.[400,446,593] Modifications of the technique do not seem to result in substantial improvement in the efficacy, cost, or safety of the procedure; for example, suture anchors do not have strength equal to that of sutures passed through holes in the glenoid lip.[220,248,268] Furthermore, when suture anchors are placed in the ideal location for capsulolabral reattachment, they have a substantial risk of rubbing on the articular surface of the humerus. In addition, it is difficult to restore the effective glenoid depth when suture anchors are used (see Fig. 14–34D).

Although some have advocated the addition of a capsular shift or capsulorrhaphy to the Bankart repair,[8,667] it does not seem necessary or advisable in the usual case of traumatic instability. Some believe that stretching of the capsular ligaments occurs at the time of injury as well and contend that these ligaments should be plicated, along with repair of the labrum. In a series of cadaveric simian shoulder dislocations, capsular microtears were seen in addition to a Bankart lesion in all shoulders.[114] The extent of the histologic findings was not quantified. Examination of the anterior band of the glenohumeral ligaments of cadaveric shoulders placed in an anterior apprehension position until ligament failure revealed a deformation of 0.04 to 0.53 mm, depending on the site of failure.[461] This finding implies that most of this deformation may be recovered with repair of the labrum to the glenoid alone in the majority of cases.

In fact, one of the outstanding features of Bankart's results was that "All these cases recovered full movement of the joint, and in no case has there been any recurrence of dislocation." Excessive tightening of the anterior capsule and subscapularis can lead to limited comfort and function, as well as to the form of secondary degenerative joint disease known as capsulorrhaphy arthropathy.[53,261,367,422] Rosenberg and colleagues[606] found that 18 of 52 patients had at least minimal degenerative changes at an average follow-up of 15 years; as a cautionary note against unnecessary capsular tightening, these authors found a correlation between loss of external rotation and the incidence of degenerative changes. To help guard against postoperative loss of motion, Rowe and associates[612] limit immobilization to just 2 to 3 days, after which the patient is instructed to gradually increase the motion and function of the extremity.

A clinical comparison has been made of the orientation of the capsulotomy performed in patients during an open Bankart repair. The group treated by horizontal capsulotomy recovered significantly more external rotation in abduction than did those treated by vertical capsulotomy, 112.9 versus 105 degrees, respectively.[319]

Thomas and Matsen described a simplified method of anatomically repairing avulsions of the glenohumeral ligaments directly to the glenoid lip without coracoid osteotomy, without splitting the capsule and the subscapularis, without metallic or other anchors, and without tightening the capsule.[441,691] This method (described in detail in the section "Authors' Preferred Method") offers excellent range of motion and stability. Subsequently, Berg and Ellison[48] again emphasized this simplified approach to capsulolabral repair.

When pathologically increased anterior laxity is combined with a Bankart lesion, the addition of capsular plication to reattachment of the capsulolabral avulsion has been recommended. Jobe and colleagues[330] and Montgomery and Jobe[483] achieved good or excellent results in athletes with shoulder pain secondary to anterior glenohumeral subluxation or dislocation. Two years after surgery, over 80% had returned to their preinjury sport and level of competition.

Wirth and colleagues reported their results in 108 patients (142 shoulders) with recurrent anterior shoulder instability.[762] All patients were managed by repair of the capsulolabral injury, when present, and reinforcement of the anteroinferior capsular ligaments by an imbrication technique that decreases the overall capsular volume. According to the grading system of Rowe and associates, 93% of the results were rated as good or excellent at an average follow-up of 5 years (range, 2 to 12 years). The incidence of recurrent instability was approximately 1%.

Athletes in collision sports who were treated with open Bankart repair and capsulorrhaphy had a 3% redislocation rate. Eight percent had recurrent subluxation and 12% had rare subluxation, thus indicating the difficulty in treating instability in contact athletes.[710]

Other Anterior Repairs

Many other anterior repairs have been described, but most are of historical interest only. The reader is also referred to a review of glenohumeral capsulorrhaphy by Friedman.[194]

Staple Capsulorrhaphy

In the DuToit staple capsulorrhaphy, the detached capsule is secured back to the glenoid with staples.[154,657] Actually, the staple repair had been described 50 years earlier by Perthes. Rao and associates[581] reported the follow-up of 65 patients who underwent DuToit staple repair for avulsion of the capsule from the glenoid rim. Two patients showed radiographic evidence of loose staples. Ward and colleagues[733] reviewed 33 staple capsulorrhaphies at an average of 50 months postoperatively. Fifty percent continued to have apprehension and 12 had staple malposition. O'Driscoll and Evans[531,532] reviewed 269 consecutive DuToit capsulorrhaphies in 257 patients at a median follow-up of 8.8 years. Fifty-three percent of the patients had postoperative pain, and internal and external rotation was limited. Recurrence was reported in 28% if stapling alone was performed and in 8% if a Putti-Platt procedure was added; staple loosening, migration, or penetration of cartilage occurred in 11%. Staple complications contributed to pain, physical restriction, and osteoarthritis. Zuckerman and Matsen pointed out that the use of staples for surgical repair may be associated with major complications (Figs. 14–147 and 14–148).[797]

Subscapularis Muscle Procedures

Putti-Platt Procedure

In 1948, Osmond-Clark[539] described this procedure, which was used by Sir Harry Platt of England and Vittorio Putti of Italy. Platt first used this technique in November 1925. Some years later, Osmond-Clarke saw Putti perform essentially the same operation that had been his standard practice since 1923. Scaglietta, one of Putti's pupils, revealed that the operation may well have been performed first by Codivilla, Putti's teacher and predecessor. Neither Putti nor Platt ever described the technique in the literature.

In the Putti-Platt procedure, the subscapularis tendon is divided 2.5 cm from its insertion. The lateral stump of the tendon is attached to the "most convenient soft-tissue structure along the anterior rim of the glenoid cavity." If the capsule and labrum have been stripped from the anterior glenoid and neck of the scapula, the tendon is sutured to the deep surface of the capsule, and "it is advisable to raw the anterior surface of the neck of the scapula, so that the sutured tendo-capsule will adhere to it." After the lateral tendon stump is secured, the medial muscle stump is lapped over the lateral stump to produce substantial shortening of the capsule and subscapularis muscle. The

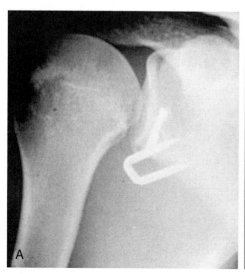
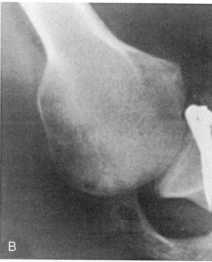

■ Figure 14–147
Complications of staple capsulorrhaphy. **A,** Anteroposterior radiograph showing a prominent staple on the inferior glenoid rim. **B,** Axillary view showing impingement of a staple on the head of the humerus.

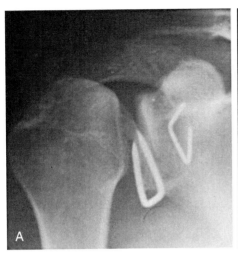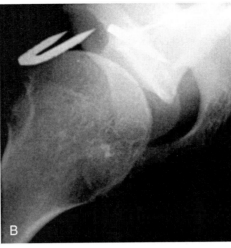

■ **Figure 14–148**
A loose staple after staple capsulorrhaphy. **A,** Anteroposterior radiograph showing a loose staple in the glenohumeral joint. **B,** Axillary view.

exact placement of the lateral stump into the anterior soft tissues and the medial stump into the greater tuberosity is determined so that after conclusion of the procedure, the arm should externally rotate to the neutral position. Variations on the Putti-Platt procedure have been described by Blazina and Satzman,[56] Watson-Jones,[743] Müller,[495] and Symeonides.[685]

Quigley and Freedman[576] reported the results of 92 Putti-Platt operations; of these patients, 11 had more than 30% loss of motion. Seven had recurrent instability after their surgery. Leach and coworkers[388] in 1982 reported a series of 78 patients who had been treated with a modified Putti-Platt procedure. Loss of external rotation averaged between 12 and 19 degrees. Collins and associates[111] reviewed a series of 58 Putti-Platt procedures and 48 Putti-Platt–Bankart procedures. The redislocation rate was 11% (some because of significant trauma), 20% had residual pain, and the average restriction of external rotation was 20 degrees. Hovelius and colleagues,[297] in a follow-up of 114 patients who underwent either a Bankart or Putti-Platt reconstruction, found a recurrence rate of 2% in 46 patients treated with the Bankart procedure and 19% in 68 patients treated with a Putti-Platt procedure. Follow-up was between 1.5 and 10 years. Fredriksson and Tegner[193] reviewed 101 patients who had had a Putti-Platt procedure with a mean follow-up of approximately 8 years (range, 5 to 14 years). Recurrent instability occurred in 20% of cases, and all patients demonstrated a decrease in the range of all measured movements, especially external rotation. Additionally, a significant decrease in strength and power was noted by Cybex dynamometer assessment. The authors stated that the restricted motion after this procedure did not improve with time as previous reports had suggested and concluded that this method of reconstruction should not be recommended for young active patients.

It is important to recognize that if this operation is carried out as described, a 2.5-cm lateral stump of subscapularis tendon is attached to the anterior glenoid. Because the radius of the humerus is approximately 2.5 cm, a 2.5-cm stump of subscapularis fused to the anterior glenoid would limit total humeral rotation to 1 radian, or 57 degrees. Angelo and Hawkins[13,261] presented

a series of patients in whom osteoarthritis developed an average of 15 years after a Putti-Platt repair. It is now recognized that limitation of external rotation after repair for anterior instability is a factor predisposing to capsulorrhaphy arthropathy.[367,422]

Magnuson-Stack Procedure

Transfer of the subscapularis tendon from the lesser tuberosity across the bicipital groove to the greater tuberosity was originally described by Paul Magnuson and James Stack in 1940.[347,429-431,473,581] In 1955, Magnuson recommended that in some cases the tendon should be transferred not only across the bicipital groove but also distally into an area between the greater tuberosity and the upper shaft. DePalma[137] recommended that the tendon be transferred to the upper shaft below the greater tuberosity. Karadimas and colleagues,[347] in the largest single series of Magnuson-Stack procedures (154 patients), reported a 2% recurrence rate. Badgley and O'Connor[26] and Bailey[29] reported on a combination of the Putti-Platt and the Magnuson-Stack operations; they used the upper half of the subscapularis muscle to perform the Putti-Platt procedure and the lower half of the muscle to perform the Magnuson-Stack procedure.

Complications of the Magnuson-Stack procedure include excessive anterior tightening with posterior subluxation or dislocation (Fig. 14–149), damage to the biceps (Fig. 14–150), and recurrent instability.

Bone Block

Eden-Hybbinette Procedure

The Eden-Hybbinette procedure was performed independently by Eden[156] in 1918 and by Hybbinette[306] in 1932. Eden first used tibial grafts, but both authors finally recommended the use of iliac grafts. This procedure is supposed to extend the anterior glenoid. It has been used by Palmer and Widen,[548] Lavik,[384] and Hovelius and colleagues[293] to treat shoulder subluxation and dislocation. Lavik modified the procedure by inserting the graft into the substance of the anterior glenoid rim. Lange[379] inserted the bone graft into an osteotomy on the anterior

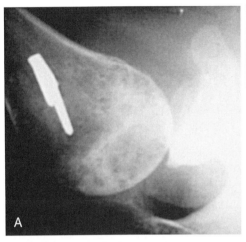

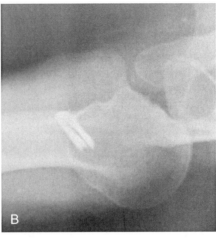

■ **Figure 14–149**
The Magnuson-Stack procedure.
A, This axillary view shows posterior subluxation of the humeral head on the glenoid as a result of excessive anterior tightening with the Magnuson-Stack procedure. **B,** Another patient's axillary view shows excessive anterior tightening from the Magnuson-Stack procedure that resulted in posterior glenohumeral displacement of the humeral head.

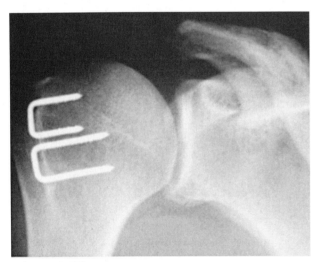

■ **Figure 14–150**
Impingement of a staple on the long head of the biceps tendon. This anteroposterior radiograph shows the position of the staple resulting in tendon impingement. The patient's anterior shoulder pain resolved when the staple was removed.

glenoid. Hehne and Hubner[269] reported a comparison of the Eden-Hybbinette–Lange and the Putti-Platt procedures in 170 patients; their results seemed to favor the latter. Paavolainen and coworkers[544] reported on 41 patients treated with the Eden-Hybbinette procedure; 3 had recurrent instability, and external rotation was diminished an average of 10%. They found the results to be similar to those in their series of Putti-Platt operations. Degenerative joint disease developed in 10% in each group!

Niskanen and coworkers[518] reported a series of 52 shoulders with a mean follow-up of 6 years that had been treated with a modification of the Eden-Hybbinette procedure. The operation involved the creation of a trough through the capsule and into the anteroinferior aspects of the scapula neck. A tricortical iliac crest bone graft was then wedged into the trough without fixation. A 21% recurrence rate was attributed to 1 spontaneous dislocation and 10 traumatic redislocations. Postoperative arthrosis was noted in 9 shoulders and early degenerative changes in an additional 18 shoulders.

Oudard Procedure

In 1924, Oudard[540] described a method in which the coracoid process was prolonged with a bone graft from the tibia. The graft (4 × 3 × 1 cm) was inserted between the sawed-off tip and the remainder of the coracoid and was directed laterally and inferiorly. The graft acted as an anterior buttress that served to prevent recurrent dislocations. Oudard also shortened the subscapular tendon. Later, he published another method of achieving elongation of the coracoid: oblique osteotomy of the coracoid with displacement of the posterolateral portion to serve as a bone block.

Bone blocks are not the procedure of choice for routine cases of recurrent anterior glenohumeral instability. One must be concerned about procedures that may bring the humeral head into contact with bone that is not covered by articular cartilage because of the high risk of degenerative joint disease. Soft tissue repairs and reconstructions are safer and more effective for dealing with the usual case of recurrent traumatic instability. However, when a major anterior glenoid deficiency reduces the anterior or anteroinferior balance stability angle to an unacceptably small value, reconstruction of the anterior glenoid lip may be necessary. Matsen and Thomas[442] described a technique for using a contoured bone graft covered with joint capsule or other soft tissue to replace the missing glenoid bone in order to offer a smooth surface to articulate with the humeral head.

Coracoid Transfer

In transfer of the coracoid process to the anterior glenoid, an attempt is made to create an anteroinferior musculotendinous sling. Some authors also refer to a bone block effect and intentional tethering of the subscapularis in front of the glenohumeral joint. Thus, it is apparent that these procedures do not address the usual pathology of traumatic instability. Redislocation rates after coracoid transfer for the usual case of traumatic instability are no lower than those for soft tissue reconstructions, but the rate of serious complications is substantially higher (Figs. 14–151 to 14–156). Furthermore, in contrast to soft tissue procedures, coracoid transfer procedures are extremely difficult and hazardous to revise: the subscapularis,

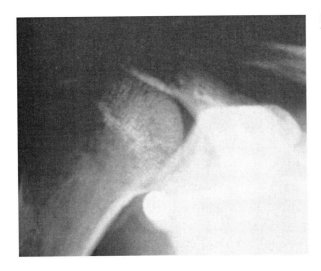

■ **Figure 14–151**
This anteroposterior radiograph shows impingement of a screw on the humeral head after the Bristow procedure.

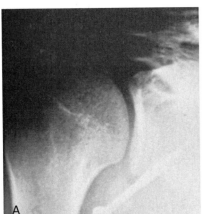
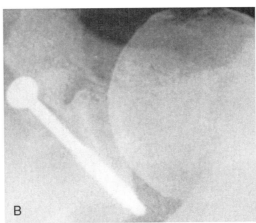

■ **Figure 14–152**
Nonunion of the coracoid process after the Bristow procedure. **A,** An anteroposterior radiograph shows nonunion of the coracoid process. **B,** An axillary view in a different patient shows nonunion of the coracoid process after the Bristow procedure.

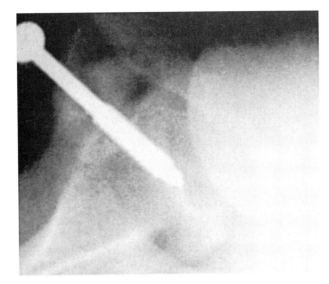

■ **Figure 14–153**
This axillary view shows the screw backing out of the glenoid after the Bristow procedure.

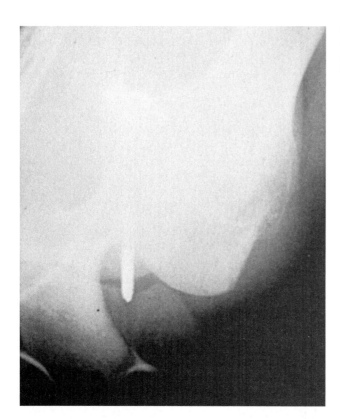

■ **Figure 14–154**
Axillary view showing an excessively long screw used during the Bristow procedure. The patient had an infraspinatus palsy as a result of injury to the nerve to this muscle.

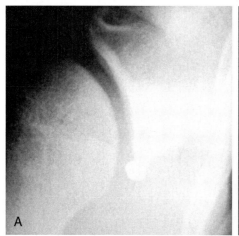
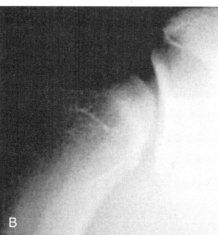

■ **Figure 14–155**
Anteroposterior radiographs showing broken screws with the humerus in external rotation (**A**) and internal rotation (**B**).

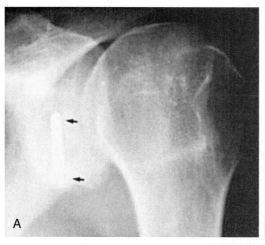
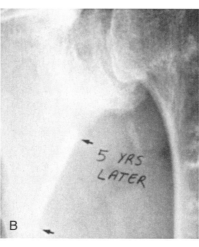

■ **Figure 14–156**
Late screw loosening after the Bristow procedure. **A,** An anteroposterior radiograph shows the position of the screw in the transferred coracoid process. **B,** An anteroposterior radiograph taken 5 years later shows the screw backed out and significant glenohumeral arthropathy.

musculocutaneous, and axillary nerves are scarred in abnormal positions; the subscapularis muscle is scarred and tethered; and the axillary artery may be displaced in scar tissue.

Trillat Procedure

Trillat and Leclerc-Chalvet[59,521,705,706] performed an osteotomy at the base of the coracoid process and then displaced the coracoid downward and laterally. The displaced coracoid is held in position by a special nail-pin or screw. The pin is passed into the scapula above the inferiorly displaced subscapularis muscle, which effectively shortens the muscle.

Bristow-Helfet Procedure

This procedure was developed, used, and reported by Arthur Helfet[270] in 1958 and was named the Bristow operation after his former chief at St. Thomas Hospital, W. Rowley Bristow of South Africa. Helfet originally described detaching the tip of the coracoid process from the scapula just distal to the insertion of the pectoralis minor muscle and leaving the conjoined tendons (i.e., the short head of the biceps and the coracobrachialis) attached. Through a vertical slit in the subscapularis tendon, the joint is exposed and the anterior surface of the neck of the scapula is "rawed up." The coracoid process with its attached tendons is then passed through the slit in the subscapularis and kept in contact with the raw area on the scapula by suturing the conjoined tendon to the cut edges of the subscapularis tendon. In effect, a subscapularis tenodesis is performed.

In 1958, T. B. McMurray (son of T. P. McMurray of hip osteotomy fame) visited Dr. Newton Mead[464] of Chicago and described modifications of the Bristow operation that were being used in Capetown, Johannesburg, and Pretoria. Mead and Sweeney[464] reported use of the modifications in over 100 cases. The modifications consist of splitting the subscapularis muscle and tendon unit in line with its fibers to open the joint and firmly securing the coracoid process to the anterior glenoid rim with a screw. May[445] modified the Bristow procedure further by vertically dividing the entire subscapularis tendon from the lesser tuberosity; after exploring the joint, he attaches the tip of the coracoid process with the conjoined tendon to the anterior glenoid with a screw. The subscapularis tendon is then split horizontally and reattached—half the tendon above and half below the transferred conjoined tendon—to the site of its original insertion. Again, the net effect is a tenodesis of the subscapularis.

Helfet[270] reported that the procedure not only "reinforced" the defective part of the joint but also had a "bone block" effect. Mead and Sweeney,[464] however, do not regard the bone block as being a very important part of the procedure and believe that the transfer adds a muscle reinforcement at the lower anterior aspect of the shoulder joint that prevents the lower portion of the subscapularis muscle from displacing upward as the humerus is abducted. Bonnin[60,61] modified the Bristow procedure in the following way: he does not shorten or split the subscapularis muscle tendon unit, but for exposure, he divides the subscapularis muscle at its muscle-tendon junction, and after attachment of the coracoid process to the glenoid with a screw, he reattaches the subscapularis on top of the conjoined tendon. The results of this modification in 81 patients have been reported by Hummel and associates.[302]

Torg and coworkers[703] reported their experience with 212 Bristow procedures. In their modification the coracoid was passed over the superior border rather than through the subscapularis. Their postoperative instability rate was 8.5% (3.8% redislocation and 4.7% subluxation rate). Ten patients required reoperation for screw-related problems; 34% had residual shoulder pain, and 8% were unable to do overhead work. Only 16% of athletes were able to return to their preinjury level of throwing. Carol and associates[85] reported on the results of the Bristow procedure performed for 32 recurrently dislocating shoulders and 15 "spontaneous" shoulder instabilities. At an average follow-up of 3.7 years, only one patient had recurrent instability, and the average limitation of external rotation was 12 degrees. Banas and coworkers[31] reported a 4% recurrence rate with a 8.6-year follow-up; however, additional surgery was required in 14%. Wredmark and colleagues[778] found only 2 of 44 recurrent dislocations at an average follow-up of 6 years, but 28% of patients complained of pain. Hovelius and coworkers[293] reported follow-up on 111 shoulders treated with the Bristow procedure. At 2.5 years their postoperative instability rate was 13% (6% dislocation and 7% subluxation rate). External rotation was limited an average of 20 degrees, and 6% required a reoperation because of screw-related complications. Muscle strength was 10% less in the operated shoulder. Chen and colleagues[95] found that after the Bristow procedure, the reduced strength of the short head of the biceps was compensated for by increased activity in the long head. Other series of Bristow procedures have been reported, each of which emphasizes the potential risks.[745]

Lamm and coworkers[376] and Lemmens and de Waal Malefijt[392] described four special x-ray projections to evaluate the position of the transplanted coracoid process: anteroposterior, lateral, oblique lateral, and modified axial. Lower and coworkers[419] used CT scans to demonstrate impingement of a Bristow screw on the head of the humerus. Collins and Wilde[110] and Nielsen and Nielsen[517] reported that although they had minimal problems with recurrence of dislocation, they did encounter problems with screw breakage, migration, and nonunion of the coracoid to the scapula. Hovelius and colleagues[291,295] reported only a 50% union rate of the coracoid to the scapula.

Norris and associates[523] evaluated 24 patients with failed Bristow repairs; only 2 had union of the transferred coracoid. Causes of failure included residual subluxation and osteoarthritis from screw or bone impingement or an overtight repair. They pointed to the difficulty of reconstructing a shoulder after a failed Bristow procedure. Singer and colleagues[656] conducted a 20-year follow-up study of the Bristow-Latarjet procedure; in spite of an average Constant-Murley score of 80 points, radiographic evidence of degenerative joint disease was detected in 71%.

Ferlic and DiGiovine[182] reported on 51 patients treated with the Bristow procedure. They had a 10% incidence of redislocation or subluxation and a 14% incidence of complications related to the screw. An additional surgical procedure was required in 14% of the patients. In a long-term follow-up study of 79 shoulders, Banas and colleagues[31] also reported complications necessitating reoperation in 14% of patients. Seventy-three percent of reoperations were for hardware removal secondary to persistent shoulder pain.

Recurrent subluxation after the Bristow procedure also appears to be a significant problem.[182,295,428,448,523] Hill and coworkers[284] and MacKenzie[427] noted failure to manage subluxation with this procedure. Schauder and Tullos[634] reported 85% good or excellent results with a modified Bristow procedure in 20 shoulders at a minimum of 3 years of follow-up. Interestingly, the authors attributed the success to healing of the Bankart lesion because in many instances, the position of the transferred coracoid precluded it from containing the humeral head. The authors suggested that the 15% fair or poor results were secondary to persistent or recurrent subluxation.

In 1989, Rockwood and Young[601,784] reported on 40 patients who had previously been treated with the Bristow procedure. They commented on the danger and the technical difficulty of these repairs. Thirty-one underwent subsequent reconstructive procedures: 10 had a capsular shift reconstruction, 4 required capsular release, 4 had total shoulder arthroplasty, 1 had an arthrodesis, and 6 had various combined procedures. The authors concluded the Bristow procedure was nonphysiologic and associated with too many serious complications and recommended that it not be performed for routine anterior reconstruction of the shoulder.

Latarjet Procedure

The Latarjet procedure,[382,383,555] described in 1954, involves the transfer of a larger portion of the coracoid process than used with the Bristow procedure, with the biceps and coracobrachialis tendons transferred to the anteroinferior aspect of the neck of the scapula. Instead of the raw cut surface of the tip of the coracoid process being attached to the scapula as is done in the Bristow-Helfet procedure, the coracoid is laid flat on the neck of the scapula and held in place with one or two screws. Tagliabue and Esposito[686] reported on the Latarjet procedure in 94 athletes.

Wredmark and colleagues[778] analyzed 44 patients at an average follow-up of 6 years after a Bristow-Latarjet procedure for recurrent shoulder dislocation. Seventy-two percent of patients had no discomfort, but the remaining 28% complained of moderate exertional pain. Vittori has modified the procedure by turning the subscapularis tendon downward and holding it displaced downward with the transferred coracoid. Pascoet and associates[555] reported on use of the Vittori modification in 36 patients and noted one recurrence.

Other Open Repairs

Gallie Procedure

Gallie and LeMesurier[197,198] originally described the use of autogenous fascia lata to create new ligaments between the anteroinferior aspect of the capsule and the anterior

neck of the humerus in 1927. Bateman[41] of Toronto has also used this procedure. Although fascia lata may not be the ideal graft material, the use of exogenous autograft or allograft to reconstruct deficient capsulolabral structures may be necessary in the management of failed previous surgical repairs.

Nicola Procedure

Toufick Nicola's name is usually associated with this operation, but the procedure was first described by Rupp[622] in 1926 and Heymanowitsch[281] in 1927. In 1929, Nicola[512] published his first article in which he described the use of the long head of the biceps tendon as a checkrein ligament. The procedure has been modified several times.[511,513-515] Recurrence rates have been reported to be between 30% and 50%.[86,342,746]

Saha Procedure

A. K. Saha[624-628] has described transfer of the latissimus dorsi posteriorly into the site of the infraspinatus insertion on the greater tuberosity. He reported that during abduction, the transferred latissimus reinforces the subscapularis muscle and the short posterior steering and depressor muscles by pulling the humeral head backward. He has used the procedure for traumatic and atraumatic dislocations, and in 1969 he reported 45 cases with no recurrence.

Boytchev Procedure

Boytchev first described this procedure in 1951 in the Italian literature,[64,65] and later modifications were developed by Conforty.[112] The muscles that attach to the coracoid process along with the tip of the coracoid are rerouted deep to the subscapularis muscle between it and the capsule. The tip of the coracoid with its muscles is then reattached to its base in the anatomic position. Conforty[112] reported on 17 patients, none of whom had a recurrence of dislocation. Ha'eri and Maitland[242] reported 26 cases with a minimum of 2 years' follow-up.

Osteotomy of the Proximal Humerus

Debevoise and associates[131,367] stated that humeral torsion is abnormal in a repeatedly dislocating shoulder. B. G. Weber[350,473,581,746,747] of Switzerland reported a rotational osteotomy whereby he increased the retroversion of the humeral head and simultaneously performed an anterior capsulorrhaphy. The indications were a moderate to severe posterior lateral humeral head defect, which he found in 65% of his patients with recurrent anterior instability. By increasing the retroversion, the posterolateral defect is delivered more posteriorly and the anterior undisturbed portion of the articular surface of the humeral head then articulates against the glenoid. It is recognized that the effective articular surface of the humerus is reduced by the posterior lateral head defect and that the osteotomy realigns the remaining articular surface in a position more compatible with activities of daily living. Weber and colleagues[747] reported a redislocation rate of 5.7%, with good to excellent results in 90%. Most patients required a reoperation for plate removal.

Osteotomy of the Neck of the Glenoid

In 1933, Meyer-Burgdorff reported on decreasing the anterior tilt of the glenoid with a posterior closing wedge osteotomy.[624] Saha has written[624] about an anterior opening wedge osteotomy with a bone graft placed into the neck of the glenoid to decrease the tilt.

Complications of Anterior Repairs

Complications of surgical repairs for anterior glenohumeral instability may be grouped into several categories.[386]

The first includes complications that may follow any surgical procedure. Of primary importance in this category is postoperative infection. Thorough skin preparation, adhesive plastic drapes, and prophylactic antibiotics are useful in reducing contamination by axillary bacterial flora. It is also important to prevent the accumulation of significant hematoma by achieving good hemostasis, obliterating any dead space, and using a suction drain if significant bleeding persists. Finally, it is important to keep the axilla clean and dry postoperatively by using a gauze sponge as long as the arm is held at the side.

The second category of complications consists of postoperative recurrent instability. The published incidence of recurrent dislocation after anterior repairs ranges from 0% to 30%. It is noteworthy that many of the reports included in their tally only recurrent dislocation rather than recurrent subluxation or recurrent apprehension. A 1975 review of 1634 reconstructions compiled from the literature revealed that the incidence of redislocation averaged 3%.[597] In a 1983 review of 3076 procedures, the incidence was unchanged.[595] This review included 432 Putti-Platt operations, 571 Magnuson-Stack operations or modifications, 513 Bankart operations or modifications, 45 Saha operations, 203 Bankart–Putti-Platt combinations, 639 Bristow operations, 115 Badgley combined procedures, 254 Eden-Hybbinette operations, 277 Gallie operations or modifications, and 27 Weber operations.

The incidence of recurrence is underestimated by studies with only 2 years of follow-up. Morrey and Janes,[488] in a long-term follow-up study of 176 patients that averaged 10.2 years, found a redislocation rate of 11%. The operative reconstructions were of the Bankart and Putti-Platt types. In 7 of the 20 patients, redislocation occurred 2 or more years after surgery. The need for long-term follow-up was further emphasized in a study by O'Driscoll and Evans,[531] who monitored 269 consecutive patients undergoing staple capsulorrhaphy for a minimum of 8.8 years. Twenty-one percent of 204 shoulders demonstrated redislocation; this incidence increased progressively with the length of follow-up.

Factors that have been shown to be significantly associated with a poor outcome after open surgical anterior stabilization are workers' compensation, voluntary instability, previous instability surgery, age of the patient, and shorter periods of postoperative immobilization.[257]

Immobilization less than 6 weeks and age 32 years or older were associated with significantly lower Rowe scores. The sex of the patient, Hill-Sachs lesions, the type of instability, labral tears, and the surgeon's experience were not statistically significant. The majority of these patients had Bankart repairs or capsular shifts.

Rowe and colleagues[618] reported on the management of 39 patients with recurrence of instability after various surgical repairs. Of 32 who underwent reoperation, 84% did not have an effective repair of the Bankart lesion at the initial surgery. When the previously unrepaired Bankart lesion was repaired at revision surgery, almost all (22 of 24) the shoulders became stable and remained so for at least 2 years. Excessive laxity was thought to be the primary cause of instability in only four shoulders. Ungersbock and associates[713] also found that rounded or deficient glenoid rims and large unhealed Bankart lesions were associated with failure of surgical repair for anterior instability. Zabinski and coauthors reported similar findings: over half of their failed instability repairs were associated with unhealed Bankart lesions; most regained stability after revision repair.[789] By contrast, only 9 of the 21 shoulders with recurrent multidirectional instability obtained a good/excellent result from revision surgeries.

All 17 patients who had a significant traumatic event subsequent to instability surgery had excellent results after revision open stabilization. Of 33 patients with recurrent instability and no significant trauma after initial surgery, only 67% had good or excellent results.[399]

Refractory instability can be a major problem, whether caused by bone deficiency, poor-quality soft tissue, musculotendinous failure, or decompensation of neuromuscular control (Fig. 14–157). Richards and colleagues[591] described the challenges associated with trying to manage such cases of refractory or "terminal" instability by glenohumeral arthrodesis.

The third major category of complications arises from failure of diagnosis. It is essential to differentiate traumatic unidirectional instability (TUBS syndrome) from atraumatic multidirectional instability (AMBRII syndrome) before carrying out any surgical repair. The consequences of mistaking multidirectional instability for pure anterior instability are substantial. In this situation, if only the anterior structures are tightened, limited external rotation along with the resulting obligate posterior subluxation may lead to rapid loss of glenohumeral articular cartilage and capsulorrhaphy arthropathy.[261,367,422] This complication can be prevented only by accurate preoperative diagnosis and appropriate surgery that avoids unnecessary capsular tightening.

The importance of an accurate diagnosis and subsequent treatment cannot be overemphasized: 20 shoulders (53%) in the study of Cooper and Brems[115] and 22 shoulders (15%) in the report of Wirth and Rockwood[769] had previously been operated on for a mistaken diagnosis. In the latter report, diagnostic errors included (in order of decreasing frequency) rotator cuff disease, biceps tendinitis, thoracic outlet syndrome, and cervical disk herniation.

The fourth category of operative complications consists of neurovascular injuries. The musculocutaneous

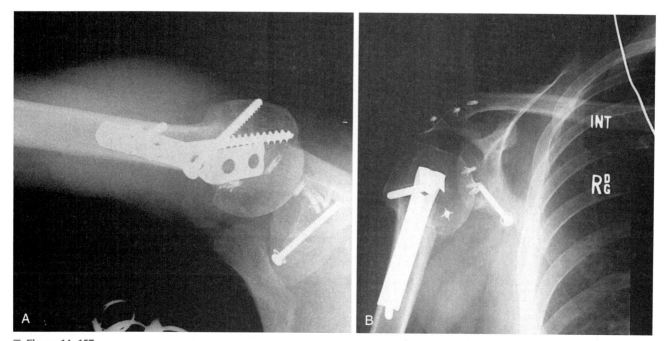

■ **Figure 14–157**

A and **B,** Anteroposterior and axillary radiographs of the shoulder of a young woman. The shoulder remained unstable after six surgeries for glenohumeral instability, including Bankart repairs, capsular shifts, and a Bristow and derotational osteotomy.

nerve runs as a single or multipartite structure obliquely through the coracobrachialis, a variable distance distal to the coracoid process. In this location it may be injured by (1) dissection to free up the coracoid process, (2) retraction, or (3) inclusion in sutures.[649] Helfet[270] described one case in which the nerve had high penetration into the coracobrachialis and became injured where the conjoined tendon entered the slit made in the subscapularis tendon for a Bristow procedure. The axillary nerve may be injured during dissection and suture of the inferior capsule and subscapularis.[417] Richards and associates[592] presented nine patients sustaining nerve injuries during anterior shoulder repair (three Bristow and six Putti-Platt procedures). Seven involved the musculocutaneous nerve and two involved the axillary nerve. Two of the nerves were lacerated, five were injured by suture, and two were injured by traction. These nerve injuries are relatively more common during reoperation after a previous repair; in this situation, the nerves are tethered by scar tissue and are thus more difficult to mobilize out of harm's way. Neurovascular complications can best be avoided by good knowledge of local anatomy (including the possible normal variations), good surgical technique, and a healthy respect for the change in position and mobility of the neurovascular structures after a previous surgical procedure in the area. The authors recommend that the axillary nerve be routinely palpated and protected during all anterior reconstructions.[441,597]

The fifth category of complications includes those related to hardware inserted about the glenohumeral joint.[93,264] The screw used to fix the coracoid fragment in Bristow procedures has a particular potential for being problematic.[517,576] Loosening of the screw may result from rotation of the coracoid fragment as the arm is raised and lowered (Fig. 14–158). Artz and Huffer[22] and Fee

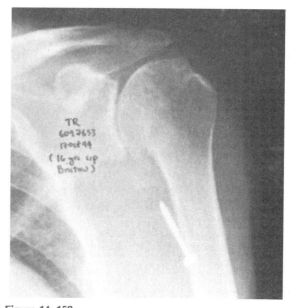

■ **Figure 14–158**

This patient experienced a pop while externally rotating the shoulder 5 months after a Bristow procedure. Shortly after this episode, he palpated a bump in his axilla while applying deodorant. *(From Rockwood CA Jr, Green DP, and Bucholz RW [eds] : Fractures in Adults. Philadelphia: JB Lippincott, 1991.)*

and coauthors[179] reported a devastating complication in which the screw became loose and caused a false aneurysm of the axillary artery with subsequent compression of the brachial plexus and paralysis of the upper extremity. Similar complications have been reported as late as 3 years after surgery.[179] In other instances, the Bristow screw has damaged the articular surface of the glenoid and humeral

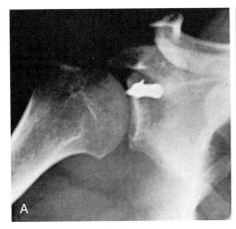
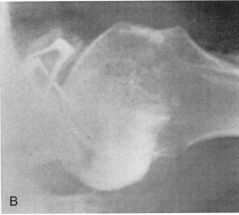

Figure 14–159
A, An anteroposterior radiograph shows the position of an arthroscopically placed staple. Impingement on the humeral head is suggested by this view. **B,** An axillary view with contrast material demonstrates impingement of the staple on the humeral head.

head when placed too close to the glenoid lip, irritated the infraspinatus or its nerve when too long, or affected the brachial plexus when it became loose (Figs. 14-151 to 14-156).

Staples used to attach the capsule to the glenoid may miss their target and damage the humeral or glenoid articular cartilage (Figs. 14-147 to 14-149 and 14-159). Staples also may become loose from repeated pull of the muscles and capsule during shoulder use, particularly if they were not well seated in the first place. O'Driscoll and Evans[531] reported an 11% incidence of staple complications after the DuToit procedure. If screws and staples migrate into the intra-articular region, significant damage to the joint surfaces may result (Fig. 14-160). Metal fixation may injure the biceps tendon in a Magnuson-Stack procedure (see Fig. 14-150).

Zuckerman and Matsen[797] reported a series of patients with problems related to the use of screws and staples about the glenohumeral joint; 21 had problems related to the Bristow procedure and 14 to the use of staples (either for capsulorrhaphy or subscapularis advancement). The time between placement and symptom onset ranged from 4 weeks to 10 years. Screws and staples had been incorrectly placed in 10 patients, had migrated or loosened in 24, and had fractured in 3. Almost all patients required reoperation, at which time 41% had a significant injury to one or both of the joint surfaces.

Recent attempts to "soften" the potential complications of hardware by using bioabsorbable implants have been described. However, Edwards and colleagues[157] reported the adverse effects of a polyglyconate polymer in six shoulders after repair of the glenoid labrum. All patients had increasing pain and loss of motion requiring arthroscopic débridement. Dual-contrast arthrotomography revealed bony cystic changes around the implant, and histologic evaluation was consistent with a granulomatous reaction.

Taken together, these data suggest that primary repairs with hardware are more risky, yet no more effective than anatomic soft tissue repairs to bone with suture alone; the recurrence rates of techniques using screws and staples are no better than those with hardware-free repairs. Risks are incurred with hardware that simply do not exist with other repair techniques. The depth and variable

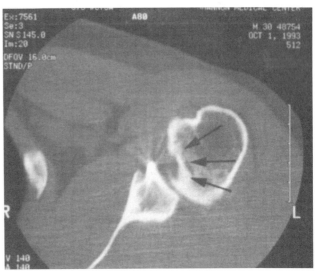

Figure 14–160
Significant humeral head erosion *(arrows)* secondary to intra-articular placement of an anterior capsular staple.

orientation of the glenoid at surgery provide substantial opportunity for hardware misplacement (into the joint, under the articular cartilage, subperiosteally, out the back, too high, too low, too medial, too prominent anteriorly, and too insecurely). The large range of motion of the shoulder with frequent vigorous challenge to its stability creates an opportunity for loosening of hardware and for irreversible surface and neurovascular damage.

The sixth category of complications is limited motion. Limited range of motion, especially external rotation, has been reported after the Magnuson-Stack and the Putti-Platt procedures. It has also been noted after the Bristow procedure, which was supposed to be free of this problem.[36,67,286] Hovelius and colleagues[297] reported an average loss of external rotation of 21 degrees with the arm in abduction. In their series of 46 patients with continuing problems after shoulder reconstruction, Hawkins and Hawkins[260] found that 10 had stiffness related to limited external rotation.

MacDonald and colleagues[425] described release of the subscapularis muscle in 10 patients who had an internal rotation contracture after shoulder reconstruction for recurrent instability. At an average follow-up of 3 years, all patients reported less pain and demonstrated an average increase of 27 degrees of external rotation.

Lazarus and Harryman[386] pointed out that each centimeter of surgical lengthening of excessively tightened capsule regains approximately 20 degrees of rotation.

Lusardi and associates reported on 19 patients (20 shoulders) who had been treated for severe loss of external rotation of the glenohumeral joint after a previous anterior capsulorrhaphy for recurrent instability.[422] All 20 shoulders were managed by release of the anterior soft tissue. The average increase in external rotation was 45 degrees (range, 25 to 65 degrees).

The seventh complication is that of capsulorrhaphy arthropathy, or secondary degenerative joint disease resulting from surgery for recurrent instability.[13,367,386,422,441] This condition most commonly arises from excessive surgical tightening of the anterior capsule causing obligate posterior translation with secondary degenerative joint disease (see Figs. 14–47 and 14–49). The condition can be prevented by ensuring that the shoulder has a functional range of motion after repair for instability and by performing a surgical release of shoulders with major limitations in external rotation. Severe capsulorrhaphy may require shoulder arthroplasty with normalization of the posteriorly inclined glenoid version.[367,386,422,423]

Angelo and Hawkins[13] reported eight patients with disabling degenerative arthritis seen an average of 15.1 years after a Putti-Platt procedure. None of the patients had ever gained external rotation beyond 0 degrees after their repair. Lusardi and colleagues[422] described 20 shoulders with severe loss of external rotation after anterior capsulorrhaphy and spoke about the risk of posterior subluxation and secondary degenerative joint disease in these circumstances.

Lusardi and coworkers[422] also reported on 7 shoulders in which the humeral head had been subluxated or dislocated posteriorly and 16 shoulders that had been affected by mild to severe degenerative joint disease after surgical repair for recurrent anterior dislocation. Nine required shoulder arthroplasty because of severe joint surface destruction. At a mean follow-up of 48 months, all shoulders had an improvement in ratings for pain and range of motion.

The eighth complication after surgical repair is failure of the subscapularis. As pointed out by Lazarus and Harryman,[386] the clinical manifestations of subscapularis failure may include pain, weakness of abdominal press and lumbar pushoff, apprehension, and frank instability. A failed subscapularis can sometimes be repaired directly and on other occasions may require a hamstring autograft, allograft, or transfer of the pectoralis major tendon.

Wirth and coauthors[771] reported a series of failed repairs in which the subscapularis was completely disrupted and contracted medially into a dense connective tissue scar that precluded mobilization. Most of the shoulders had undergone multiple previous procedures. The subscapularis deficiency was reconstructed by transfer of either the upper portion of the pectoralis major or the pectoralis minor in five shoulders.

■ MATSEN AND LIPPITT'S PREFERRED METHOD OF MANAGEMENT OF RECURRENT TRAUMATIC SHOULDER INSTABILITY

A patient with traumatic anterior glenohumeral instability usually has symptoms primarily when the arm is elevated near the coronal plane, extended, and externally rotated. Characteristically, the shoulder is relatively asymptomatic in other extreme positions or in midrange positions. Thus, appropriate management for some patients may consist solely of education about the nature of the lesion and identification of the positions and activities that need to be avoided.

Strengthening the shoulder musculature may help prevent the shoulder from being forced into positions of instability. The exercise program previously described for atraumatic instability may be considered as an option for traumatic instability as well.

The option of surgical repair is discussed when careful clinical evaluation has documented the diagnosis of refractory anterior instability after an initial episode that was sufficiently traumatic to tear the anterior inferior glenohumeral ligament and produce significant functional deficits (recurrent apprehension, subluxation, or dislocation) when the arm is in abduction, external rotation, and extension.

A patient desiring surgical stabilization is presented with a frank discussion of the alternatives and the risks of infection, neurovascular injury, stiffness, recurrent instability, pain, and the need for revision surgery.

Preoperative radiographs are obtained, including an anteroposterior view in the plane of the scapula, an apical oblique (Garth) view, and an axillary view. A preoperative rotator cuff ultrasound is obtained if cuff disease is suspected, for example, in an individual older than 40 years with pain between episodes of dislocation or weakness of internal rotation, external rotation, or elevation. An electromyogram is performed if clinical evaluation suggests the possibility of nerve injury.

SURGICAL TECHNIQUE

The goal of surgical management of traumatic anterior inferior glenohumeral instability is safe, secure, and anatomic repair of the traumatic lesion and restoration of the attachment of the glenohumeral ligaments, capsule, and labrum to the rim of the glenoid from which they were avulsed. (V14-1) By ensuring that reattachment to the rim occurs, the effective depth of the glenoid is restored (see Fig. 14–34). This anatomic reattachment should reestablish not only the capsuloligamentous checkrein but also the fossa-deepening effect of the glenoid labrum. Unnecessary steps are avoided, such as coracoid osteotomy and splitting the subscapularis from the capsule. No attempt is made to modify the normal laxity of the anterior capsule in the usual case of traumatic instability. The repair must be secure from the time of surgery so that it will allow the patient to resume activities of daily living while the repair is healing. Such a secure repair allows controlled mobilization, thereby minimizing

V14-1

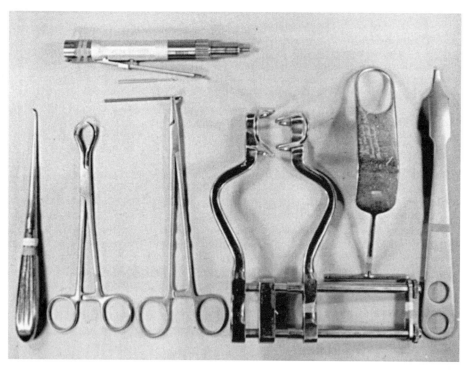

■ **Figure 14–161**
Instruments for surgical repair of recurrent glenohumeral instability. *Top,* A high-speed drill is used for drilling holes in the glenoid rim. *Left to right,* 000-angled curet and reaming tenaculum for connecting the holes drilled in the glenoid rim, curved-nosed needle holder for passing a No. 5 Mayo needle through these holes, self-retaining retractor, humeral head retractor, and sharp-tipped levering retractor.

the possibility of unwanted stiffness. The tools needed for this repair are simple and commonly available (Fig. 14–161).

The procedure is performed with a brachial plexus block or general anesthetic. The glenohumeral joint is examined under anesthesia. Although this examination rarely changes the procedure performed, it provides helpful confirmation of the diagnosis.

The patient is positioned in a slight head-up position (approximately 20 degrees) with the shoulder off the edge of the operating table. This position provides a full range of humeral and scapular mobility and, if necessary, access to the posterior aspect of the shoulder. The neck, chest, axilla, and entire arm are prepared with iodine solution.

The shoulder is approached through the dominant anterior axillary crease (Fig. 14–162), which is marked before the application of an adherent, transparent plastic drape to facilitate a cosmetically acceptable scar.[249] If the incision is confined to the axillary crease, it is less noticeable than the scars from arthroscopic portals. **(V14-2)**

The skin is incised and the subcutaneous tissue is undermined up to the level of the coracoid process, which is then used as a guide to the cephalic vein and the deltopectoral groove (Fig. 14–163). The groove is opened by spreading with the two index fingers medial to the cephalic vein. A neurovascular bundle (a branch of the thoracoacromial artery and the lateral pectoral nerve) is commonly identified in the upper third of the groove[227]; this bundle is cauterized and transected. It is not necessary to release the upper pectoralis major unless a prominent falciform border extends up to the superior extent of the bicipital groove.

The clavipectoral fascia is incised just lateral to the short head of the biceps, up to but not through the coracoacromial ligament (Fig. 14–164); the incision then enters the humeroscapular motion interface and exposes

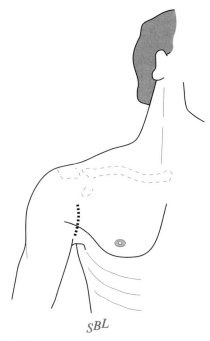

SBL

■ **Figure 14–162**
An incision in the major axillary crease.

the subjacent subscapularis tendon and lesser tuberosity. The axillary nerve is routinely palpated as it crosses the anteroinferior border of the subscapularis. At this point it is useful to insert a self-retaining retractor, with one blade on the deltoid muscle and the other on the coracoid muscles. Care must be taken to ensure that the medial limb of this retractor does not compress the brachial plexus. Rotating the arm from internal to external rotation reveals, in succession, the greater tuberosity, the bicipital groove, the lesser tuberosity, and the subscapu-

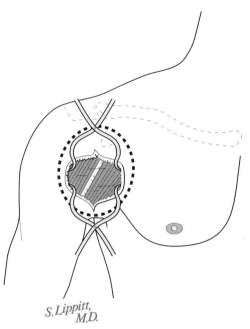

Figure 14–163
Subcutaneous tissue is undermined to the level of the coracoid. The cephalic vein is identified.

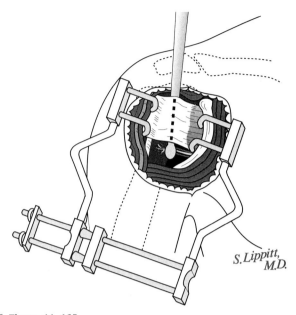

Figure 14–165
A blunt dissector is passed through the rotator interval and deep to subscapularis tendon. The tendon is divided so that strong tissue remains on either side for later repair.

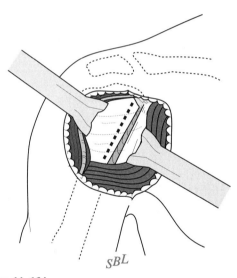

Figure 14–164
The deltopectoral groove is entered medial to the cephalic vein. An incision is made in the clavicopectoral fascia just lateral to the coracoid muscles and up to the level of the coracoacromial ligament.

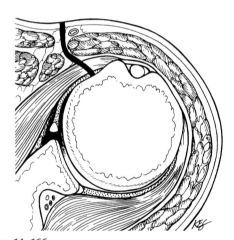

Figure 14–166
Transverse plane section from a superior view showing the incision and the plane for exposure. Note that the deltopectoral interval is used. The subscapularis tendon and the underlying joint capsule are incised as a unit 1 cm medial to the insertion. *(From Matsen FA and Thomas SC: Glenohumeral instability. In Evarts CM [ed]: Surgery of the Musculoskeletal System, 2nd ed. New York: Churchill Livingstone, 1989.)*

laris. **(V14-3)** The anterior humeral circumflex vessels can usually be protected by bluntly dissecting them off the subscapularis muscle at its inferior border. The interval between the supraspinatus and subscapularis tendons is identified by palpation, and a blunt elevator is inserted through this interval into the joint. This elevator brings the upper subscapularis into the incision (Fig. 14–165). With care taken to protect the tendon of the biceps, the subscapularis tendon and subjacent capsule are then incised together approximately 1 cm medial to the lesser tuberosity (Fig. 14–166), beginning at the superior rounded edge of the tendon. **(V14-4)** A tag suture is placed in the upper rolled border of the subscapularis to mark it for subsequent repair. The incision is then extended infe-

riorly to the level of the anterior circumflex humeral vessels, which are not transected, cauterized, or ligated. It is important that the incision through the subscapularis tendon leave strong tendinous material on both sides of the incision to facilitate a secure repair at the conclusion of the procedure.

Without separating them, the subscapularis tendon and anterior shoulder capsule are retracted medially to provide an excellent view of the joint. If necessary for greater exposure, the joint capsule may be further divided parallel to the upper rolled border of the subscapularis. The biceps tendon is inspected and note taken of the integrity of the transverse humeral ligament. Particularly in patients older than 40 years, the shoulder is inspected for evidence of rotator cuff tears. In traumatic anterior instability, a posterolateral humeral head defect is usually palpable by passing an index finger over the top of the humeral head (see Fig. 14-3). If the humeral head defect is so large that it contributes to instability in functional positions, anterior capsular tightening may be necessary to keep the defect from entering the joint on external rotation.

The capsule and subscapularis are retracted together medially, and a humeral head retractor is placed so that it leans on the posterior glenoid lip and pushes the humeral head posterolaterally. **(V14-5)** This technique reveals the anterior inferior glenoid lip from which the labrum and capsule are avulsed in the great majority of patients with anterior traumatic instability (see Figs. 14-3, 14-34B, and 14-101). The labrum usually remains attached to the capsular ligaments, but it may remain on the glenoid side of the rupture, may be a separate ("bucket handle") fragment, or may be absent. Occasionally, flimsy attempts to heal the lesion will temporarily obliterate the defect. However, in these cases a blunt elevator will easily separate the capsule from the glenoid lip and reveal the typical lesion in the anteroinferior quadrant of the glenoid. A spiked retractor is then placed through the capsular avulsion to expose the glenoid lip. The glenohumeral joint is inspected thoroughly for loose bodies, defects of the bony glenoid, and loss of cartilage from the remaining anterior glenoid.

Reconstruction of the capsulolabral detachment from the glenoid is necessary and sufficient for the surgical management of most cases of traumatic instability. Additional tightening jeopardizes the shoulder's range of motion. This repair is carried out from inside the joint, without needing to separate the capsule from the subscapularis muscle and tendon. The glenoid is well exposed by a humeral head retractor laterally and a sharp-tipped levering retractor inserted through the capsular defect onto the neck of the glenoid (Fig. 14-167). Bucket handle or flap tears of the glenoid labrum[2,37] are preserved for incorporation into the reconstruction of the glenoid lip.

The anterior, nonarticular aspect of the glenoid lip is roughened with a curet or a motorized bur, with care taken to not compromise the bony strength of the glenoid lip (Fig. 14-168). **(V14-6)** A 1.8-mm drill bit is used to make holes on the articular aspect of the glenoid 3 to 4 mm back from the edge of the lip to ensure a sufficiently strong bony bridge (Fig. 14-169). We place these holes 5 to 6 mm apart; thus the size of the defect dictates the number of holes used for the reconstruction (Fig. 14-170). **(V14-7)** Corresponding slots are placed on the anterior nonarticular aspect of the glenoid (Fig. 14-169). A 000-angled curet is used to establish continuity between the corresponding slots and holes (Fig. 14-171).

A strong No. 2 absorbable braided suture is passed through the holes in the glenoid lip with a trocar needle and an angled needle holder (Fig. 14-172). **(V14-8)** After each suture is placed through the glenoid lip, the integrity of the bony bridge is checked by a firm pull on the suture.

When sufficient sutures have been placed to span the capsular defect, the spiked retractor is removed and replaced with a right-angled retractor positioned to reveal the trailing medial edge of the avulsed capsule and labrum. This edge is most easily identified by tracing the

intact labrum around the glenoid to its point of detachment at the Bankart defect. Next, by using the trocar needle, the anterior end of the suture (the limb exiting the anterior nonarticular aspect of the glenoid lip) is passed through the trailing medial edge of the capsule, with care taken to incorporate the glenoid labrum, if present, and the strong medial edge of the capsule (Fig. 14-173). **(V14-9)** To prevent unwanted tightening of the anteroinferior capsule, no more capsule is taken than necessary to obtain firm purchase. In larger glenohumeral ligament avulsions, the detached medial edge of the capsule tends to sag inferiorly; in this situation an effort is made to pass each suture through the capsule slightly inferior to the corresponding bony hole in the glenoid lip. Thus, when the sutures are tied, the inferiorly sagging medial capsule is repositioned anatomically (Fig. 14-174).

Once the sutures have been passed through the capsule, they are tied so that the labrum and medial edge of the capsule are brought up on the glenoid lip to restore the fossa-deepening effect of the labrum.[387] The knots are tied so that they come to rest over the capsule rather than on the articular surface of the glenoid (Fig. 14-174). Because they lie over soft tissue, these sutures do not present a mechanical problem, even though they lie within the joint (Fig. 14-175).

Once these sutures are tied, the smooth continuity between the articular surface of the glenoid fossa and the capsule should be re-established along with a reconstructed labrum-like structure (see Figs. 14-34C and 14-175). No stepoff or discontinuity in the capsule should be present when the concavity is palpated. If a substantial anterior capsular defect exists anywhere but at the normal subcoracoid recess, it is closed.

Approximately 10% of TUBS patients have fractures or deficiencies of the anterior bony lip of the glenoid. It is reasonable to attempt to attach the avulsed anterior capsule to the lip of the remaining glenoid articular surface. Anterior glenoid deficiencies greater than 33% or

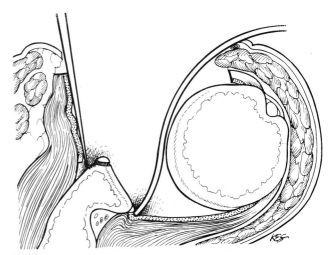

■ **Figure 14–167**
Transverse plane section showing the placement of retractors and the location of drill holes. Note the area roughened by a curet along the anterior glenoid neck; also note the position of the drill hole relative to the anterior glenoid rim. *(From Matsen FA and Thomas SC: Glenohumeral instability. In Evarts CM [ed]: Surgery of the Musculoskeletal System, 2nd ed. New York: Churchill Livingstone, 1989.)*

V14-5
or
V14-9

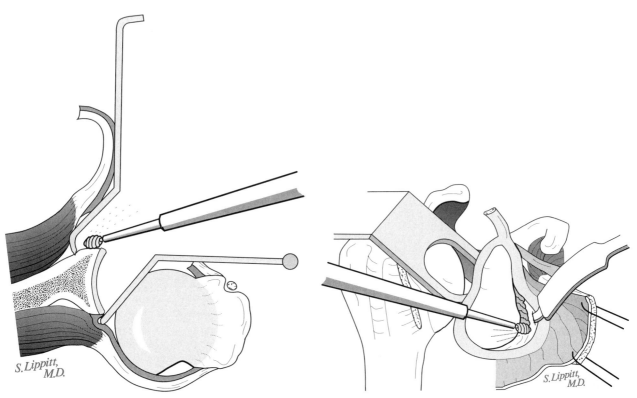

■ Figure 14–168

Roughening of the anterior, nonarticular surface of the glenoid with a pine cone bur. The capsule and subscapularis are retracted medially with a sharp-tipped retractor. The humeral head is retracted laterally with a humeral head retractor. *(Modified from Matsen FA III, Lippitt SB, Sidles JA, and Harryman DT II: Practical Evaluation and Management of the Shoulder. Philadelphia: WB Saunders, 1994.)*

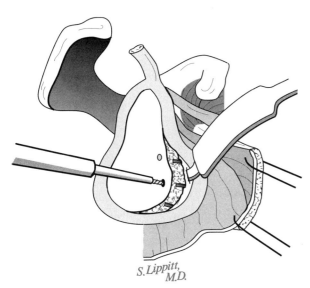

■ Figure 14–169

Holes are drilled in the lip of the articular glenoid 4 mm from the edge and 6 mm apart. *(Modified from Matsen FA III, Lippitt SB, Sidles JA, and Harryman DT II: Practical Evaluation and Management of the Shoulder. Philadelphia: WB Saunders, 1994.)*

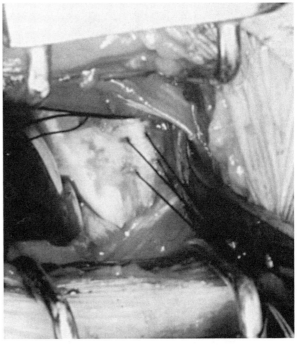

■ Figure 14–170

Intraoperative photograph of the Bankart procedure showing the placement of sutures through holes in the glenoid rim.

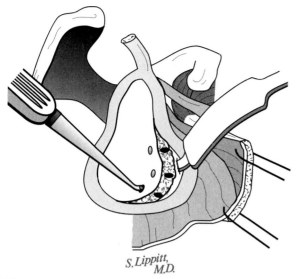

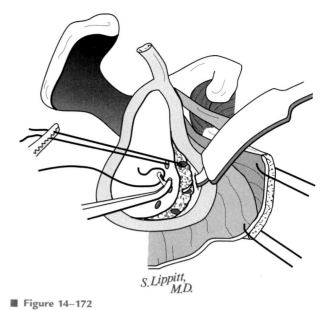

■ Figure 14–171
These drill holes are completed to the bony groove with a 000-angled curet. *(Modified from Matsen FA III, Lippitt SB, Sidles JA, and Harryman DT II: Practical Evaluation and Management of the Shoulder. Philadelphia: WB Saunders, 1994.)*

■ Figure 14–172
A nonabsorbable suture is passed through the drill holes. *(Modified from Matsen FA III, Lippitt SB, Sidles JA, and Harryman DT II: Practical Evaluation and Management of the Shoulder. Philadelphia: WB Saunders, 1994.)*

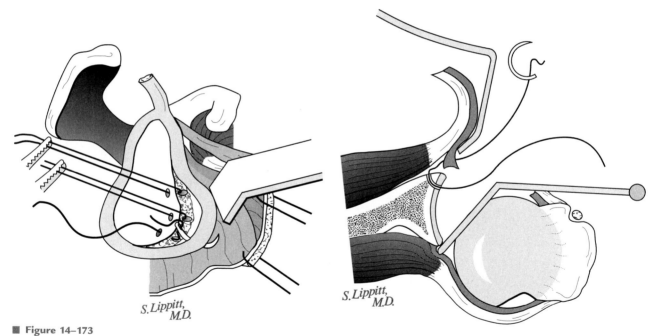

■ Figure 14–173
The sutures are then passed through the trailing medial edge of the capsule and the labrum. *(Modified from Matsen FA III, Lippitt SB, Sidles JA, and Harryman DT II: Practical Evaluation and Management of the Shoulder. Philadelphia: WB Saunders, 1994.)*

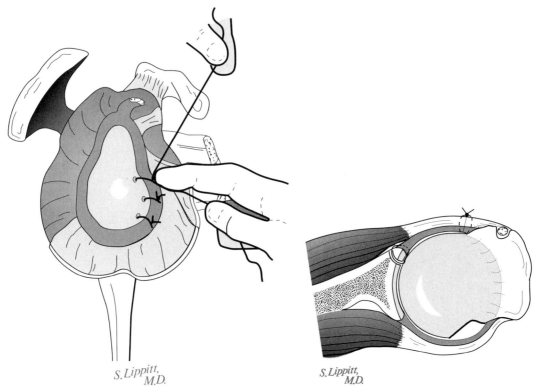

V14-10

■ Figure 14–174
The suture is tied over the capsule, which securely reapproximates the detached tissues to the roughened glenoid edge and restores the fossa-deepening effect of the capsule and labrum. The subscapularis and subjacent capsule are then repaired anatomically to their mates at the lesser tuberosity. *(Modified from Matsen FA III, Lippitt SB, Sidles JA, and Harryman DT II: Practical Evaluation and Management of the Shoulder. Philadelphia: WB Saunders, 1994.)*

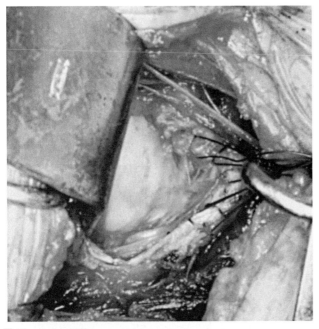

■ Figure 14–175
Intraoperative photograph during re-exploration of a Bankart repair. This patient ruptured the subscapularis tendon repair in a fall 2 months after a Bankart procedure. At the time of reoperation for repair of the subscapularis tendon, the anterior glenoid rim was explored and the Bankart repair was intact. The repair sutures were covered by synovium. The reconstructed labrum is strong.

those associated with previous surgical failure may require that repair of the capsule to the edge of the remaining articular cartilage be backed up by reconstruction of the lip of the glenoid with an iliac bone block. The iliac bone block is contoured flush with the normal glenoid curvature and held to the anterior glenoid with two screws placed securely and well away from the humeral joint surface. By placing the graft outside the repaired capsule, it becomes covered with periosteum or joint capsule, thereby preventing direct contact with the humeral head (Figs. 14–176 and 14–177). This technique is described in detail by Churchill and colleagues.[98]

At the conclusion of the surgical repair, the capsule and subscapularis tendon are anatomically repaired to their mates at the lesser tuberosity (see Fig. 14–174) by using the upper rolled border of the subscapularis as a reference. **(V14-10)** At least six sutures of No. 2 braided nonabsorbable suture are used in this repair to ensure a good bite in both the medial and lateral aspects of the repair. If the tissue on the lateral side is insufficient, the tendon and capsule are repaired via drill holes at the base of the lesser tuberosity. A strong subscapularis and capsular repair is essential to early rehabilitation. The shoulder should have at least 30 degrees of external rotation at the side after the subscapularis/capsular repair. Once this repair has been completed, shoulder stability is examined. If excessive anterior laxity remains, for example, external rotation in excess of 45 degrees (which is rarely the case), the lateral capsular and subscapularis reattachment may be advanced laterally or superolaterally as desired.

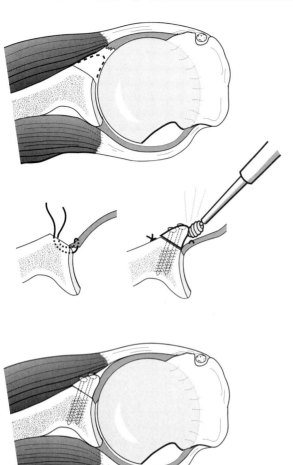

■ **Figure 14–176**
Bone-reinforced Bankart repair. When major anterior glenoid lip bone loss complicates a Bankart lesion, the Bankart repair can be backed up by an extracapsular bone block screwed to the anterior aspect of the glenoid neck and carefully contoured to provide a congruent surface separated from the humeral head by the repaired capsule.

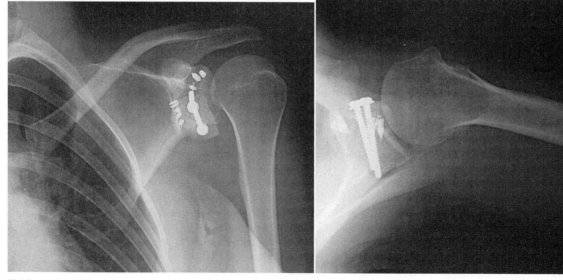

■ **Figure 14–177**
Anteroposterior and axillary radiographs show a bone-reinforced Bankart repair performed for recurrent instability and anterior glenoid lip deficiency after multiple previous anterior repairs that used the suture anchors seen. In this procedure, the capsule is repaired to the lip of the remaining glenoid articular cartilage. The contoured iliac crest graft is then secured to the anterior glenoid outside the capsule, which provides a smooth covering for articulation with the humeral head. Final smoothing of the graft is carried out after it is in position to ensure that it presents the optimal congruent extension of the bony glenoid.

In the highly unusual situation in which a shoulder with the TUBS syndrome is found to not have capsular detachment, the shoulder should be inspected carefully for midsubstance capsular defects. If none are found, the anterior instability may be treated by reefing the anterior capsule and the subscapularis tendon (Fig. 14–178). Shortening these structures by 1 cm limits external rotation of the humerus by approximately 20 degrees. The goal of this restriction is to limit positions of the arm to those in which the net humeral joint reaction force will lie within the balance stability angle. Generally, restricting external rotation to 30 degrees at the operating table will permit a very functional shoulder after rehabilitation is complete. If the patient has marked anterior ligamentous laxity, proportionately greater anterior tightening may be necessary, although the surgeon must be certain that the patient does not have multidirectional laxity before unidirectional tightening is carried out.

Standard wound closure is performed with a subcuticular suture, which is removed in 3 days.

After surgery, most patients are started on a self-conducted "90-0" rehabilitation program with instructions from a physical therapist or physician. We move the shoulder soon after surgery because (1) the repair is strong enough that motion is safe for reliable patients and (2) early motion can increase the ultimate strength of a ligament repair.[191] On the day after surgery, exercises five times daily are started, including assisted flexion to 90 degrees and external rotation to 0 degrees. The contralateral arm is used as the "assistant" until the operated arm can conduct the exercises alone. Patients are allowed to perform many activities of daily living as comfort permits within the 90-degree/0-degree range, as long as they avoid lifting anything heavier than a glass of water. Allowed activities include eating and personal hygiene, as well as certain vocational activities such as writing and keyboarding. Gripping, isometric external rotation, and isometric abduction exercises are started immediately after surgery to minimize the effects of disuse. If a patient does not appear to be able to comply with this restricted-use program, the arm is kept in a sling for 3 weeks; otherwise,

a sling is used only for comfort between exercise sessions and to protect the arm when the patient is out in public and at night while sleeping. Driving is allowed as early as 2 weeks after surgery if the arm can be used actively and comfortably, particularly if the patient's car has an automatic transmission and the operated arm is not used to set the emergency brake. This rapid return to functional activities is made possible because of the strength of the repair and is encouraged to maintain the shoulder's strength and neuromuscular control. It minimizes the immediate postoperative disability and discomfort without jeopardizing the healing process.

At 2 weeks after surgery the patient should return for an examination and should have at least 90 degrees of elevation and external rotation to 0 degrees. From 2 weeks to 6 weeks postoperatively, the patient is instructed to increase the range of motion to 140 degrees of elevation and 40 degrees of external rotation. At 6 weeks after surgery, if there is good evidence of active control of the shoulder, controlled repetitive activities such as swimming and using a rowing machine are instituted to help rebuild coordination, strength, and endurance of the shoulder. More vigorous activities such as basketball, volleyball, throwing, and serving in tennis should not be started until 3 months—and then only if the patient has excellent strength, endurance, range of motion, and coordination of the shoulder.

Vigilance must be exercised in patients older than 35 years to be sure that unwanted postoperative stiffness does not develop. Thus, particularly for these patients, the 2-week and 6-week checkups are very important to make sure that the range of elevation and external rotation are 90 and 0 degrees at 3 weeks and 140 and 40 degrees at 6 weeks, respectively.

In a 5.5-year follow-up of the first group of these repairs, we found 97% good to excellent results based on Rowe's[610] grading system. One of 39 shoulders had a single redislocation 4 years after repair while the patient was practicing karate. He became asymptomatic after completing a strengthening program and is back to full activities, including karate. The average range of motion at follow-up was 171 degrees of elevation, 68 degrees of external rotation with the arm at the side, and 85 degrees of external rotation at 90 degrees of abduction. Ninety-five percent of these patients reported that their shoulder felt stable with all activities; 80% had no shoulder pain, whereas 20% had occasional pain with activity. None had complications of posterior subluxation as a result of excessive anterior tightness, nor did any patient have complications related to hardware!

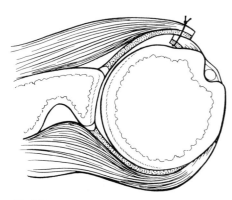

■ **Figure 14–178**
Transverse plane section showing reefing of the subscapularis tendon and capsule in a situation in which no Bankart lesion or other capsular defect is found with isolated anterior instability. Note the intact anterior glenoid rim and the strong repair of the subscapularis tendon. *(From Matsen FA and Thomas SC: Glenohumeral instability. In Evarts CM [ed]: Surgery of the Musculoskeletal System, 2nd ed. New York: Churchill Livingstone, 1989.)*

■ ROCKWOOD AND WIRTH'S PREFERRED METHOD FOR MANAGEMENT OF TRAUMATIC SHOULDER INSTABILITY

Before surgery, all our patients are instructed in a series of exercises designed to strengthen the rotator cuff, deltoid, and scapular stabilizers (see Fig. 14–146). For the past 15 years, our preferred method of surgical repair has been an anatomic reconstruction—that is, repair of the Perthes/Bankart lesion or double-breasting of the capsule. We rarely have to overlap, and thus shorten, the subscapularis tendon.

SURGICAL INCISION

The standard anterior axillary incision begins in the anterior axillary crease and extends up toward and usually stops at the coracoid process (Fig. 14–179A). **(V14-11)** In large muscular men, the incision may extend proximally as far as the clavicle. In women, we use the modified axillary incision described by Leslie and Ryan.[396] The skin is undermined subcutaneously in the proximal medial and distal lateral corners to expose the deltopectoral interval (see Fig. 14–179B). Usually, this interval is identified by the presence of the cephalic vein (see Fig. 14–179C), which may either be absent or lying deep in the interval out of sight. When the vein is not present, we can define the deltopectoral interval proximally because in this area, it is easier to see the difference in angles of the muscle fibers between the pectoralis major and the deltoid. The interval should be very carefully opened, with the vein taken laterally with the deltoid muscle. Routine ligation of the vein produces venous congestion in the area and in the upper extremity and increases postoperative discomfort. Preservation of the vein contributes to an easier postoperative course (i.e., less pain and swelling). We use 8-0 nylon suture to repair any inadvertent nicks in the vein. The deltopectoral interval is developed all the way up to the clavicle without any need to detach any of the deltoid from the clavicle. We usually detach the upper 2 cm of the pectoralis major tendon to allow better visualization of the inferior capsule and make it easier to locate and protect the axillary nerve, which passes just inferior to the capsule. We do not find it necessary to detach the coracoid process or the conjoined tendons (see Fig. 14–179D). With the deltopectoral muscles retracted out of the way, the clavipectoral fascia is seen covering the conjoined tendons. This fascia is divided vertically along the lateral border of the conjoined tendons. Proximally, the clavipectoral fascia blends into the coracoacromial ligament.

IDENTIFICATION OF THE MUSCULOCUTANEOUS NERVE

Before a Richardson retractor is placed in the medial side of the incision to retract the conjoined muscles and pectoralis major muscle, we palpate for the musculocutaneous nerve as it enters the conjoined tendon. Ordinarily, the nerve enters the coracobrachialis and biceps muscles from the medial aspect approximately 5 cm distal to the tip of the coracoid process. However, it must be remembered that it might penetrate immediately below the tip of the coracoid. We have even seen the nerve visible on the lateral aspect of the conjoined tendon (Fig. 14–180). Usually, by palpating just medial to the conjoined tendon and muscles, one can feel the entrance of the musculocutaneous nerve.

IDENTIFICATION AND PROTECTION OF THE AXILLARY NERVE

Next, we locate the axillary nerve—an especially important step when performing the capsular shift procedure—by passing the finger down and along the lower and intact subscapularis muscle-tendon unit (see Fig. 14–179E). The right index finger should be used to locate the nerve in the left shoulder, and the left index finger should be used to locate the nerve in the right shoulder. When the finger is as deep as it will go, the volar surface of the finger should be on the anterior surface of the muscle. Then, the distal phalanx is flexed and rotated anteriorly, which will hook under the axillary nerve before it dives back posteriorly under the inferior capsule. With the arm in external rotation, the nerve is displaced medially and difficult to locate. This large nerve can easily be located with the arm in adduction and neutral rotation. With the upper 2 cm of the pectoralis major tendon taken down, not only can the nerve be palpated, it can also be visualized. The nerve is at least 5/32 inch in size.

DIVISION OF THE SUBSCAPULAR TENDON AND PRESERVATION OF THE ANTERIOR HUMERAL CIRCUMFLEX VESSELS

With the arm in external rotation, the upper and lower borders of the subscapularis tendon can be visualized and palpated. The "soft spot" at the superior border of subscapularis tendon is the interval between the subscapularis and supraspinatus tendons. The lower border of the tendon is identified by the presence of the anterior humeral circumflex artery and veins (see Fig. 14–179F). The upper three fourths of the subscapularis tendon will be vertically transected usually $\frac{3}{4}$ to 1 inch medial to its insertion into the lesser tuberosity. We cut only the upper two thirds of the subscapularis tendon and prefer to do so with the electric cautery (see Fig. 14–179F and G). We are very careful to divide only the tendon and usually try to leave a little of the subscapularis tendon on the capsule to add to its strength (see Fig. 14–179H). We avoid transecting the lower third of the subscapularis tendon and leave it in place to prevent injury to the anterior humeral circumflex artery and veins, to preserve a portion of the tendon's proprioceptive capability, and to protect the axillary nerve. The anterior humeral circumflex artery is the primary blood supply to the head of the humerus, and we believe that it should be preserved. Once the vertical cut in the tendon has been completed, we very carefully reflect the medial part of the tendon off the capsule with curved Mayo scissors until there are no further connections between the tendon and the capsule. When applying lateral traction on the tendon, it should have a rubbery bounce to it. Three or four stay sutures of No. 2 cottony Dacron are placed in the medial edge of the tendon; these sutures are used initially for retraction and later at the time of tendon repair. The lateral stump of the subscapularis tendon is reflected off the capsule with a small sharp knife. This step is easy with the capsule intact when the arm is in external rotation and difficult when the capsule

Text continued on p. 758

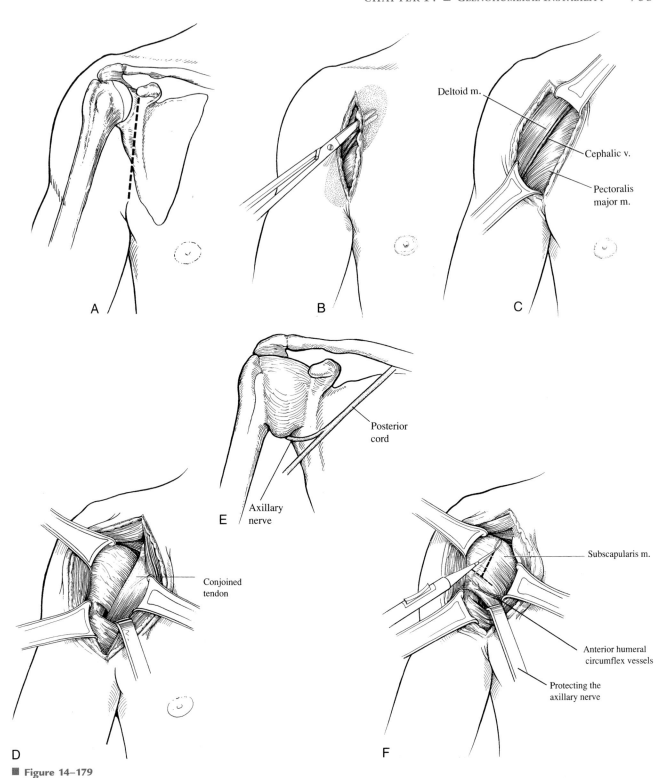

Deltoid m.

Cephalic v.

Pectoralis
major m.

Posterior
cord

Axillary
nerve

Conjoined
tendon

Subscapularis m.

Anterior humeral
circumflex vessels

Protecting the
axillary nerve

A

B

C

E

D

F

■ **Figure 14–179**
The precise details of the operative procedure can be followed in the detailed description of the authors' preferred method of operative treatment in the text. **A-BB,** The procedure used if the anterior capsule is not stripped off the scapula. *(From Wirth MA, Blatter G, and Rockwood CA Jr: The capsular imbrication procedure for recurrent anterior instability of the shoulder. J Bone Joint Surg Am 78:246-259, 1996.)*

Continued

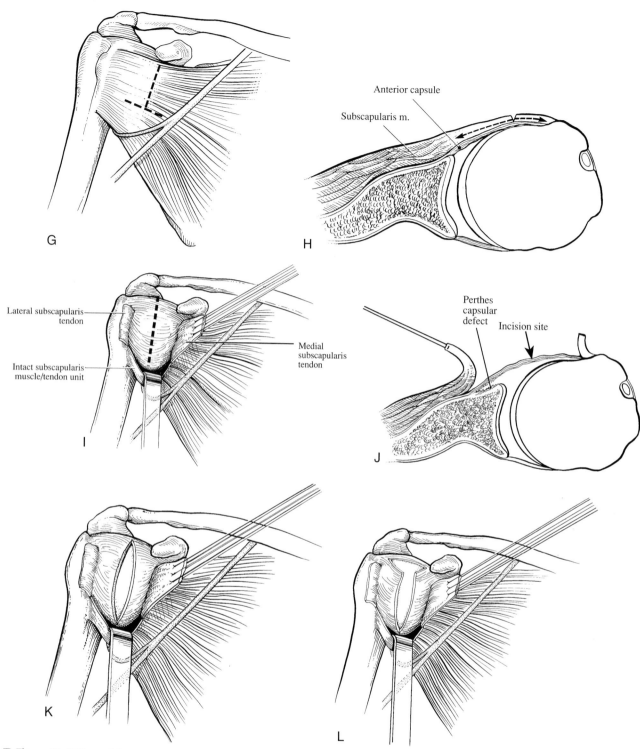

G

H

Anterior capsule

Subscapularis m.

I

Lateral subscapularis tendon

Intact subscapularis muscle/tendon unit

Medial subscapularis tendon

J

Perthes capsular defect

Incision site

K

L

■ **Figure 14–179, cont'd**

The precise details of the operative procedure can be followed in the detailed description of the authors' preferred method of operative treatment in the text. **A-BB,** The procedure used if the anterior capsule is not stripped off the scapula. *(From Wirth MA, Blatter G, and Rockwood CA Jr: The capsular imbrication procedure for recurrent anterior instability of the shoulder. J Bone Joint Surg Am 78:246-259, 1996.)*

Continued

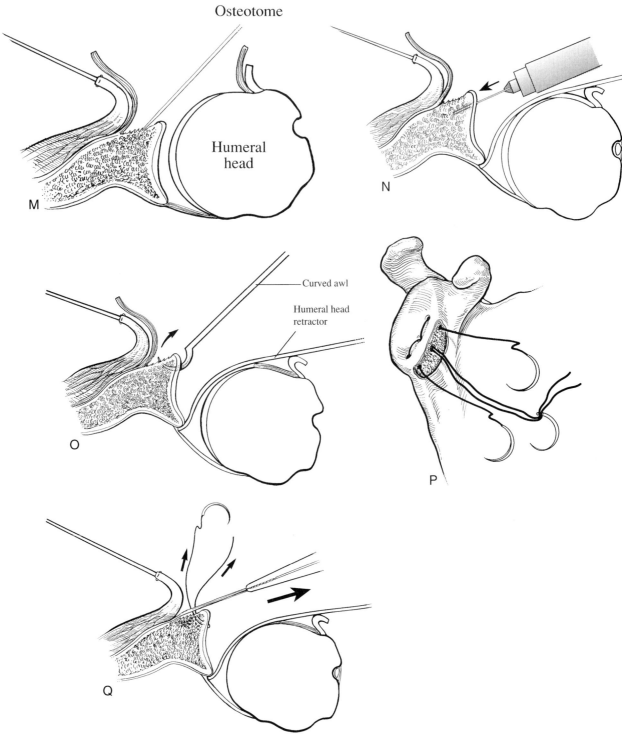

■ Figure 14–179, cont'd

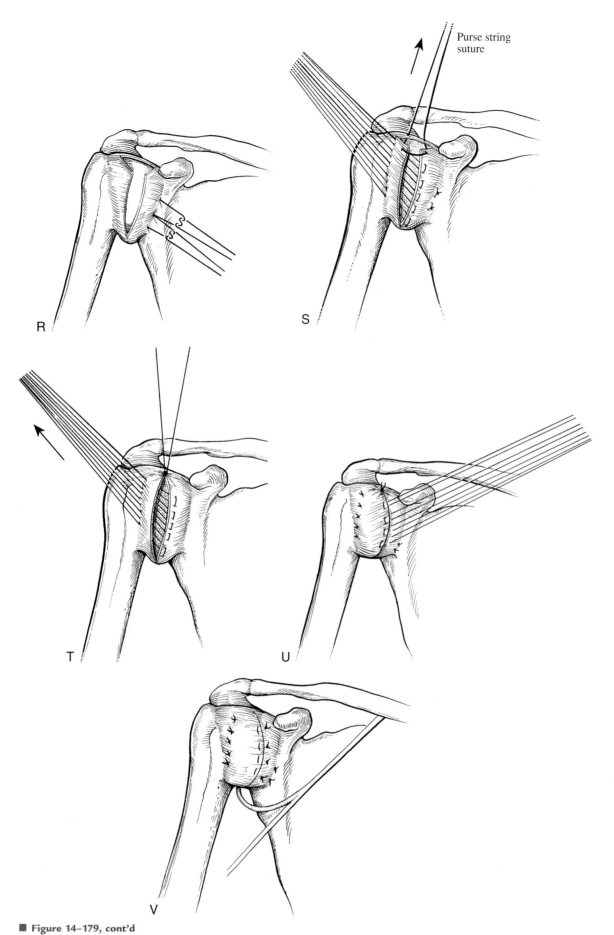

■ Figure 14–179, cont'd
The precise details of the operative procedure can be followed in the detailed description of the author's preferred method of operative treatment in the text. **A-BB,** The procedure used if the anterior capsule is not stripped off the scapula. *(From Wirth MA, Blatter G, and Rockwood CA Jr: The capsular imbrication procedure for recurrent anterior instability of the shoulder. J Bone Joint Surg Am 78:246-259, 1996.)*

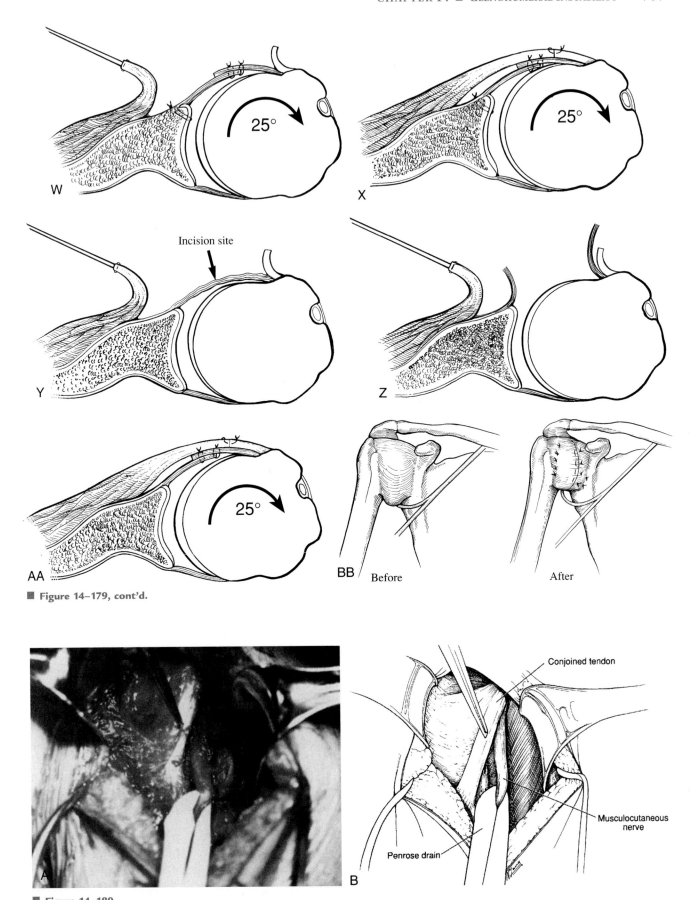

W

X

Incision site

Y

Z

AA

BB   Before   After

■ Figure 14–179, cont'd.

Conjoined tendon

Musculocutaneous nerve

Penrose drain

A

B

■ Figure 14–180

A and **B**, Intraoperative photograph and correlative diagram demonstrating the path of the musculocutaneous nerve as it courses lateral to the conjoined tendons. *(From Rockwood CA Jr, Green DP, and Bucholz RW [eds]: Fractures in Adults. Philadelphia: JB Lippincott, 1991.)*

has been divided. Failure to perform this step will make the two-layer closure of the capsule and the subscapularis tendon more difficult.

With the divided portions of the subscapularis tendon reflected medially and laterally and with the arm in mild external rotation, we use an elevator to gently strip the intact lower fourth of the subscapularis muscle-tendon unit off the anteroinferior capsule. A narrow deep retractor (e.g., Scofield) should be used to retract the lower part of the subscapularis muscle anteriorly and distally, which allows for easy visualization of the inferior capsule. The retractor holds not only the lower part of the subscapularis muscle but also the axillary nerve anteriorly and distally out of the way to prevent injury when the inferior capsule is opened, divided, and repaired (see Fig. 14–179L).

DIVISION OF THE CAPSULE

Next, the capsule is divided vertically midway between its usual attachment on the glenoid rim and the humeral head (see Fig. 14–179I-K). **(V14-12)** Division of the capsule at this location is easier and allows for repair of the capsule if a Perthes-Bankart lesion is present. Furthermore, after the medial capsule is reattached to the glenoid rim, we have plenty of room to add strength to the anteroinferior capsule by double-breasting it with the planned capsular reconstruction. This vertical incision begins at the superior glenohumeral ligament and extends all the way down to the most inferior aspect of the capsule. Occasionally, the superior capsular region is deficient, but such deficiency does not alter the vertical capsular incision (see Fig. 14–179L). We prefer to insert horizontal mattress sutures in the medial capsule just as we complete the division of the most inferior portion of the capsule. We explore the joint carefully and remove loose bodies and glenoid labrum tears. Close attention should be paid to stripping of the labrum, capsule, and periosteum from their normal attachments on the glenoid rim and neck of the scapula (i.e., the Perthes-Bankart lesion).

CAPSULAR SHIFT AND RECONSTRUCTION

If the capsule has secure fixation on the glenoid rim, capsular reconstruction can then be performed. However, if the capsule and periosteum have been stripped from the glenoid rim and neck of the scapula, the capsule must first be reattached before proceeding to capsular reconstruction. Formerly, the senior author believed that if the capsule was stripped from the neck of the scapula, all that was needed was to roughen this area up with a curet or osteotome to create bleeding and then the capsule would spontaneously reattach or heal itself back to the glenoid rim. However, because of failures that required reoperation, it was obvious that this area had not healed and the capsule was still stripped off the glenoid neck. Most likely, synovial fluid within this area inhibits the usual healing process and prevents consistent firm reattachment of the capsule and periosteum to the bony glenoid rim.

In some situations, it may be necessary to horizontally split the medial part of the capsule in its midportion to better visualize and decorticate the anterior rim and neck of the scapula with an osteotome or an air bur. A special retractor developed by Dr. Carter Rowe, which we call the "dinner fork" because of its shape and three sharp teeth, is used to retract the capsule and muscles out of the way while the anterior glenoid rim and neck of the scapula are decorticated and drill holes are being placed in the glenoid rim. We have tried a number of devices, including angled dental drills and Hall drills, curved cutting gouges, clamps, and the Ellison glenoid rim punch; no matter what instrument is used, it always seems to be difficult to place these holes in the dense glenoid rim. With the Bowen, Rowe, or Fukuda retractor holding the humeral head out of the way and the "dinner fork" holding the medial capsule and muscles out of the way, an osteotome is used to decorticate the anterior surface of the neck of the scapula down to raw cancellous bone (see Fig. 14–179M). Usually, three holes are then made between 3 and 6 o'clock on the anterior articular surface of the glenoid. These holes are made with a small drill bit approximately 1/8 inch in from the rim of the glenoid on the articular surface (see Fig. 14–179N). Next, a curved Carter Rowe awl and tenaculum are used to connect the drill holes with the decorticated neck of the anterior glenoid (see Fig. 14–179O). We pass the No. 2 nonabsorbable cottony Dacron sutures through these holes so that two loops of intra-articular suture pass through the three holes (the center hole has two sutures through it) (see Fig. 14–179P).

The medial capsule is then pulled laterally and the needles on the intra-articular loops of suture are passed up and through the medial capsule so that when they are tied, the capsule is reapproximated to the raw bone of the glenoid rim (see Fig. 14–179Q and R). **(V14-13)** We believe that this step is absolutely critical to eliminate the abnormal pouch in the capsule.

With the medial capsule secured back to the glenoid rim, we proceed with capsular reconstruction. Before closure of the capsule, the joint is thoroughly irrigated with saline. The medial capsule will be double-breasted laterally and superiorly under the lateral capsule after closing the superior capsular defect, when present, with a "purse-string" ligature (see Fig. 14–179S and T). All sutures should be placed and tied while being sure that the arm is held in 25 to 30 degrees of external rotation. To carry out this step, the lateral stump of the subscapularis tendon must have been separated from the lateral portion of the capsule. It is critical that the capsular reconstruction sutures be placed under proper tension so that the arm may rotate easily to the desired position. Next, the lateral capsule is double-breasted by taking it medially and superiorly and suturing it down to the anterior surface of the medial capsule (see Fig. 14–179U and V). These sutures are also placed with the arm in the desired rotation. Not only does this type of capsular reconstruction eliminate all laxity in the anterior and inferior capsular ligaments, but because of the double-breasting, the capsule is much stronger. The wound is again carefully irrigated with several liters of saline.

With the arm held in 25 degrees of external rotation, the medial subscapularis tendon is brought into view by pulling on the previously placed sutures (see Fig. 14–179W). The two borders of the tendon are easily approximated with gentle traction, and the tendon is repaired without any overlapping (see Fig. 14–179X). If the tendon is loose with the arm in 25 degrees of external rotation, double-breasting or overlapping of the tendon can be performed by using a two-layer closure with No. 2 Dacron horizontal mattress sutures.

If the capsule has a secure foundation on the glenoid rim, it will only be necessary to perform the capsular shift (Fig. 14–179AA and BB).

WOUND CLOSURE

Before closure of the wound, we carefully irrigate with antibiotic solution and then infiltrate the joint, muscles, and subcutaneous tissue with 25 to 30 mL of 0.5% bupivacaine (Marcaine). This agent aids in decreasing the immediate postoperative pain. We are convinced that the use of bupivacaine before wound closure gives the patient an easier postoperative recovery period. The effect of the bupivacaine will last 6 to 8 hours, which allows the patient to have relatively little pain on awakening; later in the day, as the anesthesia begins to wear off, the patient can request pain medications. Care should be taken to not overuse the bupivacaine or inject it directly into vessels. It is usually unnecessary to put any sutures in the deltopectoral interval. The deep subcutaneous layer is closed with 2-0 nonabsorbable suture, which help prevents widening of the scar. Subcutaneous fat is closed with absorbable sutures, and a running subcuticular nylon suture is used in the skin.

SURGICAL TECHNIQUE SUMMARY

In contrast to a number of previously reported reconstructions for anterior shoulder instability, the procedure that we advocate is an anatomic method of reconstruction that affords great latitude in correcting any pathology encountered at the time of surgery. The anatomic capsular shift procedure is a physiologic repair that includes repair of capsulolabral injury, when present, and reinforcement of the anteroinferior capsular ligaments by a double-breasting technique that decreases overall capsule volume. This reconstruction is a modification of the published reports of the Putti-Platt, Bankart, and Neer capsular shift procedures, and several points deserve emphasis. First, only the upper two thirds of the subscapularis tendon is detached and the inferior third of the tendon is left intact because of the theoretical advantages of preserving a portion of the tendon's proprioceptive capability and protecting the anterior humeral circumflex vessels, which are the primary blood supply to the humeral head. The intact portion of the tendon is also gently stripped and retracted from the underlying capsule to allow visualization of the inferior-most part of the capsule while protecting the axillary nerve and vessels. Second, the deltopectoral interval should be carefully developed and the cephalic vein taken laterally with the deltoid because the majority of tributaries in this region arise from this muscle. In our experience, preservation of the vein contributes to an easier postoperative course, whereas routine ligation produces venous congestion in the upper extremity and increases postoperative

discomfort. Third, it is unnecessary to detach the coracoid or conjoined tendons to gain adequate exposure, but occasionally, we will release the upper 1 cm of the pectoralis major tendon to allow better visualization of the inferior capsule. Such release also facilitates identification of the axillary nerve, which passes just inferior to the capsule as it exits the quadrilateral space. Fourth, proper identification of the musculocutaneous and axillary nerves cannot be overemphasized. Identification of the axillary nerve is especially critical so that it can be protected when opening and repairing the inferior capsule. Fifth, the capsule is divided in a vertical fashion midway between its glenoid and humeral site of attachment. Division in this location provides excellent intra-articular exposure to repair a Perthes-Bankart lesion, and it is easy to perform and facilitates subsequent imbrication, which reinforces the capsular reconstruction. Sixth, the upper two thirds of the subscapularis tendon is repaired anatomically to itself to help minimize the development of undesirable internal rotation contractures of the glenohumeral joint.

POSTOPERATIVE MANAGEMENT

Postoperatively we prefer to use a commercial shoulder immobilizer because it is comfortable, quick, and simple to apply and it prevents abduction, flexion, and external rotation. Regardless of the type of immobilization, it is very important to temporarily remove the device when the patient is seen on the afternoon or evening of the day of surgery. For some reason, a patient who awakens from surgery with the arm in the "device" does not want to wiggle any part of the arm—almost as though it were frozen in the sling-and-swathe position. The commercial immobilizer can easily be removed to allow the patient to move the hand and wrist and then gradually extend the elbow down to the side and lay it on the bed. Such movement almost always relieves the aching pain in the arm and the muscle tension pain. We then tell the patient to flex and extend the elbow several times, which also relieves the generalized arm and shoulder discomfort. In many instances, a patient has related that the vague ache in the shoulder and elbow is more of a problem than pain at the operative site and that this simple release of the immobilizer to allow movement of the elbow and wrist eliminates the discomfort. We allow the patient to remove the immobilizer three to four times a day to exercise the elbow, but otherwise we instruct the patient to always keep the immobilizer in place. Specific instructions are given to the patient to avoid abduction, flexion, and external rotation when the device is removed.

Patients are usually dismissed on the second or third postoperative day, and we allow them to remove the immobilizer two or three times a day while at home when sitting, reading, or watching television. The patient can return to school or work any time after discharge from the hospital. Five days after surgery, the patient can remove the small dressing, take a shower, and reapply the new bandage. We usually delay removing the running subcuticular nylon stitch for 2 weeks because such delay seems to help prevent a wide scar.

As a general rule, the older the patient, the shorter the postoperative immobilization; the younger the patient, the longer the immobilization. In patients younger than 20 years or in a competitive, aggressive athlete, we immobilize the shoulder for 3 to 4 weeks; in young, semiathletic people younger than 30 years, shoulders are immobilized for 3 weeks; the shoulders of patients younger than 50 are immobilized for 2 weeks; and the shoulders of patients older than 50 years are immobilized for 1 to 2 weeks. After removal of the shoulder immobilizer, we allow the patient to gently use the arm for everyday living activities but do not allow any rough use (e.g., lifting, moving furniture, pushing, pulling). At the end of the immobilization period, we start the patient on a stretching exercise program using an overhead pulley and rope set. After the return of motion, we institute a resisted weight exercise and shoulder-strengthening program to strengthen the deltoid, internal rotators, external rotators, and scapular stabilizers (see Fig. 14-146). Athletes are not permitted to return to competitive sports until they have reached a full and functional range of motion and have regained normal muscle strength, which usually requires 4 to 6 months.

RESULTS

In our series,[762] 93% of the results were rated as good or excellent at an average follow-up of 5 years, with a high degree of patient satisfaction and marked improvement in ratings for pain, strength, stability, and function. The average loss of external rotation was 7 degrees, and the average loss of elevation was 6 degrees, which represents physiologic preservation of motion and compares favorably with other reports. The results after revision surgery were encouraging, with 45 (87%) good to excellent results and 7 (13%) fair to poor results. Despite this success, revision anterior shoulder surgery is a formidable challenge with a less predictable outcome inasmuch as 7 of 10 patients graded as fair or poor had failed previous reconstructive efforts. Although progressive symptoms of discomfort were noted in the subset of patients with previous surgery and degenerative changes in the glenohumeral joint, no relationship was found between symptomatic instability after the index procedure and the length of follow-up.

Arthroscopic Repair for Traumatic Anterior Instability

Arthroscopic surgery for Bankart lesions was pioneered by Johnson and Bayley as early as 1982.[337] In their initial procedure, a metal staple was used to reattach the torn labrum or capsule to the roughened edge of the glenoid. In 106 patients so treated, the instability recurred in 21%.[598] Lane and colleagues[378] reported a 33% recurrence rate within 3 years after 54 arthroscopic staple capsulorrhaphies; 15% of asymptomatic patients were found to have loose staples. Detrisac and Johnson[142] found a 12% incidence of recurrence after staple capsulorrhaphy, along with complications related to erosion of the humeral head and subscapularis tendon. Warner and associates[739] reviewed a series of instability repairs with arthroscopically inserted suture anchors and concluded that the failure rate remains "unacceptably high." In a companion

paper[738] they pointed to the technical difficulty of the procedure. Concern about the safety of using staples and the high redislocation rate gave rise to other arthroscopic techniques (see Fig. 14-159).

Wolf[772] reported the use of a screw to reattach the labrum. Biodegradable fixation was introduced by Warren[740] and Johnson.[339] Speer and colleagues[668] reported 52 patients who had undergone arthroscopic shoulder surgery and repair with a bioabsorbable tack. Eleven of the patients exhibited some degree of anterior instability at an average follow-up of 42 months. Warme and coauthors reported that the use of absorbable suture anchors in open Bankart reconstructions resulted in no significant difference from those treated with standard suture anchors at a follow-up ranging from 17 to 45 months.[734]

Caspari[87-89] reported 100 consecutive arthroscopic suture repairs for recurrent anterior instability, with good results in 86%. Other reports of suture methods have been provided by Landsiedl,[377] Goldberg and colleagues,[222] and Morgan and Bodenstab.[486] Grana and associates[226] reviewed 27 patients after arthroscopic suturing for anterior shoulder instability; 12 of these surgeries failed because of pain and recurrent instability.

Arthroscopic Bankart repair has been shown to produce a successful outcome in 97% of all patients and in 93% of those with high physical demands.[752] In young athletes with initial shoulder dislocations, arthroscopic stabilization has been shown to reduce the incidence of subsequent dislocations from 75% to 11% in a group of 21 patients.[62] In a group of 49 shoulders of military personnel with initial anterior shoulder dislocations treated by arthroscopic Bankart repair with an absorbable tack, 12% had continued instability.[131] Other studies using absorbable tacks for arthroscopic Bankart repair report the rate of subsequent dislocation or subluxation to be 15% to 23% versus a 9% to 12% recurrence rate with open repair.[109,349,669]

Recurrence rates of 16% to 33% have been reported after the use of staples for capsulorrhaphy, 0% to 60% after transglenoid suturing, 0% to 37% after labral repair with absorbable tacks, and 0% to 30% after labral repair with suture anchors.[646,750]

In a retrospective, nonrandomized study comparing arthroscopic and open Bankart repair with suture anchors, a redislocation rate of 6.7% was noted in the open group and 3.4% in the arthroscopic group. Apprehension was higher in the arthroscopic group than in the open group, 6.8% versus 3.3%. The arthroscopic group had significantly higher UCLA and Rowe scores than the open group did at a minimum of 2 years' follow-up. The open group received two to three anchors whereas the arthroscopic group received three to six anchors for labral repair.[355] Another study with a minimum of 2 years of follow-up showed a 4% rate of recurrent instability after capsulolabral repair with suture anchors.[210]

The use of a knotless suture anchor in arthroscopic Bankart repair to eliminate arthroscopic knot tying has been described by Thal. The pullout strength of this anchor has been shown to be higher than that of a standard suture anchor, but no clinical studies have been published.[689]

Revision of instability by labral repair in addition to capsular shift and plication has been attempted arthroscopically. Although 82% of patients had good or excellent results based on UCLA shoulder scores, 21% had recurrent instability at a minimum of 24 months' follow-up.[358]

During the Open Meeting of the Arthroscopic Association of North America, which was held in February 2003 in New Orleans, Rockwood[599] added some unpublished material indicating that the failure rate of arthroscopic procedures was two to three times that of open procedures, the so-called gold standard of repairing recurrent anterior dislocations of the shoulder. He reviewed the literature on the subject between 1980 and 1994; in 24 series, the average failure rate for arthroscopic procedures was 27%, with a range of 0% to 39%. In a second review of 32 series between 1994 and 1999, the average failure rate was 19%, with a range of 0% to 40%. In contrast to the arthroscopic procedures, in the 24 series of open anterior reconstructions performed between 1950 and 1999, the average failure rate was 7%, with a range of 0% to 24%. He then reviewed seven series in which the authors compared their own results of open versus arthroscopic repair and found that the average failure with scope procedures was 18% with a range of 0% to 70% versus a failure rate of 7% with a range of 0% to 17% for open procedures. He concluded from the material reviewed that the failure rate of arthroscopic procedures was roughly three times that of open repairs.[599]

For treatment of bidirectional instability, arthroscopic capsulolabral repair with suture anchors was performed in a group of 54 patients. At least 36 of these patients were simultaneously treated with rotator interval tightening, limited thermal tightening, or both. With at least a 2-year follow-up, 7.4% experienced recurrent instability.[209]

Andrews,[12] Ellman,[160-162] Hawkins,[260,262] Esch,[168,169] Jobe,[328-333] and Gartsman[206-208] and their colleagues have provided additional reports of arthroscopic surgery for instability.

Suggested advantages of arthroscopic repair include shorter hospitalization, lower morbidity, less postoperative pain, early recovery of strength, and minimal to no loss of motion.[263,444,485]

Green and Christensen reported a 1.8-fold decrease in operative time, a 10-fold decrease in blood loss, and a 2.5-fold decrease in postoperative narcotic use when compared with the open procedure ($P < .001$).[230] Hospital stay averaged 3.1 days with the open procedure versus 1.1 days with the arthroscopic method ($P < .001$). Time lost from work was 25.5 and 15.3 days for the open and arthroscopic procedures, respectively ($P < .001$).

Others have reported low complication rates after arthroscopic Bankart repair.[46,232,485,587,684,715] Arthroscopic repair avoids incision of the tendon. Ziegler and coauthors reported on the diagnostic and functional deficits in 30 patients with postoperative subscapularis failure, 26 of which followed repairs for anterior instability.[792]

The potential complications after arthroscopic repair are similar in type to those of open repair. Of particular concern are hardware loosening and migration, staple or suture anchor abrasion of the cartilage of the humeral head, and recurrent instability.[89,141,196,340,658,769] Although the use of suture anchors is associated with more

successful outcomes than with previous devices, they are not without complications. Kaar reported a series of eight patients with complications referable to suture anchors, three of whom had articular damage from intra-articular anchors.[345] Infection after arthroscopic shoulder surgery has been reported to occur in 0% to 3.4% of arthroscopies.[750] Recurrence rates after arthroscopic stabilization have been variable in the literature and somewhat dependent on the techniques and devices used.

Published reports of arthroscopic methods for management of glenohumeral instability indicate that (1) many different approaches are being explored with as yet no clear consensus on the best method, (2) the learning curve is long for these procedures, (3) return to physical activity is no more rapid than after open repairs, and (4) rates of recurrent instability after repair are substantially higher than with open repairs.*

At open revision of arthroscopic failures, most have been found to have a detached inferior glenohumeral ligament at the anteroinferior labrum.[444] The open Bankart approach affords direct fixation of the detached structures to bone, whereas the majority of arthroscopic approaches do not. Resch and colleagues described an anteroinferior approach to the glenoid to deal with this deficiency.[586] The authors dissected 87 cadavers to confirm the safety of their direct approach to repair through the substance of the subscapularis. In 264 clinical cases, they report a 5.7% recurrence rate after excluding the first 30 cases.

A consistent challenge for arthroscopic repair is security of the repair to bone. In an attempt to characterize the initial failure strength of Bankart repairs, McEleney used a canine model to compare eight common fixation techniques in current use for both open and arthroscopic repair.[446] The open and arthroscopic two-suture repairs were statistically equivalent in holding strength, and two-suture repairs were significantly stronger than one-suture or absorbable rivet repairs ($P < .01$). In a similar study, Shea and colleagues demonstrated that suture repair had significantly better strength than staple fixation did.[648]

Green and Christensen[232] found significant or complete degeneration of the glenoid labrum–inferior glenohumeral ligament complex (type IV or V labra) in 13 of 15 failed cases. These findings indicate that redislocation after an arthroscopic Bankart procedure may be influenced by the degree of damage to the glenoid labrum–inferior glenohumeral ligament complex and by the presence of articular surface defects.

Warner and coworkers postulated that the success rate of an arthroscopic procedure might be improved by selecting only patients with unidirectional, post-traumatic anterior instability who are found to have a discrete Bankart lesion and well-developed ligamentous tissue.[739] Grana and associates[226] concluded that contact sports appeared to predispose his patients to a high risk of

---

*See references 8, 16, 30, 118, 123, 211, 230, 234, 259, 263, 275, 339, 377, 421, 444, 450, 482, 484-486, 585, 598, 605, 632, 644, 659, 660, 662, 666, 668, 696, 711, 715, 728, 748, 749, 755, 773, 774, 782, 785.

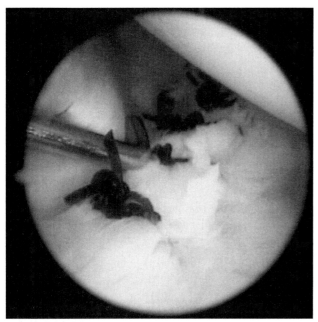

■ Figure 14–181
Arthroscopic intra-articular suture repair of a large Bankart lesion on the glenoid rim performed with the Seattle Bankart guide without suture anchors. Note the attachment of the labrum to reconstitute the glenoid depth. *(Courtesy of Douglas T. Harryman II, MD, Department of Orthopaedics, University of Washington.)*

recurrence and recommended caution in the use of arthroscopic procedures for competitive athletes.

In an attempt to permit secure restoration of the labrum and capsular ligaments to the low anteroinferior rim of the glenoid, Harryman and colleagues developed a posterior approach using a direct arthroscopic glenoid suture guide.[251] This technique does not rely on risky approaches, transosseous sutures adjacent to neurovascular structures, or implanted devices (Fig. 14–181). Though still in the development stages, the early results are encouraging, with a redislocation rate of 6% and elimination of symptoms in all but 11%.[250]

Although all surgical repairs are dependent on excellent knot technique, optimizing knots is particularly challenging in arthroscopic surgery. It is possible that the relatively high rate of recurrent instability after arthroscopic repair is due in part to the difficulty of tying secure knots arthroscopically. In a most important study, Loutzenheiser and coworkers[418] pointed to the arthroscopic challenge of avoiding tying knots that will slip. By using rigorous criteria and mechanical testing, these authors determined that the most secure knot configurations were achieved by reversing the half-hitch throws and by alternating the strands about which the throws were made.

Because of persisting concern about substantial recurrence rates after arthroscopic repairs, arthroscopists are using longer periods of postoperative immobilization and adjunctive steps not necessary with open repairs, such as closure of the rotator interval and capsular tightening.

Thermal Capsulorrhaphy

Thermal capsulorrhaphy was originally a very popular procedure that was used for the treatment of patients with instability. It appeared to be a quick, simple arthroscopic procedure to shrink the capsule of patients with shoulder instability. However, beginning in 2001 throughout 2002, its popularity has lessened because of a high recurrence rate and irreparable injury to the capsular articular surface and in some instances to the brachial plexus. We believe that it is safe to say that thermal capsulorrhaphy is still being carefully investigated.

Thermal energy disorganizes the intramolecular cross-links of collagen by denaturing its triple helical structure. The intermolecular bonds are maintained, which results in shortening and thickening of the collagen molecules. The optimal temperature at which this effect occurs is 65° C to 75° C.[20] The fibers contract approximately 10% to 60% of their length.[266,526] In areas of fiber organization, such as ligaments, the fibers contract more than in disorganized areas. The tissues are weakened, initially up to 90%, with 60% of the strength regained at 6 to 8 weeks and 80% at 12 weeks.[177,267] In the rabbit medial collateral ligament, creep strain was still significantly higher 12 weeks after thermal shrinkage,[732] which suggests that prolonged protection is needed after laser or radiofrequency cauterization of the capsule.

After thermal capsulorrhaphy, translation of the humeral head was significantly reduced in the anterior and posterior directions in a cadaveric study.[698] This study could not, of course, explore biologic healing after cauterization; it is healing of the burn that will determine its effect on shoulder mechanics in patients.

In military personnel with multidirectional instability, some with traumatic mechanisms, 76% returned to full activity after thermal capsulorrhaphy.[187] Thermal capsulorrhaphy alone has been shown to relieve the symptoms of instability in 81% to 96% of patients.[178,424] A survey of orthopaedic surgeons revealed recurrence of instability in 7.1% to 8.4% after thermal capsulorrhaphy[776]; 1.4% of cases in this series resulted in axillary neuropathy, 93% of which were purely sensory and 95% recovered fully. Other series report much higher failure rates. A comparison of radiofrequency and laser thermal capsulorrhaphy showed that 24.5% of the laser group and 23.7% of the radiofrequency group redislocated.[402] In 15 failed thermal capsulorrhaphies from a group of 106 patients, the average time to failure was 6.3 months. Factors associated with failure were previous surgery and multiple dislocations.[9]

Thermal capsulorrhaphy has been used to limit external rotation in baseball players in an attempt to manage internal abutment. A comparison of baseball players treated with arthroscopic surgery with and without thermal capsulorrhaphy showed that 97% returned to play after thermal capsulorrhaphy, 87% at the same level. Patients receiving arthroscopy but not thermal capsulorrhaphy returned to play 80% of the time, only 61% at the same level.[401]

Thermal capsulorrhaphy has been combined with other procedures such as an arthroscopic Bankart repair. In 42 patients with a minimum of 24 months of follow-up, 7% (3 patients) had a subsequent dislocation after combined arthroscopic Bankart repair and thermal capsulorrhaphy.[479]

The unpredictability of healing after thermal injury, the requirement for prolonged restriction of activities, the risk of complications, and the lack of defined indications are reducing the enthusiasm for thermal interventions in the management of shoulder problems.[213]

Operative Management of Posterior Instability

Considerations in the Decision for Surgery

The choice of management for recurrent posterior instability is complicated by the facts that (1) most often recurrent posterior instability is atraumatic, in contrast to the situation with anterior instability, in which only a small percentage of cases are obviously traumatic in etiology; (2) the pathogenesis of recurrent posterior instability is multifactorial, complex, and less well understood than for anterior instability; and (3) the results of the methods for posterior repair are at least 10 times worse than the average for anterior repair. As an example, Hawkins and coworkers[260, 263, 365] presented 50 shoulders in 35 patients treated for recurrent posterior instability. Only 11 of the 50 followed a traumatic event, and 41 demonstrated voluntary and involuntary instability. Of those operated on, 17 patients had a glenoid osteotomy, 6 had a reverse Putti-Platt procedure, and 3 had biceps tendon transfers. The dislocation rate after surgery was 50%, with complications occurring in 20% of the operated cases. Substantial degenerative osteoarthritis developed in two patients after glenoid osteotomy.

Many shoulders with posterior instability can be well managed by education, muscle strengthening, and neuromuscular retraining. Surgical stabilization of posterior glenohumeral instability may be considered when recurrent involuntary posterior subluxation or dislocation occurs in spite of a concerted effort at a well-structured rehabilitation program.[570] Before surgery it is essential to identify all directions of instability and any anatomic factors that may predispose the joint to recurrent instability, such as humeral head or glenoid defect, abnormal glenoid version, rotator cuff tears, neurologic injuries, or generalized ligamentous laxity.[768,769] It is important for the patient to understand the high recurrence and complication rates associated with attempted surgical correction of posterior instability. Because the functional limitations and pain with recurrent posterior instability can be minimal, they suggested that some of these patients may do better without reconstructive procedures. Tibone and coworkers[699] stated that recurrent posterior dislocation of the shoulder is not a definite indication for surgery and stressed the need for careful patient selection before surgical reconstruction.

Posterior Surgical Approaches

Several surgical approaches have been described for the treatment of recurrent posterior glenohumeral instability,

including the posterior deltoid-splitting approach (see Fig. 14–9).[763] Shaffer and colleagues[645] described a surgical approach to the posterior glenohumeral joint through an infraspinatus-splitting incision that they found to offer safe and excellent exposure of the posterior capsule, labrum, and glenoid without requiring tendon detachment or causing neurologic compromise. Most surgeons prefer to split the deltoid at the posterior corner of the acromion and incise the infraspinatus tendon near its attachment to the greater tuberosity.

Posterior Soft Tissue Repairs

The goal of these procedures is to tighten the posterior capsule (the infraspinatus and posterior capsule) to restrict the range of positions attainable by the humerus in relation to the scapula.[221,298,403,504,618,716] In some cases, the infraspinatus and teres minor tendons may be used together in the plication. Boyd and Sisk[63] described transplanting the long head of the biceps tendon posteriorly around the humerus to the posterior glenoid rim.

One of the difficulties with these procedures is that the repair tends to stretch out as the shoulder resumes normal use. Hurley and associates[304] retrospectively reviewed 50 patients with recurrent posterior shoulder instability. Of the 25 patients treated surgically, 72% experienced recurrent instability. Tibone and Bradley[697] reported a failure rate of 30% after posterior staple capsulorrhaphy. Bayley and Kessel[42] stated that failure to distinguish between traumatic and habitual (atraumatic) types of instability led to inappropriate surgery and was a major cause of recurrence after operative repair. Bigliani and colleagues[51] reported a 20% failure rate for management of recurrent posteroinferior instability with a posterior capsular shift; most of the failures were in patients who had undergone previous attempts at surgical stabilization.

Tibone and Bradley[697] reviewed their experience with the management of posterior subluxation in athletes. They pointed out the difficulty in diagnosis, the unclear pathology, the importance of nonoperative management with exercises, and a 40% failure rate of surgical management with a posterior capsular shift. Eleven of the failures were secondary to instability, with 8 having a recurrence of their posterior instability and 3 demonstrating anterior subluxation. These cases of conversion of posterior instability to anterior instability emphasize the importance of recognition and the challenge of management of multidirectional instability.

Arthroscopic capsular shift to the posterior and inferior labrum with closure of the rotator interval resulted in conversion of a positive to a negative jerk test in 85% of patients at a minimum of 12 months' follow-up.

Rotation Osteotomy of the Humerus[574,685,749]

Sunn and colleagues[683] evaluated 12 shoulders that had recurrent posterior shoulder instability treated by external rotation osteotomy of the humerus. Recurrent instability developed in one shoulder with multidirectional instability.

Glenoid Osteotomy and Bone Blocks

Kretzler and Blue,[365,366] Scott,[640] English and Macnab,[167] Bestard,[50] Vegter and Marti,[722] and Ahlgren and associates[6] and others[174,214,221,238,500] have reported using a posterior, opening wedge glenoid osteotomy for recurrent posterior dislocations of the shoulder. In 1966, Kretzler and Blue[366] reported the use of this procedure in six patients with cerebral palsy. They used the acromion as the source of the graft to hold the wedge open. Kretzler[365] reported on 31 cases of posterior glenoid osteotomy in patients with voluntary (15 cases) and involuntary (16 cases) posterior dislocations, with recurrence in 4 patients, 2 from each category.

Extreme care must be taken during this procedure to prevent the osteotome from entering the glenoid, although cracks in subchondral bone are often experienced as the osteotomy is opened (Fig. 14–182). The suprascapular nerve above and the axillary nerve below are also at risk. English and Macnab[167] pointed out that the humeral head may have a tendency to subluxate anteriorly after osteotomy of the glenoid. Gerber and associates[213] demonstrated that with major angular changes, posterior glenoid osteotomy can thrust the humeral head forward and potentially cause abutment of the humeral head against the coracoid and produce pain and dysfunction. Their cadaver studies demonstrated that glenoplasty consistently resulted in squeezing of the subscapularis between the coracoid tip and the humeral head. In cadaveric shoulders, posteroinferior glenoplasty increased the posteroinferior glenoid depth from 3.8 to 7.0 mm and shifted the center of the humeral head anteriorly and superiorly by an average of 2.2 and 1.8 mm, respectively. This, along with an increase in the posterior slope, resulted in an increase in the stability ratio in the posteroinferior direction from 0.47 to 0.81.[468]

The posterior bone block, or glenoid osteotomy, has been combined with various soft tissue reconstructions.[145]

Mowery and associates[494] reported a series of five patients treated with a bone block for recurrent posterior dislocation. One patient had a subsequent anterior dislocation.

Wirth and colleagues[770] reported the use of glenoid osteotomy to manage recurrent posterior glenohumeral instability (Fig. 14–183).

Complications of Posterior Repairs

The principal cause of failure after a posterior soft tissue repair is recurrent instability.[263,506] Unless excellent dynamic stabilization is regained so that concavity compression rather than capsular restraint is the dominant mechanism of stability, the tightened posterior soft tissues are likely to stretch out as motion is regained. Even in its normal state, the posterior capsule is thin, often translucent. Its stretching out after surgical tightening is hastened if the posterior soft tissues are of poor quality, if the patient voluntarily or habitually tries to translate the shoulder posteriorly, or if large bony defects cause unphysiologic dependency on soft tissues for stability.

Occasionally, the opposite outcome can occur: posterior repair may produce a shoulder that is too tight, which may push the shoulder out anteriorly. Insufficient posterior laxity can limit flexion, cross-body adduction, and internal rotation.

Complications may also result from bony procedures for posterior instability. Attempted posterior opening wedge osteotomy of the glenoid may result in an intra-articular fracture, in avascular necrosis of the osteotomized fragment, or in excessive anterior inclination and anterior instability. Posterior bone blocks placed in an excessively prominent position may cause severe degenerative joint disease.

Neurovascular injuries may also complicate posterior instability surgery. The axillary nerve may be injured as it exits the quadrangular space, or the nerve to the infraspinatus may be injured in the spinoglenoid notch.[310,504]

■ MATSEN'S PREFERRED METHOD FOR TREATMENT OF RECURRENT POSTERIOR GLENOHUMERAL INSTABILITY

Care is taken to identify the circumstances and directions of instability, the presence of generalized ligamentous laxity, and any anatomic factors that might potentially compromise the surgical result. We evaluate the possibilities of multidirectional and voluntary instability in each patient with posterior instability. All patients with posterior instability are started on the rehabilitation program described previously for atraumatic instability. A substantial number of patients with recurrent posterior instability respond to this program, particularly those with relatively atraumatic initiation of their condition. Straightforward patients who continue to have major symptomatic posterior instability after a reasonable rehabilitation effort may be considered for surgery. The type of posterior repair is influenced by the pathophysiology:

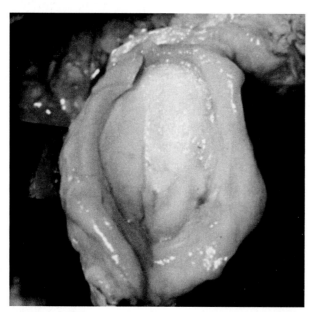

■ **Figure 14–182**
The articular surface of the glenoid after a posterior opening wedge osteotomy in a cadaver specimen.

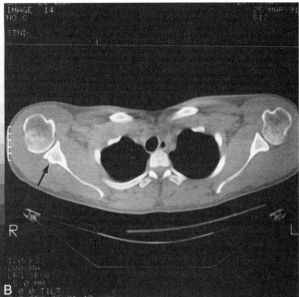

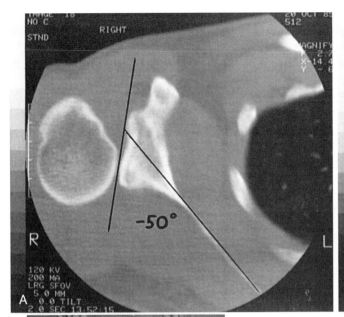

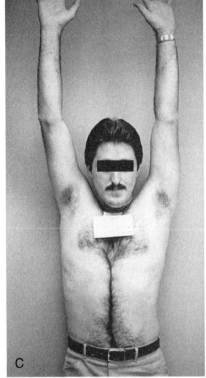

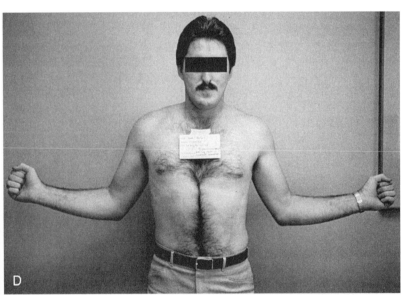

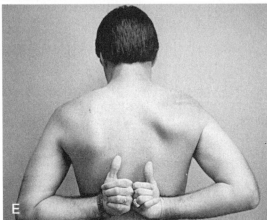

■ **Figure 14–183**

A, Preoperative computed tomographic (CT) scan demonstrating moderate glenoid retrotilt. **B,** Postoperative CT scan revealing a significant degree of correction of the glenoid version and incorporation of the tricortical bone graft after a posterior opening wedge osteotomy of the glenoid. **C-E,** Clinic photographs demonstrating full and symmetric motion. *(From Wirth MA, Seltzer DG, and Rockwood CA Jr: Recurrent posterior glenohumeral dislocation associated with increased retroversion of the glenoid. Clin Orthop 308:98-101, 1994.)*

- Those with traumatic posterior instability may in fact have pathology very similar to that of traumatic anterior instability (avulsion of the capsule and labrum from the glenoid rim or a capsular tear), which is amenable to primary repair. This condition must be diagnosed primarily from a history of an initial forcible posterior displacement of the humeral head on the glenoid, but it may be corroborated by a painful snap on the posterior drawer test.

- Those with lax posterior capsules may be managed with posterior capsulorrhaphy, but this capsular tightening is subject to stretching out again postoperatively with resultant recurrent instability. This condition is suggested if the shoulder has an excessive range of cross-body adduction or internal rotation in abduction. If atraumatic multidirectional laxity is present, an inferior capsular shift may be performed from an anterior approach so that the rotator interval can be closed at the same procedure.

- Shoulders without an effective posterior glenoid lip may require augmentation of the posterior lip with a labral reconstruction or posterior glenoid osteotomy. This situation is suggested if little resistance to posterior translation occurs when the humeral head is pressed into the glenoid whein performing the posterior load and shift test.

- Those with major anteromedial humeral head defects (for example, over one third of the humeral articular surface), may require insertion of a proximal humeral prosthesis. This situation needs to be identified preoperatively because the preferred surgical approach for this procedure is anterior.

Preoperatively, patients are informed of the alternatives and the risks of recurrent instability, excessive tightness with limited flexion and internal rotation, pain, neurovascular injury, infection, and the need for revision surgery.

Before the patient is placed prone, the shoulder is examined under anesthesia, with particular attention paid to resistance to posterior translation with the humeral head pressed into the glenoid—such resistance indicates the degree of competence of the posterior glenoid lip. The patient is then placed prone with the shoulder off the operating table to allow a full range of humeral and scapular motion. After routine preparation of the arm, shoulder, neck, and back, a 10-cm incision is made in the extended line of the posterior axillary crease (see Fig. 14–9). The deltoid muscle is split for a distance of 4 cm between its middle and posterior thirds. If necessary, additional exposure may be obtained by carefully dissecting the muscle for a short distance from the scapular spine and posterior acromion (Fig. 14–184). Retraction of the deltoid muscle inferiorly and laterally reveals the infraspinatus muscle, the teres minor muscle, and the axillary nerve emerging from the quadrangular space. The spinoglenoid notch is palpated to determine the location of the important nerve to the infraspinatus.

The infraspinatus, teres minor, and attached capsule are incised 1 cm from the greater tuberosity to expose the posterior glenohumeral joint (Fig. 14–184). Excessive traction on the axillary nerve and the nerve to the infraspina-

tus is carefully avoided. The joint is inspected for humeral head defects, wear of the anterior or posterior glenoid, tears in the glenoid labrum, loose bodies, and tears of the rotator cuff. Traumatic posterior capsular avulsions are repaired to the lip of the glenoid by a technique similar to that described for anterior repair. Excessive capsular laxity may be managed by reefing the capsule along with the attached infraspinatus and teres minor tendons. Such reefing is accomplished by overlapping the medial and lateral flaps by the desired amount or by advancing the capsule and tendon into a bony groove at the desired length. We usually try to limit internal rotation of the adducted humerus to 45 degrees. Internal rotation is limited by approximately 20 degrees for each centimeter of shortening of the posterior capsule and tendon. Greater tightening may be used in patients with generalized ligamentous instability.

If the patient demonstrates excessive posteroinferior capsular laxity, the capsule is released from the inferior neck of the humerus under direct visualization as the humerus is progressively internally rotated. The capsule and muscle tendons are then advanced superiorly as well as laterally to tighten the axillary recess. If significant multidirectional instability is present, a formal inferior capsular shift may be performed; however, this situation should be recognized preoperatively because a capsular shift is preferably performed from the front so that (1) the rotator interval can be closed and (2) the posterior inferior capsule becomes tightened with flexion (Figs. 14–185 and 14–186).[502]

Anteromedial humeral head defects of moderate size are managed by tightening the posterior capsule so that internal rotation is limited to 30 degrees. A shoulder with an anterior humeral head defect constituting more than a third of the articular surface often cannot be stabilized by soft tissue surgery. In these instances, insertion of a prosthetic head through the anterior approach will be required to restore stability and function to the glenohumeral joint. Because it changes the surgical approach, a lesion of this size needs to be identified preoperatively.

In patients with deficiency of the posterior glenoid lip, increased glenoid retroversion, or undependable posterior soft tissues, a posteroinferior glenoid osteotomy can be considered. This osteotomy increases the effective glenoid arc and balances the stability angles posteriorly and inferiorly. It is most safely performed by exposing the posterior inferior glenoid neck and joint surface simultaneously and inserting an osteotome parallel to the joint surface and about 6 mm medial to it. The depth of the osteotomy needs to be judged carefully to avoid excessive anterior penetration of the osteotome. The osteotome is advanced slowly and the posterior inferior glenoid lip is pried laterally with each advancement. This technique optimizes reconstruction of the posterior inferior glenoid lip. The opening wedge osteotomy is held open by a wedge-shaped bone graft from the posterior acromion inserted so that its cortex is tucked just anterior to that of the posterior glenoid. Posterior humeral head displacement is attempted while the head is pressed into the glenoid to ensure that the correction is sufficient and the bone graft is secure. If the amount of correction needs

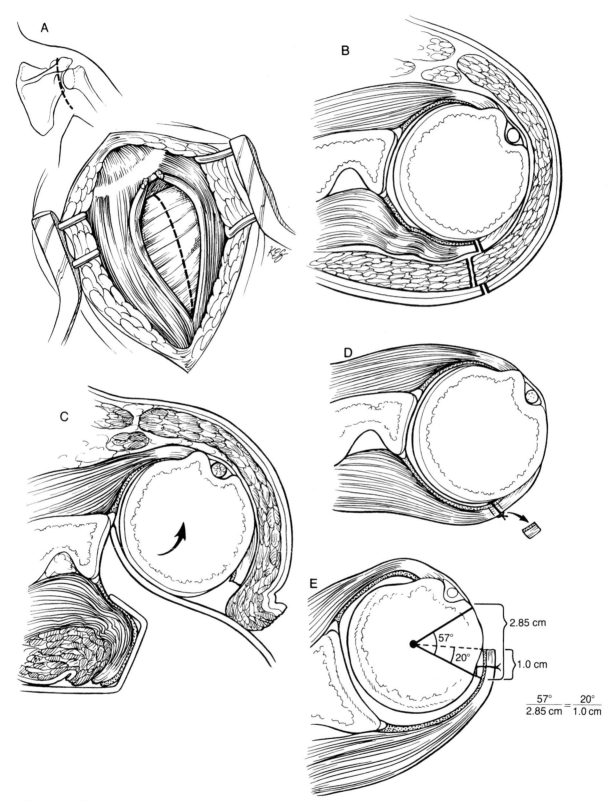

■ **Figure 14–184**

Operative repair for recurrent posterior glenohumeral instability. **A,** A 10-cm skin incision is made in the extended line of the posterior axillary crease *(inset)*. The deltoid muscle is split between its middle and posterior thirds. **B,** A transverse plane section shows the interval through the deltoid muscle and the infraspinatus tendon. **C,** A transverse plane section shows placement of the retractors to expose the glenoid. **D,** A transverse plane section shows repair of the infraspinatus tendon after resecting the desired amount for capsular and tendon advancement. Shortening the posterior capsule and tendon by 1 cm will limit internal rotation by approximately 20 degrees. **E,** The effect of shortening of capsular structures on limitation of rotation. The average radius of the humerus is 2.85 cm, which is the length of an arc equal to 1 radian, or approximately 57 degrees. If the capsule was shortened by 2.85 cm, rotation would be restricted by 57 degrees. Proportionally, a 1-cm shortening of the capsule would restrict rotation by 20 degrees. Posterior reefing of approximately 1 cm, which decreases internal rotation by approximately 20 degrees, is shown here.

CAPSULAR SHIFT TO FRONT

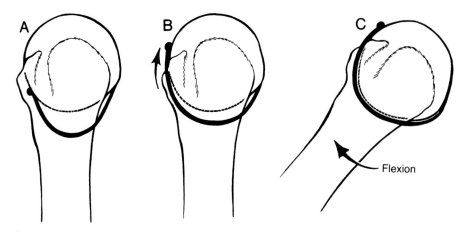

■ Figure 14–185
An inferior capsular shift, when performed from the anterior approach, advances the capsule anteriorly on the humerus. Such advancement produces additional posterior capsular tightening with shoulder flexion. **A,** Lax inferior capsule. **B,** Inferior capsule brought anteriorly on the humerus in an anterior approach. **C,** With humeral flexion, the posterior and inferior portion of the capsule is further tightened.

CAPSULAR SHIFT TO BACK

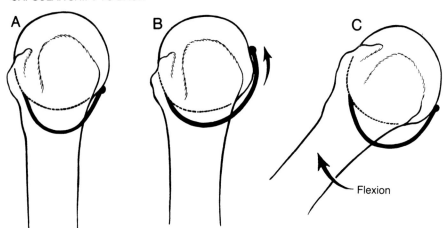

■ Figure 14–186
When an inferior capsular shift is performed from the posterior approach and the capsule is advanced posteriorly on the humerus, the tightened capsule loosens with shoulder flexion. **A,** Lax inferior capsule. **B,** From the posterior approach, the lax inferior capsule is advanced posteriorly on the humerus. **C,** Humeral flexion loosens the posterior and inferior portion of the capsule.

to be modified, it can easily be accomplished at this time. After the osteotomy, routine soft tissue repair is carried out.

When the indicated procedure is complete with maximal strength of the soft tissue reattachments, the deltoid is carefully repaired to the scapular spine and acromion, with the use of drill holes as necessary. After surgery, the patient is immobilized in a "handshake" cummerbund cast (see Fig. 14–116) or orthotic (see Fig. 14–117) with the shoulder in adduction, neutral rotation, and slight extension for 3 weeks, during which time internal rotation isometric exercises are instituted. After the immobilization is discontinued, the patient is allowed to perform more vigorous rotator-strengthening exercises and to use the shoulder below the horizontal plane. The patient is encouraged to regain motion in abduction, where stability against posterior displacement is optimal, and avoid forward flexion and internal rotation. As strength of external rotation and confidence are developed, more anterior planes of elevation are used. Vigorous shoulder activity is prohibited until normal rotator strength, coordination, and confidence in anterior planes are achieved. The patient is advised to continue rotator-strengthening exercises on a daily basis to optimize dynamic shoulder stability.

■ ROCKWOOD AND WIRTH'S TECHNIQUE OF POSTERIOR RECONSTRUCTION FOR TRAUMATIC INSTABILITY[763]

STANDARD POSTERIOR REPAIR

The patient is placed in the lateral decubitus position with the operative shoulder upward. The best way to support the patient in this position is to use kidney supports and the "bean bag."

The incision begins 1 inch medial to the posterolateral corner of the acromion and extends downward 3 inches toward the posterior axillary creases (Fig. 14–187).[79] If a bone graft is to be taken from the acromion, the incision extends a little farther superiorly so that the acromion can be exposed. Next, the subcutaneous tissues are dissected medially and laterally so that the skin can be retracted to visualize the fibers of the deltoid.

A point 1 inch medial to the posterior corner of the acromion is selected, and the deltoid is then split distally for 4 inches in the line of its fibers. The deltoid can be easily retracted medially and laterally to expose the

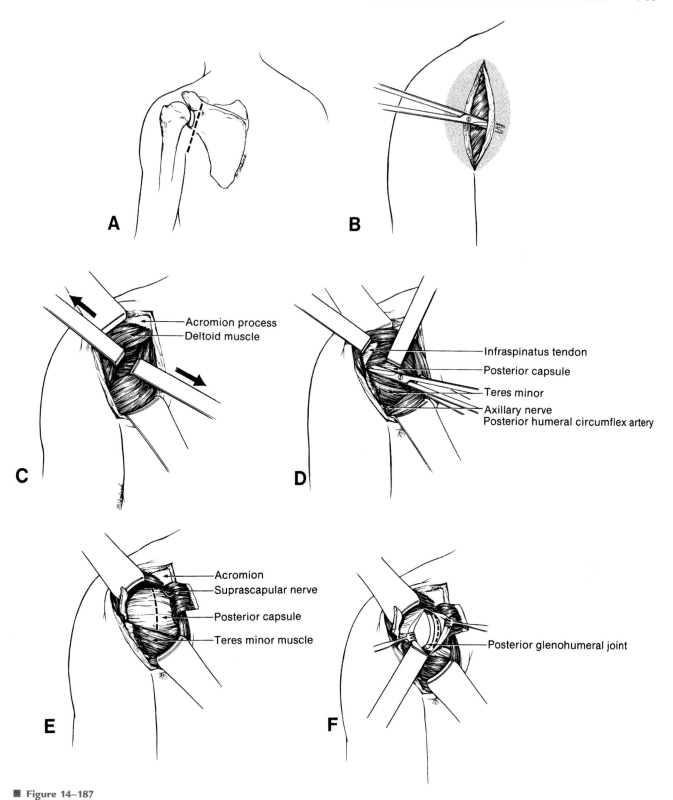

■ Figure 14–187

A-R, Rockwood's preferred posterior shoulder reconstruction. (See text for a detailed description of each step of the procedure.)
(From Rockwood CA and Green DP [eds]: Fractures, 3 vols, 2nd ed. Philadelphia: JB Lippincott, 1984.)

Continued

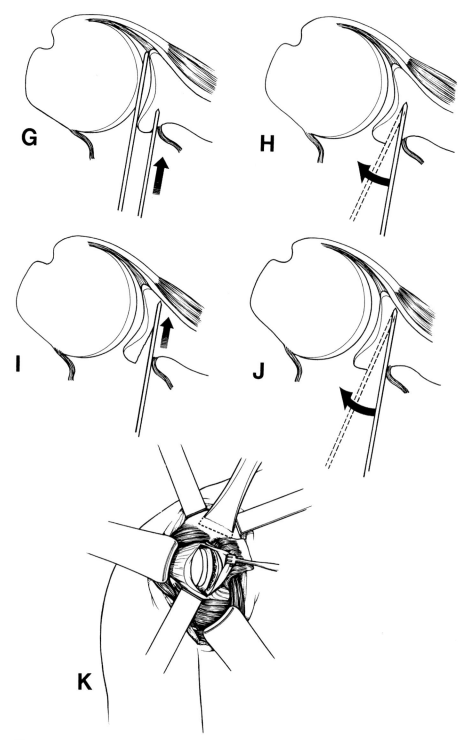

■ **Figure 14–187, cont'd**
A-R, Rockwood's preferred posterior shoulder reconstruction. (See text for a detailed description of each step of the procedure.) *(From Rockwood CA and Green DP [eds]: Fractures, 3 vols, 2nd ed. Philadelphia: JB Lippincott, 1984.)*

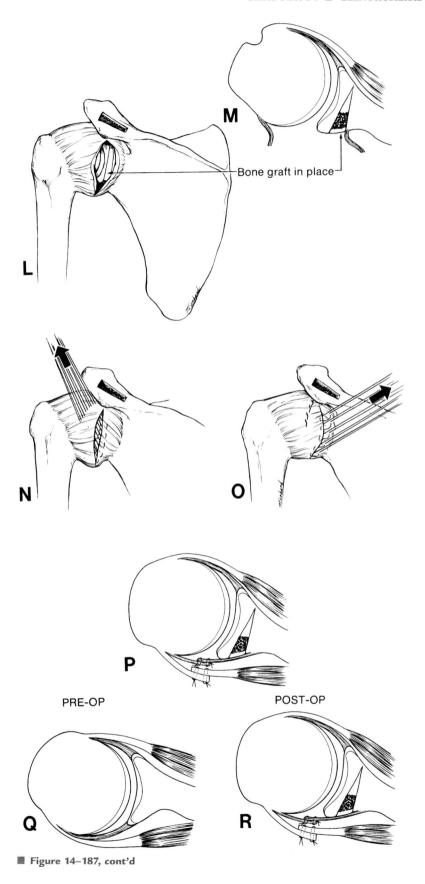

Bone graft in place

■ Figure 14–187, cont'd

underlying infraspinatus and teres minor muscles. This deltoid split can be made down to the midportion of the teres minor muscle. Remember that the axillary nerve exits the quadrangular space at the lower border of the teres minor muscle.

When performing a posterior reconstruction, the teres minor tendon should be reflected inferiorly down to the level of the inferior joint capsule. If the infraspinatus tendon is divided and reflected medially and laterally, care should be taken to not injure the suprascapular nerve. When the infraspinatus tendon is very lax, it can be reflected off the capsule and retracted superiorly without having to divide the tendon.

With the infraspinatus and teres minor muscles retracted out of the way, a vertical incision can be made in the posterior capsule to expose and explore the joint. We prefer to make the incision midway between the humeral and glenoid attachment so that at closure we can double-breast it and make it stronger. When performing the posterior capsular shift procedure, it is essential to have the teres minor muscle reflected sufficiently inferior so that the vertical cut in the capsule will go all the way down to the most inferior recess of the capsule. If the capsule is thin and friable and it appears that a capsular shift alone will be insufficient, the infraspinatus tendon can be divided so that it can be double-breasted to shorten it.

With the capsule divided all the way down inferiorly, horizontal mattress sutures of No. 2 cottony Dacron are inserted in the edge of the medial capsule. The arm should be held in neutral rotation and the medial capsule sutured laterally and superiorly under the lateral capsule. Next, the lateral capsule is reflected and sutured medially and superiorly over the medial capsule and again held in place with horizontal mattress sutures. This capsular shift procedure has effectively eliminated any of the posterior and inferior capsular redundancy.

The infraspinatus tendon is repaired next; this repair should also be performed with the arm in neutral rotation. If laxity exists, the tendon can be double-breasted. The wound is thoroughly irrigated, and the muscle and subcutaneous tissues are infiltrated with 25 to 30 mL of 0.5% bupivacaine. Care must be taken to not overuse the bupivacaine or inject it directly into vascular channels.

When the retractors are withdrawn, the deltoid falls nicely together and subcutaneous closure is performed. Care must be taken throughout closure of the capsule, infraspinatus tendon, and skin to maintain the arm in neutral rotation. The patient is then gently rolled into the supine position while making sure that the arm is in neutral rotation. When the anesthesia is completed, the patient is transferred to a bed, where the arm is maintained in neutral position and supported by skin traction. Usually within 24 hours after surgery the patient can stand, and a modified shoulder immobilizer cast is applied.

POSTERIOR GLENOID OSTEOTOMY

We do not use this procedure as a routine part of posterior reconstruction. Occasionally, when posterior glenoid deficiency is present or in patients with congenital retrotilt of the glenoid (i.e., greater than 30 degrees),

posterior osteotomy should be considered. We recently reported a patient who had failed two previous attempts at posterior capsulorrhaphy for recurrent posterior shoulder instability.[770] The patient had a previously unrecognized unilateral increase in glenoid fossa retrotilt and was successfully treated with a posterior opening wedge osteotomy of the scapular neck (Fig. 14–183).

When performing a posterior glenoid osteotomy, care must be taken to not overcorrect the retroversion because overcorrection may force the head out anteriorly. If a posterior osteotomy is to be performed, it is absolutely essential to know the anatomy and angle of the slope of the glenoid, which can best be determined by placing a straight, blunt instrument into the joint so that it lies on the anterior and posterior glenoid rim (Fig. 14–187). Next, the osteotome is placed intracapsularly and directed parallel to the blunt instrument. If one is unsure of the angle and does not have a guide instrument in place, it is possible that the osteotomy may enter the joint (see Fig. 14–182). The osteotomy site is not more than $\frac{1}{4}$ inch medial to the articular surface of the glenoid. If the osteotomy is more medial than $\frac{1}{4}$ inch, the suprascapular nerve may be injured as it passes around the base of the spine of the scapula to supply the infraspinatus muscle. Each time that the osteotome is advanced, the osteotomy site is pried open (Fig. 14–187) to help create a lateral plastic deformation of the posterior glenoid. The osteotomy should not exit anteriorly but should stop just at the anterior cortex of the scapula (Fig. 14–187). The intact anterior cortex periosteum and soft tissue will act as a hinge and allow the graft to be secure in the osteotomy without any need for internal fixation. We generally use an osteotome that is 1 inch wide to make the original cut and then use smaller $\frac{1}{2}$-inch osteotomes superiorly and inferiorly to complete the posterior division of bone. Osteotomes are used to open up the osteotomy site, and the bone graft is placed into position (Fig. 14–187). If the anterior cortex is partially intact, internal fixation of the graft is not necessary because it is held securely in place by the osteotomy. We prefer to take the bone graft from the acromion (Fig. 14–187). Either a small piece (8 × 30 mm) for the osteotomy or a large piece (15 × 30 mm) for a posteroinferior bone block can be taken from the top or the posterior edge of the acromion. If a larger piece of graft is required, it should be taken from the ilium. After completion of the osteotomy, a capsular shift, as described earlier, is performed.

After surgery, the patient lies supine with the forearm supported by the overhead bed frame and the arm held in neutral rotation. We usually let the patient sit up on the bed the evening of surgery while maintaining the arm in neutral rotation. We let the patient sit up in a chair the next day, again holding the arm in neutral rotation. Either 24 or 48 hours after surgery, when the patient can stand comfortably, we apply a lightweight long arm cast. Next, a well-padded iliac crest band that sits around the abdomen and iliac crest is applied. The arm is then connected to the iliac crest band with a broom handle support to maintain the arm in 10 to 15 degrees of abduction and neutral rotation. The cast is left in place for 6 to 8 weeks. After removal of the plaster, the patient is allowed to use the arm for 4 to 6 weeks for everyday living activities. A rehabilitation program is begun that includes pendulum exercises, isometric exercises, and stretching of the shoulder with the use of an overhead pulley, after which resistive exercises are gradually increased.

ANTERIOR CAPSULAR SHIFT RECONSTRUCTION

We have used a capsular shift reconstruction in patients whose primary pathology is posterior shoulder instability if a recognizable component of multidirectional shoulder laxity is present (Fig. 14–188).[764] This procedure is indicated when instability or apprehension repeatedly compromises shoulder comfort or function in spite of an adequate trial of rotator cuff–strengthening and coordination exercises. The mainstay of the capsular shift procedure is reduction of excessive joint volume through symmetric and anatomic plication of the redundant capsule. We have found it unnecessary to perform a combined anterior and posterior approach but, instead, reserve posterior capsular reconstruction for patients with recurrent traumatic posterior shoulder instability who do not have concomitant generalized ligamentous laxity and multidirectional laxity of the shoulder. Open anterior capsular shift procedures for posterior instability resulted in 10 of 11 patients having a stable shoulder at a minimum of 2 years of follow-up.[765] The patients lost motion in internal as well as external rotation.[15]

One explanation for the difficulties encountered with traditional posterior reconstructions has been the poor quality and unsubstantial nature of the posterior capsule, which precludes a strong surgical reconstruction. Additionally, surgically addressable lesions known to contribute to recurrent instability, such as associated fractures involving the posterior glenoid rim or anteromedial humeral head, are less frequent. In contrast to the capsulolabral injuries seen with traumatic anterior

shoulder instability, posterior glenoid lateral pathology is often limited to degenerative changes rather than capsulolabral avulsions, which lend themselves to stable surgical repair. Finally and perhaps the most subtle reason for poor surgical results is failure to recognize that some shoulders demonstrate multidirectional laxity even though the patient may have a history, physical examination, and radiographs consistent with symptomatic posterior shoulder instability.

The basis for this seemingly unorthodox approach is supported by several reports in the literature. In 1988, Schwartz and colleagues[639] performed arthroscopically assisted selective sectioning of the shoulder capsule to quantitate the relative contribution of specific structures to glenohumeral stability. The superior glenohumeral ligament was found to provide secondary restraint to posterior shoulder instability. In addition, posterior glenohumeral dislocation did not occur after incision of the posterior capsule until the anterosuperior capsular structures were also sectioned. More recently, Harryman and associates[254] investigated the role of selective capsular sectioning and imbrication of the rotator interval capsule. Surgical modifications were found to alter several different parameters of shoulder motion, including rotation and translation, which ultimately affected the stability of the shoulder joint. Specifically, the intrarotator interval was found to be a major component of stability against posterior and inferior glenohumeral displacement. Posterior and inferior glenohumeral dislocations usually occurred after sectioning of the rotator interval capsule, whereas imbrication of this structure increased the resistance to translation in these directions. These authors concluded that patients with inferior or posterior shoulder instability may benefit from anterior reconstruction of the interval capsule.

Nonoperative Treatment of the AMBRII Syndrome: Recurrent Multidirectional Instability

The goal of treatment of patients with atraumatic instability is restoration of shoulder function by increasing the effectiveness of concavity compression. Many patients with the AMBRII syndrome have simply become deconditioned from their normal state of dynamic glenohumeral stability. They have lost the proper neuromuscular control of humeroscapular positioning, and concavity compression has become dysfunctional. Neuromuscular control cannot be restored surgically; rather, it requires prolonged adherence to a well-constructed reconditioning program. The patient may need to be convinced that training and exercises constitute a reasonable therapeutic approach. Many would prefer a surgical "cure." It is often useful to demonstrate that the contralateral shoulder has substantial laxity on examination, yet is clinically stable. In this way the patient and family can appreciate that a loose shoulder is not necessarily unstable; for example, gymnasts usually have very lax, but very stable shoulders.

Nonoperative management of glenohumeral instability has been discussed earlier in this chapter. In general,

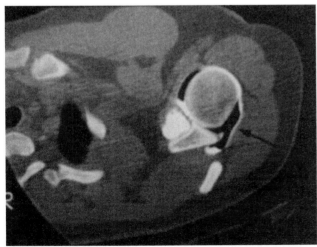

■ Figure 14–188
Computed tomographic arthrogram in a patient with symptomatic posterior shoulder instability and multidirectional glenohumeral laxity. Note the overall capsular volume and the posterior capsular redundancy *(arrow)*. *(From Rockwood CA Jr, Green DP, and Bucholz RW [eds]: Fractures in Adults. Philadelphia: JB Lippincott, 1991.)*

but particularly in atraumatic instability, glenohumeral stability is dependent on dynamic compression of the humeral head into the glenoid concavity (concavity compression) and excellence of neuromuscular control. Thus, the nonoperative and postoperative programs for an AMBRII shoulder need to optimize both.

Operative Treatment of Atraumatic Instability

Presurgical Considerations

The ability of surgery alone to *cure* atraumatic instability is limited. Usually, there is no single lesion that can be repaired. Most of the factors providing midrange stability cannot be enhanced by surgical reconstruction. Problems of neuromuscular control or relative glenoid flatness do not have easy surgical solutions. Even after a snug capsulorrhaphy, the midrange stabilizing mechanisms of balance and concavity compression must be optimized through muscle strengthening and kinematic training. Otherwise, excessive loads will be applied to the surgically tightened glenohumeral capsule and result in stretching and failure of the surgical reconstruction.

In this light, indications for surgical treatment of atraumatic instability need to be carefully considered. First, the patient must have major functional problems that are clearly related to atraumatic glenohumeral instability. Second, the patient must clearly understand that good strength and kinematic technique are the primary stabilizing factors for the shoulder rather than capsular tightness. Third, the patient must have conscientiously participated in a strengthening and training program and recognize that strength and proper technique will continue to be major stabilizing factors for the shoulder even after reconstructive surgery is performed. The patient must also recognize that capsulorrhaphy is designed to stiffen the shoulder: the surgery will compromise range of motion in the hope of gaining stability. If attempts to regain totally normal range are made in the first postoperative year, instability is likely to recur. Thus, the limitations imposed by surgical capsulorrhaphy may be incompatible with the goals of normal or supernormal range of motion. Therefore, gymnasts, dancers, and baseball pitchers may not be good candidates for this surgical procedure. Similarly, this procedure has a limited ability to hold up under the demands of heavy physical labor unless it is accompanied by a superb strength and kinematic rehabilitation program. The patient must understand that rehabilitation after a capsular shift procedure is protracted. It is important that the shoulder be immobilized in a brace for a month, during which time muscles get weak and normal kinematics is lost. After this month of immobilization, many months are required for the reestablishment of good strength and shoulder kinematics. In spite of the best operative and postoperative management, the success of this procedure in re-establishing normal shoulder function is substantially less than that of procedures for traumatic instability. Finally, the shoulder must have an identified mechanical problem for which surgery is the answer. The presence of shoulder pain and

laxity does not indicate that the patient will be better after a surgical procedure.

The foregoing is a large amount of very important information about the surgical procedure that must be understood by the patient. The situation is further complicated by the fact that many patients with atraumatic midrange instability are young and may have difficulty understanding and accepting the ramifications of this information. Thus, during preoperative discussions with young patients it may be important that parents participate actively. We find that many families who request that "the shoulder be fixed" are prepared to work more diligently on the nonoperative program after this discussion.

When the history and physical examination indicate that the shoulder is loose in all directions and when the patient has failed to respond to vigorous exercises for internal and external rotator strengthening, endurance, and coordination, an inferior capsular shift procedure may be considered as originally described by Neer and Foster.[503] The principle of the procedure is to symmetrically tighten the anterior, inferior, and posterior aspects of the capsule by advancing its humeral attachment.

However, it is now recognized that capsular laxity may not be the essential lesion in atraumatic instability. Procedures designed to improve the quality of the glenoid concavity may provide a more physiologic solution. Capsulolabral augmentation of the posteroinferior labrum without capsular shift significantly increased glenoid depth (1.9 mm inferiorly, 2 mm posteroinferiorly, and 0.9 mm posteriorly) and the stability ratios posteroinferiorly and inferiorly (0.24 increase in both directions).[471]

Results of Reconstructions for Atraumatic Instability

A capsular shift procedure is often considered in the surgical management of atraumatic instability. However, most of the existing reports of inferior capsular shift surgery include patients with both traumatic and atraumatic forms of instability.[8,115,503] Therefore, the results are substantially better than would be expected in the treatment of atraumatic instability. Cooper and Brems[115] reported a 2-year follow-up of inferior capsular shift procedures and found that 9% continued to have significant instability. Altchek and colleagues[8] used a T-plasty modification of the Bankart procedure for multidirectional instability on 42 shoulders injured during athletics. Four patients experienced episodes of instability after the procedure, and throwing velocity decreased in the throwing athletes. Despite these shortcomings, patient satisfaction was noted to be excellent in 95% of shoulders. Bigliani and associates[51] used an inferior capsular shift procedure to manage 68 shoulders in 63 athletes with anterior and inferior instability. Fifty-eight patients returned to their major sports, 75% at the same competitive level, but only 50% of elite throwing athletes returned to their previous level of competition. In contact sport athletes, 92% had no further dislocations after an anterior-based capsular shift, and 88% of patients who underwent a posterior-based capsular shift had no further dislocations. Eighty-two percent and 75% of athletes were able to return to their sport after an anterior or posterior procedure, respectively. Only 17% of patients with bilateral procedures were able to return to their sport, however.[96] American football players were able to return to their sport 89% of the time after open anterior capsulorrhaphy along with repair of a Bankart lesion if present.[547]

At an average 61-month follow-up, 94% patients with primarily anterior multidirectional instability remained stable after the anterior capsular shift procedure, and all 15 patients with primarily posterior instability remained stable after posterior capsular shift.[568]

In general, better results are obtained with surgery whenever trauma is a contributing factor. In an attempt to evaluate the effectiveness of a homogeneous series of primary capsular shift surgery for purely atraumatic instability, Obremskey and coworkers[524] reviewed 26 patients with no history or radiographic or surgical evidence of a traumatic etiology. The patients in this series had failed an average of 17 months of vigorous physical rehabilitation before proceeding with surgery. Fifty-seven percent of the patients had bilateral symptoms. The average age was 22 ± 6 years (range, 13 to 34). Twenty-nine percent had generalized ligamentous laxity, and 15% had an industrial claim. At an average of 27 months after a standard capsular shift was performed,[503] 74% of the patients were satisfied with the condition of their shoulder; 46% were able to return to recreation and 69% to their previous job. Thirty-nine percent had persistent pain and 57% had night pain that interfered with sleeping. Sixty-eight percent had at least occasional symptoms of instability and 10% required further surgery. By regression analysis, the most important correlate of patient dissatisfaction was not recurrent instability, but rather persistent pain and stiffness. These results suggest that a key in the management of patients with atraumatic multidirectional instability is not the degree of surgical tightness achieved but rather restoration of comfort and motion.

■ MATSEN'S APPROACH TO CAPSULAR SHIFT IN THE TREATMENT OF RECURRENT ATRAUMATIC MULTIDIRECTIONAL GLENOHUMERAL INSTABILITY

Our use of capsular shift surgery is diminishing. We recognize that most patients with atraumatic instability can best be managed with a rehabilitation program.

The goals of the surgery are to tighten the capsule symmetrically around the joint, close the rotator interval, and create a new, stronger rotator interval capsule and coracohumeral ligament (Fig. 14–189). These goals can be accomplished only through an anterior surgical approach. Thus, we routinely approach a repair for atraumatic instability from the front, even if the predominant direction of instability appears to be posterior. In addition, the anterior approach is cosmetically superior to the posterior approach. Furthermore, it can be accomplished without incising the critical external rotator cuff musculature. Finally, when the capsule is advanced anterosuperiorly on the humeral side, elevation of the arm anteriorly results in desirable additional tightening of the inferior and posterior capsule (Fig. 14–185). In contrast, when the procedure is performed from a posterior approach, the capsule is advanced posterosuperiorly on the humerus so that it loosens as the humerus is flexed (Fig. 14–186).

The shoulder is approached through a low anterior axillary incision, with the deltopectoral groove entered medial to the cephalic vein (Fig. 14–190). The clavipectoral fascia is divided up to the level of the coracoacromial ligament to provide access to the humeroscapular motion interface. The axillary nerve is palpated medially as it courses across the subscapularis and passes inferiorly toward the quadrangular space. The superior edge of the

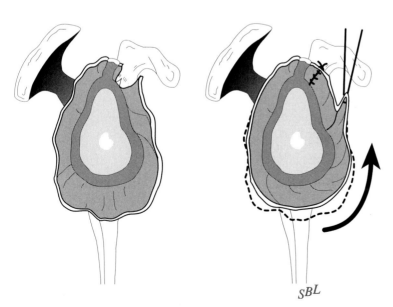

■ **Figure 14–189**

The essence of reconstruction of atraumatic instability is reduction of the posteroinferior recess by anterosuperior advancement of the capsule combined with closure of the rotator interval capsule. This reconstruction has the advantage of becoming additionally tight as the arm is elevated in anterior planes (see Fig. 14–185). *(From Matsen FA III, Lippitt SB, Sidles JA, and Harryman DT II: Practical Evaluation and Management of the Shoulder. Philadelphia: WB Saunders, 1994.)*

subscapularis is then identified by palpating the rotator interval lateral to the coracoid process and medial to the bicipital groove. The triad of anterior humeral circumflex vessels marks the inferior border of the subscapularis, where they can be prospectively cauterized. The subscapularis tendon is sharply and carefully dissected from the capsule while ensuring that the thickness of the capsule is not compromised.

A substantial defect in the rotator interval is seen consistently in the AMBRII syndrome. This defect is bordered by the capsule adjacent to the supraspinatus overlying the biceps tendon superiorly, the anterior capsule and subscapularis anteroinferiorly, the coracoid process medially, and the transverse humeral ligament laterally. The defect is accentuated by pushing the humeral head posteriorly. Sutures of No. 2 nonabsorbable material are securely placed in the superior edge of the defect and then passed across to the inferior edge of the defect (Figs. 14–190 and 14–191). When these sutures are tied, a strong rotator interval capsule is reconstructed.

The anterior capsule is incised from the humeral neck, and as it is released, traction sutures are placed in the incised margin. The axillary nerve is identified and protected during this dissection. The dissection is continued until superiorly directed traction on the capsular flap causes the capsule to tighten on a finger placed in the posteroinferior capsular recess (Fig. 14–192). Usually, this point is reached when the capsule is released just past the inferior (6 o'clock) position on the humeral neck by sectioning the posterior band of the inferior glenohumeral ligament.

After capsular release, a bony trough is created in the anteroinferior humeral neck adjacent to the articular surface with a power bur (Fig. 14–193). Holes are made in the humeral neck lateral to the groove, and sutures are passed through these holes into the groove for reattachment of the capsule securely to bone. With the arm at the side and in neutral rotation and with strong anterior superior traction on the sutures to obliterate the posterior inferior recess, the sutures from the groove are passed through the lateral edge of the capsule (Fig. 14–194). Tying these sutures securely fixes the capsule in its advanced position (Fig. 14–195). This step needs to be accomplished under excellent direct vision to be sure that the bites in the capsule are sufficiently inferior to tighten it to the groove and ensure the safety of the axillary nerve. The surgeon must make sure that pulling up on these sutures obliterates the posterior inferior recess. If such is not the case, either the inferior capsular release was insufficient or the sutures were not placed sufficiently inferior.

This repair to the groove is continued anteriorly up the humeral neck.

Redundant anterior superior capsule is folded down over the previous repair to reinforce it (Fig. 14–196).

At this point the shoulder is checked to ensure that internal rotation of the abducted arm is limited to 45 degrees, that the posterior drawer is less than 50% of the humeral head diameter, and that external rotation of the arm at the side is 30 degrees. Excessive internal rotation of the abducted arm indicates that the inferior capsule was not advanced sufficiently anteriorly. Excessive translation on the sulcus test indicates that the rotator interval capsule was insufficiently tightened. Excessive limitation of external rotation is an indication that the anterior capsule was tightened too much.

The subscapularis is then repaired to its normal anatomic insertion. After standard wound closure, the arm is placed in a prefitted "handshake" orthosis (see Fig. 14–117) or cast (see Fig. 14–116) with the arm in neutral rotation and slight abduction.

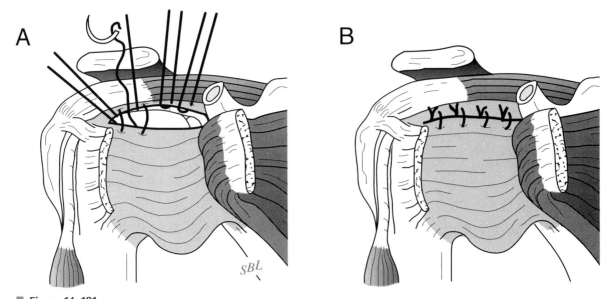

■ Figure 14–191

Identification of the superior edge of the rotator interval defect and placement of sutures, with care taken to protect the long head of the biceps tendon (**A**). When these sutures are tied, they securely reconstruct the coracohumeral–rotator interval capsular mechanism (**B**). *(Modified from Matsen FA III, Lippitt SB, Sidles JA, and Harryman DT II: Practical Evaluation and Management of the Shoulder. Philadelphia: WB Saunders, 1994.)*

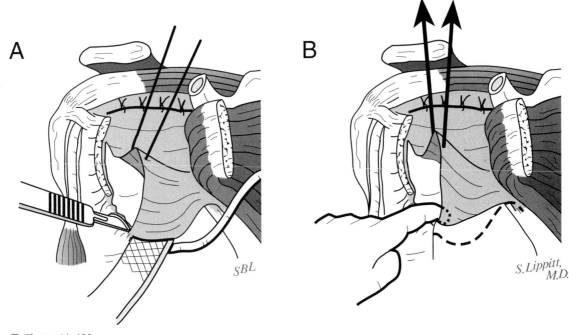

■ Figure 14–192

Release of the capsule from the humeral neck laterally. This dissection is carried beyond the inferior (6 o'clock) position (**A**) until traction on the anterior capsular flap reduces the posteroinferior recess (**B**). *(From Matsen FA III, Lippitt SB, Sidles JA, and Harryman DT II: Practical Evaluation and Management of the Shoulder. Philadelphia: WB Saunders, 1994.)*

With the arm in the orthosis or cast, the patient is started on shoulder exercises for grip strengthening, elbow range of motion, isometric external rotation, and isometric abduction. Immobilization is usually continued for 1 month, although longer periods may be used for individuals who are extremely lax and shorter periods for individuals older than 25 years because of the potential for excessive stiffness.

The patient is then weaned from immobilization over a period of a week. During this time the patient is instructed to elevate the arm in the plane of the scapula (the plane of maximal stability), to continue the exercises for cuff and deltoid strengthening, and to avoid any activities that may challenge the repair. From this point, range of motion is gained only with active exercises; no passive stretching is used. Lifting of more than 10 lb is delayed for 6 months.

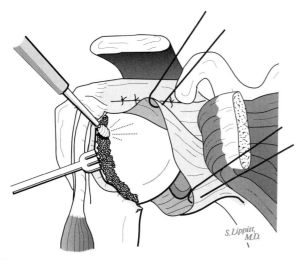

■ Figure 14–193

Preparation of the humeral neck with a groove at the margin of the articular surface. (*Modified from Matsen FA III, Lippitt SB, Sidles JA, and Harryman DT II: Practical Evaluation and Management of the Shoulder. Philadelphia: WB Saunders, 1994.*)

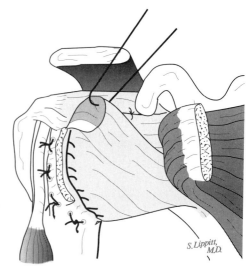

■ Figure 14–195

Tying the sutures fixes the advanced capsule to the groove. (*From Matsen FA III, Lippitt SB, Sidles JA, and Harryman DT II: Practical Evaluation and Management of the Shoulder. Philadelphia: WB Saunders, 1994.*)

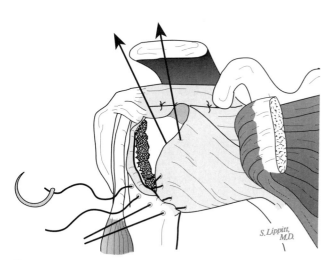

■ Figure 14–194

Sutures are placed through drill holes so that they exit the groove and pass through the advanced capsule and then back through adjacent drill holes. (*Modified from Matsen FA III, Lippitt SB, Sidles JA, and Harryman DT II: Practical Evaluation and Management of the Shoulder. Philadelphia: WB Saunders, 1994.*)

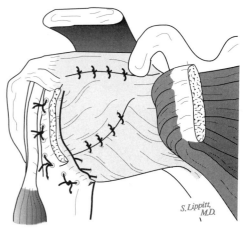

■ Figure 14–196

Any redundant anterosuperior capsule is folded down to reinforce the previous repair. (*From Matsen FA III, Lippitt SB, Sidles JA, and Harryman DT II: Practical Evaluation and Management of the Shoulder. Philadelphia: WB Saunders, 1994.*)

Sports are delayed for at least 1 year after surgery and are permitted only if the patient has excellent strength and dynamic control of the shoulder. The patient is asked to learn and maintain the program for nonoperative management of glenohumeral instability.

■ ROCKWOOD'S APPROACH TO TREATMENT OF ATRAUMATIC AND MULTIDIRECTIONAL GLENOHUMERAL INSTABILITY

Treatment of patients with atraumatic instability requires that the physician differentiate between the voluntary and the involuntary types. Certainly, a patient with voluntary instability who has psychiatric problems should never be treated surgically. Rowe and Yee[615] reported on disasters in patients with psychiatric problems who had been treated with surgical reconstruction. Patients with emotional disturbances and psychiatric problems should be referred for psychiatric help. Rowe and Yee also pointed out that there are patients with voluntary instability who do not have psychiatric problems and can be significantly improved with a rehabilitation program.

Consistent with this recommendation, we place all patients with atraumatic instability problems on a very specific rehabilitation program to strengthen the three parts of the deltoid, the rotator cuff, and the scapular stabilizers. If the patient has an obvious psychiatric or emotional problem, we do our best to explain the problem to the patient and family and help them seek psychiatric help. Under no circumstances do we ever tell the patient or family that surgery is a possibility for an emotionally disturbed patient. When we have ruled out congenital or developmental causes of the instability problem, we personally teach the patient how to perform the shoulder-strengthening exercises and give the patient a copy of the exercise diagrams (see Fig. 14–146). We give the patient a set of TheraBands, which includes yellow, red, green, blue, and black bands, and diagrams of the exercises to be performed. Each TheraBand is a strip 3 inches wide and 5 ft long that is tied into a loop. The loop can be fastened over a doorknob or any fixed object to offer resistance to pull. The patient does five basic exercises to strengthen the deltoid and the rotator cuff. The yellow TheraBand is the weakest and offers 1 lb of resistance to pull; the red, 2 lb; the green, 3 lb; the blue, 4 lb; and finally, the black, 5 lb. The patient is instructed to perform the five exercises two to three times a day. Each exercise should be performed five to ten times and each held for a count of five to ten. The patient is instructed to gradually increase the resistance (i.e., yellow to red and green, and so on) every 2 to 4 weeks. After the black TheraBand becomes easy to use, the patient is given a pulley kit and is instructed to do the same five basic exercises, but now lifting weights, as shown in Figure 14–146. The pulley kit consists of a pulley, an open-eye screw hook, a handle, and a piece of rope, all in a plastic bag. The patient begins by attaching 7 to 10 lb of weight to the end of the rope and proceeds to the five basic exercises. Gradually over several months, the patient increases the weights of resistance, up to 15 lb for women and 20 to 25 lb for men. When we start the basic strengthening of the rotator cuff and the deltoid, we also instruct the patient how to perform the exercises to strengthen the scapular stabilizer muscles. Pushups (i.e., wall pushups, knee pushups, and regular pushups) are used to strengthen the serratus anterior, rhomboids, and other muscles, and shoulder-shrugging exercises are performed to strengthen the trapezius muscles. We have learned that the rehabilitation program is 80% successful in managing anterior instability problems and 90% successful in managing atraumatic posterior instability problems.[603] Regardless of any previous "rehabilitation program" that the patient has participated in, we always start the patient on our strengthening routine.

If the patient still has signs and symptoms of instability after 6 months of exercises, a very specific capsular shift procedure is performed. One must always remember that it is possible for a patient with laxity of the major joints to have a superimposed traumatic episode, which ordinarily does not respond to a rehabilitation program. A patient with atraumatic instability who has a history of significant trauma, pain, swelling, and so forth will probably require surgical reconstruction, but only after a trial with the rehabilitation program.

The details of the incision, surgical approach, protection of the axillary nerve, and preservation of the anterior humeral circumflex vessels are essentially the same as we use for management of a recurrent traumatic anterior instability problem (Fig. 14–197). The main difference is noted after the capsule is opened and the surgeon does not find a Perthes-Bankart lesion. The deficiency is simply a very redundant capsule anteriorly, inferiorly, or posteroin-

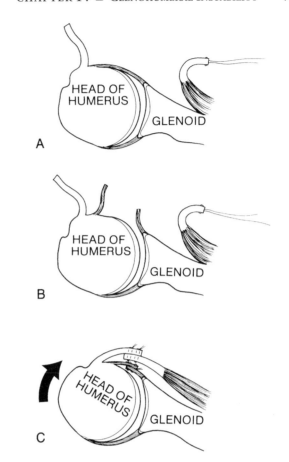

Procedure if anterior capsule is not stripped off scapula.

Capsular Repair

D   Before   E   After

■ **Figure 14–197**
Capsular shift reconstruction for atraumatic anterior subluxation or dislocation. The Bankart-Perthes lesion is not present, and the capsule is shifted to eliminate the anterior inferior laxity.

feriorly. The principle of the capsular shift is to divide the capsule all the way down inferiorly, midway between its attachment on the humerus and the glenoid rim. The joint is carefully inspected and then the shift is performed. As demonstrated in Figure 14–179P and Q, we prefer to take the medial capsule superiorly and laterally under the lateral capsule and then take the lateral capsule superiorly and medially over the medial capsule. We are careful that placement and tying of the sutures are done with the arm in approximately 15 to 20 degrees of external rotation for an anterior reconstruction and in neutral rotation for a posterior reconstruction. Ordinarily, the subscapularis is simply repaired to itself, but should there be laxity of the subscapularis with the arm in 15 to 20 degrees of external rotation, the subscapularis can be double-breasted. Normally, when performing a posterior capsular shift, the infraspinatus tendon can be reflected superiorly and the teres minor reflected inferiorly off the posterior capsule. As with the anterior shift, the posterior capsule is divided midway between its attachments, thus allowing a double-breasting or strengthening of the midportion of the capsule. The reader must remember, however, that posterior shifts are rarely required because most patients do so well with the rehabilitation program.

Surgical management of patients with atraumatic instability demands that the shoulder not be put up too tight, as can occur with the Magnuson-Stack, Putti-Platt, or Bristow procedure. If the surgeon fails to recognize that the patient has an atraumatic instability problem and if a routine muscle-tightening procedure is performed, the result may be that the humeral head will be pushed out in the opposite direction. The surgeon must also be careful, even in patients with atraumatic instability, to not perform a capsular shift that is so tight that it forces the head out in the opposite direction. As mentioned, we prefer to place and tie the sutures in the anterior capsular shift procedure with the arm in 15 to 20 degrees of external rotation and held in neutral rotation during the posterior capsular shift reconstruction. The reader must also be warned that it is essential to isolate and protect the axillary nerve when performing an anterior or posterior capsular shift.

Arthroscopic Repair of Atraumatic Instability

Arthroscopists have described redundancy in shoulders with atraumatic instability.[142,153,687,696,697] Methods of intra-articular plication, shifting and suturing the capsule or actually shrinking the redundant tissue by thermal energy have been reported.[153,176,247,250,435]

Arthroscopic examination of shoulders with atraumatic instability frequently reveal insufficient posterior and inferior labral tissue. In the laboratory, Lippitt and colleagues and Lazarus and coworkers have documented the essential stabilizing effect of the glenoid labrum by increasing stability ratios.[387,413] Snyder, Wolf, and Harryman have relied on this principle clinically and have augmented the depth of the glenoid at surgery.[250] This procedure has been called arthroscopic capsular plication and capsulolabral augmentation.

Recently, Doug Harryman, Johnathan Pond, Mike Metcalf, Kevin Smith, and John Sidles have quantitated the effect of arthroscopic posteroinferior capsulolabral reconstruction in six cadavers. Although the shoulders were elderly, these investigators were able to demonstrate substantial increases in glenoid depth (Fig. 14–198) and stability ratios (Fig. 14–199).

Reports in the literature of arthroscopic management of atraumatic instability have been few and preliminary. Tauro and Carter described a modification of the arthroscopic Bankart repair that includes an inferior capsular split and shift to remove capsular redundancy for patients with anterior instability–associated inferior laxity.[687] Duncan and Savoie reported on 10 consecutive patients

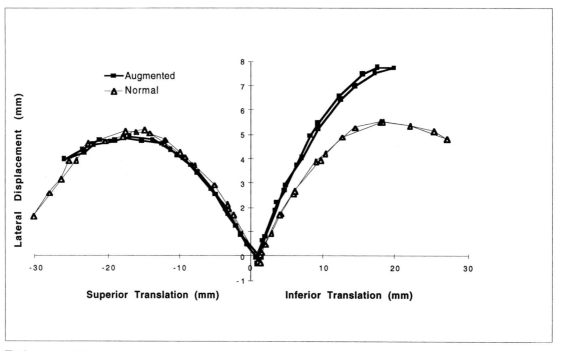

■ **Figure 14–198**
Glenoidograms indicate the path of the center of the humeral head as it is translated across the face of the glenoid superiorly (left abscissa) and inferiorly (right abscissa). The height of the *curves* indicates the effective depth of the glenoid in the respective directions. Results are shown before (normal) and after (augmented) arthroscopic capsulolabral reconstruction, a procedure that increases the effective glenoid depth inferiorly.

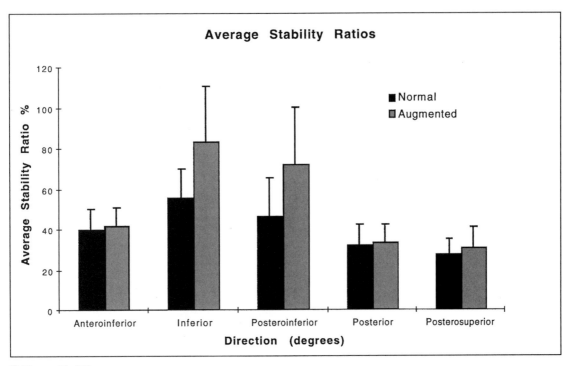

■ Figure 14–199
Stability ratios are ratios of the force necessary to displace the head from the glenoid divided by the compressive load pressing the humeral head into the glenoid. These ratios are different for different directions of displacement because of differences in effective glenoid depth. This graph shows the variations in stability ratio for different directions of displacement in the intact cadaver shoulder (normal), as well as variations in the increment in inferior and posteroinferior stability ratios seen after arthroscopic posteroinferior capsulolabral reconstruction (*crosshatched*).

with involuntary multidirectional instability who were managed by an arthroscopic modification of the inferior capsular shift procedure performed with the Caspari suture punch.[153] All their patients had a satisfactory result according to Neer's outcome scoring.

Early studies that mixed atraumatic and traumatized shoulders attempted to address posterior and multidirectional instability arthroscopically by using a staple to shift and repair the capsule.[142,696,697] Detrisac and Johnson reported a 12% failure rate and attributed problems to inadequate immobilization, lack of sufficient posterior capsule, and the presence of a metal staple.[142] Tibone and colleagues also used a metal staple in 40 athletes with posterior instability.[696,697] They reported a 40% failure rate and a high number of complications that were attributed to ligamentous laxity and unrecognized and untreated multidirectional instability. They found that the higher the competitive level of the athlete, the worse the overall results. They concluded that staple capsulorrhaphy was not acceptable treatment of posterior instability of the shoulder.

At the University of Washington, Doug Harryman started a prospective study of patients who failed a thorough nonoperative treatment course for functionally incapacitating atraumatic instability. All patients were treated with (1) education regarding activities to be avoided and (2) a conditioning exercise program of rotator cuff and periscapular muscle strengthening.[4413] Patients met specific diagnostic criteria. The operative goals were to stabilize the glenohumeral joint by

removing capsular redundancy and deepening the glenoid concavity by performing capsulolabral augmentation.

■ HARRYMAN'S SURGICAL TECHNIQUE FOR ARTHROSCOPIC ATRAUMATIC INSTABILITY REPAIR

Each shoulder was compared with the opposite side under anesthesia. All patients demonstrated a positive jerk test[443] with either displacement over the glenoid rim or frank dislocation posteroinferiorly.

Only a single anterior and posterior portal is necessary for scope and instrument access. Arthroscopic inspection revealed posterior and inferior labral flattening or rounding or partial or complete detachment from the articular cartilage, but no anteroinferior labral detachments were found (Fig. 14–200). The synovium and capsule were typically redundant and partially stripped away from the labrum, which resulted in a large posterior and inferior recess. Only three patients were found to have a deficient rotator interval capsule.

The peripheral rim of the glenoid labrum was roughened with a motorized shaver. Next, a suture hook was used to bring up approximately 1 cm of the inferior capsule in a posterosuperior direction to buttress the glenoid labrum. Additionally, the posterior and anterior capsule was shifted in a similar manner about the labrum.

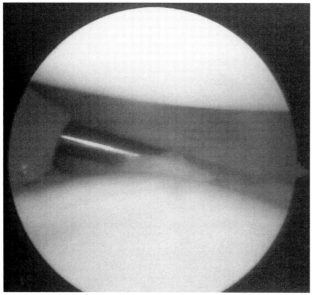

■ **Figure 14–200**
A shoulder with chronic posteroinferior atraumatic instability. Notice the synovial stripping adjacent to the labrum (glenoid on the bottom with flaps of synovium in the center) and the appearance of labral flattening to the right of center. The posteroinferior capsular recess is enlarged. *(Courtesy of Douglas T. Harryman II, MD, Department of Orthopaedics, University of Washington.)*

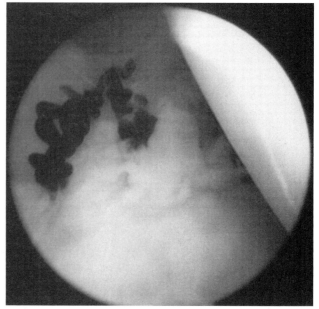

■ **Figure 14–201**
Posteroinferior capsulolabral augmentation. Notice how the capsule is bunched up and attached to the peripheral annular fibers of the labrum to increase the glenoid depth and reduce the capsular redundancy. *(Courtesy of Douglas T. Harryman II, MD, Department of Orthopaedics, University of Washington.)*

Five to nine sutures were placed through the capsule and between the deepest annular fibers of the glenoid labrum adjacent to the articular cartilage (Fig. 14–201). When necessary, plication of the rotator interval capsule was performed with a 30-degree straight suture hook by working within the subacromial space. Postoperative management must avoid capsular stretching and emphasize a program of early active rotator cuff, deltoid, and scapular strengthening.

Twenty patients with a mean follow-up of 21 months (range, 12 to 52) are included in this review. At present, recurrent instability has developed in two patients (10%) who had failed a previous open instability repair; no primary repairs have failed to date.

Doug Harryman has passed away. It is our sincere hope that others will pursue this most promising approach to the essential pathology in atraumatic instability.

Treatment of Other Types of Recurrent Instability

The AMBRII and TUBS syndromes represent clearly defined clinical pathologic entities, each of which has specific diagnostic features and treatment strategies. Together, they account for the great majority of patients with glenohumeral instability. Patients who do not fit into one of these two categories have highly individualized problems and cannot be grouped together effectively. In evaluating these patients, a meticulous history and physical examination take on even greater importance. When an initiating injury has occurred, it is essential to determine the position of the arm and the direction and

magnitude of the force producing the injury so that the likelihood of a capsular tear can be determined. Unless this is clearly the case, the default assumption is that the shoulder has become dysfunctional without a substantial anatomic lesion and therefore needs to be managed with a rehabilitative approach that emphasizes strength, balance, endurance, and good technique. Unless a functionally significant instability can be determined by the history and physical examination, the emphasis on rehabilitation must continue. When the history and physical examination do not indicate the nature of the shoulder problem, "studies" such as contrast CT, MRI, examination under anesthesia, and arthroscopy are unlikely to be helpful in determining the treatment. "Findings" on these tests, such as "increased translation," "increased laxity," "a large axillary pouch," or "labral fraying," may be identified even in functionally normal shoulders and as such may have no relationship to the patient's functional problem. The risk, therefore, is that findings on these tests may distract the clinician from findings on the history and physical examination. Unless functional instability can be rigorously characterized by the history and physical examination, it is unlikely that surgical attempts to increase stability will be curative.

In summary, the history and physical examination constitute the most efficient and cost-effective methods for identifying treatable problems of glenohumeral instability. When these clinical tools do not clearly define the nature of the patient's functional problem, surgical management is unlikely to be effective. The use of expensive diagnostic approaches can be reduced to a minimum. Surgery is reserved for those with clearly defined mechanical stability. This highly selective approach improves

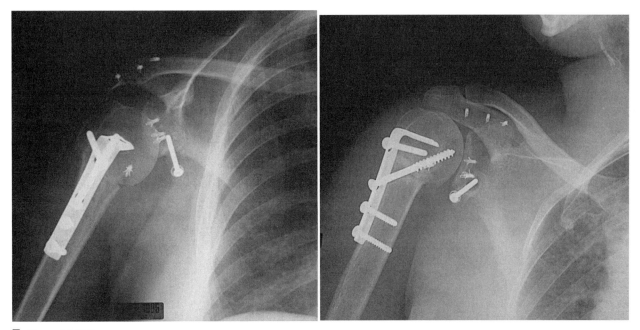

■ **Figure 14–202**
Radiographs of a shoulder with continued instability after five operations, including a capsular shift, a Bristow procedure, and a rotational osteotomy.

the overall results of surgical treatment of instability by helping minimize situations in which an operation fails to restore the patient's function (Fig. 14–202).

Superior Labral Lesions

Superior labral anterior and posterior (SLAP) lesions are sometimes encountered along with other labral pathology in patients with instability. The mechanism of injury is typically indirect compression of the humeral head into the glenoid through an outstretched hand. Symptoms are often manifested as pain and are exacerbated with diagnostic maneuvers that produce stress on the long head of the biceps tendon, as well as its attachment to the superior labrum.

In addition to the history and physical examination, the diagnosis may be facilitated with imaging studies. The sensitivity of MR arthrography in diagnosing SLAP lesions has ranged from 82% to 92% with a specificity of 69% to 91%.[44,322]

Arthroscopic treatment of superior labral lesions has been the most common surgical intervention. Such treatment generally consists of one to two suture anchors at the biceps root. The results of arthroscopic treatment have been successful in 91% of patients. Patients who were involved in overhead sports had less optimal outcomes, however.[356]

The reader is directed to the chapter in this text on SLAP lesions for more detailed information.

REFERENCES AND BIBLIOGRAPHY

1. Adams FL: The Genuine Works of Hippocrates, vols 1 and 2. New York: William Woods, 1886.
2. Adams F: The Genuine Works of Hippocrates, vol 2. New York: William Woods, 1891.
3. Adams JC: Recurrent dislocation of the shoulder. J Bone Joint Surg Br *30*:26, 1948.
4. Adams JC: The humeral head defect in recurrent anterior dislocations of the shoulder. Br J Radiol *23*:151-156, 1950.
5. Ahlgren O, Lorentzon R, and Larsson SE: Posterior dislocation of the shoulder associated with general seizures. Acta Orthop Scand *52*:694-695, 1981.
6. Ahlgren SA, Hedlund T, and Nistor L: Idiopathic posterior instability of the shoulder joint. Acta Orthop Scand *49*:600-603, 1978.
7. Albert E: Arthodese bei einer habituellen Luxation der Schultergelenkes. Klin Rundschau *2*:281-283, 1898.
8. Altchek DW, Warren RF, Skyhar MJ, and Ortiz G: T-plasty modification of the Bankart procedure for multidirectional instability of the anterior and inferior types. J Bone Joint Surg Am *73*:105-112, 1991.
9. Anderson D, Zvirbulis R, and Ciullo J: Scapular manipulation for reduction of anterior shoulder dislocations. Clin Orthop *164*:181-183, 1982.
10. Anderson K, Warren RF, Altchek DW, et al: Risk factors for early failure after thermal capsulorrhaphy. Am J Sports Med *30*:103-107, 2002.
11. Anderson L, Rush R, Sherer L, and Highes CJ: The effects of a TheraBand exercise program on shoulder internal rotation strength. Phys Ther *72*(suppl):40, 1992.
12. Andrews J, Carson WCM, and Hughston JC: Operative Shoulder Arthroscopy. Homestead, VA: American Orthopaedics Association, 1983.
13. Angelo RN and Hawkins RJ: Osteoarthritis following an excessively tight Putti-Platt repair. Paper presented at the 4th Open Meeting of the American Shoulder and Elbow Surgeons, 1988, Atlanta.
14. Antal CS, Conforty B, and Engelberg M: Injuries to the axillary due to anterior dislocation of the shoulder. J Trauma *13*:564, 1973.
15. Antoniou J, Duckworth DT, and Harryman DT II: Capsulolabral augmentation for the management of posteroinferior instability of the shoulder. J Bone Joint Surg Am *82*:1220-1230, 2000.
16. Arciero RA: Arthroscopic stabilization of initial anterior shoulder dislocations. Paper presented at the American Academy of Orthopaedic Surgeons Specialty Day, Arthroscopy Association of North America, 1994, New Orleans.
17. Arciero RA: Arthroscopic stabilization of acute, initial anterior shoulder dislocation. *In* Current Techniques in Arthroscopy, 2nd ed. New York: Churchill Livingstone, 1996, pp 117-124.
18. Arciero RA, Taylor DC, Snyder RJ, and Uhorchak JM: Arthroscopic bioabsorbable tack stabilization of initial anterior shoulder dislocations: A preliminary report. Arthroscopy *2*:410-417, 1995.
19. Arciero RA, Wheeler JH, Ryan JB, and McBride JT: Arthroscopic Bankart repair vs. nonoperative treatment for acute, initial, anterior shoulder dislocations. Am J Sports Med *22*:589-594, 1994.
20. Arnoczky SP and Aksan A: Thermal modification of connective tissues: Basic science considerations and clinical implications. J Am Acad Orthop Surg *8*:305-313, 2000.
21. Aronen JG and Regan K: Decreasing the incidence of recurrence of first time anterior shoulder dislocations with rehabilitation. Am J Sports Med *12*:283-291, 1984.

22. Artz T and Huffer JM: A major complication of the modified Bristow procedure for recurrent dislocation of the shoulder: A case report. J Bone Joint Surg Am 54:1293-1296, 1972.

23. Assmus H and Meinel A: Schulterverletzung und Axillarparese. Hefte Unfallheilkd 79:183-187, 1976.

24. Aston JW and Gregory CF: Dislocation of the shoulder with significant fracture of the glenoid. J Bone Joint Surg Am 55:1531-1533, 1973.

25. Atwater AE: Biomechanics of overarm throwing movements and of throwing injuries. Exerc Sports Sci Rev 71:43-85, 1980.

26. Badgley CE and O'Connor GA: Combined procedure for the repair of recurrent anterior dislocation of the shoulder. J Bone Joint Surg Am 47:1283, 1965.

27. Baeyens JP, Van Roy P, De Schepper A, et al: Glenohumeral joint kinematics related to minor anterior instability of the shoulder at the end of the late preparatory phase of throwing. Clin Biomech (Bristol, Avon) 16:752-757, 2001.

28. Bailey PL and Stanley TH: Pharmacology of the intravenous narcotic anesthetics. In Miller R (ed): Anesthesia. New York: Churchill Livingstone, 1986, pp 745-797.

29. Bailey RW: Acute and recurrent dislocation of the shoulder. Instr Course Lect 18:70-74, 1962-1969.

30. Baker CL, Uribe JW, and Whitman C: Arthroscopic evaluation of acute initial anterior shoulder dislocations. Am J Sports Med 18:25-28, 1990.

31. Banas MP, Dalldorf PG, Sebastianelli WJ, and DeHaven KE: Long-term followup of the modified Bristow procedure [see comments]. Am J Sports Med 21:666-671, 1993.

32. Bankart ASB: Recurrent or habitual dislocation of the shoulder joint. BMJ 2:1132-1133, 1923.

33. Bankart ASB: The pathology and treatment of recurrent dislocation of the shoulder joint. Br J Surg 26:23-29, 1938.

34. Bankart ASB: The pathology and treatment of recurrent dislocation of the shoulder joint. Br J Surg 26:23-29, 1939.

35. Baratta JB, Lim V, Mastromonaco E, and Edillon E: Axillary artery disruption secondary to anterior dislocation of the shoulder. J Trauma 23:1009-1011, 1983.

36. Bardenheuer BA: Die Verletzungen der oberen Extremitaten. Dtsch Chir 63:268-418, 1886.

37. Barrett J: The clavicular joints. Physiotherapy 57:268-269, 1971.

38. Basmajian JV and Bazant FJ: Factors preventing downward dislocation of the adducted shoulder joint. J Bone Joint Surg Am 41:1182-1186, 1959.

39. Basmajian JV and DeLuca CJ: Muscles Alive, 5th ed. Baltimore: Williams & Wilkins, 1985, pp 270-271.

40. Bassett RW, Browne AO, Morrey BF, and An KN: Glenohumeral muscle force and moment mechanics in a position of shoulder instability. J Biomech 23:405-415, 1990.

41. Bateman JE: Gallie technique for repair of recurrent dislocation of the shoulder. Surg Clin North Am 43:1655-1662, 1963.

42. Bayley JIL and Kessel L: Posterior dislocation of the shoulder: The clinical spectrum. J Bone Joint Surg Br 60:440, 1978.

43. Beattie TF, Steedman DJ, McGowan A, and Robertson CE: A comparison of the Milch and Kochner techniques for acute anterior dislocation of the shoulder. Injury 17:349-352, 1986.

44. Bencardino JT, Beltran J, Rosenberg ZS, et al: Superior labrum anterior-posterior lesions: Diagnosis with MR arthrography of the shoulder. Radiology 214:267-271, 2000.

45. Benechetrit E and Friedman B: Fracture of the coracoid process associated with subglenoid dislocation of the shoulder. J Bone Joint Surg Am 61:295-296, 1979.

46. Benedetto KP and Glotzer W: Arthroscopic Bankart procedure by suture technique: Indications, technique, and results. Arthroscopy 8:111-115, 1992.

47. Bennett GE: Old dislocations of the shoulder. J Bone Joint Surg 18:594-606, 1936.

48. Berg EE and Ellison AE: The inside-out Bankart procedure. Am J Sports Med 18:129-133, 1990.

49. Bertrand JC, Maestro M, Pequignot JP, and Moviel J: Les complications vasculaires des luxations artérieures fermes de l'épaule. Ann Chir 36:329-333, 1981.

50. Bestard EA: Glenoplasty: A simple reliable method of correcting recurrent posterior dislocation of the shoulder. Orthop Rev 5:29-34, 1976.

51. Bigliani LU, Pollock RG, McIlveen SJ, et al: Shift of the posteroinferior aspect of the capsule for recurrent posterior glenohumeral instability. J Bone Joint Surg Am 77:1011-1020, 1995.

52. Bigliani LU, Pollock RG, Soslowsky LJ, et al: Tensile properties of the inferior glenohumeral ligament. J Orthop Res 10:187-197, 1992.

53. Bigliani LU, Weinstein DM, Glasgow MT, et al: Glenohumeral arthroplasty for arthritis after instability surgery. J Shoulder Elbow Surg 4:87-94, 1995.

54. Blasier RB, Carpenter JE, and Huston LJ: Shoulder proprioception: Effect of joint laxity, joint position, and direction of motion. Orthop Rev 23:45-50, 1994.

55. Blasier RB, Guldberg RE, and Rothman ED: Anterior shoulder stability: Contributions of rotator cuff forces and the capsular ligaments in a cadaver model. J Shoulder Elbow Surg 1:140-150, 1992.

56. Blazina ME and Satzman JS: Recurrent anterior subluxation of the shoulder in athletes—a distinct entity. J Bone Joint Surg Am 51:1037-1038, 1969.

57. Blom S and Dahlback LO: Nerve injuries in dislocations of the shoulder joint and fractures of the neck of the humerus. Acta Chir Scand 136:461-466, 1970.

58. Bloom MH and Obata WG: Diagnosis of posterior dislocation of the shoulder with use of Velpeau axillary and angle-up roentgenographic views. J Bone Joint Surg Am 49:943-949, 1967.

59. Bodey WN and Denham RA: A free bone block operation for recurrent anterior dislocation of the shoulder joint. Injury 15:184, 1983.

60. Bonnin JG: Transplantation of the tip of the coracoid process for recurrent anterior dislocation of the shoulder. J Bone Joint Surg Br 51:579, 1969.

61. Bonnin JG: Transplantation of the coracoid tip: A definitive operation for recurrent anterior dislocation of the shoulder. R Soc Med 66:755-758, 1973.

62. Bottoni CR, Wilckens JH, DeBerardino TM, et al: A prospective, randomized evaluation of arthroscopic stabilization versus nonoperative treatment in patients with acute, traumatic, first-time shoulder dislocations. Am J Sports Med 30:576-580, 2002.

63. Boyd HB and Sisk TD: Recurrent posterior dislocation of the shoulder. J Bone Joint Surg Am 54:779, 1972.

64. Boytchev B: Treatment of recurrent shoulder instability. Minerva Orthop 2:377-379, 1951.

65. Boytchev B, Conforty B, and Tchokanov K: Operatiunaya Ortopediya y Travatologiya, 2nd ed. Meditsina y Fizkultura, Sofia, Bulgaria, 1962.

66. Bradley JP and Tibone JE: Electromyographic analysis of muscle action about the shoulder. Clin Sports Med 10:789-805, 1991.

67. Braly WG and Tullos HS: A modification of the Bristow procedure for recurrent anterior shoulder dislocation and subluxation. Am J Sports Med 13:81, 1985.

68. Braunstein EM and O'Conner G: Double-contrast arthrotomography and the shoulder. J Bone Joint Surg Am 64:192-195, 1982.

69. Brav EA: Ten years' experience with Putti-Platt reconstruction procedure. Am J Surg 100:423-430, 1960.

70. Brewer BJ, Wubben RC, and Carrera GF: Excessive retroversion of the glenoid cavity: A cause of non-traumatic posterior instability of the shoulder. J Bone Joint Surg Am 68:724-731, 1986.

71. Bridle SH and Ferris BD: Irreducible acute anterior dislocations of the shoulder: Interposed scapularis. J Bone Joint Surg Br 72:1078-1079, 1990.

72. Broca A and Hartmann H: Contribution a l'étude des luxations de l'épaule. Bull Soc Anat Paris 4:312-336, 1890.

73. Brockbank W and Griffiths DL: Orthopaedic surgery in the 16th and 17th centuries. J Bone Joint Surg Br 30:365-375, 1948.

74. Brostrom LA, Kronberg M, Nemeth G, and Oxelback U: The effect of shoulder muscle training in patients with recurrent shoulder dislocations. Scand J Rehabil Med 24:11-15, 1992.

75. Brown FW and Navigato WJ: Rupture of the axillary artery and brachial plexus palsy associated with anterior dislocation of the shoulder—report of a case with successful vascular repair. Clin Orthop 60:195-199, 1968.

76. Brown JT: Nerve injuries complicating dislocation of the shoulder. J Bone Joint Surg Br 34:526, 1952.

77. Burkhart SS, Debeer JF, Tehrany AM, and Parten PM: Quantifying glenoid bone loss arthroscopically in shoulder instability. Arthroscopy 18:488-491, 2002.

78. Burkhead WZ and Rockwood CA Jr: Treatment of instability of the shoulder with an exercise program. J Bone Joint Surg Am 74:890-896, 1992.

79. Butters KP, Curtis RJ, and Rockwood CA Jr: Posterior deltoid splitting shoulder approach. J Bone Joint Trans 11:233, 1987.

80. Cain PR, Mischler T, Fu FH, and Lee SK: Anterior stability of the glenohumeral joint: A dynamic model. Am J Sports Med 15:144-148, 1987.

81. Caird FM: The shoulder joint in relation to certain dislocations and fractures. Edinb Med J 32:708-714, 1887.

82. Calandra JJ, Baker CL, and Uribe J: The incidence of Hill-Sachs lesions in initial anterior shoulder dislocations. Arthroscopy 5:254-257, 1989.

83. Calvet J, Leroy M, and Lacroix L: Luxations de l'épaule et lesions vasculaires. J Chir 58:337-346, 1942.

84. Carew-McColl M: Bilateral shoulder dislocations caused by electrical shock. Br J Clin Pract 34:251-254, 1980.

85. Carol EJ, Falke LM, Kortmann JH, et al: Bristow-Laterjet repair for recurrent anterior shoulder instability; an 8 year study. Neth J Surg 37:109-113, 1985.

86. Carpenter GI and Millard PH: Shoulder subluxation in elderly inpatients. J Am Geriatr Soc 30:441-446, 1982.

87. Caspari RB: Shoulder arthroscopy: A review of the present state of the art. Contemp Orthop 4:523-531, 1982.

88. Caspari RB: Arthroscopic reconstruction for anterior shoulder instability. Tech Orthop 3:59-66, 1988.

89. Caspari RB: Arthroscopic reconstruction of anterior shoulder instability. Paper presented at the Fourth International Conference on Surgery of the Shoulder, 1989, New York.

90. Cautilli RA, Joyce MF, and Mackell JV Jr: Posterior dislocation of the glenohumeral joint. Jefferson Orthop J 7:15-20, 1978.

91. Cautilli RA, Joyce MF, and Mackell JV Jr: Posterior dislocations of the shoulder: A method of postreduction management. Am J Sports Med 6:397-399, 1978.

92. Cave EF, Burke JF, and Boyd RJ: Trauma Management. Chicago: Year Book, 1974, p 437.

93. Cayford EH and Tees FJ: Traumatic aneurysm of the subclavicular artery as a late complication of fractured clavicle. Can Med Assoc J 25:450-452, 1931.

94. Chandnani VP, Yeager TD, DeBerardino T, et al: Glenoid labral tears: Prospective evaluation with MRI imaging, MR arthrography, and CT arthrography. AJR Am J Roentgenol 161:1229-1235, 1993.

95. Chen SK, Perry J, Jobe FW, et al: Elbow flexion analysis in Bristow patients: A preliminary report. Am J Sports Med 12:347-350, 1984.

96. Choi CH and Ogilvie-Harris DJ: Inferior capsular shift operation for multidirectional instability of the shoulder in players of contact sports. Br J Sports Med 36:290-294, 2002.

97. Churchill RS, Brems JJ, and Kotschi H: Glenoid size, inclination, and version: An anatomic study. J Shoulder Elbow Surg 10:327-332, 2001.

98. Churchill RS, Moskal M, Lippitt SB, and Matsen FA III: Extracapsular anatomically contoured anterior glenoid bone grafting for complex glenohumeral instability. Tech Shoulder Elbow Surg 2:210-218, 2001.

99. Ciccone WJ 2nd, Hunt TJ, Lieber R, et al: Multiquadrant digital analysis of shoulder capsular thickness. Arthroscopy 16:457-461, 2000.

100. Clairmont P and Ehrlich H: Ein neues Operations—Verfahren zur Behandlung der habituellen Schulterluxation mittels Muskelplastik. Verh Dtsch Ges Chir 38:79-103, 1909.

101. Clark JM and Harryman DT II: Tendons, ligaments, and capsule of the rotator cuff. Gross and microscopic anatomy. J Bone Joint Surg Am 74:713-725, 1992.

102. Clark JM, Sidles JA, and Matsen FA III: The relationship of the glenohumeral joint capsule to the rotator cuff. Clin Orthop 254:29-34, 1990.

103. Clark KC: Positioning in Radiography, 2nd ed. London: William Heinemann, 1941.

104. Cleaves EN: A new film holder for roentgen examination of the shoulder. AJR Am J Roentgenol 45:288-290, 1941.

105. Clotteau JE, Premont M, and Mercier V: A simple procedure for reducing dislocations of the shoulder without anesthesia. Nouv Presse Med 11:127-128, 1982.

106. Codman EA: Rupture of the Supraspinatus Tendon and Other Lesions in or about the Subacromial Bursa. Boston: Thomas Todd, 1934.

107. Cofield RH: Physical examination of the shoulder: Effectiveness in assessing shoulder stability. In Matsen FA III, Fu F, and Hawkins R (eds): The Shoulder: A Balance of Mobility and Stability. Rosemont, IL: American Academy of Orthopaedic Surgeons, 1993, pp 331-344.

108. Cofield RH, Nessler JP, and Weinstabl R: Diagnosis of shoulder instability by examination under anesthesia. Clin Orthop 291:45-53, 1993.

109. Cole BJ, L'Insalata J, Irrgang J, and Warner JJ: Comparison of arthroscopic and open anterior shoulder stabilization. A two- to six-year follow-up study. J Bone Joint Surg Am 82:1108-1114, 2000.

110. Collins HR and Wilde AH: Shoulder instability in athletes. Orthop Clin North Am 4:759-773, 1973.

111. Collins KA, Capito C, and Cross M: The use of the Putti-Platt procedure in the treatment of recurrent anterior dislocation, with special reference to the young athlete. Am J Sports Med 14:380-382, 1986.

112. Conforty B: The results of the Boytchev procedure for treatment of recurrent dislocation of the shoulder. Int Orthop 4:127-132, 1980.

113. Cooper A: On the dislocation of the os humeri upon the dorsum scapula, and upon fractures near the shoulder joint. Guys Hosp Rep 4:265-284, 1839.

114. Cooper ME and Hutchinson MR: The microscopic pathoanatomy of acute anterior shoulder dislocations in a simian model. Arthroscopy 18:618-623, 2002.

115. Cooper RA and Brems JJ: The inferior capsular-shift procedure for multidirectional instability of the shoulder. J Bone Joint Surg Am 74:1516-1521, 1992.

116. Costigan PS, Binns MS, and Wallace WA: Undiagnosed bilateral anterior dislocation of the shoulder. Injury 21:409, 1990.

117. Cotton FJ: Subluxation of the shoulder downward. Boston Med Surg J 185:405-407, 1921.

118. Coughlin L, Rubinovich M, Johansson J, et al: Arthroscopic staple capsulorrhaphy for anterior shoulder instability. Am J Sports Med 20:253-256, 1992.

119. Cramer F: Resection des Oberamkopfes wegen habitueller Luxation (nach einem im arzlichen Verein zu Wiesbaden gehaltenen Vortrage). Berl Klin Wochenschr 19:21-25, 1882.

120. Cramer F, Von BM, and Kramps HA: CT diagnosis of recurrent subluxation of the shoulder. Fortschr Rontgenstr 136:440-443, 1982.

121. Cranley JJ and Krause RF: Injury to the axillary artery following anterior dislocation of the shoulder. Am J Surg 95:524-526, 1958.

122. Crockett HC, Gross LB, Wilk KE, et al: Osseous adaptation and range of motion at the glenohumeral joint in professional baseball pitchers. Am J Sports Med 30:20-26, 2002.

123. Cuckler JM, Bearcroft J, and Asgian CM: Femoral head technologies to reduce polyethylene wear in total hip arthroplasty. Clin Orthop 317:57-63, 1995.

124. Curr JF: Rupture of the axillary artery complicating dislocation of the shoulder. Report of a case. J Bone Joint Surg Br 52:313-317, 1970.

125. Cyprien JM, Vasey HM, and Burdet A: Humeral retrotorsion and glenohumeral relationship in the normal shoulder and in recurrent anterior dislocation. Clin Orthop 175:8-17, 1983.

126. D'Angelo D: Luxacaorecidivante Anterior de Ombro. Rio de Janeiro: Brazil University of Rio de Janeiro, 1970.

127. Danzig LA, Greenway G, and Resnick D: The Hill-Sachs lesion: An experimental study. Am J Sports Med 8:328-332, 1980.

128. Danzig LA, Resnick D, and Greenway G: Evaluation of unstable shoulders by computed tomography. Am J Sports Med 10:138-141, 1982.

129. Das SP, Roy GS, and Saha AK: Observations on the tilt of the glenoid cavity of scapula. J Anat Soc India 15:114, 1966.

130. DeBerardino TM, Arciero RA, Taylor DC, and Uhorchak JM: Prospective evaluation of arthroscopic stabilization of acute, initial anterior shoulder dislocations in young athletes. Two- to five-year follow-up. Am J Sports Med 29:586-592, 2001.

131. Debevoise NT, Hyatt GW, and Townsend GB: Humeral torsion in recurrent shoulder dislocation. Clin Orthop 76:87-93, 1971.

132. de Laat EA, Visser CP, Coene LN, et al: Nerve lesions in primary shoulder dislocations and humeral neck fractures: A prospective clinical and EMG study. J Bone Joint Surg Br 76:381-383, 1994.

133. Delorme D: Die Hemmungsbander des Schultergelenks und ihre Bedeutung fur die Schulterluxationen. Arch Klin Chir 92:79-101, 1910.

134. DePalma AF: Recurrent dislocation of the shoulder joint. Ann Surg 132:1052-1065, 1950.

135. DePalma AF: Surgery of the Shoulder. Philadelphia: JB Lippincott, 1950.

136. DePalma AF: The Management of Fractures and Dislocations: An Atlas, vol 1, 2nd ed. Philadelphia: WB Saunders, 1970.

137. DePalma AF: Surgery of the Shoulder, 2nd ed. Philadelphia: JB Lippincott, 1973.

138. DePalma AF: Surgery of the Shoulder, 3rd ed. Philadelphia: JB Lippincott, 1983.

139. DePalma AF, Callery G, and Bennett GA: Variational Anatomy and Degenerative Lesions of the Shoulder Joint, vol 6. Ann Arbor, MI: 1949, pp 255-281.

140. DePalma AF, Cooke AJ, and Prabhakar M: The role of the subscapularis in recurrent anterior dislocations of the shoulder. Clin Orthop 54:35-49, 1967.

141. Detrisac DA: Arthroscopic Shoulder Staple Capsulorrhaphy for Traumatic Anterior Instability. New York: Raven Press, 1991.

142. Detrisac DA and Johnson LL: Arthroscopic shoulder capsulorrhaphy using metal staples. Orthop Clin North Am 24:71-88, 1993.

143. Dhinakharan SR, and Ghosh A: Towards evidence based emergency medicine: Best BETs from the Manchester Royal Infirmary. Intra-articular lidocaine for acute anterior shoulder dislocation reduction. Emerg Med J 19:142-143, 2002.

144. Dias JJ, Mody BS, Finlay DB, and Richardson RA: Recurrent anterior glenohumeral joint dislocation and torsion of the humerus. J Orthop Sports Phys Ther 18:379-385, 1993.

145. Dick W and Baumgartner R: Hypermobilitat und wilkurliche hintere Schulterluxation. Orthop Prax 16:328-330, 1980.

146. Didiee J: Le radiodiagnostic dans la luxation récidivante de l'épaule. J Radiol Electrol 14:209-218, 1930.

147. Doege KW: Irreducible shoulder joint dislocations. Lancet 49:191-195, 1929.

148. Dolk T and Stenberg B: Arterial injury in fracture dislocation of the shoulder. Acta Orthop Scand 62(suppl 246):17, 1991.

149. Dorgan JA: Posterior dislocation of the shoulder. Am J Surg 89:890-900, 1955.

150. Dowdy PA and O'Driscoll SW: Shoulder instability: An analysis of family history. J Bone Joint Surg Br 75:782-784, 1993.

151. Dowdy PA and O'Driscoll SW: Recurrent anterior shoulder instability. Am J Sports Med 22:489-492, 1994.

152. Drury JK and Scullion JE: Vascular complications of anterior dislocation of the shoulder. Br J Surg 67:579-581, 1980.

153. Duncan R and Savoie FHD: Arthroscopic inferior capsular shift for multidirectional instability of the shoulder: A preliminary report. Arthroscopy 9:24-27, 1993.

154. DuToit GT and Roux D: Recurrent dislocation of the shoulder: A 24 year study of the Johannesburg stapling operation. J Bone Joint Surg Am 38:1-12, 1956.

155. Eberly VC, McMahon PJ, and Lee TQ: Variation in the glenoid origin of the anteroinferior glenohumeral capsulolabrum. Clin Orthop 400:26-31, 2002.

156. Eden R: Zur Operation der habituellen Schulterluxation unter Mitteilung eines neuen Verfahrens bei Abriss am inneren Pfannenrande. Dstch Ztschr Chir 144:269, 1918.

157. Edwards DJ, Hoy G, Saies AD, and Hayes MG: Adverse reactions to an absorbable shoulder fixation device. J Shoulder Elbow Surg 3:230-233, 1994.

158. Ehgartner K: Has the duration of cast fixation after shoulder dislocations had an influence on the frequency of recurrent dislocation? Arch Orthop Unfallchir 89:187-190, 1977.

159. El-Khoury GY, Kathol MH, Chandler JB, and Albright JP: Shoulder instability: Impact of glenohumeral arthrotomography on treatment. Radiology 160:669-673, 1986.

160. Ellman H: Arthroscopic subacromial decompression: Analysis of one to three year results. Arthroscopy 3:173-181, 1987.

161. Ellman H: Arthroscopic subacromial decompression: New techniques and result. Paper presented at the 8th Annual Meeting of the Arthroscopy Association of North America, Instructional Course, 1989, Seattle.

162. Ellman H and Kay SP: Arthroscopic treatment of calcific tendinitis [abstract]. Orthop Trans 13:240, 1989.

163. Emery RJ and Mullaji AB: Glenohumeral joint instability in normal adolescents. Incidence and significance. J Bone Joint Surg Br 73:406-408, 1991.

164. Endo S, Kasai T, Fujii N, et al: Traumatic anterior dislocation of the shoulder in a child. Arch Orthop Trauma Surg 112:201-202, 1993.

165. Engebretsen L and Craig EV: Radiologic features of shoulder instability. Clin Orthop 291:29-44, 1993.
166. Engelhardt MB: Posterior dislocation of the shoulder: Report of six cases. South Med J 71:425-427, 1978.
167. English E and Macnab I: Recurrent posterior dislocation of the shoulder. Can J Surg 17:147-151, 1974.
168. Esch JC: Shoulder arthroscopy: Treatment of rotator cuff pathology. Paper presented at the 8th Annual Meeting of the Arthroscopy Association of North America, Instructional Course, 1989, Seattle.
169. Esch JC, Ozerkis LR, Helgager JA, et al: Arthroscopic subacromial decompression: Results according to the degree of rotator cuff tear. Arthroscopy 4:241-249, 1988.
170. Eve FS: A case of subcoracoid dislocation of the humerus with the formation of an indentation on the posterior surface of the head. Medico-Chirurg Trans Soc Lond 63:317-321, 1880.
171. Eyre-Brook AL: The morbid anatomy of a case of recurrent dislocation of the shoulder. Br J Surg 29:32-37, 1943.
172. Eyre-Brook AL: Recurrent dislocation of the shoulder: Lesions discovered in seventeen cases. Surgery employed, and intermediate report on results. J Bone Joint Surg Br 30:39, 1948.
173. Eyre-Brook AL: Recurrent dislocation of the shoulder. Physiotherapy 57:7-13, 1971.
174. Fairbank HAT: Birth palsy: Subluxation of the shoulder joint in infants and young children. Lancet 1:1217-1223, 1913.
175. Fairbank TJ: Fracture-subluxations of the shoulder. J Bone Joint Surg Br 30:454-460, 1948.
176. Fanton GS: Shoulder arthroscopy using the holmium-YAG laser method. State of the art 1994. Orthopade 25:79-83, 1996.
177. Fanton GS and Khan AM: Monopolar radiofrequency energy for arthroscopic treatment of shoulder instability in the athlete. Orthop Clin North Am 32:511-523, 2001.
178. Favorito PJ, Langenderfer MA, Colosimo AJ, et al: Arthroscopic laser-assisted capsular shift in the treatment of patients with multidirectional shoulder instability. Am J Sports Med 30:322-328, 2002.
179. Fee HJ, McAvoy JM, and Dainko EA: Pseudoaneurysm of the axillary artery following a modified Bristow operation: Report of a case and review. Cardiovasc Surg 19:65, 1978.
180. Fehringer EV, Schmidt GR, Boorman RS, et al: The anteroinferior labrum helps center the humeral head on the glenoid. J Shoulder Elbow Surg 12:53-58, 2003.
181. Ferkel RD, Hedley AK, and Eckardt JJ: Anterior fracture-dislocations of the shoulder: Pitfalls in treatment. J Trauma 24:363-367, 1984.
182. Ferlic DC and DeGiovine NM: A long-term retrospective study of the modified Bristow procedure. Am J Sports Med 16:469-474, 1988.
183. Ferrari DA: Capsular ligaments of the shoulder: Anatomical and functional study of the anterior superior capsule. Am J Sports Med 18:20-24, 1990.
184. Fick R: Handbuch der Anatomie und Mechanik der Gelenke unter Berucksichtigung der Bewegenden Muskeln. Jena, Germany, Fischer, 1904.
185. Finsterer H: Die operative Behandlung der habituellen Schulterluxation. Dtsch Z Chir 141:354-497, 1917.
186. Fipp GJ: Simultaneous posterior dislocation of both shoulders. Clin Orthop 44:191-195, 1966.
187. Fitzgerald BT, Watson BT, and Lapoint JM: The use of thermal capsulorrhaphy in the treatment of multidirectional instability. J Shoulder Elbow Surg 11:108-113, 2002.
188. Fitzgerald JF and Keates J: False aneurysm as a late complication of anterior dislocation of the shoulder. Ann Surg 181:785-786, 1975.
189. Flatow EL, Raimondo RA, Kelkar R, et al: Active and passive restraints against superior humeral translation: The Contributions of the rotator cuff, the biceps tendon, and the coracoacromial arch. Paper presented at the Annual Meeting of the American Academy of Orthopaedic Surgeons, 1996, Atlanta.
190. Flower WH: On pathologic changes produced in the shoulder joint by traumatic dislocation. Trans Pathol Soc Lond 12:179-200, 1861.
191. Frank CB: Ligament healing: Current knowledge and clinical applications. J Am Acad Orthop Surg 4:74-83, 1996.
192. Francke GH: Dislocations of shoulder. Dtsch Z Chir 48:399, 1898.
193. Fredriksson AS and Tegner Y: Results of the Putti-Platt operation for recurrent anterior dislocation of the shoulder. Int Orthop 15:185-188, 1991.
194. Friedman RJ: Glenohumeral capsulorrhaphy. In Matsen FA III, Fu FH, and Hawkins RJ (eds): The Shoulder: A Balance of Mobility and Stability. Rosemont, IL: American Academy of Orthopaedic Surgeons, 1993, pp 445-458.
195. Frizziero L, Zizzi F, and Facchini A: Arthroscopy of the shoulder joint: A review of 23 cases. Rheumatologie 11:267-276, 1981.
196. Fu FH and Klein BS: Shoulder Arthroscopy: Complications and Pitfalls. Gaithersburg, MD: Aspen, 1991.
197. Gallie WE and LeMesurier AB: An operation for the relief of recurring dislocations of the shoulder. Trans Am Surg Assoc 45:392-398, 1927.
198. Gallie WE and LeMesurier AB: Recurring dislocation of the shoulder. J Bone Joint Surg Br 30:9-18, 1948.
199. Ganel A, Horoszowski H, and Heim M: Persistent dislocation of the shoulder in elderly patients. J Am Geriatr Soc 28:282-284, 1980.
200. Gardham JRC and Scott JE: Axillary artery occlusion with erect dislocation of the shoulder. Injury 11:155-158, 1980.
201. Gardner E: The prenatal development of the human shoulder joint. Surg Clin North Am 43:1465-1470, 1963.
202. Gariepy R, Derome A, and Laurin CA: Brachial plexus paralysis following shoulder dislocation. Can J Surg 5:418-421, 1962.
203. Garneau RA, Renfrew DL, Moore TE, et al: Glenoid labrum: Evaluation with MR imaging. Radiology 179:519-522, 1991.
204. Garth WP Jr, Allman FL, and Armstrong WS: Occult anterior subluxations of the shoulder in noncontact sports. Am J Sports Med 15:579-585, 1987.
205. Garth WP Jr, Slappey CE, and Ochs CW: Roentgenographic demonstration of instability of the shoulder: The apical oblique projection. A technical note. J Bone Joint Surg Am 661:1450-1453, 1984.
206. Gartsman GM: Arthroscopic acromioplasty for rotator cuff lesions. Unpublished paper, 1989.
207. Gartsman GM: Arthroscopic subacromial decompression for advanced rotator cuff disease [abstract]. Orthop Trans 13:240, 1989.
208. Gartsman GM, Blair M, Bennett JB, et al: Arthroscopic subacromial decompression: An anatomical study. Am J Sports Med 16:48-50, 1988.
209. Gartsman GM, Roddey TS, and Hammerman SM: Arthroscopic treatment of bidirectional glenohumeral instability: Two- to five-year follow-up. J Shoulder Elbow Surg 10:28-36, 2001.
210. Gartsman GM, Roddey TS, and Hammerman SM: Arthroscopic treatment of multidirectional glenohumeral instability: 2- to 5-year follow-up. Arthroscopy 17:236-243, 2001.
211. Geiger DF, Hurley JA, Tovey JA, and Rao JP: Results of arthroscopic versus open Bankart suture repair. Paper presented at the American Academy of Orthopaedic Surgeons Specialty Day, 1993, San Francisco.
212. Gerber C, Ganz R, and Vinh TS: Glenoplasty for recurrent posterior shoulder instability. Clin Orthop 216:70-79, 1987.
213. Gerber A and Warner JJ: Thermal capsulorrhaphy to treat shoulder instability. Clin Orthop 400:105-116, 2002.
214. Ghormley RK, Black JR, and Cherry JH: Ununited fractures of the clavicle. Am J Surg 51:343-349, 1941.
215. Gibb TD, Harryman DT II, Sidles JA, et al: The effect of capsular venting on glenohumeral laxity. Clin Orthop 268:120-127, 1991.
216. Gibson JMC: Rupture of the axillary artery following anterior dislocation of the shoulder. J Bone Joint Surg Br 44:114-115, 1962.
217. Glessner JR: Intrathoracic dislocation of the humeral head. J Bone Joint Surg Am 42:428-430, 1961.
218. Gleyze P and Habermeyer P: Aspects arthroscopiques et évolution chronologique des lesions du complexe labro-ligamentaire dans l'instabilite antero-inférieure post-traumatique de l'épaule. Rev Chir Orthop 82:288-298, 1996.
219. Glousman R, Jobe F, and Tibone J: Dynamic electromyographic analysis of the throwing shoulder with glenohumeral instability. J Bone Joint Surg Am 70:220-226, 1988.
220. Gohlke F, Schneider P, Siegel K, and Balzer C: Tensile strength of various anchor systems in surgical correction of instability of the shoulder joint. Unfallchirurg 96:546-550, 1993.
221. Gold AM: Fractured neck of the humerus with separation and dislocation of the humeral head (fracture-dislocation of the shoulder, severe type). Bull Hosp Jt Dis 32:87-99, 1971.
222. Goldberg BJ, Nirschl RP, McConnell JP, and Pettrone FA: Arthroscopic transglenoid suture capsulolabral repairs: Preliminary results. Am J Sports Med 21:656-664, 1993.
223. Gonzalez D and Lopez R: Concurrent rotator-cuff tear and brachial plexus palsy associated with anterior dislocation of the shoulder: A report of two cases. J Bone Joint Surg Am 73:620-621, 1991.
224. Gosset J: Une technique de greffe coraco-glenordienne dans le traitement des luxations récidivantes de l'épaule. Mem Acad Chir 86:445-447, 1960.
225. Gould R, Rosenfield AT, and Friedlaender GE: Loose body within the glenohumeral joint in recurrent anterior dislocation: CT demonstration. J Comput Assist Tomogr 9:404-405, 1985.
226. Grana WA, Buckley PD, and Yates CK: Arthroscopic Bankart suture repair. Am J Sports Med 21:348-353, 1993.
227. Grant JCB: Grant's Atlas of Anatomy, 6th ed. Baltimore: Williams & Wilkins, 1972.
228. Grashey R: Atlas Typischer Rontgenfilder. 1923.
229. Grasshoff H, Buhtz C, Gellerich I, and von Knorre C: CT diagnosis in instability of the shoulder joint. Rofo Fortschr Geb Rontgenstr Neuen Bildgeb Verfahr 155:523-526, 1991.
230. Green MR and Christensen KP: Arthroscopic versus open Bankart procedures: A comparison of early morbidity and complications. Arthroplasty 9:371-374, 1993.
231. Green MR and Christensen KP: Magnetic resonance imaging of the glenoid labrum in anterior shoulder instability. Am J Sports Med 22:493-498, 1994.
232. Green MR and Christensen KP: Arthroscopic Bankart procedure: Two- to five-year followup with clinical correlation to severity of glenoid labral lesion. Am J Sports Med 23:276-281, 1995.
233. Gross ML, Seeger LL, Smith JB, et al: Magnetic resonance imaging of the glenoid labrum. Am J Sports Med 18:229-234, 1990.
234. Gross RM: Arthroscopic shoulder capsulorrhaphy: Does it work? Am J Sports Med 17:495-500, 1989.
235. Guanche C, Knatt T, Solomonow M, et al: The synergistic action of the capsule and the shoulder muscles. Am J Sports Med 23:301-306, 1995.

236. Gugenheim S and Sanders RJ: Axillary artery rupture caused by shoulder dislocation. Surgery 95:55, 1984.
237. Guibe M: Des lesions des vaisseaux de l'aiselle qui compliquent les luxations de l'épaule. Rev Chir 4:580-583, 1911.
238. Guilfoil PH and Christiansen T: An unusual vascular complication of fractured clavicle. JAMA 200:72-73, 1967.
239. Haaker RG, Eickhoff U, and Klammer HL: Intraarticular autogenous bone grafting in recurrent shoulder dislocations. Mil Med 158:164-169, 1993.
240. Habermeyer P and Schuller U: Significance of the glenoid labrum for stability of the glenohumeral joint: An experimental study. Unfallchirurg 93:19-26, 1990.
241. Habermeyer P, Schuller U, and Wiedemann E: The intra-articular pressure of the shoulder: An experimental study on the role of the glenoid labrum in stabilizing the joint. J Arthrosc 8:166-172, 1992.
242. Ha'eri GB and Maitland A: Arthroscopy findings in the frozen shoulder. J Rheumatol 8:149-152, 1981.
243. Halder A, Zobitz ME, Schultz E, and An KN: Structural properties of the subscapularis tendon. J Orthop Res 18:829-834, 2000.
244. Halder AM, Halder CG, Zhao KD, et al: Dynamic inferior stabilizers of the shoulder joint. Clin Biomech (Bristol, Avon) 16:138-143, 2001.
245. Halder AM, Kuhl SG, Zobitz ME, et al: Effects of the glenoid labrum and glenohumeral abduction on stability of the shoulder joint through concavity-compression: An in vitro study. J Bone Joint Surg Am 83:1062-1069, 2001.
246. Hall RH, Isaac F, and Booth CR: Dislocations of the shoulder with special reference to accompanying small fractures. J Bone Joint Surg Am 41:489-494, 1959.
247. Hardy P, Thabit GR, Fanton GS, et al: Arthroscopic management of recurrent anterior shoulder dislocation by combining a labrum suture with antero-inferior holmium: YAG laser capsular shrinkage. Orthopade 25:91-93, 1996.
248. Harner CD and Fu FH: The Bankart lesion of the shoulder: A biochemical analysis following repair. Knee Surg Sports Traumatol Arthrosc 3:117-120, 1995.
249. Harryman DT II: Common surgical approaches to the shoulder. Instr Course Lect 41:3-11, 1992.
250. Harryman DT II: Arthroscopic management of shoulder instability. Univ Washington Res Rep 1:24-26, 1996.
251. Harryman DT II, Ballmer FP, Harris SL, and Sidles JA: Arthroscopic labral repair to the glenoid rim. J Arthrosc 10:20-30, 1994.
252. Harryman DT II, Lazarus MD, Sidles JA, and Matsen FA III: Pathophysiology of Shoulder Instability, vol 2, McGinty JB (ed). 1996, pp 677-693.
253. Harryman DT II, Sidles JA, Clark JM, et al: Translation of the humeral head on the glenoid with passive glenohumeral motion. J Bone Joint Surg Am 72:1334-1343, 1990.
254. Harryman DT II, Sidles JA, Harris S, and Matsen FA III: The role of the rotator interval capsule in passive motion and stability of the shoulder. J Bone Joint Surg Am 74:53-66, 1992.
255. Harryman DT II, Sidles JA, and Matsen FA III: Laxity of the normal glenohumeral joint: A quantitative in vivo assessment. J Shoulder Elbow Surg 1:66-76, 1992.
256. Hashimoto T, Hamada T, Sasaguri Y, and Suzuki K: Immunohistochemical approach for the investigation of nerve distribution in the shoulder joint capsule. Clin Orthop 305:273-282, 1994.
257. Hattrup SJ, Cofield RH, and Weaver AL: Anterior shoulder reconstruction: prognostic variables. J Shoulder Elbow Surg 10:508-513, 2001.
258. Hauser EDW: Avulsion of the tendon of the subscapularis muscle. J Bone Joint Surg Am 36:139-141, 1954.
259. Hawkins RB: Arthroscopic stapling repair for shoulder instability: A retrospective study of 50 cases. Arthroscopy 5:122-128, 1989.
260. Hawkins RH and Hawkins RJ: Failed anterior reconstruction for shoulder instability. J Bone Joint Surg Br 67:709-714, 1985.
261. Hawkins RJ and Angelo RL: Glenohumeral osteoarthritis: A late complication of the Putti-Platt repair. J Bone Joint Surg Am 72:1193-1197, 1990.
262. Hawkins RJ, Koppert G, and Johnston G: Recurrent posterior instability (subluxation) of the shoulder. J Bone Joint Surg Am 66:169, 1984.
263. Hawkins RJ and Mohtadi NGH: Controversy in anterior shoulder instability. Clin Orthop 272:152-161, 1991.
264. Hawkins RJ, Neer CS II, Pianta R, and Mendoza FX: Missed posterior dislocations of the shoulder. Paper presented at the Annual Meeting of the American Academy of Orthopaedic Surgeons, 1982, New Orleans.
265. Hawkins RJ, Neer CS II, Pianta RM, and Mendoza FX: Locked posterior dislocation of the shoulder. J Bone Joint Surg Am 69:9, 1987.
266. Hayashi K, Thabit G 3rd, Massa KL, et al: The effect of thermal heating on the length and histologic properties of the glenohumeral joint capsule. Am J Sports Med 25:107-112, 1997.
267. Hayashi K, Thabit G 3rd, Vailas AC, et al: The effect of nonablative laser energy on joint capsular properties. An in vitro histologic and biochemical study using a rabbit model. Am J Sports Med 24:640-646, 1996.
268. Hecker AT, Shea M, Hayhurst JO, et al: Pull-out strength of suture anchors for rotator cuff and Bankart lesion repairs. Am J Sports Med 21:874-879, 1993.
269. Hehne HJ and Hubner H: Die Behandlung der rezidivieremden Schulterluxation nach Putti-Platt-Bankart und Eden-Hybinette-Lange. Orthop Prax 16:331-335, 1980.
270. Helfet AJ: Coracoid transplantation for recurring dislocation of the shoulder. J Bone Joint Surg Br 40:198-202, 1958.
271. Heller KD, Forst J, Forst R, and Cohen B: Posterior dislocation of the shoulder. Arch Orthop Trauma Surg 113:228-231, 1994.
272. Helm AT and Watson JS: Compression of the brachial plexus in a patient with false aneurysm of the axillary artery as a result of anterior shoulder dislocation. J Shoulder Elbow Surg 11:278-279, 2002.
273. Henderson MS: Habitual or recurrent dislocation of the shoulder. Surg Gynecol Obstet 33:1-7, 1921.
274. Henderson MS: Tenosuspension operation for recurrent or habitual dislocation of the shoulder. Surg Clin North Am 5:997-1007, 1949.
275. Henderson WD: Arthroscopic stabilization of the anterior shoulder. Clin Sports Med 6:581-586, 1987.
276. Henry JH and Genung JA: Natural history of glenohumeral dislocation—revisited. Am J Sports Med 10:135-137, 1982.
277. Henson GF: Vascular complications of shoulder injuries: A report of two cases. J Bone Joint Surg Br 38:528-531, 1956.
278. Hermodsson I: Rontgenologische Studein uber die Traumatischen und habituellen Schultergelenk-Verrenkungen nach Vorn und nach Unten. Acta Radiol Suppl 20:1-173, 1934.
279. Hertz H, Kwasny O, and Wohry G: Therapeutic procedure in initial traumatic shoulder dislocation (arthroscopy-limbus refixation). Unfallchirurgie 17:76-79, 1991.
280. Hertz H, Weinstabl R, Grundschober F, and Orthner E: Macroscopic and microscopic anatomy of the shoulder joint and the limbus glenoidalis. Acta Anat (Basel) 125:96-100, 1986.
281. Heymanowitsch Z: Ein Beitrag zur operativen Behandlung der habituellen Schulterluxationen. Zentralbl Chir 54:648-651, 1927.
282. Hildebrand: Zur operativen Behandlung der habituellen Schulterluxation. Arch Klin Chir 66:360-364, 1902.
283. Hill HA and Sachs MD: The grooved defect of the humeral head. A frequently unrecognized complication of dislocations of the shoulder joint. Radiology 35:690-700, 1940.
284. Hill JA, Lombardo SJ, Kerlan RK, et al: The modified Bristow-Helfet procedure for recurrent anterior shoulder subluxations and dislocations. Am J Sports Med 9:283-287, 1981.
285. Hill NA and McLaughlin HL: Locked posterior dislocation simulating a "frozen shoulder." J Trauma 3:225-234, 1963.
286. Hintermann B and Gachter A: Theo van Rens Prize. Arthroscopic assessment of the unstable shoulder. Knee Surg Sports Traumatol Arthrosc 2:64-69, 1994.
287. Hippocrates: Works of Hippocrates with an English Translation. London: William Heinemann, 1927.
288. Hirakawa M: On the etiology of the loose shoulder—biochemical studies on collagen from joint capsules. Nippon Seikeigeka Gakkai Zasshi 65:550-560, 1991.
289. Hirschfelder H and Kirsten U: Biometric analysis of the unstable shoulder. Z Orthop Ihre Grenzgeb 129:516-520, 1991.
290. Honner R: Bilateral posterior dislocation of the shoulder. Aust N Z J Surg 38:269-272, 1969.
291. Hovelius L: Incidence of shoulder dislocation in Sweden. Clin Orthop 166:127-131, 1982.
292. Hovelius L: Anterior dislocation of the shoulder in teenagers and young adults. Five-year prognosis. J Bone Joint Surg Am 69:393, 1987.
293. Hovelius L, Akermark C, and Albrektsson B: Bristow-Latarjet procedure for recurrent anterior dislocation of the shoulder. Acta Orthop Scand 54:284-290, 1983.
294. Hovelius L, Augustini BG, Fredin H, et al: Primary anterior dislocation of the shoulder in young patients. J Bone Joint Surg Am 78:1677-1684, 1996.
295. Hovelius L, Eriksson K, Fredin H, et al: Recurrences after initial dislocation of the shoulder. Results of a prospective study of treatment. J Bone Joint Surg Am 65:343-349, 1983.
296. Hovelius L, Malmqvist B, and Augustini BG: Ten year prognosis of primary anterior dislocation of the shoulder in young [abstract 2]. Paper presented at the 10th Open Meeting of the American Shoulder and Elbow Surgeons, 1994, New Orleans.
297. Hovelius L, Thorling J, and Fredin H: Recurrent anterior dislocation of the shoulder: Results after the Bankart and Putti-Platt operations. J Bone Joint Surg Am 61:566-569, 1979.
298. Howard FM and Shafer SJ: Injuries to the clavicle with neurovascular complications. J Bone Joint Surg Am 47:1335-1346, 1965.
299. Howell SM and Galinat BJ: The glenoid-labral socket: A constrained articular surface. Clin Orthop 43:122-125, 1989.
300. Howell SM, Galinat BJ, Renzi AJ, and Marone PJ: Normal and abnormal mechanics of the glenohumeral joint in the horizontal plane. J Bone Joint Surg Am 70:227-232, 1988.
301. Huber H and Gerber C: Voluntary subluxation of the shoulder in children. J Bone Joint Surg Br 76:118-122, 1994.
302. Hummel A, Bethke RO, and Kempf L: Die Behandlung der habituellen Schulterluxation nach dem Bristow-Verfahren. Unfallheilkunde 85:482-484, 1982.
303. Humphry GM: A Treatise on the Human Skeleton (Including the Joints), Vol 410. London: Macmillan, 1858, pp 73-74.
304. Hurley JA, Anderson TE, Dear WA, et al: Posterior shoulder instability. Surgical versus conservative results with evaluation of glenoid version. Am J Sports Med 20:396-400, 1992.
305. Hussein MK: Kocher's method is 3,000 years old. J Bone Joint Surg Br 50:669-671, 1968.

306. Hybbinette S: De la transplantation d'un fragment osseux pour remedier aux luxations récidivantes de l'épaule; constations et résultats operatoires. Acta Chir Scand 71:411-445, 1932.

307. Iannotti JP, Zlatkin MB, Esterhai JL, et al: Magnetic resonance imaging of the shoulder. Sensitivity, specificity, and predictive value. J Bone Joint Surg Am 73:17-29, 1991.

308. Imazato Y: Etiological considerations of the loose shoulder from a biochemical point of view—biochemical studies on collagen from deltoid and pectoral muscles and skin. Nippon Seikeigeka Gakkai Zasshi 66:1006-1015, 1992.

309. Inao S, Hirayama T, and Takemitsu Y: Irreducible acute anterior dislocation of the shoulder: Interposed bicipital tendon. J Bone Joint Surg Br 72:1079-1080, 1990.

310. Inman VT, Saunders JB, and Abbott LC: Observations on the function of the shoulder joint. J Bone Joint Surg Am 26:1-30, 1994.

311. Itoi E, Kuechle DK, Newman SR, et al: Stabilizing function of the biceps in stable and unstable shoulders. J Bone Joint Surg Br 75:546-550, 1993.

312. Itoi E, Lee SB, Berglund LJ, et al: The effect of a glenoid defect on anteroinferior stability of the shoulder after Bankart repair: A cadaveric study. J Bone Joint Surg Am 82:35-46, 2000.

313. Itoi EA, Motzkin NE, Browne AO, et al: Intraarticular pressure of the shoulder. Arthroscopy 9:406-413, 1993.

314. Itoi E, Motzkin NE, Morrey BP, and An KN: Scapular inclination and inferior stability of the shoulder. J Shoulder Elbow Surg 1:131-139, 1992.

315. Itoi E, Motzkin NE, Morrey BF, and An K: Bulk effect of rotator cuff on inferior glenohumeral stability as function of scapular inclination angle: A cadaver study. Tohoku J Exp Med 171:267-276, 1993.

316. Itoi E, Newman SR, Kuechle DK, et al: Dynamic anterior stabilizers of the shoulder with the arm in abduction. J Bone Joint Surg Br 76:834-836, 1994.

317. Itoi E, Sashi R, Minagawa H, et al: Position of immobilization after dislocation of the glenohumeral joint. A study with use of magnetic resonance imaging. J Bone Joint Surg Am 83:661-667, 2001.

318. Itoi E and Tabata S: Rotator cuff tears in anterior dislocation of the shoulder. Int Orthop 16:240-244, 1992.

319. Itoi E, Watanabe W, Yamada S, et al: Range of motion after Bankart repair. Vertical compared with horizontal capsulotomy. Am J Sports Med 29:441-445, 2001.

320. Janecki CJ and Shahcheragh GH: The forward elevation maneuver for reduction of anterior dislocations of the shoulder. Clin Orthop 164:177-180, 1982.

321. Jardon OM, Hood LT, and Lynch RD: Complete avulsion of the axillary artery as a complication of shoulder dislocation. J Bone Joint Surg Am 55:18-192, 1973.

322. Jee WH, McCauley TR, Katz LD, et al: Superior labral anterior posterior (SLAP) lesions of the glenoid labrum: Reliability and accuracy of MR arthrography for diagnosis. Radiology 218:127-132, 2001.

323. Jens J: The role of the subscapularis muscle in recurring dislocation of the shoulder [abstract]. J Bone Joint Surg Br 34:780, 1964.

324. Jerosch J, Castro WH, Grosse-Hackman A, and Clahsen H: Function of the glenohumeral ligaments in active protection of shoulder stability. Z Orthop Ihre Grenzgeb 133:67-71, 1995.

325. Jerosch J, Goertzen M, and Marquardt M: Possibilities of diagnostic sonography in assessment of instability of the shoulder joint. Unfallchirurg 94:88-94, 1991.

326. Jerosch J, Marquardt M, and Winklemann W: Ultrasound documentation of translational movement of the shoulder joint: Normal values and pathologic findings. Ultraschall Med 12:31-35, 1991.

327. Jerosch J, Moersler M, and Castro WH: The function of passive stabilizers of the glenohumeral joint—a biomechanical study. Z Orthop Ihre Grenzgeb 128:206-212, 1990.

328. Jobe FW: Unstable shoulders in the athletes. Instr Course Lect 34:228-231, 1985.

329. Jobe FW, Giangarra CE, Glousman RE, and Kvitne RS: Anterior capsulolabral reconstruction in throwing athletes [abstract]. Orthop Trans 13:230, 1989.

330. Jobe FW, Giangarra CE, Kvitne RS, and Glousman RE: Anterior capsulolabral reconstruction of the shoulder in athletes in overhand sports. Am J Sports Med 19:428-434, 1991.

331. Jobe FW, Moynes DR, and Brewster CE: Rehabilitation of shoulder joint instabilities. Orthop Clin North Am 18:473-482, 1987.

332. Jobe FW, Tibone JE, Perry J, and Moynes D: An EMG analysis of the shoulder in throwing and pitching. Am J Sports Med 11:3-5, 1983.

333. Jobe FW and Zeman B: How to detect and manage an unstable shoulder. J Musculoskel Med 2:60-68, 1985.

334. Joessel D: Ueber die recidine der humerus-luxationen. Dtsch Z Chir 13:167-184, 1880.

335. Johnson HF: Unreduced dislocation of the shoulder. Nebr State Med J 16:220-224, 1931.

336. Johnson JR and Bayley JIL: Loss of shoulder function following acute anterior dislocation. J Bone Joint Surg Br 63:633, 1981.

337. Johnson JR and Bayley JIL: Early complications of acute anterior dislocation of the shoulder in the middle-aged and elderly patient. Injury 13:431-434, 1982.

338. Johnson LL: Arthroscopy of the shoulder. Orthop Clin North Am 11:197-204, 1980.

339. Johnson LL: Symposium: The controversy of arthroscopic versus open approaches to shoulder instability and rotator cuff disease: A new perspective, a new opportunity, a new challenge. Paper presented at the 4th Open Meeting of the American Shoulder and Elbow Surgeons, 1988, Atlanta.

340. Johnson LL, Schneider DA, Austin MD, et al: Two percent glutaraldehyde: A disinfectant in arthroscopy and arthroscopic surgery. J Bone Joint Surg Am 64:237, 1982.

341. Johnston GW and Lowry JH: Rupture of the axillary artery complicating anterior dislocation of the shoulder. J Bone Joint Surg Br 44:116-118, 1962.

342. Jones FW: Attainment of upright position of man. Nature 146:26-27, 1940.

343. Jordan H: New technique for the roentgen examination of the shoulder joint. Radiology 25:480-484, 1935.

344. Jorgensen U and Bak K: Shoulder instability: Assessment of anterior-posterior translation with a knee laxity tester. Acta Orthop Scand 66:398-400, 1995.

345. Kaar TK, Schenck RC Jr, Wirth MA, and Rockwood CA Jr: Complications of metallic suture anchors in shoulder surgery: A report of 8 cases. Arthroscopy 17:31-37, 2001.

346. Kaltsas DS: Comparative study of the properties of the shoulder joint capsule with those of other joint capsules. Clin Orthop 173:20-26, 1983.

347. Karadimas J, Rentis G, and Varouchas G: Repair of recurrent anterior dislocation of the shoulder using transfer of the subscapularis tendon. J Bone Joint Surg Am 62:1147-1149, 1980.

348. Karlsson D and Peterson B: Towards a model for force predictions in the human shoulder. J Biomech 25:189-199, 1992.

349. Karlsson J, Magnusson L, Ejerhed L, et al: Comparison of open and arthroscopic stabilization for recurrent shoulder dislocation in patients with a Bankart lesion. Am J Sports Med 29:538-542, 2001.

350. Kavanaugh JH: Posterior shoulder dislocation with ipsilateral humeral shaft fracture. A case report. Clin Orthop 131:168-172, 1978.

351. Kazar B and Relovszky E: Prognosis of primary dislocation of the shoulder. Acta Orthop Scand 40:216, 1969.

352. Kelley JP: Fractures complicating electroconvulsive therapy and chronic epilepsy. J Bone Joint Surg Br 36:70-79, 1954.

353. Keppler P, Holz U, Thieleman FW, and Meinig R: Locked posterior dislocation of the shoulder. J Orthop Trauma 8:286-292, 1994.

354. Kiett GJ, Bloem JL, Rozing PM, et al: MR Imaging of recurrent anterior dislocation of the shoulder: Comparison with CT arthrography. AJR Am J Roentgenol 150:1083-1087, 1988.

355. Kim SH and Ha KI: Bankart repair in traumatic anterior shoulder instability: Open versus arthroscopic technique. Arthroscopy 18:755-763, 2002.

356. Kim SH, Ha KI, and Choi HJ: Results of arthroscopic treatment of superior labral lesions. J Bone Joint Surg Am 84:981-985, 2002.

357. Kim SH, Ha KI, Kim HS, and Kim SW: Electromyographic activity of the biceps brachii muscle in shoulders with anterior instability. Arthroscopy 17:864-868, 2001.

358. Kim SH, Ha KI, and Kim YM: Arthroscopic revision Bankart repair: A prospective outcome study. Arthroscopy 18:469-482, 2002.

359. Kinnard P, Gordon D, Levesque RY, and Bergeron D: Computerized arthrotomography in recurring shoulder dislocations and subluxations. Can J Surg 27:487-488, 1984.

360. Kirker JR: Dislocation of the shoulder complicated by rupture of the axillary vessels. J Bone Joint Surg Br 34:72-73, 1952.

361. Kiviluoto O, Pasila M, Jaroma H, and Sundholm A: Immobilization after primary dislocation of the shoulder. Acta Orthop Scand 51:915-919, 1980.

362. Kleinman PD, Kanzaria PK, Goss TP, and Pappas AM: Axillary arthrotomography of the glenoid labrum. AJR Am J Roentgenol 142:993-999, 1984.

363. Kocher T: Eine neue reductions Methode fur Schulterverrenkung. Berl Klin Wochenschr 7:101-105, 1870.

364. Koppert G and Hawkins RJ: Recurrent posterior dislocating shoulder. J Bone Joint Surg 62:127-128, 1980.

365. Kretzler HH: Posterior glenoid osteotomy. Paper presented at a meeting of the American Academy of Orthopaedic Surgeons, 1944, Dallas.

366. Kretzler HH and Blue AR: Recurrent posterior dislocation of the shoulder in cerebral palsy. J Bone Joint Surg Am 48:1221, 1966.

367. Kronberg M and Brostrom LA: Humeral head retroversion in patients with unstable humeroscapular joints. Clin Orthop 260:207-211, 1990.

368. Kronberg M, Brostrom LA, and Nemeth G: Differences in shoulder muscle activity between patients with generalized joint laxity and normal controls. Clin Orthop 269:181-192, 1991.

369. Kubin Z: Luxatio humeri erecta: Kasuisticke sdeleni. Acta Chir Orthop Traumatol Cech 31:565, 1964.

370. Kuboyama M: The role of soft tissues in downward stability of the glenohumeral joint—an experimental study with fresh cadavers. Igaku Kenkyu 61:20-33, 1991.

371. Kuhnen W and Groves RJ: Irreducible acute anterior dislocation of the shoulder: Case report. Clin Orthop 139:167-168, 1979.

372. Kumar VP and Balasubramaniam P: The role of atmospheric pressure in stabilizing the shoulder. An experimental study. J Bone Joint Surg Br 67:719-721, 1985.

373. Kuster E: Ueber habituelle schulter Luxation. Verh Dtsch Ges Chir 11:112-114, 1882.

374. Lacey T II: Reduction of anterior dislocation of the shoulder by means of the Milch abduction technique. J Bone Joint Surg Am 34:108-109, 1952.

375. Lam SAS: Irreducible anterior dislocation of the shoulder. J Bone Joint Surg Br 48:132, 1966.

376. Lamm CR, Zaehrisson BE, and Korner L: Radiography of the shoulder after Bristow repair. Acta Radiol Diagn 23:523-528, 1982.

377. Landsiedl F: Arthroscopic therapy of recurrent anterior luxation of the shoulder by capsular repair. Arthroscopy 8:296-304, 1992.
378. Lane JG, Sachs RA, and Riehl B: Arthroscopic staple capsulorrhaphy: A long-term follow-up. Arthroscopy 9:190-194, 1993.
379. Lange M: Die operative Behandlung der gewohnheitsmabigen Verrenkung an Schulter. Knie Fub Z Orthop 75:162, 1944.
380. Langfritz HV: Die doppelseitige traumatische Luxatio Humeri Erecta eine seltene Verletzungsform. Monatschr Unfallheilkunde 59, 1956.
381. Laskin RS and Sedlin ED: Luxatio erecta in infancy. Clin Orthop 80:126-129, 1971.
382. Latarjet M: Technique de la butée coracoidienne preplenoidienne dans le traitement des luxations récidivantes de l'épaule. Lyon Chir 54:604-607, 1958.
383. Latarjet M: Résultat du traitement des luxations récidivantes de l'épaule par le procédé de Latarjet, à propos de 42 cas. Lyon Chir 64, 1968.
384. Lavik K: Habitual shoulder luxation. Acta Orthop Scand 30:251-264, 1961.
385. Lawrence WS: New position in radiographing the shoulder joint. AJR Am J Roentgenol 2:728-730, 1915.
386. Lazarus MD and Harryman DT II: Complications of open anterior repairs for instability and their solutions. In Warner J, Iannotti J, and Gerber R (eds): Complex and Revision Problems in Shoulder Surgery. Philadelphia: Lippincott-Raven, 1996.
387. Lazarus MD, Sidles JA, Harryman DT II, and Matsen FA III: Effect of a chondral-labral defect on glenoid concavity and glenohumeral stability: A cadaveric model. J Bone Joint Surg Am 78:94-102, 1996.
388. Leach RE, Corbett M, Schepsis A, and Stockel J: Results of a modified Putti-Platt operation for recurrent shoulder dislocation and subluxation. Clin Orthop 164:20-25, 1982.
389. Lee AJ, Garraway WM, Hepburn W, and Laidlaw R: Influence of rugby injuries on players' subsequent health and lifestyle: Beginning a long term follow up. Br J Sports Med 35:38-42, 2001.
390. Lee SB and An KN: Dynamic glenohumeral stability provided by three heads of the deltoid muscle. Clin Orthop 400:40-47, 2002.
391. Leffert RD and Seddon H: Infraclavicular brachial plexus injuries. J Bone Joint Surg Br 47:9-22, 1965.
392. Lemmens JA and de Waal Malefijt J: Radiographic evaluation of the modified Bristow procedure for recurrent anterior dislocation of the shoulder. Diagn Imaging Clin Med 53:221-225, 1984.
393. L'Episcopo JB: Restoration of muscle balance in the treatment of obstetrical paralysis. N Y J Med 39:357-363, 1939.
394. Lerat JL, Chotel F, Besse JL, et al: Dynamic anterior jerk of the shoulder. A new clinical test for shoulder instability: Preliminary study. Rev Chir Orthop Reparatrice Appar Mot 80:461-467, 1994.
395. Lescher TJ and Andersen OS: Occlusion of the axillary artery complicating shoulder dislocation: Case report. Mil Med 144:621-622, 1979.
396. Leslie JT and Ryan TJ: The anterior axillary incision to approach the shoulder joint. J Bone Joint Surg Am 44:1193-1196, 1962.
397. Lev-El A and Rubinstein Z: Axillary artery injury in erect dislocation of the shoulder. J Trauma 21:323-325, 1981.
398. Levick JR: Joint pressure-volume studies: Their importance, design and interpretation. J Rheumatol 10:353-357, 1983.
399. Levine WN, Arroyo JS, Pollock RG, et al: Open revision stabilization surgery for recurrent anterior glenohumeral instability. Am J Sports Med 28:156-160, 2000.
400. Levine WN, Richmond JC, and Donaldson WR: Use of the suture anchor in open Bankart reconstruction: A follow-up report. Am J Sports Med 22:723-726, 1994.
401. Levitz CL, Dugas J, and Andrews JR: The use of arthroscopic thermal capsulorrhaphy to treat internal impingement in baseball players. Arthroscopy 17:573-577, 2001.
402. Levy O, Wilson M, Williams H, et al: Thermal capsular shrinkage for shoulder instability. Mid-term longitudinal outcome study. J Bone Joint Surg Br 83:640-645, 2001.
403. Leyder P, Augereau B, and Apoil A: Traitement des luxations postérieures inveterées de l'épaule par double abord et butée osseuse retro-glenoidienne. Ann Chir 34:806-809, 1980.
404. Lieber R: Skeletal Muscle Structure and Function. Baltimore: Williams & Wilkins, 1992, p 314.
405. Liedelmeyer R: External rotation method of shoulder dislocation reduction [letter]. Ann Emerg Med 10:228, 1981.
406. Lilleby H: Arthroscopy of the shoulder joint. Acta Orthop Scand 53:708-709, 1982.
407. Lindholm TS and Elmstedt E: Bilateral posterior dislocation of the shoulder combined with fracture of the proximal humerus. Acta Orthop Scand 51:485-488, 1980.
408. Lippert FG: A modification of the gravity method of reducing anterior shoulder dislocations. Clin Orthop 165:259-260, 1982.
409. Lippitt SB, Harris SL, Harryman DT II, et al: In vivo quantification of the laxity of normal and unstable glenohumeral joints. J Shoulder Elbow Surg 3:215-223, 1994.
410. Lippitt SB, Harryman DT II, Sidles JA, and Matsen FA III: Diagnosis and management of AMBRI syndrome techniques. Tech Orthop 6:61-73, 1991.
411. Lippitt SB, Kennedy JP, and Thompson TR: Intraarticular lidocaine versus intravenous analgesia in the reduction of dislocated shoulders. Orthop Trans 15:804, 1991.
412. Lippitt SB, Kennedy JP, and Thompson TR: Intraarticular lidocaine versus intravenous analgesia in the reduction of dislocated shoulders. Orthop Trans 16:230, 1992.
413. Lippitt SB, Vanderhooft JE, Harris SL, et al: Glenohumeral stability from concavity-compression: A quantitative analysis. J Shoulder Elbow Surg 2:27-35, 1993.
414. Liu SH and Boynton E: Posterior superior impingement of the rotator cuff on the glenoid rim as a cause of shoulder pain in the overhead athlete. Arthroscopy 9:697-699, 1993.
415. Liu SH and Henry MH: Anterior shoulder instability. Clin Orthop 323:327-337, 1996.
416. Löbker K: Einige Präparate von habitueller Schulterluxation. Arch Klin Chir 34:658-667, 1887.
417. Loomer R and Graham B: Anatomy of the axillary nerve and its relation to inferior capsular shift. Clin Orthop 243:100-105, 1989.
418. Loutzenheiser TD, Harryman DT II, Yung SW, et al: Optimizing arthroscopic knots. Arthroscopy 11:199-206, 1995.
419. Lower RF, McNiesh LM, and Callaghan JJ: Computed tomographic documentation of intra-articular penetration of a screw after operations on the shoulder: A report of two cases. J Bone Joint Surg Am 67:1120-1122, 1985.
420. Lucas GL and Peterson MD: Open anterior dislocation of the shoulder. J Trauma 17:883-884, 1977.
421. Luetzow WF, Atkin DM, and Sachs RA: Arthroscopic versus open Bankart repair of the shoulder for recurrent anterior dislocations. Paper presented at the American Academy of Orthopaedic Surgeons Specialty Day, American Shoulder and Elbow Surgeons Annual Open Meeting, 1995.
422. Lusardi DA, Wirth MA, Wurtz D, and Rockwood CA Jr: Loss of external rotation following anterior capsulorrhaphy of the shoulder. J Bone Joint Surg Am 75:1185-1192, 1993.
423. Lynn FS: Erect dislocation of the shoulder. Surg Gynecol Obstet 39:51-55, 1921.
424. Lyons TR, Griffith PL, Savoie FH III, and Field LD: Laser-assisted capsulorrhaphy for multidirectional instability of the shoulder. Arthroscopy 17:25-30, 2001.
425. MacDonald PB, Hawkins RJ, Fowler PJ, and Miniaci A: Release of the subscapularis for internal rotation contracture and pain after anterior repair for recurrent dislocation of the shoulder. J Bone Joint Surg Am 74:734-737, 1992.
426. Mack LA, Matsen FA III, and Kilcoyne RF: Ultrasound: US evaluation of the rotator cuff. Radiology 157:205, 1985.
427. Mackenzie DB: The Bristow-Helfet operation for recurrent anterior dislocation of the shoulder. J Bone Joint Surg Br 62:273-274, 1980.
428. Mackenzie DB: The treatment of recurrent anterior shoulder dislocation by the modified Bristow-Helfet procedure. S Afr Med J 65:325, 1984.
429. Magnuson PB: Treatment of recurrent dislocation of the shoulder. Surg Clin North Am 25:14-20, 1945.
430. Magnuson PB and Stack JK: Bilateral habitual dislocation of the shoulder in twins, a familial tendency. JAMA 144:2103, 1940.
431. Magnuson PB and Stack JK: Recurrent dislocation of the shoulder. JAMA 123:889-892, 1943.
432. Maki S and Gruen T: Anthropomorphic studies of the glenohumeral joint. Trans Orthop Res Soc 1:173, 1976.
433. Malgaigne JF: Traite des Fractures et des Luxations. Paris: JB Bailliere, 1855.
434. Manes HR: A new method of shoulder reduction in the elderly. Clin Orthop 147:200-202, 1980.
435. Markel MD, Hayashi K, Thabit GR, and Thielke RJ: Changes in articular capsular tissue using holmium:YAG laser at non-ablative energy densities. Potential application in non-ablative stabilization procedures. Orthopade 25:37-41, 1996.
436. Marquardt M and Jerosch J: Ultrasound evaluation of multidirectional instability of the shoulder. Unfallchirurg 94:295-301, 1991.
437. Martin B, Javelot T, and Vidal J: Long-term results obtained with the Bankart method for the treatment of recurring anterior instability of the shoulder. Chir Organi Mov 76:199-207, 1991.
438. Martin SS, and Limbird TJ: The terrible triad of the shoulder. J South Orthop Assoc 8:57-60, 1999.
439. Marx RG, McCarty EC, Montemurno TD, et al: Development of arthrosis following dislocation of the shoulder: A case-control study. J Shoulder Elbow Surg 11:1-5, 2002.
440. Matsen FA III, Fu FH, and Hawkins RJ (eds): The Shoulder: A Balance of Mobility and Stability. Rosemont, IL: American Academy of Orthopaedic Surgeons, 1993.
441. Matsen FA III, Lippitt SB, Sidles JA, and Harryman DT II: Practical Evaluation and Management of the Shoulder. Philadelphia: WB Saunders, 1994.
442. Matsen FA III and Thomas SC: Glenohumeral instability. In Evarts CMC (ed): Surgery of the Musculoskeletal System, vol 3. New York: Churchill Livingstone, 1990, pp 1439-1469.
443. Matsen FA III, Thomas SC, and Rockwood CA Jr: Glenohumeral instability. In Rockwood CA Jr and Matsen FA III (eds): The Shoulder, vol 1. Philadelphia: WB Saunders, 1990, pp 547-551.
444. Matthews L, Vetter W, Oweida S, et al: Arthroscopic staple capsulorrhaphy for recurrent anterior shoulder instability. Arthroscopy 4:106-111, 1988.
445. May VR: A modified Bristow operation for anterior recurrent dislocation of the shoulder. J Bone Joint Surg Am 52:1010-1016, 1970.
446. McEleney ET, Donovan MJ, Shea KP, and Nowak MD: Initial failure strength of open and arthroscopic Bankart repairs. Arthroscopy 11:426-431, 1995.

447. McFarland EG, Neira CA, Gutierrez MI, et al: Clinical significance of the arthroscopic drive-through sign in shoulder surgery. Arthroscopy 17:38-43, 2001.
448. McFie J: Bilateral anterior dislocation of the shoulders: A case report. Injury 8:67-69, 1976.
449. McGlynn FJ, El-Khoury G, and Albright JP: Arthrotomography of the glenoid labrum in shoulder instability. J Bone Joint Surg Am 64:506-518, 1982.
450. McIntyre LF and Caspari RB: The rationale and technique for arthroscopic reconstruction of anterior shoulder instability using multiple sutures. Orthop Clin North Am 24:55-58, 1993.
451. McKenzie AD and Sinclair AM: Axillary artery occlusion complicating shoulder dislocation. Am Surg 148:139-141, 1958.
452. McLaughlin HL: Discussion of acute anterior dislocation of the shoulder by Toufick Nicola. J Bone Joint Surg Am 31:172, 1949.
453. McLaughlin HL: On the "frozen" shoulder. Bull Hosp Jt Dis 12:383-393, 1951.
454. McLaughlin HL: Posterior dislocation of the shoulder. J Bone Joint Surg Am 34:584, 1952.
455. McLaughlin HL: Trauma. Philadelphia: WB Saunders, 1959.
456. McLaughlin HL: Recurrent anterior dislocation of the shoulder. I. Morbid anatomy. Am J Surg 99:628-632, 1960.
457. McLaughlin HL: Dislocation of the shoulder with tuberosity fractures. Surg Clin North Am 43:1615-1620, 1963.
458. McLaughlin HL: Locked posterior subluxation of the shoulder—diagnosis and treatment. Surg Clin North Am 43:1621, 1963.
459. McLaughlin HL and Cavallaro WU: Primary anterior dislocation of the shoulder. Am J Surg 80:615-621, 1950.
460. McLaughlin HL and MacLellan DI: Recurrent anterior dislocation of the shoulder. II. A comparative study. J Trauma 7:191-201, 1967.
461. McMahon PJ, Dettling JR, Sandusky MD, and Lee TQ: Deformation and strain characteristics along the length of the anterior band of the inferior glenohumeral ligament. J Shoulder Elbow Surg 10:482-488, 2001.
462. McMaster WC: Anterior glenoid labrum damage: A painful lesion in swimmers. Am J Sports Med 14:383-387, 1986.
463. McMurray TB: Recurrent dislocation of the shoulder (Proceedings). J Bone Joint Surg Br 43:402, 1961.
464. Mead NC and Sweeney HJ: Bristow procedure. Spectator Letter 1964.
465. Meadowcroft JA and Kain TM: Luxatio erecta shoulder dislocation: Report of two cases. Jefferson Orthop J 6:20-24, 1977.
466. Merrill V: Atlas of Roentgenographic Positions and Standard Radiologic Procedures, vol 1, 4th ed. St Louis: CV Mosby, 1975.
467. Mestdagh H, Maynou C, Delobelle JM, et al: Traumatic posterior dislocation of the shoulder in adults. A propos of 25 cases. Ann Chir 48:355-363, 1994.
468. Metcalf MH, Duckworth DG, Lee SB, et al: Posteroinferior glenoplasty can change glenoid shape and increase the mechanical stability of the shoulder. J Shoulder Elbow Surg 8:205-213, 1999.
469. Metcalf MH, Pond JD, Harryman DT 2nd, et al: Capsulolabral augmentation increases glenohumeral stability in the cadaver shoulder. J Shoulder Elbow Surg 10:532-538, 2001.
470. Meyer SJ and Dalinka MK: Magnetic resonance imaging of the shoulder. Orthop Clin North Am 21:497-513, 1990.
471. Middeldorpf M and Scharm B: De Nova Humeri Luxationis Specie. Clinique Europenne, Inaugural Dissertation, vol 2. Breslau, Poland, 1859.
472. Milch H: Treatment of dislocation of the shoulder. Surgery 3:732-740, 1938.
473. Miller LS, Donahue JR, Good RP, and Staerk AJ: The Magnuson-Stack procedure for treatment of recurrent glenohumeral dislocation. Am J Sports Med 12:133, 1984.
474. Mills KLG: Simultaneous bilateral posterior fracture dislocation of the shoulder. Injury 6:39-41, 1974-1975.
475. Milton GW: The mechanism of circumflex and other nerve injuries in dislocation of the shoulder and the possible mechanism of nerve injuries during reduction of dislocation. Aust N Z J Surg 23:24-30, 1953-1955.
476. Milton GW: The circumflex nerve and dislocation of the shoulder. Br J Phys Med 17:136-138, 1954.
477. Minkoff J and Cavaliere G: Glenohumeral instabilities and the role of magnetic resonance imaging techniques. The orthopedic surgeon's perspective. Magn Reson Imaging Clin N Am 1:105-123, 1993.
478. Mirick MJ, Clinton JE, and Ruiz E: External rotation method of shoulder dislocation reduction. J Am Coll Emerg Physicians 8:528-531, 1979.
479. Mishra DK and Fanton GS: Two-year outcome of arthroscopic Bankart repair and electrothermal-assisted capsulorrhaphy for recurrent traumatic anterior shoulder instability. Arthroscopy 17:844-849, 2001.
480. Mital MA and Karlin LI: Diagnostic arthroscopy in sports injuries. Orthop Clin North Am 11:771-785, 1980.
481. Moeller JC: Compound posterior dislocation of the shoulder. J Bone Joint Surg Am 57:1006-1007, 1975.
482. Mologne TS, Lapoint JM, Morin WD, and Zilberfarb J: Arthroscopic anterior labral reconstruction using a transglenoid suture technique: Results in the active duty military patient. Paper presented at the American Academy of Orthopaedics Surgeons Specialty Day, American Shoulder and Elbow Surgeons, 1995, Orlando, FL.
483. Montgomery WH and Jobe FW: Functional outcomes in athletes after modified anterior capsulolabral reconstruction. Am J Sports Med 22:352-357, 1994.
484. Moran MC and Warren RF: Development of a synovial cyst after arthroscopy of the shoulder. A brief note. J Bone Joint Surg Am 71:127-129, 1989.
485. Morgan CD: Arthroscopic transglenoid Bankart suture repair. Oper Tech Orthop 1:171-179, 1991.
486. Morgan CD and Bodenstab AB: Arthroscopic Bankart suture repair: Technique and early results. Arthroscopy 3:111-122, 1987.
487. Morgan CD, Rames RD, and Snyder SJ: Arthroscopic assessment of anatomic variants of the glenohumeral ligaments associated with recurrent anterior shoulder instability. Orthop Trans 15:727, 1992.
488. Morrey BF and Janes JM: Recurrent anterior dislocation of the shoulder: Long-term follow-up of the Putti-Platt and Bankart procedures. J Bone Joint Surg Am 58:252-256, 1976.
489. Moseley HF: Shoulder Lesions. Springfield, IL: Charles C Thomas, 1945.
490. Moseley HF: Recurrent Dislocations of the Shoulder. Montreal: McGill University Press, 1961.
491. Moseley HF: The basic lesions of recurrent anterior dislocation. Surg Clin North Am 43:1631-1634, 1963.
492. Moseley HF: Shoulder Lesions. Edinburgh: Churchill Livingstone, 1972.
493. Moseley HF and Overgaard B: The anterior capsular mechanism in recurrent anterior dislocation of the shoulder: Morphological and clinical studies with special reference to the glenoid labrum and glenohumeral ligaments. J Bone Joint Surg Br 44:913-927, 1962.
494. Mowery CA, Garfin SR, Booth RE, and Rothman RH: Recurrent posterior dislocation of the shoulder: treatment using a bone block. J Bone Joint Surg Am 67:777-781, 1985.
495. Müller W: Über den negativen Luftdruck im Gelenkraum. Dtsch Z Chir 217:395-401, 1929.
496. Mumenthaler M and Schliack H: Lasionen Peripherer Nerven. Stuttgart, Germany: Georg Thieme Verlag, 1965.
497. Murrard J: Un cas de luxatio erecta de l'épaule double et symmétrique. Rev Orthop 7:423, 1920.
498. Myers JB and Lephart SM: Sensorimotor deficits contributing to glenohumeral instability. Clin Orthop 400:98-104, 2002.
499. Mynter H: Subacromial dislocation from muscular spasm. Ann Surg 36:117-119, 1902.
500. Neer CS II: Degenerative lesions of the proximal humeral articular surface. Clin Orthop 20:116-124, 1961.
501. Neer CS II: Fractures of the distal third of the clavicle. Clin Orthop 58:43-50, 1968.
502. Neer CS II: Displaced proximal humeral fractures. I. Classification and evaluation. J Bone Joint Surg Am 52:1077-1089, 1970.
503. Neer CS II and Foster CR: Inferior capsular shift for involuntary inferior and multidirectional instability of the shoulder: A preliminary report. J Bone Joint Surg Am 62:897-908, 1980.
504. Neer CS II and Horwitz BS: Fracture of the proximal humeral epiphyseal plate. Clin Orthop 41:24-31, 1965.
505. Neer CS II, Satterlee CC, Dalsey RM, and Flatow EL: On the value of the coracohumeral ligament release. Orthop Trans 13:235-236, 1989.
506. Neumann CH, Petersen SA, and Jahnke AH: MR imaging of the labral capsular complex: Normal variation. AJR Am J Roentgenol 157:1015-1021, 1991.
507. Neviaser RJ, Neviaser TJ, and Neviaser JS: Concurrent rupture of the rotator cuff and anterior dislocation of the shoulder in the older patient. J Bone Joint Surg Am 70:1308-1311, 1988.
508. Neviaser RJ, Neviaser TJ, and Neviaser JS: Anterior dislocation of the shoulder and rotator cuff rupture. Clin Orthop 291:103-106, 1993.
509. Neviaser TJ: The anterior labroligamentous periosteal sleeve avulsion lesion: A cause of anterior instability of the shoulder. Arthroscopy 9:17-21, 1993.
510. Ng KC, Singh S, and Low YP: Axillary artery damage from shoulder trauma—a report of 2 cases. Chirurgie 116:190-193, 1990.
511. Nicola FG, Ellman H, Eckardt J, and Finerman G: Bilateral posterior fracture-dislocation of the shoulder treated with a modification of the McLaughlin procedure. J Bone Joint Surg Am 63:1175-1177, 1981.
512. Nicola T: Recurrent anterior dislocation of the shoulder. J Bone Joint Surg 11:128-132, 1929.
513. Nicola T: Recurrent dislocation of the shoulder—its treatment by transplantation of the long head of the biceps. Am J Surg 6:815, 1929.
514. Nicola T: Anterior dislocation of the shoulder: The role of the articular capsule. J Bone Joint Surg 24:614-616, 1942.
515. Nicola T: Acute anterior dislocation of the shoulder. J Bone Joint Surg Am 31:153-159, 1949.
516. Nicola T: Recurrent dislocation of the shoulder. Am J Surg 86:85-91, 1953.
517. Nielsen AB and Nielsen K: The modified Bristow procedure for recurrent anterior dislocation of the shoulder. Acta Orthop Scand 53:229-232, 1982.
518. Niskanen RO, Lehtonen JY, and Kaukonen JP: Alvik's glenoplasty for humeroscapular dislocation. Acta Orthop Scand 62:279-283, 1991.
519. Nobel W: Posterior traumatic dislocation of the shoulder. J Bone Joint Surg Am 44:523-538, 1962.
520. Nobuhara K and Ikeda H: Rotator interval lesion. Clin Orthop 223:44-50, 1987.
521. Noesberger B and Mader G: Die modifizierte Operation nach Trillat bei habitueller Schulterluxation. Z Unf Med Berufskr 69:34-36, 1976.
522. Norris TR: C-Arm Fluoroscopic Evaluation under Anesthesia for Glenohumeral Subluxations. Philadelphia: BC Decker, 1984, pp 22-25.

523. Norris TR, Bigliani LU, and Harris E: Complications following the modified Bristow repair for shoulder instability. Paper presented at the American Shoulder and Elbow Surgeons 3rd Open Meeting, 1987, San Francisco.

524. Obremskey WT, Lippitt SB, Harryman DT II, and Matsen FA III: Follow-up of the inferior capsular shift procedure for atraumatic multidirectional instability. Submitted to Clin Orthop 1995.

525. O'Brien SJ, Neves MC, Arnoczky SP, et al: The anatomy and histology of the inferior glenohumeral ligament complex of the shoulder. Am J Sports Med 18:449-456, 1990.

526. Obrzut SL, Hecht P, Hayashi K, et al: The effect of radiofrequency energy on the length and temperature properties of the glenohumeral joint capsule. Arthroscopy 14:395-400, 1998.

527. O'Connell PW, Nuber GW, Mileski RA, and Lautenschlager E: The contribution of the glenohumeral ligaments to anterior stability of the shoulder joint. Am J Sports Med 18:579-584, 1990.

528. O'Conner SJ: Posterior dislocation of the shoulder. Arch Surg 72:479-491, 1956.

529. O'Conner SJ and Jacknow AS: Posterior dislocation of the shoulder. J Bone Joint Surg Am 37:1122, 1955.

530. O'Driscoll SW: Atraumatic instability: Pathology and pathogenesis. In Matsen III FA, Fu FH, and Hawkins RJ (eds): The Shoulder: A Balance of Mobility and Stability. Rosemont, IL: American Academy of Orthopaedic Surgeons, 1993, pp 305-318.

531. O'Driscoll SW and Evans DC: The DuToit Staple Capsulorrhaphy for Recurrent Anterior Dislocation of the Shoulder: Twenty Years of Experience in Six Toronto Hospitals. Paper presented at the American Shoulder and Elbow Surgeons 4th Open Meeting, 1988, Atlanta.

532. O'Driscoll SW and Evans DC: Long-term results of staple capsulorrhaphy for anterior instability of the shoulder. J Bone Joint Surg Am 75:249-258, 1993.

533. Older MWJ: Arthroscopy of the shoulder joint. J Bone Joint Surg Br 58:253, 1976.

534. Olsson O: Degenerative changes of the shoulder joint and their connection with shoulder pain. Acta Chir Scand Suppl 181:1-130, 1953.

535. Onabowale BO and Jaja MOA: Unreduced bilateral synchronous shoulder dislocations. Niger Med J 9:267-271, 1979.

536. Onyeka W: Anterior shoulder dislocation: An unusual complication. Emerg Med J 19:367-368, 2002.

537. Oppenheim WL, Dawson EG, Quinlan C, and Graham SA: The cephaloscapular projection: A special diagnostic aid. Clin Orthop 195:191-193, 1985.

538. Orlinsky M, Shon S, Chiang C, et al: Comparative study of intra-articular lidocaine and intravenous meperidine/diazepam for shoulder dislocations. J Emerg Med 22:241-245, 2002.

539. Osmond-Clarke H: Habitual dislocation of the shoulder. The Putti-Platt operation. J Bone Joint Surg Br 30:19-25, 1948.

540. Oudard P: La luxation reécidivante de l'épaule (variete anterointerne) procédé opératoire. J Chir 23:13, 1924.

541. Ovesen J and Nielsen S: Experimental distal subluxation in the glenohumeral joint. Arch Orthop Trauma Surg 104:82-84, 1985.

542. Ovesen J and Nielsen S: Stability of the shoulder joint: Cadaver study of stabilizing structures. Acta Orthop Scand 56:149-151, 1985.

543. Ozaki J: Glenohumeral movement of the involuntary inferior and multidirectional instability. Clin Orthop 238:107-111, 1989.

544. Paavolainen P, Bjorkenheim JM, Ahovuo J, and Slatis P: Recurrent anterior dislocation of the shoulder. Results of Eden-Hybinette and Putti-Platt operations. Acta Orthop Scand 55:556-560, 1984.

545. Pagden D, Halaburt AS, Wiroszo R, and Karyn A: Posterior dislocation of the shoulder complicating regional anesthesia. Anesth Analg 65:1063-1065, 1986.

546. Pagnani MJ, Deng XH, Warren RF, et al: Effect of lesions of the superior portion of the glenoid labrum on glenohumeral translation. J Bone Joint Surg Am 77:1003-1010, 1995.

547. Pagnani MJ, and Dome DC: Surgical treatment of traumatic anterior shoulder instability in American football players. J Bone Joint Surg Am 84:711-715, 2002.

548. Palmer I and Widen A: The bone block method for recurrent dislocation of the shoulder joint. J Bone Joint Surg Br 30:53, 1948.

549. Palmer WE and Caslowitz PL: Anterior shoulder instability: Diagnostic criteria determined from prospective analysis of 121 MR arthrograms. Radiology 197:819-825, 1995.

550. Pappas AM, Goss TP, and Kleinman PK: Symptomatic shoulder instability due to lesions of the glenoid labrum. Am J Sports Med 11:279-288, 1983.

551. Parisien JS: Shoulder arthroscopy technique and indications. Bull Hosp Jt Dis 43:56-69, 1983.

552. Parisien VM: Shoulder dislocation: An easier method of reduction. J Maine Med Assoc 70:102, 1979.

553. Parrish GA and Skiendzielewski JJ: Bilateral posterior fracture-dislocations of the shoulder after convulsive status epilepticus. Ann Emerg Med 14:264-266, 1985.

554. Parsons SW and Rowley DI: Brachial plexus lesions in dislocations and fracture dislocation of the shoulder. J R Coll Surg Edinb 31:85-87, 1986.

555. Pascoet G, Jung F, Foucher G, and Kehr P: Treatment of recurrent dislocation of the shoulder by preglenoid artificial ridge using the Latarjet-Vittori technique. J Med Strasbourg 6:501-504, 1975.

556. Pasila M, Jaroma H, and Kiviluoto O: Early complications of primary shoulder dislocations. Acta Orthop Scand 49:260-263, 1978.

557. Pasila M, Kiviluoto O, Jaroma H, and Sundholm A: Recovery from primary shoulder dislocation and its complications. Acta Orthop Scand 51:257-262, 1980.

558. Patel MR, Pardee ML, and Singerman RC: Intrathoracic dislocation of the head of the humerus. J Bone Joint Surg Am 45:1712-1714, 1963.

559. Pavlov H, Warren RF, Weiss CBJ, and Dines DM: The roentgenographic evaluation of anterior shoulder instability. Clin Orthop 194:153-158, 1985.

560. Peiro A, Ferrandis R, and Correa F: Bilateral erect dislocation of the shoulders. Injury 6:294, 1975.

561. Percy LR: Recurrent posterior dislocation of the shoulder. J Bone Joint Surg Br 42:863, 1960.

562. Perniceni B and Augereau A: Treatment of old unreduced anterior dislocations of the shoulder by open reduction and reinforced rib graft: Discussion of three cases. Ann Chir 36:235-239, 1983.

563. Perry J and Glousman RE: Biomechanics of Throwing. St Louis: CV Mosby, 1989, pp 727-751.

564. Perthes G: Uber Operationen bei habitueller Schulterluxation. Dtsch Z Chir 85:199-222, 1906.

565. Pettersson G: Rupture of the tendon aponeurosis of the shoulder joint in anterior inferior dislocation. Acta Chir Scand Suppl 77:1-187, 1942.

566. Pilz W: Zur Rontgenuntersuchung der habituellen Schulterverrenkung. Arch Klin Chir 135:1-22, 1925.

567. Pollock RG and Bigliani LU: Recurrent posterior shoulder instability: Diagnosis and treatment. Clin Orthop 291:85-96, 1993.

568. Pollock RG, Owens JM, Flatow EL, and Bigliani LU: Operative results of the inferior capsular shift procedure for multidirectional instability of the shoulder. J Bone Joint Surg Am 82:919-28, 2000.

569. Poppen NK and Walker PS: Normal and abnormal motion of the shoulder. J Bone Joint Surg Am 58:195, 1976.

570. Poppen NK and Walker PS: Forces at the glenohumeral joint in abduction. Clin Orthop 135:165-170, 1978.

571. Porteous MJL and Miller AJ: Humeral rotation osteotomy for chronic posterior dislocation of the shoulder. J Bone Joint Surg Br 72:181-186, 1990.

572. Post M: The Shoulder. Surgical and Non-surgical Management. Philadelphia: Lea & Febiger, 1978.

573. Prodromos CC, Ferry JA, Schiller AL, and Zarins B: Histological studies of the glenoid labrum from fetal life to old age. J Bone Joint Surg Am 72:1344-1348, 1990.

574. Protzman RR: Anterior instability of the shoulder. J Bone Joint Surg Am 62:909-918, 1980.

575. Prozorovskii VF, Khvisiuk NI, and Gevorkian AD: Surgical treatment of anterior instability of the shoulder joint. Ortop Traumatol Protez 4:14-18, 1991.

576. Quigley TB and Freedman PA: Recurrent dislocation of the shoulder. Am J Surg 128:595-599, 1974.

577. Rafii M, Firooznia H, and Bonamo JJ: CT arthrography of capsular structures of the shoulder. AJR Am J Roentgenol 146:361-367, 1986.

578. Rafii M, Firooznia H, and Bonamo JJ: Athlete shoulder injuries: CT arthrographic findings. Radiology 162:559-564, 1987.

579. Rafii M, Firooznia H, Golimbu C, and Weinreb J: Magnetic resonance imaging of glenohumeral instability. Magn Reson Imaging Clin N Am 1:87-104, 1993.

580. Randelli M and Gambrioli PL: Glenohumeral osteometry by computed tomography in normal and unstable shoulders. Clin Orthop 208:151, 1986.

581. Rao JP, Francis AM, Hurley J, and Daczkewycz R: Treatment of recurrent anterior dislocation of the shoulder by duToit staple capsulorrhaphy: Results of long-term follow-up study. Clin Orthop 204:169, 1986.

582. Reeves B: Arthrography in acute dislocation of the shoulder. J Bone Joint Surg Br 48:182, 1968.

583. Reeves B: Experiments on the tensile strength of the anterior capsular structures of the shoulder in man. J Bone Joint Surg 50:858-865, 1968.

584. Reeves B: Acute anterior dislocation of the shoulder. Ann R Coll Surg Engl 43:255, 1969.

585. Resch H: Current aspects in the arthroscopic treatment of shoulder instability. Orthopade 20:273-281, 1991.

586. Resch H, Wykypiel HF, Maurer H, and Wambacher M: The antero-inferior (transmuscular) approach for arthroscopic repair of the Bankart lesion: An anatomic and clinical study. J Arthrosc 12:309-319, 1996.

587. Rhee KJ, Ahn SR, and Lee JK: Arthroscopic capsular suture for anterior instability of the shoulder. Orthopedics 15:217-224, 1992.

588. Rhee YG, Harryman DT II, Romeo AA, et al: Translational laxity of the glenohumeral joint. Submitted to Am J Sports Med, 1994.

589. Ribbans WJ, Mitchell R, and Taylor GJ: Computerized arthrotomography of primary anterior dislocation of the shoulder. J Bone Joint Surg Br 72:181-185, 1990.

590. Richards RD, Sartoris DJ, Pathria MN, and Resnick D: Hill-Sachs lesion and normal humeral groove: MR imaging features allowing their differentiation. Radiology 190:665-668, 1994.

591. Richards RR, Beaton D, and Hudson AR: Shoulder arthrodesis with plate fixation: Functional outcome analysis. J Shoulder Elbow Surg 2:225-239, 1993.

592. Richards RR, Waddell JP, and Hudson MB: Shoulder Arthrodesis for the treatment of brachial plexus palsy: A review of twenty-two patients. Paper presented at the American Shoulder and Elbow Surgeons 3rd Open Meeting, 1987, San Francisco.

593. Richmond JC, Donaldson WR, Fu F, and Harner CD: Modification of the Bankart reconstruction with a suture anchor: Report of a new technique. Am J Sports Med 19:343-346, 1991.

594. Rob CG and Standeven A: Closed traumatic lesions of the axillary and brachial arteries. Lancet 1:597-599, 1956.

595. Roca LA and Ramos-Vertiz JR: Luxacion erecta de hombro. Rev San Mil Arg 61:135, 1962.

596. Rockwood CA Jr: Subluxation of the shoulder—the classification, diagnosis and treatment. Orthop Trans 4:306, 1979.

597. Rockwood CA Jr: Part 2: Dislocations about the Shoulder, vol 1. In Rockwood CA and Green DP (eds): Fractures, 2nd ed. Philadelphia: JB Lippincott, 1984.

598. Rockwood CA Jr: Shoulder arthroscopy. J Bone Joint Surg Am 70:639-640, 1988.

599. Rockwood, CA: Comparison of arthroscopic and open repairs for recurrent anterior dislocation of the shoulder. Paper presented at an open meeting of Arthroscopic Sssociation of North America, Feb 8, 2003, New Orleans.

600. Rockwood CA Jr, Burkhead WZ Jr, and Brna J: Subluxation for the gleno-humeral joint; response to rehabilitative exercise in traumatic vs. atraumatic instability. Paper presented at the American Shoulder and Elbow Surgeons 2nd Open Meeting, 1986, New Orleans.

601. Rockwood CA Jr and Young DC: Complications and management of the failed Bristow shoulder reconstructions. Orthop Trans 13:232, 1989.

602. Rodosky MW, Harner CD, and Fu FH: The role of the long head of the biceps muscle and superior glenoid labrum in anterior stability of the shoulder. Am J Sports Med 22:121-130, 1994.

603. Rokous JR, Feagin JA, and Abbott HG: Modified axillary roentgenogram. A useful adjunct in the diagnosis of recurrent instability of the shoulder. Clin Orthop 82:84-86, 1972.

604. Romanes GJ(ed): Cunningham's Textbook of Anatomy, 11th ed. London: Oxford University Press, 1972.

605. Rose DJ: Arthroscopic suture capsulorrhaphy for recurrent anterior and anteroinferior shoulder instability: 2-6 year followup. Paper presented at the American Academy of Orthopaedic Surgeons Specialty Day, Arthroscopy Association of North America, 1994.

606. Rosenberg BN, Richmond JC, and Levine WN: Long-term follow up of Bankart reconstruction. Am J Sports Med 23:538-544, 1995.

607. Rossi F, Ternamian PJ, Cerciello G, and Walch G: Posterosuperior glenoid rim impingement in athletes: The diagnostic value of traditional radiology and magnetic resonance. Radiol Med (Torino) 87:22-27, 1994.

608. Roston JB and Haines RW: Cracking in the metacarpo-phalangeal joint. J Anat 81:165-173, 1947.

609. Rowe CR: Prognosis in dislocations of the shoulder. J Bone Joint Surg Am 38:957-977, 1956.

610. Rowe CR: Instabilities of the glenohumeral joint. Bull Hosp Joint Dis 39:180-186, 1978.

611. Rowe CR, Patel D, and Southmayd WW: The Bankart procedure—a study of late results (Proceedings). J Bone Joint Surg Br 59:122, 1977.

612. Rowe CR, Patel D, and Southmayd WW: The Bankart procedure: A long-term end-result study. J Bone Joint Surg Am 60:1-16, 1978.

613. Rowe CR, Pierce DS, and Clark JG: Voluntary dislocation of the shoulder: A preliminary report on a clinical, electromyographic, and psychiatric study of 26 patients. J Bone Joint Surg Am 55:445-460, 1973.

614. Rowe CR and Sakellarides HT: Factors related to recurrences of anterior dis-locations of the shoulder. Clin Orthop 20:40, 1961.

615. Rowe CR and Yee LBK: A posterior approach to the shoulder joint. J Bone Joint Surg Am 26:580, 1944.

616. Rowe CR and Zarins B: Recurrent transient subluxation of the shoulder. J Bone Joint Surg Am 63:863-872, 1981.

617. Rowe CR and Zarins B: Chronic unreduced dislocations of the shoulder. J Bone Joint Surg Am 64:494-505, 1982.

618. Rowe CR, Zarins B, and Ciullo JV: Recurrent anterior dislocation of the shoul-der after surgical repair: Apparent causes of failure and treatment. J Bone Joint Surg Am 66:159, 1984.

619. Rozing PM, De Bakker HM, and Obermann WR: Radiographic views in recur-rent anterior shoulder dislocation: Comparison of six methods for identifi-cation of typical lesions. Acta Orthop Scand 57:328-330, 1986.

620. Rubin SA, Gray RL, and Green WR: Scapular Y—a diagnostic aid in shoulder trauma. Radiology 110:725-726, 1974.

621. Runkel M, Kreitner KF, Wenda K, et al: Nuclear magnetic tomography in shoulder dislocation. Unfallchirurg 96:124-128, 1993.

622. Rupp F: Ueber ein vereinfachtes Operationsverfahren bei habitueller Schul-terluxatuion. Dtsch Z Chir 198:70-75, 1926.

623. Russell JA, Holmes EMI, and Keller DJ: Reduction of acute anterior shoulder dislocations using the Milch technique: A study of ski injuries. J Trauma 21:802-804, 1981.

624. Saha AK: Theory of Shoulder Mechanism. Springfield, IL: Charles C Thomas, 1961.

625. Saha AK: Anterior recurrent dislocation of the shoulder. Acta Orthop Scand 39:479-493, 1967.

626. Saha AK: Dynamic instability of the glenohumeral joint. Acta Orthop Scand 42:491-505, 1971.

627. Saha AK: Mechanics of elevation of glenohumeral joint: Its application in rehabilitation of flail shoulder in upper brachial plexus injuries and poliomyelitis and in replacement of the upper humerus by prosthesis. Acta Orthop Scand 44:668, 1973.

628. Saha AK, Das NN, and Chakravarty BF: Treatment of recurrent dislocation of shoulder: Past, present, and future: Studies on electromyographic changes of muscles acting on the shoulder joint complex. Calcutta Med J 53:409-413, 1956.

629. Sarma A, Savanchak H, Levinson ED, and Sigman R: Thrombosis of the axil-lary artery and brachial plexus injury secondary to shoulder dislocation. Conn Med 45:513-514, 1981.

630. Sarrafian AK: Gross and functional anatomy of the shoulder. Clin Orthop 173:11-19, 1983.

631. Savarsee JJ and Covino BG: Basic and clinical pharmacology of local anes-thetic drugs. In Miller RD (ed): Anesthesia. New York: Churchill Livingstone, 1986.

632. Savoie FH III: Arthroscopic reconstruction of recurrent traumatic anterior instability. Paper presented at the American Academy of Orthopaedic Sur-geons Specialty Day, American Shoulder and Elbow Surgeons, 1995.

633. Saxena K and Stavas J: Inferior glenohumeral dislocation. Ann Emerg Med 12:718-720, 1983.

634. Schauder KS and Tullow HS: Role of the coracoid bone block in the modi-fied Bristow procedure. Am J Sports Med 20:31-34, 1992.

635. Schiffern SC, Rozencwaig R, Antoniou J, et al: Anteroposterior centering of the humeral head on the glenoid in vivo. Am J Sports Med 30:382-387, 2002.

636. Schlemm F: Ueber die Verstarkungsbander am Schultergelenk. Arch Anat Physiol Wissenschaft Med 22:45, 1853.

637. Schüller M: Berl Klin Wochenschr 33:760, 1896.

638. Schulz TJ, Jacobs B, and Patterson RL: Unrecognized dislocations of the shoulder. J Trauma 9:1009-1023, 1969.

639. Schwartz RE, O'Brien SJ, Warren RF, and Torzilli PA: Capsular restraints to anterior-posterior motion in the shoulder. Orthop Trans 12:727, 1988.

640. Scott DJJ: Treatment of recurrent posterior dislocations of the shoulder by glenoplasty. J Bone Joint Surg Am 49:471, 1967.

641. Scougall S: Posterior dislocation of the shoulder. J Bone Joint Surg Br 39:726-732, 1957.

642. Segal D, Yablon IG, Lynch JJ, and Jones RP: Acute bilateral anterior disloca-tion of the shoulders. Clin Orthop 140:21-22, 1979.

643. Seltzer SE and Weissman BN: CT findings in normal and dislocating shoul-ders. J Can Assoc Radiol 36:41-46, 1985.

644. Sever JW: Obstetrical paralysis. Surg Gynecol Obstet 44:547-549, 1927.

645. Shaffer BS, Conway J, Jobe FW, et al: Infraspinatus muscle-splitting incision in posterior shoulder surgery: An anatomic and electromyographic study. Am J Sports Med 22:113-120, 1994.

646. Shaffer BS, and Tibone JE: Arthroscopic shoulder instability surgery. Com-plications. Clin Sports Med 18:737-767, 1999.

647. Shea KP and Lovallo JL: Scapulothoracic penetration of a Beath pin: An unusual complication of arthroscopic Bankart suture repair. Arthroscopy 7:115-117, 1991.

648. Shea KP, O'Keefe RM Jr, and Fulkerson JP: Comparison of initial pull-out strength of arthroscopic suture and staple Bankart repair techniques. Arthroscopy 8:179-82, 1992.

649. Shively J and Johnson J: Results of modified Bristow procedure. Clin Orthop 187:150, 1984.

650. Shuman WP, Kilcoyne RF, Matsen FA III, et al: Double-contrast computed tomography of the glenoid labrum. AJR Am J Roentgenol 141:581-584, 1983.

651. Sidles JA, Harryman DT, and Simkin PA: Passive and active stabilization of the glenohumeral joint. Submitted to J Bone Joint Surg, 1989.

652. Silliman JF and Hawkins RJ: Classification and physical diagnosis of insta-bility of the shoulder. Clin Orthop 291:7-19, 1993.

653. Simkin PA: Structure and function of joints. In Schumacher HR (ed): Primer on the Rheumatic Diseases, 9th ed. Atlanta: Arthritis Foundation, 1988.

654. Simonet WT and Cofield RH: Prognosis in Anterior Shoulder Dislocation. Homestead, VA: American Orthopaedic Society for Sports Medicine, 1983.

655. Simons P, Joekes E, Nelissen RG, and Bloem JL: Posterior labrocapsular periosteal sleeve avulsion complicating locked posterior shoulder dislocation. Skeletal Radiol 27:588-590, 1998.

656. Singer GC, Kirkland PM, and Emery RJH: Coracoid transposition for recur-rent anterior instability of the shoulder. J Bone Joint Surg Br 77:73-76, 1995.

657. Sisk TD and Boyd HB: Management of recurrent anterior dislocation of the shoulder. DuToit-type or staple capsulorrhaphy. Clin Orthop 103:150, 1974.

658. Small NC: Complications in arthroscopy: The knee and other joints. Arthroscopy 2:253, 1986.

659. Small NC: Complications in arthroscopic surgery performed by experienced arthroscopists. Arthroscopy 4:215-221, 1988.

660. Small NC: Complications in arthroscopic surgery of the knee and shoulder. Orthopedics 16:985-988, 1993.

661. Snyder SJ, Banas MP, and Karzel RP: An analysis of 140 injuries to the supe-rior glenoid labrum. J Shoulder Elbow Surg 4:243-248, 1995.

662. Snyder SJ and Strafford BB: Arthroscopic management of instability of the shoulder. Orthopedics 16:993-1002, 1993.

663. Sonnabend DH: Treatment of primary anterior shoulder dislocation in patients older than 40 years of age. Clin Orthop 304:74-77, 1994.

664. Soslowsky LJ, Bigliani LU, Flatow EL, and Mow VC: Articular geometry of the glenohumeral joint. Clin Orthop 285:181-190, 1992.

665. Speed K: Fractures and Dislocation, 4th ed. Philadelphia: Lea & Febiger, 1942.

666. Speer KP, Deng X, Borrero S, et al: A biomechanical evaluation of the Bankart lesion. Paper presented at the American Academy of Orthopaedic Surgeons Specialty Day, American Shoulder and Elbow Surgeons, 1995.

667. Speer KP, Deng X, Torzilli PA, et al: Strategies for an anterior capsular shift of the shoulder: A biomechanical comparison. Rev Chir Orthop Reparatice Appar Mot 80:602-609, 1994.
668. Speer KP, Pagnani M, and Warren RF: Arthroscopic anterior shoulder stabilization: 2-5 year follow-up using a bioabsorbable tac. Paper presented at the American Shoulder and Elbow Surgeons 10th Open Meeting, 1994 New Orleans.
669. Sperber A, Hamberg P, Karlsson J, et al: Comparison of an arthroscopic and an open procedure for posttraumatic instability of the shoulder: A prospective, randomized multicenter study. J Shoulder Elbow Surg 10:105-108, 2001.
670. Sperber A and Wredmark T: Capsular elasticity and joint volume in recurrent anterior shoulder instability. Arthroscopy 10:598-601, 1994.
671. Staffel F: Verh Dtsch Ges Chir 24:651-656, 1895.
672. Steenburg RW and Ravitch MM: Cervicothoracic approach for subclavian vessel injury from compound fracture of the clavicle: Considerations of subclavian axillary exposures. Ann Surg 157:839-846, 1963.
673. Stefko JM, Tibone JE, McMahon PJ, et al: Strain of the anterior band of the glenohumeral ligament at the time of capsular failure. Paper presented at the American Shoulder and Elbow Surgeons Closed Meeting, 1995, LaQuinta, CA.
674. Stein E: Case report 374: Posttraumatic pseudoaneurysm of axillary artery. Skeletal Radiol 15:391-393, 1986.
675. Steiner D and Hermann B: Collagen fiber arrangement of the human shoulder joint capsule—an anatomical study. Acta Anat (Basel) 136:300-302, 1989.
676. Stener B: Dislocation of the shoulder complicated by complete rupture of the axillary artery. J Bone Joint Surg Br 39:714-717, 1957.
677. Stevens JH: Brachial Plexus Paralysis. New York: G. Miller, 1934.
678. Stimson LA: Fractures and Dislocations, 3rd ed. Philadelphia: Lea Brothers, 1900.
679. Stimson LA: A Practical Treatise on Fractures and Dislocations, 7th ed. Philadelphia: Lea & Febiger, 1912.
680. Stromsoe K, Senn E, Simmen B, and Matter P: Rezidivhaufigkeit nach erstmaliger traumatischer Schulterluxation. Helv Chir Acta 47:85-88, 1980.
681. Stufflesser H and Dexel M: The treatment of recurrent dislocation of the shoulder by rotation osteotomy with internal fixation. Ital J Orthop Traumatol 39:191, 1977.
682. Sudarov Z: The results of the modified Nosske-Oudard-Bazy-Savic operation for recurrent dislocation of the shoulder [abstract]. J Bone Joint Surg Br 48:855, 1966.
683. Surin V, Blader S, Markhede G, and Sundholm K: Rotational osteotomy of the humerus for posterior instability of the shoulder. J Bone Joint Surg Am 72:181-186, 1990.
684. Swenson TM and Warner JJ: Arthroscopic shoulder stabilization: Overview of indications, technique, and efficacy. Clin Sports Med 14:841-862, 1995.
685. Symeonides PP: The significance of the subscapularis muscle in the pathogenesis of recurrent anterior dislocation of the shoulder. J Bone Joint Surg Br 54:476-483, 1972.
686. Tagliabue D and Esposito A: L'intervento di Latarjet nella lussazione recidivante di spalla-dello sportivo. Ital J Orthop Traumatol 2:91-100, 1980.
687. Tauro JC and Carter FMN: Arthroscopic capsular advancement for anterior and anterior-inferior shoulder instability: A preliminary report. Arthroscopy 10:513-517, 1994.
688. Terry GC, Hammon D, and France P: The stabilizing function of passive shoulder restraints. Am J Sports Med 19:26-34, 1991.
689. Thal R: Knotless suture anchor: Arthroscopic Bankart repair without tying knots. Clin Orthop 390:42-51, 2001.
690. Thomas MA: Posterior subacromial dislocation of the head of the humerus. AJR Am J Roentgenol 37:767-773, 1937.
691. Thomas SC and Matsen FA III: An approach to the repair of glenohumeral ligament avulsion in the management of traumatic anterior glenohumeral instability. J Bone Joint Surg Am 71:506-513, 1989.
692. Thomas TT: Habitual or recurrent anterior dislocation of the shoulder. Am J Med Sci 137:229-246, 1909.
693. Thomas TT: Habitual or recurrent dislocation of the shoulder: Forty-four shoulder operations in 42 patients. Surg Gynecol Obstet 32:291-299, 1921.
694. Thompson FR and Winant WM: Unusual fracture-subluxations of the shoulder joint. J Bone Joint Surg Am 32:575-582, 1950.
695. Thompson FR and Winant WM: Comminuted fractures of the humeral head with subluxation. Clin Orthop 20:94-96, 1961.
696. Tibone J and Ting A: Capsulorrhaphy with a staple for recurrent posterior subluxation of the shoulder. J Bone Joint Surg Am 72:999-1002, 1990.
697. Tibone JE and Bradley JP: The treatment of posterior subluxation in athletes. Clin Orthop 291:124-137, 1993.
698. Tibone JE, McMahon PJ, Shrader TA, et al: Glenohumeral joint translation after arthroscopic, nonablative, thermal capsuloplasty with a laser. Am J Sports Med 26:495-498, 1998.
699. Tibone JE, Prietto C, Jobe FW, et al: Staple capsulorrhaphy for recurrent posterior shoulder dislocation. Am J Sports Med 9:135-139, 1981.
700. Tietjen R: Occult glenohumeral interposition of a torn rotator cuff. J Bone Joint Surg Am 64:458-459, 1982.
701. Tijmes J, Loyd HM, and Tullos HS: Arthrography in acute shoulder dislocations. South Med J 72:564-567, 1979.
702. Toolanen G, Hildingsson C, Hedlund T, et al: Early complications after anterior dislocation of the shoulder in patients over 40 years: An ultrasonographic and electromyographic study. Acta Orthop Scand 64:549-552, 1993.
703. Torg JS, Balduini FC, Bonci C, et al: A modified Bristow-Helfet-May procedure for recurrent dislocations and subluxation of the shoulder: Report of two hundred and twelve cases. J Bone Joint Surg Am 69:904-913, 1987.
704. Townley CO: The capsular mechanism in recurrent dislocation of the shoulder. J Bone Joint Surg Am 32:370-380, 1950.
705. Trillat A: Traitement de la luxation récidivante de l'épaule: Considerations, techniques. Lyon Chir 49:986, 1954.
706. Trillat A and Leclerc-Chalvet F: Luxation Récidivante de L'Épaule. Paris: Masson, 1973.
707. Trimmings NP: Hemarthrosis aspiration in treatment of anterior dislocation of the shoulder. J R Soc Med 78:1023-1027, 1985.
708. Turkel SJ, Panio MW, Marshall JL, and Girgis FG: Stabilizing mechanisms preventing anterior dislocation of the glenohumeral joint. J Bone Joint Surg Am 63:1208-1217, 1981.
709. Tuszynski W and Dworczyndki W: [Anterior shoulder dislocation complicated by transient paralysis of the brachial plexus. Chir Narzadow Ruchu Ortop Pol 46:129-131, 1981.
710. Uhorchak JM, Arciero RA, Huggard D, and Taylor DC: Recurrent shoulder instability after open reconstruction in athletes involved in collision and contact sports. Am J Sports Med 28:794-799, 2000.
711. Uhorchak JM, Arciero RA, and Taylor DC: recurrent instability after open shoulder stabilization in athletes. Paper presented at the American Academy of Orthopaedic Surgeons Specialty Day, American Shoulder and Elbow Surgeons, 1995.
712. Uhthoff HK and Piscopo M: Anterior capsular redundancy of the shoulder: Congenital or traumatic? An embryological study. J Bone Joint Surg Br 67:363-366, 1985.
713. Ungersbock A, Michel M, and Hertel R: Factors influencing the results of a modified Bankart procedure. J Shoulder Elbow Surg 4:365-369, 1995.
714. Unsworth A, Dowson D, and Wright V: "Cracking joints": A bioengineering study of cavitation in the metacarpophalangeal joint. Ann Rheum Dis 30:348, 1971.
715. Uribe JW and Hechtman KS: Arthroscopically assisted repair of acute Bankart lesion. Orthopedics 16:1019-1023, 1993.
716. Valls J: Acrylic prosthesis in a case with fracture of the head of the humerus. Bal Soc Orthop Trauma 17:61, 1952.
717. Van der Helm FC: A finite element musculoskeletal model of the shoulder mechanics. J Biomech 27:551-569, 1994.
718. Van der Helm FC, Veeger HE, Pronk GM, et al: Geometry parameters for musculoskeletal modeling of the shoulder system. J Biomech 25:129-144, 1992.
719. Van der Spek K: Rupture of the axillary artery as a complication of dislocation of the shoulder. Arch Chir Neerl 16:113-118, 1964.
720. Vangsness CTJ, Ennis M, Taylor JG, and Atkinson R: Neural anatomy of the glenohumeral ligaments, labrum, and subacromial bursa. Arthroscopy 11:180-184, 1995.
721. Veeger HE, Van der Helm FC, Van der Woude LH, et al: Inertia and muscle contraction parameters for musculoskeletal modeling of the shoulder mechanism. J Biomech 24:615-629, 1991.
722. Vegter J and Marti RK: Treatment of posterior dislocation of the shoulder by osteotomy of the neck of the scapula. J Bone Joint Surg 63:288, 1981.
723. Vellet AD, Munk PL, and Marks P: Imaging techniques of the shoulder: Present perspectives. Clin Sports Med 10:721-756, 1991.
724. Verrina F: Para-articular ossification following simple dislocation of the shoulder. Minerva Orthop 210:480-486, 1975.
725. Volpin G, Langer R, and Stein H: Complete infraclavicular brachial plexus palsy with occlusion of axillary vessels following anterior dislocation of the shoulder joint. J Orthop Trauma 4:121-123, 1990.
726. von Eisenhart-Rothe RM, Jager A, Englmeier KH, et al: Relevance of arm position and muscle activity on three-dimensional glenohumeral translation in patients with traumatic and atraumatic shoulder instability. Am J Sports Med 30:514-522, 2002.
727. Wagner SC, Schweitzer ME, Morrison WB, et al: Shoulder instability: Accuracy of MR imaging performed after surgery in depicting recurrent injury—initial findings. Radiology 222:196-203, 2002.
728. Walch G, Boileau P, Levigne C, et al: Arthroscopic stabilization for recurrent anterior shoulder dislocation. Arthroscopy 11:173-179, 1995.
729. Walch G, Liotard JP, Boileau P, and Noel E: Postero-superior glenoid impingement: Another shoulder impingement. Rev Chir Orthop Reparatrice Appar Mot 77:571-574, 1991.
730. Walch G, Liotard JP, Boileau P, and Noel E: Postero-superior glenoid impingement: Another impingement of the shoulder. J Radiol 74:47-50, 1993.
731. Waldron VD: Dislocated shoulder reduction—a simple method that is done without assistants. Orthop Rev 11:105-106, 1982.
732. Wallace AL, Hollinshead RM, and Frank CB: Creep behavior of a rabbit model of ligament laxity after electrothermal shrinkage in vivo. Am J Sports Med 30:98-102, 2002.
733. Ward WG, Bassett FHI, and Garrett WEJ: Anterior staple capsulorrhaphy for recurrent dislocation of the shoulder: A clinical and biomechanical study. South Med J 83:510-518, 1990.
734. Warme WJ, Arciero RA, Savoie FH 3rd, et al: Nonabsorbable versus absorbable suture anchors for open Bankart repair. A prospective, randomized comparison. Am J Sports Med 27:742-746, 1999.
735. Warner JJ, Deng XH, Warren RF, and Torzilli PA: Static capsuloligamentous restraints to superior-inferior translation of the glenohumeral joint. Am J Sports Med 20:675-685, 1992.

736. Warner JJ, Kann S, and Marks P: Arthroscopic repair of combined Bankart and superior labral detachment anterior and posterior lesions: Technique and preliminary results. Arthroscopy 10:383-391, 1994.
737. Warner JJ, Micheli LJ, Arslanian LE, et al: Scapulothoracic motion in normal shoulders and shoulders with glenohumeral instability and impingement syndrome: A study using Moir'e topographic analysis. Clin Orthop 285:191-199, 1992.
738. Warner JJ, Miller MD, and Marks P: Arthroscopic Bankart repair with the Suretac device. Part II. Experimental observations. Arthroscopy 11:14-20, 1995.
739. Warner JJ, Miller MD, Marks P, and Fu FH: Arthroscopic Bankart repair with the Suretac device. Part I. Clinical observations. Arthroscopy 11:2-13, 1995.
740. Warren RF: The Role of Shoulder Arthroscopy. Minneapolis, MN: American Academy of Orthopaedic Surgeons Instructional Course, 1989.
741. Warren RF, Kornblatt IB, and Marchand R: Static factors affecting posterior shoulder stability. Orthop Trans 8:89, 1984.
742. Watson-Jones R: Dislocation of the shoulder joint. Proc R Soc Med 29:1060-1062, 1936.
743. Watson-Jones R: Recurrent dislocation of the shoulder. J Bone Joint Surg Br 30:6-8, 1948.
744. Watson-Jones R: Fractures and Joint Injuries, 4th ed. Baltimore: Williams & Wilkins, 1957.
745. Weaver JK and Derkash RS: Don't forget the Bristow-Latarjet procedure. Clin Orthop 308:102-110, 1994.
746. Weber BG: Operative treatment for recurrent dislocation of the shoulder. Injury 1:107-109, 1969.
747. Weber BG, Simpson LA, and Hardegger F: Rotational humeral osteotomy for recurrent anterior dislocation of the shoulder associated with a large Hill-Sachs lesion. J Bone Joint Surg Am 66:1443, 1984.
748. Weber S: The gold standard revisited: Recent experience with the open Bankart repair for recurrent anterior glenohumeral dislocation. Paper presented at the American Academy of Orthopaedic Surgeons Specialty Day, American Shoulder and Elbow Surgeons, 1995.
749. Weber SC: Open versus arthroscopic repair of traumatic anterior glenohumeral instability. Paper presented at the American Academy of Orthopaedic Surgeons Specialty Day Meeting, Arthroscopy Association of North America, 1995.
750. Weber SC, Abrams JS, and Nottage WM: Complications associated with arthroscopic shoulder surgery. Arthroscopy 18(suppl 1):88-95, 2002.
751. Weishaupt D, Zanetti M, Nyffeler RW, et al: Posterior glenoid rim deficiency in recurrent (atraumatic) posterior shoulder instability. Skeletal Radiol 29:204-210, 2000.
752. Weiss KS, and Savoie FH 3rd: Recent advances in arthroscopic repair of traumatic anterior glenohumeral instability. Clin Orthop 400:117-122, 2002.
753. Weitbrecht J: Syndesmology; or, a Description of the Ligaments of the Human Body (trans EB Kaplan). Philadelphia: WB Saunders, 1969.
754. West EF: Intrathoracic dislocation of the humerus. J Bone Joint Surg Br 31:61-62, 1949.
755. Wheeler JH, Ryan JB, Arciero RA, and Molinari RN: Arthroscopic versus nonoperative treatment of acute shoulder dislocations in young athletes. Arthroscopy 5:213-217, 1989.
756. White ADN: Dislocated shoulder—a simple method of reduction. Med J Aust 2:726-727, 1976.
757. Wickstrom J: Birth injuries of the brachial plexus: Treatment of defects in the shoulder. Clin Orthop 23:187-196, 1962.
758. Wiley AM and Austwick DH: Shoulder Surgery through the Arthroscope. Toronto: Department of Surgery, University of Toronto and Toronto Wester Hospital, 1982.
759. Wiley AM and Older MWJ: Shoulder arthroscopy. J Sports Med 8:31-38, 1980.
760. Williams MM, Snyder SJ, and Buford DJ: The Buford complex—the cord-like middle glenohumeral ligament and absent anterosuperior labrum complex: In a normal anatomic capsulolabral variant. Arthroscopy 10:241-247, 1994.
761. Wilson JC and McKeever FM: Traumatic posterior (retroglenoid) dislocation of the humerus. J Bone Joint Surg Am 31:160-172, 1949.
762. Wirth MA, Blatter G, and Rockwood CA Jr: The capsular imbrication procedure for recurrent anterior instability of the shoulder. J Bone Joint Surg Am 78:246-259, 1996.
763. Wirth MA, Butters KP, and Rockwood CA Jr: The posterior deltoid-splitting approach to the shoulder. Clin Orthop 296:92-98, 1993.
764. Wirth MA, Groh GI, and Rockwood CA Jr: the treatment of symptomatic posterior glenohumeral instability with an anterior capsular shift. Paper presented at the 58th Annual Meeting of the Western Orthopaedic Association, 1994.
765. Wirth MA, Groh GI, and Rockwood CA Jr: Capsulorrhaphy through an anterior approach for the treatment of atraumatic posterior glenohumeral instability with multidirectional laxity of the shoulder. J Bone Joint Surg Am 80:1570-1578, 1998.
766. Wirth MA, Jensen KL, Agarwal A, et al: Fracture-dislocation of the proximal part of the humerus with retroperitoneal displacement of the humeral head. J Bone Joint Surg Am 79:763-766, 1997.
767. Wirth MA, Lyons FR, and Rockwood CA Jr: Hypoplasia of the glenoid: A review of sixteen patients. J Bone Joint Surg Am 75:1175-1184, 1993.
768. Wirth MA and Rockwood CA Jr: Traumatic glenohumeral instability. In Matsen FA III, Fu FH, and Hawkins RJ (eds): The Shoulder: A Balance of Mobility and Stability. Rosemont, IL: American Academy of Orthopaedic Surgeons, 1993, pp 279-304.
769. Wirth MA and Rockwood CA Jr: Complications of treatment of injuries of the shoulder. In Epps CH (ed): Complications in Orthopaedic Surgery. Philadelphia: JB Lippincott, 1994, pp 229-255.
770. Wirth MA, Seltzer DG, and Rockwood CA Jr: Recurrent posterior glenohumeral dislocation associated with increased retroversion of the glenoid. Clin Orthop 308:98-101, 1994.
771. Wirth MA, Seltzer DG, and Rockwood CA Jr: Replacement of the subscapularis with pectoralis muscle in anterior shoulder instability. Paper presented at the 62nd Annual Meeting of the American Academy of Orthopaedics Surgeons, 1995, Orlando, FL.
772. Wolf EM: Arthroscopic anterior shoulder capsulorrhaphy. Tech Orthop 3:67-73, 1988.
773. Wolf EM: Arthroscopic capsulolabral repair using suture anchors. Orthop Clin North Am 24:59-69, 1993.
774. Wolf EM: Arthroscopic capsulolabral reconstruction using suture anchors. Paper presented at the American Academy of Orthopaedic Surgeons Specialty Day, American Shoulder and Elbow Surgeons Annual Meeting, 1994.
775. Wolf EM, Cheng JC, and Dickson K: Humeral avulsion of glenohumeral ligaments as a cause of anterior shoulder instability. Arthroscopy 11:600-607, 1995.
776. Wong KL and Williams GR: Complications of thermal capsulorrhaphy of the shoulder. J Bone Joint Surg Am 83(suppl 2):151-155, 2001.
777. Wong-Pack WK, Bobechko PE, and Becker EJ: Fractured coracoid with anterior shoulder dislocation. J Can Assoc Radiol 31:278-279, 1980.
778. Wredmark T, Tornkvist H, Johansson C, and Brobert B: Long-term functional results of the modified Bristow procedure for recurrent dislocations of the shoulder. Am J Sports Med 20:157-161, 1992.
779. Wulker N, Rossig S, Korell M, and Thren K: Dynamic stability of the glenohumeral joint: A biomechanical study. Sportverletz Sportschaden 9:1-8, 1995.
780. Wulker N, Sperveslage C, and Brewe F: Passive stabilizers of the glenohumeral joint: A biomechanical study. Unfallchirurg 96:129-133, 1993.
781. Yadav SS: Bilateral simultaneous fracture-dislocation of the shoulder due to muscular violence. J Postgrad Med 23:137-139, 1977.
782. Yahiro MA and Matthews LS: Arthroscopic stabilization procedures for recurrent anterior shoulder instability. Orthop Rev 18:1161-1168, 1989.
783. Yoneda B, Welsh RP, and MacIntosh DL: Conservative treatment of shoulder dislocation in young males (Proceedings). J Bone Joint Surg Br 64:254-255, 1982.
784. Young DC and Rockwood CA Jr: Complications of a failed Bristow procedure and their management. J Bone Joint Surg Am 73:969-981, 1991.
785. Youssef JA, Carr CF, Walther CE, and Murphy JM: Arthroscopic Bankart suture repair for recurrent traumatic unidirectional anterior shoulder dislocations. Arthroscopy 11:561-563, 1995.
786. Yu JS, Ashman CJ, and Jones G: The POLPSA lesion: MR imaging findings with arthroscopic correlation in patients with posterior instability. Skeletal Radiol 31:396-399, 2002.
787. Yuen MC, Yap PG, Chan YT, and Tung WK: An easy method to reduce anterior shoulder dislocation: The Spaso technique. Emerg Med J 18:370-372, 2001.
788. Yung SW and Harryman DT II: The Surgical anatomy of the subscapular nerves. Paper presented at the 62nd Annual Meeting of the American Academy of Orthopaedic Surgeons, 1995, Orlando, FL.
789. Zabinski SJ, Callaway GH, Cohen S, and Warren RF: Long term results of revision shoulder stabilization. Paper presented at the American Shoulder and Elbow Surgeons Closed Meeting, 1995, La Quinta, CA.
790. Zachary RB: Transplantation of teres major and latissimus dorsi for loss of external rotation at the shoulder. Lancet 2:757-761, 1947.
791. Ziegler DW, Harrington RM, and Matsen FA III: The superior rotator cuff tendon and acromion provide passive superior stability to the shoulder. Submitted to J Bone Joint Surg, 1996.
792. Ziegler DW, Harryman DT II, and Matsen FA III: Subscapularis insufficiency in the previously operated shoulder. Paper presented at the American Shoulder and Elbow Surgeons 12th Open Meeting, 1996, Atlanta.
793. Zimmerman LM and Veith I: Great Ideas in the History of Surgery: Clavicle, Shoulder, Shoulder Amputations. Baltimore: Williams & Wilkins, 1961.
794. Zizzi F, Frizziero L, Facchini A, and Zini GL: Artroscopia della spalla: Indicazioni e limiti. Reumatismo 33:429-432, 1981.
795. Zorowitz RD, Idank D, Ikai T, et al: Shoulder subluxation after stroke: A comparison of four supports. Arch Phys Med Rehabil 76:763-771, 1995.
796. Zuckerman JD, Gallagher MA, Cuomo F, and Rokito AS: Effect of instability and subsequent anterior shoulder repair on proprioceptive ability. Paper presented at the American Shoulder and Elbow Surgeons 12th Open Meeting, 1996, Atlanta.
797. Zuckerman JD and Matsen FAI: Complications about the glenohumeral joint related to the use of screws and staples. J Bone Joint Surg Am 66:175, 1984.

CHAPTER 15

ROTATOR CUFF

Frederick A. Matsen III, M.D., Robert M. Titelman, M.D., Steven B. Lippitt, M.D.,
Michael A. Wirth, M.D., and Charles A. Rockwood, Jr., M.D.

• • • •

Ay, there's the rub.

- Hamlet, III. i. 47, Shakespeare

The coracoacromial ligament has an important duty and should not be thoughtlessly divided at any operation.

- E. A. Codman, 1934

The wise surgeon, realizing that he may find little but rotten cloth to sew, will operate only by necessity and make a carefully guarded prognosis.

- H. L. McLaughlin, 1962

HISTORICAL REVIEW

Rotator Cuff Tears

It is often difficult to tell where concepts actually begin. It is certainly not obvious who first used the term rotator or musculotendinous cuff. Credit for first describing ruptures of this structure is often given to J. G. Smith, who in 1834 described the occurrence of tendon ruptures after shoulder injury in the *London Medical Gazette.*[415] In 1924 Meyer published his attrition theory of cuff rupture.[280] In his 1934 classic monograph, Codman summarized his 25 years of observations on the musculotendinous cuff and its components and discussed rupture of the supraspinatus tendon.[66] Beginning 10 years after the publication of Codman's book and for the next 20 years, McLaughlin wrote on the etiology of cuff tears and their management.[273,277] Arthrography with air used as the contrast medium was first carried out by Oberholtzer in 1933.[325] Lindblom and Palmer[251] used radiopaque contrast and described partial-thickness, full-thickness, and massive tears of the cuff.

Codman recommended early operative repair for complete cuff tears and carried out what may have been the first cuff repair in 1909.[65] Current views of cuff tear pathogenesis, diagnosis, and treatment are quite similar to those that he proposed over 50 years ago.

Pettersson has provided an excellent summary of the early history of published observations on subacromial pathology. Because of its completeness, his account is quoted here.[354]

> As already mentioned, the tendon aponeurosis of the shoulder joint and the subacromial bursa are intimately connected with each other. An investigation on the pathological changes in one of these formations will necessarily concern the other one also. A historical review shows that there has been a good deal of confusion regarding the pathological and clinical observations on the two.
>
> The first to observe morbid processes in the subacromial bursa was Jarjavay,[199] who on the basis of a few cases gave a general description of subacromial bursitis. His views were modified and elaborated by Heineke[183] and Vogt.[464] Duplay[105] introduced the term "periarthritis humeroscapularis" to designate a disease picture characterized by stiffness and pain in the shoulder joint following a trauma. Duplay based his observations on cases of trauma to the shoulder joint and on other cases of stiffness in the shoulder following dislocation, which he had studied at autopsy. The pathological foundation for the disease was believed by Duplay to lie in the subacromial and subdeltoid bursa. He thought that the cause was probably destruction or fusion of the bursa.
>
> Duplay's views, which were supported by his followers Tillaux[445] and Desché,[97] were hotly disputed. His opponents, Gosselin and his pupil Duronea[106] and Desplats,[98] Pingaud and Charvot,[357] tried to prove that the periarthritis should be regarded as a rheumatic affection, neuritis, etc.

In Germany, Colley[76] and Küster[228] were of practically the same opinion regarding periarthritis humeroscapularis as Duplay. Roentgenography soon began to contribute to the problem of humeroscapular periarthritis. It was not long before calcium shadows began to be observed in the soft parts between the acromion and the greater tuberosity.[340] The same finding was made by Stieda,[426] who assumed that these calcium masses were situated in the wall and in the lumen of the subacromial bursa. These new findings were indiscriminately termed "bursitis calcarea subacromialis" or "subdeltoidea." The term "bursoliths" was even used by Haudek[173] and Holzknecht.[187] Later, however, as the condition showed a strong resemblance to humeroscapular periarthritis, it became entirely identified with the latter.

In America, Codman[68] made a very important contribution to the question when he drew attention to the important role played by changes in the supraspinatus in the clinical picture of subacromial bursitis. Codman was the first to point out that many cases of inability to abduct the arm are due to incomplete or complete ruptures of the supraspinatus tendon.

With Codman's findings it was proved that humeroscapular periarthritis was not only a disease condition localized in the subacromial bursa, but that pathological changes also occurred in the tendon aponeurosis of the shoulder joint. This theory was further supported by Wrede,[490] who, on the basis of one surgical case and several cases in which roentgenograms had revealed calcium shadows in the region of the greater tuberosity, was able to show that the calcium deposits were localized in the supraspinatus tendon.

More and more disease conditions in the region of the shoulder joint have gradually been distinguished and separated from the general concept, periarthritis humeroscapularis. For example, Sievers[410] drew attention to the fact that arthritis deformans in the acromioclavicular joint may give a clinical picture reminiscent of periarthritis humeroscapularis. Bettman[27] and Meyer and Kessler[282] pointed to the occurrence of deforming changes in the intertubercular sulcus, the canal in which the biceps tendon glides. Payr[349] attempted to isolate the clinical picture which appears when the shoulder joint without any previous trauma is immobilized too long in an unsuitable position. Julliard[208] demonstrated apophysitis in the coracoid process (coracoiditis) as forming a special subdivision of periarthritis. Wellisch[481] described apophysitis at the insertion of the deltoid muscle on the humerus, giving it the name of "deltoidalgia." Schár and Zweifel[399] described deforming changes in connection with certain cases of os acromiale.

In addition to this excellent review, Pettersson himself made a number of important contributions to study of the rotator cuff, as will be seen subsequently in this chapter.

The cuff story continues with recognition of subacromial abrasion as a possible element in rotator cuff disease by a number of well-known surgeons, including Codman,[68] Armstrong,[5] Hammond,[166,167] McLaughlin,[273] Moseley,[296] Smith-Petersen and colleagues,[417] and Watson-Jones.[475] Some of these surgeons proposed complete acromionectomy for relief of these symptoms,[5,99,166,167,475]

whereas others advocated lateral acromionectomy.[273,417] The term "impingement syndrome" was popularized by Charles Neer in 1972.[304] In 100 dissected scapulas, Neer found 11 with a "characteristic ridge of proliferative spurs and excrescences on the undersurface of the anterior process (of the acromion), apparently caused by repeated impingement of the rotator cuff and the humeral head, with traction of the coracoacromial ligament. . . . Without exception it was the anterior lip and undersurface of the anterior third that was involved." It is surely of relevance that the spurs were thought to be the result of impingement rather than its cause. Neer emphasized that the supraspinatus insertion to the greater tuberosity and the bicipital groove lie anterior to the coracoacromial arch with the shoulder in the neutral position and that with forward flexion of the shoulder, these structures must pass beneath the arch, thereby providing the opportunity for abrasion. He suggested a continuum from chronic bursitis and partial tears to complete tears of the supraspinatus tendon that may extend to involve rupture of other parts of the cuff. He pointed out that the physical examination and plain radiographic findings were not reliable in differentiating chronic bursitis and partial tears from complete tears. Importantly, he emphasized that patients with partial tears seemed more prone to increased shoulder stiffness and that surgery in this situation was inadvisable until the stiffness had resolved. He described the use of a subacromial lidocaine injection to help localize the clinical problem and before acromioplasty as a "useful guide of what the procedure would accomplish."

Neer described three different stages of the "impingement syndrome." In stage 1, reversible edema and hemorrhage are present in a patient younger than 25 years. In stage 2, fibrosis and tendinitis affect the rotator cuff of a patient typically in the 25- to 40-year-old age group. Pain often recurs with activity. In stage 3, bone spurs and tendon ruptures are present in an individual older than 40 years. He emphasized the importance of nonoperative management of cuff tendinitis. If surgery was performed, Neer pointed out the importance of preserving a secure acromial origin of the deltoid, performing a smooth resection of the undersurface of the anteroinferior acromion, making a careful inspection for other sources of abrasion (such as the undersurface of the acromioclavicular joint), and ensuring careful postoperative rehabilitation.[304,306,309]

In 1972 Neer[304] described the indications for acromioplasty as (1) long-term disability from chronic bursitis and partial tears of the supraspinatus tendon or (2) complete tears of the supraspinatus. He pointed out that the physical and roentgenographic findings in these two categories were indistinguishable and included crepitus and tenderness over the supraspinatus with a painful arc of active elevation from 70 to 120 degrees and pain at the anterior edge of the acromion on forced elevation. Neer's 1983 report[306] described candidates for acromioplasty as (1) patients with an arthrographically demonstrated cuff tear; (2) patients older than 40 years with negative arthrograms but persistent disability for 1 year despite adequate conservative treatment (including efforts to eliminate stiffness), provided that the pain can be temporarily eliminated by the subacromial injection of lidocaine; (3) certain patients younger than 40 years with refractory stage II impingement lesions; and (4) patients undergoing other procedures for conditions in which impingement is likely (such as total shoulder replacement in those with rheumatoid arthritis or old fractures). The proposed goal of acromioplasty was to relieve mechanical wear at the critical area of the rotator cuff. Surgery was not considered until any stiffness had resolved and the disability had persisted for at least 9 months. Even in patients with continuing symptoms after lateral acromionectomy, Neer considered anterior acromioplasty because he found that many still had problems related to subacromial impingement. Neer also reported that the rare patient with an irreparable tear in the rotator cuff could be made more comfortable and could gain surprising function if the impingement were relieved, as long as the deltoid origin was preserved.[306]

Neer[306] recommended resection of small unfused acromial growth centers and internal fixation of larger unfused segments in a manner that tilted the acromion upward to avoid impingement. His indications for resection of the lateral aspect of the clavicle included (1) arthritis of the acromioclavicular joint, (2) a need for greater exposure of the supraspinatus in a cuff repair, and (3) nonarthritic enlargement of the acromioclavicular joint resulting in impingement on the supraspinatus (in this situation, only the undersurface of the joint was resected).[306]

Additional approaches to subacromial abrasion have been proposed, including section of the coracoacromial ligament,[177,198,216,351] resection arthroplasty of the acromioclavicular joint,[200] extensive acromionectomy,[5,99,166,167,273,283,296,417,475] and combined procedures such as acromioplasty, incision of the coracoacromial ligament, acromioclavicular resection arthroplasty, and excision of the intra-articular portion of the biceps tendon with tenodesis of the distal portion of the bicipital groove.[160,318,364]

Comparison of the results of these procedures is difficult because of the heterogeneous patient groups and varying methods of evaluation. In 16 patients with chronic bursitis and fraying or a partial tear of the supraspinatus, Neer[304] found that 15 attained satisfactory results (no significant pain, less than 20 degrees of limitation in overhead extension, and at least 75% of normal strength). Thorling and coworkers[442] found good to excellent results in 33 of 51 patients after acromioplasty (in 11, resection of the acromioclavicular joint was performed as well).

More recently, arthroscopic acromioplasty has been introduced. The frequency with which this procedure is performed has increased dramatically as the strictness of Neer's original indications for acromioplasty has been allowed to relax. Ellman[109] presented the initial results of 50 consecutive cases of arthroscopic acromioplasty for stage II impingement without a cuff tear (40 cases) and for full-thickness cuff tears (20 cases). Eighty-eight percent of the patients had excellent or good results, and the rest were unsatisfactory at a 1- to 3-year follow-up. He pointed out that the technique was technically demanding. Difficulties with arthroscopic acromioplasty range from inadequate subacromial smoothing on the one hand to transection of the acromion or virtually total acromionectomy on the other. In his early series of 100 arthroscopic acromioplasties, Gartsman[136] found that at an average of 18.5 months' follow-up, 85 shoulders were improved and 15 were failures, 9 of which required subsequent open acromioplasty. The procedure took longer than open acromioplasty and did not speed the patient's return to work or sports. A comparison between open and arthroscopic acromioplasties by Spangehl and colleagues showed no significant differences in outcome based on UCLA scores and patient satisfaction. Open acromioplasty patients had significantly more pain relief at a minimum of 1-year follow-up.[421] Morrison[293] reported a series of arthroscopic acromioplasties in which the quality of the result was closely correlated with conversion of a curved or hooked acromion to a flat undersurface.

Even though the indications for its performance are still unresolved, arthroscopic acromioplasty is currently one of the most common of all orthopaedic procedures in that it is used to treat shoulder pain, bursal hypertrophy, partial-thickness cuff tears, calcific tendinitis, and reparable and irreparable rotator cuff tears.

RELEVANT ANATOMY AND MECHANICS

The Skin

Rotator cuff surgery can usually be accomplished through cosmetically acceptable incisions in the lines of the skin (Fig. 15–1). These skin lines run obliquely in a superolateral-to-inferomedial direction. The usual "superior" approach to the cuff is made through such an oblique incision that runs over the anterior corner of the acromion. In most cases, this incision heals with a scar less noticeable than those resulting from arthroscopic portals.

The Deltoid Muscle

The deltoid arises from the lateral half of the clavicle, the acromion, and posteriorly from the scapular spine. Because the origin of the deltoid is over the entire anterior height of the acromion, a substantial amount of the deltoid origin must be detached when performing an acromioplasty, whether the procedure is carried out by open means or arthroscopically.[450] The deltoid has an important and constant tendon of origin separating its anterior and lateral thirds. This tendon attaches to the anterolateral corner of the acromion, in which location it provides the key to the anterior deltoid-splitting approach to the cuff. By making the deltoid split down the center of the tendon, the surgeon can be ensured of having strong tendinous "handles" on the muscle for use in closure of the deltoid (Fig. 15–1). Although it is often said that the location of the axillary nerve is on average 5 cm distal to the acromion, its anterior branches swoop upward, so it is desirable to limit the inferior extent of the deltoid split to minimize the risk of injury to the axillary nerve branches (Fig. 15–1).

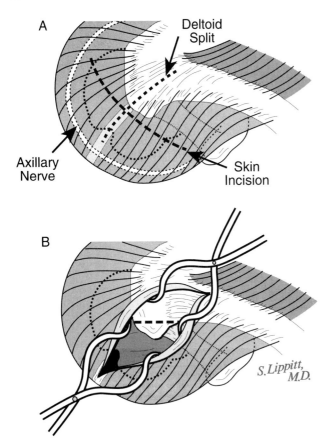

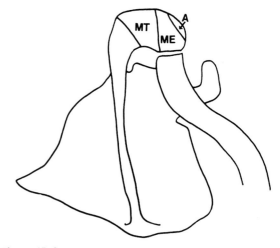

■ Figure 15–1
The deltoid on approach. **A,** Skin incision in Langer's lines across the front of the acromion. The deltoid is split along the tendon at the junction of the anterior and middle thirds. **B,** The deltoid origin can be sharply dissected from the acromion for greater exposure. It is desirable to preserve Sharpey's fibers of origin on the muscle and continuity of the medial and lateral flaps with the insertion of the trapezius. *(Modified from Matsen FA III, Lippitt SB, Sidles JA, and Harryman DT II: Practical Evaluation and Management of the Shoulder. Philadelphia: WB Saunders, 1994.)*

The Acromion, the Coracoid, and the Coracoacromial Ligament

The *acromion* is a scapular process arising from three separate centers of ossification—a pre-acromion, a meso-acromion, and a meta-acromion.[60,299,395] These centers of ossification are usually united by 22 years of age. When these centers fail to unite, the ununited portion is referred to as an *os acromiale* (Fig. 15–2). This condition may have first been recognized by Schár and Zweifel[399] in 1936, as was mentioned by Pettersson.[354] Grant[157] found that 16 of 194 cadavers older than 30 years demonstrated incomplete fusion of the acromion; the condition was bilateral in 5 subjects and unilateral in 11. In a large review of 1000 radiographs, Liberson[244] found unfused acromia in 2.7%; of these, 62% were bilateral. Most commonly the lesion is a failure of fusion of the meso-acromion to the meta-acromion. He found the axillary view to be most helpful in revealing the condition. The size of the unfused fragment may be substantial, up to 5 × 2 cm.[304] Resection of a fragment this large creates a serious challenge for deltoid reattachment.

■ Figure 15–2
A superior view of the scapula and clavicle. A, acro-os acromiale; ME, meso-os acromiale; MT, meta-os acromiale. *(From Iannotti JP: Rotator Cuff Disorders: Evaluation and Treatment. Rosemont, IL: American Academy of Orthopaedic Surgeons, 1991.)*

Norris and coworkers[324] and Bigliani and associates[31] pointed to an association of cuff degeneration and an unfused acromial epiphysis. Mudge and coworkers[299] found that 6% of 145 shoulders with cuff tears had an os acromiale, whereas Liberson found a 2.7% incidence of this finding in unselected scapulas.[244] The statistical and clinical significance of this association remains unclear. Warner and associates studied 14 patients with os acromiale who were treated by open reduction and internal fixation. Overall, 50% achieved union, but 86% achieved union with a tension band and cannulated screw fixation versus 14% with a tension band alone. Eighty-six percent of patients who achieved union had good results, but only 14% of patients with nonunion were considered to have a good result.[469]

An additional anatomic feature of importance is the acromial branch of the thoracoacromial artery. This artery runs in a close relationship with the coracoacromial ligament and is often transected in the course of acromioplasty and section of the coracoacromial ligament.

The *coracoid* arises from two or three ossification centers.[395] It provides the medial attachment site for both the coracohumeral and coracoacromial ligaments. In that their muscle bellies lie medial to it, the neighboring supraspinatus and subscapularis tendons must be able to glide by the coracoid with their full excursion during shoulder movement. Scarring of one or both these tendons to the coracoid can inhibit passive and active shoulder motion. Although the coracoid does not normally contact the anterior subscapularis tendon, forced internal rotation, particularly in the presence of a tight posterior capsule, can produce such contact as a result of the obligate translation.[145,171]

The *coracoacromial ligament* spans from the undersurface of the acromion to the lateral aspect of the coracoid and is continuous with the less dense clavipectoral fascia. It forms a substantial part of the superficial aspect of the humeroscapular motion interface (Figs. 15–3 and 15–4). This ligament may be thought of as the "spring" ligament of the shoulder in that it maintains the normal

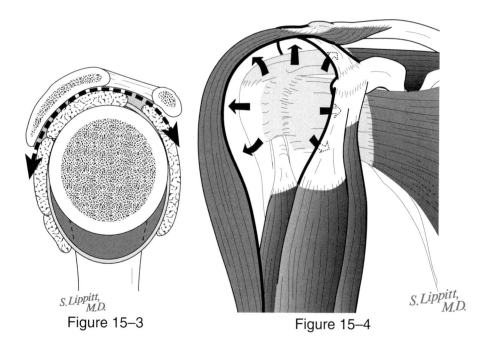

Figure 15–3   Figure 15–4

■ **Figures 15–3 and 15–4**
The humeroscapular motion interface is an important location of motion between the humerus and the scapula. The deltoid, acromion, coracoacromial ligament, coracoid process, and tendons attaching to the coracoid lie on the superficial side of this interface, whereas the proximal end of the humerus, rotator cuff, and biceps tendon sheath lie on its deep side. These two groups of structures are essentially in contact and separated only by lubricating bursal surfaces.

relationships between the coracoid and the acromion. Separation of these two scapular processes has been observed on sectioning this ligament in cadavers.[123] Calcification in the acromial end of this ligament may give the appearance of a subacromial spur.

The *coracoacromial arch* is the inferiorly concave smooth surface consisting of the anterior undersurface of the acromion and the coracoacromial ligament. It provides a strong ceiling for the shoulder joint, along which the cuff tendons must glide during all shoulder movements (Figs. 15–3 and 15–4). Passage of the cuff tendons and the proximal end of the humerus under this arch is facilitated by the subacromial-subdeltoid bursa, which is not normally a space, as often shown on diagrams, but rather two serosal surfaces in contact with each other, one on the undersurface of the coracoacromial arch and deltoid and the other on the cuff. These sliding surfaces are lubricated by the bursal surfaces and synovial fluid.

Recognition of the gliding articulation between the arch and the cuff is not new. Renoux and colleagues credited Ludkewitch, who in 1900 recognized that proper functioning of the "scapulohumeral articulation" requires the presence of a "secondary socket" that extends the glenoid fossa of the scapula above, in front, and behind, with the coracoacromial arch forming the ceiling.[373] In 1934, Codman stated that the coracoacromial arch was an auxiliary joint of the shoulder and that its roughly hemispheric shape was "almost a counterpart in the size and curvature of the articular surface of the true joint." He referred to the "gleno-coraco-acromial socket."[66] His belief in the importance of the coracoacromial arch was great enough to state that "the coracoacromial ligament has an important duty and should not be thoughtlessly divided at any operation." Wiley has pointed to the severe superior instability that results when the ceiling of the shoulder is lost in association with cuff deficiency.[484] Kernwein and associates in 1961 stressed the importance of the "suprahumeral gliding mechanism"

consisting of the coracoacromial arch on one side and the rotator cuff and biceps tendon on the other separated by the subacromial bursa.[214] They believed that these two opposing, gliding surfaces and interposed bursa constituted a fifth joint that contributed to shoulder motion. DePalma, in 1967, also recognized the intimate relationship between the arch and the structures below it.[92] He referred to the arch, together with the head of the humerus, the rotator cuff, and the subacromial bursa, as the "superior humeral articulation."

Matsen and colleagues described the humeroscapular motion interface as an articulation (Figs. 15–3 and 15–4) between the cuff, the humeral head, and the biceps on the inside and the coracoacromial arch, the deltoid, and the coracoid muscles on the outside[269]; they measured up to 4 cm of gliding at this articulation in normal shoulders in vivo.

More recent investigations[53,123,124,371,491,502] have pointed to the importance of contact and load transfer between the rotator cuff and the coracoacromial arch in the function of normal shoulders, including the provision of superior stability. Because there is normally no gap between the superior cuff and the coracoacromial arch, the slightest amount of superior translation compresses the cuff tendon between the humeral head and the arch. Superior displacement is opposed by a countervailing force exerted by the coracoacromial arch through the cuff tendon to the humeral head. Ziegler and collaborators[502] demonstrated this "passive resistance" effect in cadavers by showing that the acromion bent upward when a superiorly directed force was applied to the humerus in the neutral position. The amount of acromial deformation was directly related to the amount of superior force applied to the humerus, the load being transmitted through the intact superior cuff tendon. Furthermore, these authors found that the amount of superior humeral displacement resulting from a superiorly directed humeral load of 80 N was increased from 1.7 to 5.4 mm when the cuff tendon was excised

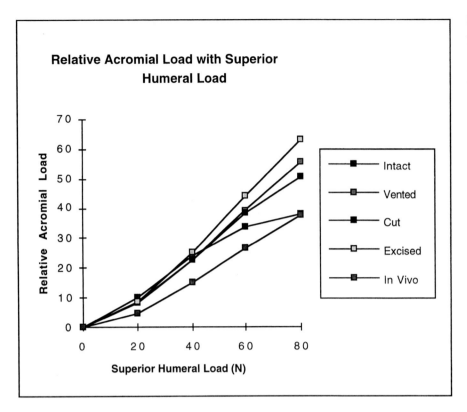

Figure 15-5
Superiorly directed humeral loads are transmitted to the acromion. If the superior cuff is intact, the load is transferred through the cuff tendon. If the cuff tendon is not interposed, the humeral head loads the acromion directly. The chart compares the relative acromial load as a function of the superiorly directed humeral load for intact specimens (1), after venting of the joint to air (2), after cutting (but not excising) the cuff tendon (3), and after excising the superior cuff tendon (4); also included are data from a single in vivo experiment performed with the identical instrumentation (5). Note the minimal difference in these acromial load–humeral load relationships, even when the cuff tendon has been excised.

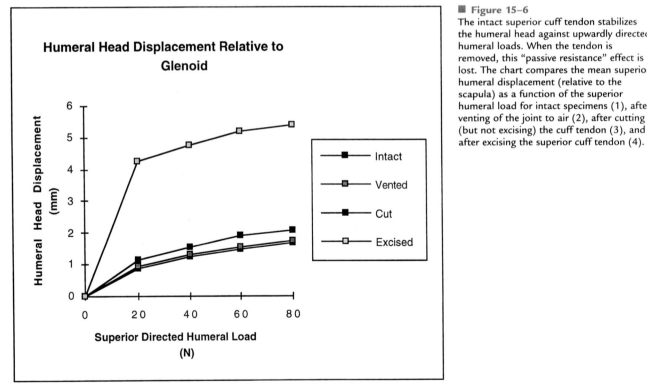

Figure 15-6
The intact superior cuff tendon stabilizes the humeral head against upwardly directed humeral loads. When the tendon is removed, this "passive resistance" effect is lost. The chart compares the mean superior humeral displacement (relative to the scapula) as a function of the superior humeral load for intact specimens (1), after venting of the joint to air (2), after cutting (but not excising) the cuff tendon (3), and after excising the superior cuff tendon (4).

($P < .0001$) (Figs. 15-5 and 15-6). These results indicate that an intact superior cuff tendon is subject to compressive loading between the humeral head and the coracoacromial arch and that the presence of this tendon provides passive resistance against superior displacement of the humeral head when superiorly directed loads are applied.

Flatow and coauthors[123] also noted in a dynamic cadaver model that the presence of the supraspinatus tendon limited superior translation of the humeral head, even when no tension was placed on the tendon from simulated muscle action.

The spacer effect of the superior cuff tendon is evident when comparing shoulders with intact cuffs (Fig. 15-7)

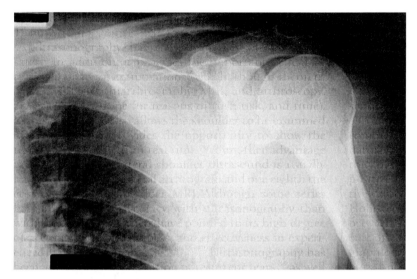

■ **Figure 15–7**
Passive resistance effect of an intact cuff tendon. The acromiohumeral interval of the left shoulder is preserved by the interposed superior cuff tendon in a 58-year-old man.

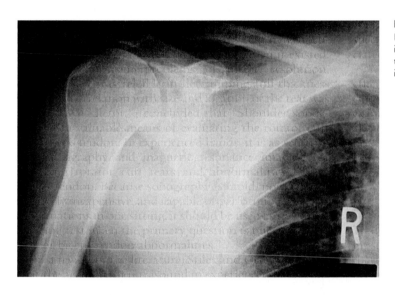

■ **Figure 15–8**
Loss of the passive resistance effect. The acromiohumeral interval of the right shoulder is narrowed because of loss of the interposed superior cuff tendon in the same individual as in Figure 15-7.

with those in which the superior tendon is deficient (Fig. 15–8).

Both Ziegler and colleagues and Flatow and coworkers cautioned that superior stability of the shoulder is dependent on an intact coracoacromial arch. Surgical sacrifice of the arch can lead to severe superior instability (Fig. 15–9).

Changes in the coracoacromial arch have been described in association with cuff disease[420] along with variations in acromial shape.[31,304] Two percent to 4% of asymptomatic college athletes with an average age of 19.9 years were found to have type III acromial morphology, whereas 12% to 14% and 84% to 85% had type I and II acromial morphology, respectively.[424] Another study of asymptomatic individuals showed no correlation of acromial morphology with age, but acromial and clavicular spurring was significantly associated with increasing age in persons without shoulder symptoms.[35] Bigliani and colleagues[30] studied 140 shoulders in 71 cadavers. The average age was 74.4 years. They identified three acromial shapes: type I (flat) in 17%, type II (curved) in 43%, and type III (hooked) in 40%. Fifty-eight percent of the cadavers had the same type of acromion on each side. Thirty-

three percent of the shoulders had full-thickness tears, 73% of which were seen in association with type III acromia, 24% with type II, and 3% with type I. The anterior slope of the acromion in shoulders with cuff tears averaged 29 degrees, slightly more than the slope of those without cuff tears, which averaged 23 degrees. The clinical significance of this relatively small difference is not known. A number of other authors have reported that patients with cuff defects are more likely to have hooked or angled acromia.[294,448,451] Nicholson and coworkers[320] demonstrated in a review of 420 scapulas that spur formation on the anterior acromion was an age-related process such that individuals younger than 50 years had less than one fourth the prevalence of those older than 50 years. The status of the cuffs of these shoulders is unknown. Another study by Gill and associates[147] showed that in patients older than 50 years, no significant association between acromial morphology and rotator cuff pathology could be found. However, there was a significant correlation with age and rotator cuff tears. Older patients were more likely to have type II and III acromia, although this study did not comment on whether this

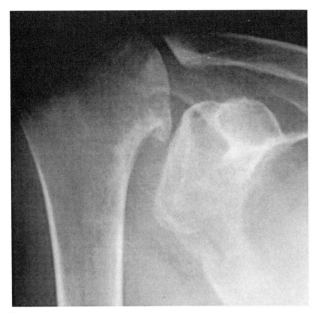

■ **Figure 15–9**
Anteroposterior roentgenogram after radical acromionectomy. This procedure removes the origin of the deltoid muscles and may fail to provide complete subacromial smoothing. This patient's symptoms were much more severe after surgery than before.

trend was significant. These findings imply that apparent correlations between acromial morphology and rotator cuff tears may be exaggerated because of the confounding variable of age.

A study of contact geometry between the undersurface of the coracoacromial arch and the rotator cuff revealed no significant differences in cadaveric shoulders with and without rotator cuff tears.[234]

A rotator cuff tear subsequently developed in 20% of patients who underwent an acromioplasty, thus suggesting that acromioplasty does not prevent the occurrence of rotator cuff tears.[189]

In a remarkable study, Ozaki and colleagues[336] correlated the histology of the acromial undersurface with the status of the rotator cuff in 200 cadaver shoulders. Cuff tears that did not extend to the bursal surface were associated with normal acromial histology, whereas those that extended to the bursal surface were associated with pathologic changes in the acromial undersurface. They concluded that most cuff tears are related to tendon degeneration and that acromial changes are secondary to pathology of the bursal side of the cuff. These results are similar to those reported Fukuda and coauthors.[133] The contact geometry of the rotator cuff and the undersurface of the coracoacromial arch was not significantly different between cadaveric shoulders with and without rotator cuff tears.[234]

Recent studies suggest that type II and III acromia are acquired rather than developmental.[500] In that most acromial "hooks" lie within the coracoacromial ligament (Figs. 15–10 and Fig. 15–11), it seems likely that they are actually traction spurs in this ligament (analogous to the traction spur seen in the plantar ligament at its attachment to the calcaneus) (Fig. 15–12). The traction loads producing this "hook" may result from loading of the arch by the cuff and may be increased with increasing dependency on the coracoacromial arch for superior stability in the presence of cuff degeneration.[123,124,502] The concept of the "hook" as a traction phenomenon was first forwarded by Neer over 30 years ago.[304] More recently, Putz and Reichelt[365] reported that three quarters of 133 operative specimens of the coracoacromial ligament showed chondroid metaplasia near the acromial insertion, thus

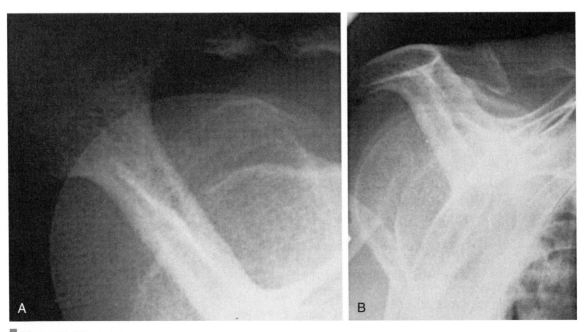

■ **Figure 15–10**
A, Variations in acromial shape are commonly observed in patients with cuff disease. The supraspinatus outlet view is helpful in defining this anatomy. **B,** In this arthrogram (lateral view), one can see indentation of the supraspinatus by the anteroinferior acromion.

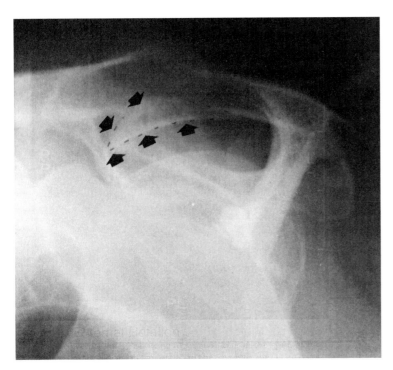

■ **Figure 15–11**
Supraspinatus outlet radiograph demonstrating a large
anterior inferior osteophyte *(arrows)*. *(From Iannotti JP:
Rotator Cuff Disorders: Evaluation and Treatment. Rosemont, IL:
American Academy of Orthopaedic Surgeons, 1991.)*

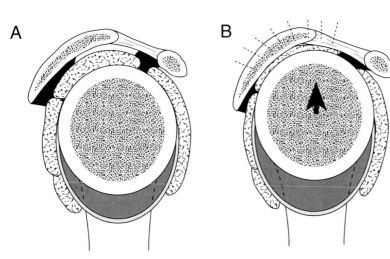

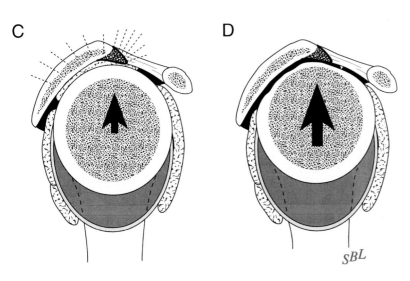

■ **Figure 15–12**
Progression of cuff fiber failure. **A,** Normal
relationships of the cuff and coracoacromial arch.
B, Upward displacement of the head, with the cuff
squeezed against the acromion and the coracoacromial
ligament. **C,** Greater contact and abrasion giving rise to
a traction spur in the coracoacromial ligament. **D,** Still
greater upward displacement resulting in abrasion
of the humeral articular cartilage and cuff tear
arthropathy. *(Modified from Matsen FA III, Lippitt SB,
Sidles JA, and Harryman DT II: Practical Evaluation and
Management of the Shoulder. Philadelphia: WB Saunders,
1994.)*

suggesting that this metaplastic area becomes the acromial "hook" by enchondral bone formation.[326] Because this "hook" lies within the ligament and points toward the coracoid (Fig. 15–11), it seems unlikely that it would jeopardize passage of the cuff beneath the coracoacromial arch (Fig. 15–12). Even in the severest cases of cuff tear arthropathy, the undersurface of the coracoacromial arch commonly presents a smooth articulating concavity (Figs. 15–12 and 15–13). The smoothness of the undersurface of the coracoacromial arch can be verified by palpation at surgery—even in cases in which an acromial spur is suggested by radiographs.

In view of the forgoing, it is instructive to consider the humeroscapular articulation as consisting of two concentric spheres, the glenohumeral sphere and the sphere represented by the articulation between the inferior surface of the coracoacromial arch and the proximal humeral convexity. Together, these two spheres enhance both shoulder stability and the surface available for scapulohumeral load transfer (Fig. 15–14).[66] Normally, the spheres of the humeral head and the coracoacromial arch share the same center. The difference in radius of the two spheres (R and r in Fig. 15–14) is provided by the thickness of the rotator cuff, which serves as a spacer. In the presence of posterior capsular tightness, shoulder flexion and/or internal rotation causes obligate anterosuperior translation of the humeral head and loss of the concentricity of the two spheres (Fig. 15–15).[73,171] As a result, the proximal humeral convexity is forced against the anterior undersurface of the concave coracoacromial arch rather than rotating concentrically beneath it (Fig. 15–14). In the presence of degeneration of the cuff tendon, the shoulder may lose the concentricity of the humeral head and coracoacromial arch spheres (Figs. 15–16 and 15–17). Taken together, these observations reinforce the shoulder's need for (1) normal posterior capsular laxity; (2) a smooth, concentric, and congruent coracoacromial undersurface; and (3) a normally thick and uniform cuff interposed between the humeral head and the coracoacromial arch.

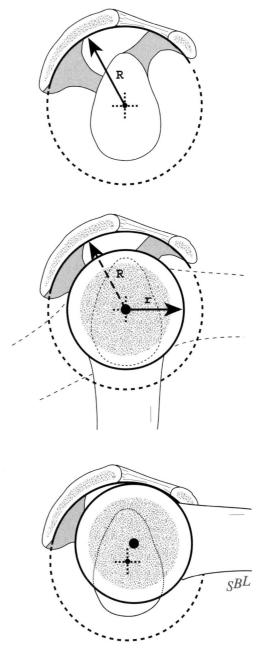

■ **Figure 15–14**
The two concentric spheres of the humeroscapular articulation. The coracoacromial arch sphere has a somewhat larger radius (R) than the humeral head sphere (r) does. In normal shoulder movement, these two spheres share the same center. When the posterior capsule is tight, obligate translation of the humeral head occurs in the anterosuperior direction as the shoulder is flexed. In this situation the centers no longer coincide, and the cuff (not shown) is squeezed between the humeral head and the anterior undersurface of the coracoacromial arch.

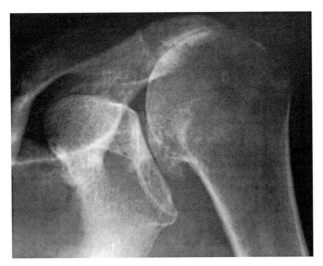

■ **Figure 15–13**
Chronic massive tears result in upward displacement of the humeral head until it articulates with the acromion. Humeral osteophytes result from an abnormal glenohumeral articulation. Note the smooth undersurface of the coracoacromial arch.

THE ACROMIOCLAVICULAR JOINT. Theoretically, osteophytes from the acromioclavicular joint may encroach on the space normally occupied by the cuff tendons (Fig. 15–18). However, these spurs are usually too medial to contact the tendons. In a series of 47 patients with arthrographically confirmed supraspinatus tendon rupture, Peterson and Gentz[353] found that 51% had distally pointing acromioclavicular joint osteophytes. A

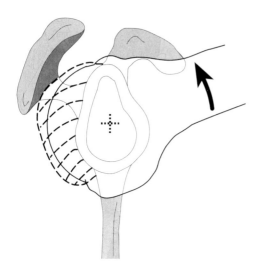

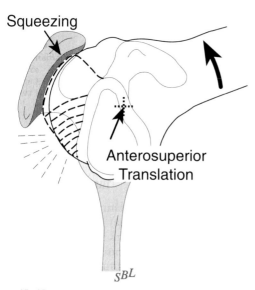

Squeezing

Anterosuperior
Translation

SBL

■ **Figure 15–15**
Normal capsular laxity allows the humeral head to remain centered
during elevation. Tightness of the posterior capsule can create obligate
anterosuperior translation with shoulder flexion. Such translation may
cause squeezing of the cuff (not shown) between the humerus and the
undersurface of the coracoacromial arch. *(Modified from Matsen FA III,
Lippitt SB, Sidles JA, and Harryman DT II: Practical Evaluation and
Management of the Shoulder. Philadelphia: WB Saunders, 1994.)*

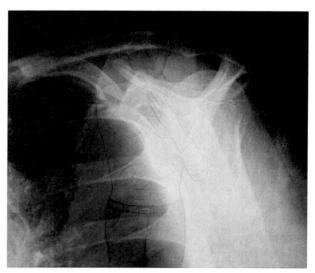

■ **Figure 15–16**
Concentricity of the humeral head and coracoacromial arch spheres
in a scapular lateral radiograph of the normal left shoulder of a
58-year-old man.

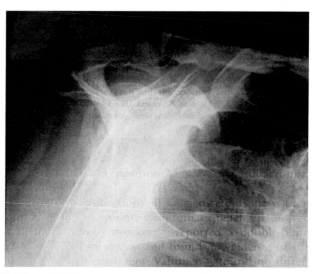

■ **Figure 15–17**
Scapular lateral radiograph of a right shoulder (same patient as in
Figure 15–16) that has a full-thickness tear of the supraspinatus
tendon. Note the loss of concentricity of the humeral head and the arc
of the coracoacromial undersurface.

similar incidence was found in their series of 170 autopsy
specimens with cuff defects. The incidence of distally
pointing acromioclavicular osteophytes in normal shoulders was 14% and 10% in the clinical and cadaver studies,
respectively. It is recognized, however, that degenerative
changes in the cuff and degenerative changes in the
acromioclavicular joint may coexist in the aging population without the former being causally related to the
latter. Again, it is recognized that acromioclavicular osteophytes are usually sufficiently medial that they do not
jeopardize the cuff.

The Rotator Cuff

The rotator cuff is a complex of four muscles that arise
from the scapula and whose tendons blend in with the
subjacent capsule as they attach to the tuberosities of the
humerus. The *subscapularis* arises from the anterior aspect
of the scapula and attaches over much of the lesser
tuberosity. It is innervated by the upper and lower subscapular nerves.[501] The *supraspinatus* muscle arises from
the supraspinatus fossa of the posterior portion of the
scapula, passes beneath the acromion and the acromioclavicular joint, and attaches to the superior aspect of the
greater tuberosity. It is innervated by the suprascapular
nerve after it passes through the suprascapular notch. The
infraspinatus muscle arises from the infraspinous fossa of
the posterior portion of the scapula and attaches to the
posterolateral aspect of the greater tuberosity. It is innervated by the suprascapular nerve after it passes through
the spinoglenoid notch. The *teres minor* arises from the

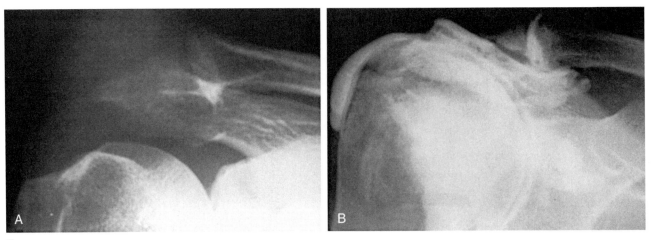

■ **Figure 15-18**
A, This anteroposterior roentgenogram shows acromioclavicular joint arthritis. **B,** An arthrogram in the same patient reveals leakage of dye into the acromioclavicular joint ("geyser sign"), thereby confirming the clinical suspicion of a rotator cuff tear. Note the indentation of the cuff caused by the acromioclavicular joint osteophytes.

lower lateral aspect of the scapula and attaches to the lower portion of the greater tuberosity. It is innervated by a branch of the axillary nerve.

The insertion of these tendons as a continuous cuff around the humeral head (Fig. 15-3) permits the cuff muscles to provide an infinite variety of moments to rotate the humerus and oppose unwanted components of deltoid and pectoralis muscle force.

The cross-sectional area of the anterior belly of the supraspinatus was found to be larger than its posterior belly. The tendon of the anterior muscle belly was found to have a smaller cross-sectional area than that of its posterior belly, however.[383] This increase in muscle strength-to-tendon area ratio may explain why rotator cuff tears often begin in the anterior portion of the supraspinatus. The superior portion of the subscapularis was found to be stiffer than its inferior portion.[163]

Bey and associates[28] found that the strain within the rotator cuff increased in positions of greater abduction, even when the same force was applied through the rotator cuff. No significant difference in strain on the superficial and deep portions of the cuff was detected. The compressive stiffness of the articular side of the supraspinatus tendon was found to be significantly less than that of its bursal side.[236] This difference in stiffness may contribute to the fact that most tears begin on the articular surface.

For an excellent review of the anatomy and histology of the rotator cuff, the reader is referred to the works of Clark and Harryman[61-63] and Warner's chapter on shoulder anatomy in *The Shoulder: A Balance of Mobility and Stability.*[470]

The long head of the biceps tendon may be considered a functional part of the rotator cuff. It attaches to the supraglenoid tubercle of the scapula, runs between the subscapularis and the supraspinatus, exits the shoulder through the bicipital groove under the transverse humeral ligament, and attaches to its muscle in the proximal part of the arm. Slátis and Aalto[413] point out that the coracohumeral ligament and the transverse humeral ligament keep the biceps tendon aligned in the groove. Tension in the long head of the biceps can help compress the

humeral head into the glenoid. Furthermore, this tendon has the potential for guiding the head of the humerus as it is elevated, with the bicipital groove traveling on the biceps tendon like a monorail on its track. This mechanism helps explain why the humerus is capable of substantial rotation when it is adducted and allows very little rotation when it is maximally abducted (in which position the tuberosities are constrained as they straddle the biceps tendon near its attachment to the supraglenoid tubercle).

The *mechanics of cuff action* is complex. The humeral torque resulting from contraction of a cuff muscle is determined by the moment arm (the distance between the effective point of application of this force and the center of the humeral head) and the component of the muscle force that is perpendicular to it (Fig. 15-19).[493]

The magnitude of force that can be delivered by a cuff muscle is determined by its size, health, and condition, as well as the position of the joint. The cuff muscles'

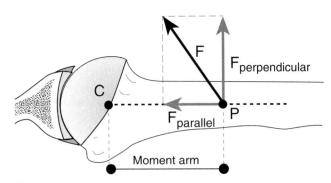

■ **Figure 15-19**
The moment arm is the distance between the point of application of a force (P) and the center of movement (C). Torque is the product of the moment arm and the component of the muscle force perpendicular to it (F perpendicular). The component of the muscle force that is parallel to the moment arm (F parallel) can contribute to joint stability through compression of the concavity. *(Modified from Matsen FA III, Lippitt SB, Sidles JA, and Harryman DT II: Practical Evaluation and Management of the Shoulder. Philadelphia: WB Saunders, 1994.)*

contribution to shoulder strength has been evaluated by Colachis and associates,[74,75] who used selective nerve blocks and found that the supraspinatus and infraspinatus provide 45% of abduction and 90% of external rotation strength. Howell and coworkers[188] measured the torque produced by the supraspinatus and deltoid muscles in forward flexion and elevation. They found that the supraspinatus and deltoid muscles are equally responsible for producing torque about the shoulder joint in the functional planes of motion. Generation of force in abduction of the arm decreased only 5% after a simulated tear of one third and two thirds of the supraspinatus. Detachment of the entire tendon resulted in a 17% loss of strength. Simulation of retraction of tears of one third, two thirds, and the entire supraspinatus resulted in losses of 19%, 36%, and 58%, respectively. These losses were almost completely regained with side-to-side repair.[164] Other estimates of the relative contributions of the rotator cuff to shoulder strength have been published.[30,71,462]

At least three factors complicate analysis of the contribution of a given muscle to shoulder strength:

1. The force and torque that a muscle can generate vary with the position of the joint: muscles are usually stronger near the middle of their excursion and weaker at the extremes (Fig. 15–20).[246]
2. The direction of a given muscle force is determined by the position of the joint. For example, the supraspinatus can contribute to abduction and/or external rotation, depending on the initial position of the arm.[333]
3. The effective humeral point of application for a cuff tendon wrapping around the humeral head is not its anatomic insertion, but rather the point at which the tendon first contacts the head, a point that usually lies on the articular surface (Fig. 15–21).

The cuff muscles may be thought of as having three functions:

1. They *rotate the humerus* with respect to the scapula.
2. They *compress the head into the glenoid fossa*, thereby providing a critical stabilizing mechanism to the shoulder known as concavity compression. Although in the past the cuff muscles were referred to as head depressors, it is evident that the inferiorly directed components of

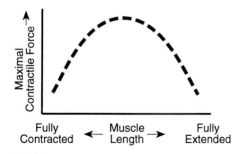

■ Figure 15–20
Typical relationship between a muscle's length and the maximal force that it can produce. The muscle's length is determined by its origin, insertion, and the position of the joint or joints that it spans. *(From Matsen FA III, Lippitt SB, Sidles JA, and Harryman DT II: Practical Evaluation and Management of the Shoulder. Philadelphia: WB Saunders, 1994.)*

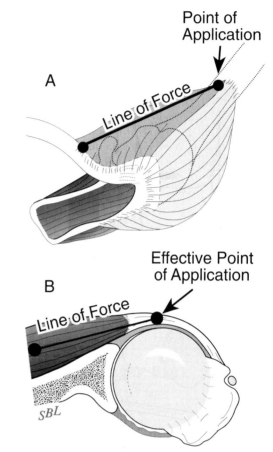

■ Figure 15–21
Point of application of muscle force. **A,** Determination of the point of application of force is simple when the line of force is colinear with its origin and insertion. **B,** However, the rotator cuff tendons wrap around the head of the humerus, so their effective point of attachment usually lies on the humeral articular surface. *(Modified from Matsen FA III, Lippitt SB, Sidles JA, and Harryman DT II: Practical Evaluation and Management of the Shoulder. Philadelphia: WB Saunders, 1994.)*

cuff muscle force are small; instead, the primary stabilizing function of the cuff muscles is through head compression into the glenoid (Fig. 15–22).[406,492]
3. They *provide muscular balance,* a critical function that will be discussed in some detail here. In the knee, the muscles generate torque primarily about a single axis: that of flexion-extension. If the quadriceps pull is a bit off center, the knee still extends. By contrast, in the shoulder, no fixed axis exists. In a specified position, activation of a muscle creates a unique set of rotational moments. For example, the anterior deltoid can exert moments in forward elevation, internal rotation, and cross-body movement (Fig. 15–23). If forward elevation is to occur without rotation, the cross-body and internal rotation moments of this muscle must be neutralized by other muscles, such as the posterior deltoid and infraspinatus (Fig. 15–24).[406] As another example, use of the latissimus dorsi in a movement of pure internal rotation requires that its adduction moment be neutralized by the superior cuff and deltoid. Conversely, use of the latissimus in a movement of pure adduction requires that its internal rotation moment be

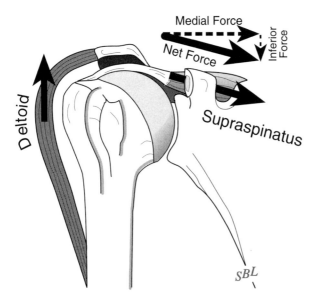

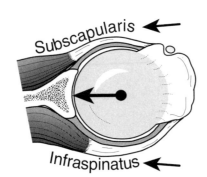

■ Figure 15–22
Concavity compression. The supraspinatus muscle is not optimally oriented to depress the head of the humerus against upward pull of the deltoid because the inferiorly directed component of the supraspinatus force is small. Instead, the humeral head is stabilized in the concave glenoid fossa by the compressive action of the cuff muscles. *(Modified from Matsen FA III, Lippitt SB, Sidles JA, and Harryman DT II: Practical Evaluation and Management of the Shoulder. Philadelphia: WB Saunders, 1994.)*

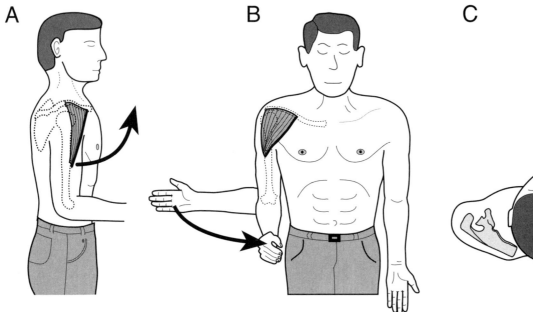

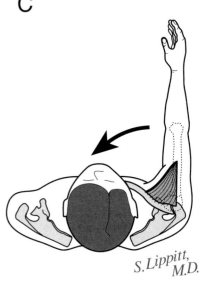

■ Figure 15–23
The anterior deltoid generates moments in forward elevation (**A**), internal rotation (**B**), and cross-body movement (**C**). (Modified from Matsen FA III, Lippitt SB, Sidles JA, and Harryman DT II: Practical Evaluation and Management of the Shoulder. Philadelphia: WB Saunders, 1994.)

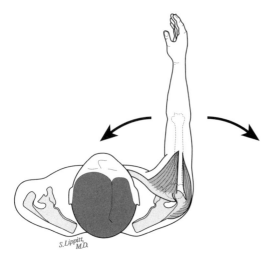

■ **Figure 15–24**
Pure elevation requires that the internal rotation and cross-body moments of the anterior deltoid be opposed by other muscle action. For example, even though it is an antagonist to the anterior deltoid, the posterior deltoid must contract during elevation in a plus 90-degree thoracic plane to resist the cross-body moment of the anterior deltoid. *(From Matsen FA III, Lippitt SB, Sidles JA, and Harryman DT II: Practical Evaluation and Management of the Shoulder. Philadelphia: WB Saunders, 1994.)*

neutralized by the posterior cuff and posterior deltoid muscles.

The timing and magnitude of these balancing muscle effects must be precisely coordinated to avoid unwanted directions of humeral motion. For gymnasts to hold their arms motionless above their head, all the force and torque exerted by each of the shoulder muscles must add up to zero. Thus, the simplified view of muscles as isolated motors, or as members of "force couples," must give way to an understanding that all shoulder muscles function together in a precisely coordinated way: opposing muscles canceling out undesired elements and leaving only the net torque that is needed to produce the desired action.[389]

This degree of coordination requires a preprogrammed strategy of muscle activation or engram that must be established before the motion is carried out. The rotator cuff muscles are critical elements of this shoulder muscle balance equation.*

The vascular anatomy of the cuff tendons has been described by a number of investigators.[43,256,297,369,388] Lindblom[249,250] described an area of relative avascularity in the supraspinatus tendon near its insertion. Rothman and Parke[388] found contributions to the cuff vessels from the suprascapular, anterior circumflex, and posterior circumflex arteries in all cases. The thoracoacromial contributed in 76% to the cuff's blood supply, the suprahumeral in 59%, and the subscapular in 38%. These authors found the area of the supraspinatus just proximal to its insertion to be markedly undervascularized in comparison to the remainder of the cuff. Uhthoff and coworkers[454] observed

relative hypovascularity of the deep surface of the supraspinatus insertion as compared with its superficial aspect.

By contrast, Moseley and Goldie studied the vascular pattern in the cuff tendons, including the "critical zone" of the supraspinatus (i.e., the anterior corner of the tendon near its insertion, which is prone to rupture and calcium deposits). They found a vascular network that received contributions from the anterior humeral circumflex, the subscapular, and the suprascapular arteries.[297] They concluded that the critical zone was not much less vascularized than other parts of the cuff; rather, it was rich in anastomoses between the osseous and tendinous vessels. Rathbun and Macnab[369] found that filling of cadaveric cuff vessels was dependent on the position of the arm at the time of injection. They noted a consistent zone of poor filling near the tuberosity attachment of the supraspinatus when the arm was adducted; with the arm in abduction, however, there was almost full filling of vessels to the point of insertion. They suggested that some of the previous data suggesting hypovascularity were, in fact, due to this artifact of positioning. Nixon and DiStefano[321] suggested that the "critical zone" of Codman corresponds to the area of anastomoses between the osseous vessels (the anterolateral branch of the anterior humeral circumflex and the posterior humeral circumflex) and the muscular vessels (the suprascapular and the subscapular vessels).

More recently, the vascularity of the supraspinatus tendon has been reconfirmed by the laser Doppler studies of Swiontkowski and colleagues.[432] The laser Doppler assesses red cell motion at a depth of 1 to 2 mm. These investigators found substantial flow in the "critical zone" of normal tendon and increased flow at the margins of cuff tears. Furthermore, Clark and associates,[61-63] found no avascular areas in their extensive histologic studies of the supraspinatus tendon.

Uhthoff and Sarkar[456] examined biopsy specimens obtained during surgery on 115 patients with complete rotator cuff rupture. They found vascularized connective tissue covering the area of rupture and proliferating cells in the fragmented tendons. They concluded that the main source of fibrovascular tissue for tendon healing was the wall of the subacromial bursa.

The *histology* of the supraspinatus insertion has been studied in some detail. Codman[66] observed that there were "transverse fibers in the upper portion of the tendon." He stated that "the insertion of the infraspinatus overlaps that of the supraspinatus to some extent. Each of the other tendons also interlaces its fibers to some extent with its neighbor's tendons." In detailed anatomic studies, Clark and colleagues[61-63] studied the tendons and capsule of the rotator cuff from shoulders aged 17 to 72 years. They found that the tendons splayed out and interdigitated to form a common continuous insertion on the humerus. The biceps tendon was unsheathed by interwoven fibers derived from the subscapularis and supraspinatus. Blood vessels were noted throughout the tendons with no avascular zones. When dissecting what initially appeared to be an intact cuff, the authors frequently encountered a deep substance tear in which fibers were avulsed from the humerus.

*See references 15, 92, 122, 159, 192, 200, 205, 247, 393, 422, 433, 466.

Benjamin and coworkers[23] analyzed four zones of the supraspinatus attachment to the greater tuberosity: (1) the tendon itself, (2) uncalcified fibrocartilage, (3) calcified fibrocartilage, and (4) bone. Whereas blood vessels were present in the other three zones, the zone of uncalcified fibrocartilage appeared to be avascular. A tidemark existed between the uncalcified and calcified fibrocartilage that was continuous with the tidemark between the uncalcified and calcified portions of articular cartilage. The collagen fibers often meet this tidemark at approximately right angles. The tendon of the supraspinatus had an abrupt change in fiber angle just before the tendon becomes fibrocartilaginous and only a slight change in angle within fibrocartilage. In interpreting the significance of these findings, these authors point out that the angle between the humerus and the tendon of the supraspinatus changes constantly in shoulder movement (Fig. 15–25). While the belly of the muscle remains parallel to the spine of the scapula, the tendon must bend to reach its insertion. This bending appears to take place above the level of the fibrocartilage so that the collagen fibers meet the tidemark at right angles. The fibrocartilage provides a transitional zone between hard and soft tissues, and this zone protects the fibers from sharp angulation at the interface between bone and tendon. The fibrocartilage pad keeps the tendon of the supraspinatus from rubbing on the head of the humerus during rotation, as well as

keeping it from bending, splaying out, kinking, or becoming compressed at the interface with hard tissue.

The *loading environment* of the cuff tendon fibers is complex, even in a normal shoulder. These fibers sustain concentric tension loads when the humerus is moved actively in the direction of action of the cuff muscle (Fig. 15–26). They sustain eccentric tension loads as they resist humeral motion or displacement in directions opposite the direction of action of the cuff muscles (Fig. 15–27). The tendon fibers are subjected to bending loads when the humeral head rotates with respect to the scapula (Fig. 15–25). As observed by Matsen and colleagues[269] in magnetic resonance imaging (MRI) with the arm positioned at the limits of motion, the glenoid rim can apply a sheering load to the deep surface of the tendon insertion (Fig. 15–28). This abutment of the labrum of the cuff

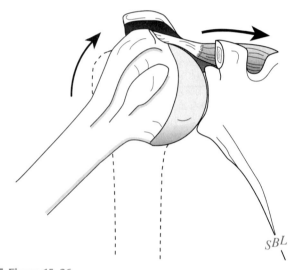

■ **Figure 15–26**
Concentric action of the cuff muscles: the muscle shortens under active tension. *(Modified from Matsen FA III, Lippitt SB, Sidles JA, and Harryman DT II: Practical Evaluation and Management of the Shoulder. Philadelphia: WB Saunders, 1994.)*

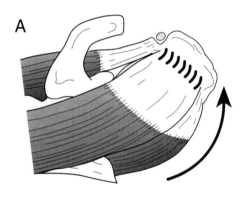

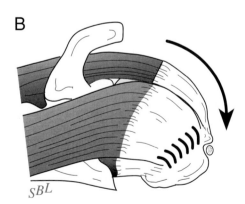

■ **Figure 15–25**
The cuff fibers bend at their insertion as the humerus rotates from internal rotation (**A**) to external rotation (**B**). *(Modified from Matsen FA III, Lippitt SB, Sidles JA, and Harryman DT II: Practical Evaluation and Management of the Shoulder. Philadelphia: WB Saunders, 1994.)*

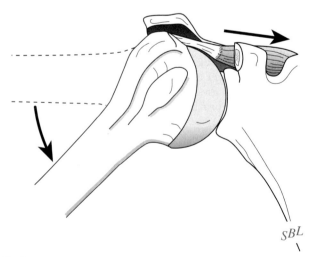

■ **Figure 15–27**
Eccentric action of the cuff muscles: the muscle lengthens under active tension. *(Modified from Matsen FA III, Lippitt SB, Sidles JA, and Harryman DT II: Practical Evaluation and Management of the Shoulder. Philadelphia: WB Saunders, 1994.)*

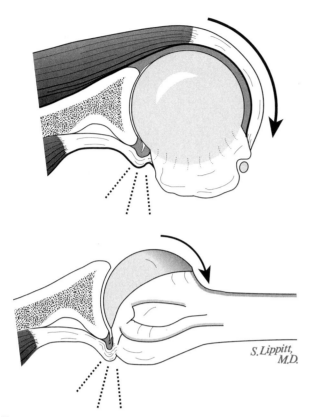

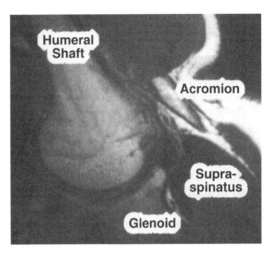

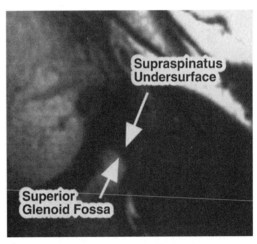

■ **Figure 15–28**
Abutment of the deep surface of the cuff insertion against the glenoid rim at the extremes of motion. *(Modified from Matsen FA III, Lippitt SB, Sidles JA, and Harryman DT II: Practical Evaluation and Management of the Shoulder. Philadelphia: WB Saunders, 1994.)*

■ **Figure 15–29**
This magnetic resonance image of the glenohumeral joint at maximal elevation shows abutment of the acromion against the humerus, which limits elevation. Note, however, that the supraspinatus tendon has cleared the acromion, so the acromion contacts the humerus distal to the cuff insertion rather than impinging on the tendon. *(From Matsen FA III, Lippitt SB, Sidles JA, and Harryman DT II: Practical Evaluation and Management of the Shoulder. Philadelphia: WB Saunders, 1994.)*

■ **Figure 15–30**
In the same shoulder as shown in Figure 15–29, abutment of the undersurface of the supraspinatus tendon against the superior glenoid fossa occurs at the extremes of motion. *(From Matsen FA III, Lippitt SB, Sidles JA, and Harryman DT II: Practical Evaluation and Management of the Shoulder. Philadelphia: WB Saunders, 1994.)*

against the cuff insertion may be a better explanation than acromial impingement for the deep surface cuff defects seen in throwers (Figs. 15–29 and 15–30).[121,202,255,386,447,465]

Recently, Ziegler and coauthors[502] suggested that the superior cuff tendon also experiences *compressive loads* as it is squeezed between the humeral head and the coracoacromial arch when superiorly directed loads are applied to the humerus. In a cadaver model, they found that the preponderance of an upwardly directed humeral load was transmitted through the cuff tendon to the overlying acromion. When the cuff tendon was excised, the humeral head moved cephalad 6 mm until the superior humeral load was applied directly to the acromion (Figs. 15–5 and 15–6). Using completely different methodologies, Lazarus and coworkers[231] and Poppen and Walker[358] also found that the humeral head translated 6 mm superiorly when the cuff tendon was absent. Flatow and colleagues[124] referred to this phenomenon as the "spacer" effect of the cuff tendon. Kaneko and associates[209] found that superior displacement of the humeral head was one of the most significant plain radiographic signs of massive cuff deficiency (Figs. 15–7 and 15–8). Sigholm and colleagues[411] found evidence of this normal tendon compression in vivo. Using a micropipette infusion technique, they found that the normal subacromial resting pressure of 8 mm Hg was elevated to 39 mm Hg by active shoulder flexion to 45 degrees and to 56 mm Hg by the addition of a 1-kg weight to the hand in the elevated position.

Morphologic evidence has emerged to support the concept of compressive loading of the supraspinatus tendon. Okuda[330] described fibrocartilaginous areas in regions of tendons subjected to compression. Riley and coworkers[377] found such areas in the supraspinatus tendon and noted that they had the proteoglycan/glycosaminoglycan of tendon fibrocartilage. They indicated that these morphologic features were an adaptation to mechanical forces, including compression. It has been questioned whether compression of the cuff by the acromion could produce the type of cuff defects commonly seen in clinical practice. Recent investigations in a rat model[402] demonstrated that increasing the loading and abrasion of the cuff tendon by the addition of bone plates between the acromion and the tendon produced only bursal-side lesions and never the intratendinous or articular-side cuff tendon defects that are most frequently seen clinically.

Although young healthy tendons seem to tolerate their complex loading situation without difficulty, structurally inferior tissue,[227,377] tissue with compromised repair potential,[87,165] or tendons frequently subjected to unusually large loads (as in an individual with paraplegia)[19] may degenerate in their hostile mechanical environment.[148,336,376]

TENDON DEGENERATION. Normal tendon is exceedingly strong. The work of McMaster[278] is frequently quoted in this regard. He conducted experiments showing that loads applied to normal rabbit Achilles tendons produced failure at the musculotendinous junction, at the insertion into bone, at the muscle origin, or at the bone itself, but not at the tendon midsubstance. In his preparation, half of the tendon's fibers had to be severed before the tendon failed in tension. If the tendon was crushed with a Kocher clamp, pounded, and then doubly ligated above and below the injury, rupture could be produced in half the specimens when tested over 4 weeks later. Normal tendon is obviously tough stuff!

It is estimated that in normal activities, the force transmitted through the cuff tendon is in the range of 140 to 200 N.[230,244,256,395] The ultimate tensile load of the supraspinatus tendon in specimens from the sixth or seventh decade of life has been measured to be between 600 and 800 N.[194]

Although cuff strength may be compromised by inflammatory arthritis[72,272] and steroids,[111,212] the primary cause of tendon degeneration is aging. Like the rest of the body's connective tissues, rotator cuff tendon fibers become weaker with disuse and age; as they become weaker, less force is required to disrupt them (Fig. 15–31).[60,305,369,432] Hollis and associates[185] showed that the anterior cruciate ligament of a 70-year-old is only 20% to 25% as strong as that of a 20-year-old. Others have shown similar loss of tendon strength with age.[66,93,249-251,265,304,306,321,354,476] Uhthoff and Sarkar concluded that "aging is the single most important contributing factor in the pathogenesis of tears of the cuff tendons."[457]

Pettersson[354] provides an excellent summary of the early work on the pathology of degenerative changes in

the cuff tendons. Citing the research of Loschke, Wrede, Codman, Schaer, Glatthaar, Wells, and others, he builds a convincing case for primary, age-related degeneration of the tendon manifested by changes in cell arrangement, calcium deposition, fibrinoid thickening, fatty degeneration, necrosis, and rents. He states that "the degenerative changes in the tendon aponeurosis of the shoulder joint, except for calcification and rupture, give no symptoms, as far as is known at present. On the other hand the tensile strength and elasticity of a tendon aponeurosis that exhibits such degenerative lesions are unquestionably less than in a normal tendon aponeurosis."

The major role of tendon degeneration in the production of cuff defects was promoted by Meyer[280,281] and corroborated by the studies of DePalma and others.[80,94-96,158,307,336,455,504] Nixon and DiStefano, reviewing the literature on the microscopic anatomy of cuff deterioration,[321] found loss of the normal organizational and staining characteristics of bone, fibrocartilage, and tendon without evidence of repair. They summarized these degenerative changes as follows:

> Early changes are characterized by granularity and a loss of the normal clear wavy outline of the collagen fibers and bundles of fibers. The structures take on a rather homogenous appearance; the connective tissue cells become distorted and the parallelism of the fibers is lost. The cell nuclei become distorted in appearance—some rounded, others pyknotic or fasiculated. Some areas of the tendon have a gelatinous or edematous appearance with loosening of fibers that contain broken, frayed elements separated by a pale staining homogeneous material.

This histologic picture is reminiscent of that described for tennis elbow, Achilles tendinitis, and patellar tendinitis.

Brewer[41] has demonstrated age-related changes in the rotator cuff. These changes include diminution of fibrocartilage at the cuff insertion, diminution of vascularity, fragmentation of the tendon with loss of cellularity and staining quality, and disruption of the attachment to bone via Sharpey's fibers. The bone at the insertion becomes osteoporotic and prone to fracture.[210]

Kumagai and colleagues[227] studied the attachment zone of the rotator cuff tendons to determine how degenerative changes affect the pattern of collagen fiber distribution. Degenerative changes were found in all elderly tendons but not in tendons from younger subjects. Changes in insertional fibrocartilage included calcification, fibrovascular proliferation, and microtears. In degenerative tendons, the normal distribution of collagen fiber types was markedly altered, with fibrovascular tissue containing type III collagen instead of the usually predominant type II. The authors concluded that severe degenerative changes in the cuff tendons of elderly individuals alter the collagen characteristic of the rotator cuff and that these changes could be associated with impairment of the biomechanical properties of the attachment zone. Virtually identical findings were reported by Riley and coauthors.[376]

In all clinical reports, the incidence of cuff defects is relatively low before the age of 40, begins to rise in the 50- to 60-year-old age group, and continues to increase in

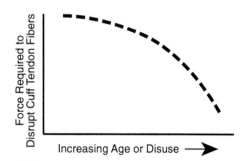

■ **Figure 15–31**
The force necessary to disrupt the rotator cuff tendon fibers diminishes with age, disuse, or both. *(From Matsen FA III, Lippitt SB, Sidles JA, and Harryman DT II: Practical Evaluation and Management of the Shoulder. Philadelphia: WB Saunders, 1994.)*

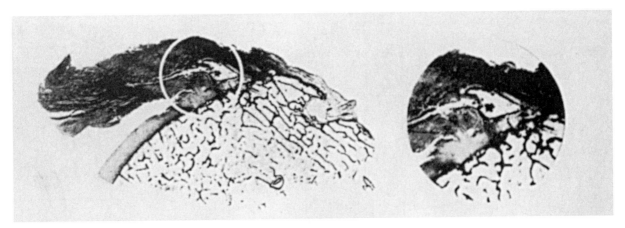

■ Figure 15–32
Codman's illustration of "A rim rent where all the tendon is torn away from the sulcus except the superficial portion which extends into the periosteum." These photomicrographs provide a convincing argument that cuff tears frequently begin on the deep surface and extend outward until they become full-thickness defects. *(From Codman EA: The Shoulder: Rupture of the Supraspinatus Tendon and Other Lesions in or about the Subacromial Bursa. Malabar, FL: Robert E Krieger, 1984.)*

the 70-year and older age group. Of 55 patients with arthrographically verified cuff tears, Bakalim and Pasila[10] found only 3 who were younger than 40 years. Yamada and Evans found no cuff tears in 42 shoulders younger than 40 years.[495] In Hawkins and coworkers' series of 100 cuff repairs, only two patients were in their third or fourth decade.[178] In their series of shoulder dislocations, Reeves[370] and Moseley[296] found the incidence of cuff tears in patients younger than 30 to be very low. These authors found that the incidence of cuff failure in dislocated shoulders rose dramatically with the age of the patient. As noted by DePalma, even massive injuries to young healthy shoulders "seem more likely to produce glenohumeral ligament tears and fractures than ruptures of the rotator cuff." Pettersson[354] states that "even in cases of traumatic rupture . . . the age distribution indicates that changes in the elasticity and tensile strength are prerequisites for the appearance of the rupture." Pettersson[354] reported further that in patients with anteroinferior dislocations, the incidence of arthrographically proven partial- or full-thickness cuff tears was 30% in the fourth decade and 60% in the sixth decade.

Many cuff defects occur in 50- to 60-year-old individuals who have led quite sedentary lives without a history of injury or heavy use. Asymptomatic people 50 years and older were found to have ultrasonographic evidence of a rotator cuff tear in 23% of shoulders. Thirteen percent of people aged 50 to 59 years, 20% of 60- to 69-year-olds, and 31% of 70- to 79-year-old people had sonographic evidence of a rotator cuff tear.[440] In one of his clinical series, Neer provided substantial evidence for a degenerative etiology of cuff defects[306]: (1) 40% of those with cuff defects have "never done strenuous physical work," (2) cuff defects are frequently bilateral, (3) cuff defects never develop in many heavy laborers, and (4) 50% of patients with cuff defects had no recollection of shoulder trauma. In their 1988 report to the American Shoulder and Elbow Surgeons, Neer and coworkers[309] found that of 233 patients with cuff defects, all but 8 were older than 40 years; 70% of the defects occurred in sedentary individuals doing light work, 27% in females, and 28% in the nondominant arm.

As expected, the deterioration in cuff quality is usually bilateral. Matsen and colleagues found that 55% of patients being evaluated for cuff tears on one side had ultrasonographic evidence of cuff defects on the contralateral side.[269] Age-related degeneration can also be observed by MRI.[453]

The pattern of degenerative cuff failure is distinctive. E. A. Codman described the "rim rent" in which the deep surface of the cuff is torn at its attachment to the tuberosity.[66] The many photomicrographs of these rim rents in Codman's wonderful book provide a convincing argument that cuff tears most frequently begin on the deep surface and extend outward until they become full-thickness defects (see Fig. 15-32). Codman pointed out that "it would be hard to explain this . . . by erosion from contact with the acromion process." Similarly, McLaughlin[273] observed that partial tears of the cuff "commonly involve only the deep surface of the cuff. . . ." Wilson and Duff[486] also described partial tears near the insertion of the cuff. They occurred on the articular surface, on the bursal surface, and in the substance of the tendon. Cotton and Rideout[80] described "slight" tears on the deep surface of the supraspinatus adjacent to the biceps tendon in their necropsy studies. Pettersson and DePalma noted that the innermost fibers of the cuff begin to tear away from their bony insertion to the humeral head in the fifth decade and that these partial-thickness tears increase in size over the next several decades.[93,354] The partial-thickness tears observed by Uhthoff and coworkers[454] were always on the articular side; none occurred on the bursal side in spite of the occasional presence of spurs or osteophytes on the acromion. Other authors also have described partial-thickness tears.* These observations suggest that the deep fibers of the cuff near its insertion to the tuberosity are most vulnerable to failure, either because of the loads to which they are exposed, because of their relative lack of strength, or because of their limited capacity for repair.

---

*See references 37, 38, 66, 131, 135, 229, 288, 337, 428, 434, 435, 438, 496-498.

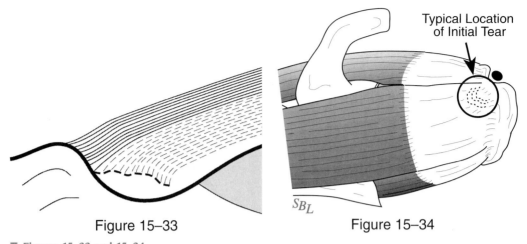

Figure 15–33   Figure 15–34

■ Figures 15–33 and 15–34
In degenerative cuff disease, the tendon fibers fail a few at a time, usually starting at the deep surface of the supraspinatus near its insertion close to the long head of the biceps. *(Modified from Matsen FA III, Lippitt SB, Sidles JA, and Harryman DT II: Practical Evaluation and Management of the Shoulder. Philadelphia: WB Saunders, 1994.)*

An important study by Fukuda and colleagues documented the patterns of intratendinous tears and observed that these lesions tend to not heal.[132] Further evidence of the nonhealing of cuff lesions was provided by Yamanaka and Matsumoto,[499] who demonstrated progression of partial-thickness tears. After initial arthrography, they monitored 40 tears (average patient age, 61 years) managed without surgery. Repeat arthrograms an average of 1 year later showed apparent healing in only 10%, a reduction in apparent tear size in 10%, and enlargement of the tear size in over 50%, with over 25% progressing to full-thickness tears. Interestingly, the clinical pain and function scores of these patients were *improved* at follow-up. These observations lend "proof" to Codman's statement 60 years earlier, "It is my unproved opinion that many of these lesions never heal, although the symptoms caused by them usually disappear after a few months. Otherwise, how could we account for their frequent presence at autopsy?"[66] These studies also demonstrate the critical point that scores based on clinical symptoms are an unreliable way of determining the integrity of the cuff tendon.

The traumatic and the degenerative theories of cuff tendon failure can be synthesized into a unified view of pathogenesis. Throughout its life the cuff is subjected to various adverse factors such as traction, compression, contusion, subacromial abrasion, inflammation, injections, and, perhaps most importantly, age-related degeneration. Lesions of the cuff typically start where the loads are presumably the greatest: at the deep surface of the anterior insertion of the supraspinatus near the long head of the biceps (Figs. 15–33 and 15–34). Tendon fibers fail when the applied load exceeds their strength. Fibers may fail a few at a time or en masse (Fig. 15–35). Because these fibers are under load even with the arm at rest, they retract after rupture. Each instance of fiber failure has at least four adverse effects: (1) it increases the load on the neighboring, as yet unruptured fibers and gives rise to the "zipper" phenomenon; (2) it detaches muscle fibers from bone, thereby diminishing the force that the cuff muscles

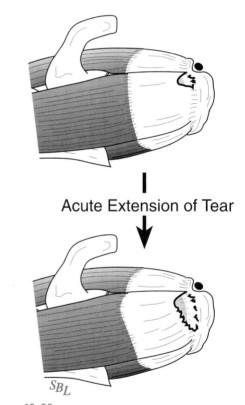

Acute Extension of Tear

■ Figure 15–35
Acute extension of a defect in the rotator cuff. *(Modified from Matsen FA III, Lippitt SB, Sidles JA, and Harryman DT II: Practical Evaluation and Management of the Shoulder. Philadelphia: WB Saunders, 1994.)*

can deliver; (3) it compromises the tendon fibers' blood supply by distorting the anatomy and thus contributes to progressive local ischemia (Fig. 15–36); and (4) it exposes increasing amounts of the tendon to joint fluid containing lytic enzymes, which remove any hematoma that could contribute to tendon healing (Fig. 15–37). Even when the tendon heals, its scar tissue lacks the normal resilience of tendon and is therefore at increased risk of failure with subsequent loading. These events weaken the

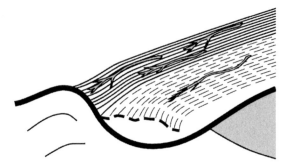

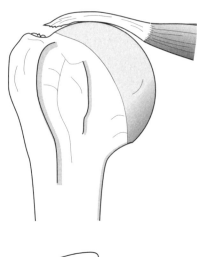

■ **Figure 15–36**
Excessive tension at the margin of the tear can compromise local tendon circulation. *(From Matsen FA III, Lippitt SB, Sidles JA, and Harryman DT II: Practical Evaluation and Management of the Shoulder. Philadelphia: WB Saunders, 1994.)*

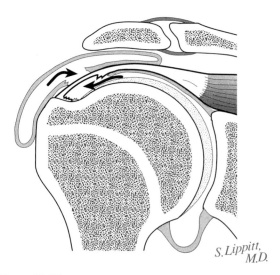

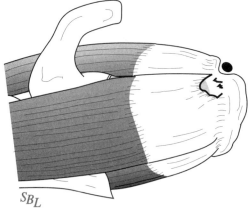

■ **Figure 15–37**
The tendon defect is bathed in joint fluid, thereby preventing the formation of a fibrin clot and further compromising the healing potential of the tear. *(Modified from Matsen FA III, Lippitt SB, Sidles JA, and Harryman DT II: Practical Evaluation and Management of the Shoulder. Philadelphia: WB Saunders, 1994.)*

■ **Figure 15–38**
Full-thickness defect in the supraspinatus tendon. *(Modified from Matsen FA III, Lippitt SB, Sidles JA, and Harryman DT II: Practical Evaluation and Management of the Shoulder. Philadelphia: WB Saunders, 1994.)*

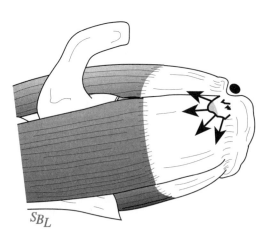

■ **Figure 15–39**
The notch phenomenon: the stress on the tendon is channeled toward the edges of the defect, thereby leading to further fiber failure. *(From Matsen FA III, Lippitt SB, Sidles JA, and Harryman DT II: Practical Evaluation and Management of the Shoulder. Philadelphia: WB Saunders,1994.)*

substance of the cuff, impair its function, and diminish its ability to effectively repair itself. In the absence of repair, the degenerative process tends to continue through the substance of the supraspinatus tendon and produce a full-thickness defect in the anterior supraspinatus tendon (Fig. 15–38). This full-thickness defect tends to concentrate loads at its margin, thereby facilitating additional fiber failure with smaller loads than those that produced the initial defect (Fig. 15–39). With subsequent episodes of loading, this pattern repeats itself and renders the cuff weaker, more prone to additional failure with less load, and less able to heal. Once a supraspinatus defect is established, it typically propagates posteriorly through the remainder of the supraspinatus and then into the infraspinatus (Fig. 15–40).

With progressive dissolution of the cuff tendon, the spacer effect of the cuff tendon is lost and the humeral head can become displaced superiorly (Figs. 15–8 and 15–12), thus placing increased load on the biceps tendon. As a result, the breadth of the tendon of the long head of the biceps is often greater in patients with cuff tears than

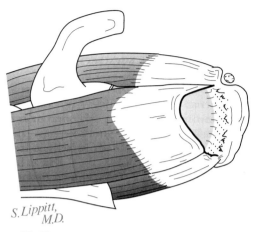

■ Figure 15–40
The defect propagates through the remainder of the supraspinatus and into the infraspinatus tendon. *(Modified from Matsen FA III, Lippitt SB, Sidles JA, and Harryman DT II: Practical Evaluation and Management of the Shoulder. Philadelphia: WB Saunders, 1994.)*

in uninjured shoulders (Fig. 15–41).[446] In chronic cuff deficiency, the tendon of the long head of the biceps is frequently ruptured.

Further propagation of the cuff defect crosses the bicipital groove to involve the subscapularis, starting at the top of the lesser tuberosity and extending inferiorly. As the defect extends across the bicipital groove, it may be associated with rupture of the transverse humeral ligament and destabilization of the tendon of the long head of the biceps, thereby allowing medial displacement of the tendon (Fig. 15–42).[413]

The concavity compression mechanism of glenohumeral stability (Fig. 15–22) is compromised by cuff disease. Rotator cuff muscles are important in shoulder stability in the mid and end ranges of motion. In the mid

ranges, the supraspinatus and subscapularis were most important for glenohumeral stability. In the apprehension position, however, the subscapularis, infraspinatus, and teres minor were more important in providing glenohumeral stability.[235]

Beginning with the early stages of cuff fiber failure, compression of the humeral head becomes less effective in resisting upward pull of the deltoid. Partial-thickness cuff tears cause pain on muscle contraction similar to that seen with other partial tendon injuries (such as those of the Achilles tendon or extensor carpi radialis brevis). This pain produces reflex inhibition of the muscle's action. In turn, this reflex inhibition along with the absolute loss of strength from fiber detachment makes the muscle less effective in balance and stability. However, as long as the glenoid concavity is intact, the compressive action of the residual cuff muscles may stabilize the humeral head (Fig. 15–43). When the weakened cuff cannot prevent the humeral head from rising under the pull of the deltoid, the residual cuff becomes squeezed between the head and the coracoacromial arch. Under these circumstances, abrasion occurs with humeroscapular motion, thus further contributing to cuff degeneration (Fig. 15–44). Degenerative traction spurs develop in the coracoacromial ligament, which is loaded by pressure from the humeral head (analogous to the calcaneal traction spur that occurs with chronic strains of the plantar fascia) (see Fig. 15–12). Upward displacement of the head also wears on the upper glenoid lip and labrum (Fig. 15–45) and thereby reduces the effectiveness of the upper glenoid concavity. Further deterioration of the cuff allows the tendons to slide down below the center of the humeral head and produce a "boutonnière" deformity (Fig. 15–46).[324] The cuff tendons become head elevators rather than head compressors. Just as in a boutonnière deformity of the finger, a shoulder with a buttonholed cuff is victimized by the conversion of balancing forces into

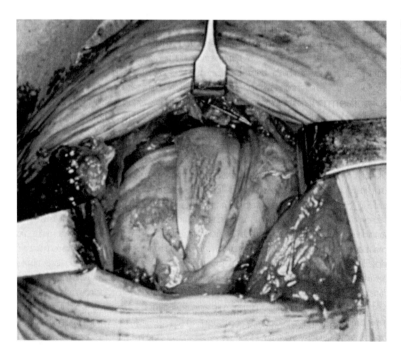

■ Figure 15–41
Rotator cuff tears are frequently accompanied by changes in the tendon of the long head of the biceps as it exits the bicipital groove. In many cases, the biceps is seen to be hypertrophied and flattened to the contour of the humeral head—almost as though it were trying to become a substitute cuff.

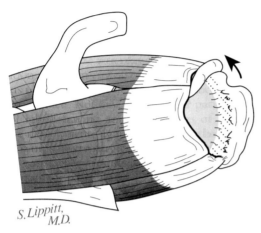

■ **Figure 15–42**
Further propagation of the defect across the bicipital groove to the subscapularis destabilizes the tendon of the long head of the biceps. *(Modified from Matsen FA III, Lippitt SB, Sidles JA, and Harryman DT II: Practical Evaluation and Management of the Shoulder. Philadelphia: WB Saunders, 1994.)*

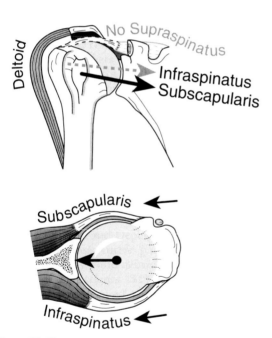

■ **Figure 15–43**
Compression by the infraspinatus and the subscapularis can help stabilize the humeral head in the absence of a supraspinatus, provided that the glenoid concavity is intact. *(From Matsen FA III, Lippitt SB, Sidles JA, and Harryman DT II: Practical Evaluation and Management of the Shoulder. Philadelphia: WB Saunders, 1994.)*

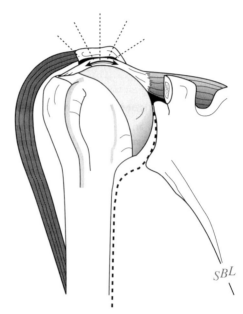

■ **Figure 15–44**
Abrasion of the superficial surface of the cuff by the coracoacromial arch associated with superior displacement of the head relative to the glenoid. *(Modified from Matsen FA III, Lippitt SB, Sidles JA, and Harryman DT II: Practical Evaluation and Management of the Shoulder. Philadelphia: WB Saunders, 1994.)*

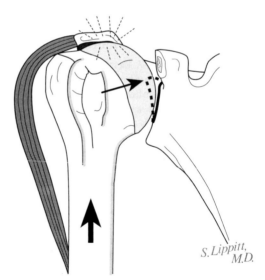

■ **Figure 15–45**
Erosion of the superior glenoid concavity compromises the concavity compression stability mechanism and allows upward translation. The destabilizing effect of this permanent loss of the effective glenoid concavity cannot be offset by rotator cuff repair (see also Fig. 15–47). *(Modified from Matsen FA III, Lippitt SB, Sidles JA, and Harryman DT II: Practical Evaluation and Management of the Shoulder. Philadelphia: WB Saunders, 1994.)*

unbalancing forces. Erosion of the superior glenoid lip may thwart attempts to keep the humeral head centered after cuff repair (Fig. 15–47). Once the full thickness of the cuff has failed, abrasion of the humeral articular cartilage against the coracoacromial arch may lead to a secondary degenerative joint disease known as cuff tear arthropathy (see Figs. 15–12 and 15–48).[308]

The cuff muscle deterioration that inevitably accompanies chronic cuff tears is one of the most important limiting factors in cuff repair surgery. Atrophy, fatty degeneration, retraction, and loss of excursion are all commonly associated with chronic cuff tendon defects.[239,302]

To a large extent, these factors are irreversible.[154] These changes increase with the duration of the tear and do not rapidly reverse after cuff repair.[155]

CLINICAL CONDITIONS INVOLVING THE CUFF

The requisites for normal cuff function are stringent and include healthy, strong cuff muscles, normal capsular

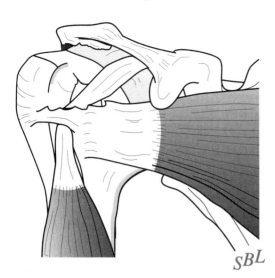

■ **Figure 15–46**

The boutonnière deformity, in which the subscapularis and infraspinatus tendons slide below the center of the humeral head. *(Modified from Matsen FA III, Lippitt SB, Sidles JA, and Harryman DT II: Practical Evaluation and Management of the Shoulder. Philadelphia: WB Saunders, 1994.)*

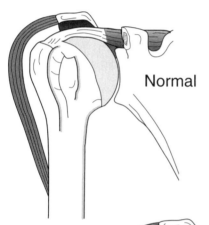

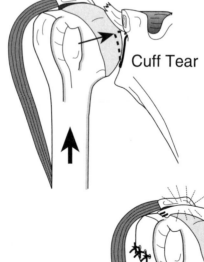

Normal

Cuff Tear

Cuff Repair

■ **Figure 15–47**

In chronic cuff deficiency, erosion of the upper glenoid may leave the shoulder with a permanent tendency toward superior subluxation that cannot be reversed by cuff repair surgery.

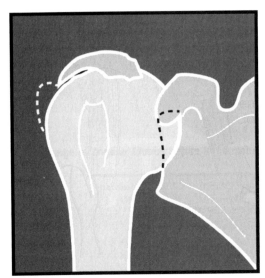

■ **Figure 15–48**
Radiographic appearance of cuff tear arthropathy with acetabularization of the upper glenoid and the coracoacromial arch and femoralization of the proximal end of the humerus. *(Modified from Matsen FA III, Lippitt SB, Sidles JA, and Harryman DT II: Practical Evaluation and Management of the Shoulder. Philadelphia: WB Saunders, 1994.)*

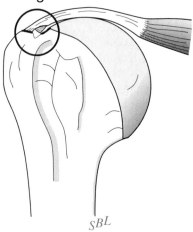

Avulsion with Bone Fragment

■ **Figure 15–49**
Partial-thickness cuff tear with avulsion of a bony fragment from the tuberosity. *(Modified from Matsen FA III, Lippitt SB, Sidles JA, and Harryman DT II: Practical Evaluation and Management of the Shoulder. Philadelphia: WB Saunders, 1994.)*

laxity, intact cuff tendons, a smooth contour of the under-surface of the coracoacromial arch, a thin, lubricating bursa, a smooth upper surface of the cuff and tuberosities, and concentricity of the glenohumeral and cuff-coracoacromial spheres of rotation (see Figs. 15–3, 15–4, 15–14, 15–15, and 15–22). Disorders of this complex mechanism are the most common source of shoulder problems.[57,190]

Cuff disruption may be partial or full thickness, acute or chronic, and traumatic or degenerative.[71,269] The magnitude of cuff disruption ranges from the mildest strain to total absence of the cuff tendons. In younger patients, partial-thickness cuff lesions may include avulsion of a small chip of bone from the tuberosity, the radiographic appearance of which should not be confused with that of calcific tendinitis (Fig. 15–49). Contributing factors may include trauma,[65,67] attrition,[95,218,280,295] ischemia,[249,251,297,369,388] and subacromial abrasion.[81,304,306,316,353,473]

Degenerative cuff failure almost always starts with a partial-thickness defect on the deep surface near the attachment of the supraspinatus to the greater tuberosity. Codman's view of the frequency of this lesion and the potential range of pathology is indicated by the following passage[66]:

Figure 15–50 shows an extensive tear so that the rent has come through to the most superficial fibers of the tendon. The reader should visualize this vertical section so as to understand that the rent also extends along the curve of the edge of the joint cartilage to a considerable extent, leaving the sulcus bare, perhaps for an inch or more. This condition I like to call a "rim rent," and I am confident that these rim rents account for the great majority of sore shoulders. It is my unproved opinion that many of these lesions never heal, although the symptoms caused by them usually disappear after a few months. Otherwise, how could we account for their frequent presence at autopsy?

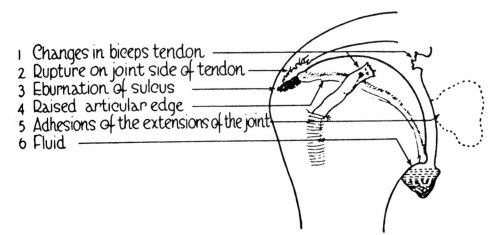

1 Changes in biceps tendon
2 Rupture on joint side of tendon
3 Eburnation of sulcus
4 Raised articular edge
5 Adhesions of the extensions of the joint
6 Fluid

■ **Figure 15–50**
In 1934, Codman described the "rim rent" wherein the deep surface of the cuff is torn at its attachment to the tuberosity. *(From Codman EA: The Shoulder: Rupture of the Supraspinatus Tendon and Other Lesions in or about the Subacromial Bursa. Malabar, FL: Robert E Krieger, 1984.)*

The anatomically observed prevalence of partial-thickness cuff lesions leads one to Codman's suggestion that the commonly diagnosed conditions involving shoulder pain, referred to as "cuff tendinitis," "bursitis," or "impingement syndrome," may actually represent failure of the deep surface fibers of the rotator cuff.[132] The degree to which the fibers that remain intact may hypertrophy, strengthen, or adapt[50] to stabilize the tear and take up the function of the damaged fibers is not known. It appears likely that repeated failure of small groups of fibers leads not only to self-limited, acute symptoms (perhaps interpreted as "tendinitis" or "bursitis"[178]) but also to progressive weakness of the rotator cuff that makes it increasingly susceptible to damage from lesser loads. This scenario gives rise to the "creeping tendon ruptures" described by Pettersson.[354] The observation by Pettersson[354] and others that major cuff defects may occur without symptoms or recognized injury suggests that previous minor, often subclinical fiber failure leaves the shoulder weaker and the cuff tendons progressively less able to withstand the loads encountered in daily living.

Incidence of Rotator Cuff Defects

The frequency of rotator cuff tendon defects has been described in various reports of cadaver dissections: Smith[415] found an incidence of 18%; Keyes,[217] 19%; Wilson,[485,486] 20% in a series of autopsy dissections and 26.5% in a series of cadaver dissections; Cotton and Rideout,[80] 8%; Yamanaka and coworkers,[498] 7%; Fukuda and associates,[135] 7%; and Uhthoff and colleagues,[454] 20%. Neer found that the incidence of complete cuff tears in more than 500 cadaver shoulders was less than 5%.[306] Lehman and colleagues[238] stated that the incidence of full-thickness rotator cuff tears in 235 male and female cadavers ranging in age from 27 to 102 years (average, 64.7 years) was 17% (53 female, 26 male). The average age of cadavers with tears was 77.8 years versus 64.7 years in the intact group. Recognizing the importance of age in the prevalence of cuff lesions, these authors noted that in cadavers younger than 60 years, the incidence of rotator cuff tears was 6% as opposed to 30% in those older than 60 years.

Partial-thickness tears appear to be about twice as common as full-thickness defects. Yamanaka and coworkers[498] and Fukuda and colleagues[131,134,135] reported on 249 cadaver left shoulders in which they found a 13% incidence of partial-thickness tears. Thirty percent of shoulders older than 40 years had cuff tears, whereas no tears were seen in those younger than 40. Three percent had tears on the bursal side, 3% had tears on the joint side, and 7% had intratendinous tears. In another clinical series of partial-thickness cuff tears, Fukuda and associates[134] found 9 tears on the bursal side, 11 on the joint side, and 1 that was intratendinous. The bursal-side tears had the most severe symptoms. All these tears were localized in the critical area of the supraspinatus tendon. In his studies of 96 shoulders in patients ranging in age from 18 to 74 years, DePalma found a 37% incidence of partial-thickness tears of the supraspinatus and infraspinatus, a 21% incidence of partial-thickness tears of the subscapularis, and

a 9% incidence of full-thickness tears. Uhthoff and associates[454] found a 32% incidence of partial-thickness tears in 306 autopsy cases with a mean age of 59 years. Other studies report partial-thickness tears in approximately 20% to 30% of cadaver shoulders.[67,71,80,134,158,178,217,249-251,454] Data from studies in which the cuff was sectioned to demonstrate the prevalence of intrasubstance lesions indicate that cadaver or clinical examinations confined to the bursal and articular sides of the tendon will overlook the common intratendinous form of cuff defect.

The incidence of cuff defects in living subjects is more difficult to study. In a community survey of 644 individuals older than 70 years, Chard and coworkers[58] found shoulder symptoms in 21% (25% in women, 17% in women), the majority of which were attributed to the rotator cuff. However, less than 40% of these subjects sought medical attention for these symptoms.

Distorted views of the incidence of cuff disease and the relationship of cuff tears to clinical symptoms are obtained if only *symptomatic* patients are studied. Thus, some of the most important studies have concerned the prevalence of cuff lesions in *asymptomatic* patients. Pettersson[354] performed arthrography on 71 apparently healthy, asymptomatic shoulders ranging in age from 15 to 85 years. He found that of 27 asymptomatic, untraumatized shoulders in patients aged 55 to 85, 13 had arthrographically proven partial- or full-thickness rotator cuff defects, most of which were observed between the ages of 70 and 75 years. All these shoulders were symptom free and without a history of trauma. Repeated episodes of fiber failure lead to progressive cuff weakness but not necessarily to pain. Milgrom and colleagues[289] found that the prevalence of partial- or full-thickness tears increased markedly after 50 years of age: over 50% in subjects in their seventh decade and over 80% in subjects older than 80 years. They concluded that "rotator-cuff lesions are a natural correlate of aging, and are often present with no clinical symptoms." Sher and associates[408] used MRI to evaluate asymptomatic shoulders over a wide age range and found that 15% had full-thickness tears and 20% had partial-thickness tears. The frequency of full-thickness and partial-thickness tears increased significantly with age ($P < .001$ and .05, respectively). Twenty-five (54%) of the 46 individuals who were older than 60 years had a tear of the rotator cuff: 13 (28%) had a full-thickness tear and 12 (26%) had a partial-thickness tear. Of the 25 individuals who were 40 to 60 years old, 1 (4%) had a full-thickness tear and 6 (24%) had a partial-thickness tear. Of the 25 individuals who were 19 to 39 years old, none had a full-thickness tear and 1 (4%) had a partial-thickness tear. They concluded that (1) MRI identified a high prevalence of tears of the rotator cuff in asymptomatic individuals, (2) these tears were increasingly frequent with advancing age, and (3) these defects were compatible with normal, painless functional activity.

In another most important study, Yamanaka and Matsumoto[499] demonstrated the progression of partial-thickness tears. After initial arthrography, they monitored 40 tears (average patient age, 61 years) managed without surgery and repeated the arthrogram at an average of more than a year later. Although at follow-up the patients had improved average shoulder scores, arthrography revealed apparent resolution of the tear in only 4 instances, reduction of the tear size in only 4, enlargement of the tear in 21, and progress to a full-thickness cuff tear in 11 patients. The authors concluded that tears were likely to progress with increasing age in the absence of a history of trauma.

Thus, it must be concluded that cuff defects become increasingly common after the age of 40 and that many of these defects occur without substantial clinical manifestations.

Certain occupations seem to be particularly problematic for the rotator cuff, including tree pruning, fruit picking, nursing, grocery clerking, longshoring, warehousing, carpentry, and painting.[259] Some patients relate the onset to some type of athletic activity such as throwing, tennis, skiing, and swimming. Richardson and associates[375] reviewed 137 of the best swimmers in the United States. The incidence of shoulder problems was 42%. These authors calculated that the average national-level swimmer puts the shoulder through about 500,000 cycles per season. Although subluxation is a recognized problem in this group, many were found to have symptoms and signs suggesting cuff involvement. The technique that an athlete uses has a major relationship to the development of or freedom from symptoms, as discussed by Richardson and coworkers,[375] Albright and colleagues,[2] Cofield and Simonet[73] Penny and Welsh,[351] Neer and Welsh,[311] and Penny and Smith.[350]

CLINICAL FINDINGS

Duckworth and associates[104] and Harryman and colleagues[168] have demonstrated substantial variability in the clinical manifestations of rotator cuff tears. Importantly, considerable variation is observed between the genders and among the practices of different physicians.

The clinical manifestations of the various clinical forms of cuff disease include difficulties with shoulder stiffness, weakness, instability and roughness.[269,396]

1. *Stiffness* limits passive range of motion and frequently causes pain at the end point of motion, as well as difficulty sleeping. Stiffness is most common in partial-thickness cuff lesions, but it may also be associated with full-thickness cuff defects.[198] Stiffness may be demonstrable as limitations in (1) internal rotation with the arm in abduction (degrees from the neutral position) (Fig. 15–51), (2) reaching up the back (posterior segment reached with the thumb) (Fig. 15–52), (3) cross-body adduction (centimeters from the ipsilateral antecubital fossa to the contralateral acromion or coracoid) (Fig. 15–53), (4) flexion (degrees from the neutral position) (Fig. 15–54), or (5) external rotation (degrees from the neutral position) (Fig. 15–55).

2. *Weakness or pain on muscle contraction* limits the function of a shoulder with cuff disease. Tendon fibers weakened by degeneration may fail without clinical manifestations or may produce only transient symptoms interpreted as "bursitis" or "tendinitis." A greater injury is required to tear the cuff of individuals at the younger end of the age distribution. Traumatic glenohumeral dislocations in individuals older than 40 have a strong association with rotator cuff tears. These traumatic cuff tears commonly involve the subscapularis and produce weakness in internal rotation. Neviaser and coauthors[317] reported on 37 patients older than 40 years in whom the diagnosis of cuff rupture was initially missed after an anterior dislocation of the shoulder. The weakness from the cuff rupture was often erroneously attributed to axillary neuropathy. Recurrent anterior instability caused by rupture of the subscapularis and anterior capsule from the lesser tuberosity developed in 11 of these patients. None of

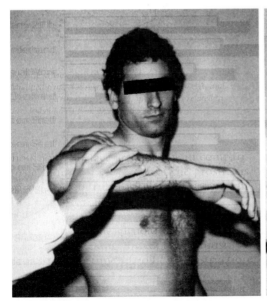
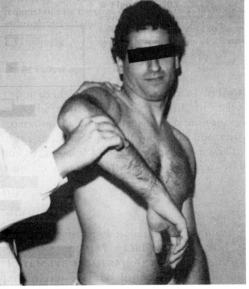

■ **Figure 15–51**
Internal rotation in abduction is limited when the posterior capsule is tight. *(From Iannotti JP: Rotator Cuff Disorders: Evaluation and Treatment. Rosemont, IL: American Academy of Orthopaedic Surgeons, 1991.)*

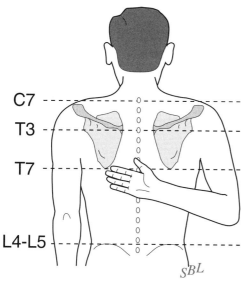

■ Figure 15-52

Maximal internal rotation is measured by the highest segment of posterior anatomy reached with the thumb, for example, L4-L5, T3, T7, or C7. *(From Matsen FA III, Lippitt SB, Sidles JA, and Harryman DT II: Practical Evaluation and Management of the Shoulder. Philadelphia: WB Saunders, 1994.)*

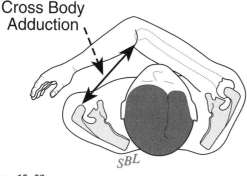

■ Figure 15-53

Maximal cross-body adduction is measured as the minimal distance from the antecubital fossa to the contralateral acromion when the arm is adducted horizontally across the body. *(From Matsen FA III, Lippitt SB, Sidles JA, and Harryman DT II: Practical Evaluation and Management of the Shoulder. Philadelphia: WB Saunders, 1994.)*

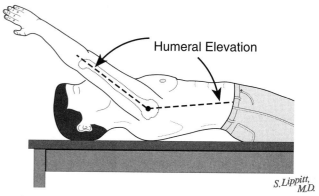

■ Figure 15-54

Maximal elevation (flexion) is measured with the patient supine and the opposite arm assisting in elevation, if necessary, to gain maximal range. *(From Matsen FA III, Lippitt SB, Sidles JA, and Harryman DT II: Practical Evaluation and Management of the Shoulder. Philadelphia: WB Saunders, 1994.)*

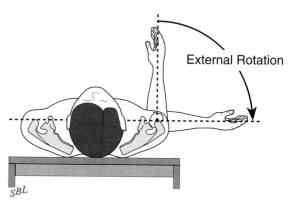

■ Figure 15-55

Maximal external rotation is measured with the arm at the side (zero degrees being the position in which the forearm of the flexed elbow points straight ahead). We prefer to make this measurement with the patient supine to help fix the thorax. *(From Matsen FA III, Lippitt SB, Sidles JA, and Harryman DT II: Practical Evaluation and Management of the Shoulder. Philadelphia: WB Saunders, 1994.)*

these shoulders had a Bankart lesion. Repair of the capsule and subscapularis restored stability in all the patients with recurrence.

Sonnabend reported a series of primary shoulder dislocations in patients[419] older than 40 years. Of the 13 patients who had complaints of weakness or pain after 3 weeks, 11 had rotator cuff tears. Toolanen found sonographic evidence of rotator cuff lesions in 24 of 63 patients older than 40 years at the time of anterior glenohumeral dislocation.[449]

Even though patients with full-thickness cuff defects may still retain the ability to actively abduct the arm,[313] significant tendon fiber failure is usually manifested by weakness on manual muscle testing.[39,178,240,241] *Isometric* testing of muscle strength prevents confusion with symptoms that may arise from shoulder movement (such as those associated with subacromial abrasion). Although individual cuff muscles cannot be specifically isolated, the following isometric tests are reasonably selective (Fig. 15-56):

- *Supraspinatus*—isometric elevation of the arm held in 90 degrees of elevation in the plane of the scapula and in mild internal rotation
- *Subscapularis*—isometric internal rotation of the arm with the elbow flexed to 90 degrees and the hand held posteriorly just off the waist
- *Infraspinatus*—isometric external rotation of the arm held at the side in neutral rotation with the elbow flexed to 90 degrees

These simple manual tests are helpful in characterizing the size of the tendon defect, from single tendon tears involving only the supraspinatus, to two tendon tears involving the supraspinatus and infraspinatus, to three tendon tears involving the subscapularis as well.

Individuals with partial-thickness cuff lesions have substantially more pain on resisted muscle action than do those with full-thickness lesions. This phenomenon

Some have suggested that weakness from pain inhibition can be distinguished from weakness from a tendon defect by subacromial injection of a local anesthetic.[24,251] If cuff dysfunction has been present for more than a month or so, it may be accompanied by supraspinatus and infraspinatus muscle atrophy. Subtle atrophy can be seen most easily by casting a shadow from a light over the head of the patient.

As pointed out by Codman,[66] defects in the cuff can often be palpated by rotating the proximal end of the humerus under the examiner's finger placed at the anterior corner of the acromion. The perimeters of the "divot" left by a defect in the supraspinatus are particularly easy to palpate. The defect is usually just posterior to the bicipital groove and medial to the greater tuberosity (Fig. 15–57).

3. *Instability.* An inability to keep the head centered in the glenoid may result from cuff disease. Acute tears of the subscapularis may contribute to recurrent anterior instability.[317, 419, 449]

Chronic loss of the normal compressive effect of the cuff mechanism and the stabilizing effect of the superior cuff tendon interposed between the humeral head and the coracoacromial arch may contribute to superior glenohumeral instability.[123,124,231,358,502] Superior instability is magnified in the presence of wear of the upper glenoid rim (see Figs. 15-12, 15-13, and 15-45)[308] and when the normal supportive function of the coracoacromial arch is lost because of erosion or surgical removal.[484]

4. *Roughness* associated with cuff disease is manifested as symptomatic crepitus on passive glenohumeral

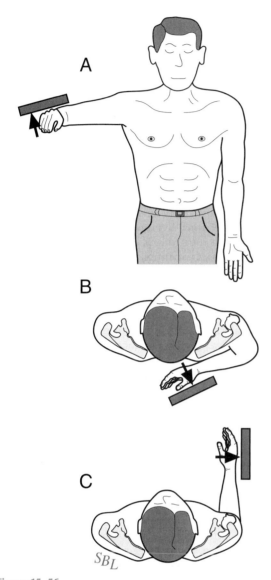

■ Figure 15–56

Tendon signs. **A,** Supraspinatus tendon sign: pain and weakness on isometric elevation of the arm when it is internally rotated and elevated to the horizontal position in the plane of the scapula. **B,** Subscapularis tendon sign: pain and weakness on isometric internal rotation of the arm with the hand held away from the body at the posterior of the waist. **C,** Infraspinatus tendon sign: pain and weakness on isometric external rotation with the arm at the side and the forearm pointing ahead. *(Modified from Matsen FA III, Lippitt SB, Sidles JA, and Harryman DT II: Practical Evaluation and Management of the Shoulder. Philadelphia: WB Saunders, 1994.)*

is analogous to the observation that partial tears of the Achilles tendon, partial tears of the patellar tendon, and partial tears of the origin of the extensor carpi radialis brevis are more painful on muscle contraction than when the complete structure is ruptured or surgically released. Fukuda and coworkers[135] characterized patients with partial-thickness cuff tears as having pain on motion, crepitus, and stiffness. They observed that patients with bursal-side tears seemed more symptomatic than those with deeper tears because of the resulting problems with roughness of the articulation between the upper surface cuff and the undersurface of the coracoacromial arch.

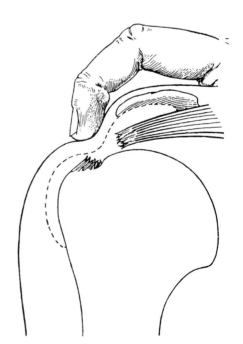

■ Figure 15–57

Tip of the finger pressing on the eminence and on the sulcus. The plane of this diagram is halfway between the coronal and sagittal planes. The *dotted line* represents the contour of the bursa. *(From Codman EA: Rupture of the Supraspinatus Tendon and Other Lesions in or about the Subacromial Bursa. Malabar, FL: Robert E Krieger, 1984.)*

motion. Bursal hypertrophy, secondary changes in the undersurface of the coracoacromial arch, loss of integrity of the upper aspect of the cuff tendons, and degenerative changes of the tuberosities may all contribute to *subacromial abrasion*. Crepitus from subacromial abrasion is easily detected by placing the examiner's thumb and fingers on the anterior and posterior aspects of the acromion while the humerus is moved relative to the scapula (Figs. 15–58 and 15–59). Because many shoulders demonstrate asymptomatic subacromial crepitus, it is important during the examination to ask whether the crepitus noted by the examiner is directly related to the patient's complaints.

Rotator cuff tear arthropathy is another cause of roughness associated with cuff disease. This term, coined by Neer and coworkers,[308] denotes loss of the glenohumeral articular surface in association with a massive rotator cuff deficiency (Fig. 15–60). These authors described 26 such shoulders, over 75% of which were in female patients. The average age was 69 years; 20% had evidence of contralateral cuff arthropathy, and 75% had no history of trauma. Typically, the shoulders were swollen, the muscles atrophic, and the long head of the biceps ruptured. Passive elevation was limited to an average of 90 degrees of elevation and 20 degrees of external rotation (a degree of limitation atypical of uncomplicated cuff tears). Often, the shoulder demonstrated anteroposterior instability. Collapse of the proximal humeral subchondral bone was a common observation. Glenoid, greater tuberosity, acromial, and lateral clavicular erosion was also commonly observed. The authors hypothesized that the arthropathy resulted from both mechanical factors (such as anteroposterior instability and superior migration of the

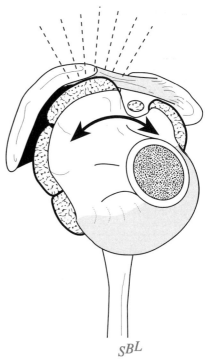

■ Figure 15–59
Abrasion sign: symptomatic subacromial crepitance on rotation of the arm elevated to 90 degrees with respect to the thorax, a position in which the capsule and ligaments are normally not under tension. *(Modified from Matsen FA III, Lippitt SB, Sidles JA, and Harryman DT II: Practical Evaluation and Management of the Shoulder. Philadelphia: WB Saunders, 1994.)*

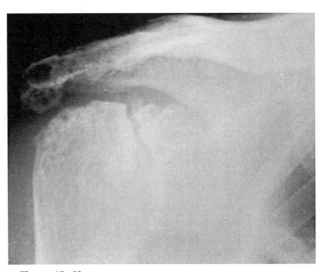

■ Figure 15–60
Collapse of the humeral head in combination with massive cuff deficiency as a result of cuff tear arthropathy.

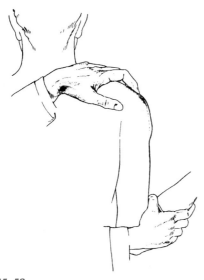

■ Figure 15–58
Position of the hands for examination of the shoulder. The left thumb lies along the depression below the spine of the scapula, and the tip of the forefinger is just anterior to the acromion. The other three fingers cross and hold the clavicle. Thus, the shoulder girdle is held firmly, and any motion of the scapulohumeral joint is detected immediately. *(From Codman EA: Rupture of the Supraspinatus Tendon and Other Lesions in or about the Subacromial Bursa. Malabar, FL: Robert E Krieger, 1984.)*

humeral head) (see Figs. 15–12, 15–13, 15–45, 15–46, and 15–48) and nutritional factors (such as loss of a closed joint space, lack of normal diffusion of nutrients to the joint surface, and disuse). To this list could be added disruption of the tendinous-osseous circulation entering through the subscapular, anterior humeral circumflex, and suprascapular vessels. This condition is distinct from osteoarthritis, rheumatoid arthritis, avascular necrosis, and neurogenic arthropathy.[277]

CLINICAL CONDITIONS RELATED TO THE ROTATOR CUFF

In discussing the broad spectrum of clinical involvement of the rotator cuff, it is useful to speak of eight clinical entities that can be easily identified by simple criteria:

1. *Asymptomatic cuff failure*—The shoulder does not bother the patient, but imaging studies document a full-thickness defect in the cuff tendon.
2. *Posterior capsular tightness*—The shoulder is limited in its range of internal rotation in abduction (see Fig. 15–51), cross-body adduction (Fig. 15–53), internal rotation up the back (Fig. 15–52), and flexion (Fig. 15–54) (in approximate order of decreasing frequency).
3. *Subacromial abrasion (without a significant defect in the cuff tendon)*—The shoulder demonstrates symptomatic crepitus as the humerus is rotated beneath the acromion (see Figs. 15–58 and 15–59); isometric testing of the cuff muscles (Fig. 15–56) reveals no pain or weakness.
4. *Partial-thickness cuff lesion*—Resisted isometric contraction of the involved cuff muscles is painful or weak (Fig. 15–56); associated posterior capsular tightness is common (Figs. 15–51 to 15–53). Imaging studies may indicate cuff tendon thinning, but the lesion does not extend through the full thickness of the tendon.
5. *Full-thickness cuff tear*—Resisted isometric contraction of one or more of the cuff muscles is painful or weak (Fig. 15–56); a full-thickness defect of one or more of the cuff tendons is demonstrated on ultrasonography, arthrography, MRI, arthroscopy, or open surgery.
6. *Cuff tear arthropathy*—Resisted isometric contraction of the cuff muscles is weak (Fig. 15–56); acromiohumeral (Figs. 15–58 and 15–59) and often glenohumeral movements produce crepitance. Radiographs demonstrate superior translation of the head of the humerus with respect to the acromion, loss of the articular cartilage of the superior humeral head, direct articulation of the head with the coracoacromial arch, "femoralization" of the proximal end of the humerus, and "acetabularization" of the upper glenoid and coracoacromial arch (see Figs. 15–12, 15–13, 15–45, 15–46, and 15–48).
7. *Failed acromioplasty*—The patient is dissatisfied with the result from a previous arthroscopic or open acromioplasty and seeks evaluation for additional surgery.
8. *Failed cuff surgery*—The patient is dissatisfied with the result from a previous arthroscopic or open operation on the rotator cuff and seeks evaluation for additional surgery.

SHOULDER FUNCTION AND HEALTH STATUS IN CLINICAL CONDITIONS OF THE ROTATOR CUFF

To better understand the function and health status of patients with various conditions involving the rotator

TABLE 15–1. Prevalence and Average Age of Patients with Six Types of Cuff Lesions

	No. of Patients	Age at Initial Evaluation
Subacromial abrasion	18	43
Partial-thickness cuff lesion	104	48
Rotator cuff tear	133	62
Failed acromioplasty	29	49
Failed cuff repair	47	60
Cuff tear arthropathy	24	74

cuff, the Simple Shoulder Test (SST)[269] and the Short Form-36 (SF-36)[468] self-assessments were completed by 355 consecutive patients with subacromial abrasion, partial-thickness cuff lesions, full-thickness cuff tears, failed acromioplasties, failed cuff repairs, and cuff tear arthropathy evaluated by one of us (F.A.M.). The number and average age of patients with each diagnosis are shown in Table 15–1.

The SST and SF-36 data for these patients are shown in Figures 15–61 and 15–62, respectively. The SST data indicate that individuals with rotator cuff problems have difficulty with most of the standardized shoulder functions questioned by the SST, especially sleeping comfortably, lifting 8 lb to a shelf, and throwing. Over half the patients with full-thickness tears are unable to lift 1 lb to a shelf, toss underhand, wash the back of the opposite shoulder, or do their usual work. The severity of functional loss is least for subacromial abrasion, followed by partial-thickness cuff lesions, full-thickness cuff tears, failed acromioplasties, failed cuff repairs, and finally, the most severely limiting of this family of conditions, cuff tear arthropathy.

The SF-36 data indicate that patients with cuff disease are most severely compromised with respect to their physical role function and comfort. Even though the differences among diagnoses are not large, those with cuff tear arthropathy and failed surgery have worse scores than those with unoperated cuff lesions and subacromial abrasion.

IMAGING TECHNIQUES

Plain Radiographs

Standard radiographs can provide limited assistance in evaluating shoulder weakness. Small avulsed fragments of the tuberosity may be seen in younger patients with cuff lesions (Fig. 15–49) (not to be confused with calcific deposits). The presence of a notch of the greater tuberosity had a statistically significant association with articular surface, partial rotator cuff tears in throwers. Not all the notches seen on arthroscopy were detected with plain radiographs, but the association between the radiographic and arthroscopic presence of a notch was statistically significant.[303] Chronic cuff disease may be accompanied by sclerosis of the undersurface of the acromion (the "sourcil" or eyebrow sign) (Fig. 15–63), traction spurs in the coracoacromial ligament from forced contact with the

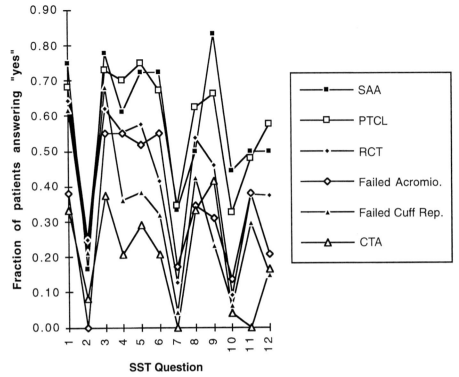

■ **Figure 15–61**

Self-assessed shoulder function of 355 patients with six different rotator cuff diagnoses: (1) subacromial abrasion (SAA), (2) partial-thickness cuff lesion (PTCL), (3) complete-thickness cuff tear (RCT), (4) failed acromioplasty, (5) failed cuff repair, and (6) cuff tear arthropathy (CTA). Simple Shoulder Test questions: (1) Is your shoulder comfortable with your arm at rest by your side? (2) Does your shoulder allow you to sleep comfortably? (3) Can you reach the small of your back to tuck in your shirt with your hand? (4) Can you place your hand behind your head with the elbow straight out to the side? (5) Can you place a coin on a shelf at the level of your shoulder without bending your elbow? (6) Can you lift 1 lb (a full pint container) to the level of your shoulder without bending your elbow? (7) Can you lift 8 lb (a full gallon container) to the level of the top of your head without bending your elbow? (8) Can you carry 20 lb (a bag of potatoes) at your side with the affected extremity? (9) Do you think you can toss a softball underhand 10 yards with the affected extremity? (10) Do you think you can throw a softball overhand 20 yards with the affected extremity? (11) Can you wash the back of your opposite shoulder with the affected extremity? and (12) Would your shoulder allow you to work full-time at your regular job?

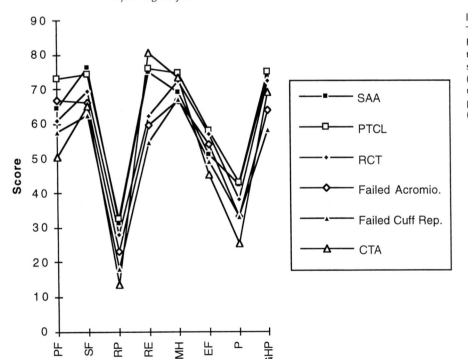

■ **Figure 15–62**

The patient population is the same as for Figure 15–61. The SF-36 parameters on this graph include physical function (PF), social function (SF), physical role function (RP), emotional role function (RE), mental health (MH), energy/fatigue (EF), pain (P), and general health perception (GHP).

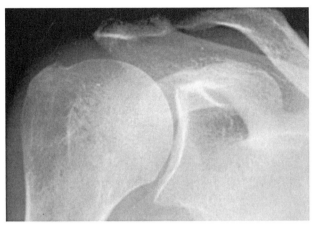

■ **Figure 15–63**
Roentgenogram demonstrating subacromial sclerosis, the so-called sourcil or eyebrow sign, from chronic loading of the undersurface of the acromion by the rotator cuff. Corresponding sclerosis or cystic changes involving the greater tuberosity may also occur.

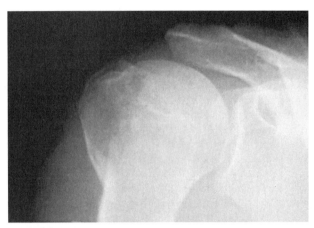

■ **Figure 15–65**
Anteroposterior roentgenogram showing malunion of a fractured greater tuberosity and malunion associated with abrasion, loss of motion, and weakness.

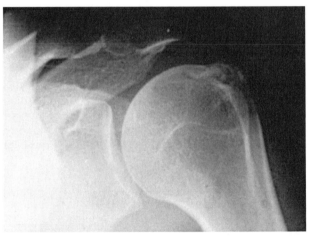

■ **Figure 15–64**
Even with small rotator cuff tears, radiographs may reveal bony cysts at the normal cuff insertion, subacromial sclerosis, and acromial spurs.

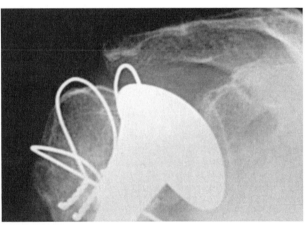

■ **Figure 15–66**
Refractory subacromial abrasion and stiffness developed in this patient because of the relative prominence of fracture fixation wires. The symptoms resolved after the subacromial wires were removed.

cuff and the humeral head, and changes at the cuff insertion to the humerus (see Figs. 15-10, 15-11, 15-12, and 15-64).[99,192,206,281,479] Radiographs may also reveal evidence of some of the conditions possibly associated with cuff disease, such as acromioclavicular arthritis, chronic calcific tendinitis, displacement of the tuberosity, and the like (Figs. 15-18 and 15-65 to 15-67). With larger tears, radiographs reveal upward displacement of the head of the humerus with respect to the glenoid and acromion (see Figs. 15-7, 15-8, 15-13, and 15-68).[74,99,193,208,248,479] Kaneko and colleagues[209] found that superior migration of the humerus and deformity of the greater tuberosity were the most sensitive in specific manifestations of massive cuff deficiency. In cuff tear arthropathy, the humeral head may have lost the prominence of the tuberosities (become "femoralized"), and the coracoid, acromion, and glenoid may have formed a deep spherical socket (become "acetabularized") (see Figs. 15-12, 15-48, 15-69, and 15-70).

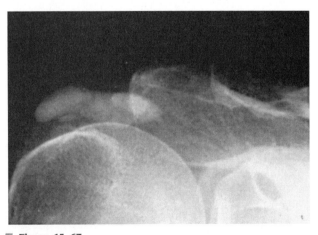

■ **Figure 15–67**
This anteroposterior roentgenogram shows chronic calcific deposits in the supraspinatus tendon. These deposits may increase the thickness of the tendon and thus contribute to subacromial abrasion and loss of motion.

Cuff Tendon Imaging

A number of different studies are available for imaging the rotator cuff. Each of these tests adds both information and expense to the evaluation of a patient; health care resources can be conserved by ordering imaging tests only if the results are likely to change management of the patient. Patients younger than 40 years without a major injury or weakness are unlikely to have significant cuff defects; thus, cuff imaging is less likely to be helpful in their evaluation. At the other extreme, patients with weak external rotation and atrophy of the spinatus muscles whose plain radiographs show the head of the humerus to be in contact with the acromion (see Figs. 15–69 and

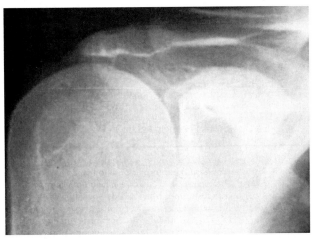

■ **Figure 15–68**
With larger cuff tears, radiographs reveal upward displacement of the humeral head with marked narrowing of the interval between the humeral head and the acromion. Note the marked cystic changes and sclerosis involving the undersurface of the acromion.

15–70) do not need cuff imaging to establish the diagnosis of a rotator cuff defect. Finally, the initial management of patients with nonspecific shoulder symptoms and an unremarkable physical examination is unlikely to be changed by the results of a cuff imaging test. Cuff imaging is strongly indicated when it would affect treatment, such as in the case of a 47-year-old with immediate weakness in flexion and external rotation after a major fall on the outstretched arm or shoulder dislocation. Imaging the cuff is also important when symptoms and signs of cuff involvement do not respond as expected, for example, symptoms of "tendinitis" or "bursitis" that do not respond to 3 months of rehabilitation.

A review of the literature suggests that in experienced hands, arthrography, MRI, ultrasound, and arthroscopy can each contribute to making the diagnosis of a full-thickness cuff tear.*

Arthrography

For many years the single-contrast shoulder arthrogram has been the standard technique for diagnosing rotator cuff tears. In this test, contrast material is injected into the glenohumeral joint (Fig. 15–71); after brief exercise, radiographs are taken to reveal intravasation of dye into the tendon (Figs. 15–72 and 15–73) or extravasation of contrast agent through the cuff into the subacromial subdeltoid bursa (Fig. 15–74). In 1933, Oberholtzer[325] used air as a contrast agent and injected it into the glenohumeral joint before radiographic evaluation. Air contrast is still useful in patients allergic to iodine. In 1939, Lindblom used opaque contrast medium.[249-251] Since then, iodinated

---

*See references 59, 85, 91, 156, 264, 334, 338, 342, 366, 378, 452, 463, 467.

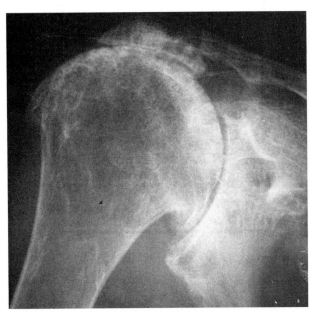

Figure 15–69

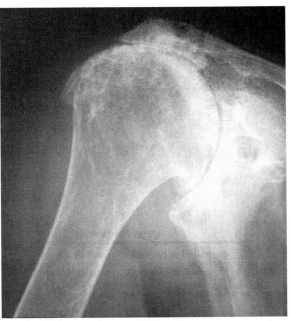

Figure 15–70

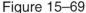

■ **Figures 15–69 and 15–70**
Cuff tear arthropathy showing "femoralization" of the proximal end of the humerus and "acetabularization" of the coracoacromial arch and glenoid.

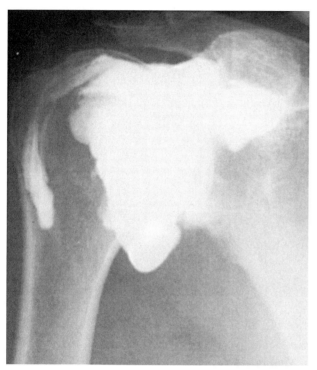

■ **Figure 15–71**
Arthrogram of a normal shoulder in neutral position. Note the normal extension of dye beneath the coracoid into the subscapularis bursa. Also note the normal extension of dye beneath the transverse humeral ligament and into the biceps sheath. The superolateral extension of dye is limited by the normal cuff attachment.

contrast media have been the standard for single-contrast arthrography. A number of extensions of the basic technique have been published.[1,215,221,306,315,374,397]

Pettersson[354] and Neviaser and coworkers[319] demonstrated the effectiveness of arthrography in revealing deep surface partial-thickness cuff tears (see Figs. 15–72 and

15–73); however, arthrography cannot reveal isolated midsubstance tears or superior surface tears. Craig[81] described the "geyser sign," in which dye leaks from the shoulder joint through the cuff into the acromioclavicular joint. The presence of this sign suggests a large tear with erosion of the undersurface of the acromioclavicular joint (see Figs. 15–18 and 15–75). Double-contrast arthrography using both air and iodinated material may enhance the resolution of arthrography.[1,111,146 215] Berquist and associates[25] reported on the use of single- and double-contrast arthrograms to evaluate the size of cuff tears seen at surgery. Their ability to accurately predict one of four cuff tear sizes (small, medium, large, and massive) was just over 50%. The reported incidence of false-negative arthrograms in the presence of surgically proven cuff tears ranges from 0% to 8%.[178,180,290,313,362,396,489] The anatomic resolution of shoulder arthrography can be enhanced to a certain degree by performing tomography with contrast material in place to give information about the size and location of the tear and the quality of the remaining tissue. Further resolution can be obtained by performing double-contrast arthrotomography.[130, 151, 152, 220] Kilcoyne and Matsen[220] used arthropneumotomography to evaluate the size of the cuff tear and the quality of the residual tissue. They found good correlation with the surgical appearance.

The accuracy of arthrography does not seem to be enhanced by digital subtraction.[119]

Subacromial injection of contrast material (bursography) has been used to evaluate the subacromial zone and the upper surface of the rotator cuff.[131,135,245,249-251,288,312,428] Fukuda reported six patients with normal arthrograms and positive bursograms, which he defined as pooling of the subacromially injected contrast material in cuff tissue. He reported an overall accuracy of 67% for bursography when compared with operative findings. Although lesions can be identified by this type of examination, criteria for making diagnoses have not been rigorously defined.

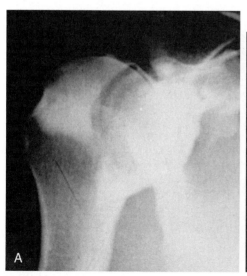
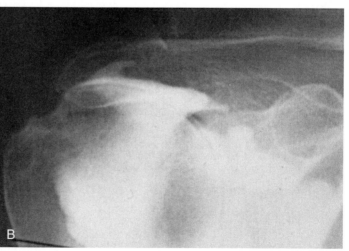

■ **Figure 15–72**
Arthrograms of two different shoulders showing partial-thickness, deep surface tears of the cuff. **A,** Note the "feathered" edge of the contrast material laterally, indicative of loss of the normal insertion at the base of the tuberosity. The absence of filling of the bursa suggests that the tendon defect is not full thickness. These findings were confirmed at surgery. **B,** Another patient had a falciform-shaped deep surface tear.

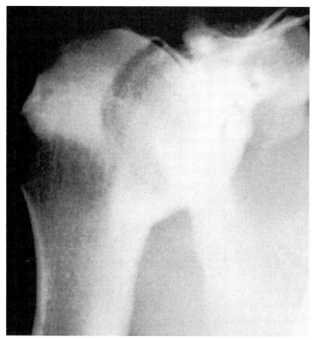

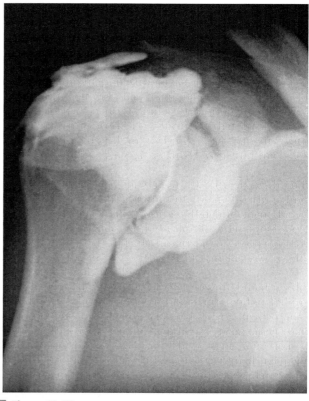

■ Figure 15–73
This arthrogram shows evidence of a partial-thickness rotator cuff tear originating at the articular surface of the cuff. Leakage of dye is seen to extend beyond the normal deep surface cuff attachment and is restrained by the more superficial cuff fibers that insert further laterally (see Fig. 15–50). These findings were confirmed at surgery.

■ Figure 15–74
This arthrogram shows leakage of dye into the subacromial space and beyond the normal cuff attachment at the greater tuberosity. This finding indicates a full-thickness cuff defect.

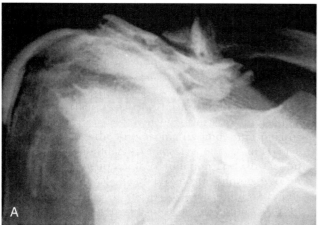

■ Figure 15–75
A, This arthrogram shows leakage of dye into the subacromial space and beyond the normal cuff attachment at the greater tuberosity. Note the dye leakage into the acromioclavicular joint, the "geyser" sign. Also note the marked inferior displacement of the cuff outline caused by this arthritic acromioclavicular joint. B, Plain radiograph of the same joint.

Magnetic Resonance Imaging

MRI can reveal information about the tendon and muscle. Seeger and coworkers[404] and Kneeland and associates[224] provided initial information on the use of MRI to image the cuff; however, they did not document the sensitivity and selectivity of this method. Crass and Craig[82] concluded that the accuracy of MRI in diagnosing cuff pathology is unknown. Kieft and associates[219] reported on

10 patients with shoulder symptoms evaluated by MRI and arthrography. Arthrography showed a tear in three patients, whereas MRI detected none of them.

In a retrospective study by Robertson and colleagues,[378] the authors found that full-thickness tears of the rotator cuff can be accurately identified by MRI with little observer variation; however, consistent differentiation of normal rotator cuff, tendinitis, and partial-thickness tears is difficult. Iannotti and coworkers in 1991 described the sensitivity, specificity, and predictive value of MRI for different clinical conditions.[191]

MRI was found to have 89% sensitivity and 100% specificity in detecting rotator cuff tears in shoulders without previous surgery. The missed tears were all partial-thickness tears.[407] MRI of shoulders after repair showed a 91% sensitivity in diagnosing recurrent tears.[298]

MRI can also image the cuff musculature. Atrophy and fatty infiltration indicate a poor prognosis for return of rotator cuff function.

Schaefer used MRI to assess atrophy of the supraspinatus muscle in patients with full-thickness rotator cuff tears and in a control group. Atrophy was deemed significant if the supraspinatus muscle belly occupied less than 50% of the supraspinatus fossa and if the supraspinatus muscle was not large enough to cross a line drawn from the apices of the coracoid process and the scapular spine. These findings were termed the *occupation ratio* and the *tangent sign,* respectively. Patients with tears of less than 25 mm in width had a mean occupation ratio of 51.6%, those with tears of 25 to 50 mm had a mean occupation ratio of 46%, and those with larger tears had a ratio of 29.3%. After repair, the small and medium-sized groups had no significant change in the mean occupation ratio, but the group with large tears had a significant increase at 12 months. Improvements in the occupation ratio and tangent sign had a significantly positive correlation with the Constant score.[398]

These findings were contradictory to those of Matsumoto and associates, who determined that reattachment of a supraspinatus tear in rabbits did not reverse atrophy, but actually mildly increased atrophy of the supraspinatus tendon.[270] The amount of degeneration was 14.9%, which was significantly less than Fabis and colleagues found after the same 12 weeks in rabbits following detachment of the supraspinatus without repair; they reported a 65.5% loss of muscle volume in comparison to controls.[117]

Ultrasonography

In experienced hands, *ultrasonography* can noninvasively and nonradiographically reveal not only the integrity of the rotator cuff but also the thickness of its various component tendons. In 1982, one of us (F.A.M.) observed during prenatal ultrasonography that movement dramatically enhanced resolution during real-time imaging of a fetal hand. Similarly, adding a dynamic element to sonographic evaluation of the rotator cuff significantly improves its resolution; moving the shoulder through even a small arc helps distinguish the cuff tendons from the humeral head, deltoid, and acromion. The importance of movement during ultrasound examination was more recently re-emphasized by Drakeford and coauthors.[102] Our initial series of ultrasound examinations of the shoulder was presented in 1983.[120] Since that time, the criteria for diagnosing cuff lesions have evolved, as have the quality of the equipment and the technique. Much of this work was carried out by and advanced as a result of the inspiration of the late Lawrence Mack.[261,262,264] He demonstrated that by careful positioning and by knowledge of the dynamic anatomy of the cuff, an experienced ultrasonographer can selectively image the upper and lower subscapularis, the biceps tendon, the anterior and posterior supraspinatus, the infraspinatus, and the teres minor. Defects are revealed as absence of the normal tissue echoes and failure of the tissue to move appropriately with defined humeral movements (Figs. 15–76 to 15–78). In his series of 141 patients from the University of Washington Shoulder Clinic,[262] Mack and associates demonstrated a specificity of 98% and a sensitivity of 91% in comparison to surgical findings. Most of the false-negative results

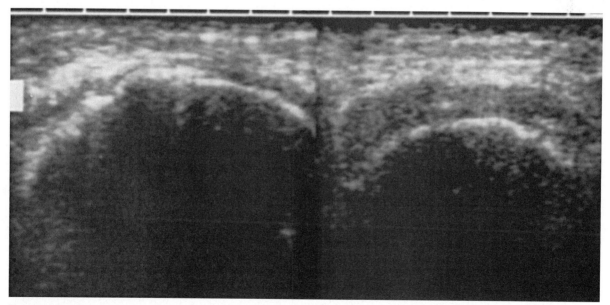

■ Figure 15–76

A sonogram with the transducer perpendicular to the long axis of the supraspinatus demonstrates the tendon as an arc of soft tissue overlying the humeral head on the normal side *(right)* and absent on the side with a large cuff tear *(left)*.

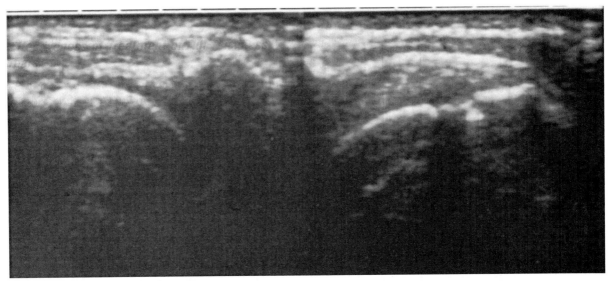

■ **Figure 15–77**

A sonogram in the plane of the supraspinatus. The normal attachment to the greater tuberosity is shown on the *right*. An absent supraspinatus insertion is shown in the shoulder with a large cuff tear *(left)*.

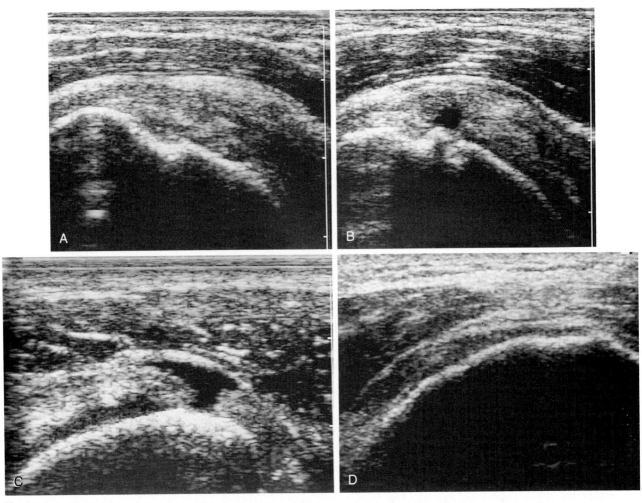

■ **Figure 15–78**

Spectrum of rotator cuff appearance in four different patients. All images are of the right supraspinatus tendon and were obtained with linear, high-frequency (10 MHz), broad-bandwidth transducers. **A,** A normal tendon. The hyperechoic line at the deep portion of the image represents the humeral cortex, whereas the nearly parallel hyperechoic curve approximately 1 cm superficial to that represents the subdeltoid bursa. The intermediate-density echoes between these two lines represent the normal supraspinatus tendon. **B,** A small (5 mm) tear is seen best along the inferior surface of the supraspinatus tendon. The tear is well delineated because it is filled with anechoic (black) fluid. **C,** An approximately 1-cm full-thickness tear. Note the tendon remnants at either side of the tear, which are again well outlined by fluid. **D,** A massive rotator cuff tear. No normal supraspinatus tendon is seen. Instead, the thickened subdeltoid bursa is directly opposed to the humeral cortex. *(Ultrasound images courtesy of Dr. Tom Winter, Department of Radiology, University of Washington.)*

occurred in patients found to have tears smaller than 1 cm.[262]

Ultrasonography has the advantages of speed and safety. In addition, it provides the important benefit of practical bilateral examinations (which, though theoretically possible with arthrography, MRI, and arthroscopy, are not usually done for reasons of cost, risk, and time). Ultrasonography also allows the shoulder to be examined dynamically and provides the opportunity to show the results to the patient in real time. Yet another advantage is its low cost: a bilateral shoulder ultrasound is usually half the cost of a unilateral arthrogram and one eighth the cost of unilateral shoulder MRI. Although some series have reported less accuracy with ultrasonography than with arthrography, others have pointed to its high degree of accuracy, noninvasiveness, and effectiveness in experienced hands.[40,77,82,85,285-287,331,338,436,482] Ultrasonography has been applied to the evaluation of recurrent tears,[84] as well as incomplete tears.[83] Seitz and coworkers[405] compared arthrography, ultrasonography, and MRI for the detection of cuff tears in 25 patients. They found that ultrasonography was the most helpful study in accurately documenting the size and location of the tear when it existed. MRI suffered from problems of image resolution. Arthrography was reliable in determining full-thickness tears, but correlation with size and location of the tear was difficult. Middleton[284] concluded that "Shoulder sonography is a valuable means of evaluating the rotator cuff and biceps tendon. In experienced hands, it is as sensitive as arthrography and magnetic resonance imaging for detecting rotator cuff tears and abnormalities of the biceps tendon. Because sonography is rapid, noninvasive, relatively inexpensive, and capable of performing bilateral examinations in one sitting, it should be used as the initial imaging test when the primary question is one of rotator cuff or biceps tendon abnormalities."

In a review of the literature, Stiles and Otte concluded that the accuracy of ultrasound in experienced hands was at least as good as that of MRI.[427]

Recent investigations have again confirmed the value of sonography. In a study of 4588 shoulders, Hedtmann and Fett[181] found that the overall sensitivity in diagnosing cuff tears was 97% for full-thickness tears and 91% for partial-thickness tears. The false-negative rate was less than 2%, for an overall accuracy of 95%. The supraspinatus was involved in 96%, the infraspinatus in 39%, the subscapularis in 10%, and the long head of the biceps in 34%. The authors also developed an approach for measuring the degree of retraction of the torn tendon. Farin and Jaroma[118] examined 184 patients for possible acute traumatic tears. Ultrasonography demonstrated 42 (91%) of 46 full-thickness tears and 7 (78%) of 9 partial-thickness tears. Ultrasonography showed more extensive tears than were found at surgery in 4 (4%) of 98 patients and less extensive tears in 7 (7%) of 98 patients. Sonographic patterns consisted of a defect in 31 (63%), focal thinning in 10 (21%), and nonvisualization in 8 (16%).

Ultrasound determination of full-thickness rotator cuff tears has a sensitivity of 58% to 100% and a specificity of 85% to 100%. Location of the tear, in terms of which tendon the tear was in, as well as the size of the tear, was accurately predicted in 87% of cases when compared with surgical findings.[52,81,93] In a comparison of imaging modalities, ultrasound was found to underestimate the area of the tear by an average of 33%, whereas MRI underestimated the size of the tear by 30%. Interestingly, arthroscopy underestimated the size of the tear by 12%.[47] Ultrasonography of partial-thickness tears resulted in a sensitivity of 67% and a specificity of 85%.[439]

Van Holsbeeck and colleagues[461] found that a 7.5-MHz commercially available linear-array transducer and a standardized study protocol yielded a sensitivity for partial-thickness tears of 93% and a specificity of 94%. The positive predictive value was 82%, with a negative predictive value of 98%. Similar results are reported by others.[463] Hollister and coworkers[186] studied the association between sonographically detected joint fluid and rotator cuff disease. In 163 shoulders they found that the sonographic finding of intra-articular fluid alone (without bursal fluid) has both low sensitivity and low specificity for the diagnosis of rotator cuff tears. However, the finding of fluid in the subacromial/subdeltoid bursa, especially when combined with a joint effusion, is highly specific and has a high positive predictive value for associated rotator cuff tears.

We find that expert ultrasonography provides the most efficient and cost-effective approach to imaging of the cuff tendons. The real-time, dynamic, and interactive examination of the rotator cuff provides the physician and the patient with the information needed to make the necessary management decisions in both primary and postsurgical cuff conditions.

DIFFERENTIAL DIAGNOSIS

Traditionally, it has been stated that rotator cuff tears must be differentiated from cuff *tendinitis* and *bursitis* and that tests such as arthrography and ultrasonography are necessary to make this distinction. Perhaps a more realistic view is that many of the symptoms often attributed to tendinitis and bursitis are, in actuality, episodes of acute fiber failure that are not clinically detected.

Patients with a *frozen shoulder* demonstrate, by definition, a restricted range of passive motion with normal glenohumeral radiographs. Patients with partial-thickness cuff defects may similarly demonstrate motion restriction, whereas patients with major full-thickness defects usually have a good range of passive shoulder motion but may be limited in strength or range of active motion. An arthrogram in the case of frozen shoulder shows a diminished volume and obliteration of the normal recesses of the joint.

A *snapping scapula* may produce shoulder pain on elevation and a catching sensation somewhat reminiscent of the subacromial snap of a cuff tear. However, the latter can usually be elicited with the scapula stabilized while the arm is rotated in the flexed and somewhat abducted position. Scapular snapping generally arises from the superomedial corner of the scapula and produces local discomfort; it is elicited by scapular movement without glenohumeral motion.

Glenohumeral arthritis may also produce shoulder pain, weakness, and catching. This diagnosis can be reliably differentiated from rotator cuff disease by a careful history, physical examination, and roentgenographic analysis (Fig. 15–79).

Acromioclavicular arthritis may imitate cuff disease. Characteristically, however, the shoulder is most painful with cross-body movements and with activities requiring strong contraction of the pectoralis major. Tenderness is commonly limited to the acromioclavicular joint. Relief of pain on selective lidocaine injection and coned-down radiographs may help establish the diagnosis of acromioclavicular arthritis.

Suprascapular neuropathy and cervical radiculopathy are common imitators of cuff disease. The suprascapular nerve and the fifth and sixth cervical nerve roots supply two of the most important cuff muscles: the supraspinatus and infraspinatus. Thus, patients with involvement of these structures may have lateral shoulder pain and lack strength of elevation and external rotation.

In the presence of weakness, the neurologic examination should test the cutaneous distribution of the nerve roots from C5 to T1. The biceps reflex and the triceps reflex help screen C5-C6 and C7-C8, respectively. The next component of the neurologic examination requires verifying the integrity of the segmental innervation of joint motion: abduction, C5; adduction, C6, C7, and C8; external rotation, C5; internal rotation, C6, C7, and C8; elbow flexion, C5 and C6; elbow extension, C7 and C8; wrist extension and flexion, C6 and C7; finger flexion and extension, C7 and C8; and finger adduction/abduction, T1.

A set of screening tests checks the motor and sensory components of the major peripheral nerves: (1) the axillary nerve—the anterior, middle, and posterior parts of the deltoid and the skin just above the deltoid insertion; (2) the radial nerve—the extensor pollicis longus and the skin over the first dorsal web space; (3) the median nerve—the opponens pollicis and the skin over the pulp of the index finger; (4) the ulnar nerve—the first dorsal interosseous and the skin over the pulp of the little finger; and (5) the musculocutaneous nerve—the biceps muscle and the skin over the lateral aspect of the forearm. The long thoracic nerve is checked by having the patient elevate the arm 60 degrees in the anterior sagittal plane while the examiner pushes down on the arm and looks for winging of the scapula posteriorly. The nerve of the trapezius is checked by observing the strength of the shoulder shrug. Lesions of the suprascapular nerve produce weakness of elevation and external rotation without sensory loss.

Clinical conditions affecting these structures include (1) cervical spondylosis involving C5 and C6, (2) brachial plexopathy involving the suprascapular nerve, (3) traction injuries (as in the mechanism of Erb's palsy), (4) suprascapular nerve entrapment at the suprascapular notch, (5) pressure on the inferior branch of the suprascapular nerve from a ganglion cyst at the spinoglenoid notch, (6) traumatic severance in fractures, or (7) iatrogenic injury.*

Cervical spondylosis involving the fifth and sixth cervical nerve root may imitate or mask rotator cuff involvement by producing pain in the lateral aspect of the shoulder as well as weakness of shoulder flexion, abduction, and external rotation. Cervical radiculopathy is suggested if the patient has pain on neck extension or on turning the chin to the affected side. Pain of cervical origin more commonly includes the area of the trapezius muscle along with the area of the deltoid and may radiate down the arm to the hand. Sensory, motor, or reflex abnormalities in the distribution of the fifth or sixth cervical nerve root provide additional support for the diagnosis of cervical radiculopathy. Inasmuch as many asymptomatic patients have degenerative changes at the C5-C6 area, cervical spine radiographs are not a specific diagnostic tool. When mild cervical spondylosis is suspected, it is practical to implement a rehabilitation program without an extensive diagnostic workup. This program includes gentle neck mobility exercises, isometric neck-strengthening exercises, home traction, and protection of the neck from positions that aggravate the condition during sleep. If the condition is unresponsive or severe, additional evaluation by electromyography and/or MRI may be indicated.

Suprascapular neuropathy is characterized by dull pain over the shoulder that is exacerbated by movement of the shoulder, weakness in overhead activities, wasting of the supraspinatus and infraspinatus muscles, weakness of external rotation, and normal radiographic evaluation. This condition may arise from suprascapular nerve traction injuries, suprascapular nerve entrapment, brachial neuritis affecting the suprascapular nerve, or a ganglion cyst in the spinoglenoid notch. The first three should involve the nerve supply to both the supraspinatus and infraspinatus and are most easily differentiated by the history. Traction injuries to the suprascapular nerve are usually associated with a history of a violent downward pull on the shoulder and may be a part of a larger Erb palsy–type injury to the brachial plexus. Suprascapular nerve entrapment may produce chronic recurrent pain and weakness aggravated by shoulder use. Finally, brachial neuritis often produces a rather intense pain lasting for several weeks, with the onset of weakness being noted as the pain subsides. A ganglion cyst in the spinoglenoid notch usually arises from a defect in the posterior shoulder joint capsule and may press on the nerve to the

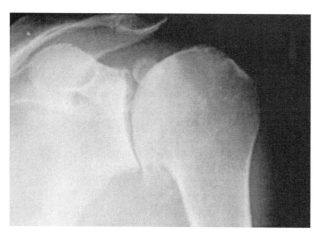

■ **Figure 15–79**
Degenerative joint disease may produce pain, stiffness, weakness, and catching. This condition can be readily diagnosed with radiographs.

*See references 9, 18, 42, 64, 101, 103, 108, 116, 142, 197, 225, 226, 265, 266, 300, 356, 368, 372, 401, 403, 418, 429, 477.

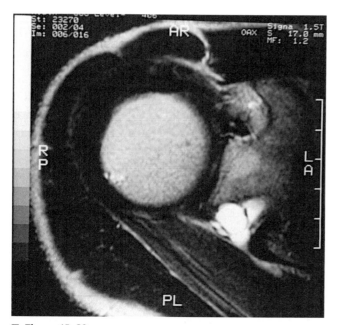

■ Figure 15–80
Magnetic resonance image showing a ganglion cyst in the spinoglenoid notch. Cysts in this location can press on the nerve to the infraspinatus, which runs through this notch. Symptoms can include pain and weakness of external rotation, somewhat similar to the symptoms of cuff disease.

infraspinatus as it passes through the notch. These cysts are well seen on MRI (Fig. 15–80). Depending on the site of the suprascapular nerve lesion, electromyography may indicate involvement of the infraspinatus alone or involvement of this muscle along with the supraspinatus. None of these conditions should produce cuff defects on shoulder ultrasonography or arthrography.

TREATMENT

The discussion of treatment will be divided in terms of the eight clinical entities previously identified: asymptomatic cuff failure, posterior capsular tightness, subacromial abrasion, failed acromioplasty, partial-thickness cuff lesions, full-thickness cuff tears, failed cuff repair, and cuff tear arthropathy.

Asymptomatic Cuff Failure

In this condition, the shoulder does not bother the patient, but imaging studies document a full-thickness defect in the cuff tendon.[169,269,289,354,408]

The realization that full-thickness cuff tears may be asymptomatic poses substantial questions regarding the prevalence of cuff tears in the general population and the indications for rotator cuff surgery. It is difficult to improve patients who have minimal symptoms. A case for surgery to prevent future problems in such patients has not been convincingly made.

Our approach is to offer surgical exploration and repair to healthy, active individuals with asymptomatic cuff tears if they think that the potential benefit of increased strength merits their investment in surgery.

Posterior Capsular Tightness

In this condition, the shoulder is limited in its range of internal rotation in abduction, cross-body adduction, internal rotation up the back, and flexion (in approximate order of decreasing frequency). The symptoms and results of physical examination of this "slightly frozen shoulder" may be similar to those attributed in the past to "impingement syndrome."[73]

A patient with posterior capsular tightness is informed that this condition is a common result of a mild injury to the rotator cuff, but that in the absence of weakness or pain on isometric muscle testing, nonoperative management is usually successful. The most effective program is one taught by the surgeon or therapist but carried out by the patient. The recommended treatment consists of gentle stretches performed five times a day by the patient (Figs. 15–81 to 15–86). Each stretch is performed to the point at which the patient feels a pull against the shoulder tightness, but not to the point of pain. Each stretch is performed for 1 minute, so the patient invests about 30 minutes per day in stretching the shoulder. Obvious improvement commonly occurs within the first month, but 3 months may be required to completely eliminate the condition. The rare refractory case may be considered for an arthroscopic capsular release as described by Harryman and colleagues.[170]

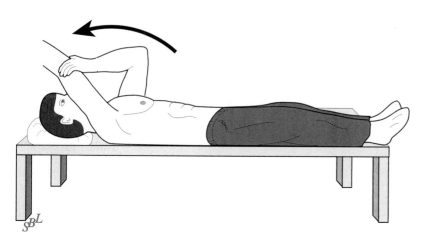

■ Figure 15–81
Stretching in overhead reach with the opposite arm used as the therapist. *(From Matsen FA III, Lippitt SB, Sidles JA, and Harryman DT II: Practical Evaluation and Management of the Shoulder. Philadelphia: WB Saunders, 1994.)*

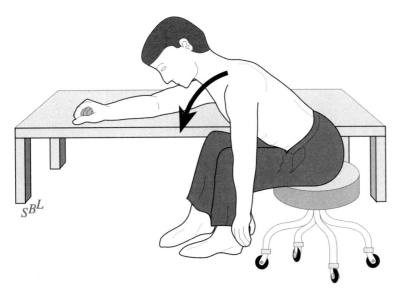

■ **Figure 15–82**
Stretching in overhead reach with a progressive forward lean used to apply a gentle elevating force to the arm. *(From Matsen FA III, Lippitt SB, Sidles JA, and Harryman DT II: Practical Evaluation and Management of the Shoulder. Philadelphia: WB Saunders, 1994.)*

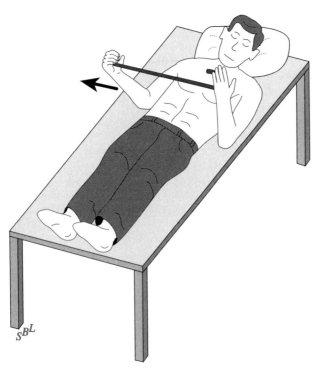

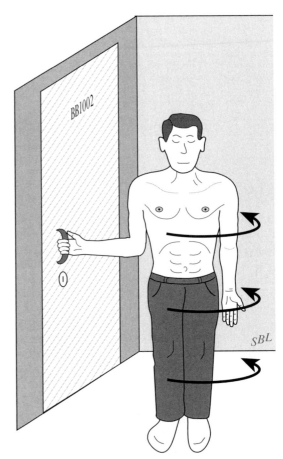

■ **Figure 15–83**
Stretching in external rotation with the opposite hand used as the therapist. *(From Matsen FA III, Lippitt SB, Sidles JA, and Harryman DT II: Practical Evaluation and Management of the Shoulder. Philadelphia: WB Saunders, 1994.)*

Subacromial Abrasion (without a Significant Defect in the Cuff Tendon)

In this condition, the shoulder demonstrates symptomatic crepitus as the humerus is rotated beneath the acromion; isometric testing of the cuff muscles reveals no pain or weakness. Maneuvers to stress the tendon against the undersurface of the coracoacromial arch are often used in the diagnosis. The sensitivity of the Neer and Hawkins impingement signs for the diagnosis of subacromial bursitis seen during arthroscopy was 75% and

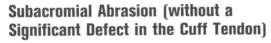

■ **Figure 15–84**
Stretching in external rotation by turning the body away from a fixed object to apply a gentle stretching force. *(From Matsen FA III, Lippitt SB, Sidles JA, and Harryman DT II: Practical Evaluation and Management of the Shoulder. Philadelphia: WB Saunders, 1994.)*

92%, respectively. Specificities were not much higher than the pretest probability.[260] A positive preoperative impingement test was shown to have no correlation with improved outcome after arthroscopic subacromial decompression on either the Western Ontario Rotator

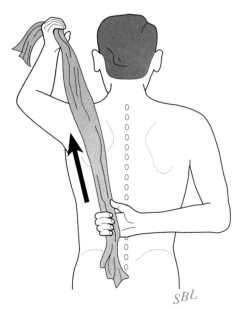

■ **Figure 15–85**
Stretching in internal rotation with a towel used to apply a gentle stretching force. *(From Matsen FA III, Lippitt SB, Sidles JA, and Harryman DT II: Practical Evaluation and Management of the Shoulder. Philadelphia: WB Saunders, 1994.)*

Cuff Index or the American Shoulder and Elbow Surgeons form.[222]

Nonoperative Treatment

Patients in whom the primary complaint is symptomatic subacromial crepitance (see Fig. 15–59) will usually benefit from reassurance and a home program of gentle stretching and strengthening exercises. Various nonoperative rotator cuff programs have been described for the general population and for athletes, including throwers.* Exercises must specifically address any shoulder stiffness that may cause obligate translation and loss of concentricity on shoulder movement (see Figs. 15–14 and 15–60). The effectiveness of nonoperative treatment was recognized many years ago by Neer, who in his initial article on anterior acromioplasty pointed out that "Many patients . . . were suspected of having impingement, but responded well to conservative treatment."[304] Furthermore, he stated that patients were advised to not undergo an acromioplasty until the stiffness of the shoulder had disappeared and the disability had persisted for at least 9 months. As a result of these conservative surgical indications, during the period covered by his report, this most active shoulder surgeon operated on an average of only 10 shoulders a year with this diagnosis; the effectiveness of nonoperative management is worthy of emphasis!

The low success rate in returning athletes to competition after acromioplasty[444] reinforces the importance of nonoperative management in this population. Similar principles apply to workers who are required to use

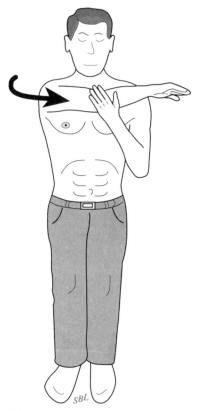

■ **Figure 15–86**
Stretching in cross-body reach with the opposite arm used as the therapist. *(From Matsen FA III, Lippitt SB, Sidles JA, and Harryman DT II: Practical Evaluation and Management of the Shoulder. Philadelphia: WB Saunders, 1994.)*

their shoulders in positions aggravating subacromial abrasion.

Subacromial injections of corticosteroids have been found by some to produce symptomatic relief.[184] However, Withrington and coworkers[487] reported a double-blind trial of steroid injections and found no evidence of the efficacy of such treatment. Valtonen[459] found no difference between subacromial and gluteal injections of steroids. Berry and colleagues[26] compared acupuncture, physiotherapy, steroid injections, and anti-inflammatory medications and found no difference among these treatments.

Steroid injections in or near the cuff and biceps tendons may produce tendon atrophy or may reduce the ability of damaged tendons to repair themselves. Such changes have been well documented in other tissues.[257,387,458] Uitto and colleagues[458] demonstrated corticosteroid-induced inhibition of the biosynthesis of collagen in human skin. The harmful effects of repetitive intra-articular injection of steroids have been noted.[21,86,267,394,431]

Ford and DeBender[126] reported 13 patients in whom 15 ruptured tendons developed subsequent to nearby injection of steroids. Other authors have reported spontaneous rupture of the Achilles tendon and patellar tendon after steroid injection.[20,193,232,279,414] Although Matthews and colleagues[271] failed to find a deleterious effect of corticosteroid injections on rabbit patellar tendons,

---

*See references 2, 8, 26, 32, 71, 73, 127, 177, 204, 213, 306, 318, 343, 344, 375, 379, 399.

Kennedy and Willis[212] found a substantial effect in the rabbit Achilles tendon. They concluded that physiologic doses of local steroid placed directly in a normal tendon weakened it significantly for up to 14 days after the injection.

Watson[474] reviewed the surgical findings in 89 patients with major ruptures of the cuff. He found that all seven patients who had not received any local steroid injections had strong residual cuff tissue. Thirteen of 62 patients who had received one to four steroid injections had soft cuff tissue that held suture poorly, and 17 of the 20 patients who had received more than four steroid injections had very weak cuff tissue; these shoulders with weak cuff tissue had poorer results after surgical repair. In this light, one can appreciate the potential hazard of making a diagnosis of "bursitis" or "bicipital tendinitis" and treating the shoulder with repeated steroid injections until the reality of a major cuff tendon deterioration becomes inescapable.[88,212]

A patient with subacromial abrasion is informed that this condition can usually be resolved with nonoperative management directed toward restoration of normal mobility, strength, coordination, and fitness.

■ AUTHORS' PREFERRED METHOD OF NONOPERATIVE MANAGEMENT OF SUBACROMIAL ABRASION

In our approach to subacromial abrasion, we recognize the important interplay between cuff weakness, stiffness of the posterior capsule, and subacromial roughness. We use a program designed by Sarah Jackins, a physical therapist who has worked with the University of Washington Shoulder and Elbow Service since its inception in 1975. This treatment regimen is analogous to one that would be used for managing a tennis elbow or Achilles tendinitis and includes (1) avoidance of repeated injury, (2) restoration of normal flexibility, (3) restoration of normal strength, (4) aerobic exercise, and (5) modification of work or sport. The emphasis is on simple, low-tech exercises that the patient can perform unassisted.

THE JACKINS PROGRAM
STEP 1: AVOIDANCE OF REPEATED INJURY

Although it seems obvious that an affected shoulder must be rested, we see patients each week who are trying to continue vigorous overhead work or swimming hundreds of miles per week in the presence of cuff symptoms. It is difficult to treat these symptoms when the affected area is repeatedly irritated; activities may need to be temporarily modified—light duty, reducing mileage, less throwing, using the kickboard for a major part of the workout rather than continuing to try to "swim through" the problem, or working on the forehand and footwork rather than beating away at the serve. Once symptoms have subsided, activity is progressively resumed with an emphasis on proper technique and paced resumption of normal levels of performance.

STEP 2: RESTORATION OF NORMAL FLEXIBILITY

The goal of step 2 is to stretch out all directions of tightness. Shoulders with subacromial abrasion are frequently stiff, especially in the posterior capsule (Fig. 15-60). As described earlier for posterior capsular tightness, the most effective program is one that is taught by the surgeon or therapist but is carried out by the patient. The goal of the flexibility program is to restore range of motion to that of the unaffected shoulder. The recommended treatment consists of gentle stretches performed five times a day by the patient (Figs. 15-81 to 15-86). Each stretch is performed to the point at which the patient feels a pull against the shoulder tightness, but not to the point of pain. Each stretch is performed for 1 minute, so the patient invests about 30 minutes per day in stretching the shoulder. Obvious improvement commonly occurs within the first month, but 3 months may be required to completely eliminate the condition.

STEP 3: RESTORATION OF NORMAL STRENGTH

When near-normal passive flexibility of the shoulder is restored, the patient's attention is directed toward regaining muscle strength. As is the case in managing tennis elbow, it is most effective to delay strengthening exercises until normal range of motion is achieved. As with the flexibility exercises, the patient is given the responsibility for strengthening the shoulder. Internal and external rotator strengthening exercises are carried out with the arm at the side (Figs. 15-87 and 15-88) to strengthen the anterior and posterior cuff muscles without the potential for subacromial grinding that exists with exercises in abduction and flexion. These exercises are most conveniently performed against the resistance of rubber tubing, sheet rubber, bike inner tubes, springs, or weights. It is convenient if the resistance device can be carried in a pocket or purse for frequent use through the day. As strength increases, the patient is advanced to more resistance: thicker tubing, tougher rubber sheets, or more springs. Deltoid strengthening is added when it can be performed comfortably (Fig. 15-89), as are exercises to strengthen the scapular motors (Figs. 15-90 and 15-91). Athletes are not returned to full activity until the shoulder has complete mobility and strength.

It is essential that these exercises be comfortable. Any discomfort during or after strengthening exercises indicates that the vigor of the exercise should be reduced.

STEP 4: AEROBIC EXERCISE

If a patient has gotten out of shape as a result of the shoulder problem, it is important to emphasize the need to regain normal fitness. To get back in shape and improve the sense of well-being, a half-hour of "sweaty" exercise 5 days a week is recommended. Brisk walking may be the safest and most effective type of aerobic exercise, but other suitable forms include jogging, biking, stationary biking, and rowing. Aerobic calisthenics as usually defined must be carefully reviewed to ensure that they do not require arm positions that aggravate the patient's symptoms.

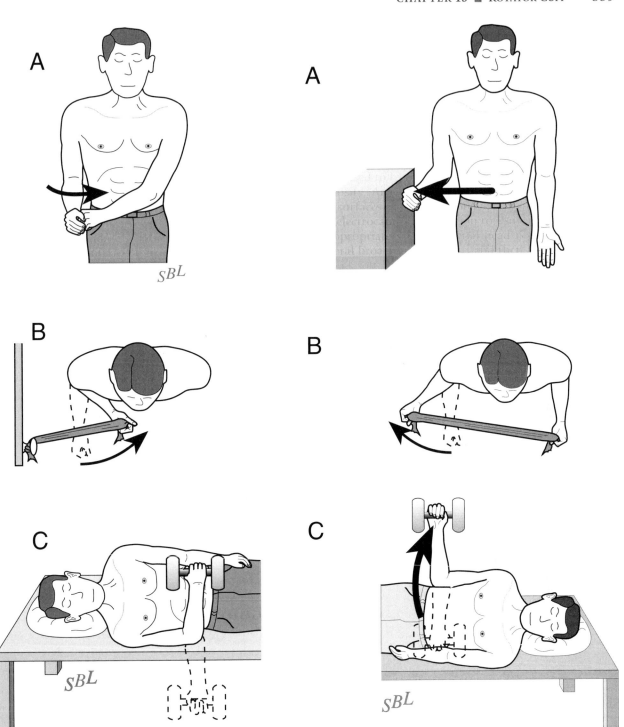

■ **Figure 15–87**
Internal rotation can be strengthened with isometrics (**A**), rubber tubing (**B**), or free weights (**C**). *(From Matsen FA III, Lippitt SB, Sidles JA, and Harryman DT II: Practical Evaluation and Management of the Shoulder. Philadelphia: WB Saunders, 1994.)*

■ **Figure 15–88**
External rotation strengthening using isometrics (**A**), rubber tubing (**B**), or free weights (**C**). *(From Matsen FA III, Lippitt SB, Sidles JA, and Harryman DT II: Practical Evaluation and Management of the Shoulder. Philadelphia: WB Saunders, 1994.)*

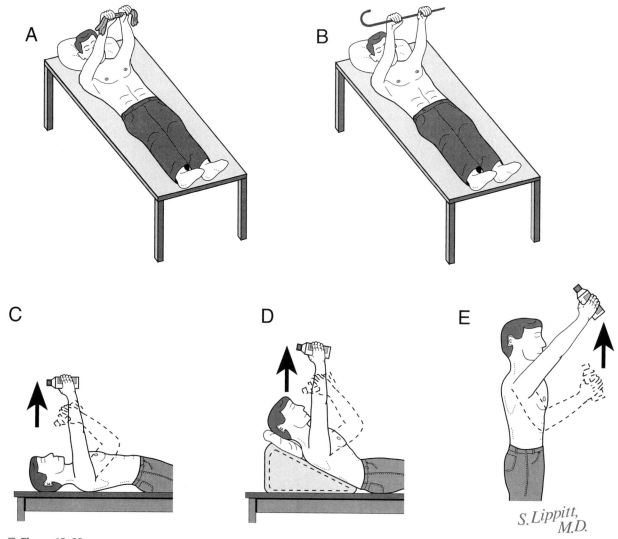

■ Figure 15–89

Progressive supine press exercises to strengthen flexion. The motion is always pushing up toward the ceiling and ends with a lift of the shoulder blade off the bed. **A,** Start with two hands together holding a wash cloth; **B,** then two hands apart; **C,** then one hand with a 1-pint (i.e., 1 lb) weight; **D,** then one hand with a 1-pint weight with greater degrees of sitting up; and finally, **E,** one hand with a 1-pint weight while standing. *(Modified from Matsen FA III, Lippitt SB, Sidles JA, and Harryman DT II: Practical Evaluation and Management of the Shoulder. Philadelphia: WB Saunders, 1994.)*

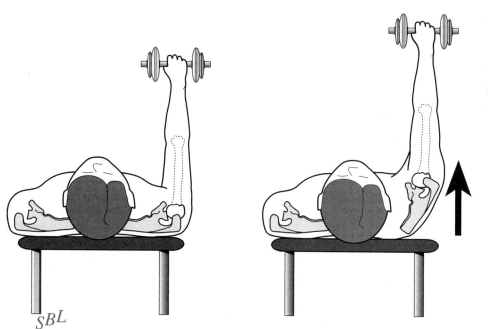

■ Figure 15–90

In the press plus, the arm is pushed upward until the shoulder blade is lifted off the table or bed. *(From Matsen FA III, Lippitt SB, Sidles JA, and Harryman DT II: Practical Evaluation and Management of the Shoulder. Philadelphia: WB Saunders, 1994.)*

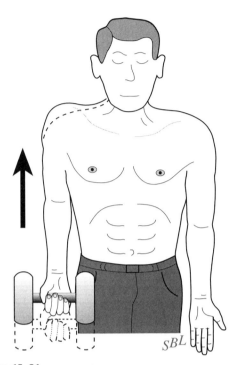

■ **Figure 15–91**

Shoulder shrug exercise. Lift the tip of the shoulder toward the ear while holding the elbow straight. *(From Matsen FA III, Lippitt SB, Sidles JA, and Harryman DT II: Practical Evaluation and Management of the Shoulder. Philadelphia: WB Saunders, 1994.)*

STEP 5: MODIFICATION OF WORK OR SPORT

Obviously, the purpose of the program is to return the patient to the comfortable pursuit of normal activities. Not infrequently, some analysis of working and recreational techniques is required. Occasionally, the answer is as simple as having a short grocery clerk stand on a platform at work. The technique of swimmers is reviewed to ensure, for example, adequate roll on the freestyle stroke. Throwers are taught the importance of body position and rotator cuff strength. Adequate knee bend and lumbar extension are reinforced in execution of the tennis serve. If the patient has an occupation that requires vigorous or repeated use of the shoulder in painful positions, vocational rehabilitation to a different job may be required.

SUBSEQUENT STEPS

It may take 6 weeks before substantial benefit is realized. As long as the patient is making progress, we continue this program. If improvement is not forthcoming, the program is reviewed to be sure that it is being conducted in an ideal way. The shoulder and the patient are also re-evaluated to ensure that no other factors are interfering with recovery. If repeat clinical evaluation indicates positive tendon signs (see Fig. 15–56) or other evidence of cuff fiber failure, tendon imaging studies may be considered if their results would change the patient's management. If a well-motivated patient continues to have symptomatic subacromial abrasion after 6 months of a well-conducted program, subacromial smoothing may be discussed as an alternative to continued nonoperative management. Poor compliance with an exercise program may foretell an equally poor result from surgical treatment.

Operative Treatment

Open Acromioplasty

In his classic description of acromioplasty, Neer[304] described approaching the shoulder through a 9-cm incision made in Langer's lines from the anterior edge of the acromion to a point just lateral to the coracoid. The deltoid is split for 5 cm distal to the acromioclavicular joint in the direction of its fibers. It is then dissected from the front of the acromion and the acromioclavicular joint capsule. The stump of the deltoid's tendinous origin is elevated upward and preserved for the deltoid repair. With an osteotome, a wedge-shaped piece of bone (0.09 by 2.0 cm) is resected from the anterior undersurface of the acromion, along with the entire attachment of the coracoacromial ligament. If acromioclavicular osteophytes are present, the distal 2.5 cm of the clavicle is also excised along with any prominences on the acromial side of the joint. After the procedure, the deltoid is carefully repaired to the acromioclavicular joint capsule, the trapezius, and its tendon of origin.

Many reports regarding the results of open acromioplasty have been published.* However, interpretation of these reports is made difficult by the admixture of patients with intact cuffs, partial-thickness cuff lesions, and full-thickness cuff tears, as well as by the inclusion of a wide range of additional elements to the surgery. Stuart and coauthors[430] reported a series that included acromioplasty with or without cuff repair, distal clavicle excision, and biceps tenodesis; 23% were still painful. Rockwood and Lyons[381] reported on a series of 71 patients who underwent a modified acromioplasty with or without cuff repair and concluded that cuff repair did not influence the percentage of excellent results. Bosley[36] reported on 35 patients treated by total acromionectomy, including patients with and without long-standing massive cuff tears; most failures were attributed to either the underlying pathology or failure of deltoid reattachment. Bjorkenheim and colleagues[33] reported a failure rate of over 25% and attributed the failures to "associated bony as well as soft-tissue subacromial lesions." Oglvie-Harris and associates[329] evaluated 67 shoulders in 65 patients who had pain and dysfunction for more than 2 years after an initial acromioplasty for impingement syndrome without a rotator cuff tear. In almost half the cases there were "diagnostic errors," and even in those with a correct diagnosis and no operative errors, the failure rate was almost 20%.

Arthroscopic Acromioplasty

Ellman,[109] in 1987, published the first large series of 50 patients (average age, 50 years) with mixed shoulder pathology who underwent arthroscopic acromioplasty; 10 had full-thickness tears. At an average follow-up of 17 months, 88% had good or excellent outcomes. These results persisted at a 2.5-year follow-up of the same treatment group.[112]

*See references 5, 99, 160, 166, 167, 177, 198, 216, 273, 283, 296, 304, 306, 318, 351, 364, 412, 417, 442, 475.

Since then, others have reported the results of arthroscopic acromioplasty.[109,115] Gartsman,[137] Speer and colleagues,[423] Altchek and coworkers,[3] and Roye and associates[390] reported series of arthroscopic acromioplasties on shoulders without cuff tears, with each finding that 83% to 94% of the results were satisfactory. Approximately 75% of the patients were able to return to sports activity. Recovery times in these series ranged from 2 to 4 months. Most authors describe the procedure as technically demanding. Control of bleeding and determination of the amount of bone to resect are two common technical difficulties when performing arthroscopic subacromial decompression. Many describe a learning curve associated with this technique and have recommended that this procedure be performed on cadaver shoulders before it is used clinically.

In the early years, after introduction of the arthroscopic technique of acromioplasty, controversy arose regarding whether a subacromial decompression performed arthroscopically was technically equivalent to that performed by open means. Gartsman and colleagues,[137,138] in a cadaver study, were able to perform arthroscopic bony resection with release of the coracoacromial ligament equivalent to the open technique described by Neer. He suggested criteria for the technical adequacy of acromioplasty: (1) the entire anterior acromial protuberance is resected, (2) the undersurface of the acromion is flattened, (3) the deltoid fibers are visible from the acromioclavicular joint to the lateral edge of the acromion, (4) the inferior aspect of the acromioclavicular joint is débrided to remove any downward protrusion, (5) the coracoacromial ligament is completely released from the anterior portion of the acromion and the acromioclavicular joint, (6) a portion of the ligament is resected, (7) an adequate subacromial bursectomy is performed to allow complete inspection of the bursal surface of the rotator cuff, and finally (8), no subacromial abrasion is observed when the arm is taken through a range of motion at the completion of the procedure.

Most authors state that the *indications* for arthroscopic acromioplasty should be identical to those for the open procedure described by Neer in 1972. However, when compared with the rate at which Neer used open acromioplasty in his practice, it is apparent that arthroscopic acromioplasty is performed much more commonly with broader indications. Although overall "satisfactory" results were obtained in the majority of reports, some authors were uncertain whether relief was obtained from the modification in acromial shape or other aspects of the treatment.

To keep things in perspective, Brox and coworkers[46] compared the effectiveness of arthroscopic acromioplasty, an exercise program, and placebo in a randomized clinical trial. The study group consisted of 125 patients 18 to 66 years of age who had had rotator cuff disease for at least 3 months and whose condition was resistant to treatment. The authors concluded that surgery or a supervised exercise regimen significantly and equally improved rotator cuff disease when compared with placebo; however, the surgical treatment was substantially more costly.

Comparison of Open and Arthroscopic Acromioplasty

In 1994, Sachs and coauthors[392] reported on a series of 44 patients with stage II impingement prospectively randomized into open (22 patients, average age of 49) and arthroscopic treatment groups (19 patients, average age of 51). In both groups, full recovery took at least 1 year for the majority of patients. Over 90% of patients in both groups achieved a satisfactory result (good or excellent). Final analysis showed that the main benefits of arthroscopic acromioplasty were evident in the first 3 months postoperatively, with the arthroscopic patients regaining flexion and strength more rapidly than patients treated with open decompression. Furthermore, because the arthroscopic treatment group had shorter hospitalization, used less narcotics, and returned more quickly to both work and activities of daily living, the authors suggested that arthroscopic acromioplasty may have significant economic advantages.

In 1992, van Holsbeeck and colleagues[460] compared their results of 53 patients treated by arthroscopic acromioplasty and 53 treated by open acromioplasty. Based on the UCLA rating scale, good or excellent results were identical for both groups at a 2-year follow-up. The authors suggested that arthroscopic acromioplasty was associated with a shorter recovery time; however, in the long term, no difference in strength of forward flexion was noted between the open and arthroscopic groups.

Hawkins and coauthors[179] reported 40% satisfactory results with arthroscopic subacromial decompression and 87% satisfactory results in a concurrent series of open acromioplasty. Hawkins was later involved in a direct comparison of open and arthroscopic acromioplasty, with no significant differences in outcomes. Open acromioplasty patients had significantly more pain relief at a minimum of a 1-year follow-up.[421]

Roye and associates[390] reported a series of 90 arthroscopic acromioplasties and found that most of the patients who were not throwing athletes obtained satisfactory results and that the presence or absence of a cuff tear did not affect the result.

Lindh and coworkers, in 1993, reported on a series of 20 patients who were randomly selected for either open or arthroscopic acromioplasty (10 patients in each group). The average duration of symptoms before surgery was over 5 years. Functional results in both the arthroscopic and open surgery groups were good and similar. Patients in the arthroscopic group were observed to demonstrate earlier restoration of full range of motion and reduction in time away from work.

Proponents of arthroscopic acromioplasty have argued that this procedure requires less surgical dissection and produces less scarring and less postoperative morbidity. In most instances, the procedure can be performed on an outpatient basis. Postoperative discomfort is moderate and can usually be controlled with oral analgesics. Additionally, cosmesis is good, and patient acceptance is high.

A countervailing benefit of an open procedure is the advantage of being able to directly observe the subacromial space during motions that preoperatively caused the patient's symptomatic subacromial crepitance, as well as the ability to ensure that the crepitance is resolved before the procedure is concluded.

Deltoid retraction can be a significant problem after open procedures that require detachment and subsequent reattachment of the deltoid to the anterior acromion.[29] Arthroscopic acromioplasty has the theoretical advantage of leaving the deltoid origin almost totally undisturbed. However, in a recent report, Torpey and collaborators[450] pointed out that much of the deltoid arose from the anterior acromion. Their analysis indicated that a 4-mm anterior acromioplasty would detach approximately half the deltoid fibers, whereas a 6-mm anterior acromioplasty would detach approximately 75% of the fibers. They concluded that neither an open nor an arthroscopic acromioplasty can be performed without substantial compromise of the anterior deltoid origin.

Arthroscopy offers the ability to directly inspect the glenohumeral joint as well as the subacromial space. During an open procedure, the deep surface of the cuff (where most cuff lesions begin) is not visible. By contrast, at arthroscopy, partial- or complete-thickness tears of either surface of the rotator cuff, as well as other findings, can be identified by an experienced observer. However, even with arthroscopy, common intratendinous lesions remain inaccessible. Paulos and Franklin,[346] in their series of 80 arthroscopic acromioplasties, reported a high number of unsuspected diagnoses that were made during arthroscopy. These diagnoses included 26 partial rotator cuff tears, 12 labral tears, 8 instances of humeral chondrosis, 4 cases of biceps tendon fraying, and 2 loose bodies in the glenohumeral joint. They reported that for most of these shoulders, such findings would have been missed with the open technique.

In their series of 44 patients treated by arthroscopic acromioplasty, Altchek and associates[3] reported that 11 patients had lesions of the glenoid labrum. Preoperatively, these patients had no evidence of instability, either by history or physical examination in action. Five of these patients had a tear involving the inferior part of the labrum; they failed to recover completely after the acromioplasty and were unable to return to full participation in sports. The authors thought that undetected slight instability may have played a role in the production of these patients' symptoms. The authors argued that arthroscopic inspection of the glenohumeral joint makes it possible to detect such problems and thus provide information that is important for prognosis. Others have reported a higher than anticipated percentage of unsuspected associated lesions in shoulders being treated arthroscopically for impingement symptoms.[203] Burns and Turba[52] reported on their findings in 29 patients treated by arthroscopic acromioplasty; conditions included anterior glenoid labrum tear (15), undersurface rotator cuff tear (8), chondromalacia of the humerus (3), biceps rupture (1), posterior glenoid labrum tear (1), and acromioclavicular arthritis (1).

These results indicate that the preoperative diagnosis of "impingement syndrome" has been associated with a wide range of shoulder pathologies. They leave unanswered the question of the prevalence of these same findings in asymptomatic shoulders and the role played by each of the findings in producing clinical symptoms. One hopes that in the future, methodical clinical-pathologic correlation will lead to improved accuracy in preoperative diagnosis and greater specificity in treatment.

The primary difficulty in interpreting these studies on open and arthroscopic acromioplasty is that although the *outcome* of the procedure is characterized in terms such as "good" or "excellent," the *effectiveness* of the procedure is often undetermined because the preoperative status, or *ingo,* was not characterized in the same way. Ideally, a "good" result from surgery would indicate the change in the patient's condition as a result of the procedure rather than the status of the shoulder postoperatively.

Definition of the indications for and the effectiveness of acromioplasty must await multipractice studies that accurately define the pretreatment clinical findings and functional status of the shoulder, the nature of and compliance with a nonoperative program, the type of surgery, and the change in shoulder function realized after the procedure with the same parameters of comfort and function used before and after surgery. The effectiveness of a treatment is the difference between the outcome and the ingo.

Subacromial Decompression without Acromioplasty

Budoff and colleagues evaluated their results in patients with partial rotator cuff tears after débridement and arthroscopic subacromial decompression without acromioplasty. They found that 89% of patients had a good or excellent UCLA score 2 to 5 years after the procedure, with 81% good or excellent results after 5 years.[48] These results are comparable to those reported for arthroscopic subacromial decompression with acromioplasty. Two percent of patients progressed to a full-thickness tear. Three patients subsequently underwent arthroscopy, at which time it was determined that their partial-thickness tears had not healed.

■ AUTHORS' PREFERRED METHOD OF SUBACROMIAL SMOOTHING

We now recognize that the surface irregularities producing subacromial roughness are almost always on the humeral side rather than the side of the coracoacromial arch. The goal of surgery is to therefore smooth the surface of the proximal humeral convexity while preserving the integrity of the coracoacromial arch and deltoid.

In our experience, the results of subacromial smoothing are likely to be best in the following circumstances: (1) a well-motivated patient older than 40 years; (2) absence of posterior capsular stiffness; (3) presence of symptomatic subacromial crepitus (see Fig. 15–59), which the patient agrees is the dominant clinical problem; (4) absence of tendon signs (see Fig. 15–56) and other shoulder pathology; and (5) symptoms that are not associated with a work-related injury. Poor prognostic signs include (1) age younger than 40, (2) stiffness, (3) absence of subacromial crepitus, (4) presence of tendon signs or evidence of other shoulder pathology, (5) attribution of problem by the patient to occupation, (6) concomitant evidence of glenohumeral instability, and (7) neurogenic cuff muscle weakness.

We use an open approach to subacromial smoothing so that we can directly observe passage of the proximal humeral convexity beneath the coracoacromial arch. The patient is positioned with the head up at 30 degrees and the arm draped free so that full motion is possible. Before making the incision, we note the positions and motions in which subacromial crepitus can be palpated through the acromion. The shoulder is approached through an incision in the skin lines over the anterolateral corner of the acromion (see Fig. 15-1). The acromion is exposed while striving to maintain continuity of the deltoid fascia, the acromial periosteum, and the trapezius fascia. The deltoid tendon is split in line with its fibers along the strong tendon of origin that divides the anterior and middle deltoid. This technique allows two strong "handles" on the deltoid for repair. In most cases, no detachment of the deltoid origin is needed. This split is deepened under direct vision until the bursa is entered. Rotating the humerus provides easy differentiation between the deltoid surface of the bursa (which does not move with humeral rotation) and the superficial surface of the cuff (which does).

On entering the subacromial aspect of the humeroscapular motion interface (see Figs. 15-3 and 15-4), the subacromial space is observed while the preoperatively identified crepitus-producing movements are carried out. This step reveals the cause of the crepitance, which is usually some combination of hypertrophic bursa, adhesions between the cuff and acromion, roughness of the superior surface of the rotator cuff, and prominence of the greater tuberosity. By gently rotating the arm, most of the cuff can be brought to the incision as pointed out by Codman (Figs. 15-92 and 15-93). The rotator cuff is thoroughly explored and palpated for evidence of superior surface blisters, partial tears, thinning, or full-thickness defects. Although deep surface cuff fiber failure cannot be seen through this approach, it is also true that such fiber disruption cannot be causing the subacromial crepitance. The methylene blue "dye test" of Hiro Fukuda[134] or, more recently, the "Fukuda-lite" test with saline is used to evaluate shoulders with suspicious cuff integrity. In this test, fluid is injected to distend the glenohumeral joint to further explore suspected thinning or small cuff defects.

Hypertrophic bursa is resected. Superior surface cuff defects are smoothed either by resecting their protruding aspects or, occasionally, by reattaching a superior surface cuff flap. Prominences of the tuberosity are smoothed so that the tuberosity passes easily beneath the coracoacromial arch. The undersurface of the coracoacromial arch is palpated to identify areas of roughness or prominence. It is of great interest to note that roughness of the undersurface of the coracoacromial arch is actually rare in spite

■ **Figure 15–92**

A, Operative position, superior view. **B,** Rotation of the humerus beneath the incision. *(From Codman EA: Rupture of the Supraspinatus Tendon and Other Lesions in or about the Subacromial Bursa. Malabar, FL: Robert E Krieger, 1984.)*

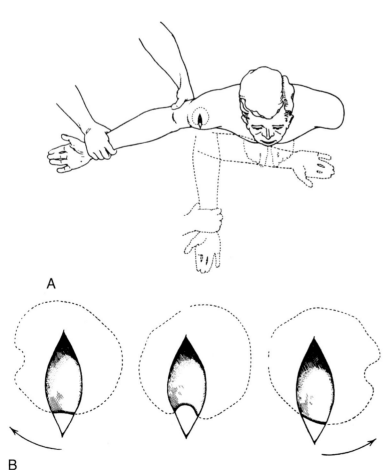

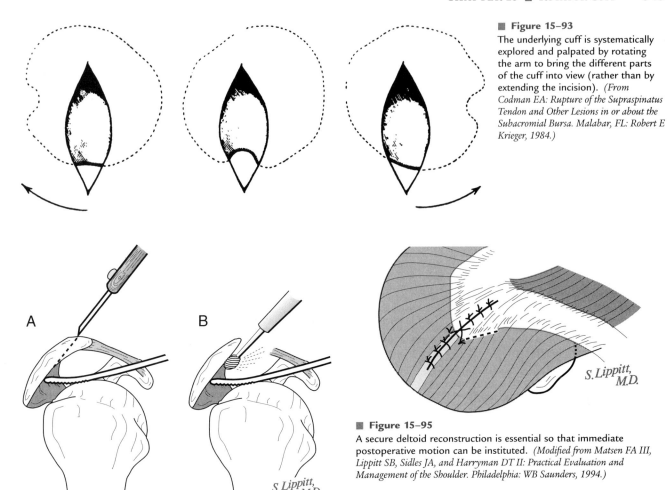

■ **Figure 15–93**
The underlying cuff is systematically explored and palpated by rotating the arm to bring the different parts of the cuff into view (rather than by extending the incision). *(From Codman EA: Rupture of the Supraspinatus Tendon and Other Lesions in or about the Subacromial Bursa. Malabar, FL: Robert E Krieger, 1984.)*

■ **Figure 15–94**
A thin-bladed osteotome is used to resect the anteroinferior surface of the acromion. The coracoacromial ligament is resected along with the acromial fragment. The osteotomy is oriented in line with the extrapolated undersurface of the posterior acromion. Exposure and access are facilitated by using a Darrach retractor to gently depress the humeral head. *(Modified from Matsen FA III, Lippitt SB, Sidles JA, and Harryman DT II: Practical Evaluation and Management of the Shoulder. Philadelphia: WB Saunders, 1994.)*

■ **Figure 15–95**
A secure deltoid reconstruction is essential so that immediate postoperative motion can be instituted. *(Modified from Matsen FA III, Lippitt SB, Sidles JA, and Harryman DT II: Practical Evaluation and Management of the Shoulder. Philadelphia: WB Saunders, 1994.)*

of radiographic suggestions of "spurs." If irregularities are identified by palpation, they can be smoothed with a "pinecone" bur. Very rarely, an osteotome or rongeur may be needed for larger lesions (Fig. 15–94). The coracoacromial ligament is preserved unless it is seen to be the cause of crepitance on motion.

Additional surgery is avoided unless clearly indicated. Inferiorly directed acromioclavicular osteophytes are resected if they scrape on the cuff. The biceps is left undisturbed unless it appears to be seriously inflamed, obviously unstable, or partially torn, in which case we perform a tenotomoy or tenodesis to the proximal part of the humerus.

The shoulder is gently manipulated through a complete range of motion to ensure the absence of stiffness or additional adhesions. The entire humeroscapular motion interface (see Figs. 15–3 and 15–4) is inspected to ensure the absence of adhesions and other pathology. Before the procedure is concluded, the upper surface of the cuff and

tuberosities and the undersurface of the coracoacromial arch are carefully palpated to ensure the absence of residual roughness. The entire range of passive shoulder motion must be free of subacromial crepitance.

On closure, a secure deltoid reconstitution is top priority so that early postoperative motion may be instituted. The deltoid is repaired by side-to-side closure of the medial and lateral aspects of the tendon split with No. 2 nonabsorbable suture (Fig. 15–95). If the deltoid origin has been partially detached, the area of detachment is secured to the acromion by suturing to bone as necessary. Suture from the medial hole is passed through the lateral part of the deltoid tendon and suture from the lateral hole is passed through the medial part of the deltoid tendon to effect a crisscross closure. Such technique avoids the "telltale V" defect indicative of poor deltoid closure. All knots are placed on the superficial aspect to avoid re-creating the subacromial roughness.

Postoperative Program

After any type of subacromial surgery, there is great potential for adhesions between the cuff and the arch. In cases of failed acromioplasty, such scarring seems to be a dominant feature and appears to often be related to delay in the institution of motion after surgery. To avoid these problems, we begin motion as soon as possible, preferably with continuous passive motion in the recovery room (Fig. 15–96). Continuous passive motion is set to move the arm slowly through an arc of 0 to 90 degrees of elevation

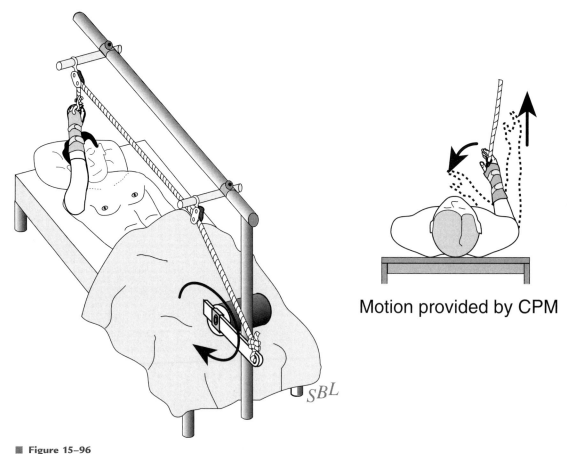

Motion provided by CPM

■ **Figure 15–96**
Continuous passive motion (CPM) is helpful for the first 24 to 48 hours after a procedure to mobilize the shoulder. Elevation to 90 degrees is easily achieved by using a simple pulley system with a motor-driven eccentric cam. *(Modified from Matsen FA III, Lippitt SB, Sidles JA, and Harryman DT II: Practical Evaluation and Management of the Shoulder. Philadelphia: WB Saunders, 1994.)*

and from 50 to 0 degrees of internal rotation. It is applied whenever the patient is in bed during the hospitalization, but it is not continued after discharge. On the day of surgery, the patient is instructed in the "140/40 passive program," in which the opposite hand is used to assist the operated shoulder in achieving 140 degrees of elevation (see Fig. 15–81) and 40 degrees of external rotation (Fig. 15–83). Emphasis is also placed on posterior capsular stretching, including cross-body adduction (Fig. 15–86), reaching up the back (Fig. 15–85), and internal rotation of the abducted arm.

Early implementation of passive motion is facilitated if the procedure is performed under a brachial plexus block,[441] which lasts for 12 to 18 hours. The postoperative exercises are already familiar to the patient because they have been performed as part of the preoperative trial of the Jackins program. The patient is allowed active use of the shoulder within the realm of comfort, unless strength of the deltoid reattachment is a concern. Exercises for strengthening internal (Fig. 15–87) and external rotation (Fig. 15–88) are also begun immediately. Deltoid strengthening is initiated at 6 weeks after the repair is secure (Fig. 15–89). As soon as they can be performed comfortably, exercises to strengthen the scapular motors are added (Figs. 15–90 and 15–91). Athletic activity is not allowed for 3 months after surgery and until normal motion and strength are regained.

Failed Acromioplasty

In this condition, the patient is dissatisfied with the result after a previous arthroscopic or open acromioplasty and requests that additional surgery be considered. Such results occur in every series of acromioplasty, even if the technique of the procedure seems appropriate. The incidence of these failures ranges from 3% to 11%.[304,360,367,442] In Post and Cohen's series, 11% continued to have significant pain after surgery.[360,361] Fifty-six percent of those with weakness before surgery still had weakness postoperatively; 29% of those with preoperative limitation of motion still had limitation of motion after surgery. The rate of return to high-level athletics or challenging occupations is lower. Tibone and colleagues[444] found that of 35 athletes who had impingement syndrome treated by anterior acromioplasty, 20% still had moderate to severe pain and 9% had pain at rest and with activities of daily living. Only 43% returned to their preinjury level of competitive athletics, and only 4 of 18 returned to competitive throwing. Hawkins and coworkers[176] have shown that it is difficult for patients injured on the job to return to their original occupations after acromioplasty.

Why is this? Failure to achieve complete relief of symptoms through acromioplasty may indicate (1) a problem other than acromial pathology, (2) failure to achieve subacromial smoothness, (3) failure of deltoid reattachment, (4) excessive acromial resection, (5) postoperative complications such as dense scarring between the cuff and acromion, (6) failure of rehabilitation, or (7) destabilization of the glenohumeral joint.[237] Many of these problems can leave the patient more symptomatic than before the surgery (see Fig. 15-9).

Acromioclavicular joint problems were thought to be responsible for five failures in Post and Cohen's series, were a "frequent cause of failure of surgical treatment" in the series of Penny and Welsh,[351] and were the cause of the only unsatisfactory result in Neer's series. Co-planing of the acromioclavicular joint during arthroscopic subacromial decompression without distal clavicular excision resulted in no statistically significant increase in acromioclavicular joint symptoms when compared with patients who underwent distal clavicular excision with co-planing or those who had no co-planing.[12] Arthroscopic subacromial decompression with combined excision of the distal end of the clavicle was reported to produce results comparable to those of open techniques, with 81% noting complete relief of pain.[268] In their series of patients with persisting problems after acromioplasty, Hawkins and colleagues[176] reported that 45% of the patients had a diagnosis other than continuing impingement, including acromioclavicular joint problems, cervical spondylosis, reflex sympathetic dystrophy, rotator cuff tear, thoracic outlet syndrome, glenohumeral osteoarthritis, and glenohumeral instability. Thirty-three percent were thought to have continuing subacromial abrasion. The striking finding in this series was the relative lack of improvement in patients receiving workers' compensation after revision acromioplasty. Even in these authors' series of primary acromioplasties, 22% of the workers' compensation cases had an unsatisfactory result versus an 8% failure rate in non–workers' compensation cases.[175] Post and Cohen[361] also observed that worse results were obtained after surgery performed for work-related impingement syndrome. This inability to return to work may be due to partial-thickness cuff tears, residual tendon scarring, and residual weakness. Post and Cohen emphasized the need for recovery of muscle strength before the laborer is returned to work; otherwise, recurrence can be anticipated. The difficulty of returning workers to their jobs after acromioplasty is reminiscent of the problems described by Tibone and coworkers[444] in returning athletes to a competitive level of function.

Bosley[36] reported that most failures were attributed to either the underlying pathology or failure of deltoid reattachment. Bjorkenheim and associates[33] reported a failure rate of over 25% and attributed the failures to "associated bony as well as soft-tissue subacromial lesions." Ogilvie-Harris and colleagues[329] evaluated 67 shoulders in 65 patients who had pain and dysfunction for more than 2 years after an initial acromioplasty for impingement syndrome without a rotator cuff tear. In almost half the cases there were "diagnostic errors," and even in those with a correct diagnosis and no operative errors, the failure rate was almost 20%.

Radical acromionectomy may worsen a patient's comfort and function (see Fig. 15-9). This procedure removes the origin of the deltoid muscle and facilitates scar formation between the deltoid muscle and the rotator cuff. Neer and Marberry pointed out that radical acromionectomy may seriously compromise shoulder function without achieving subacromial smoothness.[310] In their series of 30 patients, all had marked shoulder weakness and almost all had persistent pain. In the 20 shoulders reoperated on, all had a retracted and scarred middle deltoid that was adherent to the cuff and humerus. Fifteen of the patients had residual cuff tears. Attempts to reconstruct these severely damaged shoulders were disappointing. The effects of loss of the deltoid attachment and the permanent contracture could not be reversed. In addition, these authors observed a high incidence of wound problems and infection after radical acromionectomy, which further complicated their attempts at revision.

To help understand some of the other causes of unsuccessful acromioplasty, Flugstad and coworkers[125] reviewed 19 patients referred to the University of Washington Shoulder and Elbow Service because of persistent pain and stiffness after open acromioplasty performed elsewhere. The average age was 42 years, and 16 were male. Eleven patients had a traumatic onset of their shoulder problem, 8 of which were work related. The average time of postoperative immobilization was 4 weeks. At the time of initial evaluation, the patients complained of pain and stiffness. Physical examination revealed an average of 126 degrees of forward flexion and 36 degrees of external rotation and internal rotation, with the thumb being able to touch T12. In 13 of these patients, revision surgery was performed after an exercise program failed to improve their symptoms. The average interval between the initial surgery and revision surgery was 15 months. At revision surgery, 10 patients were found to have roughness of the undersurface of the acromion. Five patients had distinct spurs protruding from the lateral or medial acromion; eight patients had large amounts of subacromial scarring in which heavy bands of cicatrix connected the undersurface of the acromion to the rotator cuff. Three patients had acromioclavicular joint spurs, one had a large ununited acromial fragment, and another had an os acromiale. Although no patient had a full-thickness cuff tear, the incidence of partial-thickness deep surface or midsubstance cuff tears is unknown. The revision surgical procedure included excision of scar tissue, revision of the acromioplasty to ensure adequate resection of the anterior and inferior acromion, resection of acromioclavicular spurs, inspection of the rotator cuff, and careful deltoid repair. Immediately after surgery, gentle range-of-motion exercises were initiated to minimize restriction from postoperative scarring. Follow-up at an average of 10 months postoperatively revealed substantial, though incomplete improvement in comfort, range of motion, and ability to work.

This report emphasizes the importance of accurate diagnosis and effective subacromial smoothing. However, the key lesson was the importance of rapid restoration of full joint motion before restricting adhesions have the opportunity to form; the average patient in this series had a 1-month delay between surgery and the implementation of motion.

■ AUTHORS' PREFERRED METHOD FOR THE MANAGEMENT OF FAILED ACROMIOPLASTY

Patients who have previously undergone acromioplasty with unsatisfactory results need to be carefully re-evaluated to determine the presence of stiffness, weakness, instability, or persisting roughness. The social and vocational context of the shoulder problem must be re-evaluated as well.

The Jackins nonoperative program is instituted, even if the patient has already "had therapy"; because surgery has failed once already, there is plenty of time for conservatism and a period of observation.

Patients with positive tendon signs (see Fig. 15-56) may be considered for cuff imaging studies if these signs are refractory to rehabilitation. Vocational rehabilitation may be essential; if one procedure has not returned the patient back to work, the odds would not seem much better the second go-round.

Reoperation is considered in well-motivated patients with evidence of residual subacromial roughness or stiffness that is attributable to postoperative scarring in the humeroscapular motion interface (see Figs. 15-3 and 15-4). In contrast to primary acromioplasty, we are willing to reoperate on patients with refractory shoulder stiffness because this stiffness may be due to dense scarring between the cuff and the acromion that cannot be managed nonoperatively. Our revision procedure is based on the same principles as the primary subacromial smoothing described in the previous section.

Partial-Thickness Cuff Lesions

In this condition, partial-thickness disruption of the cuff is manifested by pain or weakness on resisted isometric contraction of the involved cuff muscles. The shoulder commonly has associated posterior capsular tightness. Imaging studies may indicate cuff tendon thinning or partial-thickness defects, but the lesion does not extend through the full thickness of the tendon.

Judging from the cadaver studies reviewed earlier in this chapter, intrasubstance and articular surface partial-thickness cuff tears represent the most common forms of cuff involvement. These lesions usually involve the supraspinatus tendon near its anterior insertion, but they may also involve the infraspinatus and subscapularis. Clinical observation of patients with documented partial-thickness cuff lesions suggests that these lesions produce symptoms analogous to other partial-thickness tendon lesions, such as a partial Achilles tear, a partial tear of the patellar tendon, or a partial tear of the tendon of origin of the extensor carpi radialis brevis ("tennis elbow"). Symptoms of partial tendon lesions include *stiffness* of the joint on passive motion in a direction that stretches the tendon and *tendon signs* such as pain or weakness on isometric contraction of the tendon's muscle (see Fig. 15-56). These partial tendon lesions are often much more painful than full-thickness tears because in contrast to full-thickness tears, partial-thickness defects of the cuff

give rise to stiffness and unphysiologic tension on the remaining fibers.

In its less common form involving the bursal aspect of the cuff tendon, partial-thickness cuff lesions may be associated with *subacromial abrasion* producing subacromial crepitance on passive joint motion.

Not a lot of information has been published regarding the results of operative treatment of partial-thickness cuff lesions. Fukuda and colleagues[134,135] described the management of six patients with partial-thickness bursal-side tears by acromioplasty and/or wedge resection with tendon repair to bone. They used an intraoperative "color test" in which dye was injected into the shoulder joint to indicate the extent of joint-side tears. The results were satisfactory in 90% of cases. Itoi and Tabata[195] reported their results in managing 38 shoulders with partial-thickness cuff lesions. The average follow-up period was 4.9 years, and the average age at surgery was 52.2 years. Three types of lesions were identified: superficial (12 shoulders), intratendinous (3), and deep surface tears (23). The authors performed full-thickness resection of the cuff, including the lesion, and repaired the defect with side-to-side suture (13 shoulders), side-to-bone suture (8), fascial patch grafting (16), or side-to-bone suture with fascial patch grafting (1). The overall results were satisfactory in 31 shoulders (82%). The results were not affected by the type of tear, the operative method, or the follow-up period.

Arthroscopic Treatment

Andrews and colleagues[4] presented 36 patients with partial-thickness tears of the supraspinatus portion of the cuff treated by arthroscopic débridement of the rotator cuff defect. No acromioplasty was performed. The average age was 22.5 years, and 64% of the patients were baseball pitchers. Of the 34 patients available for follow-up, 85% had an excellent (26 patients) or good (3 patients) result and were able to return to sports. The authors suggested that débridement may initiate a healing response. Arthroscopy revealed a tear of some part of the glenoid labrum in all patients. Six had partial tears of the long head of the biceps tendon. These observations point to the difficulty of deciding which surgical findings are responsible for the patient's symptoms.

Ogilvie-Harris and Wiley[328] reported on the arthroscopic treatment of 57 incomplete tears of the rotator cuff with symptoms of impingement. These tears were débrided, and no acromioplasty was performed. Half the patients improved.

Wiley[483] reported on 33 patients treated arthroscopically for partial tears of the rotator cuff. Only three patients achieved a satisfactory result.

Ellman and Kay reported good results from arthroscopic acromioplasty performed in conjunction with arthroscopic débridement of partial-thickness tears of the rotator cuff.[113]

Esch and colleagues,[115] in 1988, reported on 34 patients with stage II rotator cuff disease and partial-thickness rotator cuff tears treated by arthroscopic acromioplasty and tear débridement. Twenty-eight patients were satisfied with their results; 16 patients were rated excellent, 10 were good, 6 were fair, and 2 were rated as poor.

Gartsman[137] presented 40 patients with partial-thickness rotator cuff tears in a group of 125 patients treated by arthroscopic acromioplasty. Of these partial-thickness tears, 32 involved the articular surface of the supraspinatus tendon and 4 tears involved the bursal side. Four infraspinatus tears were identified, three of which involved the articular surface. Notably, in these 40 patients were 27 cases of labral fraying and 6 instances of biceps/labral complex detachment, again indicating the difficulty of relating symptoms to surgical findings. Of the 40 patients, 33 (83% satisfactory results) had major improvement in their ratings for pain, activities of daily living, work, and sports at an average of 28.9 months after arthroscopic débridement. Two patients who had an unsatisfactory result underwent a second operation: one, open acromioplasty, and the other, repair of the rotator cuff, with satisfactory results. Of the 30 patients in this group engaged in sports preoperatively, 10 returned to those sports at the same level of performance as before the symptoms had started.

Altchek and coauthors[3] reported four of six good or excellent results in patients with partial-thickness rotator cuff tears treated by arthroscopic acromioplasty and débridement of the rotator cuff defect.

Roye and coworkers[390] presented 38 patients with partial-thickness rotator cuff tears (32 involving the supraspinatus) treated with arthroscopic acromioplasty. A satisfactory result was achieved in 95%.

As part of a larger series, Ryu[391] reported on 35 patients with partial-thickness rotator cuff tears treated with arthroscopic acromioplasty. Thirty of 35 patients (86%) were rated as having excellent or good results (5 fair, no poor) at a minimal follow-up of 12 months. Of the group with partial tears, four were found to involve only the articular surface. Three of these four were considered failures.

In 1994, Olsewki and Depew[332] reported on their experience with 61 consecutive patients treated by arthroscopic acromioplasty and débridement of the rotator cuff defect (17 of 21 patients [81%] with a partial-thickness rotator tear were deemed to have a satisfactory result [UCLA rating scale]). This result was identical to that achieved in 27 patients treated by arthroscopic acromioplasty for rotator cuff "tendonitis" with an intact rotator cuff. As was the case in the series of Roye and associates,[390] the extent of the tear did not statistically affect the result.

From this group of reports it is difficult to define (1) the indications for surgery, (2) which aspects of the patients' pathology were responsible for their symptoms, (3) why 15% to 50% of patients failed to achieve a satisfactory result, and (4) which aspect of the surgery (acromioplasty or débridement) was responsible for improvement after surgery. It seems likely that patients benefiting from this procedure were able to resolve the insertional mechanism of the cuff in a way that evenly distributed the loads and thus avoided localized areas of increased fiber tension.

■ AUTHORS' PREFERRED METHOD OF TREATING PARTIAL-THICKNESS CUFF LESIONS

NONOPERATIVE TREATMENT

The nonoperative management of partial-thickness cuff tears is similar to that for subacromial abrasion described earlier in this chapter. Just as with partial lesions of the Achilles, patellar, or extensor radialis brevis tendons, the program must emphasize stretching against all directions of tightness, including internal rotation (Fig. 15–85), cross-body adduction (Fig. 15–86), elevation (Figs. 15–81 and 15–82), and occasionally, external rotation (Fig. 15–83). As in a tennis elbow rehabilitation program, when a comfortable normal range of passive motion is re-established, gentle progressive muscle strengthening is instituted (see Figs. 15–87 and 15–88). Emphasis is always placed on gentle and comfortable progress of this rehabilitation program. The goal of this program is to ensure that the scar collagen that forms in the defect will become as supple as normal tendon; otherwise, scar contracture will tend to concentrate the loads of the cuff on the lesion and lead to recurrence and propagation of injury.

OPERATIVE TREATMENT
OPEN SURGERY

Just as in the case of partial Achilles, patellar, and extensor carpi radialis brevis tendon lesions, no surgical treatment reliably restores the tendon to its normal condition. Preoperatively, it is important to determine whether the patient's primary problem is due to stiffness or to difficulties during active muscle contraction so that the procedure can be biased accordingly. On the one hand, sectioning of the fibers that remain intact (as in a tennis elbow release) may worsen the problem of weakness, although this technique may be the basis of the arthroscopic "débridement" advocated by some surgeons for this lesion. On the other hand, excision of the defect and repair may exacerbate the problems of stiffness.[505] Furthermore, such surgical tightening of the involved part of the cuff would cause the area of damage and repair to bear the majority of the load when the cuff muscles contract (reminiscent of the "quadregia" phenomenon in hand surgery). Thus, during excision and repair of partial-thickness cuff lesions, surgeons must ensure that the tendon load is distributed evenly at the insertion by carrying out a repair that is isometric to allow uniform load distribution and by carrying out a release of the capsule tightened in the repair.[170]

The surgical exposure to a partial-thickness cuff lesion is identical to that described for management of subacromial roughness (see Fig. 15–1). If symptoms are related to subacromial abrasion (i.e., symptomatic subacromial crepitance), subacromial smoothing is performed as described previously in this chapter.

If the tendon insertion is basically strong and if the deep surface tear is small, curettage of the defect through a minimal tenotomy can be performed. No repair is

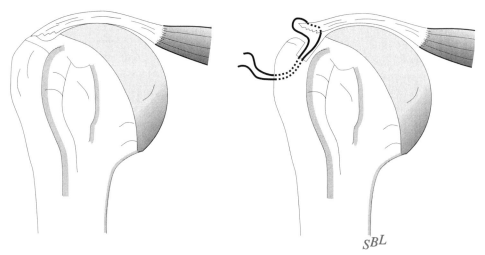

performed, and a full-motion program is implemented after surgery.

The decision to convert a partial-thickness cuff defect to a full-thickness defect and to then repair it (Fig. 15-97) is based on the patient's preoperative evaluation and surgical findings. Such an approach is favored if the tendon tear is almost complete, yet the quality of the remaining tissue is good. The thickness of the cuff can be determined at surgery by inspection, palpation, and the Fukuda test described earlier. A depth gauge or calibrated nerve hook inserted into the area of the lesion may help determine the percentage of the tendon that remains intact. If a decision is made to perform an open repair, a tenotomy is performed in the most suspicious area along the line of the tendon fibers to explore the full thickness of the tissue. If, as is usually the case, the defect is within the substance of the tendon or on its deep surface near the anterior insertion of the supraspinatus, a longitudinal tenotomy and capsulotomy are performed along the anterior aspect of the supraspinatus near the rotator interval. This cut is then extended at right angles posteriorly through the partially detached cuff at its insertion to the greater tuberosity, with the flap of cuff turned back until normal tendon of full thickness is encountered. Next, an attempt is made to retrieve and consolidate any split laminations of cuff that may have retracted medially (Fig. 15–97). These laminations are usually on the deep articular surface where the cuff lesion begins and may have retracted up to 1 cm. Release of the coracohumeral ligament and the rotator interval capsule from the base of the coracoid (Figs. 15–98 and 15–99), as well as release of the capsule from the glenoid lip (Fig. 15–100), will minimize tension on the repair. The full-thickness defect is then repaired (Figs. 15–101 and 15–102), with care taken to render the cuff insertion isometric with respect to all its fibers and smooth on its superior surface. Finally, with the anterior undersurface of the acromion in full view, the shoulder is put through a full range of motion to verify the elimination of any subacromial abrasion (see Fig. 15–59) and to ensure that the repair has not restricted shoulder motion.

Postoperative management is the same as for repair of full-thickness defects, with particular emphasis on continuous passive motion (Fig. 15–96) and early restitution

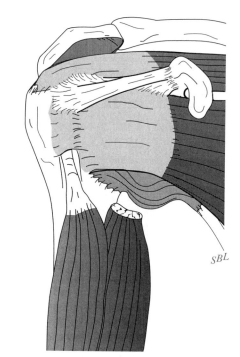

■ **Figure 15–98**
The rotator interval capsule–coracohumeral ligament complex lies between the coracoid process, the bicipital groove, the subscapularis tendon, and the supraspinatus tendon. This complex is not a separate structure but rather a particular area of the glenohumeral capsule. Tightness of this structure can limit external rotation of the adducted arm, adduction, and humeral elevation in the anterior and posterior scapular planes. *(From Matsen FA III, Lippitt SB, Sidles JA, and Harryman DT II: Practical Evaluation and Management of the Shoulder. Philadelphia: WB Saunders, 1994.)*

of full range of motion to prevent stiffness and adhesions (Figs. 15–81 to 15–86).

Full-Thickness Cuff Tear

Characteristically, full-thickness cuff tears cause pain or weakness on resisted isometric contraction of one or more of the cuff muscles. Age older than 65 years, night pain, and weakness of external rotation were most predictive of rotator cuff tears.[252] Three tests were evaluated for the

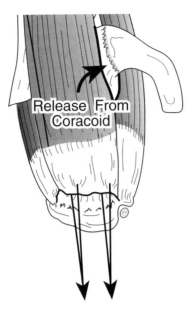
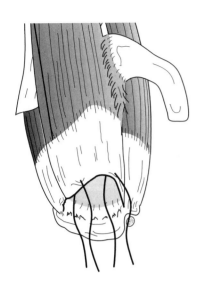

■ **Figure 15–99**
Release of the cuff tendons from the coracoid allows lateral advancement of them. *(Modified from Matsen FA III, Lippitt SB, Sidles JA, and Harryman DT II: Practical Evaluation and Management of the Shoulder. Philadelphia: WB Saunders, 1994.)*

Release From Coracoid

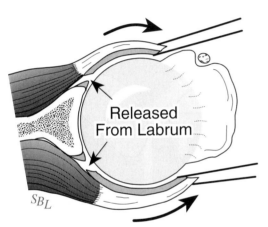

Released From Labrum

SBL

■ **Figure 15–100**
Release of the capsule from the labrum allows further lateral advancement. *(Modified from Matsen FA III, Lippitt SB, Sidles JA, and Harryman DT II: Practical Evaluation and Management of the Shoulder. Philadelphia: WB Saunders, 1994.)*

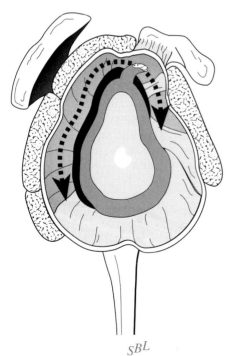

SBL

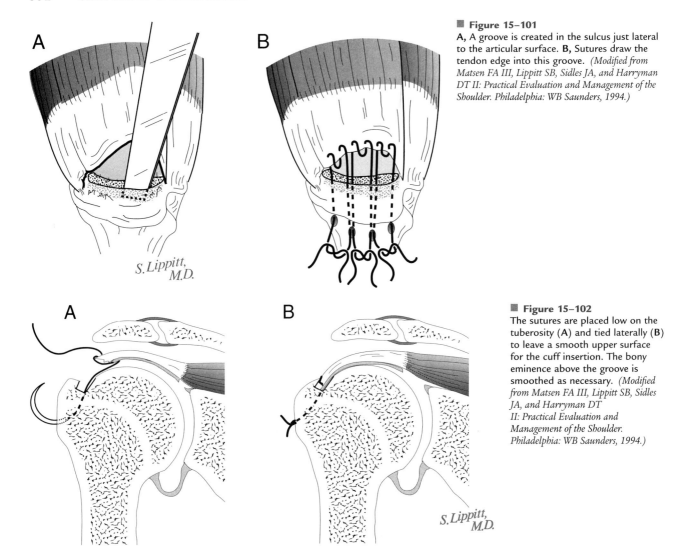

■ **Figure 15–101**
A, A groove is created in the sulcus just lateral to the articular surface. **B,** Sutures draw the tendon edge into this groove. *(Modified from Matsen FA III, Lippitt SB, Sidles JA, and Harryman DT II: Practical Evaluation and Management of the Shoulder. Philadelphia: WB Saunders, 1994.)*

■ **Figure 15–102**
The sutures are placed low on the tuberosity (**A**) and tied laterally (**B**) to leave a smooth upper surface for the cuff insertion. The bony eminence above the groove is smoothed as necessary. *(Modified from Matsen FA III, Lippitt SB, Sidles JA, and Harryman DT II: Practical Evaluation and Management of the Shoulder. Philadelphia: WB Saunders, 1994.)*

diagnosis of rotator cuff tears: supraspinatus weakness, external rotation weakness, and impingement signs. In patients with three of three positive tests or in patients with two of three and 60 years or older, 98% had a rotator cuff tear.[301] Palpation of rotator cuff tears had a 95.7% sensitivity and 96.8% specificity in the diagnosis of full-thickness rotator cuff tears; in contrast, MRI had a 90.9% sensitivity and 89.5% specificity.[488]

A full-thickness defect of one or more of the cuff tendons can be demonstrated by ultrasonography, arthrography, MRI, arthroscopy, or open surgery.

Although the diagnosis is not difficult, a number of key factors must be considered in selecting the appropriate management for cuff defects. Some defects cannot be repaired because as McLaughlin pointed out, they offer only "rotten cloth to sew."[273-275,277] The recognition that full-thickness cuff tears may exist without clinical symptoms[169,269,289,354,408] cautions that cuff defects need not be repaired just because they are there.

Nonoperative Treatment

Substantial data are available on the results of nonoperative treatment of full-thickness cuff defects. The programs generally include some combination of "compound tincture of time" along with physical therapy, administration of nonsteroidal anti-inflammatory medications, rest, avoidance of aggravating activities, and steroid injections.

The physiology of the rotator cuff muscles may not be significantly improved after repair. Delayed reattachment of a supraspinatus tear 12 weeks after detachment did not reverse the muscle atrophy in a rabbit model. Fat accumulation was actually worse in the reattached muscle than in muscle in which the tendons were detached and not repaired.[270]

Clinical improvement with nonoperative management was noted in 33% of Wolfgang's series,[489] 44% of Takagishi's series,[437] 59% of Samilson and Binder's series,[396] and 90% of Brown's series.[44] Goldberg and colleagues reported that 59% of patients had improved outcomes after at least 12 months of nonoperative management of a rotator cuff tear, as measured with the SF-36 and SST.[150] Nonoperative management consisted of four-quadrant stretching, as well as strengthening exercises of the rotator cuff, deltoid, and surrounding musculature.

Steroid injections do not seem to be a major enhancement to the nonoperative management program. Although Weiss[480] presented some evidence that patients with arthrographically proven cuff tears are symptomatically improved by intra-articular injections, there is little evidence for a protracted benefit from this method. Other observers have found that steroid injections offer no benefit to patients with cuff tears. Coomes and Darlington,[79,88] Lee and colleagues,[233] and Connolly[78] compared steroid and local anesthetic injections in patients with tendinitis and tendon tears. They found a small subjective benefit in relief of pain but no effect on function in the steroid-treated group. A comparison of sodium hyaluronate with steroid (dexamethasone) injection in patients with rotator cuff tears revealed no significant difference in patient satisfaction.[409] No control group was used for comparison.

A recent resurgence of reports have confirmed the value of nonoperative management for chronic cuff tears. Bartolozzi and coworkers[14] studied the factors predictive of outcome in 136 patients with cuff disease who were treated nonoperatively. The mean follow-up was 20 months (range, 6 to 41 months). The authors found 66% to 75% good or excellent results, along with an indication that the clinical result improved significantly as the follow-up duration increased. Prognostic factors associated with an unfavorable clinical outcome included a rotator cuff tear larger than 1 cm², a history of pretreatment clinical symptoms for over 1 year's duration, and significant functional impairment at initial evaluation.

Hawkins and Dunlop[174] found that over half the patients with full-thickness cuff tears treated with a supervised nonoperative program of rotator-strengthening exercises obtained satisfactory results at an average of 4 years' follow-up. Bokor and associates[34] managed 53 patients (average age, 62 years) with full-thickness cuff tears documented arthroscopically by using a program of nonsteroidal medications, stretching, strengthening, and occasional steroid injections. At an average of 7.6 years

later, 39 of the 53 patients (74%) had only slight or no shoulder discomfort. Of the 28 shoulders seen within 3 months of injury, 24 (86%) were rated as satisfactory at the time of latest evaluation. Of the 16 patients who initially had shoulder pain for over 6 months, only 9 (56%) were rated as satisfactory. Most patients showed improvement with regard to their ability to perform activities of daily living. The average active total elevation was 149 degrees versus 121 degrees at initial evaluation. Thirty-two of the 34 patients examined (94%) had evidence of weakness on muscle testing, and 19 (56%) had demonstrable muscle atrophy.

Itoi and Tabata[196] monitored 62 shoulders with complete rotator cuff tears that were treated conservatively from 1980 until 1989. The follow-up period averaged 3.4 years. Fifty-one shoulders (82%) were rated satisfactory. The overall scores of pain, motion, and function improved significantly. The authors concluded that conservative treatment affords satisfactory results when given to patients with well-preserved motion and strength, although in some cases function may deteriorate with time.

In our own practice we have follow-up data on 56 patients (23 women, 33 men) with full-thickness cuff tears managed nonoperatively. The average age was 61 ± 10 years (range, 45 to 84), and the mean follow-up was 25 months. The initial and final responses to the questions on the SST are shown in Table 15–2 and Figure 15–103.

Taken together, these results clearly offer encouragement for a trial of nonoperative management for chronic full-thickness cuff tears, particularly when the prospect of achieving a durable cuff repair appears doubtful, such as with atraumatic tears, large long-standing tears, tears associated with spinatus atrophy, tears that have been treated with repeated steroid injections, and tears in smokers or those who are debilitated.

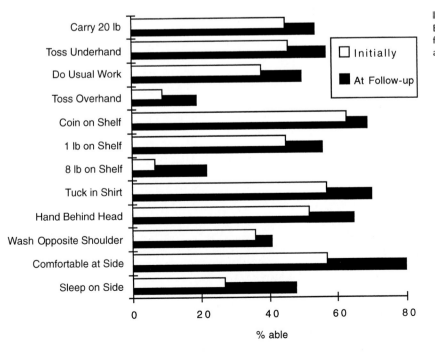

■ **Figure 15–103**
Effectiveness of nonoperative management of full-thickness cuff tears (56 patients with an average follow-up time of 25 months).

TABLE 15-2. Effectiveness of Nonoperative Management of Full-Thickness Cuff Tears (56 Patients with an Average Follow-up of 25 Months)

Function	% Able Initially	% Able at Follow-up
Sleep on side	27	48
Arm comfortable at side	57	80
Wash back of opposite shoulder	36	41
Place hand behind head	52	65
Tuck in shirt	57	70
Place 8 lb on shelf	7	22
Place 1 lb on shelf	45	56
Place coin on shelf	63	69
Toss overhand	9	19
Do usual work	38	50
Toss underhand	46	57
Carry 20 lb	45	54

Operative Treatment

Cuff Repair

Patient Selection

Substantial information bearing on the potential reparability of a rotator cuff defect can be obtained from the history along with the physical examination and plain radiographs (Table 15-3). Acute traumatic tears in younger, healthy individuals without previous shoulder disease are more likely to be reparable. Long-standing

TABLE 15-3. Prognostic Factors Related to the Durability of Rotator Cuff Repair

Encouraging	Discouraging
History	
Age younger than 55 yr	Age older than 65 yr
Acute traumatic onset	Insidious atraumatic onset
No relationship to work	Affrition of tear to work
Short duration of weakness	Weakness over 6 mo
No history of smoking	Many smoking pack-years
No steroid injections	Repeated steroid injections
No major medications	Systemic steroids or antimetabolites
No concurrent disease	Inflammatory joint disease; other chronic illnesses
No infections	History of previous shoulder infection
No previous shoulder surgery	Previous cuff repair attempts
Benign surgical history	History of failed soft tissue repairs (e.g., dehiscence, infections complicating herniorrhaphy)
Physical Examination	
Good nutrition	Poor nutrition
Mild to moderate weakness	Severe weakness
No spinatus atrophy	Severe spinatus atrophy
Stable shoulder	Anterior superior instability
Intact acromion	Previous acromial resection
No stiffness	Stiffness
Radiographs	
Normal radiographs	Upward displacement of head against the coracoacromial arch; cuff tear arthropathy

tears associated with major weakness in older patients carry a poorer prognosis. The prognosis for a durable repair is even worse if the history reveals the administration of local or systemic steroids, smoking, or difficulty in healing of previous injuries or surgeries.

These guidelines are derived from our experience, but they are also supported by the literature. In a study of 73 cuff repairs, Postacchini and colleagues[363] found that although 73% of cases had satisfactory results, rotator cuff repair is almost always successful in patients with more than 60 degrees of active arm flexion and either small or medium-sized tears. Less than two thirds of patients with major tears and less than 60 degrees of motion achieved satisfactory results, particularly if cuff muscle atrophy was present.

Watson[474] reviewed the surgical findings in 89 patients with major ruptures of the cuff. He found that all seven patients who had not received any local steroid injections had strong residual cuff tissue. Thirteen of 62 patients who received one to four steroid injections had soft cuff tissue that held suture poorly, and 17 of the 20 patients with more than four steroid injections had very weak cuff tissue; these shoulders with weak cuff tissue had poorer results after surgical repair.

Misamore and collaborators[291] evaluated 107 consecutive cuff repairs, including 24 patients receiving workers' compensation and 79 who were not. Although other factors such as the age and sex of the patients, the size of the tear of the rotator cuff, and preoperative strength, pain, and active range of motion of the shoulder were comparable, only 54% of the shoulders covered by workers' compensation were rated good or excellent versus 92% of those not covered. Forty-two percent of the patients receiving workers' compensation returned to full activity versus 94% of those not receiving it.

Samilson and Binder listed the following indications for operative repair of nonacute cuff tears[396]: (1) a patient "physiologically" younger than 60 years, (2) clinically or arthrographically demonstrable full-thickness cuff tears, (3) failure of the patient to improve with nonoperative management for a period not less than 6 weeks, (4) patient's need to use the involved shoulder in overhead elevation for vocation or avocation, (5) full passive range of shoulder motion, (6) patient's willingness to exchange decreased pain and increased external rotator strength for some loss of active abduction, and (7) ability and willingness of the patient to cooperate.

Grana and colleagues[156] reviewed their experience with 54 patients who underwent open repair of chronic cuff tears. They concluded that prerepair arthroscopic evaluation did not affect the functional outcome, but it did increase the cost by about $2000 per patient.

Laboratory Studies on Repair Techniques

Gerber and associates[144] studied the mechanical properties of several techniques of tendon-to-bone suture used in rotator cuff repair in cadavers. Two simple stitches failed at 184 N, four simple stitches failed at 208 N, and two Mason-Allen stitches failed at 359 N. These results indicate that in addition to the quality of the bone and the quality of the cuff tissue, the number of sutures and the suture technique affect the load to failure. The quality of the bone is an important factor; in cadaveric shoulders with rotator cuff tears, a significantly less amount of trabeculae was found in the greater tuberosity than in shoulders with intact rotator cuffs. The greater tuberosities of all the shoulders with rotator cuff tears also exhibited degenerative changes.[201]

A most important study bearing on the technique of cuff repair was published by Zuckerman and coauthors.[505] These authors used a cadaver model to determine the effect of arm position and capsular release on tension in the repaired tendon as reflected by strain gauges on the greater tuberosity. They found that with repair of supraspinatus-only defects, tension in the repair increased significantly as the arm was lowered from 30 to 15 degrees of abduction. Release of the capsule from the glenoid rim (see Figs. 15–99 and 15–100) significantly reduced tension at 15 and 0 degrees of abduction. For tears involving the supraspinatus and infraspinatus, abduction of at least 30 degrees was required to reduce tension in the repair. Release of the capsule from the glenoid (Fig. 15–100) resulted in a 30% reduction in repair tension when the arm was adducted. Hatakeyama and colleagues demonstrated that release of the superior capsule reduced strain in the repaired supraspinatus by 17.2%. Additional release of the coracohumeral ligament decreased the strain by 43.1%.[172] To reduce tension on the repair, some advocate medialization of the repair site. Liu showed that medialization of the supraspinatus insertion produced no significant decrease in lifting strength in cadaveric specimens with up to 10 mm of medialization.[253]

Warner and coworkers[471] studied the relationships of the suprascapular nerve to the cuff muscles in 31 cadaveric shoulders. The suprascapular nerve ran an oblique course across the supraspinatus fossa, was relatively fixed on the floor of the fossa, and was tethered underneath the transverse scapular ligament. Eighty-four percent of the shoulders had no more than two motor branches to the supraspinatus muscle, and the first was always the larger of the two. In 84%, the first motor branch originated underneath the transverse scapular ligament or very near it. In one shoulder (3%), the first motor branch passed over the ligament. The average distance from the origin of the long tendon of the biceps to the motor branches of the supraspinatus was 3 cm. In 48%, the infraspinatus muscle had three or four motor branches of the same size. The average distance from the posterior rim of the glenoid to the motor branches of the infraspinatus muscle was 2 cm. The motor branches to the supraspinatus muscle were fewer, usually smaller, and significantly shorter than those to the infraspinatus muscle. The standard anterosuperior approach allowed only 1 cm of lateral advancement of either tendon and limited the ability of the surgeon to safely dissect beyond the neurovascular pedicle. The advancement technique of Debeyre and colleagues,[89] or a modification of that technique, permitted lateral advancement of each muscle of as much as 3 cm and was limited by tension in the motor branches of the suprascapular nerve. In some situations, the safe limit of advancement may be even less. The authors concluded that lateral advancement of the rotator cuff is limited anatomically and may place the neurovascular structures at risk.

Surgical Approaches

Many different surgical approaches to a complete cuff tear have been used in the past, including a saber cut,[65] an anterior approach through the acromioclavicular joint,[17] a posterior approach,[89] and an "extensile" approach.[161] Many authors prefer the anterior acromioplasty approach, with care taken to preserve the deltoid attachment and acromial lever arm.[69,71,304,310] This technique provides excellent exposure of the common sites of lesions—the anterior cuff, biceps groove, undersurface of the acromion, and acromioclavicular joint.

Packer and coworkers,[339] reporting on 63 cuff repairs monitored for an average of 32.7 months, found that those performed with acromioplasty yielded more pain relief than cuff repair without acromioplasty did. If greater access to the supraspinatus is needed, the acromioclavicular joint can be excised.[306] Debeyre and associates[89] described a posterior approach with acromial osteotomy. Ha'eri and Wiley described an approach that is extensile through the acromioclavicular joint to the supraspinous fossa.[161] A study by Goldberg and colleagues demonstrated that repair of the rotator cuff without acromioplasty resulted in an average increase in the SST by 62%, from a score of 6 to 10.[149] This increase was similar to the result in another study that included acromioplasty with cuff repair; the average result was also 10 on the SST.[385] These studies suggest that acromioplasty may not be a necessary component of rotator cuff surgery.

Repair Methods

Operative techniques for repairing full-thickness cuff defects include tendon-to-tendon repair and tendon advancement to bone. McLaughlin[273-277] described his approach to transverse ruptures (reinsertion into bone), longitudinal rents (side-to-side repair), and tears with retraction (side-to-side repair followed by reinsertion of the retracted portion of cuff into the head wherever it will reach with ease with the arm at the side). Although many of his principles are still applied today, most authors would not concur with his use of the transacromial approach or his belief that "distinct benefits are gained by excising and discarding the outer fragment of the divided acromion."[273,275] Hawkins and colleagues used side-to-side repair for small tears and tendon-to-bone repair for larger defects.[178] A cadaveric study demonstrated that loss of abduction strength in shoulders with supraspinatus tears was almost completely regained with side-to-side repair.[164]

Cofield has emphasized identification of the tear pattern and the use of direct repair and flaps as indicated by the tear pattern.[70,71] Nobuhara and coworkers[322] reviewed, at an average of 7 years, 187 patients (189 shoulders) treated surgically for massive rotator cuff tears with either a tendon-to-tendon repair or the McLaughlin procedure. Ninety-five percent of the patients were 45 years or older. Excellent or good functional results were attained in 93% of patients. Thirty-three percent of those who underwent tendon-to-tendon repair complained of pain after overuse versus only 18% who had the McLaughlin procedure.

A number of authors have described extensive tendon mobilization or advancement of major tendon flaps to repair large defects. Cofield recommended transposition of the subscapularis for repair of large cuff defects.[70] In this technique, the subscapularis and the anterosuperior capsule are freed from the anteroinferior capsule, with the middle and inferior glenohumeral ligaments left intact. The tendon is then transferred superiorly to the anterior aspect of the greater tuberosity. Most patients required postoperative protection in an abduction splint or cast for 4 to 5 weeks. These patients, who had severe symptoms of pain and limitation of function preoperatively, had less pain and slight improvement in active motion; 12 of 26 patients gained more than 30 degrees of active abduction, and 4 lost this amount of motion. Two patients disrupted their repair during the acute postoperative period. Of the 26, 25 were satisfied with the procedure.

Karas and Giachello[211] recently reported their results in 20 patients treated by acromioplasty and subscapularis transfer for massive (>5 cm) tears of the cuff in which direct tendon-to-bone reconstruction could not be achieved. At a mean of 30 months after surgery, 17 patients were satisfied. Nine had weakness and discomfort with overhead activities, and two had lost active elevation despite relief of pain. The authors found this procedure useful when "traditional" methods of repair were insufficient, but cautioned against its use when patients had full functional elevation preoperatively.

In less than 5% of his cuff repairs, Neer[306] shifted the infraspinatus and upper half of the subscapularis superiorly to close a defect in the supraspinatus and left the lower half of the subscapularis, the teres minor, and the intervening capsule intact. He described the use of a second incision posteriorly for better mobilization of the infraspinatus toward the top of the greater tuberosity. Neviaser and Neviaser[316] described transposition of both the subscapularis and teres minor to close the defect. Debeyre and colleagues and others described the use of a supraspinatus muscle slide to help close major cuff defects.[89,161,162] Ha'eri and Wiley[162] used the supraspinatus advancement technique of Debeyre; most of their 18 patients achieved satisfactory results.

Latissimus transfers as described for Erb's palsy[355] have been used to manage large cuff defects. Gerber[143] reported on 16 irreparable massive rotator cuff tears treated with latissimus dorsi transfer and reviewed after an average of 33 months. Pain relief was satisfactory in 94% of the shoulders at rest and in 81% on exertion. Flexion was 83 degrees preoperatively and 135 degrees postoperatively. If the subscapularis was torn and could not be adequately repaired, latissimus dorsi transfer was of no value. In patients with good subscapularis function but irreparable defects in the external rotator tendons, restoration of approximately 80% of normal shoulder function was obtained.

A flap of deltoid has been used to cover cuff defects. Thur and Julke[443] analyzed the results of shoulder reconstruction involving an anterolateral deltoid muscle flap–plasty in 100 patients with rotator cuff lesions that were at least 5 × 5 cm in size. Ninety percent of patients were satisfied. Shoulder function improved significantly, and 72% recovered their strength completely. Most of the patients were able to work after 6 months. The overall result was good to very good in 83%.

Dierickx and Vanhoof[100] reviewed 20 patients with a painful, massive irreparable rotator cuff tear treated by open partial acromionectomy and an anterior deltoid muscle inlay flap. After follow-up averaging 12 months, 17 of 20 patients were satisfied, and the UCLA score improved from an average of 9.35 to an average of 25.7. Active forward flexion improved in 17 patients, and strength of forward flexion improved in 15.

As an alternative approach to surgery for massive tears, Burkhart and associates[51] repaired the margins of the tear to restore force transmission in the belief that complete coverage of the defect was not essential. In 14 patients this procedure led to improvement in active elevation from 59.6 to 150.4 degrees. Strength improved an average of 2.3 grades on a 0- to 5-point scale. The average score on the UCLA shoulder rating scale improved from a preoperative value of 9.8 to a postoperative value of 27.6. All but one patient was very satisfied with the result.

Some authors have used biologic and prosthetic grafts to repair large cuff defects. Neviaser,[313] Bush,[54] and McLaughlin and Asherman[277] used grafts from the long head of the biceps tendon to patch cuff defects. Ting and coworkers[446] found that electromyographic activity and the size of the long head of the biceps tendon are significantly greater in shoulders with cuff tears than in uninjured shoulders. Their study suggests that the long head of the biceps may be a greater contributor to abduction and flexion in a shoulder with a cuff tear than in a normal shoulder and that sacrificing the intracapsular portion of the tendon for grafting material may not be advisable. Heikel[182] used fascia lata to close cuff defects, and both Heikel and Bateman described the use of the coracoacromial ligament. Freeze-dried rotator cuff has been used by Neviaser and coworkers.[314] In this report, 16 patients with massive tears received cadaver grafts, and nocturnal pain decreased in all 16. The change in shoulder function and strength was not reported. Post[359] reported the preliminary results of five patients in whom a carbon fiber prosthesis was used to manage massive cuff deficiencies. Three had excellent to good results and two failed, one because of possible infection. The author states that these results are no better than with conventional repairs. Finally, synthetic cuff prostheses have been used by Ozaki and colleagues[335] and by Post.[359] The former found that of 168 shoulders with cuff tears (almost all of which were "chronic" and "massive"), 25 could not be repaired with standard surgical techniques. Their defects were typically 6 × 5 cm. These patients underwent cuff reconstruction with Teflon fabric, Teflon felt, or Marlex mesh. This procedure was followed by a structured postoperative program that included the use of an abduction orthosis to keep the arm elevated in the plane of the scapula for 2 to 3 months and continued rehabilitation for 3 to 6 months. At an average of 2.1 years' follow-up, 23 of 25 patients gained 120 to 160 degrees of abduction (the other 2 having had an axillary nerve injury). Whereas 20 had reported continual or intolerable pain preoperatively, pain was absent in 23 patients at follow-up. The authors found that results were better with the thicker felt and now recommend the use of 3- to 5-mm-thick Teflon felt in their patients with massive defects.

■ AUTHORS' TECHNIQUE FOR OPEN ROTATOR CUFF TEAR REPAIR WITH RESTORE ORTHOBIOLOGIC IMPLANT

More recently, the FDA recently cleared the use of a porcine small intestine submucosa (SIS) implant (DePuy Orthopaedics, Warsaw, IN) as a reabsorbable scaffold to promote the ingrowth of host tissues at the site of implantation. Introduced in 1999, the Restore Orthobiologic implant provides a new alternative to reinforce rotator cuff repairs. Dejardin, et al. used this material to tissue engineer rotator cuff defects in a canine model.[89a] Histological and mechanical evaluation established its efficacy in stimulating the regeneration of a rotator cuff tendon to replace a completely resected infraspinatus tendon in 21 adult dogs. (V15-1, V15-2)

Postoperative pain control may be improved with the use of brachial plexus blocks and continuous local infusion. Continuous intrabursal infusion of morphine and bupivacaine via a catheter after arthroscopic subacromial decompression resulted in significant pain relief at rest and less narcotic use in the first 3 postoperative days.[345] The use of narcotics was less during motion exercises in the experimental group than in the saline group, but this difference was not significant. No catheter infections occurred in this group of 60 patients. Infusion of bupivacaine for 48 hours after arthroscopic shoulder surgery resulted in significantly lower visual analog pain scores up to 8 days postoperatively.[13]

Some authors recommend postoperative immobilization in an abduction splint,[10,17,89 182] whereas others advise against such immobilization.[275, 321]

Results of Treatment

Neer and coworkers[309] reported the results of 233 primary cuff repairs with an average follow-up of 4.6 years. Results were excellent (essentially normal) in 77%, satisfactory in 14%, and unsatisfactory in 9%. The unsatisfactory ratings were usually due to lack of strength rather than pain and generally occurred in patients with long-standing, neglected tears. Hawkins and coworkers found that 86% of their patients had relief of pain after repair.[178] Recovery of strength was more common in patients with smaller tears.[178] In other series, pain relief was reported in 58%,[352] 60%,[182] 66%,[89] 74%,[148] and 85%.[396]

Gore and associates[153] reviewed the results of 63 primary cuff repairs with an average of 5.5 years' follow-up. Shoulders without a traumatic onset were repaired an average of 32 months after the onset of symptoms, whereas those with a traumatic onset were repaired an average of 6 months after the traumatic episode. The surgical approach and technique varied somewhat but usually consisted of acromioplasty and tendon repair to bone or to adjacent tendon. Six shoulders had biceps tendon grafts. Most shoulders were immobilized at the side for 4 to 6 weeks, but 12 had immobilization in abduction. Subjective improvement was seen in 95% of shoulders with repaired cuffs. Flexion averaged 126 degrees actively and 147 degrees passively. Most patients had marked relief of pain and minimal or no problems with activities of daily living. Patients with tears less than 2.5 cm long had better results than those with larger tears. The superior results with repair of smaller tears is consistent with the observations of Godsil and Linscheid[148] and Post and coworkers.[362] Watson[474] found that the results were worse in patients with larger cuff defects, multiple preoperative steroid injections, and preoperative weakness of the deltoid. Ellman and colleagues[111] reported a 3.5-year follow-up of 50 patients who underwent rotator cuff repair. Techniques of repair included tendon-to-tendon suture, reimplantation into bone, grafts, and tendon flaps. Comfort and function were usually improved by these procedures. Their report provides additional support for timely repair: patients with symptoms of longer duration had larger tears and more difficult repairs. Shoulders with grade 3 or less strength of abduction before surgery had poorer results; those with an acromiohumeral interval of 7 mm or less also had poorer results. Arthrography was not consistently accurate in estimating the size of the tear.

Hawkins found that acromioplasty and cuff repair relieved the patients' pain and restored the ability to sleep on the affected side in most patients. Seventy-eight percent were able to use the arm above shoulder level after surgery, whereas only 16% were able to do so before surgery. Hawkins and coworkers[178] found that the results of cuff repair were worse in patients receiving workers' compensation. Only 2 of 14 patients unable to work because of cuff tears could return to work after surgery, whereas 8 of 9 patients not receiving workers' compensation did return to work after surgery. Involvement of the infraspinatus in the rotator cuff tear, female sex, and workers' compensation claims were all found to have a significant correlation with lower shoulder function on the SST.[416]

Other series of cuff repairs include those of Codman,[66] Moseley,[295] Neviaser,[313] Wolfgang,[489] Bakalim and Pasila,[10] Bassett and Cofield,[16] Earnshaw and coworkers,[107] Packer and associates,[339] Post and colleagues,[362] Samilson and Binder,[396] and Weiner and Macnab.[478] Cofield[71] averaged the results of many reports in the literature and found that pain relief occurred in 87% (range, 71% to 100%) and patient satisfaction averaged 77% (range, 72% to 82%). The reader is encouraged to compare and contrast these results with those after nonoperative treatment, which was described earlier in this chapter.

Some reports focus on the results of acute repairs. Bakalim and Pasila reviewed their series of 55 patients with arthrographically verified rupture of the cuff tendons treated surgically.[10] Whereas only half the workers were able to return to their previous work, all workers operated on within 1 month of a traumatic rupture of the cuff were able to return to their jobs. Bassett and Cofield[16] presented a series of 37 patients who underwent surgical repair within 3 months of cuff rupture. At an average follow-up of 7 years, active abduction averaged 168 degrees for those undergoing repair within 3 weeks and 129 degrees for those undergoing repair within 6 to 12 weeks after injury. Patients with small tears averaged 148 degrees and those with large tears averaged 133 degrees of elevation. The authors concluded that surgical repair must be considered within 3 weeks of injury to achieve maximal return of shoulder function.

V15-1
V15-2

TABLE 15-4.   Recovery of Torque after Cuff Repair

	Flexion	Abduction	External Rotation
Preoperative	54	45	64
6 mo	78	80	79
12 mo	84	90	91

From Rokito AS, Zuckerman JD, Gallagher MA, and Cuomo F: Strength after surgical repair of the rotator cuff. J Shoulder Elbow Surg 5:12-17, 1996.

The importance of continued postoperative exercises is emphasized by the data of Walker and associates,[466] who measured the isokinetic strength of the shoulder after cuff repair. They found a significant increase in strength between 6 and 12 months after surgery. One year after surgery, abduction was 80% of normal and external rotation was 90% of normal. Brems[39] found that the strength of external rotation after cuff repair averaged 20% at 3 months, 38% at 6 months, 57% at 9 months, and 71% at 1 year.

Rokito and colleagues[384] monitored the isokinetic strength of 42 patients at 3-month intervals after repair of full-thickness defects. The torques for the operated shoulder (as a percentage of the opposite uninvolved shoulder) are shown in Table 15-4. Recovery of strength correlated primarily with the size of the tear: for small and medium-sized tears, recovery of strength was almost complete during the first year; for large and massive tears, recovery was slower and less consistent. The authors concluded that at least a year is required to regain strength after cuff repair.

Kirschenbaum and colleagues[223] came up with very similar results in their evaluation of 25 shoulders tested isokinetically with a pain-relieving subacromial lidocaine injection before and after cuff repair (Table 15-5).

Analysis of the results of cuff repair is hampered by the lack of a uniform approach to the description of (1) patient selection, (2) the shoulder's preoperative functional status, (3) the magnitude and location of the cuff defect, (4) the quality of tissue available for repair, (5) the technique of repair, (6) postoperative management, (7) anatomic integrity at follow-up, and (8) postoperative functional status. The need for correlation of anatomic and functional outcomes is demonstrated by the surprisingly good results obtained with débridement for irreparable cuff tears. Neer,[304] Rockwood,[380] and others have reported that in certain cases when the cuff cannot be repaired, comfort and function may be improved by débridement of the shreds of residual cuff and subacromial smoothing, followed by muscle-strengthening and range-of-motion exercises. The realization that patients may have good function and comfort in the presence of

major cuff defects makes the definition of "success" after a cuff repair challenging. Like studies of other conditions, rotator cuff studies are affected by sample bias, particularly in patients lost to follow-up. Patients with rotator cuff tears who were lost to follow-up were less likely to have had surgery for the rotator cuff, had lower social and mental health scores on the SF-36, and were less likely to consume alcohol.[323] Patients also gave higher SST scores on a telephone interview than at the time of last follow-up. This result points to the importance of a consistent methodology for investigation of the clinical outcomes of treatment of cuff lesions.

Interestingly, few follow-up studies have investigated the relationship of cuff integrity to the quality of the result after cuff surgery. MRI of asymptomatic patients at least 2 years after rotator cuff repair showed a 20% to 21% retear rate, with an average tear size of 8 mm. All the patients in one study had evidence of bursitis on MRI.[425,503] Patients with retears still had significantly higher Constant scores and pain relief than they did preoperatively.[207] The patients were monitored prospectively, and all were imaged regardless of symptomatology. Eighty percent of retears were smaller than the original tears, and smaller tears correlated with better outcomes. Lundberg[258] monitored 21 cuff repairs with arthrography and found leakage in seven. The results in patients with leaking cuffs were not as good as in those with sealed cuffs. Calvert and associates[55] performed double-contrast arthrography in 20 patients at an average of 30 months after operative repair of a torn cuff. In 17 of 20 shoulders, contrast leaked into the bursa, indicative of a cuff defect. These defects were estimated to be small in eight, medium in eight, and large in two. However, 17 patients had complete relief of pain, 15 had a full range of shoulder elevation, and 10 believed that they had regained full function. The authors suggest that complete closure of the cuff is not essential for a good functional result and that arthrography may not be helpful in the investigation of failure of repair.

Ultrasonography appears to offer greater potential for evaluating postoperative cuff integrity. Mack and coworkers[263] investigated the accuracy of ultrasonography in this regard. In a group of symptomatic postoperative shoulders that were subsequently operated on again, ultrasonography accurately diagnosed recurrent cuff tears in 25 of 25 cases and correctly confirmed cuff integrity in 10 of 11.

Using expert ultrasonography, Harryman and associates[169] correlated the integrity of the cuff with functional status after 105 surgical repairs of chronic rotator cuff tears in 89 patients at an average of 5 years postoperatively. The patients' ages at the time of repair averaged 60 years (range, 32 to 80). The numbers of patients in each age decade were as follows: 30 to 39—1, 40 to 49—16, 50 to 59—31, 60 to 69—42, 70 to 79—14, and 80 to 89—1. Eighty-six (82%) of the shoulders had no previous attempt at repair of the cuff. In all the surgeries, an anterior-inferior acromioplasty was carried out. The involved tendon or tendons were mobilized as necessary. A bony trough was created in the humerus to reattach the mobilized tendons. The site of reattachment was usually in the sulcus adjacent to the humeral articular surface. In some cases, the

TABLE 15-5.   Recovery of Torque after Cuff Repair

	Flexion	Abduction	External Rotation
Preoperative	33	37	36
6 mo	66	68	76
12 mo	97	104	142

From Kirschenbaum D, Coyle MPJ, Leddy JP, et al: Shoulder strength with rotator cuff tears. Pre- and postoperative analysis. Clin Orthop 288:174-178, 1993.

TABLE 15-6.   Integrity of Cuff Repairs at Follow-up

Size of Defect Repaired at Surgery (All Cases)	Primary Repairs (86)	Repeat Repairs (19)	Total No. of Repairs (105)	Size of Cuff Defect at Follow-up Examination					% Intact (0 or 1A) (65)	Years of Follow-up Average (Range): 5 (2-11)
				None (0) (40)	Partial (1A) (28)	Supraspinatus Tear (1B) (12)	Supraspinatus and Infraspinatus Tear (2) (14)	Supraspinatus, Infraspinatus, and Subscapularis Tear (3) (11)		
Partial tears (1A)	5	1	6	4	2	0	0	0	100	2.7 (2-6)
Supraspinatus tears (1B)	39	10	49	23	16	3	5	2	80	5.1 (2-10.5)
Supraspinatus and infraspinatus (2)	25	3	28	7	9	6	5	1	57	5.9 (2-6)
Supraspinatus, infraspinatus, and subscapularis (3)	17	5	22	6	1	3	4	8	32	4.1 (2-11)
Intact at follow-up	60	8	68							

From Matsen FA III, Lippitt SB, Sidles JA, and Harryman DT II: Practical Evaluation and Management of the Shoulder. Philadelphia: WB Saunders, 1994.

TABEL 15-7.   Influence of Size of Cuff Defect at Follow-up on Active Range, Comfort, and Satisfaction at Follow-up

Size of Cuff Defect at Follow-up	Number	Active Range of Motion at Follow-up				Total Painless	Total Satisfied
		Flexion	External Rotation at Side	External Rotation at 90° Abduction	Internal Rotation		
None (0)	40	132°	41°	71°	T7	37	39
Partial (1A)	28	124°	38°	68°	T7	21	23
Supraspinatus (1B)	12	107°	34°	63°	T8	8	12
Supraspinatus and infraspinatus (2)	14	109°	25°	48°	T9	10	10
Supraspinatus, infraspinatus, and subscapularis (3)	11	71°	27°	61°	T10	8	10
Total	105					84	94

From Matsen FA III, Lippitt SB, Sidles JA, and Harryman DT II: Practical Evaluation and Management of the Shoulder. Philadelphia: WB Saunders, 1994.

trough was placed somewhat more medially if after mobilization the tendons did not reach their original anatomic attachment without undue tension when the arm was at the side. The cuff was protected from active use for 3 months postoperatively. The status of the cuff at surgery and at follow-up was characterized in terms of the integrity of the different tendons: type 0 was a cuff of normally full thickness, type 1A was thinning or a partial-thickness defect of the supraspinatus tendon, type 1B was a full-thickness defect of the supraspinatus, type 2 was a full-thickness two-tendon defect involving the supraspinatus and the infraspinatus, and type 3 was a full-thickness defect involving three tendons: the supraspinatus, infraspinatus, and subscapularis. The results are summarized in Table 15-6. No patient who had a partial-thickness tear repaired had a full-thickness retear. In 80% of shoulders with repaired full-thickness supraspinatus tears, the cuff was found to be intact (no full-thickness defect) at follow-up. Only 57% of cuffs that had tears involving both the supraspinatus and infraspinatus were intact at an average follow-up of 6 years. Less than a third of the cuffs that had tears involving all three major tendons were intact after repair at an average of 4 years of follow-up. Patients were generally satisfied with the results of surgery, even when expert sonography showed that the cuff was no longer intact (see Table 15-7). Shoulders with intact repairs (no full-thickness defect) at follow-up had greater range of active flexion (129 ± 20

degrees) than did those with large recurrent defects (71 ± 41 degrees) (Fig. 15-104). Shoulders with intact repairs also demonstrated the best function in activities of daily living. When the cuff was not intact, the degree of functional loss was related to the size of the recurrent defect (Fig. 15-105). Although the chance of having an intact repair at follow-up was less for those with large tears, patients with intact repairs of large tears had just as good function as those with intact repairs of small tears. Similarly, shoulders with repeat repairs had an overall greater incidence of recurrent defects, yet shoulders with intact cuffs after repeat repairs functioned as well as those with intact primary repairs (Fig. 15-106). From this study it can be concluded that (1) the integrity of the rotator cuff at follow-up (and not the size of the tear at the time of repair) is a major determinant of the functional outcome of surgical repair, (2) the chance of a repair of a large tear remaining intact is not as good as that for a small tear, and (3) older patients tended to have larger tears and a higher incidence of recurrent defects (see Table 15-8).

In a very comparable study, Gazielly and colleagues[139-141] examined the anatomic condition by ultrasonography and the function of the rotator cuff 4 years after surgical repair in a series of 100 full-thickness rotator cuff tears. The series comprised 98 patients (62 men and 36 women) with an average age of 56 years. Sixty-nine tears of the supraspinatus were less than 2 cm in size

(39 cases) or between 2 and 4 cm (3 cases), 22 tears of the supraspinatus and infraspinatus measured between 2 and 4 cm, and 9 were massive tears. All 98 patients were operated on by the same surgeon using the same repair technique. Ultrasonography revealed intact cuffs in 65%, thinned cuffs in 11%, and recurrent full-thickness tears in

24% of cases. The risk for a recurrent tear increased with the extent of the tear to be repaired (57%), in older patients (25%), and with a higher level of postsurgical occupational use (18%). At follow-up, they noted a close correlation between the anatomic condition of the cuff by ultrasound and the Constant functional score.

Similar results have been reported by Cammerer and colleagues[56] and Bellumore and associates.[22]

Wulker and coworkers[494] monitored 97 of 116 shoulders operated on for rotator cuff lesions for an average follow-up period of 37 months. Seventy percent had a

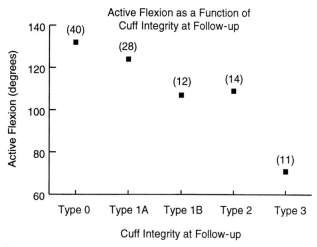

Figure 15–104
Active flexion after cuff repair as a function of cuff integrity at follow-up. The numbers of shoulders are in parentheses. Type 0 represents a cuff of normally full thickness; type 1A is thinning or partial-thickness lesions of the cuff; type 1B is a full-thickness cuff defect of the supraspinatus; type 2 is a full-thickness defect of the supraspinatus and infraspinatus; and type 3 is a full-thickness defect of the subscapularis, supraspinatus, and infraspinatus. *(From Matsen FA III, Lippitt SB, Sidles JA, and Harryman DT II: Practical Evaluation and Management of the Shoulder. Philadelphia: WB Saunders, 1994.)*

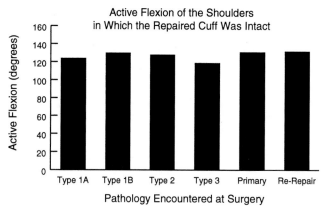

Figure 15–106
Active flexion of the shoulders in which the repaired cuff remained intact (no full-thickness recurrent defect) was independent of the pathologic conditions encountered at surgery. *(From Matsen FA III, Lippitt SB, Sidles JA, and Harryman DT II: Practical Evaluation and Management of the Shoulder. Philadelphia: WB Saunders, 1994.)*

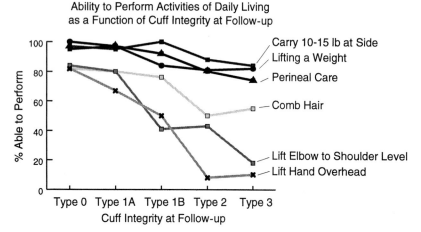

Figure 15–105
The ability to perform activities of daily living as a function of cuff integrity at follow-up. The ordinate indicates the percentage of shoulders that were functional enough for the patient to perform the activity. *(From Matsen FA III, Lippitt SB, Sidles JA, and Harryman DT II: Practical Evaluation and Management of the Shoulder. Philadelphia: WB Saunders, 1994.)*

TABLE 15–8. Influence of Size of Cuff Tear Repaired at Surgery on Active Range of Motion at Follow-up

Size of Defect Repaired at Surgery	Number	Age at Repair (Mean ± SD)	Active Range of Motion at Follow-up			
			Flexion	*External Rotation at Side*	*External Rotation at 90° Abduction*	*Internal Rotation*
Partial (1A)	6	49 ± 13	126°	38°	68°	T8
Supraspinatus (1B)	49	57 ± 8	129°	40°	70°	T7
Supraspinatus and infraspinatus (2)	28	64 ± 8	119°	28°	60°	T8
Supraspinatus, infraspinatus, and subscapularis (3)	22	64 ± 8	92°	33°	60°	T10

From Matsen FA III, Lippitt SB, Sidles JA, and Harryman DT II: Practical Evaluation and Management of the Shoulder. Philadelphia: WB Saunders, 1994.

good or excellent clinical result; however, ultrasonographic examination revealed that only 37 had a normal rotator cuff, 31 had thinning and/or hyperdensity, and 29 had a complete rupture of the cuff. The authors concluded that rotator cuff tears should be closed only if closure can be achieved without undue tension and without extensive tissue mobilization or coverage; otherwise, they recommended that the lesion be débrided and left open and only anterior acromioplasty be performed.

Taken together, these studies provide strong evidence that after cuff repair surgery, a high percentage of patients have a satisfactory clinical result in spite of recurrence of the cuff defect. Several conclusions are evident: (1) one cannot infer integrity of the repaired cuff from a "good" or "excellent" clinical result, (2) factors other than cuff integrity must contribute to the quality of the clinical result after rotator cuff surgery, and (3) if we are to learn more about the value of cuff repair, analysis of cuff integrity and change in functional status must become essential elements in outcome studies of cuff repair surgery.

Arthroscopically Assisted Repair

Some authors have reported short-term follow-up of arthroscopically assisted rotator cuff repair.[243,341] These authors suggest that required components of the repair include adequate smoothing of the undersurface of the acromion and the acromioclavicular joint; arthroscopic (or open) resection of the distal end of the clavicle in the presence of significant acromioclavicular joint arthrosis; mobilization of the entire rotator cuff with release of adhesions and scar tissue; and repair of strong tendon to a properly placed, well-prepared, bleeding bone trough.

The rotator cuff repair is often performed through a lateral deltoid muscle–splitting incision. The deltoid is not detached from the acromion. The deltoid muscle is split by blunt dissection with careful attention paid to the axillary nerve, which crosses on the deep surface of the deltoid as close as 5 cm to the lateral edge of the acromion. A bony trough is developed in the greater tuberosity. Reapposition of the torn cuff edge to the greater tuberosity is accomplished with nonabsorbable sutures passed through drill holes and tied over bone.

Alternative methods for arthroscopically assisted cuff repair include the percutaneous insertion of absorbable tacks and metallic staples. The use of fixation implants of this type carries the potential for loss of fixation, particularly in patients with soft cancellous bone. Loss of fixation can result in failure of tendon repair, as well as mechanical irritation caused by displacement of these devices in the subacromial space.

Palette and coauthors reported success in the arthroscopic management of small tears.[341] Levy and colleagues[243] in 1990 reported on 25 patients with full-thickness rotator cuff tears treated with an arthroscopically assisted rotator cuff repair. After performing an arthroscopic acromioplasty, the rotator cuff was identified, débrided, mobilized with arthroscopically placed sutures, and then repaired to a bony trough through a

limited deltoid-splitting approach. The patients, who had average age of 57.7 years (range, 21 to 74 years), were evaluated at an average of 18 months (range, 12 to 27 months). Based on the UCLA shoulder rating scale, 80% were rated as excellent or good, with reported significant improvements in pain, function, motion, and strength. Ninety-six percent of the patients were satisfied with their result. Of the 15 large tears (3 to 5 cm), 4 results were excellent, 6 were good (67% satisfactory), 4 were fair, and 1 was poor (33% unsatisfactory). Of the patients with small (<1 cm) or moderate (1 to 3 cm) tears, 100% received a satisfactory rating.

Warren and colleagues[472] reported good or excellent results in 13 of their 17 patients who underwent arthroscopic acromioplasty and arthroscopically assisted rotator cuff repair with a minimum of 2 years' follow-up (average, 25 months). Tear size was small in four, moderate in five, large in six, and massive in two. The rotator cuff was repaired into a prepared bony trough with arthroscopically placed sutures through a limited deltoid-splitting incision and, in some cases, percutaneous fixation with a cannulated tack. Eight of nine tennis players and all the golfers returned to their previous sports.

Paulos and Kody,[348] in 1994, reported their results of 18 consecutive patients who underwent arthroscopic acromioplasty and rotator cuff repair through a 4-cm deltoid-splitting approach with an average follow-up of 46 months (range, 36 to 72 months) and a mean age of 47.2 years (range, 26 to 74 years). Sixteen repairs were tendon to bone; 2 repairs were tendon to tendon. Sixteen patients (88%) scored good to excellent on the UCLA shoulder rating scale with significant improvement in pain and function scores. Two patients had poor results; both had workers' compensation cases pending. One patient with a poor result had two complications: superficial infection and failure of repair that required reoperation. Seventeen of the eighteen patients (94%) were satisfied with their result.

In 1994, Liu[254] reported on 44 patients (average age, 58 years; range, 35 to 76) with full-thickness rotator cuff tears at an average of 4.2 years (range, 2.5 to 6.1 years) after arthroscopically assisted rotator cuff repair. Eighty-five percent of the patients were discharged from the hospital immediately after the operation. The results were rated as good or satisfactory in 84% (37/44; 8/8 in those with small tears [less than 1 cm], 15/17 with moderate tears [1 to 3 cm], 12/15 with large tears [3 to 5 cm], and 2/5 with massive tears [>5 cm]). Eighty-eight percent of the patients were satisfied with the result, and 64% of the athletes returned to their previous sport. The size of the tear seemed to be a determining factor in the functional outcome: small and moderate tears did better than large and massive tears. Patient satisfaction, however, did not seem to relate to the size of the tear repair; those with small, moderate, and large tears were equally satisfied.

In 1995, Baker and Liu[11] compared the results of open and arthroscopically assisted rotator cuff repair in 36 patients with a minimal follow-up of 2 years. The open repair group (average age, 60 years) consisted of 20 shoulders with an average follow-up of 3.3 years; the arthroscopically assisted repair group (average age, 59 years) consisted of 17 shoulders with an average follow-up of 3.2

years. Overall, the open repair group had 88% good to excellent results and 88% patient satisfaction; the arthroscopically assisted repair group had 85% good to excellent results and 92% patient satisfaction (based on the UCLA rating scale). The functional outcome with regard to shoulder flexion, strength of abduction, and size of the rotator cuff tear repaired did not differ significantly between the two treatment groups. In general, however, small and moderate-sized tears (<3 cm) demonstrated earlier return to full function after arthroscopically assisted rotator cuff repair; this group was hospitalized 1.2 days less and returned to previous activities an average of 1 month earlier. In the patients with large tears, two of four patients (50%) in the arthroscopically assisted repair group and four of five (80%) in the open repair group had good to excellent results. In general, the authors found arthroscopically assisted rotator cuff repair to be as effective as open repair in the treatment of small and moderated-sized tears (<3 cm), whereas large tears did better after open repair.

These studies suggest that arthroscopic acromioplasty combined with arthroscopically assisted rotator cuff repair can provide acceptable clinical results with minimal tissue retraction and scarring in the management of small full-thickness rotator cuff tears in patients with excellent-quality tissue. These results, however, are not directly comparable to the results of traditional open surgery because studies involving open techniques include larger numbers of older patients, many of whom have large chronic tears requiring extensive soft tissue mobilization. The long-term clinical results and the integrity of the cuff after these arthroscopically assisted repairs have yet to be determined.

Open Operative Treatment When Repair Is Not Possible

Although it used to be said by some that "the term 'irreparable cuff' reflects more on the surgeon than the patient," the fact is that some rotator cuff tears may be impossible to repair. Rockwood and colleagues[380, 382] reported on their experience using a modified Neer acromioplasty and débridement of massive irreparable lesions involving the supraspinatus and infraspinatus tendons in 53 shoulders (average age, 60). At an average of 6.5 years' follow-up, comfort, function, and satisfaction were acceptable in 83%. Good prognostic findings were an intact biceps, an intact anterior deltoid, and no previous shoulder surgery. Active forward flexion improved from 105 to 140 degrees. These results indicate that subacromial smoothness and vigorous postsurgical rehabilitation can substantially improve comfort and function, even when large cuff defects are irreparable.

In a small series, Hawkins and coauthors[178] reported only 50% satisfactory results with open subacromial decompression alone in patients with massive full-thickness rotator cuff tears.

Bakalim and Pasila[10] found that acromial excision alone gave relief of night pain in certain cases.

Arthroscopic Operative Treatment When Repair Is Not Possible

Several authors have reported acceptable clinical results with full-thickness cuff defects when arthroscopic acromioplasty and débridement were performed without

rotator cuff repair, especially for sedentary, low-demand patients whose main complaint is pain.[110,115,137,179,423,460]

In one of the earliest studies, Wiley,[483] in 1985, reported on 20 patients with full-thickness rotator cuff tears who underwent arthroscopic rotator cuff débridement and shoulder manipulation without acromioplasty. Within 24 months, 16 patients had pain relief (5 complete, 11 partial), 12 had increased range of motion, and 11 were able to return to work. He concluded that arthroscopic treatment was useful in treating older patients with chronic shoulder pain associated with full-thickness rotator cuff tears.

Ellman,[109] in 1987, presented 10 patients with full-thickness tears of the rotator cuff treated with arthroscopic acromioplasty and rotator cuff débridement. Based on the UCLA shoulder rating scale, 80% were rated satisfactory (eight good) and 20% unsatisfactory (two poor). It was noted that none of the eight satisfactory results achieved an excellent objective rating.

Esch and colleagues,[115] in 1988, presented their results according to the degree of rotator cuff tendon failure. Their patients with complete tears were divided into groups with tears less than 1 cm in size, tears larger than 1 cm in size, and massive tears. The patients were treated by arthroscopic acromioplasty, coracoacromial ligament resection, and débridement of acromioclavicular spurs. All patients were monitored for a minimum of 1 year. Four patients with tears less than 1 cm in size had a satisfactory result and an excellent rating. Of the 16 patients with tears larger than 1 cm in size, 14 were satisfied, and 13 had good or excellent objective results (based on the UCLA shoulder rating scale). There were three fair objective ratings and no poor ratings. Of the six patients with massive tears, five were satisfied but only three had a satisfactory score. Thus, patients with complete rotator cuff tears had an overall patient satisfaction rate of 88% and an objective satisfaction rating of 77%. Esch and coworkers subsequently concluded that results are related to tear size. Patients with small full-thickness tears may achieve excellent results with arthroscopic acromioplasty and cuff débridement. Of the patients with large tears, only 4 of the 13 obtained an excellent objective result.

Gartsman,[137] as part of a larger series, reported on 25 patients with full-thickness rotator cuff tears treated with arthroscopic acromioplasty, resection of the coracoacromial ligament and subacromial bursa, removal of osteophytes, and minimal débridement of the rotator cuff defect. The tears were divided into four groups based on size of the tear: small tears less than 1 cm (3 total), tears between 1 and 3 cm (13 total), tears between 3 and 5 cm (6 total), and 3 massive tears larger than 5 cm. At an average of 31 months, 14 satisfactory and 11 unsatisfactory results were achieved. Seven of these patients were subsequently treated with open rotator cuff repair, six of whom had a satisfactory result. Notably, no correlation could be found between the final result and the patient's age, sex, hand dominance, or location of the tear. Only rotator cuff tear size correlated with outcome—13 of 16 patients with a tear less than 3 cm had a satisfactory result, whereas only 1 of 9 patients with a larger tear (over 3 cm) did well.

Montgomery and coauthors[292] reported on 87 patients with 89 full-thickness rotator cuff tears who failed to respond to conservative treatment. Fifty patients (group I) were treated by open rotator cuff repair and Neer acromioplasty. Thirty-eight patients (group II) were managed by arthroscopic débridement, acromioplasty, and abrasion of the greater tuberosity. With similar-size rotator cuff tears represented in each group at a 1-year follow-up, the authors found no statistically significant difference between the two groups. However, on re-evaluation 2 years after surgery, the open surgical repair group (I) was statistically much better than the arthroscopic débridement group (II) with regard to pain and function. In 4 of the 38 patients in the arthroscopic débridement group, rotator cuff tear arthropathy developed and was thought to have occurred secondary to the instability and abnormal movement of the humeral head on the glenoid.

In 1991, Levy and coworkers[242] reported on 25 patients with full-thickness tears of the rotator cuff treated by arthroscopic acromioplasty and rotator cuff tendon débridement alone. Significant improvement in pain, function, motion, and strength was achieved. Eighty-four percent of the cases were rated as excellent or good (and 88% of the patients were satisfied with the procedure). Although all tear sizes were improved significantly, small tears fared better than larger tears.

In a follow-up series,[506] Zvijac and associates re-evaluated all 25 patients from the original study group with full-thickness rotator cuff tears who underwent arthroscopic acromioplasty. At a mean follow-up of 45.8 months, 68% of the patients were rated as excellent or good, a significant decrease from the initial report of 84% satisfactory results at a mean follow-up of 24.6 months. The authors found a significant decrease in rating with regard to pain and function. Ratings for motion and strength did not change significantly with time. Large and massive rotator cuff tears fared worse over time than small and moderate-size tears did. These findings led the authors to abandon support for the use of arthroscopic acromioplasty and rotator cuff débridement alone in the treatment of reparable full-thickness rotator cuff tears.

In 1993, Ellman and colleagues[114] reported their follow-up results of 40 full-thickness rotator cuff tears treated by arthroscopic acromioplasty and débridement in a selected group of patients. The patients were divided into three groups based on the size of their tear. Small (0 to 2 cm) tears (*n* = 10) in older patients not involved in strenuous activities were rated satisfactory in 90% of cases. Patients with larger (2 to 4 cm) reparable tears (*n* = 8) did poorly (50% satisfactory results). Arthroscopic treatment in patients with massive irreparable tears (*n* = 22) did not improve range of motion or restore strength, but it did result in significant pain relief, and 86% were satisfied with the results on a "limited-goals basis." Ellman and coauthors concluded that for patients with medium-sized tears, pain relief from arthroscopic acromioplasty alone is inadequate and the "procedure probably should not be offered." In carefully selected patients described as "relatively older and very sedentary" with small rotator cuff tears (0 to 2 cm), however, arthroscopic acromioplasty can have a useful role. Ellman emphasized that even for these patients, and certainly for the majority of patients, reparable rotator cuff tears are best treated by open surgical repair.

In a series of 80 consecutive arthroscopic acromioplasties in 76 patients with stage II and III impingement syndrome, Paulos and Franklin[346] identified 7 patients with full-thickness rotator cuff tears. Three of these patients, all with small (1 cm) tears, remained symptomatic and required a reoperation for open repair of the rotator cuff tear.

In 1993, Ogilvie-Harris and Demaziere,[327] in a prospective cohort study, compared the results of arthroscopic acromioplasty plus rotator cuff débridement (22 patients) and open repair plus acromioplasty (23 patients) as treatment of tears of the rotator cuff 1 to 4 cm in size. Follow-up varied from 2 to 5 years. The two treatment groups showed no significant differences in age, size of the tear, preoperative pain, function, range of active forward flexion, and strength of forward flexion. At follow-up, both groups had similar pain relief and range of active forward flexion. The open repair group scored significantly better in function, strength, and overall status; however, patient satisfaction was similar in both groups. These authors found no significant difference in the final result with regard to the age of the patient or the size of the rotator cuff tear. On the basis of their results, the authors consider the use of arthroscopic acromioplasty and débridement in patients with demands whose main complaints are pain and loss of range of movement. For patients who need good function and strength, however, arthroscopic débridement plus acromioplasty is not sufficient, and open repair plus acromioplasty is advised.

Olsewski and Depew[332] in 1994 reported on their results of arthroscopic acromioplasty and rotator cuff débridement performed on 61 consecutive patients with a minimum of 2 years of follow-up (mean, 27.7 months). In this study, 13 full-thickness rotator cuff tears were identified. Of the 13 full-thickness tears treated, 10 were rated satisfactory (77%) and 3 unsatisfactory (23%). Of the 10 satisfactory results, 8 were in patients who were either retired or worked at sedentary jobs that did not demand above-shoulder activities and strength and whose principal preoperative complaint was pain. All 10 of these patients had relief of their pain. The three unsatisfactory results were all in active patients with demands on strength and overhead activity.

Burkhart[49] described 10 patients with massive (irreparable/>5 cm) complete rotator cuff tears primarily involving the supraspinatus treated by arthroscopic acromioplasty with débridement of redundant nonfunctional rotator cuff tissue. All patients except one had normal active motion and strength preoperatively and all had a roentgenographically normal acromiohumeral distance and an anterior-inferior acromial osteophyte. The procedure was offered to a subset of older patients with activity-limiting pain who were preoperatively found to have a full range of active shoulder motion and normal strength of external rotation. Arthroscopic débridement plus decompression was accompanied by pain relief without loss of motion or strength in all 10 patients. The follow-up period ranged from 8 to 33 months (mean, 17.6 months). Patients ranged from 53 to 77 years in age (average, 65 years). Seven excellent and three good results were reported. All patients were satisfied with their result.

Cost-Effectiveness of Treatment of Full-Thickness Cuff Tears

Rotator cuff disease is one of the most common afflictions of the shoulder. Many health care dollars are spent on its evaluation and management. It is apparent that a large number of variables have a bearing on the effectiveness of treatment of cuff lesions. The cost of various treatment methods varies substantially as well. To initiate a practical investigative method by which the cost-effectiveness might be compared among treatment methods, the authors conducted a preliminary study of 67 unmatched patients evaluated for treatment of documented, symptomatic full-thickness tears. Based on our clinical assessment and the desires of the patient, one of three treatment methods was selected for each patient: nonoperative management, subacromial smoothing without repair, and surgical repair. The number of patients, average age, gender, and length of follow-up for the patients in each of the three groups are given in Table 15–9.

All patients completed SST and SF-36 questionnaires preoperatively and at follow-up. The effectiveness of treatment was measured in terms of the postoperative-preoperative change in the number of "yes" responses on the SST and the postoperative-preoperative change in the SF-36 comfort score. This analysis indicated that the greatest improvement was found in the group undergoing surgical repair (see the solid bars in Figures 15–107 and 15–108). The changes in the SST and SF-36 comfort score results for each patient were then divided by the

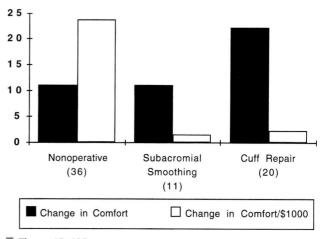

■ Figure 15–108
Median change in the SF-36 comfort score.

total hospital, office, and physician charges for the treatment to yield the average change per $1000 charge. In this analysis, nonoperative treatment was associated with the greatest change per unit charge (see the hollow bars in Figures 15–107 and 15–108).

Although no conclusions should be drawn from these preliminary results, it is hoped that further studies of this type will help determine the cost-effectiveness of different treatment methods.

■ AUTHORS' PREFERRED METHOD FOR SURGICAL TREATMENT OF FULL-THICKNESS ROTATOR CUFF TEARS

For the last decade, we have avoided acromioplasty as a routine component of rotator cuff surgery. By preserving the origin of the deltoid and the stability and smoothness of the coracoacromial arch, the patient's recovery is optimized.[149]

The goal of rotator cuff surgery is to improve comfort and function of the shoulder. Surgery is considered (1) in patients with a significant acute cuff tear and (2) in patients with a chronic cuff defect associated with significant symptoms that have been refractory to a 3-month course of nonoperative management. In the situation of an acute cuff tear in a previously normal shoulder, the quality and quantity of tendon for repair should be excellent. Repair should be carried out promptly before tissue loss, retraction, and atrophy occur.

For tears older than 6 months, surgical repair is not an emergency; there is time to explore nonoperative management, including a general program of shoulder stretching and strengthening. This nonoperative program may be the treatment of choice for patients with chronic weakness who are not candidates for surgery or for those in whom achieving a durable repair seems unlikely (see Table 15–3). This regimen has been described earlier in this chapter as the "Jackins program"; it emphasizes stretching and strengthening the muscle groups that provide elevation and rotation of the shoulder. Surgical exploration is considered for patients with functionally

TABLE 15–9. Data on 67 Patients Treated for Documented Full-Thickness Tears of the Rotator Cuff

	No. of Patients	Average Age	% Female	Average Follow-up (yr)
Nonoperative	36	62.4	36	1.7
Subacromial smoothing	11	67.8	45	1.7
Cuff repair	20	60.3	10	2.0

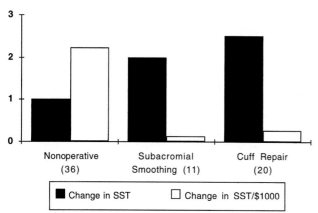

■ Figure 15–107
Median change in the number of positive Simple Shoulder Test (SST) responses.

significant symptoms from longer-standing tears refractory to nonoperative management, provided that their expectations are realistic. Although a successful cuff repair may increase the strength of the shoulder, patients with repairs of chronic tears are advised against returning to heavy lifting, pushing, pulling, or overhead work after surgery for fear of rerupturing the abnormal tendon tissue. Thus, we initiate vocational rehabilitation as soon as the diagnosis is made and inform patients that in spite of optimal treatment, they have a substantial risk of retearing the cuff if it is again subjected to major loads. It is important to remind both the patient and the employer that a cuff tear usually occurs through abnormal cuff tendon. Repairing the tear does not restore the quality of the tendon tissue; thus, the repaired cuff remains permanently vulnerable to sudden or large loads.

Critical determinants of a durable repair are the quality of the tendon and muscle and the amount of cuff tendon tissue that has been lost. The strength of the cuff tendon diminishes with age and disuse; as a result, the chance of a durable cuff repair also decreases in older and less active shoulders, particularly if the cuff defect has been long-standing.

Table 15–3 lists some of the factors that contribute to a durable repair, as well as those that predispose to failure. None of the factors in this table require special imaging of the rotator cuff; all are discernible from the history, physical examination, and plain radiographs. Although none of these factors are a contraindication to surgery, each works to some degree against the chance of a durable repair. The choice of treatment of shoulder weakness caused by cuff failure is determined by the functional needs of the patient and the likelihood of a durable surgical repair. Patients with low functional requirements and a substantial number of the "discouraging" factors from Table 15–3 are given a nonoperative program to help optimize the strength and coordination of the muscles about the shoulder that remain intact. At the opposite extreme, patients with major functional demands and mostly "encouraging" factors are presented with the option of an attempt at surgical repair and informed that the success of this repair will be determined primarily by the quality of the tendon and muscle and the amount of tissue lost.

We recall that cuff repair is a shoulder-tightening operation: in a sense, it is a capsulorrhaphy. Thus, it is not a treatment for a shoulder whose primary functional limitation is caused by tightness, even if a cuff defect is also present. If the shoulder demonstrates stiffness, a shoulder mobilization program is instituted before consideration of surgery.

For surgery, the patient is positioned in a semisitting (beach chair) position. Both the anterior and posterior aspects of the chest and the arm are prepared to allow access to the back of the shoulder and full motion of the arm. Surgery begins with an inspection of the cuff through a "deltoid-on" approach (see Fig. 15–1). This incision offers excellent exposure and the opportunity for cosmetic closure. Great care is taken to minimize the deltoid detachment and preserve the tendon fibers of the deltoid origin so that a strong repair can be achieved at the conclusion of the case. The deltoid has an important

tendon of origin between its anterior and middle thirds. Arising from the anterior lateral corner of the acromion, this tendon is not only the guide to exposure of the cuff but is also the key to reattachment of the deltoid origin at the conclusion of the surgery. This tendon is split longitudinally for 2 cm distal to the acromion in line with its fibers, with care taken to leave some of the tendon on each side of the split. If additional exposure is needed, the split is continued up over the acromion and into the trapezius insertion. Splitting the parietal layer of the bursa on the deep aspect of the deltoid provides a view of the rotator cuff. Later closure of the split is facilitated if at this point in the procedure a suture is placed on each side of the split to fix the incised bursal layer to the deltoid.

This window is used to inspect the cuff and determine its reparability without further compromising the deltoid or the coracoacromial arch. The undersurface of the coracoacromial arch is palpated to detect any points of roughness. Any rough spots are smoothed with a pinecone bur or, rarely, an osteotome (see Fig. 15–94). It is essential to preserve the integrity of the coracoacromial arch. Hypertrophic bursa and scar tissue are resected to allow a good view of cuff tendon involvement, tendon quality, and tendon tissue loss. Cuff tendon involvement is conveniently characterized by using the system introduced by Harryman and colleagues,[169] which is based on the number of tendons torn. In type 1, only one tendon (almost always the supraspinatus) is torn. In type 2, two tendons (usually the supraspinatus and infraspinatus) are torn. In type 3, the supraspinatus, infraspinatus, and subscapularis are torn. Type 1 is broken down into type 1A, or a partial-thickness tear, and type 1B, or a full-thickness tear confined to a single tendon. The quality of the cuff tissue is judged in terms of its ability to hold a strong pull applied to a suture passed through its edge. Finally, it is critical to note the amount of tissue that has been lost. The extent of tissue loss and the ability of the remaining tissue to hold suture are the major determinants of cuff reparability.

The goal of repair is strong fixation of the tendon to the humerus under normal tension with the arm at the side while leaving a smooth surface on the proximal humeral concavity to articulate with the undersurface of the coracoacromial arch. The desired attachment site is at the sulcus near the base of the tuberosity. This goal is facilitated by using three stages of sequential release. These releases are required because the cuff is usually retracted and tissue is lost in chronic cuff disease. Unless these releases are carried out, increased tension in the repaired tendon will predispose to tightness of the glenohumeral joint and will additionally challenge the repair site.[505] The humeral head is rotated to successively present the margins of the cuff defect through the incision (see Fig. 15–93) rather than enlarging the exposure to show the entire lesion at one time. The deep surface of the cuff is searched for retracted laminations. All layers of the cuff are assembled and tagged with sutures. By applying traction to these sutures, the cuff is mobilized sequentially as necessary to allow the torn tendon edge to reach the desired insertion at the base of the tuberosity. First, the humeroscapular motion interface (see Figs. 15–3 and 15–4) is freed between the cuff and the deltoid, acromion, coracoacromial ligaments, coracoid, and coracoid muscles. Next, the coracohumeral ligament/rotator interval capsule (Fig. 15-98) is sectioned around the coracoid process to eliminate any restriction to excursion of the cuff tendons and minimize tension on the repair during passive movement (Fig. 15-99). This release of the coracohumeral ligament and rotator interval capsule also contributes to comfort and ease of motion after the surgical repair by minimizing the capsular-tightening effect of cuff repair.[505] At this point the ease with which the cuff margins can be approximated to their anatomic insertion at the base of the tuberosity is evaluated. If good tissue cannot reach the sulcus, the third release is carried out. This release divides the capsule from the glenoid just outside the glenoid labrum (Fig. 15-100), which allows the capsule and tendon of the cuff to be drawn further laterally toward the desired tuberosity insertion without restricting range of motion.

After the necessary releases have been completed, a judgment is made concerning the site at which the cuff can be implanted into the bone without undue tension while the arm is at the side. Ideally, the site of implantation will be in the sulcus at the base of the tuberosity. In large cuff defects, a somewhat more medial insertion site may be necessary. Often, when a medial insertion site is required for a large cuff defect, the new insertion lies in an area where the articular cartilage has been damaged by abrasion against the undersurface of the acromion.

The repair is accomplished as a tongue-in-groove type of repair, with the cuff tendon drawn into a trough near the tuberosity to provide a smooth upper surface to glide beneath the acromion (Fig. 15-101). This groove provides the additional advantage that if some slippage occurs in the suture fixation of the cuff to bone, contact between these two structures is not lost. Nonabsorbable sutures woven through the tendon margin are passed through drill holes in the distal tuberosity so that the knots will not catch beneath the acromion (Fig. 15-102). The knots are tied over the tuberosities so that they will lie out of the subacromial space. If the bone of the tuberosities is osteopenic, the sutures can be passed through bone more distally, even down to the junction of the metaphysis and diaphysis. If the tear has a longitudinal component, it is repaired in side-to-side fashion with the knots buried out of the humeroscapular motion interface. The repair is checked throughout a range of motion to 140 degrees of elevation and 40 degrees of external rotation to ensure that it is strong, that it is not under excessive tension, and that it will permit smooth subacromial motion. If additional subacromial smoothing is required to allow smooth passage of the repaired tendon, it is performed at this time.

After a careful and robust deltoid repair using nonabsorbable sutures (Fig. 15-95) and cosmetic skin closure, the patient is returned to the recovery room with the affected arm in continuous passive motion (Fig. 15-96). Immediate postoperative motion is valuable because of the tendency for scarring between the raw undersurface of the acromion and the upper aspect of the rotator cuff or the proximal end of the humerus. Immediate postoperative continuous passive motion is facilitated if the surgery is performed under a brachial plexus block, which lasts up to 18 hours after surgery. Continuous passive motion is continued for up to 48 hours after surgery but does not

appear to be necessary after that. The patient is expected to perform passive exercises in flexion and external rotation. Before discharge from the medical center, the patient should be able to comfortably attain 140 degrees of passive flexion and 40 degrees of passive external rotation. A progress chart mounted on the patient's wall helps document progress toward these discharge goals (Fig. 15-109).

Postdischarge management must consider the magnitude of the tear and the strength of the repair. It is unlikely that the repair will have substantial strength until at least 3 months after surgery.[128] As is the case with repairs of the anterior cruciate ligament, major cuff repairs may require 6 to 12 months to regain useful strength. Thus, in the first several postoperative months, emphasis is placed on maintaining passive motion and avoiding loading of the repair. Posterior capsular stretching is not started until 3 months after surgery. Gentle progressive strengthening of the repaired cuff muscles is also started at 3 months. Work and sports are not resumed until the shoulder is comfortable, flexible, and strong.

When Cuff Repair Cannot Be Achieved

When the cuff cannot be repaired, it is essential that the coracoacromial arch be preserved. Sacrifice of the coracoacromial arch jeopardizes the secondary stabilization required in cuff deficiency. Without this secondary restraint, the shoulder is prone to anterosuperior "escape" of the humeral head when superiorly directed loads are applied to the humerus (see Fig. 15-9). The smoothness of the undersurface of the coracoacromial arch is ensured so that passage of the humeral head and residual cuff is unimpeded. Any debris, scar, useless fronds of cuff, or thickened bursa in the subacromial area is excised. It is important to also ensure smoothness of the upper surface of the uncovered proximal part of the humerus, particularly if the tuberosities are prominent or irregular. Before closure, the shoulder should demonstrate full passive motion without subacromial crepitance.

A strong repair of the deltoid is accomplished by performing a side-to-side repair of the surgical split in the deltoid tendon and secure reattachment of any detached muscle to the acromion through drill holes in the bone (Fig. 15-95). The full thickness of the deltoid, including the deltoid side of the bursa, is incorporated in the sutures to be certain that it does not impede smooth motion in the humeroscapular motion interface.

A subcuticular skin closure reinforced with paper tapes provides optimal cosmesis. The patient is returned to the recovery room with the arm in continuous passive motion to minimize the tendency to form adhesions in the humeroscapular motion interface (Fig. 15-96).

The patient is taught passive mobilization of the shoulder to 140 degrees of elevation (Figs. 15-81 and 15-82) and 40 degrees of external rotation (Fig. 15-83), as well as stretching of the posterior capsule (Figs. 15-85 and 15-86), and is discharged from the medical center when these goals are achieved. Active use of the shoulder with the arm at the side is instituted immediately. Sling immobilization is unnecessary. Strengthening of the deltoid and residual cuff muscles is started 6 weeks after surgery.

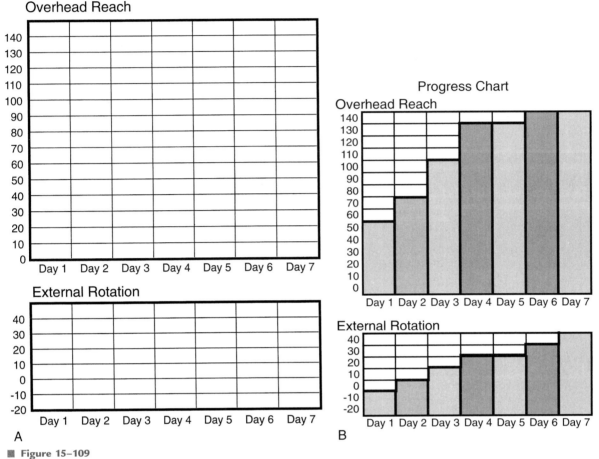

■ **Figure 15–109**

A, Wall charts are used to display the patient's overhead reach *(top)* and external rotation *(bottom)*. These charts are posted in the patient's room to provide positive feedback to the patient. With a colored marker, the physical therapist, nurse, or physician charts the range of motion achieved each day. **B,** Typical wall charts showing the improvement in overhead reach and external rotation after an open release. *(From Matsen FA III, Lippitt SB, Sidles JA, and Harryman DT II: Practical Evaluation and Management of the Shoulder. Philadelphia: WB Saunders, 1994.)*

An ideal exercise for optimizing the strength of active elevation is the progressive supine press (Fig. 15-89). In this exercise, small increments are used to train the remaining muscles to optimal advantage. Note that the scapular muscles are also put to work in these exercises (Figs. 15-90 and 15-91). This program is easy for the patient to learn and carry out alone.

Failed Cuff Surgery

In this condition, the patient is dissatisfied with the result from a previous arthroscopic or open operation on the rotator cuff and requests evaluation for additional surgery.

Causes of Failure

Rotator cuff repair may fail to yield a satisfactory result for many reasons, including failure to achieve preoperative expectations of strength and comfort, infection, deltoid denervation, deltoid detachment, loss of the acromial lever arm, adhesions in the humeroscapular motion interface, persisting subacromial roughness, denervation of the cuff,

failure of the cuff repair, retear of abnormal tendon, failure of grafts to "take," failure of rehabilitation, and loss of superior stability. Effective treatment of these failures depends on establishment of the proper diagnosis. Infection requires culture-specific antibiotics and irrigation and drainage if purulence is present. A prompt definitive approach may prevent joint surface destruction. Acute failure of the deltoid reattachment requires prompt repair before muscle retraction becomes fixed. Chronically painful and functionally limiting postoperative scarring often responds to gentle, frequent stretching at home. Shoulder manipulation in this situation is inadvisable because of the risk of cuff damage. However, in certain shoulders that are refractory to rehabilitation, substantial improvement in comfort and function can be achieved by open lysis of adhesions and subacromial smoothing, followed by early assisted motion. Weakness of shoulder elevation often responds to gentle, progressive strengthening of the anterior deltoid and external rotators. Persistent weakness requires evaluation for possible neurologic injury or cuff failure. Denervation of the deltoid is diagnosed by selective electromyography of the anterior muscle fibers. In selected cases, anterior deltoid denervation may be treated by anterior transfer of the origin of the middle deltoid with closure to the clavicular head of the pectoralis major, although consistently good results from this procedure have not been documented. Denervation of the supraspinatus and infraspinatus or subscapularis is diagnosed by selective electromyography and is difficult to manage. Postoperative cuff failure is suggested by failure of the patient to regain strength of external rotation or elevation of the shoulder, subacromial snapping, and upward instability of the humeral head. In this situation, arthrography may not be reliable; false-negative results from scarring or false-positive results from inconsequential leaks reduce its diagnostic accuracy. In our experience, expert dynamic cuff ultrasonography provides the most specific data on cuff thickness and integrity. Repeat cuff exploration with smoothing or repair may be considered, although the patient is warned that the tissue may be of insufficient quantity and quality for a durable repeat repair. Loss of superior stability can result when the coracoacromial arch has been sacrificed without re-establishing stability with a durable cuff repair. The deltoid becomes stretched so that the humeral head seems to be just below the skin. Patients who lose stability and deltoid function are some of the most unhappy we encounter after previous repair attempts.

The results of surgery for failure of previous cuff repairs are inferior to those of primary repair. DeOrio and Cofield[90] reviewed their experience with repeat repairs. At a minimum of 2 years' follow-up (average, 4 years), 76% of patients had a substantial diminution in pain; however, 63% still had moderate or severe pain. Only seven patients gained more than 30 degrees of abduction, and only four patients were thought to have a good result. The authors suggest that the main benefit of repeat cuff surgery is likely to be a reduction in discomfort.

Harryman and associates,[169] however, showed that if cuff integrity is durably established at revision surgery, the results are comparable to those of primary repair (Fig. 15–106).

Our experience indicates that if stiffness or crepitance is present and the patient is well motivated, substantial benefit may be provided by revision cuff surgery similar to the primary procedure described in the previous section.

Arthrodesis

When a shoulder has been devastated by infection, detachment or denervation of the deltoid, intractable cuff failure or denervation, and/or acromionectomy, consideration is given to shoulder arthrodesis. In these circumstances, glenohumeral arthrodesis provides a salvage option. By securing the humeral head to the scapula, the scapular motors can be used to power the humerus through a very limited range of humerothoracic motion.

The best candidates for this procedure are patients with (1) permanent and severe weakness because of loss of cuff and deltoid function, (2) good bone stock, (3) a good understanding of the limitations and potential complications of shoulder fusion, (4) intact scapular motors, (5) good motivation, (6) minimal complaints of pain, and (7) a functional contralateral shoulder.

To establish the limitations of shoulder fusion, we studied 12 patients who underwent glenohumeral

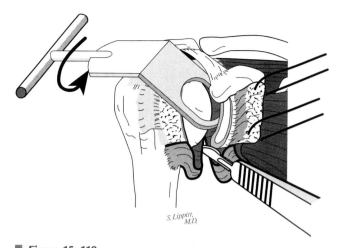

■ **Figure 15–110**

Recommended arthrodesis position: 15 degrees of humerothoracic flexion (left), 15 degrees of humerothoracic abduction (middle), and 45 degrees of internal rotation (right). (From Matsen FA III, Lippitt SB, Sidles JA, and Harryman DT II: Practical Evaluation and Management of the Shoulder. Philadelphia: WB Saunders, 1994.)

arthrodesis at least 2 years before the time of study.[269] In these patients, elevation in the plus 90-degree (anterior sagittal) plane averaged 47 degrees. Elevation in the minus 90-degree (posterior sagittal) plane averaged 22 degrees. External rotation averaged 9 degrees and internal rotation, 46 degrees. These ranges of motion were similar to the scapulothoracic motion measured in normal subjects. Only 1 of the patients could reach his hair without bending his neck forward, only 5 could reach their perineum, 6 could reach their back pocket, 7 the opposite axilla, and 10 the side pocket.

We also studied normal in vivo shoulder kinematics to predict the functions that would be allowed by various positions of glenohumeral arthrodesis, assuming that scapulothoracic motion would remain unchanged. By using normal scapulothoracic motions we were able to model the functional effects of fusion positions. We found that activities of daily living could best be performed if the joint was fused in 15 degrees of flexion, 15 degrees of abduction, and 45 degrees of internal rotation (Fig. 15–110). This low angle of elevation and relatively high degree of internal rotation facilitated reaching the face, opposite axilla, and anterior perineal region.

Cuff Tear Arthropathy

In this condition, resisted isometric contraction of the cuff muscles is weak; acromiohumeral and often glenohumeral movements produce crepitance; and radiographs demonstrate superior translation of the head of the humerus with respect to the acromion, loss of the articular cartilage of the superior humeral head, direct articulation of the head with the coracoacromial arch, "femoralization" of the proximal end of the humerus, and "acetabularization" of the upper glenoid and coracoacromial arch (Figs. 15–12, 15–13, 15–48, 15–60, 15–69, 15–70, 15–111).

The combination of glenohumeral joint surface destruction and massive cuff deficiency can be devastat-

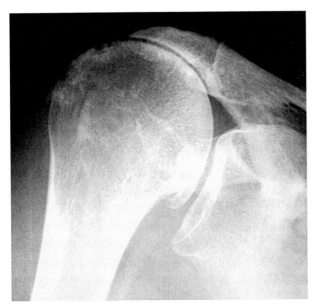

■ **Figure 15–111**
Cuff tear arthropathy.

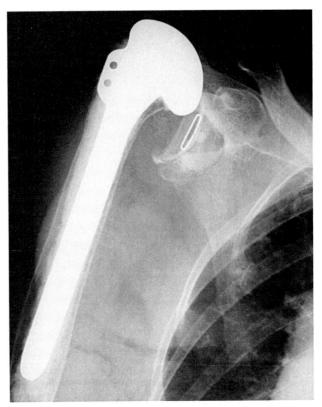

■ **Figure 15–112**
Glenoid component loosening via a "rocking horse" mechanism after shoulder replacement performed in the presence of a massive cuff deficiency (see Chapter 16).

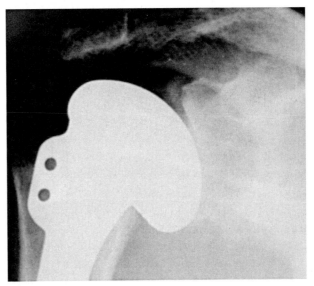

■ **Figure 15–113**
Resurfacing of the humeral head improved the comfort and function of the shoulder shown in Figure 15-60.

ing.[308] Nonetheless, each patient has an individual combination of pain and functional loss. Patients with mild pain are managed with mild analgesics and gentle, function-maintaining exercises.

When chronic cuff deficiency with upward displacement of the humeral head leads to repeated abrasive contact between the upper part of the humerus and the coracoacromial arch and symptomatic destruction of the humeral articular cartilage, reconstructive options are seriously limited. Shoulder arthrodesis is unattractive because these patients are often older and the condition may be bilateral.[306] Constrained total shoulder arthroplasty is an option, but the failure rate is very high. Secure cuff reconstruction with unconstrained total shoulder arthroplasty is usually impossible because of massive cuff tissue deficiency.[129] Unconstrained arthroplasty without a secure cuff repair carries a high incidence of eccentric loading and "rocking horse" loosening of the component (Fig. 15–112).[129,269]

In a 1986 report to the American Shoulder and Elbow Surgeons, Brownlee and Cofield reported on 20 surgical procedures for cuff tear arthropathy.[45] These procedures included Neer-type total shoulder arthroplasty, total shoulder arthroplasty using a hooded glenoid, and proximal humeral replacement without a glenoid. Extensive mobilization of tendons was attempted for repair. Pain relief was substantial in each group. Active abduction was best in the group with proximal humeral replacement. Three of the glenoid components loosened.

Arntz and associates[6] reported our results in 19 patients 54 to 84 years of age who had disabling pain attributable to a massive tear of the rotator cuff accompanied by loss of the surface of the glenohumeral joint. These patients were not considered candidates for total shoulder replacement because of the massive deficiency in the cuff and the fixed upward displacement of the humeral head (Figs. 15–12, 15–13, 15–48, 15–60, 15–69, 15–70, 15–111, and 15–113). A prerequisite for hemiarthroplasty was a functionally intact coracoacromial

arch to provide superior secondary stability for the prosthesis. One important aspect of the operative technique was the selection of a sufficiently small prosthetic head volume so that excessive tightness of the posterior aspect of the capsule could be avoided (see Chapter 16 for discussion of "overstuffing"). Eighteen shoulders in 16 patients were available for follow-up, which ranged from

25 to 122 months. Pain decreased from marked or disabling in 14 shoulders preoperatively to none or slight in 10 and to pain only after unusual activity in 4. Active forward elevation improved from an average of 66 degrees preoperatively to an average of 109 degrees postoperatively. One patient who had an excellent result fell and sustained an acromial fracture, so the functional result changed to poor. Three patients had persistent, substantial pain in the shoulder that led to a revision. Neither infection nor prosthetic loosening developed in any shoulder.

In a separate report, Arntz and colleagues[7] reviewed 23 shoulders in 23 patients with disabling pain associated with irreparable tears of the musculotendinous cuff.

Twelve shoulders with preserved passive motion, normal deltoid function, loss of glenohumeral joint surfaces, and sculpting of the coracoacromial arch underwent reconstruction with a humeral hemiarthroplasty. In another 11 shoulders that failed to meet these prerequisites or that demanded heavy use after surgery, glenohumeral arthrodesis was selected. Comfort level and overall function were improved in both groups. Active forward elevation improved an average of 44 degrees in the hemiarthroplasty group and an average of 15 degrees in the arthrodesis group. These results, coupled with the problems of glenoid loosening reported when total shoulder arthroplasty (Fig. 15-112) is performed in the presence of cuff deficiency with upward head displacement, suggest that humeral hemiarthroplasty is the preferred method for managing complex irreparable tears of the rotator cuff

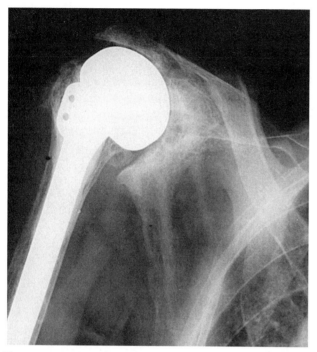

■ **Figure 15–114**
Resurfacing hemiarthroplasty for cuff tear arthropathy (same patient as in Fig. 15–69).

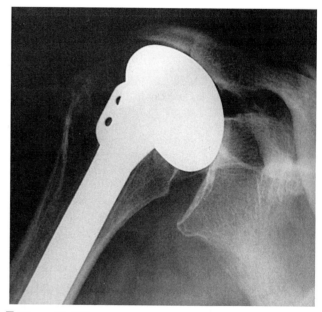

■ **Figure 15–115**
Resurfacing hemiarthroplasty for cuff tear arthropathy (same patient as in Fig. 15–111).

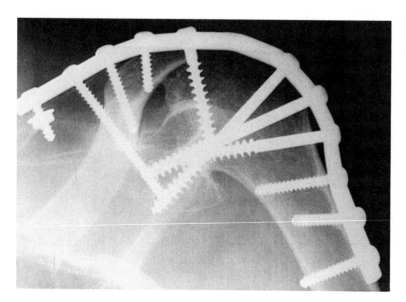

■ **Figure 15–116**
Shoulder arthrodesis for a young patient with a combined deficiency of the cuff and the deltoid.

in which the articular surface is destroyed, yet the deltoid muscle is functional (Figs. 15-69, 15-111, 15-114, and 15-115). Shoulder arthrodesis is reserved for patients who have both irreparable tears of the rotator cuff and irreparable deficiencies of the deltoid muscle or for younger patients with demands for substantial strength at low angles of flexion (Fig. 15-116).

■ MATSEN'S PREFERRED METHOD OF CUFF TEAR ARTHROPATHY

In a reconstruction for cuff tear arthropathy, we attempt to make use of "femoralization" of the proximal end of the humerus (i.e., rounding so that the prominence of the tuberosities is lost) and "acetabularization" of the glenocoracoacromial socket (i.e., erosion of the upper aspect of the glenoid and congruent concavity of the coracoacromial arch) (see Figs. 15-48, 15-69, 15-70, and 15-111). We have found that this adaptive ball-and-socket joint can be effectively and safely resurfaced by humeral hemiarthroplasty (Figs. 15-114 and 15-115). The goals of surgery are to (1) ensure a smooth coracoacromial arch (usually already created by the process itself) and avoid acromioplasty and section of the coracoacromial ligament, which would destroy the superior constraint of the humeral head; (2) débride useless fragments of cuff and bursa; and (3) anatomically resurface the destroyed humeral articular surface with a humeral endoprosthesis that will articulate with the coracoacromial arch and preserve the deltoid at all costs. We do not advocate cuff repair in this context, nor the use of double cups or oversized humeral head prostheses. Instead, the goal is to maintain normal capsular laxity and allow internal rotation of the abducted arm to approximately 60 degrees.

Postoperatively, continuous passive motion is started (Fig. 15-96), and the patient is allowed activities as comfort permits.

■ ROCKWOOD'S PREFERRED METHOD FOR CUFF TEAR ARTHROPATHY

The new Depuy Global Advantage Cuff Tear Arthropathy (CTA) humeral head prosthesis provides an extended articular surface over the greater tuberosity, which allows for articulation with the glenoid and the undersurface of the acromion. This procedure allows for a smooth functioning shoulder and obviates the need for a glenoid prosthesis or overstuffing the glenohumeral joint. **(V15-3 and V15-4)**

Refer to Rockwood's Preferred Technique for Shoulder Arthroplasty, Chapter 16 **(V16-21 to V16-23, V16-25, and V16-26)**, for a more detailed surgical technique. Once the appropriately sized humeral broach trial is inserted into the humerus, size the humeral head using standard trial heads. **(V15-5 and V15-6)** Once it is determined that the rotator cuff is irreparable, debride the frayed edges of the remaining cuff and bursa. It is important to remember not to perform an acromioplasty, or at least a coracoacromial ligament, since this may compromise postoperative prosthesis stability. With the humeral broach trial

in place, secure the CTA head resection clamp onto the humeral broach trial and attach the left or right cutting guide. The CTA head resection clamp serves as an indicator as to how much greater tuberosity will be removed. With an oscillating saw placed flat on the cutting guide, remove bone from the greater tuberosity. Exercise caution not to contact the broach with the saw blade or osteotome. Once the greater tuberosity resection has been performed, use a rasp rongeur or air bur to remove the prominent bone lateral to the CTA head. Also, a rongeur can be used to round off the edges of the resected greater tuberosity. At this point, bleeding from the cancellous bone surfaces may be encountered. This may be cauterized with electrocautery in addition to using bone wax. Next, an appropriate sized CTA trial head is placed onto the humeral broach trial. Reduce, and then assess the shoulder and soft tissue balancing as described in the aforementioned surgical technique. Next, the final head is impacted onto the final body using the impactor and a mallet. Strike the head three to four times to ensure proper seating. Lastly, insert the final component assembly into the humerus to the proper seating position.

V15-3 to V15-6

REFERENCES AND BIBLIOGRAPHY

1. Ahovou J, Paavolainen P, and Slätis P: The diagnostic value of arthrography and plain radiography in rotator cuff tears. Acta Orthop Scand 55:220-223, 1984.
2. Albright JA, Jokl P, Shaw R, and Albright JP: Clinical study of baseball pitchers: Correlation of injury to the throwing arm with method of delivery. Am J Sports Med 6:15-21, 1978.
3. Altchek DW, Warren RF, Wickiewicz TL, et al: Arthroscopic acromioplasty. J Bone Joint Surg Am 72:1198-1207, 1990.
4. Andrews JR, Broussard TS, and Carson WG: Arthroscopy of the shoulder in the management of partial tears of the rotator cuff: A preliminary report. Arthroscopy 1:117-122, 1985.
5. Armstrong JR: Excision of the acromion in treatment of the supraspinatus syndrome: Report of ninety-five excisions. J Bone Joint Surg Br 31:436-442, 1949.
6. Arntz CT, Jackins S, and Matsen FA III: Prosthetic replacement of the shoulder for the treatment of defects in the rotator cuff and the surface of the glenohumeral joint. J Bone Joint Surg Am 75:485-491, 1993.
7. Arntz CT, Matsen FA III, and Jackins S: Surgical management of complex irreparable cuff deficiency. J Arthroplasty 6:363-370, 1991.
8. Atwater AE: Biomechanics of overarm throwing movements and of throwing injuries. Exerc Sport Sci Rev 7:43-85, 1979.
9. Bacevich BB: Paralytic brachial neuritis. J Bone Joint Surg Am 58:262, 1976.
10. Bakalim G and Pasila M: Surgical treatment of rupture of the rotator cuff tendon. Acta Orthop Scand 46:751-757, 1975.
11. Baker CL and Liu SH: Comparison of open and arthroscopic assisted rotator cuff repairs. Am J Sports Med 23:99-104, 1995.
12. Barber FA: Coplaning of the acromioclavicular joint. Arthroscopy 17:913-917, 2001.
13. Barber FA and Herbert MA: The effectiveness of an anesthetic continuous-infusion device on postoperative pain control. Arthroscopy 18:76-81, 2002.
14. Bartolozzi A, Andreychik D, and Ahmad S: Determinants of outcome in the treatment of rotator cuff disease. Clin Orthop 308:90-97, 1994.
15. Basmajian JV and Bazant FJ: Factors preventing downward dislocation of the adducted shoulder joint: An electromyographic and morphological study. J Bone Joint Surg Am 41:1182-1186, 1959.
16. Bassett RW and Cofield RH: Acute tears of the rotator cuff: The timing of surgical repair. Clin Orthop 175:18-24, 1983.
17. Bateman JE: The diagnosis and treatment of ruptures of the rotator cuff. Surg Clin North Am 43:1523-1530, 1963.
18. Bauer B and Vogelsang H: Die Lähmung des N. Suprascapularis als Taumafloge. Unfallheilkunde 65:461-465, 1962.
19. Bayley JC, Cochran TP, and Seldge CB: The weight-bearing shoulder: The impingement syndrome in paraplegics. J Bone Joint Surg Am 69:676-678, 1987.
20. Bedi SS and Ellis W: Spontaneous rupture of calcaneal tendon in rheumatoid arthritis after local steroid injection. Ann Rheum Dis 29:494, 1970.
21. Behrens F, Shepherd N, and Mitchell N: Alterations of rabbit articular cartilage by intra-articular injections of glucocorticoids. J Bone Joint Surg Am 57:70-76, 1975.

22. Bellumore Y, Mansat M, and Assoun J: Results of the surgical repair of the rotator cuff. Radio-clinical correlation. Rev Chir Orthop Reparatrice Appar Mot 80:582-594, 1994.

23. Benjamin M, Evans EJ, and Copp L: The histology of tendon attachments to bone in man. J Anat 149:89-100, 1986.

24. Ben-Yishay A, Zuckerman JD, Gallagher M, and Cuomo F: Pain inhibition of shoulder strength in patients with impingement syndrome. Orthopedics 17:685-688, 1994.

25. Berquist TH, McCough PF, Hattrup SH, and Cofield RH: Arthrographic analysis of rotator cuff tear size. Paper presented at the Fourth Meeting of the American Shoulder and Elbow Surgeons, 1988, Atlanta.

26. Berry H, Fernandes L, and Bloom B: Clinical study comparing acupuncture, physiotherapy, injection and oral anti-inflammatory therapy in shoulder-cuff lesions. Curr Med Res Opin 7:121-126, 1980.

27. Bettman: Monatsschr Unfallheilk. 14, 1926.

28. Bey MJ, Song HK, Wehrli FW, and Soslowsky LJ: Intratendinous strain fields of the intact supraspinatus tendon: The effect of glenohumeral joint position and tendon region. J Orthop Res 20:869-874, 2002.

29. Bigliani LU, Cordasco FA, McIlveen SJ, et al: Operative management of failed rotator cuff repairs. Orthop Trans 12:1974, 1988.

30. Bigliani LU, Morrison D, and April EW: The morphology of the acromion and its relationship to rotator cuff tears. Orthop Trans 10:228, 1986.

31. Bigliani LU, Norris TR, and Fischer J: The relationship between the unfused acromial epiphysis and subacromial impingement lesions. Orthop Trans 7:138, 1983.

32. Binder A, Parr G, Hazleman B, and Fitton-Jackson S: Pulsed electromagnetic field therapy of persistent rotator cuff tendinitis. Lancet 1:695-698, 1984.

33. Bjorkenheim JM, Paavolainen P, Ahovuo J, and Slatis P: Subacromial impingement decompressed with anterior acromioplasty. Clin Orthop 252:150-155, 1990.

34. Bokor DJ, Hawkins RJ, Huckell GH, et al: Results of nonoperative management of full-thickness tears of the rotator cuff. Clin Orthop 294:103-110, 1993.

35. Bonsell S, Pearsall AW, Heitman RJ, et al: The relationship of age, gender, and degenerative changes observed on radiographs of the shoulder in asymptomatic individuals. J Bone Joint Surg Br 82:1135-1139, 2000.

36. Bosley RC: Total acromionectomy: A twenty-year review. J Bone Joint Surg Am 73:961-968, 1991.

37. Bosworth DM: An analysis of twenty-eight consecutive cases of incapacitating shoulder lesions, radically explored and repaired. J Bone Joint Surg 22:369-392, 1940.

38. Bosworth DM: The supraspinatus syndrome—symptomatology, pathology, and repair. JAMA 117:422, 1941.

39. Brems JJ: Digital muscle strength measurement in rotator cuff tears. Paper presented at the Third Open Meeting of the American Shoulder and Elbow Surgeons, 1987, San Francisco.

40. Brenneke SL and Morgan CJ: Evaluation of ultrasonography as a diagnostic technique in the assessment of rotator cuff tendon tears. Am J Sports Med 20:287-289, 1992.

41. Brewer BJ: Aging of the rotator cuff. Am J Sports Med 7:102-110, 1979.

42. Brogi M, Laterza A, and Neri C: Entrapment neuropathy of the suprascapular nerve. Riv Neurobiol 25:318, 1979.

43. Brooks CH, Revell WJ, and Heatley FW: A quantitative histological study of the vascularity of the rotator cuff tendon. J Bone Joint Surg Br 74:151-153, 1992.

44. Brown JT: Early assessment of supraspinatus tears: Procaine infiltration as a guide to treatment. J Bone Joint Surg Br 31:423, 1949.

45. Brownlee C and Cofield MD: Shoulder replacement in cuff tear arthropathy. Paper presented at the Second Open Meeting of the American Shoulder and Elbow Surgeons, 1986, New Orleans.

46. Brox JI, Staff PH, Ljunggren AE, and Brevik JI: Arthroscopic surgery compared with supervised exercises in patients with rotator cuff disease (stage II impingement syndrome). BMJ 307:899-903, 1993.

47. Bryant L, Shnier R, Bryant C, and Murrell GA: A comparison of clinical estimation, ultrasonography, magnetic resonance imaging, and arthroscopy in determining the size of rotator cuff tears. J Shoulder Elbow Surg 11:219-224, 2002.

48. Budoff JE, Nirschl RP, and Guidi EJ: Débridement of partial-thickness tears of the rotator cuff without acromioplasty. Long-term follow-up and review of the literature. J Bone Joint Surg Am 80:733-748, 1998.

49. Burkhart SS: Arthroscopic treatment of massive rotator cuff tears. Clin Orthop 267:45-46, 1991.

50. Burkhart SS, Fischer SP, Nottage WM, et al: Tissue fixation security in transosseous rotator cuff repairs: A mechanical comparison of simple versus mattress sutures. Arthroscopy 12:704-708, 1996.

51. Burkhart SS, Nottage WM, Ogilvie-Harris DJ, et al: Partial repair of irreparable rotator cuff tears. Arthroscopy 10:363-370, 1994.

52. Burns TP and Turba JE: Arthroscopic treatment of the shoulder impingement in athletes. Am J Sports Med 20:13-16, 1992.

53. Burns WC and Whipple TL: Anatomic relationships in the shoulder impingement syndrome. Clin Orthop 294:96-102, 1993.

54. Bush LF: The torn shoulder capsule. J Bone Joint Surg Am 57:256-259, 1975.

55. Calvert PT, Packer NP, Stoker DJ, et al: Arthrography of the shoulder after operative repair of the torn rotator cuff. J Bone Joint Surg 68:147-150, 1986.

56. Cammerer U, Habermeyer P, Plenk A, and Huber R: Ultrasound assessment of reconstructed rotator cuffs. Unfallchirurg 95:608-612, 1992.

57. Chakravarty K and Webley M: Shoulder joint movement and its relationship to disability in the elderly. J Rheumatol 20:1359-1361, 1993.

58. Chard MD, Hazleman R, Hazleman BL, et al: Shoulder disorders in the elderly: A community survey. Arthritis Rheum 34:766-769, 1991.

59. Chiodi E and Morini G: Lesions of the rotator cuff: Diagnostic validity of echography. Surgical findings. Radiol Med 88:733-735, 1994.

60. Chung SMK and Nissenbaum MM: Congenital and developmental defects of the shoulder. Orthop Clin North Am 6:382, 1975.

61. Clark JC: Fibrous anatomy of the rotator cuff. Abstract presented to the American Academy of Orthopaedic Surgeons, 1988.

62. Clark JM and Harryman DT II: Tendons, ligaments, and capsule of the rotator cuff. Gross and microscopic anatomy. J Bone Joint Surg Am 74:713-725, 1992.

63. Clark JM, Sidles JA, and Matsen FA III: The relationship of the glenohumeral joint capsule to the rotator cuff. Clin Orthop 254:29-34, 1990.

64. Clein LJ: Suprascapular entrapment neuropathy. J Neurosurg 43:337-342, 1975.

65. Codman EA: Complete rupture of the supraspinatus tendon: Operative treatment with report of two successful cases. Boston Med Surg J 164:708-710, 1911.

66. Codman EA: The Shoulder, Rupture of the Supraspinatus Tendon and Other Lesions in or about the Subacromial Bursa. Boston: Thomas Todd, 1934.

67. Codman EA: Rupture of the supraspinatus—1834-1934. J Bone Joint Surg 19:643-652, 1937.

68. Codman EA: Rupture of the supraspinatus tendon. In The Shoulder: Rupture of the Supraspinatus Tendon and Other Lesions in or about the Subacromial Bursa, suppl ed. Malabar, FL: Robert E Krieger, 1984, pp 123-177.

69. Cofield RH: Tears of rotator cuff. Instr Course Lect 30:258-273, 1981.

70. Cofield RH: Subscapular muscle transposition for repair of chronic rotator cuff tears. Surg Gynecol Obstet 154:667-672, 1982.

71. Cofield RH: Current concepts review: Rotator cuff disease of the shoulder. J Bone Joint Surg Am 67:974-979, 1985.

72. Cofield RH: Glenohumeral arthroplasty for rheumatoid arthritis: Incidence of rotator cuff tears. Paper presented at the 54th Annual Meeting of the American Academy of Orthopaedic Surgeons, 1987, San Francisco.

73. Cofield RH and Simonet WT: Symposium on sports medicine. Part 2. The shoulder in sports. Mayo Clin Proc 59:157-164, 1984.

74. Colachis SCJ and Strohm BR: Effect of suprascapular and axillary nerve blocks and muscle force in upper extremity. Arch Phys Med Rehabil 52:22, 1971.

75. Colachis SCJ, Strohm BR, and Brechner VL: Effects of axillary nerve block on muscle force in the upper extremity. Arch Phys Med Rehabil 50:647, 1969.

76. Colley F: Die Periarthritis Humeroscapularis. Rose E and Helferich von FCW. Leipzig, 1899.

77. Collins RA, Gristina AG, Carter RE, et al: Ultrasonography of the shoulder. Orthop Clin North Am 18:351, 1987.

78. Connolly JF: Humeral head defects associated with shoulder dislocations—their diagnosis and surgical significance. Instr Course Lect 21:42, 1972.

79. Coomes EN and Darlington LG: Effects of local steroid injection for supraspinatus tears: Controlled study. Ann Rheum Dis 35:943, 1976.

80. Cotton RE and Rideout D: Tears of the humeral rotator cuff: A radiological and pathological necropsy survey. J Bone Joint Surg Br 46:314-328, 1964.

81. Craig EV: The geyser sign and torn rotator cuff: Clinical significance and pathomechanics. Clin Orthop 191:213-215, 1984.

82. Crass JR and Craig EV: Noninvasive imaging of the rotator cuff. Orthopedics 11:57-64, 1988.

83. Crass JR, Craig EV, Bretzke C, et al: Ultrasonography of the rotator cuff. Radiographics 5:941-953, 1985.

84. Crass JR, Craig EV, and Feinberg SB: Sonography of the postoperative rotator cuff. AJR Am J Roentgenol 146:561-564, 1986.

85. Crass JR, Craig EV, Thompason RC, et al: Ultrasonography of the rotator cuff: Surgical correlation. J Clin Ultrasound 12:497-491, 1984.

86. Cruess RL, Blennerhassett J, and MacDonald FR: Aseptic necrosis following renal transplantation. J Bone Joint Surg Am 50:1577, 1968.

87. Dalton S, Cawston TE, Riley GP, et al: Human shoulder tendon biopsy samples in organ culture produce procollagenase and tissue inhibitor of metalloproteinases. Ann Rheum Dis 54:571-577, 1995.

88. Darlington LG and Coomes EN: The effects of local steroid injection for supraspinatus tears. Rheumatol Rehabil 16:172-179, 1977.

89. Debeyre J, Patte D, and Emelik E: Repair of ruptures of the rotator cuff with a note on advancement of the supraspinatus muscle. J Bone Joint Surg Br 47:36-42, 1965.

89a. Dejardin LM, et al: Tissue engineered rotator cuff tendon using porcine small intestine submucosa: Histological and mechanical evaluation in dogs. Am J Sports Med 29(2), 2001.

90. DeOrio JK and Cofield RH: Results of a second attempt at surgical repair of a failed initial surgical rotator cuff repair. J Bone Joint Surg Am 66:563-567, 1984.

91. D'Erme M, DeCupis V, DeMaria M, et al: Echography, magnetic resonance and double-contrast arthrography of the rotator cuff. A prospective study in 30 patients. Radiol Med 86:72-80, 1993.

92. DePalma AF: Surgical anatomy of the rotator cuff and the natural history of degenerative periarthritis. Surg Clin North Am 43:1507-1520, 1967.

93. DePalma AF: Surgery of the Shoulder, 2nd ed. Philadelphia: JB Lippincott, pp 206-210, 229, 234-235, 1973.

94. DePalma AF: Surgery of the Shoulder, 3rd ed. Philadelphia: JB Lippincott, 1983.

95. DePalma AF, Gallery G, and Bennett CA: Variational anatomy and degenerative lesions of the shoulder joint. Instr Course Lect 6:255-281, 1949.

96. DePalma AF, White JB, and Callery G: Degenerative lesions of the shoulder joint at various age groups which are compatible with good function. Instr Course Lect, 1950.

97. Desché: Contribution à l'étude au traitement de la periarthrite scapulo-humerale. Paris, 1892.

98. Desplats H: De l'atrophie musculaire dans la péri-arthrite scapulo humérale. Gazette Hebdomadaire de Médicine et de Chir 24:371, 1878.

99. Diamond B: The Obstructing Acromion. Springfield, IL: Charles C Thomas, 1964.

100. Dierickx C and Vanhoof H: Massive rotator cuff tears treated by a deltoid muscular inlay flap. Acta Orthop Belg 60:94-100, 1994.

101. Donovan WH and Kraft GH: Rotator cuff tear vs. suprascapular nerve injury. Arch Phys Med Rehabil 55:424, 1974.

102. Drakeford MK, Quinn MJ, Simpson SL, and Pettine KA: A comparative study of ultrasonography in evaluation of the rotator cuff. Clin Orthop 253:118-122, 1990.

103. Drez D: Suprascapular neuropathy in the differential diagnosis of rotator cuff injury. Am J Sports Med 4:43, 1976.

104. Duckworth DG, Smith KL, Campbell B, and Matsen FA III: Self-assessment questionnaires document substantial variability in the clinical expression of rotator cuff tears. J Shoulder Elbow Surg 8:330-333, 1999.

105. Duplay: Arch Gen Med 2:513, 1872.

106. Duronea: Essai sur la scapulalgie. 1873.

107. Earnshaw P, Desjardins D, Sarkar K, and Uhthoff HK: Rotator cuff tears: The role of surgery. Can J Surg 25:60-63, 1982.

108. Edeland HG and Zachrisson BE: Fracture of the scapular notch associated with lesion of the suprascapular nerve. Acta Orthop Scand 46:758-763, 1975.

109. Ellman H: Arthroscopic subacromial decompression: Analysis of one- to three-year results. J Arthrosc Rel Surg 3:173-181, 1987.

110. Ellman H: Arthroscopic subacromial decompression: Analysis of one- to three-year results. Arthroscopy 3:173-181, 1988.

111. Ellman H, Hanker G, and Bayer M: Repair of the rotator cuff: End-result study of factors influencing reconstruction. J Bone Joint Surg Am 68:1136-1144, 1986.

112. Ellman H and Kay SP: Arthroscopic subacromial decompression: 2-5 year results. Orthop Trans 13:239, 1989.

113. Ellman H and Kay SP: Arthroscopic subacromial decompression for chronic impingement: Two to five year results. J Bone Joint Surg Br 73:395-398, 1991.

114. Ellman H, Kay SP, and Wirth M: Arthroscopic treatment of full thickness rotator cuff tears: Two to seven year follow-up study. Arthroscopy 9:195-200, 1993.

115. Esch JC, Ozerkis LR, Helgager JA, et al: Arthroscopic subacromial decompression: Results according to degree of rotator cuff. Arthroscopy 4:241-249, 1988.

116. Esslen E, Flachsmann H, Bischoff A, et al: Die Einklemmungsneuropathie des N. Suprascapularis: Eine klinisch-therapeutische Studie. Nervenarzt 38:311-314, 1967.

117. Fabis J, Kordek P, Bogucki A, and Mazanowska-Gajdowicz J: Function of the rabbit supraspinatus muscle after large detachment of its tendon: 6-week, 3-month, and 6-month observation. J Shoulder Elbow Surg 9:211-216, 2000.

118. Farin PU and Jaroma H: Acute traumatic tears of the rotator cuff: Value of sonography. Radiology 197:269-273, 1995.

119. Farin PU and Jaroma H: Digital subtraction shoulder arthrography in determining site and size of rotator cuff tear. Invest Radiol 30:544-547, 1995.

120. Farrer IL, Matsen FAI, Rogers JV, et al: Dynamic sonographic study of lesion of the rotator cuff [abstract]. Paper presented at the 50th Annual Meeting of the American Academy of Orthopedic Surgeons, 1983, Anaheim, CA.

121. Ferrari JD, Ferrari JA, Coumas J, and Pappas AM: Posterior ossification of the shoulder: The Bennett lesion. Etiology, diagnosis, and treatment. Am J Sports Med 22:171-175, 1994.

122. Flanders M: Shoulder muscle activity during natural arm movements: What is optimized? In Matsen FA III, Fu FH, and Hawkins RJ (eds): The Shoulder: A Balance of Mobility and Stability. Rosemont, IL: American Academy of Orthopaedic Surgeons, 1993, pp 635-646.

123. Flatow EL, Raimondo RA, Kelkar R, et al: Active and passive restraints against superior humeral translation: The contributions of the rotator cuff, the biceps tendon, and the coracoacromial arch. Paper presented at the 12th Open Meeting of the American Shoulder and Elbow Surgeons, 1996, Atlanta.

124. Flatow EL, Soslowsky LJ, Ticker JB, et al: Excursion of the rotator cuff under the acromion. Patterns of subacromial contact. Am J Sports Med 22:779-788, 1994.

125. Flugstad D, Matsen FA III, Larry I, and Jackins SE: Failed acromioplasty and the treatment of the impingement syndrome. Paper presented at the 2nd Open Meeting of the American Shoulder and Elbow Surgeons, 1986, New Orleans.

126. Ford LT and DeBender J: Tendon rupture after local steroid injection. South Med J 72:827-830, 1979.

127. Fowler P: Swimmer problems. Am J Sports Med 7:141-142, 1979.

128. Frank CB: Ligament healing: Current knowledge and clinical applications. J Am Acad Orthop Surg 4:74-83, 1996.

129. Franklin JL, Barrett WP, Jackins SE, and Matsen FA III: Glenoid loosening in total shoulder arthroplasty; association with rotator cuff deficiency. J Arthroplasty 3:39-46, 1988.

130. Freiberger RH, Kaye JJ, and Spiller J: Arthrography. New York: Appleton-Century-Crofts, 1979.

131. Fukuda H: Rotator cuff tears. Geka Chiryo (Osaka) 43:28, 1980.

132. Fukuda H, Hamada K, Nakajima T, and Tomonaga A: Pathology and pathogenesis of the intratendinous tearing of the rotator cuff viewed from en bloc histologic sections. Clin Orthop 304:60-67, 1994.

133. Fukuda H, Hamada K, and Yamanada K: Pathology and pathogenesis of bursal side rotator cuff tears viewed from en bloc histologic sections. Clin Orthop 254:75-80, 1990.

134. Fukuda H, Mikasa M, Ogawa K, et al: The partial thickness tear of rotator cuff. Orthop Trans 7:137, 1983.

135. Fukuda H, Mikasa M, and Yamanaka K: Incomplete thickness rotator cuff tears diagnosed by subacromial bursography. Clin Orthop 223:51-58, 1987.

136. Gartsman GM: Arthroscopic treatment of stage II subacromial impingement. Paper presented at Fourth Meeting of the American Shoulder and Elbow Surgeons, 1988, Atlanta.

137. Gartsman GM: Arthroscopic acromioplasty for lesion of the rotator cuff. J Bone Joint Surg Am 72:169-180, 1990.

138. Gartsman GM, Blair ME, Noble PC, et al: Arthroscopic subacromial decompression: An anatomical study. Am J Sports Med 16:48-50, 1988.

139. Gazielly DF, Gleyze P, and Montagnon C: Functional and anatomical results after rotator cuff repair. Clin Orthop 304:43-53, 1994.

140. Gazielly DF, Gleyze P, Montagnon C, et al: Functional and anatomical results after surgical treatment of ruptures of the rotator cuff. 1. Preoperative functional and anatomical evaluation of ruptures of the rotator cuff. Rev Chir Orthop Reparatrice Appar Mot 81:8-16, 1995.

141. Gazielly DF, Gleyze P, Montagnon C, et al: Functional and anatomical results after surgical treatment of ruptures of the rotator cuff. 2. Postoperative functional and anatomical evaluation of ruptures of the rotator cuff. Rev Chir Orthop Reparatrice Appar Mot 81:17-26, 1995.

142. Gelmers HJ and Buys DA: Suprascapular entrapment neuropathy. Acta Neurochir (Wien) 38:121-124, 1977.

143. Gerber C: Latissimus dorsi transfer for the treatment of irreparable tears of the rotator cuff. Clin Orthop 275:152-160, 1992.

144. Gerber C, Schneeberger AG, Beck M, and Schlegel U: Mechanical strength of repairs of the rotator cuff. J Bone Joint Surg 76:371-380, 1994.

145. Gerber C, Terrier F, and Ganz R: The role of the coracoid process in the chronic impingement syndrome. J Bone Joint Surg Br 67:703-708, 1985.

146. Ghelman B and Goldman AB: The double contrast shoulder arthrogram: Evaluation of rotary cuff tears. Radiology 124:251-254, 1977.

147. Gill TJ, McIrvin E, Kocher MS, Homa K, et al: The relative importance of acromial morphology and age with respect to rotator cuff pathology. J Shoulder Elbow Surg 11:327-330, 2002.

148. Godsil RD and Linscheid RL: Intratendinous defects of the rotator cuff. Clin Orthop 69:181-188, 1970.

149. Goldberg BA, Lippitt SB, and Matsen FA III: Improvement in comfort and function after cuff repair without acromioplasty. Clin Orthop 390:142-150, 2001.

150. Goldberg BA, Nowinski RJ, and Matsen FA III: Outcome of nonoperative management of full-thickness rotator cuff tears. Clin Orthop 382:99-107, 2001.

151. Goldman AB, Dines DM, and Warren RF: Shoulder arthrography. In Technique, Diagnosis and Clinical Correlation. Boston: Little, Brown, 1982, pp 1-3.

152. Goldman AB and Gehlman B: The double-contrast shoulder arthrogram. Radiology 127:655-663, 1978.

153. Gore DR, Murray MP, Sepic SB, and Gardner GM: Shoulder-muscle strength and range of motion following surgical repair of full-thickness rotator-cuff tears. J Bone Joint Surg Am 68:266-272, 1986.

154. Goutallier D, Postel JM, Bernageau J, et al: Fatty muscle degeneration in cuff ruptures. Pre- and postoperative evaluation by CT scan. Clin Orthop 304:78-83, 1994.

155. Goutallier D, Postel JM, Bernageau J, et al: Fatty infiltration of disrupted rotator cuff muscles. Rev Rhum Engl Ed 62:415-422, 1995.

156. Grana WA, Teague B, King M, and Reeves RB: An analysis of rotator cuff repair. Am J Sports Med 22:585-588, 1994.

157. Grant JCB: Grant's Atlas of Anatomy, 6th ed. Baltimore: Williams & Wilkins, 1972.

158. Grant JCB and Smith CG: Age incidence of rupture of the supraspinatus tendon [abstract]. Anat Rec 100:666, 1948.

159. Grigg P: The role of capsular feedback and pattern generators in shoulder kinematics. In Matsen FA III, Fu FH, and Hawkins RJ (eds): The Shoulder: A Balance of Mobility and Stability. Rosemont, IL: American Academy of Orthopaedic Surgeons, 1993, pp 173-184.

160. Ha'eri GB, Orth MC, and Wiley AM: Shoulder impingement syndrome. Clin Orthop 168:128-132, 1982.

161. Ha'eri GB and Wiley AM: An extensile exposure for subacromial derangements. Can J Surg 23:458-461, 1980.

162. Ha'eri GB and Wiley AM: Advancement of the supraspinatus muscle in the repair of ruptures of the rotator cuff. J Bone Joint Surg Am 63:232-238, 1981.

163. Halder A, Zobitz ME, Schultz E, and An KN: Structural properties of the subscapularis tendon. J Orthop Res 18:829-834, 2000.

164. Halder AM, O'Driscoll SW, Heers G, et al: Biomechanical comparison of effects of supraspinatus tendon detachments, tendon defects, and muscle retractions. J Bone Joint Surg Am 84:780-785, 2002.

165. Hamada K, Okawara Y, Fryer JN, et al: Localization of mRNA of procollagen alpha 1 type I in torn supraspinatus tendons. In situ hybridization using digoxigenin labeled oligonucleotide probe. Clin Orthop 304:18-21, 1994.

166. Hammond G: Complete acromionectomy in the treatment of chronic tendinitis of the shoulder. J Bone Joint Surg Am 44:494-504, 1962.

167. Hammond G: Complete acromionectomy in the treatment of chronic tendinitis of the shoulder. A follow-up of ninety operations of eighty-seven patients. J Bone Joint Surg Am 53:173-180, 1971.

168. Harryman DT II, Hettrich C, Smith KL, et al: A prospective multipractice investigation of patients with full thickness rotator cuff tears: The importance of comorbidities, surgeon, and other covariables on self-assessed shoulder function and health status. J Bone Joint Surg Am 85:690-696, 2003.

169. Harryman DT II, Mack LA, Wang KY, et al: Repairs of the rotator cuff. J Bone Joint Surg Am 73:982-989, 1991.

170. Harryman DT II, Matsen FA III, and Sidles JA: Arthroscopic management of refractory shoulder stiffness. Arthroscopy 13:133-147, 1997.

171. Harryman DT II, Sidles JA, Clark JM, et al: Translation of the humeral head on the glenoid with passive glenohumeral motion. J Bone Joint Surg Am 72:1334-1342, 1990.

172. Hatakeyama Y, Itoi E, Urayama M, et al: Effect of superior capsule and coracohumeral ligament release on strain in the repaired rotator cuff tendon. A cadaveric study. Am J Sports Med 29:633-640, 2001.

173. Haudek: Wien Klin Wochenschr 43, 1911.

174. Hawkins RH and Dunlop R: Nonoperative treatment of rotator cuff tears. Clin Orthop 321:178-188, 1995.

175. Hawkins RJ and Brock RM: Anterior acromioplasty: Early results for impingement with intact rotator cuff. Orthop Trans 3:274, 1979.

176. Hawkins RJ, Chris AD, and Kiefer G: Failed anterior acromioplasty. Paper presented at the Third Open Meeting of the American Shoulder and Elbow Surgeons, 1987, San Francisco.

177. Hawkins RJ and Kennedy JC: Impingement syndrome in athletes. Am J Sports Med 8:151-158, 1980.

178. Hawkins RJ, Misamore GW, and Hobeika PE: Surgery of full thickness rotator cuff tears. J Bone Joint Surg Am 67:1349-1355, 1985.

179. Hawkins RJ, Saddamis S, Moor J, et al: Arthroscopic subacromial decompression: A two-to-four-year follow-up. Paper presented at the Annual Meeting of Arthroscopy Association of North America, 1992.

180. Hazlett JW: Tears of the rotator cuff. Proceedings of the Dewar Orthopaedic Club. J Bone Joint Surg Br 53:772, 1971.

181. Hedtmann A and Fett H: Ultrasonography of the shoulder in subacromial syndromes with disorders and injuries of the rotator cuff. Orthopade 24:498-508, 1995.

182. Heikel HVA: Rupture of the rotator cuff of the shoulder: Experiences of surgical treatment. Acta Orthop Scand 39:477-492, 1968.

183. Heineke: Die Anatomie und Pathologie der Schleimbeutel und Sehnenscheiden. Erlangen, 1868.

184. Hollingworth GR, Ellis RM, and Hattersley TS: Comparison of injection techniques for shoulder pain: Results of a double blind, randomized study. BMJ 287:1339-1341, 1983.

185. Hollis JM, Lyon RM, Marcin JP, et al: Effect of age and loading axis on the failure properties of the human ACL. Paper presented at the 34th Annual Meeting of the Orthopedic Research Society, 1988, Atlanta.

186. Hollister MS, Mack LA, Patten RM, et al: Association of sonographically detected subacromial/subdeltoid bursal effusion and intraarticular fluid with rotator cuff tear. AJR Am J Roentgenol 165:605-608, 1995.

187. Holzknecht G: Uber Bursitis mit Konkrementbildung. Wien Med Wochenschr 43:2757, 1911.

188. Howell SM, Imobersteg AM, Segar DH, and Marone PJ: Clarification of the role of the supraspinatus muscle in shoulder function. J Bone Joint Surg Am 68:398-404, 1986.

189. Hyvonen P, Lohi S, and Jalovaara P: Open acromioplasty does not prevent the progression of an impingement syndrome to a tear. Nine-year follow-up of 96 cases. J Bone Joint Surg Br 80:813-816, 1998.

190. Iannotti J: Full-thickness rotator cuff tears: Factors affecting surgical outcome. J Am Acad Orthop Surg 2:87-95, 1994.

191. Iannotti JP, Zlatkin MB, Esterhai JL, et al: Magnetic resonance imaging of the shoulder. Sensitivity, specificity, and predictive value. J Bone Joint Surg Am 73:17-29, 1991.

192. Inman VT, Saunders JBDCM, and Abbott LC: Observations on the function of the shoulder joint. J Bone Joint Surg Am 26:1-30, 1944.

193. Ismail AM, Balakishnan R, and Rajakumar MK: Rupture of patellar ligament after steroid infiltration. J Bone Joint Surg Br 51:503, 1969.

194. Itoi E, Berglund LJ, Grabowski JJ, et al: Tensile properties of the supraspinatus tendon. J Orthop Res 13:578-584, 1995.

195. Itoi E and Tabata S: Incomplete rotator cuff tears. Results of operative treatment. Clin Orthop 284:128-135, 1992.

196. Itoi E and Tabata S: Conservative treatment of rotator cuff tears. Clin Orthop 275:165-173, 1992.

197. Jackson DL, Farrage J, Hynninen BC, and Caborn DN: Suprascapular neuropathy in athletes: Case reports. Clin J Sports Med 5:134-136, 1995.

198. Jackson DW: Chronic rotator cuff impingement in the throwing athlete. Am J Sports Med 4:231-240, 1976.

199. Jarjavay JF: Sur la luxation du tendon de la longue portion du muscle biceps humeral; sur la luxation des tendons des muscles peroniers latéraux. Gazette Hebdomadaire de Médecine et de Chir 21:325, 1867.

200. Jens J: The role of the subscapularis muscle in recurring dislocation of the shoulder [abstract]. J Bone Joint Surg Br 34:780, 1964.

201. Jiang Y, Zhao J, Van Holsbeeck MT, et al: Trabecular microstructure and surface changes in the greater tuberosity in rotator cuff tears. Skeletal Radiol 31:522-528, 2002.

202. Jobe CM: Posterior superior glenoid impingement: Expanded spectrum. Arthroscopy 11:530-536, 1995.

203. Jobe FW and Kvitne RS: Shoulder pain in the overhand or throwing athlete. Orthop Rev 18:963-975, 1989.

204. Jobe FW and Moynes DR: Delineation of diagnostic criteria and a rehabilitation program for rotator cuff injuries. Am J Sports Med 10:336-339, 1982.

205. Joessel D: Uber die Recidine der Humerus-Luxationen. Dtsch Z Chir 13:167-184, 1880.

206. Johansson JE and Barrington TW: Coracoacromial ligament division. Am J Sports Med 12:138-141, 1984.

207. Jost B, Pfirrmann CW, Gerber C, and Switzerland Z: Clinical outcome after structural failure of rotator cuff repairs. J Bone Joint Surg Am 82:304-314, 2000.

208. Julliard: La coracoidite. Rev Med Suisse Romande 12:47, 1933.

209. Kaneko K, DeMouy EH, and Brunet ME: Massive rotator cuff tears. Screening by routine radiographs. Clin Imaging 19:8-11, 1995.

210. Kannus P, Leppala J, Lehto M, et al: A rotator cuff rupture produces permanent osteoporosis in the affected extremity, but not in the those with whom shoulder function has returned to normal. J Bone Miner Res 10:1263-1271, 1995.

211. Karas SE and Giachello TA: Subscapularis transfer for reconstruction of massive tears of the rotator cuff. J Bone Joint Surg Am 78:239-245, 1996.

212. Kennedy JC and Willis RB: The effects of local steroid injections on tendons: A biomechanical and microscopic correlative study. Am J Sports Med 4:11-21, 1976.

213. Kerlan RK, Jobe FW, and Blazina ME: Throwing Injuries of the Shoulder and Elbow in Adults, vol 6. St Louis: CV Mosby, 1975.

214. Kernwein GA, Roseberg B, and Sneed WR: Aids in the differential diagnosis of the painful shoulder syndrome. Clin Orthop 20:11-20, 1961.

215. Kerwein GH, Rosenburg B, and Sneed WR: Arthrographic studies of the shoulder joint. J Bone Joint Surg Am 39:1267-1279, 1957.

216. Kessel L and Watson M: The painful arc syndrome. Clinical classification as a guide to management. J Bone Joint Surg Br 59:166-172, 1977.

217. Keyes EL: Observations on rupture of supraspinatus tendon. Based upon a study of 73 cadavers. Ann Surg 97:849-856, 1933.

218. Keyes EL: Anatomical observations on senile changes in the shoulder. J Bone Joint Surg Am 17:953, 1935.

219. Kieft GJ, Bloem JL, Rozing PM, and Oberman WR: Rotator cuff impingement syndrome: MR imaging. Radiology 166:211-214, 1988.

220. Kilcoyne RF and Matsen FA III: Rotator cuff tear measurement by arthropneumotomography. AJR Am J Roentgenol 140:315-318, 1983.

221. Killoran PJ, Marcove RC, and Freiberger RH: Shoulder arthroscopy. AJR Am J Roentgenol 103:658-668, 1968.

222. Kirkley A, Litchfield RB, Jackowski DM, and Lo IK: The use of the impingement test as a predictor of outcome following subacromial decompression for rotator cuff tendinosis. Arthroscopy 18:8-15, 2002.

223. Kirschenbaum D, Coyle MPJ, Leddy JP, et al: Shoulder strength with rotator cuff tears. Pre- and postoperative analysis. Clin Orthop 288:174-178, 1993.

224. Kneeland JB, Middleton WD, and Carnera GF: MR imaging of the shoulder: Diagnosis of rotator cuff tears. AJR Am J Roentgenol 149:333-337, 1987.

225. Komar J: Eine wichtige Urasache des Schulterschmerzes: Incisurascapulae-Syndrom. Fortschr Neurol Psychiatr 44:644-648, 1976.

226. Kopell HP and Thompson WAL: Suprascapular nerve. In Peripheral Entrapment Neuropathies. Baltimore: Williams & Wilkins, 1963, pp 130-142.

227. Kumagai J, Sarkar K, and Uhthoff HK: The collagen types in the attachment zone of rotator cuff tendons in the elderly: An immunohistochemical study. J Rheumatol 21:2096-2100, 1994.

228. Küster E: Ueber habituelle Schutter Luxation. Verh Dtsch Ges Chir 11:112-114, 1882.

229. Kutsuma T, Akaoka K, Kinoshita H, et al: The results of surgical management of rotator cuff tear. Shoulder Joint 6:136, 1982.

230. Laing PG: The arterial supply of the adult humerus. J Bone Joint Surg 38:1105-1116, 1956.

231. Lazarus MD, Harryman DT II, Yung SW, et al: Anterosuperior humeral displacement: Limitation by the coracoacromial arch. Paper presented at the Annual Meeting of the American Association of Orthopaedic Surgeons, 1995, Orlando, FL.

232. Lee HB: Avulsion and rupture of the tendo calcaneus after injection of hydrocortisone. BMJ 2:395, 1957.

233. Lee PN, Lee M, Haq AMMM, et al: Periarthritis of the shoulder. Ann Rheum Dis 33:116-119, 1974.

234. Lee SB, Itoi E, O'Driscoll SW, and An KN: Contact geometry at the undersurface of the acromion with and without a rotator cuff tear. Arthroscopy 17:365-372, 2001.

235. Lee SB, Kim KJ, O'Driscoll SW, Morrey BF, et al: Dynamic glenohumeral stability provided by the rotator cuff muscles in the mid-range and end-range of motion. A study in cadavera. J Bone Joint Surg Am 82:849-857, 2000.

236. Lee SB, Nakajima T, Luo ZP, et al: The bursal and articular sides of the supraspinatus tendon have a different compressive stiffness. Clin Biomech (Bristol, Avon) 15:241-247, 2000.

237. Lee TQ, Black AD, Tibone JE, and McMahon PJ: Release of the coracoacromial ligament can lead to glenohumeral laxity: A biomechanical study. J Shoulder Elbow Surg 10:68-72, 2001.

238. Lehman C, Cuomo F, Kummer FJ, and Zuckerman JD: The incidence of full thickness rotator cuff tears in a large cadaveric population. Bull Hosp Jt Dis 54:30-31, 1995.

239. Leivseth G and Reikeras O: Changes in muscle fiber cross-sectional area and concentrations of Na, K-ATPase in deltoid muscle in patients with impingement syndrome of the shoulder. J Orthop Sports Phys Ther 19:146-149, 1994.

240. Leroux JL, Codine P, Thomas E, et al: Isokinetic evaluation of rotational strength in normal shoulders and shoulders with impingement syndrome. Clin Orthop 304:108-115, 1994.

241. Leroux JL, Thomas E, Bonnel F, and Blotman F: Diagnostic value of clinical tests for shoulder impingement syndrome. Rev Rhum Engl Ed 62:423-428, 1995.

242. Levy HJ, Gardner RD, and Lemak LJ: Arthroscopic subacromial decompression in the treatment of full thickness rotator tears. Arthroscopy 7:8-13, 1991.

243. Levy HJ, Urie JW, and Delaney LG: Arthroscopic-assisted rotator cuff repair: Preliminary results. Arthroscopy 6:55-60, 1990.

244. Liberson F: Os acromiale—a contested anomaly. J Bone Joint Surg 19:683-689, 1937.

245. Lie S and Mast WA: Subacromial bursography: Technique and clinical application. Tech Dev Instrum 144:626-630, 1982.

246. Lieber RL: Skeletal Muscle Structure and Function. Baltimore: Williams & Wilkins, 1992, p 314.

247. Lieber RL and Friden J: Neuromuscular stablization of the shoulder girdle. In Matsen FA III, Fu FH, and Hawkins RJ (eds): The Shoulder: A Balance of Mobility and Stability. Rosemont, IL: American Academy of Orthopaedic Surgeons, 1993, pp 91-106.

248. Lilleby H: Shoulder arthroscopy. Acta Orthop Scand 55:561-566, 1984.

249. Lindblom K: Arthrography and roentgenography in ruptures of the tendon of the shoulder joint. Acta Radiol 20:548, 1939.

250. Lindblom K: On pathogenesis of ruptures of the tendon aponeurosis of the shoulder joint. Acta Radiol 20:563, 1939.

251. Lindblom K and Palmer I: Ruptures of the tendon aponeurosis of the shoulder joint—the so-called supraspinatus ruptures. Acta Chir Scand 82:133-142, 1939.

252. Litaker D, Pioro M, El Bilbeisi H, and Brems J: Returning to the bedside: Using the history and physical examination to identify rotator cuff tears. J Am Geriatr Soc 48:1633-1637, 2000.

253. Liu J, Hughes RE, O'Driscoll SW, and An KN: Biomechanical effect of medial advancement of the supraspinatus tendon. A study in cadavera. J Bone Joint Surg Am 80:853-859, 1998.

254. Liu SH: Arthroscopically assisted rotator cuff repair. J Bone Joint Surg Br 76:592-595, 1994.

255. Liu SH and Boynton E: Posterior superior impingement of the rotator cuff on the glenoid rim as a cause of shoulder pain in the overhead athlete. Arthroscopy 9:697-699, 1993.

256. Lohr JF and Uhthoff HK: The microvascular pattern of the supraspinatus tendon. Clin Orthop 254:35-38, 1990.

257. Lund IM, Donde R, and Knudsen EA: Persistent local cutaneous atrophy following corticosteroid injection for tendinitis. Rheumatol Rehabil 18:91-93, 1979.

258. Lundberg BJ: The correlation of clinical evaluation with operative findings and prognosis in rotator cuff rupture. In Bayley I and Kessel L (eds): Shoulder Surgery. Berlin: Springer-Verlag, 1982, pp 35-38.

259. Luopajarvi T, Kuorinka I, Virolainen M, and Holmberg M: Prevalence of tenosynovitis and other injuries of the upper extremities in repetitive work. Scand J Work Environ Health 5:48-55, 1979.

260. MacDonald PB, Clark P, and Sutherland K: An analysis of the diagnostic accuracy of the Hawkins and Neer subacromial impingement signs. J Shoulder Elbow Surg 9:299-301, 2000.

261. Mack LA and Matsen FA III: Rotator cuff. Clin Diagn Ultrasound 30:113-133, 1995.

262. Mack LA, Matsen FA III, and Kilcoyne RF: Ultrasound: US evaluation of the rotator cuff. Radiology 157:205-209, 1985.

263. Mack LA, Nuberg DS, Matsen FA III, et al: Sonography of the postoperative shoulder [abstract]. Paper presented at the Annual Meeting of the American Roentgen Ray Society, 1987, Miami Beach, FL.

264. Mack LA, Nyberg DA, and Matsen FA III: Sonography of the postoperative shoulder. AJR Am J Roentgenol 150:1089-1093, 1988.

265. Macnab I: Rotator cuff tendinitis. Ann R Coll Surg Engl 53:271-287, 1973.

266. Macnab I and Hastings D: Rotator cuff tendinitis. Can Med Assoc J 99:91-98, 1968.

267. Mankin HJ and Conger KA: The acute effects of intra-articular hydrocortisone on articular cartilage in rabbits. J Bone Joint Surg Am 48:1383, 1966.

268. Martin SD, Baumgarten TE, and Andrews JR: Arthroscopic resection of the distal aspect of the clavicle with concomitant subacromial decompression. J Bone Joint Surg Am 83:328-335, 2001.

269. Matsen FA III, Lippitt SB, Sidles JA, and Harryman DT II: Practical Evaluation and Management of the Shoulder. Philadelphia: WB Saunders, 1994, pp 1-242.

270. Matsumoto F, Uhthoff HK, Trudel G, and Loehr JF: Delayed tendon reattachment does not reverse atrophy and fat accumulation of the supraspinatus—an experimental study in rabbits. J Orthop Res 20:357-363, 2002.

271. Matthews LS, Sonstegard DA, and Phelps DB: A biomechanical study of rabbit patellar tendon: Effects of steroid injection. J Sports Med 2:9, 1974.

272. McCarty DJ, Haverson PB, Carrera GF, et al: "Milwaukee Shoulder": Association of microspheroids containing hydroxyapatite crystals, active collagenase, and neutral protease with rotator cuff defects. I. Clinical aspects. Arthritis Rheum 24:353-354, 1981.

273. McLaughlin HL: Lesions of the musculotendinous cuff of the shoulder. I. The exposure and treatment of tears with retraction. J Bone Joint Surg 26:31-51, 1944.

274. McLaughlin HL: Rupture of the rotator cuff. J Bone Joint Surg 44A:979-983, 1962.

275. McLaughlin HL: Repair of major cuff ruptures. Surg Clin North Am 43:1535-1540, 1963.

276. McLaughlin HL: Lesions of the musculotendinous cuff of the shoulder. The exposure and treatment of tears with retraction. Clin Orthop 304:3-9, 1994.

277. McLaughlin HL and Asherman EG: Lesions of the musculotendinous cuff of the shoulder. IV. Some observations based upon the results of surgical repair. J Bone Joint Surg Am 33:76-86, 1951.

278. McMaster PE: Tendon and muscle ruptures: Clinical and experimental studies on the causes and location of subcutaneous ruptures. J Bone Joint Surg Am 15:705-722, 1933.

279. Melmed EP: Spontaneous bilateral rupture of the calcaneal tendon during steroid therapy. J Bone Joint Surg Br 47:104, 1965.

280. Meyer AW: Further evidence of attrition in the human body. Am J Anat 34:241-267, 1924.

281. Meyer AW: The minute anatomy of attrition lesions. J Bone Joint Surg Am 13:341, 1931.

282. Meyer AW and Kessler: Strassbourg Med 2:205, 1926.

283. Michelsson JE and Bakalim G: Resection of the acromion in the treatment of persistent rotator cuff syndrome of the shoulder. Acta Orthop Scand 48:607-611, 1977.

284. Middleton WD: Ultrasonography of rotator cuff pathology. Top Magn Reson Imaging 6:133-138, 1994.

285. Middleton WD, Edelstein G, Reinus WR, et al: Sonographic detection of rotator cuff tears. AJR Am J Roentgenol 144:349-353, 1985.

286. Middleton WD, Reinus WR, Melson GL, et al: Pitfalls of rotator cuff sonography. AJR Am J Roentgenol 146:555-560, 1986.

287. Middleton WD, Reinus WR, Totty WG, et al: Ultrasonographic evaluation of the rotator cuff and biceps tendon. J Bone Joint Surg Am 68:440-450, 1986.

288. Mikasa M: Subacromial bursography. J Jpn Orthop Assoc 53:225, 1979.

289. Milgrom C, Schaffler M, Gilbert S, and van Holsbeeck M: Rotator cuff changes in asymptomatic adults. The effect of age, hand dominance and gender. J Bone Joint Surg Br 77:296-298, 1995.

290. Mink JH, Harris E, and Rappaport M: Rotator cuff tears: Evaluation using double-contrast shoulder arthrography. Radiology 153:621-623, 1985.

291. Misamore GW, Ziegler DW, and Rushton JL II: Repair of the rotator cuff. A comparison of results in two populations of patients. J Bone Joint Surg Am 77:1335-1339, 1995.

292. Montgomery TJ, Yerger B, and Savoie FH: Management of full thickness tears of the rotator cuff: A comparison of arthroscopic débridement with open repair. Paper presented at the 8th Annual Open Meeting of the American Shoulder and Elbow Surgeons, 1992, Washington, DC.

293. Morrison DS: The use of magnetic resonance imaging in the diagnosis of rotator cuff tears. Paper presented at the Fourth Meeting of the American Shoulder and Elbow Surgeons, 1988, Atlanta.

294. Morrison DS and Bigliani LU: The Clinical Significance of Variations in Acromial Morphology. Paper presented at the 3rd Open Meeting of the American Shoulder and Elbow Surgeons, 1987, San Francisco.

295. Moseley HF: Ruptures to the Rotator Cuff. Springfield, IL: Charles C Thomas, 1952.

296. Moseley HF: Shoulder Lesions, 3rd ed. Edinburgh: Livingstone, 1969.

297. Moseley HF and Goldie I: The arterial pattern of the rotator cuff of the shoulder. J Bone Joint Surg Br 45:780, 1963.

298. Motamedi AR, Urrea LH, Hancock RE, et al: Accuracy of magnetic resonance imaging in determining the presence and size of recurrent rotator cuff tears. J Shoulder Elbow Surg 11:6-10, 2002.

299. Mudge MK, Wood VE, and Frykman GK: Rotator cuff tears associated with os acromiale. J Bone Joint Surg Am 66:427-429, 1984.

300. Murray JWG: A surgical approach for entrapment neuropathy of the suprascapular nerve. Orthop Rev 3:33-35, 1974.

301. Murrell GA and Walton JR: Diagnosis of rotator cuff tears. Lancet 357:769-770, 2001.

302. Nakagaki K, Tomita Y, Sakurai G, et al: Anatomical study on the atrophy of supraspinatus muscle belly with cuff tear. Nippon Seikeigeka Gakkai Zasshi 68:516-521, 1994.

303. Nakagawa S, Yoneda M, Hayashida K, Wakitani S, et al : Greater tuberosity notch: An important indicator of articular-side partial rotator cuff tears in the shoulders of throwing athletes. Am J Sports Med 29:762-770, 2001.

304. Neer CS II: Anterior acromioplasty for the chronic impingement syndrome in the shoulder: A preliminary report. J Bone Joint Surg Am 54:41-50, 1972.

305. Neer CS II: Unfused acromial epiphysis in impingement and cuff tears. Paper presented at the 45th Annual Meeting of the American Academy of Orthopaedic Surgeons, 1978, Dallas.
306. Neer CS II: Impingement lesions. Clin Orthop 173:70-77, 1983.
307. Neer CS II: Shoulder Reconstruction. Philadelphia: WB Saunders, 1990, pp 73-77.
308. Neer CS II, Craig EV, and Fukuda H: Cuff-tear arthropathy. J Bone Joint Surg Am 65:1232-1244, 1983.
309. Neer CS II, Flatow EL, and Lech O: Tears of the rotator cuff. Long-term results of anterior acromioplasty and repair. Paper presented at the Fourth Meeting of the American Shoulder and Elbow Surgeons, 1988, Atlanta.
310. Neer CS II and Marberry TA: On the disadvantages of radical acromionectomy. J Bone Joint Surg Am 63:416-419, 1981.
311. Neer CS II and Welsh RP: The shoulder in sports. Orthop Clin North Am 8:583-591, 1977.
312. Nelson DH: Arthrography of the shoulder. Br J Radiol 25:134, 1952.
313. Neviaser JS: Ruptures of the rotator cuff of the shoulder. New concepts in the diagnosis and operative treatment of chronic ruptures. Arch Surg 102:483-485, 1971.
314. Neviaser JS, Neviaser RJ, and Neviaser TJ: The repair of chronic massive ruptures of the rotator cuff of the shoulder by use of a freeze-dried rotator cuff. J Bone Joint Surg Am 60:681-684, 1978.
315. Neviaser RJ: Tears of the rotator cuff. Orthop Clin North Am 11:295-306, 1980.
316. Neviaser RJ and Neviaser TJ: Transfer of subscapularis and teres minor for massive defects of rotator cuff. In Bayley I and Kessel L (eds): Shoulder Surgery. Berlin: Springer-Verlag, 1982, pp 60-63.
317. Neviaser RJ, Neviaser TJ, and Neviaser JS: Anterior dislocation of the shoulder and rotator cuff rupture. Clin Orthop 291:103-106, 1993.
318. Neviaser TJ, Neviaser RJ, and Neviaser JS: The four-in-one arthroplasty for the painful arc syndrome. Clin Orthop 163:107-112, 1982.
319. Neviaser TJ, Neviaser RJ, and Neviaser JS: Incomplete rotator cuff tears. A technique for diagnosis and treatment. Clin Orthop 306:12-16, 1994.
320. Nicholson GP, Goodman DA, Flatow EA, and Bigliani LU: The acromion: Morphologic condition and age-related changes: A study of 420 scapulas. J Shoulder Elbow Surg 5:1-11, 1996.
321. Nixon JE and DiStefano V: Ruptures of the rotator cuff. Orthop Clin North Am 6:423-447, 1975.
322. Nobuhara K, Hata Y, and Komai M: Surgical procedure and results of repair of massive tears of the rotator cuff. Clin Orthop 304:54-59, 1994.
323. Norquist BM, Goldberg BA, and Matsen FA 3rd: Challenges in evaluating patients lost to follow-up in clinical studies of rotator cuff tears. J Bone Joint Surg Am 82:838-842, 2000.
324. Norris TR, Fischer J, and Bigliani LU: The unfused acromial epiphysis and its relationship to impingement syndromes. Orthop Trans 7:505, 1983.
325. Oberholtzer J: Die Arthropneumoradiographe bei habitueller Schulterluxatio. Rontgenpraxis 5:589-590, 1933.
326. Ogata S and Uhthoff HK: Acromial enthesopathy and rotator cuff tear. A radiologic and histologic postmortem investigation of the coracoacromial arch. Clin Orthop 254:39-48, 1990.
327. Ogilvie-Harris DL and Demaziere A: Arthroscopic débridement versus open repair for rotator cuff tears. J Bone Joint Surg Br 75:416-420, 1993.
328. Ogilvie-Harris DJ and Wiley AM: Arthroscopic surgery of the shoulder: A general appraisal. J Bone Joint Surg Br 68:201-207, 1986.
329. Ogilvie-Harris DJ, Wiley AM, and Sattarian J: Failed acromioplasty for impingement syndrome. J Bone Joint Surg Br 72:1070-1072, 1990.
330. Okuda Y, Gorski JP, An KN, and Amadio PC: Biochemical histological and biochemical analysis of canine tendon. J Orthop Res 5:60-68, 1987.
331. Olive RJJ and Marsh HO: Ultrasonography of rotator cuff tears. Clin Orthop 282:110-113, 1992.
332. Olsewski JM and Depew AD: Arthroscopic subacromial decompression and rotator cuff débridement for stage II and stage III impingement. Arthroscopy 10:61-68, 1994.
333. Otis JC, Jiang CC, Wickiewicz TL, et al: Changes in the moment arms of the rotator cuff and deltoid muscles with abduction and rotation. J Bone Joint Surg Am 76:667-676, 1994.
334. Owen RS, Iannotti JP, Kneeland JB, et al: Shoulder after surgery: MR imaging with surgical validation. Radiology 186:443-447, 1993.
335. Ozaki J, Fujimoto S, and Masuhara K: Repair of chronic massive rotator cuff tears with synthetic fabrics. In Bateman JE and Welsh RP (eds): Surgery of the Shoulder. Philadelphia: BC Decker, 1984, pp 185-191.
336. Ozaki J, Fujimoto S, Nakagawa Y, et al: Tears of the rotator cuff of the shoulder associated with pathological changes in the acromion. J Bone Joint Surg 70:1224-1230, 1988.
337. Ozaki J, Fujimoto S, Tomita K, and al: Non-perforated superficial surface cuff tears associated with hydrops of the subacromial bursa. Katakansetsu (Fukuoka) 9:52, 1985.
338. Paavolainen P and Ahovuo J: Ultrasonography and arthrography in the diagnosis of tears of the rotator cuff. J Bone Joint Surg 76:335-340, 1994.
339. Packer NP, Calvert PT, Bayley JIL, and Kessel L: Operative treatment of chronic ruptures of the rotator cuff of the shoulder. J Bone Joint Surg Br 65:171-175, 1983.
340. Painter: Boston Med Surg J 156:345, 1907.
341. Palette GA Jr, Warner JP, Altchek DW, et al: Arthroscopic rotator cuff repair: Evaluation of results and comparison of techniques. Paper presented at the 60th Annual Meeting of the American Academy of Orthopaedic Surgeons, 1993, San Francisco.
342. Palmer WE, Brown JH, and Rosenthal DI: Rotator cuff: Evaluation with fat-suppressed arthrography. Radiology 188:683-687, 1993.
343. Pappas AM, Zawacki RM, and McCarthy CF: Rehabilitation of the pitching shoulder. Am J Sports Med 13:223-235, 1985.
344. Pappas AM, Zawacki RM, and Sullivan TJ: Biomechanics of baseball pitching. A preliminary report. Am J Sports Med 13:216-222, 1985.
345. Park JY, Lee GW, Kim Y, and Yoo MJ: The efficacy of continuous intrabursal infusion with morphine and bupivacaine for postoperative analgesia after subacromial arthroscopy. Reg Anesth Pain Med 27:145-149, 2002.
346. Paulos LE and Franklin JL: Arthroscopic shoulder decompression development and application. Am J Sports Med 18:235-244, 1990.
347. Paulos LE, Harner CD, and Parker RD: Arthroscopic subacromial decompression for impingement syndrome of the shoulder. Tech Orthop 3:33-39, 1988.
348. Paulos LE and Kody MH: Arthroscopically enhanced "miniapproach" to rotator cuff repair. Am J Sports Med 22:19-25, 1994.
349. Payr E: Gelenk "Sperren" und "Ankylosen" Uber die "Schultersteifen verschiedener Ursache und die sogenannte "Periarthrities humero-scapularis," Ihre Behandlung. Zentralbl Chir 58:2993-3003, 1931.
350. Penny JN and Smith C: The prevention and treatment of swimmer's shoulder. Can J Appl Sport Sci 5:195-202, 1980.
351. Penny JN and Welsh RP: Shoulder impingement syndromes in athletes and their surgical management. Am J Sports Med 9:11-15, 1981.
352. Peterson C: Long-term results of rotator cuff repair. In Bayley I and Kessel L (eds): Shoulder Surgery. Berlin: Springer-Verlag, 1982, pp 64-69.
353. Peterson CJ and Gentz CF: Ruptures of the supraspinatous tendon—the significance of distally pointing acromioclavicular osteophytes. Clin Orthop 174:143, 1983.
354. Pettersson G: Rupture of the tendon aponeurosis of the shoulder joint in antero-inferior dislocation. Acta Chir Scand Suppl 77:1-187, 1942.
355. Phipps GJ and Hoffer MM: Latissimus dorsi and teres major transfer to rotator cuff for Erb's palsy. J Shoulder Elbow Surg 4:124-129, 1995.
356. Picot C: Neuropathie canalaire du nerf sus-scapulaire. Rhumatologie 21:73-75, 1969.
357. Pingaud and Charvot: Scapulalgie. In Dechambre. Dictionaire Encyclopeádique des Sciences Médicales, vol. 11. Paris, 1879, p 232.
358. Poppen NK and Walker PS: Normal and abnormal motion of the shoulder. J Bone Joint Surg Am 58:195, 1976.
359. Post M: Rotator cuff repair with carbon filament: A preliminary report of five cases. Clin Orthop 196:154-158, 1985.
360. Post M and Cohen J: Impingement syndrome—a review of late stage II and early stage III lesions. Paper presented at the First Open Meeting of the American Shoulder and Elbow Surgeons, 1985.
361. Post M and Cohen J: Impingement syndrome. Clin Orthop 207:126-132, 1986.
362. Post M, Silver R, and Singh M: Rotator cuff tear: Diagnosis and treatment. Clin Orthop 173:78, 1983.
363. Postacchini F, Perugia D, and Rampoldi M: Rotator cuff tears: Results of surgical repairs. Ital J Orthop Traumatol 18:173-188, 1992.
364. Pujadas GM: Coraco-acromial ligament syndrome. J Bone Joint Surg Am 52:1261-1262, 1970.
365. Putz R and Reichelt A: Structural findings of the coracoacromial ligament in rotator cuff rupture, tendinosis calcarea and supraspinatus syndrome. Z Orthop Ihre Grenzgeb 128:46-50, 1990.
366. Quinn SF, Sheley RC, Demlow TA, and Szumowski J: Rotator cuff tendon tears: Evaluation with fat-suppressed MR imaging with arthroscopic correlation in 100 patients. Radiology 195:497-500, 1995.
367. Raggio CL, Warren RF, and Sculco T: Surgical treatment of impingement syndrome: A four year follow-up. Paper presented at the First Open Meeting of the American Shoulder and Elbow Surgeons, 1985.
368. Rask MR: Suprascapular nerve entrapment: A report of two cases treated with suprascapular notch resection. Clin Orthop 123:73-75, 1977.
369. Rathbun JB and Macnab I: The microvascular pattern of the rotator cuff. J Bone Joint Surg Br 52:540-553, 1970.
370. Reeves B: Arthrography of the shoulder. J Bone Joint Surg Br 48:424-435, 1966.
371. Regan WD and Richards RR: Subacromial pressure pre and post acromioplasty: A cadaveric study. Orthop Trans 13:671, 1989.
372. Rengachary SS, Neff JP, Singer PA, and Brackett CE: Suprascapular entrapment neuropathy: A clinical, anatomical, and comparative study. Neurosurgery 5:441-446, 1979.
373. Renoux S, Monet J, Pupin P, et al: Preliminary note on the biometric data relating to the human coracoacromial arch. Surg Radiol Anat 8:189-195, 1986.
374. Resnick D: Shoulder arthrography. Radiol Clin North Am 19:243-252, 1981.
375. Richardson AB, Jobe FW, and Collins HR: The shoulder in competitive swimming. Am J Sports Med 8:159-163, 1980.
376. Riley GP, Harrall RL, Constant CR, et al: Tendon degeneration and chronic shoulder pain: Changes in the collagen composition of the human rotator cuff tendons in rotator cuff tendinitis. Ann Rheum Dis 53:359-366, 1994.
377. Riley GP, Harrall RL, Constant CR, et al: Glycosaminoglycans of human rotator cuff tendons: Changes with age and in chronic rotator cuff tendinitis. Ann Rheum Dis 53:367-376, 1994.

378. Robertson PL, Schweitzer ME, Mitchell DG, et al: Rotator cuff disorders: Interobserver and intraobserver variation in diagnosis with MR imaging. Radiology 194:831-835, 1995.
379. Rocks JA: Intrinsic shoulder pain syndrome. Phys Ther 59:153-159, 1979.
380. Rockwood CA Jr: Personal communication, 1983 and 1987.
381. Rockwood CA Jr and Lyons FR: Shoulder impingement syndrome: Diagnosis, radiographic evaluation, and treatment with a modified Neer acromioplasty. J Bone Joint Surg Am 75:473-474, 1993.
382. Rockwood CA Jr, Williams GR Jr, and Burkhead WZ Jr: Débridement of degenerative, irreparable lesions of the rotator cuff. J Bone Joint Surg Am 77:857-866, 1995.
383. Roh MS, Wang VM, April EW, et al: Anterior and posterior musculotendinous anatomy of the supraspinatus. J Shoulder Elbow Surg 9:436-440, 2000.
384. Rokito AS, Zuckerman JD, Gallagher MA, and Cuomo F: Strength after surgical repair of the rotator cuff. J Shoulder Elbow Surg 5:12-17, 1996.
385. Romeo AA, Hang DW, Bach BR Jr, and Shott S: Repair of full thickness rotator cuff tears. Gender, age, and other factors affecting outcome. Clin Orthop 367:243-255, 1999.
386. Rossi F, Ternamian PJ, Cerciello G, and Walch G: Posterosuperior glenoid rim impingement in athletes: The diagnostic value of traditional radiology and magnetic resonance. Radiol Med (Torino) 87:22-27, 1994.
387. Rostron PK, Orth MCH, Wigan FRCS, and Calver RF: Subcutaneous atrophy following methylprednisolone injection in Osgood-Schlatter epiphysitis. J Bone Joint Surg Am 61:627-628, 1979.
388. Rothman RH and Parke WW: The vascular anatomy of the rotator cuff. Clin Orthop 41:176-186, 1965.
389. Rowlands LK, Wertsch JJ, Primack SJ, et al: Kinesiology of the empty can test. Am J Phys Med Rehabil 74:302-304, 1995.
390. Roye RP, Grana WA, and Yates C: Arthroscopic subacromial decompression: Two-to-seven-year follow-up. Arthroscopy 11:301-306, 1995.
391. Ryu RK: Arthroscopic subacromial decompression: A clinical review. Arthroscopy 8:141-147, 1992.
392. Sachs RA, Stone ML, and Devine S: Open vs. arthroscopic acromioplasty: A prospective, randomized study. Arthroscopy 10:248-254, 1994.
393. Saha AK: Dynamic stability of the glenohumeral joint. Acta Orthop Scand 42:491-505, 1971.
394. Salter RB, Gross A, and Hall JH: Hydrocortisone arthropathy: An experimental investigation. Can Med Assoc J 97:374, 1967.
395. Samilson RL: Congenital and developmental anomalies of the shoulder girdle. Orthop Clin North Am 11:219-231, 1980.
396. Samilson RL and Binder WF: Symptomatic full thickness tears of the rotator cuff: An analysis of 292 shoulders in 276 patients. Orthop Clin North Am 6:449-466, 1975.
397. Samilson RL, Raphael RL, Post L, et al: Arthrography of the shoulder. Clin Orthop 20:21-31, 1961.
398. Schaefer O, Winterer J, Lohrmann C, Laubenberger J, et al: Magnetic resonance imaging for supraspinatus muscle atrophy after cuff repair. Clin Orthop 403:93-99, 2002.
399. Schaár W and Zweifel C: Das os acromiale und seine klinische Bedeutung. In Breitner B and Nordmann O (eds): Bruns Beiträse zur klinischen Chir. Berlin: Urban & Schwarzenberg, 1936, p 101.
400. Scheib JS: Diagnosis and rehabilitation of the shoulder impingement syndrome in the overhand and throwing athletes. Rheum Dis Clin North Am 16:971-988, 1990.
401. Schilf E: Über eine einseitige Lähmung des Nervus suprascapularis. Nervenarzt 23:306-307, 1952.
402. Schneeberger AG, Nyffeler RW, and Gerber C: Structural changes of the rotator cuff caused by experimental subacromial impingement in the rat. J Shoulder Elbow Surg 7:375-380, 1998.
403. Schneider JE, Adams OR, and Easley KJ: Scapular notch resection for suprascapular nerve decompression in 12 horses. JAMA 187:1019-1020, 1985.
404. Seeger LL, Gold RH, Bassett LW, and Ellman H: Shoulder impingement syndrome: MR findings in 53 shoulders. AJR Am J Roentgenol 150:343-347, 1988.
405. Seitz WHJ, Abram LJ, Froimson AI, et al: Rotator cuff imaging techniques: A comparison of arthrography, ultrasonography and magnetic resonance imaging. Paper presented at the Third Open Meeting of the American Shoulder and Elbow Surgeons, 1987, San Francisco.
406. Sharkey NA, Marder RA, and Hanson PB: The entire rotator cuff contributes to elevation of the arm. J Orthop Res 12:699-708, 1994.
407. Shellock FG, Bert JM, Fritts HM, et al: Evaluation of the rotator cuff and glenoid labrum using a 0.2-Tesla extremity magnetic resonance (MR) system: MR results compared to surgical findings. J Magn Reson Imaging 14:763-770, 2001.
408. Sher JS, Uribe JW, Posada A, et al: Abnormal findings on magnetic resonance images of asymptomatic shoulders. J Bone Joint Surg Am 77:10-15, 1995.
409. Shibata Y, Midorikawa K, Emoto G, and Naito M: Clinical evaluation of sodium hyaluronate for the treatment of patients with rotator cuff tear. J Shoulder Elbow Surg 10:209-216, 2001.
410. Sievers: Verh Dtsch Ges Chir 43(Kongr):243, 1914.
411. Sigholm G, Styf J, Korner L, and Herberts P: Pressure recording in the subacromial bursa. J Orthop Res 6:123-128, 1988.
412. Skoff HD: Conservative open acromioplasty. J Bone Joint Surg Br 77:933-936, 1995.
413. Slátis P and Aalto K: Medial dislocation of the tendon of the long head of the biceps brachii. Acta Orthop Scand 50:73-77, 1979.
414. Smaill GB: Bilateral rupture of Achilles tendon. BMJ 1:1657, 1961.
415. Smith JG: Pathological appearances of seven cases of injury of the shoulder joint with remarks. London Med Gazette 14:280, 1834.
416. Smith KL, Harryman DT II, Antoniou J, et al: A prospective, multipractice study of shoulder function and health status in patients with documented rotator cuff tears. J Shoulder Elbow Surg 9:395-402, 2000.
417. Smith-Petersen MN, Aufranc OE, and Larson CB: Useful surgical procedures for rheumatoid arthritis involving joints of the upper extremity. Arch Surg 46:764-770, 1943.
418. Solheim LF and Roaas A: Compression of the suprascapular nerve after fracture of the scapular notch. Acta Orthop Scand 49:338-340, 1978.
419. Sonnabend DH: Treatment of primary anterior shoulder dislocation in patients older than 40 years of age. Conservative versus operative. Clin Orthop 304:74-77, 1994.
420. Soslowsky LJ, An CH, Johnston SP, and Carpenter JE: Geometric and mechanical properties of the coracoacromial ligament and their relationship to rotator cuff disease. Clin Orthop 304:10-17, 1994.
421. Spangehl MJ, Hawkins RH, McCormack RG, and Loomer RL: Arthroscopic versus open acromioplasty: A prospective, randomized, blinded study. J Shoulder Elbow Surg 11:101-107, 2002.
422. Speer KP and Garrett WE Jr: Muscular control of motion and stability about the pectoral girdle. In Matsen FA III, Fu FH, and Hawkins RJ (eds): The Shoulder: A Balance of Mobility and Stability. Rosemont, IL: American Academy of Orthopaedic Surgeons, 1993, pp 159-172.
423. Speer KP, Lohnes J, and Garrett WE: Arthroscopic subacromial decompression: Results in advanced impingement syndrome. Arthroscopy 7:291-296, 1991.
424. Speer KP, Osbahr DC, Montella BJ, et al: Acromial morphotype in the young asymptomatic athletic shoulder. J Shoulder Elbow Surg 10:434-437, 2001.
425. Spielmann AL, Forster BB, Kokan P, et al: Shoulder after rotator cuff repair: MR imaging findings in asymptomatic individuals—initial experience. Radiology 213:705-708, 1999.
426. Stieda A: Zur Pathologie der Schulter gelenkschlembeutel. In Langebeck B (ed): Archiv für klinische Chirurgie. Berlin: Verlag von August Hirschwald, 1908, p 910.
427. Stiles RG and Otte MT: Imaging of the shoulder. Radiology 188:603-613, 1993.
428. Strizak AM, Danzig L, and Jackson DW: Subacromial bursography: An anatomic and clinical study. J Bone Joint Surg Am 64:196, 1982.
429. Strohm BR and Colachis SCJ: Shoulder joint dysfunction following injury to the suprascapular nerve. Phys Ther 45:106-111, 1965.
430. Stuart MJ, Azevedo AJ, and Cofield RH: Anterior acromioplasty for treatment of the shoulder impingement syndrome. Clin Orthop 260:195-200, 1990.
431. Sweetnam R: Corticosteroid arthropathy and tendon rupture. J Bone Joint Surg Br 51:397, 1969.
432. Swiontkowski M, Iannotti JP, Boulas JH, et al: Intraoperative Assessment of Rotator Cuff Vascularity Using Laser Doppler Flowmetry. St Louis: Mosby-Year Book, 1990, pp 208-212.
433. Symeonides PP: The significance of the subscapularis muscle in the pathogenesis of recurrent anterior dislocation of the shoulder. J Bone Joint Surg Br 54:476-483, 1972.
434. Tabata S and Kida H: Diagnosis and treatment of partial thickness tears of rotator cuff. Orthop Traumatol Surg (Tokyo) 26:1199, 1983.
435. Tabata S, Kida H, Sasaki J, et al: Operative treatment for the incomplete thickness tears of the rotator cuff. Katakansetsu (Fukuoka) 5:29, 1981.
436. Taboury J: Ultrasonography of the shoulder: Diagnosis of rupture of tendons of the rotator muscles. Ann Radiol (Paris) 35:133-140, 1992.
437. Takagishi N: Conservative treatment of the ruptures of the rotator cuff. J Jpn Orthop Assoc 52:781-787, 1978.
438. Tamai K and Ogawa K: Intratendinous tear of the supraspinatus tendon exhibiting winging of the scapula. Clin Orthop 194:159-163, 1985.
439. Teefey SA, Hasan SA, Middleton WD, et al: Ultrasonography of the rotator cuff. A comparison of ultrasonographic and arthroscopic findings in one hundred consecutive cases. J Bone Joint Surg Am 82:498-504, 2000.
440. Tempelhof S, Rupp S, and Seil R: Age-related prevalence of rotator cuff tears in asymptomatic shoulders. J Shoulder Elbow Surg 8:296-299, 1999.
441. Tetzlaff JE, Yoon HJ, and Brems J: Interscalene brachial plexus block for shoulder surgery. Reg Anesth 19:339-343, 1994.
442. Thorling J, Bjerneld H, and Hallin G: Acromioplasty for impingement syndrome. Orthop Scand 56:147-148, 1985.
443. Thur C and Julke M: The anterolateral deltoid muscle flap-plasty: The procedure of choice in large rotator cuff defects. Unfallchirurg 98:415-421, 1995.
444. Tibone JE, Jobe FW, and Kerlan RK: Shoulder impingement syndrome in athletes treated by an anterior acromioplasty. Clin Orthop 198:134-140, 1985.
445. Tillaux: Traite de la Chirurgie Clinique. Paris, 1888.
446. Ting A, Jobe FW, Barto P, et al: An EMPG analysis of the lateral biceps in shoulders with rotator cuff tears. Paper presented at the 3rd Open Meeting of the American Shoulder and Elbow Surgeons, 1987, San Francisco.
447. Tirman PF, Bost FW, Garvin GJ, et al: Posterosuperior glenoid impingement of the shoulder: Findings at MR imaging and MR arthrography with arthroscopic correlation. Radiology 193:431-436, 1994.
448. Toivonen DA, Tuite MJ, and Orwin JF: Acromial structure and tears of the rotator cuff. J Shoulder Elbow Surg 4:376-383, 1995.

449. Toolanen G, Hildingsson C, Hedlund T, et al: Early complications after anterior dislocation of the shoulder in patients over 40 years. An ultrasonographic and electromyographic study. Acta Orthop Scand 64:549-552, 1993.

450. Torpey BM, McFarland EG, Ikeda K, et al: Deltoid muscle origin: Histology and subacromial decompression. Paper presented at the 12th Open Meeting of the American Shoulder and Elbow Surgeons, 1996, Atlanta.

451. Tuite MJ, Toivonen DA, Orwin JF, and Wright DH: Acromial angle on radiographs of the shoulder: Correlation with the impingement syndrome and rotator cuff tears. AJR Am J Roentgenol 165:609-613, 1995.

452. Tuite MJ, Yandow DR, DeSmet AA, et al: Diagnosis of partial and complete rotator cuff using combined gradient echo and spin echo. Skeletal Radiol 23:541-545, 1994.

453. Tyson LL and Crues JV III: Pathogenesis of rotator cuff disorders. Magnetic resonance imaging characteristics. Magn Reson Imaging Clin N Am 1:37-46, 1993.

454. Uhthoff HK, Loehr J, and Sarkar K: The pathogenesis of rotator cuff tears. Paper presented at the Third International Conference on Surgery of the Shoulder, 1986, Fukuora, Japan.

455. Uhthoff HK and Sarkar K: Pathology of rotator cuff tendons. In Watson MS (ed): Surgical Disorders of the Shoulder. Edinburgh: Churchill Livingstone, 1991, pp 259-270.

456. Uhthoff HK and Sarkar K: Surgical repair of rotator cuff ruptures. The importance of the subacromial bursa. J Bone Joint Surg Br 73:399-401, 1991.

457. Uhthoff HK and Sarkar K: The effect of aging on the soft tissues of the shoulder. In Matsen FA III, Fu FH, Hawkins RJ (eds): The Shoulder: A Balance of Mobility and Stability. Rosemont, IL: American Academy of Orthopaedic Surgeons, 1993, pp 269-278.

458. Uitto J, Teir H, and Mustakallio KK: Corticosteroid induced inhibition of the biosynthesis of human skin collagen. Biochem Pharmacol 21:2161, 1972.

459. Valtonen EJ: Double acting betamethasone (Celestone Chronodose) in the treatment of supraspinatus tendinitis: A comparison of subacromial and gluteal single injections with placebo. J Intern Med Res 6:463-467, 1978.

460. van Holsbeeck E, DeRycke J, Declercy G, et al: Subacromial impingement: Open versus arthroscopic decompression. Arthroscopy 8:173-178, 1992.

461. Van Holsbeeck MT, Kolowich PA, Eyler WR, et al: US depiction of partial thickness tear of the rotator cuff. Radiology 197:443-436, 1995.

462. Van Linge B and Mulder JD: Function of the supraspinatus muscle and its relation to the supraspinatus syndrome: An experimental study in man. J Bone Joint Surg Br 45:750-754, 1963.

463. van-Moppes FL, Veldkamp O, and Roorda J: Role of shoulder ultrasonography in the evaluation of the painful shoulder. Eur J Radiol 19:142-146, 1995.

464. Vogt: Deutsche Chirurgie Lief 64, 1881.

465. Walch G, Liotard JP, Boileau P, and Noel E: Postero-superior glenoid impingement: Another shoulder impingement. Rev Chir Orthop Reparatrice Appar Mot 77:571-574, 1991.

466. Walker SW, Couch WH, Boester GA, and Sprowl DW: Isokinetic strength of the shoulder after repair of a torn rotator cuff. J Bone Joint Surg Am 69:1041-1044, 1987.

467. Wang YM, Shih TT, Jiang CC, et al: Magnetic resonance imaging of rotator cuff lesions. J Formos Med Assoc 93:234-239, 1994.

468. Ware JE, Snow KK, Kosinski M, and Gandek B: In Institute TH (ed): SF 36 Health Survey Manual and Interpretation Guide. Boston: New England Medical Center, 1993.

469. Warner JJ, Beim GM, and Higgins L: The treatment of symptomatic os acromiale. J Bone Joint Surg Am 80:1320-1326, 1998.

470. Warner JP: The gross anatomy of the joint surfaces, ligaments, labrum, and capsule. In Matsen FA III, Fu FH, and Hawkins RJ (eds): The Shoulder: A Balance of Mobility and Stability. Rosemont, IL: American Academy of Orthopaedic Surgeons, 1993, pp 7-28.

471. Warner JP, Krushell RJ, Masquelet A, and Gerber C: Anatomy and relationships of the suprascapular nerve: Anatomical constraints to mobilization of the supraspinatus and infraspinatus muscles in the management of massive rotator-cuff tears. J Bone Joint Surg Am 74:36-45, 1992.

472. Warren JP, Altchek DW, and Warren RF: Arthroscopic management of rotator cuff tears with emphasis on the throwing athlete. Oper Tech Orthop 1:235-239, 1991.

473. Watson M: The refractory painful arc syndrome. J Bone Joint Surg Br 0:544-546, 1978.

474. Watson M: Major ruptures of the rotator cuff: The results of surgical repair in 89 patients. J Bone Joint Surg Br 67B:618-624, 1985.

475. Watson-Jones R: Fractures and Joint Injuries, 4th ed. Baltimore: Williams & Wilkins, 1960, pp 449-451.

476. Watson-Jones R: Injuries in the region of the shoulder joint: Capsule and tendon injuries. BMJ 2:29-31, 1961.

477. Weaver HL: Isolated suprascapular nerve lesions: Injury. Br J Accident Surg 15:117-126, 1983.

478. Weiner DS and Macnab I: Ruptures of the rotator cuff: Follow-up evaluation of operative repairs. Can J Surg 13:219-227, 1970.

479. Weiner DS and Macnab I: Superior migration of the humeral head: A radiological aid in the diagnosis of tears of the rotator cuff. J Bone Joint Surg Br 52:524-527, 1970.

480. Weiss JJ: Intra-articular steroids in the treatment of rotator cuff tear: Reappraisal by arthrography. Arch Phys Med Rehabil 62:555-557, 1981.

481. Wellisch: Wien Med Wochenschr 974, 1934.

482. Wiener SN and Seitz WH Jr: Sonography of the shoulder in patients with tears of the rotator cuff: Accuracy and value for selecting surgical options. AJR Am J Roentgenol 160:103-107, 1993.

483. Wiley AM: Arthroscopic evaluation and surgery for rotator cuff disease. In Shoulder Surgery in the Athlete. Aspen, 1985, pp 83-91.

484. Wiley AM: Superior humeral dislocation. A complication following decompression and débridement for rotator cuff tears. Clin Orthop 263:135-141, 1991.

485. Wilson CL: Lesions of the supraspinatus tendon: Degeneration, rupture and calcification. Arch Surg 46:307, 1943.

486. Wilson CL and Duff GL: Pathologic study of degeneration and rupture of the supraspinatus tendon. Arch Surg 47:121-135, 1943.

487. Withrington RH, Girgis FL, and Seifert MH: A placebo-controlled trial of steroid injections in the treatment of supraspinatus tendinitis. Scand J Rheumatol 14:76-78, 1985.

488. Wolf EM and Agrawal V: Transdeltoid palpation (the rent test) in the diagnosis of rotator cuff tears. J Shoulder Elbow Surg 10:470-473, 2001.

489. Wolfgang GL: Rupture of the musculotendinous cuff of the shoulder. Clin Orthop 134:230-243, 1978.

490. Wrede L: Ueber Kalkablagerungen in der Umgebung des Schultergelenks und ihre Beziehungen zur Periarthritis. Berlin: Verlag von August Hirschwald, 1912, p 259.

491. Wuelker N, Plitz W, and Roetman B: Biomechanical data concerning the shoulder impingement syndrome. Clin Orthop 303:242-249, 1994.

492. Wuelker N, Roetman B, Plitz W, and Knop C: [Function of the supraspinatus muscle in a dynamic shoulder model.] Unfallchirurg 97:308-313, 1994.

493. Wuelker N, Wirth CJ, Plitz W, and Roetman B: A dynamic shoulder model: Reliability testing and muscle force study. J Biomech 28:489-499, 1995.

494. Wulker N, Melzer C, and Wirth CJ: Shoulder surgery for rotator cuff tears. Ultrasonographic 3 year follow-up of 97 cases. Acta Orthop Scand 62:142-147, 1991.

495. Yamada H and Evans F: Strength of Biological Materials. Baltimore: Williams & Wilkins, 1972, pp 67-70.

496. Yamamoto R: Rotator cuff rupture. J Bone Joint Surg 1:93, 1982.

497. Yamanaka K and Fukuda H: Histological study of the supraspinatus tendon. Shoulder Joint 5:9, 1981.

498. Yamanaka K, Fukuda H, Hamada K, and Mikasa M: Incomplete thickness tears of the rotator cuff. Orthop Traumatol Surg (Tokyo) 26:713, 1983.

499. Yamanaka K and Matsumoto T: The joint side tear of the rotator cuff: A followup study by arthrography. Clin Orthop 304:68-73, 1994.

500. Yazici M, Kapuz C, and Gulman B: Morphologic variants of acromion in neonatal cadavers. J Pediatr Orthop 15:644-647, 1995.

501. Yung SW and Harryman DT II: The surgical anatomy of subscapular nerves. Paper presented at the 62nd Annual Meeting of the American Academy of Orthopaedic Surgeons, 1995, Orlando, FL.

502. Ziegler DW, Matsen FA III, and Harrington RM: The superior rotator cuff tendon and acromion provide passive superior stability to the shoulder. Submitted to J Bone Joint Surg, 1996.

503. Zanetti M, Jost B, Hodler J, and Gerber C: MR imaging after rotator cuff repair: Full-thickness defects and bursitis-like subacromial abnormalities in asymptomatic subjects. Skeletal Radiol 29:314-319, 2000.

504. Zuckerman JD, Kummer FJ, Cuomo F, et al: The influence of coracoacromial arch anatomy on rotator cuff tears. J Shoulder Elbow Surg 1:4-14, 1992.

505. Zuckerman JD, Leblanc JM, Choueka J, and Kummer F: The effect of arm position and capsular release on rotator cuff repair. J Bone Joint Surg Br 73:402-405, 1991.

506. Zvijac JE, Levy HJ, and Lemak LJ: Arthroscopic subacromial decompression in the treatment of full thickness rotator cuff tears: A 3- to 6-year follow-up. Arthroscopy 10:518-523, 1994.

CHAPTER 16

GLENOHUMERAL ARTHRITIS AND ITS MANAGEMENT

Frederick A. Matsen III, M.D., Charles A. Rockwood, Jr., M.D., Michael A. Wirth, M.D.,
Steven B. Lippitt, M.D., and Moby Parsons, M.D.

• • • •

The humeral head and the glenoid normally articulate through smooth, congruent, and well-lubricated joint surfaces. Glenohumeral arthritis results when these joint surfaces are damaged by congenital, metabolic, traumatic, degenerative, vascular, septic, or nonseptic inflammatory factors. These conditions are common, especially in older populations, in whom the prevalence is approximately 20%.[72,203,413] In *degenerative joint disease,* the glenoid cartilage and subchondral bone are typically worn posteriorly, sometimes leaving the articular cartilage intact anteriorly. The cartilage of the humeral head is eroded in a pattern of central baldness that is often surrounded by a rim of remaining cartilage and osteophytes. In *inflammatory arthritis,* the cartilage is usually destroyed evenly across the humeral and glenoid joint surfaces. *Cuff tear arthropathy* occurs when a chronic large rotator cuff defect subjects the uncovered humeral articular cartilage to abrasion by the undersurface of the coracoacromial arch. Erosion of the humeral articular cartilage begins superiorly rather than centrally. *Neurotrophic arthropathy* arises in association with syringomyelia, diabetes, or other causes of joint denervation. The joint and subchondral bone are destroyed because of loss of the trophic and protective effects of its nerve supply. In *capsulorrhaphy arthropathy,* previous surgery for glenohumeral instability leads to destruction of the joint surface. In this situation, excessive anterior or posterior capsular tightening forces the head of the humerus out of its normal concentric relationship with the glenoid fossa. The eccentric glenohumeral contact increases contact pressure and joint surface wear. Most commonly, overtightening of the anterior capsule produces obligate posterior translation, posterior glenoid wear, and central wear of the humeral articular cartilage.

MECHANICS OF ARTHRITIS AND ARTHROPLASTY

Four basic mechanical characteristics are essential to shoulder function: motion, stability, strength, and smoothness. Each of these characteristics is commonly compromised in an arthritic shoulder, and each can potentially be restored by shoulder arthroplasty. Our approach to glenohumeral arthritis is guided by an understanding of the elements necessary for optimal shoulder mechanics.

Motion

The requisites of a normal range of glenohumeral motion include the following.

NORMAL CAPSULAR LAXITY. In normal shoulders, ample capsular laxity allows for full range of rotation at the glenohumeral joint. The glenohumeral capsule is normally lax through most of the functional range of shoulder motion.[177,246] As the joint approaches the limit of its range, the tension in the capsule and its ligaments increases sharply, thereby serving to check the range of rotation (Fig. 16-1). In many conditions that require shoulder arthroplasty, the capsule and ligaments are contracted, thus limiting the range of rotation. Shoulder arthroplasty may further tighten the capsule if the degenerated and collapsed humeral head is replaced by a relatively larger prosthesis and if a glenoid component is added to the surface of the glenoid bone. The prosthetic components may therefore consume more volume than the degenerated surfaces that they replace (Fig. 16-2) and consequently "stuff" the joint. Unless sufficient capsular release (Figs. 16-3 and 16-4) has been performed to accommodate this additional volume, the joint may be "overstuffed." In this situation, joint motion is further limited (Fig. 16-5), and more torque (muscle force) is required to move the arm (Fig. 16-6).

Harryman and associates determined that all motions, including flexion, external and internal rotation, and maximal elevation, are diminished when the joint is overstuffed.[176] Furthermore, this overstuffing causes obligate translation of the humeral head on the glenoid; for example, forced posterior translation occurs when external rotation is attempted against a tight anterior capsule (Figs. 16-7 and 16-8). Thus, if normal capsular laxity is lacking, unwanted translation and eccentric glenoid loading may result. Blevins and colleagues studied the effect of humeral head size on translation and rotation at the glenohumeral joint and determined that selection of head component size should be based more on restoring effective joint volume than on replicating the native head diameter.[39]

In arthroplasty surgery, the contribution of the components to joint stuffing can be estimated by adding the incremental thickness of the glenoid to the difference between the amount of intra-articular humerus replaced and the amount of humerus resected. To be comparable,

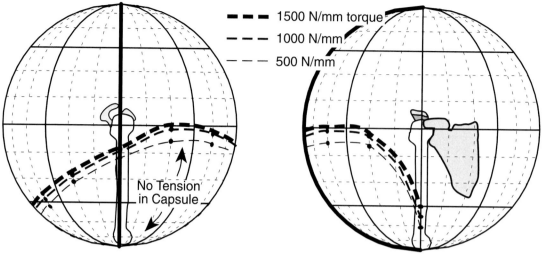

■ **Figure 16–1**

Range of humeroscapular elevation with no capsular tension. This global diagram represents data from a cadaver experiment in which the humerus was elevated in a variety of scapular planes and free axial rotation was allowed. Elevation was performed until the torque reached 500, 1000, and 1500 N/mm. The positions associated with these torque levels are indicated by the isobars. The area within the inner isobar indicates the range of positions in which there was effectively no tension in the capsuloligamentous structures. For further details, see Matsen FA III, Lippitt SB, Sidles JA, and Harryman DT II: Practical Evaluation and Management of the Shoulder. Philadelphia: WB Saunders, 1994.

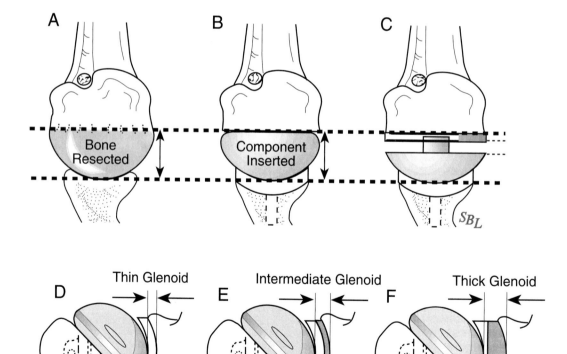

■ **Figure 16–2**

The amount of humeral stuffing is measured by comparing the amount of humerus resected (**A**) with the amount of intra-articular humeral prosthesis added (**B**). In modular systems, the amount of prosthesis added must include the collar and the exposed part of the Morse taper, as well as the prosthetic head (**C**). The amount of glenoid stuffing is determined by the distance between the bone surface and the prosthetic articular surface. This distance is greater in proportion to the thickness of the glenoid components (**D-F**). *(From Matsen FA III, Lippitt SB, Sidles JA, and Harryman DT II: Practical Evaluation and Management of the Shoulder. Philadelphia: WB Saunders, 1994.)*

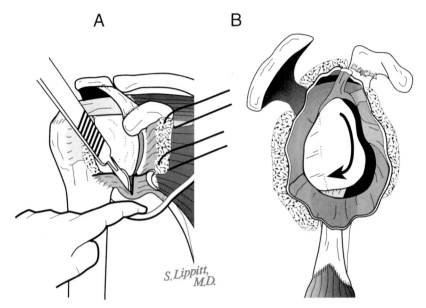

■ **Figure 16–3**
A, Division of the anteroinferior capsular attachments to the glenoid under direct vision while the axillary nerve is protected and retracted.
B, Capsular release to the 7 o'clock position on the glenoid exposes the origin of the long head of the triceps. *(Modified from Matsen FA III, Lippitt SB, Sidles JA, and Harryman DT II: Practical Evaluation and Management of the Shoulder. Philadelphia: WB Saunders, 1994.)*

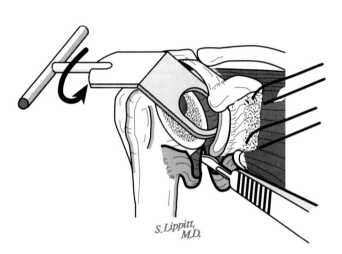

■ **Figure 16–4**
If necessary, sequential posterior release is accomplished at the glenoid rim (release at the humerus would jeopardize the cuff insertion). During this release, the capsule is tensed by twisting the humeral retractor. Care is taken to protect the axillary nerve below and the cuff behind. *(Modified from Matsen FA III, Lippitt SB, Sidles JA, and Harryman DT II: Practical Evaluation and Management of the Shoulder. Philadelphia: WB Saunders, 1994.)*

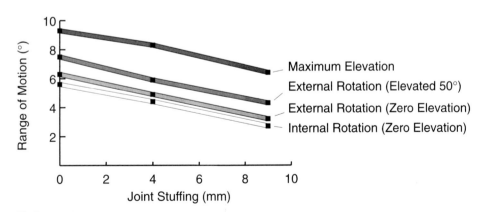

■ **Figure 16–5**
The effect of joint stuffing on range of motion. This graph compares the range of four humeroscapular motions that could be achieved with an applied torque of 1500 N/mm for (1) an anatomic joint (0 mm of joint stuffing), (2) an anatomic humeral arthroplasty with a 4-mm-thick glenoid component (4 mm of overstuffing), and (3) an arthroplasty with a 4-mm-thick glenoid and a 5-mm oversized humeral neck (total overstuffing is 9 mm). Note the sequential loss of each of the motions with increasing degrees of stuffing. *(From Matsen FA III, Lippitt SB, Sidles JA, and Harryman DT II: Practical Evaluation and Management of the Shoulder. Philadelphia: WB Saunders, 1994.)*

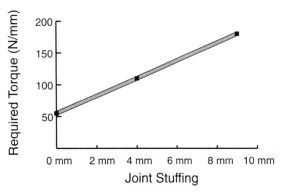

■ **Figure 16–6**
Comparison of the average torque necessary to achieve 60 degrees of elevation in the +90-degree scapular plane for an anatomic shoulder (0 mm of stuffing), an anatomic shoulder arthroplasty with 4 mm of glenoid stuffing, and an arthroplasty with 4 mm of glenoid and 5 mm of humeral overstuffing (total overstuffing is 9 mm). The required torque is almost three times higher for the joint overstuffed with 9 mm of component than for the anatomic joint. *(From Matsen FA III, Lippitt SB, Sidles JA, and Harryman DT II: Practical Evaluation and Management of the Shoulder. Philadelphia: WB Saunders, 1994.)*

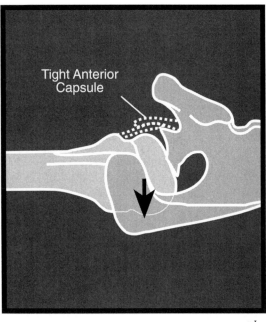

SBL

■ **Figure 16–8**
Axillary view of capsulorrhaphy arthropathy in which an excessively tight anterior capsular repair is forcing the head of the humerus posteriorly. This effect is accentuated by forced external rotation. Note also the typical posterior glenoid erosion. *(From Matsen FA III, Lippitt SB, Sidles JA, and Harryman DT II: Practical Evaluation and Management of the Shoulder. Philadelphia: WB Saunders, 1994.)*

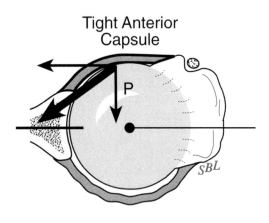

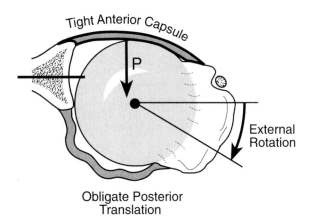

■ **Figure 16–7**
If the humerus is rotated beyond the point where the ligaments become tight, the displacing force (P) can push the humeral head out of the glenoid center—a phenomenon known as obligate translation. *(Modified from Matsen FA III, Lippitt SB, Sidles JA, and Harryman DT II: Practical Evaluation and Management of the Shoulder. Philadelphia: WB Saunders, 1994.)*

the measurement of the amount of humeral head resected and the measurement of the amount of intra-articular humeral prosthesis added must both be made from the cut surface of the humeral neck to the articular surface. In modular humeral heads, the amount of bone replaced must include the thickness of the collar and the exposed part of the Morse taper stem, in addition to the head itself (see Fig. 16–2).

The incremental thickness of the glenoid is related primarily to the thickness of the component, as well as the amount of reaming, the presence or absence of cement between the component and the bone, and the effect of bone grafts. The thickness of currently available glenoid components varies from 3 to more than 15 mm. Thicker glenoid polyethylene may help manage contact stress and may have superior wear properties.[144] Metal-backed glenoid components affect load transfer and offer opportunities for screw fixation and tissue ingrowth.[94] However, both thicker polyethylene and metal backing increase joint stuffing, which becomes particularly problematic in shoulders that remain tight even after soft tissue release. Overstuffing may also predispose a reconstructed shoulder to instability.[94]

The amount of stuffing from the humeral component is determined both by the geometry of the component and by the position in which it is placed. The size of the intra-articular aspect of the humeral component is related to its design, including its radius of curvature, the percentage of the sphere represented by its articular surface, and the distance between the base of its collar and the articular surface of the prosthesis (Fig. 16–9; see also Fig. 16–2).

The position of the component also has a major effect on the degree to which it stuffs the joint. A component inserted into varus will disproportionately stuff the joint when the arm is at the side; this outcome is more likely when the stem of the prosthesis does not fit the humeral canal snugly. A component inserted excessively high will tighten the capsule as the arm is elevated (similar to a mechanical cam) and limit the range of elevation (Fig. 16–10).

Cadaver studies[262] indicate that less than 10 mm of overstuffing can reduce normal capsular laxity by as much as 50% (Fig. 16–11). An overstuffed shoulder is predisposed to obligate translation when rotated to positions in which the capsule becomes tight (Table 16–1).

TABLE 16-1. **Range of Angular Motion before the Onset of Obligate Translation***

	Anatomic Shoulder (Degrees)	Joint Overstuffed 9 mm (Degrees)
Elevation in the plus 90-degree scapular plane	60	30
External rotation of the arm elevated 50 degrees	60	32

*Values represent the maximal elevation achieved with no more than 2 mm of obligate translation.

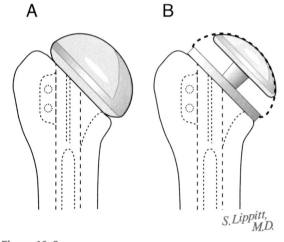

■ Figure 16–9
A, Ideally, the humeral component provides a maximal articular surface area. **B,** Significant portions of the intra-articular space can be consumed by nonarticular aspects of the prosthesis. *(From Matsen FA III, Lippitt SB, Sidles JA, and Harryman DT II: Practical Evaluation and Management of the Shoulder. Philadelphia: WB Saunders, 1994.)*

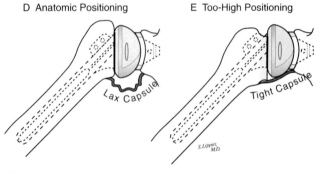

■ Figure 16–10
The position of the humeral component is an important determinant of the amount of stuffing. **A,** Anatomic positioning of the humeral component. **B,** A component placed low and in varus will disproportionately stuff the shoulder while the arm is at the side. **C,** A component placed excessively high. **D,** Normal anatomic relationships in humeral elevation. **E,** A humeral component that is too high causes tightening of the capsule as the humerus is elevated. *(From Matsen FA III, Lippitt SB, Sidles JA, and Harryman DT II: Practical Evaluation and Management of the Shoulder. Philadelphia: WB Saunders, 1994.)*

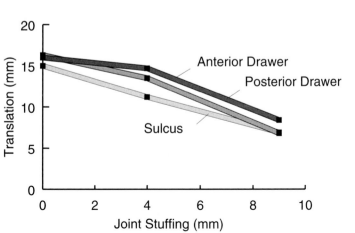

■ Figure 16–11
The effect of overstuffing on capsular laxity in eight cadaver shoulders with a mean age of 73 ± 8.5 years. The intact shoulders (0 mm of stuffing) demonstrated 15 mm of translational laxity on the anterior drawer, posterior drawer, and sulcus tests. Overstuffing by 9 mm decreased this normal joint laxity by approximately 50% in all directions. *(From Matsen FA III, Lippitt SB, Sidles JA, and Harryman DT II: Practical Evaluation and Management of the Shoulder. Philadelphia: WB Saunders, 1994.)*

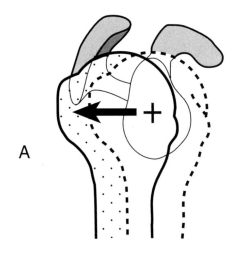

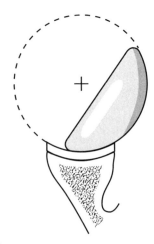

■ **Figure 16–13**

Each prosthetic head represents a portion of a sphere. Different prostheses comprise different percentages of the surface of the sphere. *(Modified from Ballmer FT, Lippitt SB, Romeo AA, and Matsen FA III: Total shoulder arthroplasty: Some considerations related to glenoid surface contact. J Shoulder Elbow Surg 3:299-306, 1994.)*

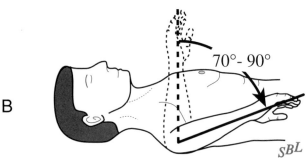

■ **Figure 16–12**

A, Proper soft tissue tension allows 50% posterior translation of the humeral head component on the glenoid and a spontaneous return to the centered position (the "springbok" test). **B,** The patient should have sufficient laxity in the posterior capsule after arthroplasty to allow internal rotation in the abducted position in the range of 70 to 90 degrees (the "scarecrow" test). *(From Pearl ML and Lippitt SB: Shoulder arthroplasty with a modular prosthesis. Tech Orthop 8:151-162, 1994. Original illustrator, S.B. Lippitt.)*

Large Head Size   Smaller Head Size
Large Arc of Motion   Smaller Arc of Motion

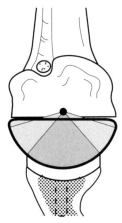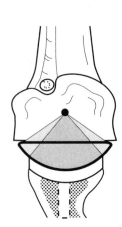

■ **Figure 16–14**

The arc of motion that can be accomplished at the glenohumeral joint before running out of humeral articular surface is determined by the difference between the angles subtended by the humeral and glenoid articular surfaces in the direction of motion. Thus, although a smaller humeral head component may increase capsular laxity, its smaller surface arc may actually diminish the glenohumeral motion allowed before the bone of the humerus makes contact with the glenoid. *(From Matsen FA III, Lippitt SB, Sidles JA, and Harryman DT II: Practical Evaluation and Management of the Shoulder. Philadelphia: WB Saunders, 1994.)*

Overstuffing can be avoided by ensuring adequate capsular laxity at the time of surgery: (1) the arm should allow 40 degrees of external rotation at the side after the anterior structures have been approximated (Fig. 16–12), (2) the humeral head should translate approximately 50% of the glenoid width on the posterior drawer test, and (3) the abducted arm should allow 60 degrees of internal rotation. These are the "40, 50, 60" guidelines.

HUMERAL ARTICULAR SURFACE. A substantial and properly located humeral articular surface area allows a large unimpeded rotational range. Humeral articular surfaces that comprise only a small portion of the sphere (Fig. 16–13) predispose to abutment of the rim of the glenoid against the tuberosities or anatomic neck of the humerus (Figs. 16–14 and 16–15).[18] The normal extent of the humeral joint surface can be restored with proper positioning of the appropriate prosthesis at the time of joint replacement (see Fig. 16–9). Williams and coworkers investigated the effect of humeral head malposition after total shoulder arthroplasty on joint translation and range of motion. An offset of 8 mm or more in any direction resulted in a significant decrease in passive range of

motion, whereas inferior malposition of greater than 4 mm led to increased subacromial contact. The authors determined that anatomic reconstruction of the humeral head–humeral shaft offset to within 4 mm is desirable for restoring normal motion and articular kinematics.[432]

GLENOID ARTICULAR SURFACE. The glenoid articular surface encompasses a relatively small portion of the sphere when compared with that of the humerus. If the

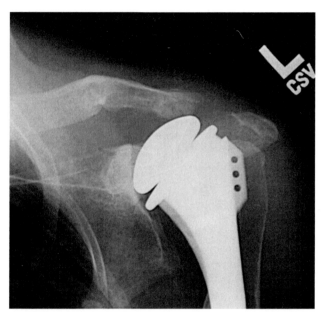

■ Figure 16–15
A humeral component with an articular surface encompassing only a small portion of the potential spherical articular surface may predispose the prosthesis to unwanted translation as well as contact between the prosthetic collar and the glenoid.

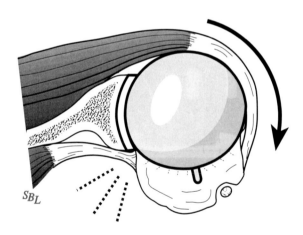

■ Figure 16–16
Motion-limiting abutment between the glenoid component and soft tissue or bone. (Modified from Ballmer FT, Lippitt SB, Romeo AA, and Matsen FA III: Total shoulder arthroplasty: Some considerations related to glenoid surface contact. J Shoulder Elbow Surg 3:299-306, 1994.)

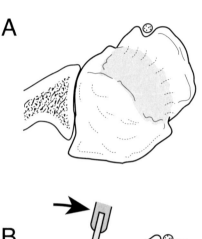

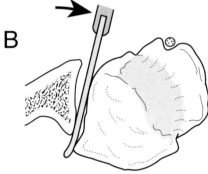

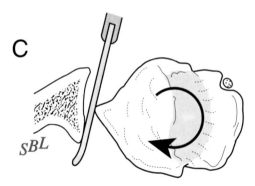

■ Figure 16–17
Osteophyte blocking range of motion. A "shoe horn" elevator may be required to ease the components into the joint at the time of surgical arthroplasty. (Modified from Matsen FA III, Lippitt SB, Sidles JA, and Harryman DT II: Practical Evaluation and Management of the Shoulder. Philadelphia: WB Saunders, 1994.)

prosthetic glenoid joint surface area is large in comparison to that of the humerus, abutment of the prosthesis against the humeral neck or tuberosities can restrict joint motion (Fig. 16–16; see also Fig. 16–14).

ABSENCE OF BLOCKING OSTEOPHYTES. Osteophytes predispose to contact with the glenoid and can impair motion (Fig. 16–17). Blocking osteophytes must be completely resected at the time of joint reconstruction (Fig. 16–18).

UNRESTRICTED HUMEROSCAPULAR MOTION INTERFACE. Normally, 4 to 5 cm of excursion takes place at the upper aspect of the interface between the coracoid muscles and the subscapularis (Fig. 16–19). Adhesions or

"spot welds" between the proximal end of the humerus and the cuff on one hand and the deltoid and coracoacromial arch on the other can limit motion, even if the intra-articular aspect of the arthroplasty is perfectly balanced. Lysis of humeroscapular spot welds is an important early step in arthroplasty of the shoulder.

Stability

The requisites of glenohumeral stability are as follows.

ANATOMICALLY ORIENTED AND SUFFICIENTLY EXTENSIVE HUMERAL ARTICULAR SURFACE AREA. The orientation of the humeral articular surface can be described in terms of the humeral head centerline, or a line passing through the center of the humeral joint surface and the center of the anatomic neck. This line

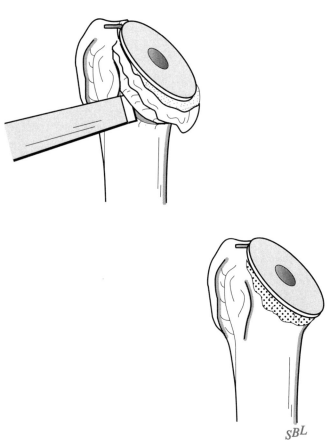

■ **Figure 16–18**
Resection of osteophytes with the rim of the prosthetic collar used as a girdle. *(From Pearl ML and Lippitt SB: Shoulder arthroplasty with a modular prosthesis. Tech Orthop 8:151-162, 1994. Original illustrator, S.B. Lippitt.)*

usually makes a valgus angle of about 130 degrees with the humeral shaft. The humeral head centerline generally makes a retroversion angle of about 30 degrees with the axis of elbow flexion.[85,99,134,145,186,298,301,357,425] Studies point out that mean humeral retroversion varies widely from 7 to 50 degrees.[230,319,348] Badet and coworkers demonstrated that humeral retroversion is decreased by as much as 8 degrees in shoulders with osteoarthritis and that humeral head subluxation is present in roughly 35% of cases.[16] Hernigou and associates pointed out the importance of clearly defining the reference system when measuring humeral version.[190] In a recent study, these authors determined that the mean angular orientation of the humeral articular surface varies by as much as 11 degrees when measured by the epicondylar axis versus a line perpendicular to the forearm axis.[191]

The extent of the humeral articular surface area is another critical determinant of stability. In an arthritic glenohumeral joint, stability can be compromised by a reduced amount of available humeral articular surface. Similarly, a prosthetic surface area that represents only a small part of the total sphere (see Figs. 16–9, 16–13, and 16–15) can predispose to instability in the same way that a Hill-Sachs defect does in traumatic instability by offering less contact area for joint surface contact (Fig. 16–20).

ANATOMICALLY ORIENTED GLENOID. The glenoid centerline, the line perpendicular to the center of the glenoid fossa, is usually within 15 degrees of the plane of the scapula (Figs. 16–21 and 16–22). In an arthritic glenohumeral joint, stability may be compromised by abnormal glenoid version (Figs. 16–23 and 16–24; see also Fig. 16–8). Friedman and colleagues,[143] Mullaji and associates,[285] and Badet and coworkers[16] have used computed tomography

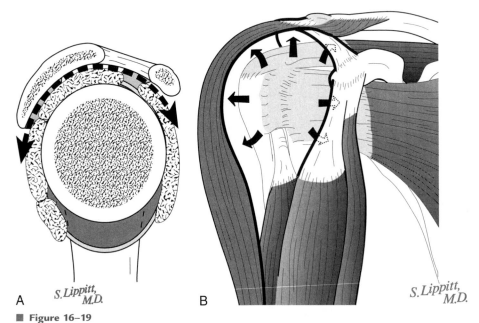

■ **Figure 16–19**
A and **B,** The humeroscapular motion interface is an important location of motion between the humerus and scapula. The deltoid, acromion, coracoacromial ligament, coracoid process, and tendons attaching to the coracoid lie on the superficial side of this interface, whereas the proximal end of the humerus, rotator cuff, and biceps tendon sheath lie on its deep side.

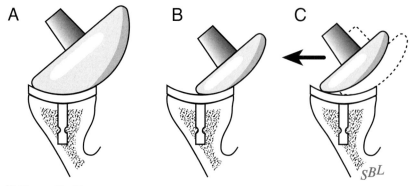

■ Figure 16–20
The effect of humeral contact area on translational stability. Full surface contact
provides maximal joint stability (**A**). When full surface contact is lacking because of a
small humeral joint surface angle (**B**), the humeral component can be translated in the
direction of the empty part of the glenoid (**C**). *(Modified from Matsen FA III, Lippitt SB,
Sidles JA, and Harryman DT II: Practical Evaluation and Management of the Shoulder.
Philadelphia: WB Saunders, 1994.)*

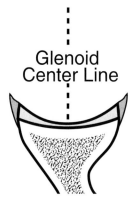

■ Figure 16–21
The glenoid centerline is a line perpendicular to the surface of the glenoid fossa at its
midpoint. *(Modified from Matsen FA III, Lippitt SB, Sidles JA, and Harryman DT II: Practical
Evaluation and Management of the Shoulder. Philadelphia: WB Saunders, 1994.)*

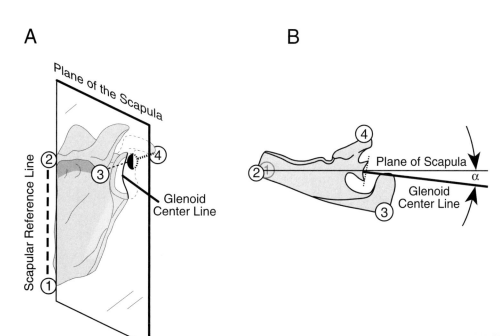

■ Figure 16–22
The glenoid centerline can be related
to scapular coordinates and to the
plane of the scapula. These reference
points are all easily palpated: **A**, the
inferior pole of the scapula (1), the
medial end of the spine of the
scapula (2), the posterior angle of
the acromion (3), and the coracoid
tip (4). The scapular reference line
connects reference points 1 and 2.
B, The plane of the scapula passes
through points 1 and 2 and halfway
between points 3 and 4. The glenoid
centerline usually makes a slightly
posterior angle (α) with the plane of
the scapula. *(Modified from Matsen FA
III, Lippitt SB, Sidles JA, and Harryman
DT II: Practical Evaluation and
Management of the Shoulder.
Philadelphia: WB Saunders, 1994.)*

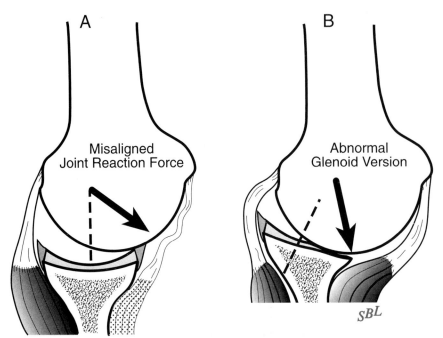

■ **Figure 16–23**
A, Stability is compromised by muscle imbalance. In this example, the humerus is aligned with the glenoid centerline, but the net humeral joint reaction force is misaligned because of weakness of the posterior cuff musculature. **B,** Balance stability is also compromised by the abnormal glenoid version. In this example, the humerus is aligned with the plane of the scapula, but severe glenoid retroversion results in a posteriorly directed glenoid centerline that is divergent from the net humeral joint reaction force. *(Modified from Matsen FA III, Lippitt SB, Sidles JA, and Harryman DT II: Practical Evaluation and Management of the Shoulder. Philadelphia: WB Saunders, 1994.)*

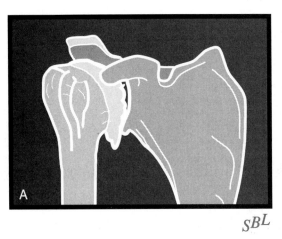
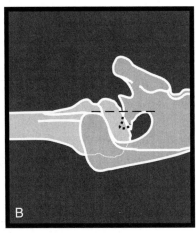

■ **Figure 16–24**
Glenohumeral degenerative joint disease. **A,** An anteroposterior view showing the typical "goat's beard" osteophyte enlarging the apparent superoinferior dimension of the head. **B,** Axillary view showing posterior subluxation and posterior rim wear. *(Modified from Matsen FA III, Lippitt SB, Sidles JA, and Harryman DT II: Practical Evaluation and Management of the Shoulder. Philadelphia: WB Saunders, 1994.)*

(CT) to document that arthritic involvement may alter glenoid version. Walch and colleagues reviewed the serial CT scans of 113 osteoarthritic shoulders to study the effect of the position of the humeral head on glenoid morphology.[418] Three main glenoid types were identified. Type A (59%) was marked by a well-centered humeral head. Symmetric erosion was explained by the absence of subluxation. Type B (32%) was denoted by posterior subluxation of the humeral head, and this morphology resulted in an exaggerated posterior wear pattern. Type C (9%) was defined by glenoid retroversion of more than 25 degrees regardless of erosion. In these cases, glenoid retroversion did not correlate with posterior wear but was primarily dysplastic in origin. The orientation of the glenoid prosthesis should be normalized as part of the arthroplasty procedure (Figs. 16–25 to 16–27).

GLENOID CONCAVITY WITH SUFFICIENTLY LARGE EFFECTIVE ARCS. The arc of the glenoid determines the maximal angles that the net humeral joint reaction force can make with the glenoid centerline before dislocation occurs (Fig. 16–28).

In an arthritic joint, the effective glenoid arc can be diminished by wear or inflammation; for example, posterior wear is typical of glenohumeral osteoarthritis (see Figs. 16–23B and 16–24) and capsulorrhaphy arthropathy (see Fig. 16–8), whereas central erosion of the glenoid is typical of rheumatoid arthritis (Fig. 16–29). One of the goals of arthroplasty is to restore effective glenoid arcs (see Fig. 16–27).

CONTROL OF THE NET HUMERAL JOINT REACTION FORCE. The direction of the net humeral joint reaction force is controlled actively by elements of the rotator cuff and other shoulder muscles (Fig. 16–30). Neural control of the magnitude of the different muscle forces provides the mechanism by which the direction of the net humeral joint reaction force is modulated. For example, by increasing the force of contraction of a muscle whose direction of force is parallel to the glenoid centerline, the body can

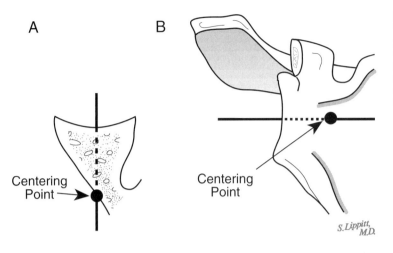

A

B

Centering
Point

Centering
Point

S. Lippitt,
M.D.

■ **Figure 16–25**

The normal glenoid centerline passes perpendicular to the center of the glenoid articular surface and exits the glenoid neck at the "centering point" between the upper and lower crura of the scapula in the lateral aspect of the subscapularis fossa. *(From Matsen FA III, Lippitt SB, Sidles JA, and Harryman DT II: Practical Evaluation and Management of the Shoulder. Philadelphia: WB Saunders, 1994.)*

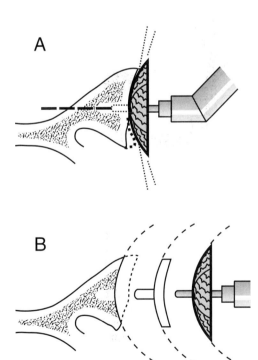

A

B

S. Lippitt,
M.D.

■ **Figure 16–26**

Use of the glenoid centering point to help orient the central hole for fixation of the glenoid component. **A,** The index finger is inserted anterior to the glenoid so that its tip palpates the centering point in the sulcus bounded by the thick upper and lower crura of the scapula and the flare of the glenoid vault. **B,** This centering point serves as a useful guide for drilling the normal glenoid centerline, particularly when the anatomic structure is distorted by eccentric glenoid wear. The normal glenoid centerline connects the center of the glenoid face with the centering point. *(Modified from Matsen FA III, Lippitt SB, Sidles JA, and Harryman DT II: Practical Evaluation and Management of the Shoulder. Philadelphia: WB Saunders, 1994.)*

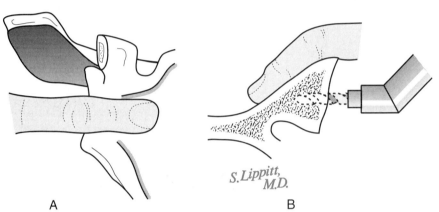

A

B

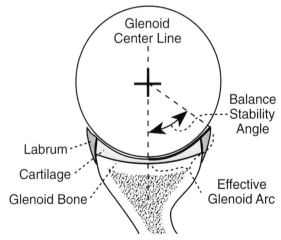

Glenoid
Center Line

Balance
Stability
Angle

Labrum

Cartilage

Glenoid Bone

Effective
Glenoid Arc

■ **Figure 16–27**

A, Reaming along the normalized glenoid centerline. The objective is to normalize the glenoid orientation and to contour the glenoid face to match the back of the glenoid component. **B,** Accurate contouring of the glenoid face improves the quality of bone support for the glenoid component. *(Modified from Matsen FA III, Lippitt SB, Sidles JA, and Harryman DT II: Practical Evaluation and Management of the Shoulder. Philadelphia: WB Saunders, 1994.)*

■ **Figure 16–28**

The effective glenoid arc is the arc of the glenoid able to support the net humeral joint reaction force. The balance stability angle is the maximal angle that the net humeral joint reaction force can make with the glenoid centerline before dislocation occurs. *(Modified from Matsen FA III, Lippitt SB, Sidles JA, and Harryman DT II: Practical Evaluation and Management of the Shoulder. Philadelphia: WB Saunders, 1994.)*

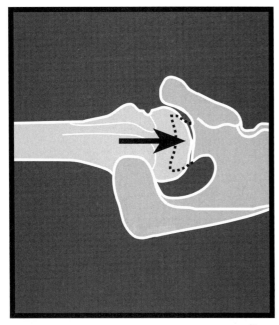

S. Lippitt,
M.D.

■ **Figure 16–29**
Axillary view of glenohumeral rheumatoid arthritis showing medial erosion of the glenoid. *(From Matsen FA III, Lippitt SB, Sidles JA, and Harryman DT II: Practical Evaluation and Management of the Shoulder. Philadelphia: WB Saunders, 1994.)*

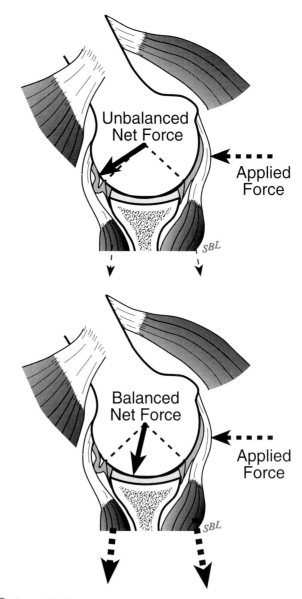

■ **Figure 16–31**
Stabilizing the glenohumeral joint against an applied translational force. Strong contraction of the cuff muscles provides an increased compression force into the glenoid concavity. As a result, the net humeral force is balanced within the glenoid concavity.

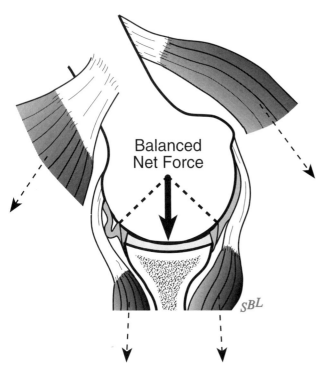

■ **Figure 16–30**
The vector sum of the deltoid and cuff muscle forces lies close to the axis of the humerus in many functional positions of the shoulder. *(Modified from Matsen FA III, Lippitt SB, Sidles JA, and Harryman DT II: Practical Evaluation and Management of the Shoulder. Philadelphia: WB Saunders, 1994.)*

change the direction of the net humeral joint reaction force to an orientation that is in closer alignment with the glenoid fossa (Fig. 16–31). Apreleva and associates demonstrated that the magnitude and direction of the net humeral joint reaction force varies according to the relative ratio of forces applied by the rotator cuff and deltoid muscles.[9]

In glenohumeral arthritis, control of the net humeral joint reaction force may be compromised by tendon rupture, tuberosity detachment, and deconditioning (see Fig. 16–23). The most striking example is in cuff tear arthropathy, where the normally stabilizing cuff muscle forces are compromised (Figs. 16–32 to 16–34).

If the net humeral joint reaction force is not centered in the glenoid fossa after glenohumeral arthroplasty, eccentric loading may produce a "rocking horse"

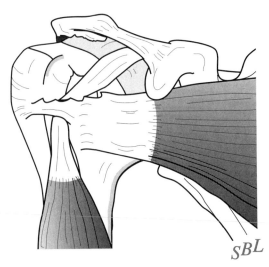

■ Figure 16–32
The boutonnière deformity, in which the subscapularis and infraspinatus tendons slide below the center of the humeral head. *(Modified from Matsen FA III, Lippitt SB, Sidles JA, and Harryman DT II: Practical Evaluation and Management of the Shoulder. Philadelphia: WB Saunders, 1994.)*

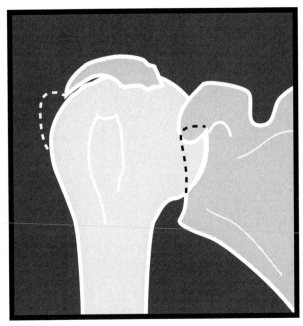

■ Figure 16–34
Radiographic appearance of cuff tear arthropathy with "acetabularization" of the upper glenoid and the coracoacromial arch and "femoralization" of the proximal part of the humerus. *(Modified from Matsen FA III, Lippitt SB, Sidles JA, and Harryman DT II: Practical Evaluation and Management of the Shoulder. Philadelphia: WB Saunders, 1994.)*

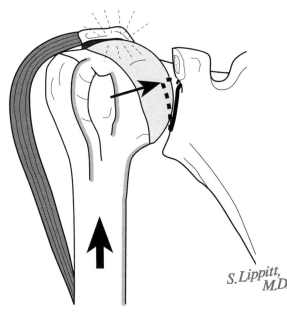

■ Figure 16–33
Erosion of the superior glenoid concavity compromises the concavity compression stability mechanism and allows upward translation when the deltoid contracts. *(Modified from Matsen FA III, Lippitt SB, Sidles JA, and Harryman DT II: Practical Evaluation and Management of the Shoulder. Philadelphia: WB Saunders, 1994.)*

basis, advocated the use of less conforming and less constrained designs. Karduna and colleagues noted that prosthetically reconstructed shoulders developed higher force for a given translation as conformity increased and that more conforming joints resulted in higher peak tensile strain just before rim loading.[214] Anglin and associates demonstrated that more conforming designs led to an increase in distraction of the glenoid component from the underlying bone during simulated edge loading.[7]

Severe degrees of mismatch may have adverse effects on the glenohumeral contact area (Fig. 16–38) and on peak stresses in the polyethylene component (Fig. 16–39). Couteau and coworkers analyzed the mechanical effect of changes in articular conformity in shoulder arthroplasty and determined that decreases in the contact area of articulation may cause high stresses that may be transferred to the glenoid fixation.[106] Thus, there must be a compromise between the arguments in favor of more mismatch between the radius of curvature of the glenoid and that of the humerus (less translational loads on the glenoid component and less risk of rim loading with translation) and those in favor of greater conformity (more stability and less contact stress).

Strength

The requisites of strength include the following:

1. A functional deltoid
2. A functional rotator cuff
3. Normal length relationships of muscle origin and insertions

loosening of the glenoid component (Fig. 16–35). A slight degree of mismatch of the glenoid and humeral diameters of curvature allows for minor amounts of force malalignment before rim contact occurs (Figs. 16–36 and 16–37). Severt and associates[379] pointed out that a high degree of conformity between the glenoid and humeral joint surfaces increases the translational force and frictional torque applied to the glenoid component and, on this

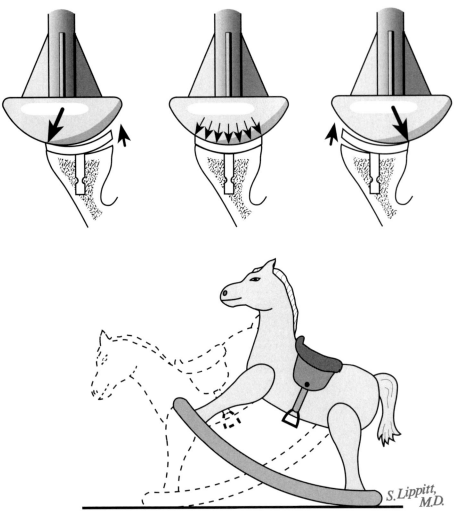

■ **Figure 16–35**
"Rocking horse" loosening of the glenoid component results when translation of the head on the glenoid produces eccentric forces on the glenoid component. *(From Matsen FA III, Lippitt SB, Sidles JA, and Harryman DT II: Practical Evaluation and Management of the Shoulder. Philadelphia: WB Saunders, 1994.)*

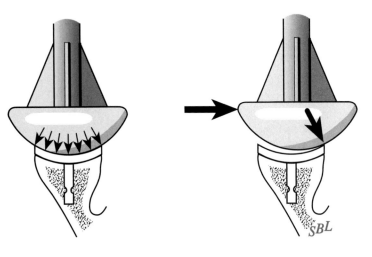

■ **Figure 16–36**
When the radii of curvature of the glenoid component and the humeral head conform, any translation results in rim loading of the glenoid component.

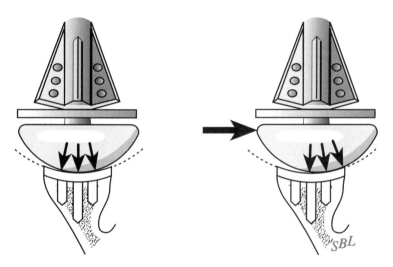

■ **Figure 16–37**
A slight increase in the diameter of curvature of the glenoid component over that of the humeral head allows some translation before rim loading occurs.

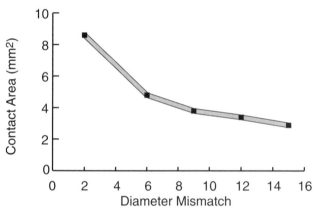

■ **Figure 16–38**
Results of a finite element model analysis of a polyethylene glenoid showing the effect of diameter mismatch on the contact area. Even a slight increase in the glenoid diameter relative to that of the humerus dramatically reduces the contact area. Any further increase in the mismatch further reduces the contact area. *(From Matsen FA III, Lippitt SB, Sidles JA, and Harryman DT II: Practical Evaluation and Management of the Shoulder. Philadelphia: WB Saunders, 1994.)*

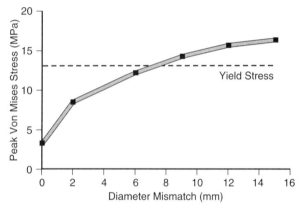

■ **Figure 16–39**
Results of a finite element model analysis of the effect of diameter mismatch on peak contact stresses (pressure-modified Von Mises stress) in a polyethylene glenoid component. The applied compressive load is 625 N (approximately one body weight). The predicted yield stress for the component is shown. A load of one body weight with diametral mismatch in excess of 6 mm is predicted to exceed the yield stress of ordinary polyethylene. *(From Matsen FA III, Lippitt SB, Sidles JA, and Harryman DT II: Practical Evaluation and Management of the Shoulder. Philadelphia: WB Saunders, 1994.)*

In an arthritic shoulder, strength can be compromised by cuff deterioration, disuse, previous injury, and previous surgery. The surgeon may be able to enhance the strength of the shoulder through muscle balancing, tendon repairs, reattachment of the tuberosity, and effective rehabilitation.[53] It is critical that the surgery not impair the function of the muscle-tendon units (Fig. 16–40).

The amount of stuffing of the joint sets the resting length of the cuff muscles and, to a lesser extent, that of the deltoid. If the components are too small, the cuff will be slack at rest and thus place the muscles at the low end of the ideal length-tension relationship. If the joint is overstuffed, the cuff muscles may be at the high end of their length-tension curve. The distance between the effective cuff insertion and the center of the humeral head establishes the moment arm for the cuff.

Jacobson and Mallon provided a method for measuring the glenohumeral offset ratio,[202] and Hsu and associates reviewed the influence of abductor lever arm changes after shoulder arthroplasty.[196]

Smoothness

The anatomic requisites of smooth motion follow.

SMOOTH JOINT SURFACES. In a normal shoulder, intact articular cartilage covering the humeral head and glenoid and lubricated with normal joint fluid provides the lowest possible resistance to motion at the joint surface. In arthritis, these factors are compromised.

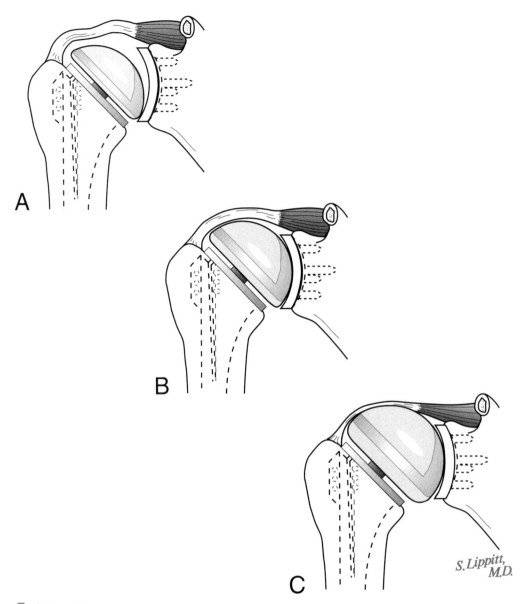

■ **Figure 16–40**
A, A humeral head that is too small leaves the joint with excessive laxity and reduced resting muscle tension.
B, The correct size of head balances the soft tissues. **C,** Overstuffing the joint places excessive tension on the
soft tissues and consequently limits their excursion, decreases range of motion, and predisposes them to
rupture. *(Modified from Matsen FA III, Lippitt SB, Sidles JA, and Harryman DT II: Practical Evaluation and*
Management of the Shoulder. Philadelphia: WB Saunders, 1994.)

Although prosthetic joint surfaces offer much less friction
than bone rubbing on bone does, they have a coefficient
of friction approximately 10 times greater than that of
normal cartilage moving on normal cartilage.

**SMOOTH AND UNIMPAIRED HUMEROSCAPULAR
MOTION INTERFACE.** The proximal end of the humerus
and rotator cuff must slide smoothly beneath the
deltoid, acromion, coracoacromial ligament, coracoid,
and coracoid muscles (see Fig. 16-19). Smoothness of
the humeroscapular motion interface is often compromised in postsurgical and post-traumatic arthritis.
The surfaces of this important interface must glide
smoothly on each other at the conclusion of the arthroplasty procedure.

CLINICAL FINDINGS AND EVALUATION

History

Patients with symptomatic glenohumeral arthritis
usually have pain and loss of function that are refractory
to rest, anti-inflammatory medications, and exercise.
The history should include a description of the onset of
the problem, the mechanism of any injuries, and the
nature and progression of functional difficulties. Systemic or polyarticular manifestations of sepsis, degenerative joint disease, or rheumatoid arthritis may provide
helpful clues. A past history of steroid medication,

fracture, or working at depths may suggest the diagnosis of avascular necrosis. Past injury or surgery suggests the possibility of secondary arthritis or capsulorrhaphy arthropathy.

Standardized methods have been developed by which patients can assess their health status and shoulder function. Bostrom and associates[46] found that standardized assessments of shoulder function are more reliable and reproducible than conventional range-of-motion measurements. As will be seen later, the Short Form-36 (SF-36) provides standardized documentation of a patient's self-assessed health status. The importance of factors such as the SF-36 scales of emotional role function, mental health, and social function is well demonstrated in the work of Summers and associates,[398] who found that objective severity of the disease showed little relationship to patients' reports of pain, whereas psychological variables were much more closely correlated with measures of pain and functional impairment.

Matsen and colleagues reported the self-assessment of 103 patients with primary glenohumeral degenerative joint disease.[262,266] More than half reported that their pain and physical role function scores were more than 1 SD below those of age- and sex-matched controls according to the SF-36 health assessment survey. These patients consistently reported an inability to perform standard shoulder functions according to the Simple Shoulder Test (SST), such as sleeping comfortably, lifting 8 lb to shoulder height, washing the back of the opposite shoulder, throwing overhand, and tucking in the back of a shirt. Gartsman and coworkers found that among other shoulder conditions, glenohumeral arthritis was comparable to diseases such as congestive heart failure, acute myocardial infarction, and diabetes in terms of its effect on health status according to the SF-36.[151] Matsen and associates used self-assessment of shoulder function (SST) and health status (SF-36) to compare patients with rheumatoid arthritis and degenerative joint disease of the shoulder.[264]

Just as poor shoulder function may affect perception of health status, comorbid conditions may similarly have an impact on shoulder function. Comorbidities may include other diseases, social or psychological factors, and work-related injuries. Rozencwaig and coworkers studied the effect of comorbidities on health status and shoulder function in 85 patients with osteoarthritis who met the criteria for shoulder arthroplasty. The number of comorbidities had a negative impact on the SST and the majority of parameters on the SF-36. The authors highlighted the importance of controlling for comorbidity when evaluating functional status and predicting the success of treatment.[362]

Physical Examination

Physical examination often reveals mild or moderate muscle wasting about the shoulder, crepitus on joint motion, and limited range of motion. The limitation in glenohumeral motion is most easily identified if one of the examiner's hands is used to stabilize the scapula while flexion/extension and internal/external rotation of the

humerus relative to the scapula are documented with the other hand.

Isometric strength is documented in flexion, extension, abduction, and rotation. Individuals being considered for prosthetic arthroplasty should have good anterior deltoid and rotator cuff strength. Strong internal and external rotators are particularly essential if a glenoid prosthesis is being considered.

It is important to emphasize that shoulder arthritis may coexist with other medical conditions, many of which will substantially alter the disability and the patient's potential to respond positively to treatment. Thus, a thorough evaluation of each individual is essential.

Radiographic Evaluation

In the evaluation of glenohumeral arthritis, standardized radiographic views are necessary to understand the disease process and its severity. Standard views include an anteroposterior view in the plane of the scapula and a true axillary view (Fig. 16–41). These views indicate the thickness of the cartilage space between the humerus and the glenoid, the relative positions of the humeral head and the glenoid, the presence of osteophytes, the degree of osteopenia, and the extent of bony deformity and erosion. Superior displacement of the humeral head relative to the scapula suggests major cuff deficiency and argues against the use of a glenoid prosthesis (see Fig. 16–34). If humeral arthroplasty is being considered, a templating anteroposterior view of the humerus in 35 degrees of external rotation relative to the x-ray beam with a magnification marker is obtained (Fig. 16–42). This view places the humeral neck in maximal profile and allows a comparison of proximal humeral anatomy with that of various humeral prostheses. If this view is taken with the arm in 45 degrees of abduction so that the middle of the humeral articular surface is placed in the middle of the glenoid fossa, it can reveal thinning of the central aspect of the humeral articular cartilage typical of degenerative joint disease (the "Friar Tuck" pattern), whereas radiographs with the arm in other positions may suggest the presence of a thicker layer of cartilage at the periphery of the head.

CT scans are obtained if there is a question about the amount or quality of bone available for reconstruction, but such questions can usually be answered from plain radiographs alone. Friedman and associates[143] and Mullaji and colleagues[285] used CT to characterize the changes in version in a group of patients with degenerative and inflammatory arthritis. The most important conclusion from these two studies is that glenoid version varies through a range of 30 degrees in these populations! Mallon and associates[253] have also conducted detailed studies of the articular surface of the glenoid and related this shape to the anatomy of the scapula.

Galinat reported variation in glenoid version, depending on the angle of the x-ray beam during positioning of the machine for the axillary radiograph.[147] Glenoid version can be measured by connecting a line drawn down the line of the body of the scapula with a line between the anterior and posterior glenoid rim. Normal version at the

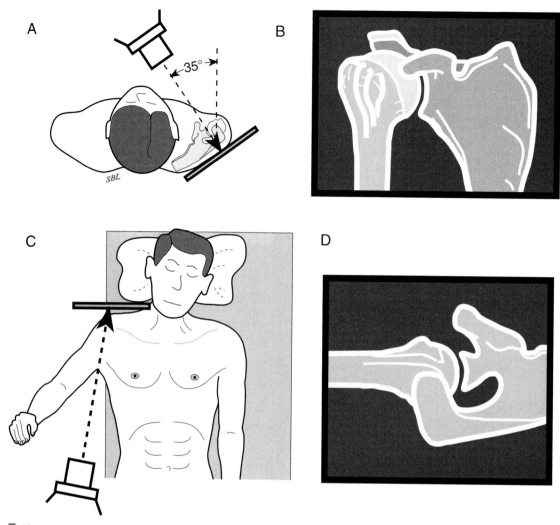

■ **Figure 16–41**
Radiographic series for a stiff shoulder. **A,** The anteroposterior view in the plane of the scapula is obtained by orienting the beam perpendicular to the plane of the scapula and centering it on the coracoid tip while the film is parallel to the plane of the scapula. **B,** The resultant radiograph should clearly reveal the radiographic joint space between the humeral head and the glenoid. **C,** The axillary view is obtained by centering the beam between the coracoid tip and the posterior angle of the acromion. **D,** The resultant radiograph should project the glenoid midway between the coracoid and the acromion and provide a clear view of the joint space. *(From Matsen FA III, Lippitt SB, Sidles JA, and Harryman DT II: Practical Evaluation and Management of the Shoulder. Philadelphia: WB Saunders, 1994.)*

level just below the coracoid process varies from 0 to −7 degrees (Fig. 16–43). In a series of 200 patients undergoing shoulder arthroplasty, Jensen and Rockwood obtained a CT scan in 78 patients to define glenoid version.[204] These 78 patients also had severe loss of external rotation and posterior subluxation of the head of the humerus. Sixty-three percent, or 49 shoulders, required specific alterations during arthroplasty (i.e., decreasing the amount of humeral retroversion or changing the version of the glenoid with special reamers). Badet and colleagues evaluated the CT findings of 113 patients with glenohumeral osteoarthritis and found that glenoid retroversion was substantially increased and humeral retroversion was decreased when compared with control shoulders without arthritis.[16]

Imaging of the rotator cuff by arthrography, magnetic resonance imaging (MRI), or ultrasound is carried out if

it will affect management of the patient. The status of the rotator cuff can usually be understood from an evaluation of the history, physical examination, and plain radiographs.

Green and Norris[158] and Slawson and associates[381] have provided a review of imaging techniques for glenohumeral arthritis and for glenohumeral arthroplasty.

Disease Characteristics

A number of different processes can destroy the glenohumeral joint surface. Clinical evaluation, management, and measurement of effectiveness are facilitated by establishing the necessary and sufficient criteria that enable us to standardize the assignment of each diagnosis.

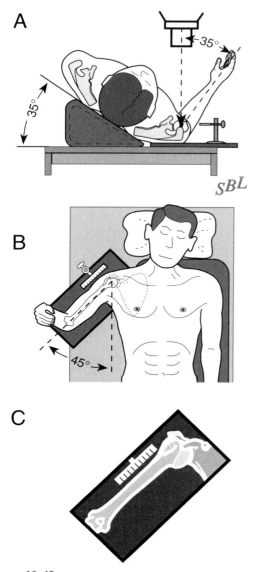

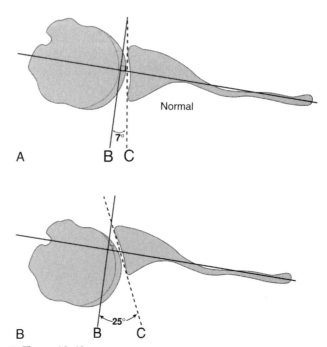

■ Figure 16–43

A, Normal glenoid version varies from 0 to –7 degrees of retroversion. In a computed tomographic scan, measurement of version is accomplished by drawing a line along the axis of the scapular body and then drawing a line perpendicular to it (B). A third line is drawn along the anterior and posterior rims of the glenoid (C). The angle between B and C is the glenoid version. B, An increase in retroversion to 25 degrees is usually accompanied by posterior subluxation of the head of the humerus.

■ Figure 16–42

Templating view, with the anteroposterior radiograph in the "centered position." The humerus is positioned in neutral rotation with respect to the thorax and is abducted 45 degrees. The anteroposterior radiograph in the plane of the scapula is obtained by positioning the scapula flat on the cassette and aiming the beam at the joint. The beam makes a 35-degree angle with the forearm, and the thorax makes a 35-degree angle with the cassette. A centimeter marker held adjacent to the lateral aspect of the humerus indicates the radiographic magnification when templates for various components are being compared. The final radiographic appearance is as shown in C. (From Matsen FA III, Lippitt SB, Sidles JA, and Harryman DT II: Practical Evaluation and Management of the Shoulder. Philadelphia: WB Saunders, 1994.)

Table 16–2 lists the necessary and sufficient criteria for six of the more common types of glenohumeral joint destruction: primary degenerative joint disease, secondary degenerative joint disease, rheumatoid arthritis, cuff tear arthropathy, capsulorrhaphy arthropathy, and avascular necrosis.

In an extension of a study on self-assessment of patients with glenohumeral osteoarthritis,[266] patients with these conditions assessed their shoulder function by using the 12 questions of the SST (Table 16–3).[262] These individuals with glenohumeral arthritis had the greatest difficulty with overhand throwing, sleeping comfortably on the affected side, washing the back of the opposite shoulder, and placing 8 lb on a shelf (Table 16–4). Interestingly, the degree of functional compromise at initial evaluation was comparable for the different diagnoses. Apparently, it is this level of functional impairment, irrespective of the diagnosis, that brings the patient in for evaluation. These functional deficits are the target of treatment of glenohumeral arthritis.

These individuals also assessed their health status with the SF-36.* The self-assessed overall health status of individuals with glenohumeral arthritis is most compromised in the domains of physical role function and overall comfort (Table 16–5). For patients with primary and secondary degenerative joint disease and cuff tear arthropathy, the other SF-36 parameters (e.g., vitality and overall health) were relatively close to population-based age- and sex-matched controls. The health status of patients with rheumatoid arthritis, capsulorrhaphy arthropathy, and

_____

*The SF-36 is a general health status self-assessment used in many fields of medicine.[337,420] It is very useful in orthopaedics for documenting the general health deficits of patients before and after reconstructive surgery. The overall comfort and physical role function scales are most commonly affected by arthritic conditions of the shoulder. Other SF-36 scores are useful for documenting the patient's vitality, mental health, general health, and social, emotional, and physical function.

TABLE 16–2. Necessary and Sufficient Diagnostic Criteria for Clinically Significant Involvement from Six Major Types of Glenohumeral Arthritis

---

Degenerative Joint Disease (Primary)

History
1. Absence of major joint trauma, previous surgery, or other known causes of secondary degenerative joint disease
2. Limited motion and function

Physical Examination
1. Limited glenohumeral motion
2. (Diagnosis is supported by bone-on-bone crepitance)

Radiographs (see Figs. 16–24, 16–44, 16–45)
1. Joint space narrowing
2. Periarticular sclerosis
3. Periarticular osteophytes
4. Absence of other pathology
5. (Diagnosis is supported by posterior glenoid erosion with posterior subluxation of the humeral head)

Secondary Degenerative Joint Disease

History
1. Evidence of major joint trauma or other known causes of secondary degenerative joint disease
2. Limited motion and function

Physical Examination
1. Limited glenohumeral motion
2. (Diagnosis is supported by bone-on-bone crepitance)

Radiographs (see Figs. 16–46 to 16–50)
1. Joint space narrowing
2. Periarticular sclerosis
3. Periarticular osteophytes
4. (Diagnosis is supported by radiographic evidence of previous trauma or other known causes of secondary degenerative joint disease)

Rheumatoid Arthritis

History
1. Established diagnosis of rheumatoid arthritis
2. Limited motion and function

Physical Examination (see Fig. 16–62)
1. Limited glenohumeral motion
2. (Diagnosis is supported by findings of muscle atrophy and weakness or bone-on-bone crepitance)

Radiographs (see Figs. 16–29, 16–51 to 16–62)
1. Joint space narrowing
2. Periarticular osteopenia
3. (Diagnosis is supported by the absence of osteophytes and sclerosis)
4. (Diagnosis is supported by the presence of periarticular erosions and medial erosion of the glenoid)

Cuff Tear Arthropathy

History
1. Limited motion and function
2. Weakness in elevation and rotation
3. (Diagnosis is supported by previously confirmed cuff tear)

Physical Examination
1. Limited glenohumeral motion
2. Evidence of large cuff defect such as
   Supraspinatus and infraspinatus atrophy
   Weakness of external rotation and elevation
   Superior position of humeral head relative to scapula
   Palpable rotator cuff defect
3. Bone-on-bone crepitance

Radiographs (see Figs. 16–33, 16–34, 16–46, 16–64, 16–65)
1. Superior displacement of humeral head relative to the glenoid leading to contact with coracoacromial arch
2. Secondary degenerative changes of the glenohumeral joint
3. (Diagnosis is supported by erosion of the greater tuberosity ("femoralization" of the proximal part of the humerus))
4. (Diagnosis is supported by a contoured coracoacromial arch and upper glenoid to produce a socket for the proximal end of the humerus ["acetabularization"])
5. (Diagnosis is supported by collapse of the superior subchondral bone of the humeral head)

Capsulorrhaphy Arthropathy

History
1. Functionally significant restricted glenohumeral motion
2. History of previous repair for glenohumeral instability

Physical Examination
1. Limited motion and function (especially external rotation)
2. (Diagnosis is supported by bone-on-bone crepitance)

Radiographs (see Figs. 16–7, 16–8, 16–46, 16–47)
1. Joint space narrowing
2. Periarticular sclerosis
3. Periarticular osteophytes
4. (Diagnosis is supported by posterior glenoid erosion with posterior subluxation of the humeral head)

Avascular Necrosis (Atraumatic)

History
1. Limited shoulder function
2. (Diagnosis is supported by the presence of risk factors such as steroid use)

Physical Examination
1. (Diagnosis is supported by glenohumeral crepitance)

Radiographs (see Figs. 16–68 to 16–71)
1. Sclerosis within the head of the humerus
2. Collapse of subchondral bone of the humeral head
3. Absence of other pathology (e.g., tumor, cuff tear arthropathy)

TABLE 16–3. Simple Shoulder Test

1. Is your shoulder comfortable with your arm at rest by your side?
2. Does your shoulder allow you to sleep comfortably?
3. Can you reach the small of your back to tuck in your shirt with your hand?
4. Can you place your hand behind your head with the elbow straight out to the side?
5. Can you place a coin on a shelf at the level of your shoulder without bending your elbow?
6. Can you lift 1 lb (a full pint container) to the level of your shoulder without bending your elbow?
7. Can you lift 8 lb (a full gallon container) to the level of the top of your head without bending your elbow?
8. Can you carry 20 lb (a bag of potatoes) at your side with the affected extremity?
9. Do you think you can toss a softball underhand 10 yards with the affected extremity?
10. Do you think you can throw a softball overhand 20 yards with the affected extremity?
11. Can you wash the back of your opposite shoulder with the affected extremity?
12. Would your shoulder allow you to work full-time at your regular job?

TABLE 16–4. Percentage of Patients with Six Different Types of Glenohumeral Arthritis Who Were Able to Perform Functions of the Simple Shoulder Test at the Time of Initial Evaluation

Function	DJD	SDJD	RA	CTA	CA	AVN
Sleep comfortably	12	13	18	8	0	29
Arm comfortable at side	67	36	61	33	65	79
Wash back of shoulder	13	20	13	0	18	7
Hand behind head	35	38	26	21	35	50
Tuck in shirt	32	33	39	38	29	50
8 lb on shelf	19	16	3	0	18	7
1 lb on shelf	54	36	26	21	53	50
Coin on shelf	59	44	29	29	53	64
Throw overhand	7	9	3	4	0	0
Do usual work	39	44	21	17	41	21
Throw underhand	53	44	13	42	29	21
Carry 20 lb	62	62	21	33	41	29

AVN, avascular necrosis; CA, capsulorrhaphy arthropathy; CTA, cuff tear arthropathy; DJD, degenerative joint disease; RA, rheumatoid arthritis; SDJD, secondary degenerative joint disease.

TABLE 16–5. Self-assessed Health Status of Patients with Six Different Types of Glenohumeral Arthritis Revealed by the SF-36*

SF-36 Parameter	DJD	SDJD	RA	CTA	CA	AVN
Physical role function	44	33	23	30	39	28
Comfort	54	47	34	39	40	47
Physical function	78	73	38	81	62	50
Emotional role function	83	76	58	100	64	40
Social function	84	73	63	81	71	62
Vitality	86	83	44	81	65	60
Mental health	92	90	87	97	76	84
General health	100	93	65	100	71	63

*Data are presented as the average percentage of age- and sex-matched population controls.[28]

AVN, avascular necrosis; CA, capsulorrhaphy arthropathy; CTA, cuff tear arthropathy; DJD, degenerative joint disease; RA, rheumatoid arthritis; SDJD, secondary degenerative joint disease.

TABLE 16–6. Pathoanatomy of Glenohumeral Osteoarthritis

Humeral head
  Cartilage loss—central, superior, or complete
  Sclerosis—central, superior
  Peripheral osteophytes—most prominent inferiorly
  Increased size
  Erosion with central flattening
  Subchondral cysts
Glenoid
  Cartilage loss—central, posterior, or complete
  Sclerosis—central or posterior
  Peripheral osteophytes—lower two thirds
  Erosion—central or posterior with flattening
  Subchondral cysts
Joint position
  Central or posterior subluxation
Capsule
  Enlarged, especially inferiorly
  Anterior contracture
Rotator cuff and biceps tendon
  Complete-thickness tearing unusual (approximately 5%)
  Degeneration or fibrosis (especially subscapularis) may be present
Loose bodies within joint or subscapularis bursa

avascular necrosis was poorer than that of controls of the same age and sex.[264] This result shows the differential impact of diagnosis on health and well-being.

Degenerative Joint Disease

In degenerative joint disease, the glenoid cartilage and subchondral bone are typically worn posteriorly, with articular cartilage often left intact anteriorly (see Fig. 16–24). The cartilage of the humeral head is eroded in a "Friar Tuck" pattern of central baldness, frequently surrounded by a rim of remaining cartilage and osteophytes. Degenerative cysts may occur in the humeral head or glenoid. Osteophytes typically surround the anterior, inferior, and posterior aspects of the humeral head and the inferior and posterior glenoid. As a result, the humeral and glenoid articular surfaces have a flattened configuration that blocks rotation (Figs. 16–44 and 16–45). Loose bodies are often found in the axillary or subscapularis recesses. The triad of anterior capsular contracture, posterior glenoid wear, and posterior humeral subluxation is common in primary degenerative joint disease. Rotator cuff defects are uncommon in patients with primary degenerative joint disease. Cofield summarized the pathoanatomy of degenerative joint disease (Table 16–6).[90]

Secondary Degenerative Joint Disease

In contrast to primary degenerative joint disease, secondary degenerative joint disease arises when previous injury, surgery, or another condition affects the joint surface and precipitates its degeneration. In chronic, unreduced dislocations,[189,335,361] the humeral head may be indented and worn (Fig. 16–46). The cartilage of the joint surfaces may be replaced with scar tissue, or the subchondral bone may be so weakened by bone atrophy that it will collapse after reduction and result in an incongruous joint surface (Fig. 16–47). Samilson and Prieto[370] identified 74 shoulders

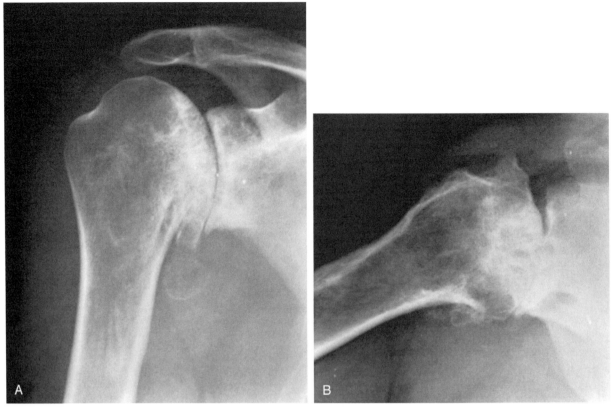

■ **Figure 16–44**
Osteoarthritis of the shoulder. **A,** A stereotypical radiographic, pathoanatomic appearance. The humeral head is somewhat enlarged and flattened. Peripheral osteophytes are particularly prominent inferiorly. There is flattening of the humeral head with subchondral sclerosis, particularly rest centrally and central-superiorly. Intraosseous cysts may be present. These cysts are best seen on the axillary projection. **B,** In the axillary view, one also sees asymmetric glenoid wear with slightly greater wear of the posterior aspect of the glenoid. In addition, the glenoid is also flattened. There is a suggestion of posterior humeral subluxation, but this feature is not striking in these radiographs.

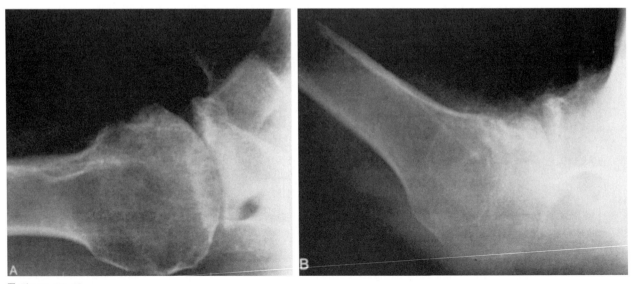

■ **Figure 16–45**
In osteoarthritis of the shoulder, varying amounts of asymmetric posterior glenoid erosion and posterior humeral instability may be present. **A,** Moderate amount of asymmetric posterior glenoid erosion and subluxation of the humeral head into the area of wear. **B,** A lesser amount of glenoid erosion but a much larger degree of posterior humeral subluxation, findings suggestive of significant elongation of the posterior shoulder capsule and the overlying rotator cuff. Reconstructive steps should take these changes—the glenoid erosion and the instability—into consideration.

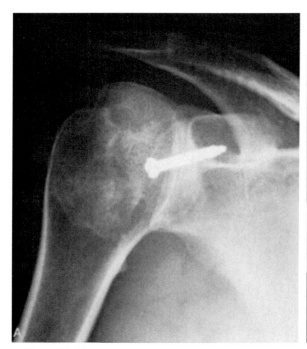
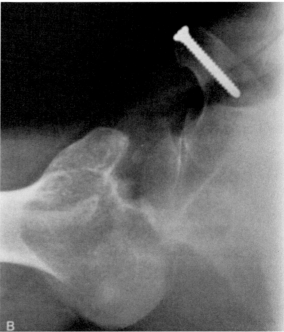

■ **Figure 16–46**

Chronic posterior shoulder dislocation in a 26-year-old man. The injury occurred approximately 1 year earlier. A recent previous anterior approach to the shoulder was ineffective in reducing the dislocation. At the time of the second surgical procedure, the shoulder was reduced, but the cartilage of the humeral head had been replaced with fibrous tissue. A proximal humeral prosthesis was placed as a part of the reconstructive procedure. **A,** A 40-degree posterior oblique radiograph illustrating the overlap between the humeral head and the glenoid. **B,** Clearly illustrated are the posterior dislocation, the slight malunion between the head and shaft fragments, and evidence of fracturing of the lesser tuberosity with healing of this tuberosity to the shaft, but somewhat displaced from the humeral head segment.

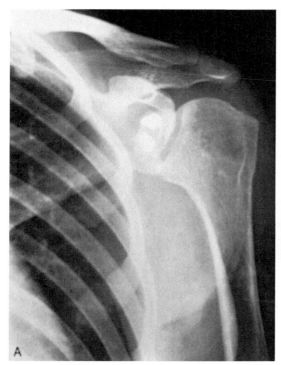
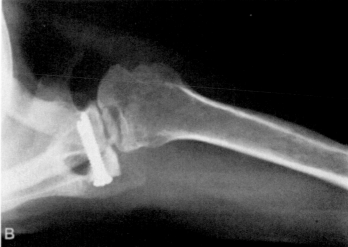

■ **Figure 16–47**

This young woman underwent open reduction of a posterior shoulder dislocation that had been unreduced for approximately 2 months. At the time of reduction, the cartilage surfaces were intact, but the humeral head was noted to be somewhat softened. A bone graft was added to the posterior aspect of the shoulder to substitute for an area of glenoid wear. Within the first month after open reduction, it was apparent on the anteroposterior view (**A**) and the axillary view (**B**) that because of its softness, the humeral head had collapsed and traumatic arthritis was developing. Subsequently, a proximal humeral prosthesis was placed.

with a history of single or multiple dislocations that exhibited radiographic evidence of glenohumeral arthritis (Fig. 16–48). The dislocations had been anterior in 62 shoulders and posterior in 11 cases, and 1 had multidirectional instability. The number of dislocations was not related to the severity of the arthrosis. Shoulders with posterior instability had a higher incidence of moderate or

TABLE 16–7. Glenohumeral Arthritis following Trauma

Potential Etiologies
Recurrent subluxation or dislocation
Chronic dislocations
Fracture malunion with joint incongruity
Osteonecrosis of the humeral head
Proximal humeral nonunion with fibrous ankylosis

severe arthritis, as did shoulders with previous surgery in which internal fixation devices intruded on the joint surface. Marx and colleagues recently suggested that the odds ratio for development of degenerative joint disease after shoulder dislocation is 10.5.[257] Hawkins and coworkers[189] suggested hemiarthroplasty if the dislocation is more than 6 months old or if the humeral head defect involves more than 45% of the articular surface. If the glenoid is destroyed, total shoulder arthroplasty may be indicated.

Tanner and Cofield reviewed 28 shoulders with chronic fracture problems that required prosthetic arthroplasty.[404] Sixteen had malunion with joint incongruity (Fig. 16–49), 8 had post-traumatic osteonecrosis (Fig. 16–50), and 4 had nonunion of a surgical neck fracture with a small, osteopenic head fragment. Cofield summarized some features of post-traumatic arthritis (Table 16–7).[90]

Shoulders with secondary degenerative joint disease often have complex pathology that entails difficult surgical management.[199,301] Difficulties may be related to a number of factors: muscle contracture, scarring, malunion requiring osteotomy, nonunion, or bone loss, especially humeral shortening. Dines and associates[115] reported their results with shoulder arthroplasty in 20 patients with post-traumatic changes. They emphasized the difficulty of these cases and the advisability of avoiding tuberosity osteotomy. Other series of arthroplasty for late sequelae of trauma include that of Norris and coworkers,[307] Habermeyer and Schweiberer,[168] and Frich and associates.[141]

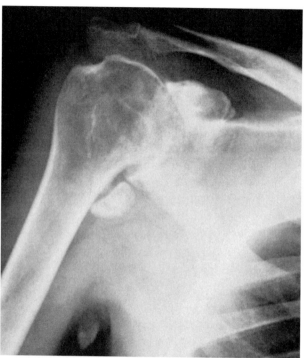

■ **Figure 16–48**
This elderly man had a 5- to 10-year history of progressively severe shoulder pain and limitation of motion. As an adolescent, he had experienced recurrent dislocations of this shoulder, and presumably his current arthritis has developed subsequent to his recurrent instability. This sequence of events certainly can occur but is surprisingly uncommon.

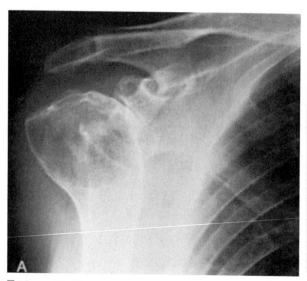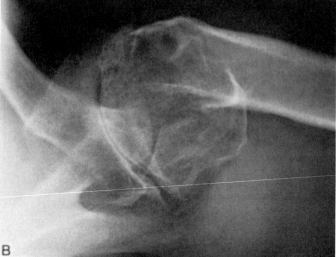

■ **Figure 16–49**
A and B, Traumatic arthritis with loss of glenohumeral cartilage has developed after malunion of a comminuted proximal humeral fracture.

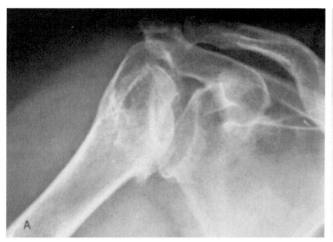
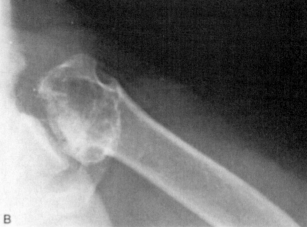

■ Figure 16–50

Traumatic arthritis with malunion and osteonecrosis of the head segment. **A,** Radiograph showing collapse of the head segment and slight malunion of the greater tuberosity relative to the shaft. **B,** Radiograph again showing collapse of the humeral head segment but reasonable positions of the tuberosities on this view. Damage to the glenoid articular surface is underestimated on these radiographic projections. At reconstructive surgery for such situations, either proximal humeral prosthetic replacement or total shoulder arthroplasty might be needed, depending on the extent of glenoid surface involvement.

Rheumatoid and Other Types of Inflammatory Arthritis

Rheumatoid arthritis is a systemic disease with highly variable clinical manifestations. It may appear to be isolated to the glenohumeral joint or may affect most of the tissues in the body. In rheumatoid arthritis and many other types of inflammatory arthritis, the cartilage is characteristically destroyed evenly across all joint surfaces. The glenoid is eroded medially (see Fig. 16-29) rather than posteriorly, such as in degenerative joint disease (see Fig. 16-24). The condition is often bilaterally symmetric. The arthritic process erodes not only cartilage but also subchondral bone and renders it osteopenic (Figs. 16-51 to 16-61). Lehtinen and coworkers evaluated the incidence of glenohumeral involvement in a prospectively monitored cohort of 74 patients with seropositive rheumatoid arthritis over a 15-year period. Erosive involvement of the glenohumeral joint occurred in 48% of patients and was most often observed on the superolateral articular surface of the humerus. Glenoid involvement was less common. Patients with the most severe destruction almost always had bilateral disease.[237]

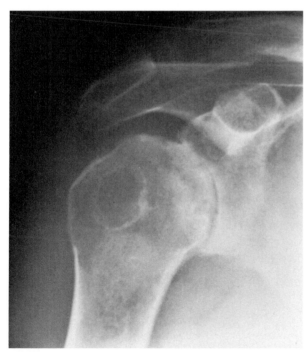

■ Figure 16–51

Rheumatoid arthritis of the shoulder with glenohumeral cartilage loss and joint stiffness, the so-called dry form of the disease.

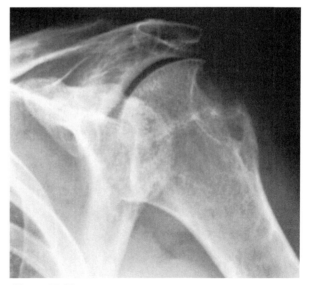

■ Figure 16–52

Rheumatoid arthritis in the shoulder with cartilage loss, extensive periarticular erosions, and an extremely hypertrophic synovitis, the so-called wet form of joint involvement.

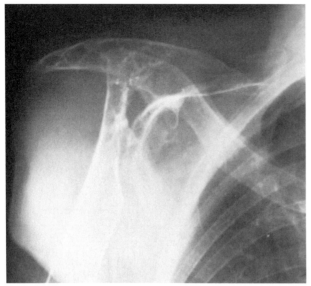

■ **Figure 16–53**
This radiograph of the shoulder of an elderly woman with long-standing rheumatoid arthritis shows extreme resorption involving the humeral head, a portion of the proximal part of the humerus, and the lateral aspect of the scapula, including the entire glenoid.

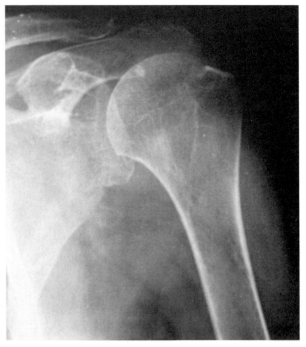

■ **Figure 16–54**
A middle-aged woman with long-standing rheumatoid arthritis and multiple joint involvement. When these radiographs were taken, the woman had severe shoulder pain and mild restriction of movement. The radiographs essentially show only osteopenia. Maintenance of the joint space is apparent, with only the slightest suggestion of marginal joint erosion. The extent of pathologic changes seen here is rather mild. Unfortunately, the patient's symptoms did not respond to conservative management. Significant synovitis was demonstrated on the arthrogram, and shoulder synovectomy was performed.

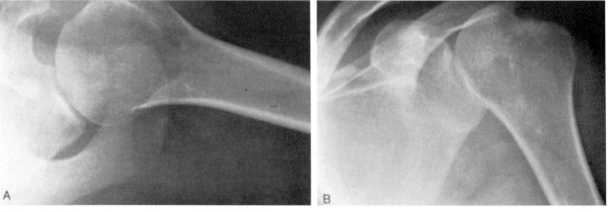

■ **Figure 16–55**
Rheumatoid arthritis involving the shoulder of a 26-year-old man with oligoarticular disease. His symptoms were moderate. The radiographs show slight cartilage loss, particularly on the axillary projection (**A**), and erosion of the humeral head near the articular surface margin on the anteroposterior radiograph (**B**). Extensive synovitis was present (see Fig. 16–60).

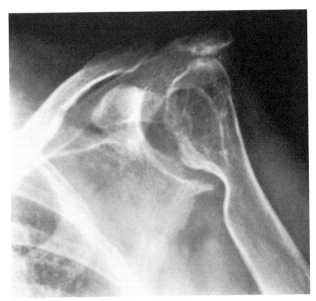

■ Figure 16–56

Long-standing rheumatoid arthritis of the shoulder with erosion of the subchondral and adjacent bone structures. This erosion is notable on the humeral head but is most pronounced in the scapula with extreme central resorption. Such patients may not have enough bone remaining to allow placement of a glenoid component at the time of reconstructive surgery.

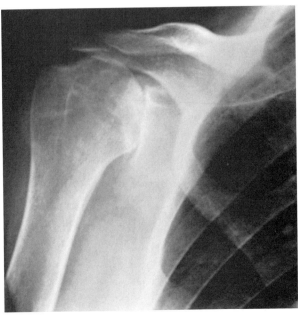

■ Figure 16–57

Rheumatoid arthritis of the shoulder. The radiograph shows a slight amount of osteopenia, cartilage loss, mild subchondral bone loss, and upward subluxation of the humeral head. In this patient, as in many with rheumatoid arthritis of the shoulder, the rotator cuff has become thin, with attrition, stretching, and fibrosis but without full-thickness rotator cuff tearing.

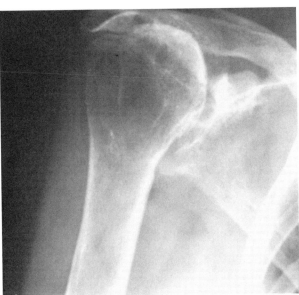

■ Figure 16–58

Rheumatoid arthritis of the shoulder in association with rotator cuff tearing. The radiograph shows cartilage loss, central-superior erosion of the glenoid, upward subluxation of the humeral head, and some erosion of the overlying acromion and distal end of the clavicle. At surgery, a large rotator cuff tear involving the infraspinatus, supraspinatus, and subscapularis was discovered.

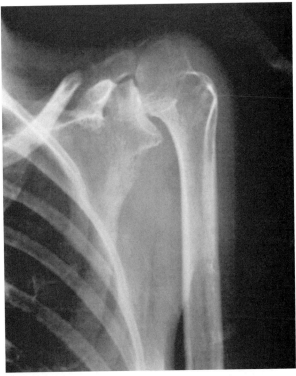

■ Figure 16–59

Juvenile rheumatoid arthritis with extreme rotator cuff and capsular involvement, even to the extent of acromial erosion. The humeral head is now beneath the skin across the superior aspect of the shoulder.

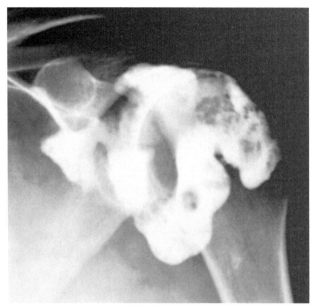

■ **Figure 16-60**
Shoulder arthrogram showing active synovitis in a patient with rheumatoid arthritis. Plain radiographs (see Fig. 16-55) showed only minor joint changes.

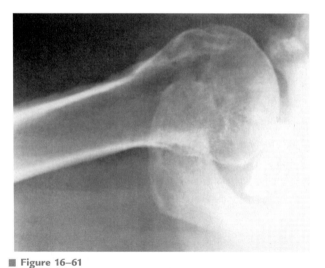

■ **Figure 16-61**
Axillary x-ray projection of the shoulder of a young woman with rheumatoid arthritis. Rheumatoid destruction of the anterior shoulder capsule and the anterior aspect of the rotator cuff has occurred such that anterior instability now exists. Enough cartilage loss had occurred that treatment included proximal humeral prosthetic replacement, glenohumeral joint synovectomy, and anterior capsule and rotator cuff repair.

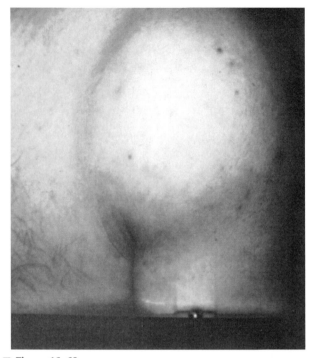

■ **Figure 16-62**
Clinical photograph of the shoulder of a young man with rheumatoid arthritis and primary rheumatoid involvement of the subacromial-subdeltoid bursa. The rotator cuff was intact, and the glenohumeral joint had minimal involvement with rheumatoid synovitis. The patient had full, minimally painful range of motion in the shoulder, with excellent shoulder strength. The hypertrophic bursitis did not respond to medical management, and surgical excision of the bursa was performed.

Rheumatoid arthritis may simultaneously involve the glenohumeral, acromioclavicular, sternoclavicular, elbow, wrist, and hand articulations, thereby greatly amplifying the resultant functional losses. Soft tissues, including the rotator cuff, may likewise be swollen, contracted, weakened, or torn (Fig. 16-62; see also Fig. 16-60). In a clinical and arthrographic study of 200 painful shoulders in patients with rheumatoid arthritis, Ennevaara found that only 26% of patients had full-thickness rotator cuff defects.[125] In two series of patients with rheumatoid

arthritis that required total shoulder arthroplasty, the rotator cuff had full-thickness tearing in 29 of 69 shoulders (42%) and in 18 of 66 shoulders (27%).[84,304] Rozing and Brand encountered a large cuff defect in 21 of 40 (52%) shoulders undergoing shoulder arthroplasty for rheumatoid arthritis. A durable repair was possible in less than half these patients, and the quality of the cuff repair correlated significantly with postoperative outcome.[363]

Even the skin may be fragile and subject to compromise in wound healing. The fragility of a patient with rheumatoid arthritis is frequently compounded by long-term use of steroids and other antimetabolic medications. Because the condition itself involves the immune system, the patient is often receiving immunosuppressive medication, and the clinical manifestations of rheumatoid arthritis are similar to those of infectious arthritis, the physician must be aware of the possible coexistence of joint infection. Cofield summarized the characteristics of rheumatoid arthritis of the shoulder (Table 16-8).[90] Petersson[323] pointed to the prevalence and progression of rheumatoid involvement of the shoulder. Winalski and Shapiro[433] and Mullaji and associates[285] used CT to characterize the rheumatoid involvement of the sternoclavicular and glenohumeral joints. Alasaarela and Alasaarela[2,3] used ultrasound to define the soft tissue changes associated with rheumatoid arthritis of the shoulder.

Other conditions may produce shoulder findings quite similar to those of rheumatoid arthritis (Fig. 16-63).

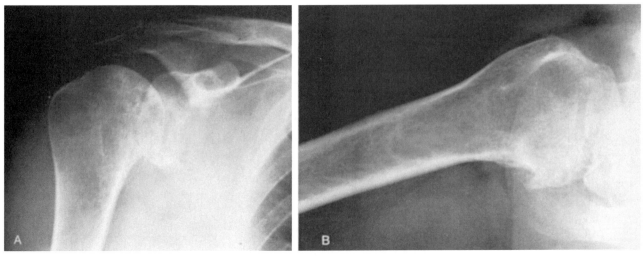

■ **Figure 16–63**

An upper-middle-aged woman with 4 years of progressively severe shoulder pain now has pain with any arm activity and at rest. She had no history of a previous injury or any history of multiple joint arthritic involvement. The sedimentation rate is slightly elevated; rheumatoid factor is negative. At surgery, the synovium exhibited histologic changes of a mild chronic synovitis but was not diagnostic of a specific type of arthritic disease. As seen on the anteroposterior (**A**) and axillary (**B**) views, this patient's disease has many of the characteristics of a nonspecific inflammatory arthritis: osteopenia, cartilage loss, granulation tissue within a cyst in the humeral head and glenoid, and minimal hypertrophic or sclerotic changes. Features such as these are somewhat uncommon but not rare.

TABLE 16–8. Rheumatoid Arthritis of the Shoulder

Tissue	Type of Pathologic Change
Subdeltoid bursa	Inflammation
	Fibrosis
	Synovial hypertrophy
Bone	Osteopenia
	Erosions
	Resorption
	Sclerosis
	Cysts
	Fracture
Cartilage	Loss, partial or complete
Rotator cuff	Inflammation
	Fibrosis
	Thinning, stretching
	Tearing
Synovial lining	Inflammation
	Fibrosis
	Synovial hypertrophy
Shoulder capsule	Inflammation
	Fibrosis
	Thinning, stretching
	Instability

Included in the list are localized processes such as pigmented villonodular synovitis,[118,119] synovial chondrometaplasia,[194] and pseudogout.[198] The shoulder may be a site of manifestation of systemic disorders such as hemophilia and hemachromatosis,[126,338] primary hyperparathyroidism,[310] acromegaly,[324] amyloid arthropathy,[112] gout,[121] chondrocalcinosis,[104] ankylosing spondylitis,[137,254] psoriasis,[138] and Lyme arthritis.[112] Sethi and associates[378] reported a "dialysis arthropathy" that affects multiple joints, including the shoulder, in individuals undergoing long-term dialysis.

Because of the fragility of the skin and other soft tissues, osteopenia, and severe bone erosion common with this condition, a patient with substantial involvement of rheumatoid arthritis or similar types of arthritis must be treated with extreme gentleness, thoroughness, and care. These admonitions are referred to as "rheumatoid rules" and guide each step of patient management.

In a review, Sneppen and associates[383] pointed to the challenges of arthroplasty in rheumatoid disease. In their series of Neer arthroplasties, at a 92-month follow-up 55% showed proximal migration of the humerus relative to the glenoid, 40% showed progressive loosening of the glenoid component, and 5 of 12 press-fit humeral components showed progressive loosening (but none in 50 cemented humeral components). Despite these problems, 89% of the patients reported good pain relief. Boyd and associates[47] found that of 111 Neer total shoulder arthroplasties with an average follow-up of 55 months, progressive proximal migration occurred in 22% of the patients (29 shoulders). Similarly Sojbjerg and colleagues noted proximal humeral migration with progressive glenoid loosening in 42% of their series of 69 patients treated for severely destructive rheumatoid arthritis by shoulder arthroplasty.[384]

As shown in Table 16-5, individuals with rheumatoid arthritis characteristically have substantially lower self-assessed vitality and overall physical function than do those with other causes of glenohumeral arthritis. The compromised general health and strength of individuals with rheumatoid arthritis must be considered in their management, as has been emphasized by a comparison study of rheumatoid arthritis and degenerative joint disease conducted by Matsen and associates.[264]

Cuff Tear Arthropathy

Cuff tear arthropathy is a compound degenerative condition of the shoulder that affects tendon, cartilage, and bone. Characteristically, chronic, massive rotator cuff

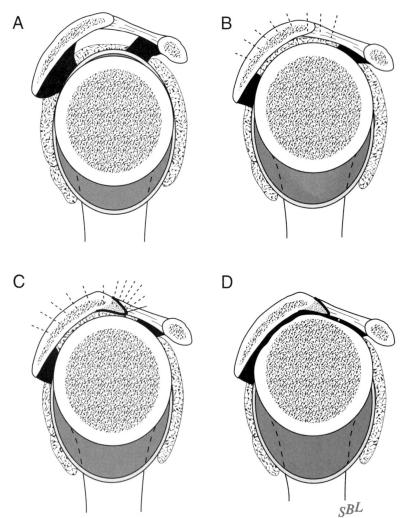

■ **Figure 16–64**
With progressive cuff fiber failure, the head moves upward against the coracoacromial arch. **A,** Normal relationships of the cuff and the coracoacromial arch. **B,** Upward displacement of the head with the cuff squeezed against the acromion and the coracoacromial ligament. **C,** Greater contact and abrasion giving rise to a traction spur in the coracoacromial ligament. **D,** Still greater upward displacement resulting in abrasion of the humeral articular cartilage and cuff tear arthropathy. *(Modified from Matsen FA III, Lippitt SB, Sidles JA, and Harryman DT II: Practical Evaluation and Management of the Shoulder. Philadelphia: WB Saunders, 1994.)*

defects are associated with loss of the superior humeral articular cartilage; such loss allows abrasion against the undersurface of the coracoacromial arch (Figs. 16-64 and 16-65). The humeral head becomes "femoralized" and the coracoacromial arch becomes "acetabularized" (see Fig. 16-34). Erosion of the humeral articular cartilage begins superiorly rather than centrally, in contrast to the situation with degenerative joint disease and capsulorrhaphy arthropathy.

In 1981, McCarty and coworkers described a shoulder condition called the "Milwaukee shoulder." This condition included significant rotator cuff disease and shoulder arthritis in older patients and often in women.[148,171,273] The synovial fluid contained aggregates of hydroxyapatite crystals, active collagenase, and neutral protease. At that time, these authors hypothesized that the crystals in the synovial fluid were phagocytized by the macrophage-like synovial cells and these cells in turn released enzymes that resulted in damage to the joint and joint-related structures. The inciting process could not be identified.

In 1983, the hypothesis was further refined. The crystals were identified as basic calcium phosphate (BCP).[272] It was thought that these crystals would form in synovial fluid by unknown mechanisms. They would subsequently be phagocytosed by the synovial lining cells. These cells

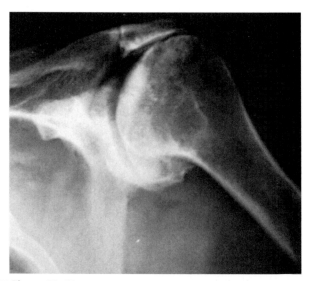

■ **Figure 16–65**
Rotator cuff tear arthropathy. The radiograph depicts the cartilage loss, mild but definite bone loss in the humeral head and glenoid, severe upward subluxation of the humeral head against the acromion with rotator cuff tearing, and some erosion of the abutting acromion. This patient has significant multitissue involvement of the cartilage, bone, capsule, and rotator cuff. Reconstructive surgery should address all these deficiencies.

would then secrete collagenase and neutral protease, which would damage the tissues and, in addition, cause the release of additional crystals. The importance of this concept may be a more universal understanding of crystal-related arthropathy and a better understanding of how multiple joint structures can be affected by an underlying problem.[170,172,173,225]

Nguyen and Nguyen[306] and Campion and colleagues[70] described an "idiopathic destructive arthritis" of the shoulder, which may be another form of the same condition.

In 1983, Neer and coworkers published an article on cuff tear arthropathy in which pathologic changes in 26 patients were described.[300] These changes included massive rotator cuff tearing, glenohumeral instability, loss of articular cartilage of the glenohumeral joint, humeral head collapse, and related bone loss. This entity was distinctly different from osteoarthritis. Neer believed that mechanical factors associated with extensive rotator cuff tearing played a prominent role in the creation of this problem and that secondary nutritional changes may augment the pathologic changes that occur.

The relationship between "Milwaukee shoulder" syndrome, crystal deposition arthritis, and cuff tear arthropathy is unclear. They may be the same process or a different process with similar end stages. For the surgeon, however, the challenge is an eroded joint lacking normal bone stock and reconstructible rotator cuff tissue. In this condition, the glenohumeral joint is deprived of several of its major stabilizing factors: (1) the normal cuff muscle force vector compressing the humeral head into the glenoid (Fig. 16–66); (2) the superior lip of the glenoid concavity, which is typically worn away by chronic superior subluxation (see Fig. 16–33); and (3) the cuff tendon interposed between the humeral head and the coracoacromial arch (Fig. 16–67). As a result of these deficits, the superior instability is usually of sufficient severity that

it cannot be reversed in a dependable way at the time of reconstructive surgery.

Arntz and associates[12] reported their results of treatment of 21 shoulders with cuff tear arthropathy. These shoulders were not candidates for glenoid replacement

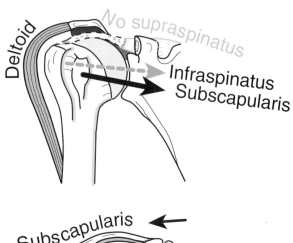
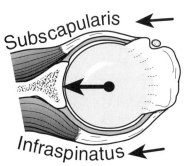

■ **Figure 16–66**

Compressive forces from the infraspinatus and subscapularis can stabilize the humeral head in the absence of a supraspinatus, provided that the glenoid concavity is intact. *(Modified from Matsen FA III, Lippitt SB, Sidles JA, and Harryman DT II: Practical Evaluation and Management of the Shoulder. Philadelphia: WB Saunders, 1994.)*

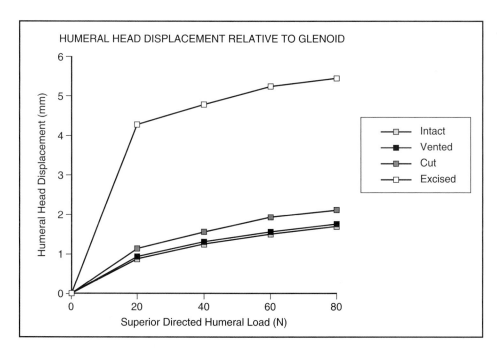

■ **Figure 16–67**

The cuff tendon interposed between the humeral head and the coracoacromial arch stabilizes the head against superiorly directed loads. This graph shows mean superior humeral displacement (relative to the scapula) as a function of superior humeral load. The chart compares displacements for (1) intact specimens, (2) after venting of the joint to air, (3) after cutting (but not excising) the cuff tendon, and (4) after excising the superior cuff tendon. Note the marked superior displacement after excision of the cuff tendon.

because of the massive deficiency in the cuff and the fixed upward displacement of the humeral head; thus, they were treated with a special hemiarthroplasty in which the prosthesis was allowed to articulate with the coracoacromial arch. The prerequisites for successful hemiarthroplasty were an intact deltoid and a functionally intact coracoacromial arch to provide superior secondary stability for the prosthesis. One important aspect of the operative technique was the selection of a sufficiently small prosthesis so that excessive tightness of the posterior aspect of the capsule could be avoided. Eighteen shoulders in 16 patients were available for follow-up, which ranged from 25 to 122 months. Pain decreased from marked or disabling in 14 shoulders preoperatively to none or slight in 10 and to pain only after unusual activity in 4. Active forward elevation improved from an average of 66 degrees preoperatively to an average of 109 degrees postoperatively. One patient, who had an excellent result, fell and sustained an acromial fracture; thus, the functional result changed to poor. Three patients had persistent, substantial pain in the shoulder that led to revision. Neither infection nor prosthetic loosening developed in any shoulder. Zuckerman and associates reported on 15 cases of shoulder hemiarthroplasty performed for cuff tear arthropathy and concluded that hemiarthroplasty can achieve favorable clinical results.[451] Sanchez-Sotelo and coworkers reviewed 33 shoulders treated by hemiarthroplasty for cuff tear arthropathy at an average follow-up of 5 years. Anterosuperior instability occurred in seven shoulders and was associated with a history of subacromial decompression. Successful results based on Neer's limited-goals criteria were achieved in 22 shoulders. The authors concluded that hemiarthroplasty remains a reconstructive option that can provide durable results but may be complicated by instability and progressive bone loss.[371] The catastrophic consequences of loss of integrity of the coracoacromial arch remind us of the need to preserve the integrity of the acromion and coracoacromial ligament.

Capsulorrhaphy Arthropathy

Capsulorrhaphy arthropathy is recognized as a special subset of secondary degenerative joint disease in which deterioration of the joint surface is related to a previous repair for recurrent dislocations. It is one of the most common causes of severe arthritis in individuals younger than 55 years (Table 16–9). Capsulorrhaphy arthropathy

may be caused by overtightening the anterior capsule; for example, in a Putti-Platt repair, overtightening limits external rotation and causes an obligate posterior translation that forces the humeral head out of its normal concentric relationship with the glenoid fossa (see Figs. 16–7, 16–8, and 16–46). The posterior glenoid is typically eroded from this chronic posterior humeral subluxation, and major posterior bone deficiencies may result (see Fig. 16–8). The converse situation may arise when obligate anterior translation results from excessive posterior capsular tightening.

Kiss and associates studied 90 primary Putti-Platt operations at an average follow-up of 9 years. Thirty-five percent of patients had pain with activity and 30% of shoulders showed moderate to severe degenerative changes.[224] Van der Zwaag and coworkers studied 66 shoulders at a mean follow-up of 22 years after a Putti-Platt operation for recurrent anterior dislocation. Osteoarthritic changes of the glenohumeral joint were observed in 61% of the shoulders and were graded as mild in 35%, moderate in 20%, and severe in 6%. The rate of glenohumeral arthritis was positively correlated with the length of time since surgery, and its severity was positively correlated with the number of preoperative dislocations.[412] Hovelius and colleagues retrospectively analyzed 26 shoulders at an average of 17.5 years after Bankart repair and compared these shoulders with a prospective series of 30 shoulders managed with a Bristow-Latarjet procedure at an average follow-up of 15.1 years. Capsulorrhaphy arthropathy was noted in 16 of 26 Bankart shoulders (62%) and in 9 of 30 Bristow-Latarjet shoulders (30%).[195]

Lusardi and associates[250] reported a retrospective study of 20 shoulders in 19 patients who had been managed for severe loss of external rotation of the glenohumeral joint after previous anterior capsulorrhaphy for recurrent instability. All patients had noted restricted range of motion, and 17 shoulders had been painful. In 7 shoulders, the humeral head had been subluxated or dislocated posteriorly, and 16 shoulders had been affected by mild to severe glenohumeral osteoarthrosis. All 20 shoulders underwent a reoperation that consisted of release of the anterior soft tissue. In addition, eight shoulders had total arthroplasties, and one was treated by hemiarthroplasty. At an average duration of 48 months of follow-up, all shoulders showed improvement in ratings for pain and range of motion. The average increase in external rotation was 45 degrees. Sperling and associates[386] reviewed the results of shoulder arthroplasty for capsulorrhaphy arthropathy in 31 patients, including 21 who underwent total shoulder arthroplasty and 10 who underwent hemiarthroplasty. At a mean follow-up of 7 years, shoulder arthroplasty was associated with significant pain relief and improvement in external rotation (from 4 to 43 degrees). According to the Neer rating system, unsatisfactory results were observed in 4 patients in the hemiarthroplasty group (40%) and in 13 patients in the total shoulder arthroplasty group (62%). The estimated survival rate of the components was 86% at 5 years and 61% at 10 years. The authors concluded that shoulder arthroplasty provides pain relief and improved function but is associated with high rates of revision surgery and unsatisfactory

TABLE 16–9. Six Diagnoses with the Relative Prevalence, Age, and Gender for 306 Patients Seen by One of Us (F.A.M.) for Evaluation and Management of Shoulder Arthritis

Diagnosis	No. of Patients		
	Age	Male	Female
Degenerative joint disease	63 ± 12	125	42
Secondary degenerative joint disease	54 ± 15	36	9
Rheumatoid arthritis	59 ± 12	7	32
Cuff tear arthropathy	75 ± 9	9	13
Capsulorrhaphy arthropathy	46 ± 9	13	4
Avascular necrosis	51 ± 15	6	8

outcomes because of component failure, instability, and pain from glenoid arthrosis.

Capsulorrhaphy arthropathy may also be related to intra-articular positioning of metallic internal fixation devices (screws or staples) or bone graft used in repairs for recurrent instability (see Fig. 16–47).[450]

Bigliani and associates,[36] Hawkins and Angelo,[184] Rockwood and Lusardi and colleagues,[250] and Green and Norris[159] reported their results of reconstruction of shoulders damaged by capsulorrhaphy arthropathy.

Avascular Necrosis

Nontraumatic avascular necrosis of the humeral head may be idiopathic or may be associated with the systemic use of steroids, dysbaric conditions, transplantation, or systemic illnesses with vasculitis. Other implicated conditions include alcoholism, sickle cell disease, hyperuricemia, Gaucher's disease, pancreatitis, familial hyperlipidemia, renal or other organ transplantation, and lymphoma.[51,110,111,358]

The pathology may first be detected by MRI before collapse is seen radiographically. Later, osteoporosis or osteosclerosis may be observed on plain radiographs. Next, evidence of a fracture through the abnormal subchondral bone superocentrally may be detected (Fig. 16–68). Subsequently, collapse of the subchondral bone occurs, often with a separated osteocartilaginous flap (Fig. 16–69). In end-stage avascular necrosis, the irregular humeral head destroys glenoid articular cartilage and thereby results in secondary degenerative joint disease (Figs. 16–70 and 16–71).[111,366]

Mont and associates studied 127 shoulders in 73 patients who were treated for atraumatic avascular necrosis of the proximal part of the humerus to define the epidemiology, clinical and radiographic findings, treatment, and prognosis of atraumatic avascular necrosis of the humeral head.[284] Clinical and radiographic characterization of this patient cohort was performed. The mean patient age was 41 years (range, 20 to 60 years). Associated factors included corticosteroid use (82%), an immunocompromising disease (58%), alcohol use (38%), moderate smoking (30%), asthma (8%), and nephrosis (3%). The severity of humeral head osteonecrosis did not correlate with the dose or duration of corticosteroid therapy. According to the modified Ficat and Arlet radiographic staging system, 20 shoulders had stage I disease, 55 shoulders had stage II disease, and 52 shoulders had stage III or IV disease. Seventy-four percent of the shoulders treated by core decompression had good to excellent clinical outcomes at a mean follow-up of 6 years. Fourteen of the 16 patients treated with hemiarthroplasty or total shoulder arthroplasty had clinically successful results at a mean follow-up of 4 years. The authors noted that avascular necrosis should be suspected in patients with shoulder pain and a history of osteonecrosis in other joints. Furthermore, early detection permitted a more conservative, joint-sparing approach as an alternative to surgical management.

Hattrup and Cofield reviewed 151 patients with 200 shoulders affected by avascular necrosis.[181] The most common associated nontraumatic factor was a history of corticosteroid use (112 shoulders). No cause could be identified in 44 shoulders. The need for replacement surgery was found to be related to the extent and stage of humeral head involvement. In a related study, Hattrup and Cofield[182] reviewed 127 shoulders treated with replacement arthroplasty for avascular necrosis, including 71 hemiarthroplasties and 56 total shoulder arthroplasties. At an average follow-up of 8.9 years, subjective improvement was noted in 80% of shoulders. Superior results were associated with patients with steroid-induced disease.

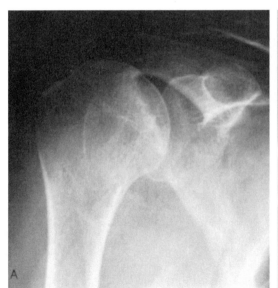 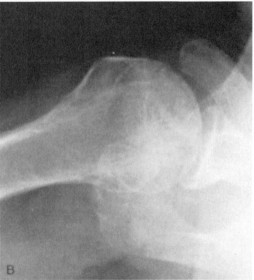

■ **Figure 16–68**
Osteonecrosis of the proximal end of the humerus. An osteochondral fracture with minimal distortion of the articular surface of the humerus has occurred. This fracture is best seen in **A**, the anteroposterior view. In **B**, the axillary view, a crescent sign can be noted in the anterocentral part of the humeral head.

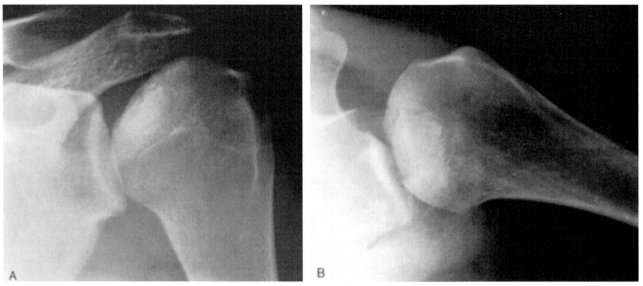

■ **Figure 16–69**

Osteonecrosis of the humeral head associated with chronic steroid use. A subchondral fracture has occurred in the past. The shape of the humeral articular surface is distorted, and early glenohumeral arthritis is present. Symptoms were significant in this young man, and treatment with a proximal humeral prosthesis was quite effective. **A,** Anteroposterior view; **B,** axillary view.

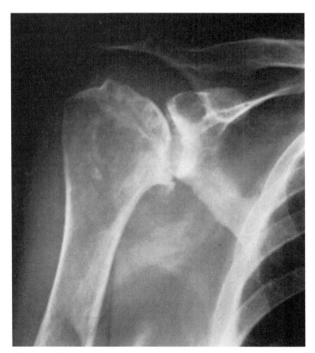

■ **Figure 16–70**

Long-standing osteonecrosis of the proximal end of the humerus with only slight distortion of the articular surface but, unfortunately, progression to significant arthritis involving both the humeral and glenoid articular surfaces.

Other Types of Arthritis

Neurotrophic arthropathy arises in association with syringomyelia, diabetes, or other causes of joint denervation. The joint and subchondral bone are destroyed because of loss of the trophic and protective effects of its nerve supply. It has been suggested that the injection of corticosteroids may contribute to the development of this condition.[314] The Charcot joint is characterized by functional limitation and pain (despite the denervation). Cervical spine trauma may have occurred in the past,[341] or unrecognized syringomyelia may exist.[268,408] Significant bone destruction and osseous debris are usually present about the joint area (Fig. 16–72). This condition may resemble infectious arthritis.[248]

Radiation therapy, especially for the treatment of breast cancer, may cause a number of shoulder problems: brachial plexopathy, osteonecrosis, malignant bone tumors, and fibrous replacement of many tissues. Glenohumeral cartilage and subchondral bone are occasionally affected by these changes and may require treatment by prosthetic arthroplasty or other alternative methods (Fig. 16–73).

Septic arthritis of the shoulder is uncommon; however, when it occurs, it is often in a person debilitated from a generalized disease,[17,63] in a person taking immunosuppressive medications, in a person who had a previous procedure on the shoulder, or in a person who has an underlying shoulder disease process such as rotator cuff tearing or rheumatoid arthritis.[10,229] In this latter setting there appears to be an exacerbation of the underlying shoulder disease, and in the absence of fever or an elevated white blood cell (WBC) count, the diagnosis will depend on a high level of suspicion, joint aspiration, and bacteriologic testing. Leslie and associates[238] reviewed 18 cases of shoulder sepsis, 11 of which were caused by *Staphylococcus aureus*. Some cases were initially confused with nonseptic arthritis and were treated with anti-inflammatory agents. The results of treatment were poor, but somewhat better with arthrotomy than with repeated aspiration.

Neoplasia develops insidiously and is often characterized by nonmechanical pain. The tumor may incite a synovial response mimicking an arthritic condition.[33,278] The pain may be more intense than the usual arthritic pain and

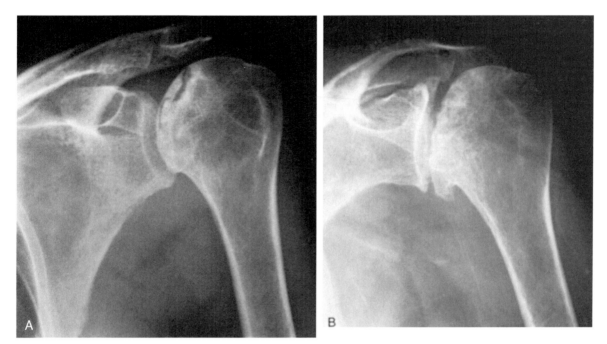

■ Figure 16–71
Steroids were used as a part of the treatment of multiple sclerosis in this middle-aged woman. **A,** Mild shoulder symptoms associated with osteonecrosis of the proximal end of the humerus and minimal distortion of the shape of the articular surface. **B,** The same shoulder is shown about 8 years later. Greater distortion of the shape of the articular surface is evident, and some glenohumeral arthritis has developed. However, her symptoms are still mild, and nonoperative treatment continues to be appropriate for this patient.

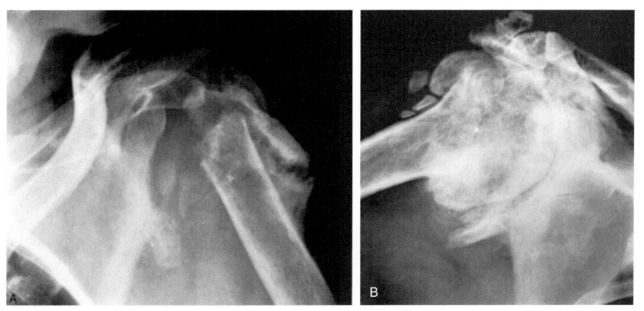

■ Figure 16–72
Occasionally, neuropathic arthritis can be confused with the more common forms of glenohumeral arthritis. **A,** Fragmentation of the proximal end of the humerus with bone debris scattered throughout the joint region. **B,** Bone fragmentation is shown, but in addition, a predominantly sclerotic response is associated with neuropathic arthritis. The underlying condition in both these patients was syringomyelia of the cervical portion of the spinal cord.

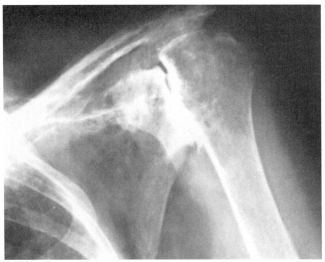

■ Figure 16–73

Cartilage loss, alteration in subchondral bone shape with segmental collapse, and change in bone texture secondary to irradiation that was performed as part of the treatment of breast cancer. Symptoms were quite significant in this elderly woman and were effectively relieved with total shoulder arthroplasty.

decidedly unresponsive to rest. The diagnosis will depend on knowledge of the patient's general health, high-quality plain radiographs, and additional imaging modes, including tomography, CT, bone scanning, or MRI. Identification of the primary lesion in metastatic disease is desirable, but sometimes biopsy of the shoulder lesion is the most direct route when making a diagnosis (Fig. 16–74).

MANAGEMENT

Nonoperative Treatment

Glenohumeral joint arthritis is commonly accompanied by stiffness related to contracture and adhesions involving the glenohumeral capsule, the cuff muscles, and the nonarticular humeroscapular motion interface. Weakness of the cuff muscles results from disuse or fiber failure. Instability patterns may also complicate glenohumeral roughness, such as the posterior subluxation characteristic of degenerative joint disease and capsulorrhaphy arthropathy or the superior subluxation characteristic of cuff tear arthropathy. There is a lot about these conditions that needs management!

Because glenohumeral roughness is usually insidious in onset and chronic in duration, one has ample opportunity for an attempt at nonoperative management. In many cases of glenohumeral arthritis, the mechanics of the shoulder can be improved by a program of patient-conducted gentle range-of-motion and strengthening exercises (Figs. 16–75 to 16–84). It is important that vigorous torque and force not be applied in an attempt to regain motion because of the possibility of causing obligate translation and accelerated wear. Nonsteroidal anti-inflammatory medication and mild analgesics may be useful adjuncts.

Surgical Treatment

Surgery is considered for well-informed, well-motivated, cooperative, sufficiently healthy, and socially supported patients with refractory and functionally significant glenohumeral roughness. Surgical reconstruction offers the potential to optimize capsular laxity and muscle mechanics, as well as the smoothness, size, shape, and orientation of the joint surface. Although prosthetic arthroplasty is the primary surgical option to be considered when major pain and functional loss result from glenohumeral arthritis, other surgical alternatives have been described in the management of arthritis. Kelly,[218,219] Bennett and Gerber,[34] Thomas and associates,[405] and Wakitani and coworkers[417] have reviewed some of the surgical options for management of a rheumatoid shoulder.

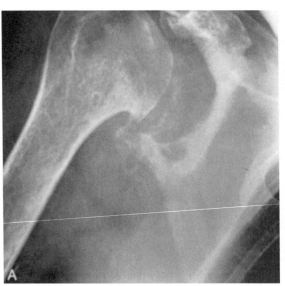
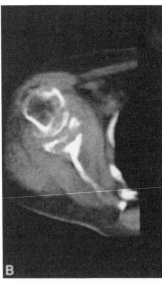

■ Figure 16–74

This upper-middle-aged woman had a gradual onset of shoulder pain and reduction in movement. The shoulder was more painful with use and was also painful at rest (often typical of shoulder arthritis). She had no known systemic illness. **A,** Arthritic involvement of the glenohumeral joint is shown with some collapse of the humeral head articular surface; however, what is more important is that it shows destruction of the bone of the glenoid. **B,** A computed tomographic image shows this bone destruction quite well. Biopsy revealed metastatic thyroid carcinoma. A neoplastic process must always be considered in the evaluation of a patient with supposed glenohumeral arthritis.

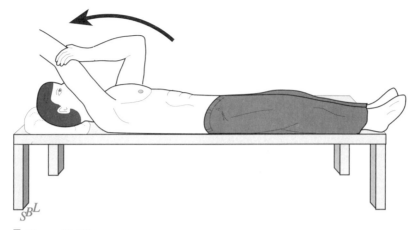

■ **Figure 16–75**
Stretching in overhead reach with the opposite arm used as the "therapist." *(From Matsen FA III, Lippitt SB, Sidles JA, and Harryman DT II: Practical Evaluation and Management of the Shoulder. Philadelphia: WB Saunders, 1994.)*

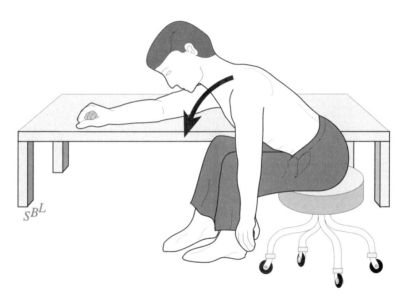

■ **Figure 16–76**
Stretching in overhead reach with progressive forward leaning used to apply gentle force to the arm. *(From Matsen FA III, Lippitt SB, Sidles JA, and Harryman DT II: Practical Evaluation and Management of the Shoulder. Philadelphia: WB Saunders, 1994.)*

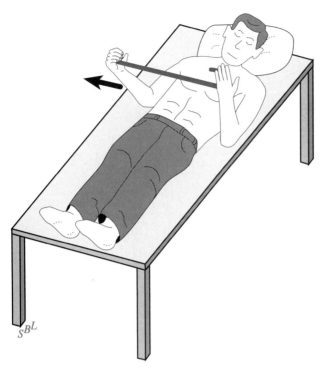

■ **Figure 16–77**
Stretching in external rotation with the opposite hand used as the "therapist." *(From Matsen FA III, Lippitt SB, Sidles JA, and Harryman DT II: Practical Evaluation and Management of the Shoulder. Philadelphia: WB Saunders, 1994.)*

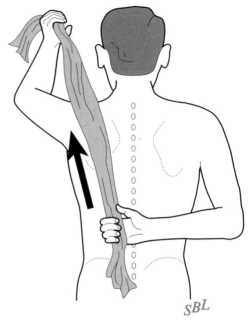

■ **Figure 16–79**
Stretching in internal rotation with a towel used to apply a gentle stretching force. *(From Matsen FA III, Lippitt SB, Sidles JA, and Harryman DT II: Practical Evaluation and Management of the Shoulder. Philadelphia: WB Saunders, 1994.)*

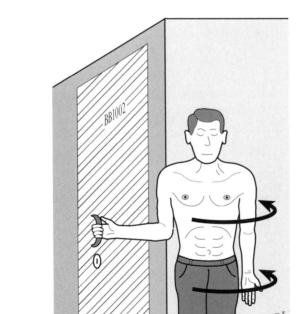

■ **Figure 16–78**
Stretching in external rotation by turning the body away from a fixed object to apply a gentle stretching force. *(From Matsen FA III, Lippitt SB, Sidles JA, and Harryman DT II: Practical Evaluation and Management of the Shoulder. Philadelphia: WB Saunders, 1994.)*

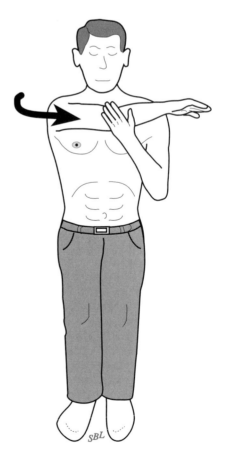

■ **Figure 16–80**
Stretching in cross-body reach with the opposite arm used as the "therapist." *(From Matsen FA III, Lippitt SB, Sidles JA, and Harryman DT II: Practical Evaluation and Management of the Shoulder. Philadelphia: WB Saunders, 1994.)*

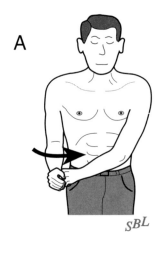

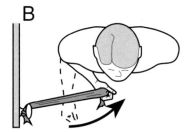

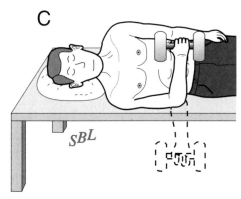

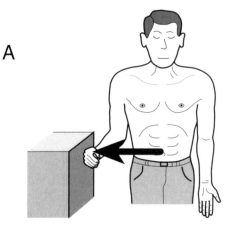

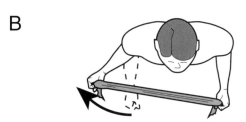

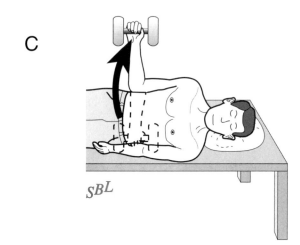

■ **Figure 16–81**
Internal rotation can be strengthened with isometrics (**A**), rubber tubing (**B**), or free weights (**C**). *(From Matsen FA III, Lippitt SB, Sidles JA, and Harryman DT II: Practical Evaluation and Management of the Shoulder. Philadelphia: WB Saunders, 1994.)*

■ **Figure 16–82**
External rotation strengthening with isometrics (**A**), rubber tubing (**B**), or free weights (**C**). *(From Matsen FA III, Lippitt SB, Sidles JA, and Harryman DT II: Practical Evaluation and Management of the Shoulder. Philadelphia: WB Saunders, 1994.)*

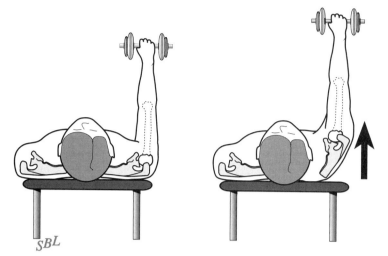

■ **Figure 16–83**
In the press plus, the arm is pushed upward until the shoulder blade is lifted off the table or bed. *(From Matsen FA III, Lippitt SB, Sidles JA, and Harryman DT II: Practical Evaluation and Management of the Shoulder. Philadelphia: WB Saunders, 1994.)*

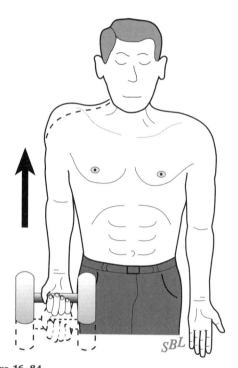

■ **Figure 16–84**
In the shoulder shrug exercise, the tip of the shoulder is lifted toward the ear while holding the elbow straight. *(From Matsen FA III, Lippitt SB, Sidles JA, and Harryman DT II: Practical Evaluation and Management of the Shoulder. Philadelphia: WB Saunders, 1994.)*

Synovectomy

Rheumatoid arthritis and other inflammatory arthropathies produce synovial tissue hyperplasia and its attendant symptoms. A benchmark article on care of rheumatoid joint problems was published in 1943.[382] This article offered great insight into the surgical care of patients with rheumatoid arthritis during the preprosthetic era. The authors observed that surgery was not always necessary or desirable and that surgery of the joint in and of itself would be unlikely to change the long-term course of the disease for the patient. When shoulder

symptoms were severe and persistent, shoulder synovectomy, bursectomy, and acromioplasty seemed to alleviate pain and allow the patient improved use of the involved limb.

Patients may be considered for synovectomy if they have chronic refractory synovitis. Clinically, this condition is evident as an enlarged, boggy-feeling shoulder, indicative of either primary bursal hypertrophy or rotator cuff tearing with extension of synovial tissue and fluid into the subdeltoid bursa (see Fig. 16-62). A shoulder arthrogram (see Fig. 16-60) may help define the severity and extent of the synovitis, as well as provide information about the presence or absence of rotator cuff tearing.

Pahle and Kvarnes[312] reported on the application and relative effectiveness of shoulder synovectomy. Their method includes subdeltoid and subacromial bursectomy, arthrotomy through the subscapularis, and synovectomy of all joint areas. In addition, any osteophytes or other joint irregularities are removed or smoothed. If tenosynovial hypertrophy is surrounding the long head of the biceps brachii, this tissue is also removed. Postoperatively, a light abduction pillow is used, and exercises are commenced 2 to 3 days after surgery. Pain relief in their patients was often quite good, with significant residual pain in only 10 of 54 shoulders (approximately half had significant joint surface irregularity). Motion in these patients was slightly improved, but not dramatically so. Lessening of the pain did improve limb function.

Currently, synovectomy is reserved for patients with intact articular cartilage or cartilage that is at least half its normal thickness. With modern rheumatologic management of synovitis, surgical synovectomy of the shoulder is becoming rare.

Synovectomy may be accomplished arthroscopically, although great care is necessary to avoid nerve damage. Open synovectomy is approached through the deltopectoral interval. The subdeltoid bursal tissue is excised carefully to protect the axillary nerve on the undersurface of the deltoid muscle. Rotator cuff defects are identified. Usually, the arthrotomy will include division of the subscapularis near its insertion and division of the anterior shoulder capsule at its humeral attachments. The capsular incision will extend up to the intra-articular portion of the long head of the biceps tendon and along this tendon to its glenoid origin. The incision will also extend inferiorly to the 6 o'clock position on the humeral head. Synovium is removed from the anterior portion of the shoulder and the subscapularis recess and then from the inferior aspect of the joint. By preserving the fibrous layer beneath the synovial tissue, the axillary nerve is protected. By working around the humeral head, the posterior synovial hypertrophy is removed. Exposure may be facilitated by partially dislocating the joint. Reparable cuff defects may be addressed by direct suturing or transposition of the subscapularis upward.[89] Drains are kept in place as long as fluid is being retrieved. Sutures are left in place for 10 days. Postoperative care includes early passive range of motion. Active exercises are delayed until healing of the tendon repairs is complete.

Resection Arthroplasty

Before prostheses were available, resection of the humeral head was used to manage severe fractures and uncontrollable infection.[108,258,393] Several authors have reported on excision of the glenoid in conjunction with synovectomy.[149,416] Milbrink and Wigren[279] reported reasonable short-term results from 13 resection arthroplasties for advanced rheumatoid arthritis. Pain relief was reported to be good.

Resection arthroplasty is useful as an adjunct to the management of septic arthritis in a shoulder with extensive humeral head and glenoid osteomyelitis. Joint resection also results after the removal of infected or mechanically compromised implants (Fig. 16–85).[83,108,239] The initial problem after resection is joint instability. Later, stiffness usually develops, and a few shoulders actually progress to bony arthrodesis.[294] Pain relief is variable.[239] Maximal active abduction is typically 60 to 80 degrees.[83,108,239,280,399] However, moderate weakness persists. Suturing the rotator cuff to the remaining portion of the upper part of the humerus may increase strength, but the results have been variable.[208,209,226,299]

Resection interposition arthroplasty has also been used in the treatment of inflammatory arthritis of the glenohumeral joint. Fink and associates[132] evaluated the therapeutic value of this procedure in 53 shoulders with rheumatoid or other inflammatory arthritis. Constant scores averaged 42% of age- and gender-matched control values and tended to worsen with time after surgery. In most cases, radiographs showed progressive medial humeral displacement, flattening of the humeral head, and joint space narrowing. The authors concluded that outcomes progressively worsened as a result of glenoid cartilage wear and osseous resorption of the humeral head.

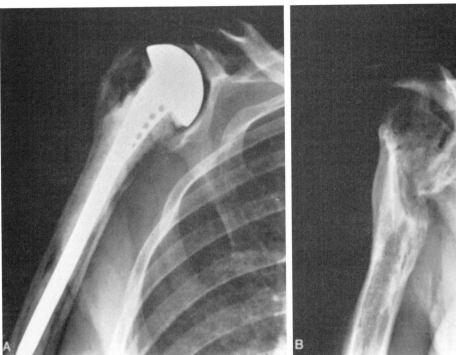
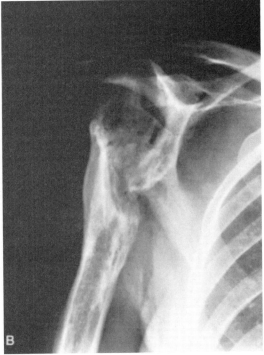

■ **Figure 16–85**
A proximal humeral prosthetic replacement had previously been placed in an elderly woman with multiple-joint osteoarthritis. Her total knee arthroplasty became infected, and the infection spread to the proximal humeral prosthetic replacement (**A**). The shoulder region was brawny and erythematous, with a draining sinus on the anterolateral aspect of the arm. The region was débrided, the prosthesis and cement were removed, and after delayed primary closure, the radiographic appearance of the joint was as seen in **B**. Fortunately, the patient had only mild pain, and the shoulder was stable because of fibrosis. She had active abduction of 65 degrees and external rotation of 10 degrees.

Glenohumeral Arthrodesis

Glenohumeral arthrodesis is usually reserved for attempts at salvaging septic arthritis or complex deficiencies of the joint surface associated with permanent loss of the cuff and deltoid. Early in this decade, there were many indications for arthrodesis of the shoulder, but now only a few are recognized.[86,93] Cofield demonstrated this trend in Table 16–10.[86,93] Most shoulder fusions today are performed for one of four reasons: (1) paralysis of the deltoid and rotator cuff, (2) infection with loss of glenohumeral cartilage, (3) refractory instability, or (4) failed reconstructive procedures.[351] Seldom, if ever is shoulder fusion undertaken for treatment of the more usual causes of shoulder arthritis, even in younger individuals who wish to be active. An exception to this trend is expressed in the article by Rybka and coworkers from Finland.[367] These authors defined the results of arthrodesis in a group of patients with rheumatoid arthritis. Thirty-seven of 41 shoulders in their series underwent glenohumeral arthrodesis. Complications were few. A brace was used for postoperative support in an attempt to avoid potential elbow stiffness. This investigation suggested that arthrodesis was easily achieved, inexpensive, and reliable for the treatment of severely involved rheumatoid shoulders.

Some consensus has been reached about the desirable position of shoulder fusion. Rowe was the first to firmly state the advantages of less abduction and flexion for shoulders treated by surgical arthrodesis: 20 degrees of abduction, 30 degrees of flexion, and internal rotation of 40 degrees (Fig. 16–86).[360] Hawkins and Neer[188] recommended 25 to 40 degrees of abduction for the arm, 20 to 30 degrees of flexion, and 25 to 30 degrees of internal rotation. In a recent review on shoulder arthrodesis, Clare and

TABLE 16–10. Indications for Shoulder Arthrodesis (at the Mayo Clinic, Rochester, Minnesota)

Diagnosis	1950–1974*	1975–1983†
Paralysis	21	20
Infection	8	15
Severe rotator cuff tearing	12	9
Traumatic arthritis or osteoarthritis	18	5
Neoplasia	0	3
Recurrent dislocation	7	0
Rheumatoid arthritis	5	0
	71	52

*From Cofield RH and Briggs BT: Glenohumeral arthritis. J Bone Joint Surg Am 61:668–677, 1979.
†From Cofield RH: Shoulder arthrodesis and resection arthroplasty. Instr Course Lect 34:268–277, 1985.

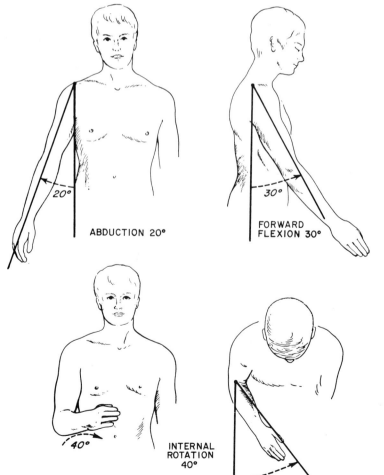

ABDUCTION 20°

FORWARD FLEXION 30°

INTERNAL ROTATION 40°

■ **Figure 16–86**
Rowe re-evaluated the position of the arm in arthrodesis of the adult shoulder. From his experience, he recommended that less abduction and forward flexion be incorporated into the fusion position and that internal rotation (not external rotation) was necessary. *(From Rowe CR: Re-evaluation of the position of the arm in arthrodesis of the shoulder in the adult. J Bone Joint Surg Am 56:913-922, 1974.)*

associates noted that excessive flexion or abduction was often associated with chronic postoperative pain.[77] When determining arm position, the trunk is commonly used as the source of reference, with the scapula being held in the anatomic position. Jónsson and associates[212] described a method for documenting the position of fusion that involved Moire photography.

The best candidates for this procedure are patients with (1) permanent and severe weakness because of loss of cuff and deltoid function, (2) good scapular motors (e.g., trapezius, levator scapulae pectoralis, serratus anterior, and rhomboids), (3) a good understanding of the limitations and potential complications of a shoulder fusion, (4) motivation to succeed, and (5) minimal complaints of pain.

To establish the limitations of shoulder fusions, Harryman and associates[178,262] studied 12 shoulders that underwent glenohumeral arthrodesis at least 2 years before the time of study. Elevation in the plus 90-degree (anterior sagittal) plane averaged 47 degrees. Elevation in the minus 90-degree (posterior sagittal) plane averaged 22 degrees. The average external rotation was 9 degrees, and the average internal rotation was 46 degrees. These ranges of motion were similar to the scapulothoracic motion measured in normal subjects.[178] Only 1 of the patients could reach his hair without bending his neck forward, only 5 patients could reach their perineum, 6 patients could reach the back pocket, 7 patients could reach the opposite axilla, and 10 patients could reach the side pocket.

These same authors studied normal in vivo shoulder kinematics to predict the functions that would be allowed by various positions of glenohumeral arthrodesis, assuming that scapulothoracic motion would remain unchanged.[262] Using normal scapulothoracic motions, they were able to model the functional effects of different fusion positions. They found that activities of daily living could best be performed if the joint was fused in 15 degrees of flexion, 15 degrees of abduction, and 45 degrees of internal rotation (Fig. 16–87). This low angle of elevation and relatively high degree of internal rotation facilitated sitting comfortably in a chair, lying flat in bed, and reaching the face, the opposite axilla, and the perineum. However, all positions represented a major compromise in normal function (Table 16–11). This compromise is the primary reason for avoiding fusion in individuals with conditions such as osteoarthritis, rheumatoid arthritis, or traumatic arthritis when adequate bone stock and muscle function are present. Function after total shoulder arthroplasty is much more favorable for performing activities of daily living (Table 16–12).

Many techniques can be used for shoulder arthrodesis (Table 16–13). These techniques are best classified as extra-articular, intra-articular, or a combination of the two. Extra-articular arthrodesis techniques, such as that of Putti,[336] Watson-Jones,[423] or Brittain,[57] had greatest usefulness as adjunctive care for infection, especially tuberculosis. With an extra-articular arthrodesis, the surgeon

TABLE 16–11. **Extremity Function following Shoulder Arthrodesis***

Function	Ability to Perform Function, No. (%)
Sleep on limb	46 (73)
Dress	45 (71)
Eat using limb	45 (71)
Toilet care	44 (70)
Lift 5 to 7.5 kg	43 (68)
Comb hair	28 (44)
Use hand at shoulder level	13 (21)

*No. of shoulders = 63.
Adapted from Cofield RH and Briggs BT: Glenohumeral arthritis. J Bone Joint Surg Am 61:668–677, 1979.

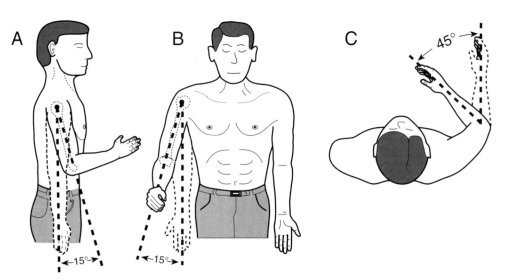

■ **Figure 16–87**
The recommended arthrodesis position: 15 degrees of humerothoracic flexion (**A**), 15 degrees of humerothoracic abduction (**B**), and 45 degrees of internal rotation (**C**). *(From Matsen FA III, Lippitt SB, Sidles JA, and Harryman DT II: Practical Evaluation and Management of the Shoulder. Philadelphia: WB Saunders, 1994.)*

TABLE 16–12. Extremity Function following Total Shoulder Arthroplasty*

Function	Ability to Perform Function, No. (%)
Sleep on limb	64 (90)
Dress	69 (97)
Eat using limb	70 (99)
Toilet care	68 (96)
Lift 5 to 7.5 kg	60 (85)
Comb hair	56 (79)
Use hand at shoulder level	53 (75)

*No. of shoulders = 71.
Adapted from Cofield RH: Total shoulder arthroplasty with the Neer prosthesis. J Bone Joint Surg Am 66:899–906, 1984.

TABLE 16–13. Techniques for Shoulder Fusion

Extra-articular	Intra-articular	Combined Extra- and Intra-articular
Acromion–humeral[206]	Suture[239]	Suture[102]
Spine of scapula–humeral[255]	Screws[20, 114, 153]	Screws[15, 50, 68, 155, 222, 251]
Axillary border of scapula or humeral plus tibial graft[32]	Pin[94]	Staples
	Tibial graft[217]	Wire[38]
	Bone bank graft[118]	Pins and tension band[29]
		Bone graft[25, 33]
		External fixator[43, 46, 123]
		Plate or plates[70, 86, 145, 212, 213, 215, 220, 256]

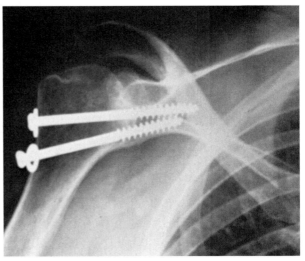

■ **Figure 16–88**
Intra-articular shoulder arthrodesis using screws for internal fixation. This young man had recurrent shoulder instability, and after anterior capsule repair, an infection developed and eventuated in cartilage loss at the glenohumeral joint. This simple form of fusion was undertaken to preserve the largely intact surrounding joint capsule and rotator cuff. His neuromuscular function is, of course, normal, and there may be a possibility in the future of reconstruction with a prosthetic joint replacement.

hoped to avoid the infectious focus and achieve fusion about the affected joint. Now, effective antimicrobial medications have essentially obviated the need for this approach.

Intra-articular fusion offers the simplest and most direct method. The joint is débrided and remaining cartilage, scar, and dense subchondral bone are removed. Cancellous bone of the humeral head and glenoid is placed against each other, and with the arm in the desired position, fixation is accomplished. Different forms of fixation have been used, including screws,[28,183,267] wires,[71] bone grafts,[197,359] and pins.[114] Currently, the use of screws seems to be favored. A cast is generally used after this technique and is continued for 3 to 6 months. This technique still seems reasonable for individuals with an excellent rotator cuff and capsule who might later be candidates for prosthetic replacement (Fig. 16–88).

Intra-articular fusion can be combined with extra-articular fusion. Extra-articular bone contact is achieved by bringing the humeral head against the acromion (Fig. 16–89) or by adding bone grafts between the humeral head and the acromion or between the humeral neck and the medial aspect of the scapula adjacent to the glenoid. Fixation is obtained by screws,[26,93,213,269,367,410] staples, bone grafts,[31,55] external fixation,[73,76,207] or bone plates.[185,233,345–347,365,424] Tension band wiring has been suggested if the bone is osteoporotic (Fig. 16–90).[37] External fixation may be preferred if the shoulder is infected or in

the presence of wound problems (Figs. 16–91 to 16–94). External fixation carries the risk of radial nerve injury.[73]

Internal fixation with one or more plates has the potential to obviate the need for long-term external cast or brace support during the postoperative period.[429] Arm position can be fixed securely in the position that the surgeon wishes without worry that the position of the arm will change during healing. Narrow dynamic compression plates are often used (Fig. 16–95). It has been suggested that pelvic reconstruction plates (either single or double) are easier to apply and may be equally effective (Fig. 16–96).[77,345]

The rate of bone fusion after many of these methods of shoulder arthrodesis is 80% to 90% (Table 16–14).

TABLE 16–14. Pseudarthrosis following Shoulder Arthrodesis

Series	No. of Shoulders	No. of Pseudarthroses
Ten series*	87	0
Hauge (1961)[183]	34	1
Cofield and Briggs (1979)[93]	71	3
Charnley and Houston (1964)[76]	19	1
Steindler (1944)[393]	82	5
Becker (1975)[28]	47	3
Rybka and coworkers (1979)[367]	41	4
De Velasco Polo and Cardoso Monterrubio (1973)[114]	31	6
Barton (1972)[23]	10	2
AOA report	102	23
Totals	524	48

*Johnson and coworkers (1986),[207] Hucherson (1959),[197] Kalamchi (1978),[213] Matsunaga (1972),[267] May (1962),[269] Richards and associates (1985),[346] Richards and associates (1988),[345] Riggins (1976),[347] Uematsu (1979),[410] Weigert and Gronert (1974).[424]
AOA, American Orthopaedic Association.

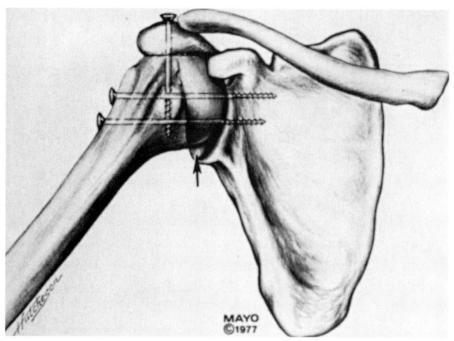

■ Figure 16–89
A technique of combined intra-articular and extra-articular shoulder arthrodesis with screws for internal fixation. *(From Cofield RH and Briggs BT: Glenohumeral arthrodesis: Operative and long-term functional results. J Bone Joint Surg Am 61:668-677, 1979. By permission of the Mayo Foundation.)*

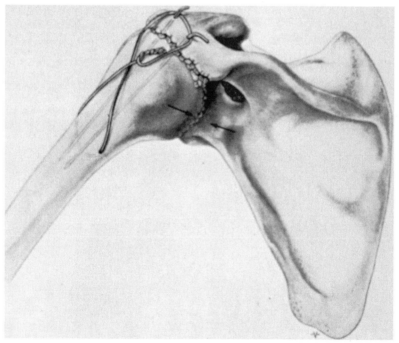

■ Figure 16–90
When the bones of the shoulder are extremely osteoporotic and one is attempting a shoulder arthrodesis, it has been suggested that pins and tension band wiring may be a satisfactory solution to obtain continued coaptation of the joint surfaces. Supplemental fixation with a cast will be necessary. *(From Blauth W and Hepp WR: Arthrodesis of the shoulder joint by traction absorbing wire. In Chapchal G [ed]: The Arthrodesis in the Restoration of Working Ability. Stuttgart, Germany: Georg Thieme, 1975, p 30.)*

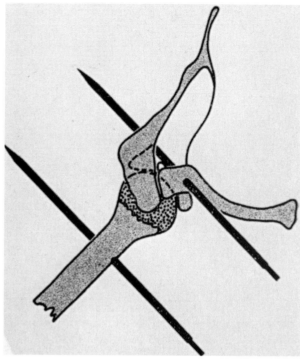

■ **Figure 16–91**
The first method of placing pins for compression arthrodesis of the shoulder as suggested by Charnley. A simple external fixator was then applied. *(From Charnley J: Compression arthrodesis of the ankle and shoulder. J Bone Joint Surg Br 33:180-191, 1951.)*

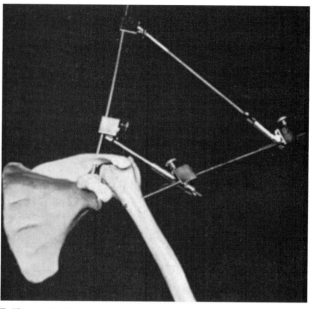

■ **Figure 16–92**
Charnley's second technique in which pins are applied as part of a shoulder arthrodesis procedure so that an external fixator might be used to apply compression across the arthrodesis site. *(From Charnley J and Houston JK: Compression arthrodesis of the shoulder. J Bone Joint Surg Br 46:614-620, 1964.)*

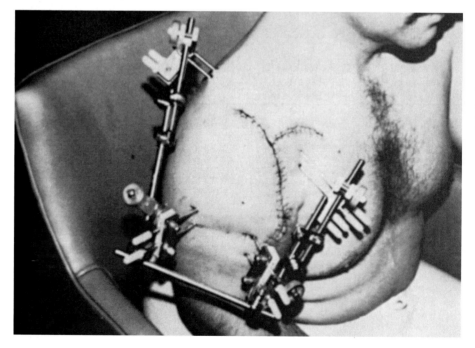

■ **Figure 16–93**
An external fixation device used for shoulder arthrodesis. Half pins are placed in the proximal part of the humerus, and then more proximal pins are inserted into the acromion and exit through the spine of the scapula. *(From Johnson CA, Healy WL, Brooker AF Jr, and Krackow KA: External fixation shoulder arthrodesis. Clin Orthop 211:219-223, 1986.)*

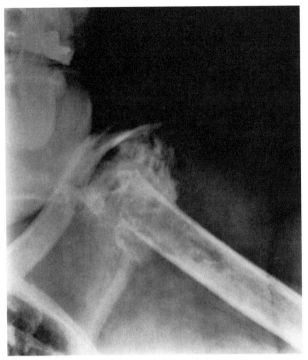

■ Figure 16–94
External fixation may prove to be a useful adjunct for achieving shoulder fusion in certain patients. Certainly, patients with open wounds who need sequential débridement might be considered for this form of support for shoulder arthrodesis. This patient had previous trauma and previous surgery, with a significant amount of bone loss. She had also lost function of her deltoid and rotator cuff. At the time of shoulder arthrodesis, pins were placed as suggested by Charnley (his revised technique). In addition, an iliac crest graft was placed around the junction of the remaining humerus and scapula. The patient went on to develop a solid bone fusion.

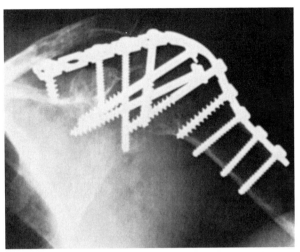

■ Figure 16–96
Radiograph of a shoulder arthrodesis involving the use of a pelvic reconstruction plate for internal fixation. This plate is more easily contoured than the standard dynamic compression plate, yet seems to offer enough rigidity for arthrodesis of the shoulder.

Shoulder fusion carries the risks of infection, reflex dystrophy, acromioclavicular arthritis, and symptomatic internal fixation that must be removed later. Fracture of the operated extremity below the fusion has been reported.[86]

Patient satisfaction can never be perfect after such a procedure, but it does approach 80%.[86] Some patients have shoulder girdle pain despite successful bone fusion.[26,86] Richards and associates[344] reviewed 57 patients who underwent fusion with a single plate to achieve glenohumeral and acromiohumeral arthrodesis. They used a 30, 30, 30 position (abduction, internal rotation, and flexion). Only two of these fusions were performed for arthritis and two for failed shoulder arthroplasty (the rest were for brachial plexus palsy, refractory instability, or sepsis). Complications occurred in 14%, and three required regrafting. Most patients, except those in the instability group, were satisfied. Persistent pain after fusion is often difficult to explain. It used to be thought that resection of the distal end of the clavicle would improve motion after shoulder fusion; however, our experience indicates that gains are minimal.

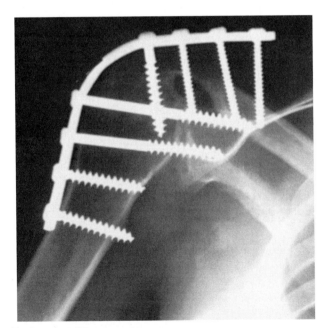

■ Figure 16–95
Radiographic illustration of a shoulder fusion incorporating both intra- and extra-articular bone contact. Fixation with a plate has provided immediate stability. Such fixation could preclude the use of cast support; however, a number of surgeons consider a 1- to 2-month period of spica cast immobilization as an adjunct to this fixation.

■ MATSEN'S TECHNIQUE FOR SHOULDER ARTHRODESIS

The patient is positioned in a beach chair position with the scapula in the field and the arm draped free. The operative approach is through an anterior deltopectoral incision with superior extension of the incision if plate fixation is used (Fig. 16–97). Recently, we have used a low anterior axillary incision when cosmesis is a concern and intra-articular fusion is planned.

Any residual articular cartilage on the humerus or glenoid is resected down to raw subchondral bone (removing subchondral bone weakens the construct and makes solid glenohumeral compression more difficult to

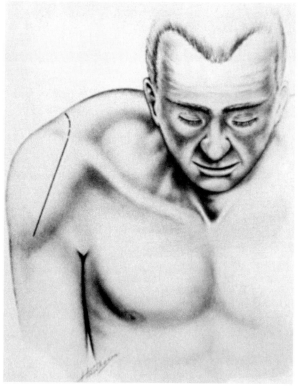

■ Figure 16–97

Anterior incision for shoulder arthrodesis. The incision can be extended over the superior aspect of the shoulder to expose the scapular spine if a plate is to be used for internal fixation. *(From Cofield RH: Shoulder arthrodesis and resection arthroplasty. Instr Course Lect 34:268-277, 1985.)*

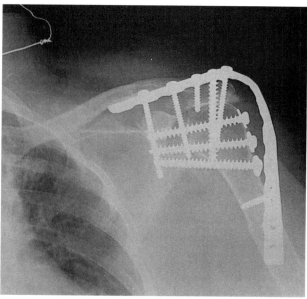

■ Figure 16–98

Glenohumeral and acromiohumeral arthrodesis using a contoured iliac crest bone graft inserted between the acromion and the humeral head. The arthrodesis is stabilized securely with three washered, fully threaded cancellous humeroglenoid screws; one fully threaded cancellous screw through the acromion, graft, and humeral head; and a contoured reconstruction plate.

achieve). The supraspinatus tendon is resected from between the humeral head and the acromion. The undersurface of the acromion is stripped down to raw bone. The soft tissues are lifted from the anterior glenoid neck so that the subscapularis fossa can be palpated. The humeral head is positioned in the glenoid in 15 degrees of abduction, 15 degrees of flexion, and 45 degrees of internal rotation position (see Fig. 16–87) and is temporarily fixed with three long 3.2-mm drills that intentionally exit the neck of the scapula anteriorly approximately 2 cm medial to the glenoid lip, where their tips can be palpated and controlled. When used in this manner, the known length of the drill bits can serve as depth gauges to determine the length of screws needed. The position of the arm is checked by making sure that the hand can reach the mouth, the anterior of the perineum, and the contralateral axilla. The 3.2-mm drill bits are sequentially replaced by fully threaded 6.5-mm cancellous screws with washers. Because the humeral head is softer than the glenoid, compression can usually be achieved without formally "lagging" the screw and without needing to use a smooth shank. An iliac crest bone graft is fashioned to fit between the humeral head and the acromion, and it rests in the position normally occupied by the supraspinatus tendon. Interposition of the iliac crest graft maximizes humeroscapular contact by preserving the normal concave-convex glenohumeral relationships while allowing for stabilizing contact between the head, the graft, and

the acromion (if the humeral head is moved upward to make contact with the acromion without a graft, the glenohumeral contact area is diminished). The graft is held in position with another screw placed from the acromion, through the graft, and out the anteromedial aspect of the humeral neck. Depending on the circumstances, a neutralization plate (usually an 8- to 12-hole dynamic compression plate or pelvic reconstruction plate) may be used (Fig. 16–98). If so, a few key points are helpful. The plate needs about a 90-degree bend at the acromion and often about a 45-degree internal rotation twist to fit on the anterior of the humerus. The strongest fixation for the plate on the scapula is obtained by a screw down the base of the spine of the scapula just medial to the spinoglenoid notch. Postoperatively, if there is concern about the fixation or the patient, a spica cast is applied and continued for 6 to 12 weeks or until fusion has occurred. When the fusion is solid, function and comfort can be enhanced by strengthening all muscle groups surrounding the fused glenohumeral joint.

■ ROCKWOOD'S TECHNIQUE FOR SHOULDER ARTHRODESIS

Rockwood prefers the anterior or oblique technique for shoulder fusion.[286] **(V16-1)** A straight skin incision is made along the spine of the scapula across the acromion and down the lateral shaft of the humerus to the insertion of the deltoid. **(V16-2)** The deltoid is elevated from the scapular spine and the acromion in a subparietal fashion, and a wide capsulotomy is performed. **(V16-3)** The shaft of the humerus is exposed, and if possible, the axillary nerve should be preserved. (V16-4) The residual portion of the rotator cuff, which lies between the humeral head and the glenoid, and the inferior acromion must be resected. (V16-5) The bursal surface of the acromion is decorticated, and all articular cartilage is resected from the humeral head and the glenoid. (V16-6) The arm is placed in 15 to 20 degrees of flexion and 15 to 20 degrees of abduction. The amount of internal rotation—usually approximately 40 to 45 degrees—should be such that the hand can easily be brought up to the level of the mouth. Once sufficient decortication has taken place, the head is jammed up under the acromion adjacent to the upper portion of the glenoid and is fixed provisionally with one or two threaded Steinmann pins. (V16-7) A malleable template is then used to match the contour of the temporarily stabilized scapula and humerus. A 4.5 pelvic reconstruction plate is then contoured to match the curve of the malleable template. The plate should be long enough to allow the purchase of three or four screws in the scapula, two screws from the plate through the humeral head and into the glenoid fossa, and at least four screws into the humeral shaft. (V16-8) With the pelvic reconstruction plate temporarily in place, a hole is selected in the plate that will allow a drill to be passed down through the acromion, down into the neck of the scapula approximately 1 to 2 cm medial to the surface of the glenoid. This is a critical anchor hole for the plate medially, and it must be accurately placed to ensure a stable, surgical construct. The plate is then laid back on the scapula and humerus, and a screw of approximate length is placed down through the plate and the acromion and then to the scapula. (V16-9) Two or three additional screws should be used to stabilize the plate through the scapula and, if possible, down into the glenoid. Three or four cortical screws are used to secure the plate to the shaft of the humerus, and then one or two cancellous screws are inserted through the plate across the head of the humerus and into the glenoid.

Periarticular Osteotomy

Benjamin and associates described the use of osteotomies adjacent to the glenohumeral joint for the relief of pain in shoulder arthritis.[32,33] In the 16 shoulders that they treated with this method, all had advanced arthritic destruction (rheumatoid arthritis in 12 and osteoarthritis in 4). The average age of the patients was 51 years; the average time for evaluation was 2 years and 11 months. Thirteen patients showed improvement in range and comfort.

Arthroplasty

Historical Review

In 1893, one of the first prosthetic shoulder replacements was performed by the French surgeon Péan.[249] As a matter of historical interest, Péan was the subject of a painting called "Une Opération de Tracheotomie" by Henri de Toulouse-Lautrec.[20] Péan asked that a platinum and rubber total joint and proximal humeral implant be fashioned for him by J. Porter Micheals, a dentist from Paris. He then inserted this implant in a 37-year-old baker with tuberculous arthritis (Fig. 16–99). The patient gained increased strength and range of the arm. However, the infection recurred. After one of the first x-ray machines documented an overwhelming reactive process, the prosthesis was removed 2 years after implantation.

In 1953, Neer and colleagues presented the option of replacement of a fractured humeral head with a Vitallium prosthesis.[299] Use of this prosthesis (Fig. 16–100) was next applied to patients with irregular articular surfaces as a result of fractures and osteonecrosis.[294] In 1971 and 1974, Neer described the results of the use of this proximal humeral implant for patients with rheumatoid arthritis and osteoarthritis of the glenohumeral joint (Table 16–15).[295,296] In these articles, Neer also described the use of a high-density polyethylene glenoid component in the management of osteoarthritis of the glenohumeral joint (Fig. 16–101). Also in 1974, Kenmore and associates published a brief article reporting on the development of a polyethylene glenoid liner to be used with a Neer humeral replacement for the treatment of degenerative joint disease of the shoulder.[221,222,304] Other early descriptions of shoulder arthroplasty components include prostheses of Vitallium as reported by Krueger[231] and acrylic as reported by Richard and Judet[342] (Fig. 16–102).

The initial Neer prosthesis had three sizes (Fig. 16–103), and two more were added. In the early 1970s, the implant was redesigned to better use the alternative of

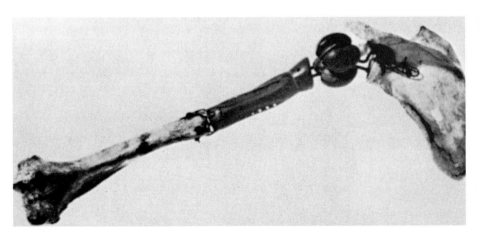

■ **Figure 16–99**

The first total shoulder arthroplasty, an artificial joint composed of platinum and rubber inserted by the French surgeon Péan in the late 1800s. *(From Lugli T: Artificial shoulder joint by Péan [1893]. The facts of an exceptional intervention and the prosthetic method. Clin Orthop 133:215-218, 1978.)*

TABLE 16–15.   Indications for Humeral Replacement Arthroplasty (1953–1963)

Diagnosis	No. of Shoulders
Arthritides	
Osteoarthritis	9
Traumatic arthritis	9
Rheumatoid arthritis	2
Radiation necrosis	1
Sickle cell infarction	1
Ochronosis	1
Trauma	
Fracture-dislocation	26
"Head-splitting" fracture	4
Displaced "shell fragment" with retracted tuberosities	2
Previous humeral head resection	1

Adapted from Neer CS II: Articular replacement of the humeral head. J Bone Joint Surg Am *46*:1607–1610, 1964.

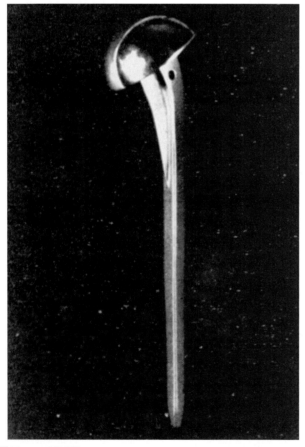

■ **Figure 16–100**
Early design of the Neer articular surface replacement for the proximal part of the humerus. This implant was used initially in the care of patients with severely comminuted fractures of the humeral head.
(From Neer CS, Brown TH Jr, and McLaughlin HL: Fracture of the neck of the humerus with dislocation of the head fragment. Am J Surg 85:252-258, 1953.)

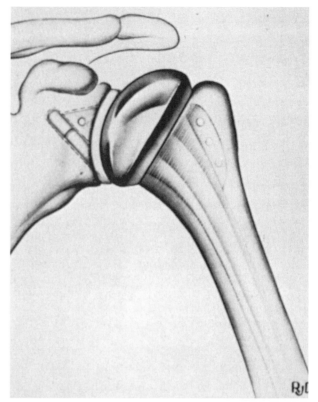

■ **Figure 16–101**
The first illustration depicting the use of a high-density polyethylene glenoid component in conjunction with a proximal humeral prosthesis—a total shoulder arthroplasty. *(From Neer CS II: Replacement arthroplasty for glenohumeral osteoarthritis. J Bone Joint Surg Am 56:1-13, 1974.)*

cement fixation, and the articular portion was made spherical.[296] This implant proved its versatility over time. It was used initially for acute fractures but subsequently has been shown to be effective in the care of patients with chronic fracture problems,[189,335,361,404] osteoarthritis,[296,448] rheumatoid arthritis,[295,448] osteonecro-

sis,[110,111,366] and a variety of the rarer forms of disease affecting the shoulder joint. A number of other shoulder implant systems include a metallic humeral component that can be used without a glenoid replacement.[4-6,25,87,88,160,162] Bipolar implants have also been described (Fig. 16–104).[13,236,401-403,443]

Some authors suggested that a cup arthroplasty might be a satisfactory alternative to prosthetic shoulder surgery.[210,211] Initially, hip cups were used,[392] and then cups were manufactured specifically for the shoulder (Fig. 16–105).[392] Rydholm and Sjogren[368] described a surface replacement for the humeral head. At an average of 4.2 years after surgery, 72 rheumatoid shoulders demonstrated substantial improvement. Twenty-five percent of the cups were loose at follow-up. However, neither cup loosening, nor proximal migration of the humerus, nor central glenoid wear apparently affected the clinical result. Levy and Copeland[242] reported on the use of cementless surface replacement arthroplasty in 103 shoulders for the treatment of osteoarthritis, rheumatoid arthritis, avascular necrosis, capsulorrhaphy arthropathy, post-traumatic arthritis, or cuff tear arthropathy. Ninety-four percent of patients considered their shoulder to be much better than before the operation. The best results were noted in patients with primary osteoarthritis, whereas those with cuff tear arthropathy and post-traumatic arthritis had less favorable outcomes. Eight shoulders required revision, two for loosening.

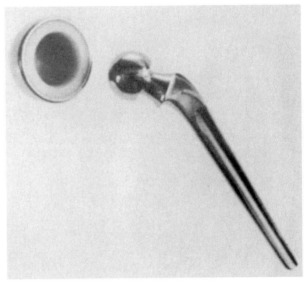

■ **Figure 16–104**
Bipolar shoulder implant system developed by Swanson. Proposed advantages include smooth concentric contact for the entire shoulder joint cavity, including the coracoacromial arch and the glenoid, a decrease in concentration of force over any one contact area, lengthening of the glenoid joint moment arm, and avoidance of abutment of the greater tuberosity against the acromion. *(From Swanson AB: Bipolar implant shoulder arthroplasty. In Bateman JE and Welsh RP [eds]: Surgery of the Shoulder. St Louis: CV Mosby, 1984, pp 211-223.)*

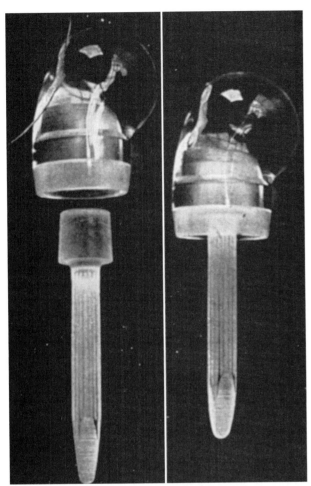

■ **Figure 16–102**
An acrylic prosthesis developed for the treatment of severe fracture-dislocations of the proximal end of the humerus. *(From Richard A, Judet R, and René L: Acrylic prosthetic reconstruction of the upper end of the humerus for fracture-luxations. J Chir 68:537-547, 1952.)*

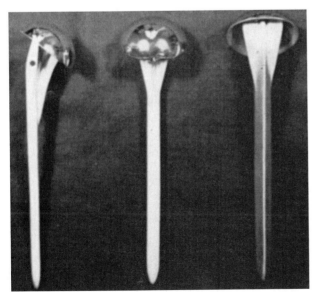

■ **Figure 16–103**
Neer replacement prosthesis for the articular surface of the humeral head. Small, medium, and large models are shown in the 1955 article. *(From Neer CS II: Articular replacement for the humeral head. J Bone Joint Surg Am 37:215-228, 1955.)*

Several plastics and other softer materials have been used as implants. Swanson designed an all–silicon rubber humeral head implant in an extension of the concept of flexible implants as an adjunct to resection arthroplasty.[400] Apparently, this design was used only rarely, and no results are available for a series of patients. Varian reported on a clinical trial of the use of a Silastic cup in patients with rheumatoid arthritis of the shoulder.[414] The early results were promising, but another series by Spencer and Skirving described a number of complications, and the authors recommended restricted use of the device.[385]

After these pioneering efforts, many additional shoulder prostheses were constructed. Some mirrored the implants used by Neer, including the St. Georg[124] (Fig. 16–106), the Bechtol,[27] the DANA,[405] the Cofield[87,88] (Fig. 16–107), and the monospherical.[160,162] Isoelastic shoulder implants have been used in Europe.[67,79,406] Other designs included a captive ball-in-socket unit to replace the stabilizing functions of the rotator cuff and shoulder capsule (Figs. 16–108 to 16–112).* Many of these designs included complex and extensive attachments to the scapula by cementing within the glenoid (Fig. 16–113) and by the use of stems (Fig. 16–114), wedges (Fig. 16–115), a screw (Fig. 16–116), and bolted flanges (Fig. 16–117). Some designs reversed the ball-and-socket configuration and attached the ball part of the implant to the glenoid (see Figs. 16–114 to 16–117).[340] Others incorpo-

Text continued on p. 936

*See references 29, 40, 62, 97, 105, 122, 129, 153, 161, 223, 227, 228, 239, 329-332, 334, 340, 427, 446.

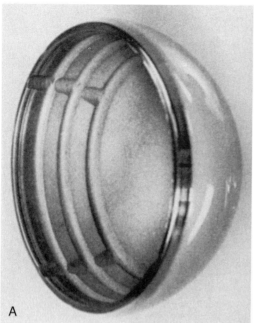

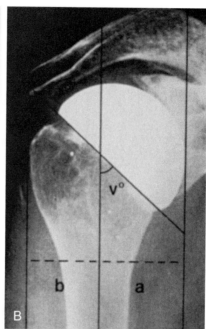

■ **Figure 16–105**
A cup arthroplasty of the shoulder. Illustrated are the cup (**A**) and a radiograph after implantation of a cup in a patient with rheumatoid arthritis (**B**). *(From Jónsson E: Surgery of the Rheumatoid Shoulder with Special Reference to Cup Hemiarthroplasty and Arthrodesis. Lund, Sweden: The University Department of Orthopaedics, 1988.)*

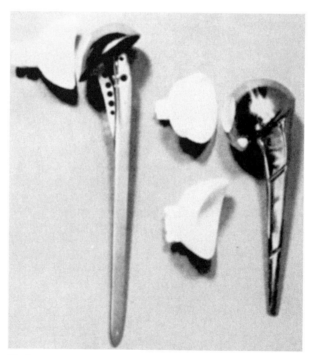

■ **Figure 16–106**
The St. Georg total shoulder prosthesis from Hamburg, Germany. Polyethylene sockets were constructed to mate with the Neer prosthesis *(left)* or the St. Georg model *(right)*. *(From Engelbrecht E and Stellbrink G: Totale Schulterendoprosthese Modell [St. Georg]. Chirurg 47:525-530, 1976.)*

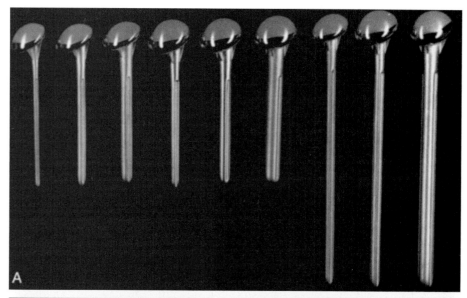

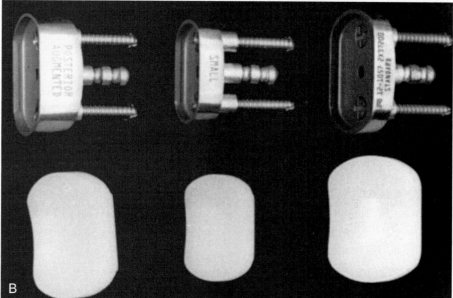

■ **Figure 16–107**

The Cofield total shoulder arthroplasty system. This system has two humeral neck lengths, four humeral stem widths, and two humeral stem lengths (**A**). Two glenoid component sizes and one glenoid component with an asymmetric construction are provided to compensate for uneven glenoid wear (**B**). The ingrowth material in the humeral head is only on the undersurface of the head and does not extend down onto the shaft. The ingrowth material on the glenoid component only abuts against the prepared face of the glenoid and does not extend into the scapular neck.

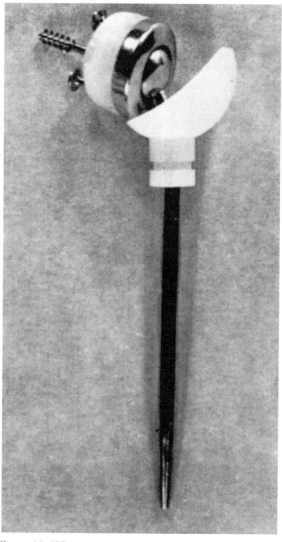

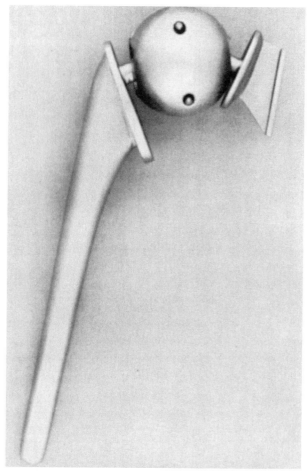

■ **Figure 16–109**
This trispherical total shoulder prosthesis was designed by Gristina and coworkers. Two spheres are held captive within a third larger sphere. The design thus allows an extremely large range of motion in a captive ball-in-socket constrained implant system. *(From Gristina AG and Webb LX: The trispherical total shoulder replacement. In Bayley I and Kessel L [eds]: Shoulder Surgery. New York: Springer-Verlag, 1982, pp 153-157.)*

■ **Figure 16–108**
Model BME total shoulder arthroplasty designed by Zippel of Hamburg, Germany. This implant is an early captive ball-in-socket type of total shoulder arthroplasty. *(From Zippel J: Luxationssichere Schulterendoprosthese Modell BME. Z Orthop 113:454-457, 1975.)*

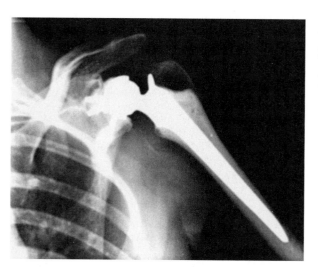

■ **Figure 16–110**
The Stanmore total shoulder replacement. The glenoid component was cemented and relied on a large amount of methylmethacrylate for support. The two components snapped together after being implanted. *(From Cofield RH: Status of total shoulder arthroplasty. Arch Surg 112:1088-1091, 1977. Copyright 1977, American Medical Association.)*

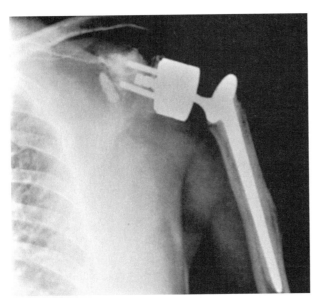

■ **Figure 16–111**

Michael Reese total shoulder replacement, perhaps the most widely used constrained total shoulder system in North America. Placement of the device requires more proximal humerus resection than with many alternative prosthetic designs. *(From Cofield RH: Status of total shoulder arthroplasty. Arch Surg 112:1088-1091, 1977. Copyright 1977, American Medical Association.)*

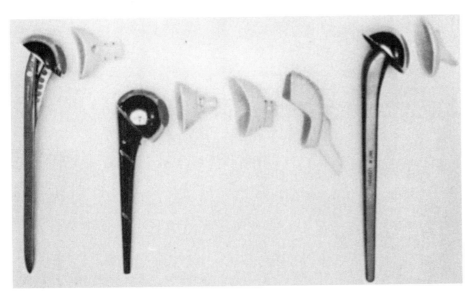

■ **Figure 16–112**

With more than 10 years' experience using unconstrained shoulder replacement, Engelbrecht and coworkers have continued to use unconstrained systems. Initially, the Neer prosthesis was used in conjunction with a high-density polyethylene component of these workers' design *(left)*. This replacement evolved to the St. Georg implant with various glenoid components, including some with rather deep hoods *(center)*. Currently, these workers have returned to a proximal humeral prosthetic replacement *(right)* with a rather simple and unconstrained polyethylene glenoid component. *(From Engelbrecht E and Heinert TK: More than ten years' experience with unconstrained shoulder replacement. In Kölbel R, Helbig B, and Blauth W [eds]: Shoulder Replacement. New York: Springer-Verlag, 1987, pp 85-91.)*

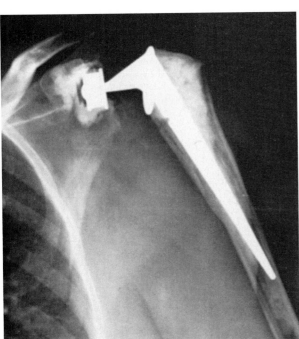

■ **Figure 16–113**

The Bickel glenohumeral prosthesis. The design included a very small ball to decrease friction between components, and the glenoid component was designed to be incorporated entirely within the glenoid cavity and, ideally, to maximize prosthesis-bone contact area. *(From Cofield RH: Status of total shoulder arthroplasty. Arch Surg 112:1088-1091, 1977. Copyright 1977, American Medical Association.)*

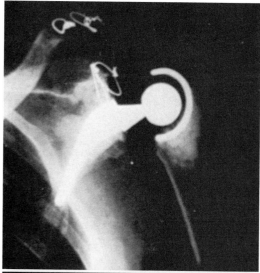

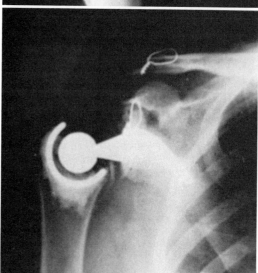

■ **Figure 16–114**

The Liverpool shoulder replacement, a reverse ball-in-socket design. The glenoid component has a stem that is inserted into the medullary cavity of the axillary border of the scapula to a depth of approximately 50 mm. *(From Beddow FH and Elloy MA: Clinical experience with the Liverpool shoulder replacement. In Bayley I and Kessel L [eds]: Shoulder Surgery. New York: Springer-Verlag, 1982, pp 164-167.)*

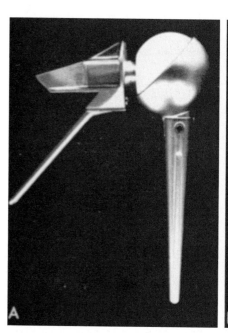

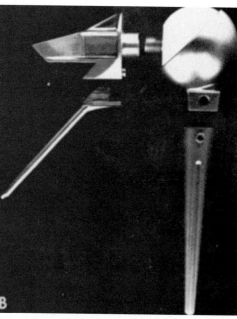

■ **Figure 16–115**

Reverse ball-in-socket total shoulder arthroplasty designed by Fenlin. **A,** The prosthesis has been assembled. **B,** The prosthesis has been disassembled. A wedge is driven into the bone of the scapula for fixation, and a column is placed down the axillary border of the scapula. *(From Fenlin JM Jr: Total glenohumeral joint replacement. Orthop Clin North Am 67:565-583, 1975.)*

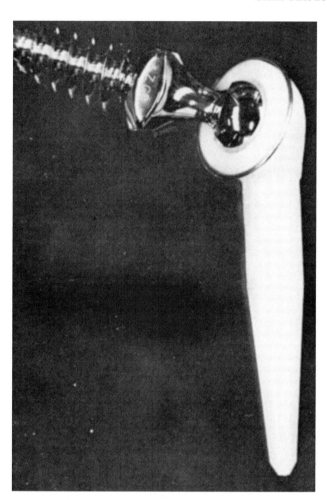

■ **Figure 16–116**

The Kessel total shoulder replacement, a reversed ball-in-socket design. The glenoid component is screwed into the glenoid, and the humeral stem is cemented in place. The components then snap together. *(From Bayley JIL and Kessel L: The Kessel total shoulder replacement. In Bayley I and Kessel L [eds]: Shoulder Surgery. New York: Springer-Verlag, 1982, pp 160-164.)*

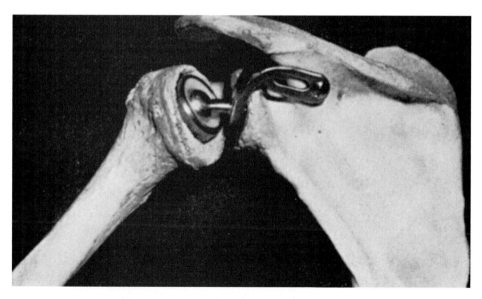

■ **Figure 16–117**

The total shoulder arthroplasty designed by Kölbel. This replacement is a reversed ball-in-socket unit. Scapular component fixation includes a flange bolted to the base of the spine of the scapula. *(From Wolff R and Kölbel R: The history of shoulder joint replacement. In Kölbel R, Helbig B, and Blauth W [eds]: Shoulder Replacement. New York: Springer-Verlag, 1987, pp 2-13.)*

rated two ball-in-socket units (Fig. 16–118; see also Fig. 16–109).[62,161] Engelbrecht and Heinert suggested a hemiarthroplasty with modification of the glenoid by osteotomy and a bone graft to buttress the humeral prosthesis (Fig. 16–119).[122] Burkhead and Hutton[65] performed biologic resurfacing of the glenoid in association with humeral hemiarthroplasty.

Some designs had a hood on the glenoid component in an attempt to prevent upward humeral subluxation associated with rotator cuff weakness or absence (Figs. 16–120 and 16–121).[4-6,124,271,275,304] Implants could be classified as anatomic, semiconstrained (hooded glenoid), or constrained (ball and socket) (Fig. 16–122). Some of the early investigators of these designs are listed in Table 16–16.

The nonretentive prosthesis of Mazas and de la Caffiniére also included a superiorly placed hood on the glenoid component. Of 38 shoulders operated on, instability developed in 9, and 14 remained stiff after surgery.[271] A third early system that included a hooded component was the English-Macnab. This system also has a nonhooded glenoid implant and incorporates porous ingrowth surfaces on the glenoid component and the humeral stem (Fig. 16–123).[127,275]

The Neer system originally included 200% and 600% enlarged glenoid components. These components were used in only 12 of 273 shoulders reported,[304] thus suggesting that the need for them was quite uncommon. The DANA total shoulder arthroplasty (Fig. 16–124) includes a semiconstrained hooded component designed to enhance stability in shoulders with irreparable rotator cuff tears.[4] The monospherical total shoulder replacement also incorporated a slight hood on the glenoid

TABLE 16–16.   Variations in Total Shoulder Arthroplasty Design

Unconstrained (Anatomic)	Semiconstrained (Hooded or Cup-Shaped Glenoid)	Constrained (Ball-in-Socket)
Bechtol[27]	DANA[4-6]	Bickel[97]
Bipolar[25]	English-Macnab[127,275]	Fenlin[129]
Cofield[87,88]	Mazas[271]	Floating-socket[62]
DANA[4-6]	Neer[304]	Gerard[153]
Kenmore[222]	St. Georg[122-124]	Kessel[223]
Monospherical[160]		Kölbel[227,228]
Neer[304]		Liverpool[29,40]
Saha[369]		Michael Reese[329-333]
St. Georg[122-124]		Reeves[340]
		Stanmore[97,105,239]
		Trispherical[162]
		Wheble-Skorecki[427]
		Zippel[446]
		Zimmer

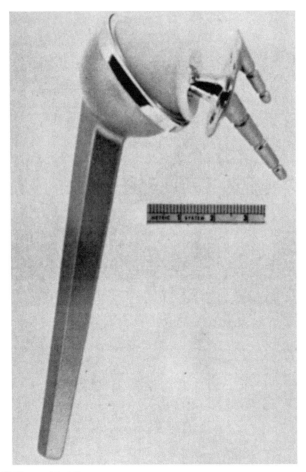

■ **Figure 16–118**
The floating-socket total shoulder replacement. This implant contains a dual spherical bearing system to provide a "floating fulcrum." This configuration allows the prosthesis to have motion in excess of normal anatomic limits. (*From Buechel FF, Pappas MJ, and DePalma AF: "Floating socket" total shoulder replacement: Anatomical, biomechanical, and surgical rationale. J Biomed Mater Res 12:89-114, 1978.*)

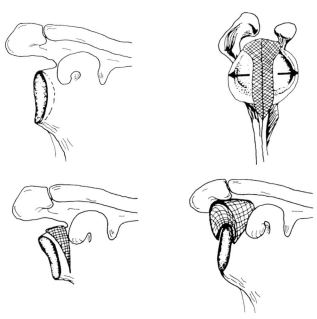

■ **Figure 16–119**
In the face of unusually frequent glenoid loosening, Engelbrecht and coworkers have tended to treat patients with shoulder arthritis by glenoid reshaping (*upper left*), glenoid osteotomies (*upper right and lower left*), or glenoid bone grafting (*upper right and lower left and right*) as an adjunct to proximal humeral prosthetic replacement rather than using a cemented glenoid component. (*From Engelbrecht E and Heinert TK: More than ten years' experience with unconstrained shoulder replacement. In Kölbel R, Helbig B, and Blauth W [eds]: Shoulder Replacement. New York: Springer-Verlag, 1987, pp 85-91.*)

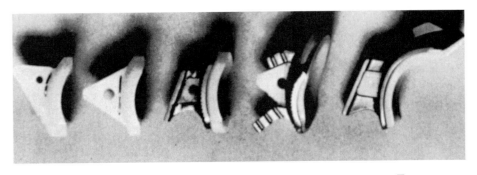

A   B   C   D   E

■ **Figure 16–120**

The Neer design of total shoulder arthroplasty includes a number of types of glenoid components. Five glenoid components were used in the series of patients reported in 1982, including (**A**) the original 1973 polyethylene component, (**B**) a standard polyethylene component, (**C**) a metal-backed standard-sized glenoid component, (**D**) a metal-backed 200% larger glenoid component, and (**E**) a metal-backed 600% larger glenoid component. These latter two hooded components were designed for additional joint constraint against superior humeral subluxation. (From Neer CS II, Watson KC, and Stanton FJ: Recent experience in total shoulder replacement. J Bone Joint Surg Am *64*:319-337, 1982.)

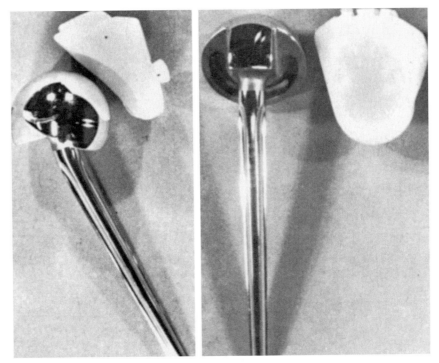

■ **Figure 16–121**

The nonretentive total shoulder arthroplasty designed by Mazas. *(From Mazas F and de la Caffiniére JY: Un prothèse totale d'épaule non rétentive: A propos de 38 cas. Rev Chir Orthop 68:161-170, 1982.)*

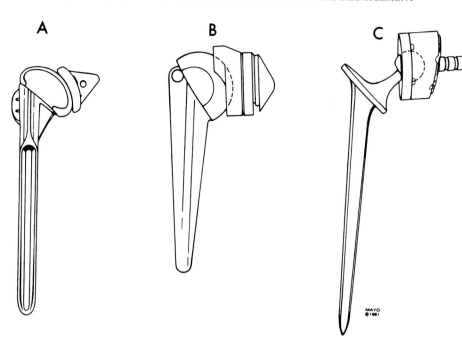

A   **B**   **C**

■ **Figure 16–122**
A variable amount of constraint is
incorporated in the various designs of
total shoulder replacement. Many
implants have their articular surfaces
shaped much like a normal joint
surface (**A**). The system may be
partially constrained by virtue of a
hooded or more cup-shaped socket
(**B**), or the components may be
secured to one another as in a ball-in-
socket prosthesis (**C**). *(From Cofield
RH: The shoulder and prosthetic
arthroplasty. In Evarts CM [ed]: Surgery of
the Musculoskeletal System. New York:
Churchill Livingstone, 1983, pp 125-143.)*

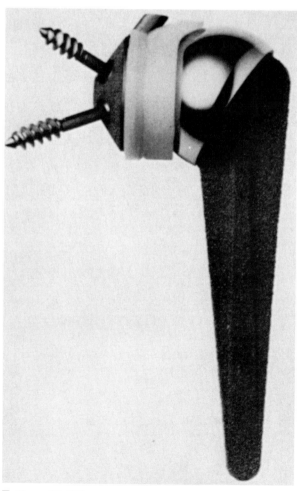

■ **Figure 16–123**
English-Macnab cementless total shoulder arthroplasty. *(From
Faludi DD and Weiland AJ: Cementless total shoulder arthroplasty:
Preliminary experience with 13 cases. Orthopedics 6:431-437, 1983.)*

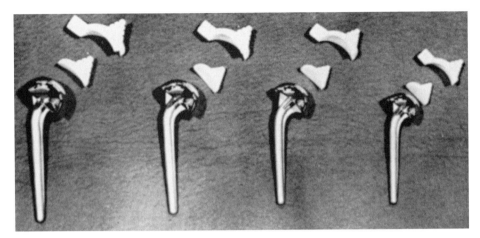

■ **Figure 16–124**
The DANA total shoulder arthroplasty. Illustrated are the four available sizes with the standard and "hooded" glenoid components. *(From Amstutz HC, Thomas BJ, Kabo JM, et al: The DANA total shoulder arthroplasty. J Bone Joint Surg Am 70:1174-1182, 1988.)*

component (Fig. 16–125) that imparted somewhat greater stability to the articulation.[146,160] Laurence[234] has described a "snap-fit" prosthesis for arthroplasty in a cuff-deficient shoulder; the cup is secured to the glenoid and the acromion.

Neer and colleagues defined many of the challenges of shoulder reconstruction, including management of malversion of the glenoid (Fig. 16–126), cementing the glenoid (Fig. 16–127), and proximal humeral deficiency (Fig. 16–128).[304] They expanded the diagnoses that could be managed by prosthetic shoulder reconstruction (Table 16–17). Cofield also pioneered the extended application of shoulder arthroplasty with an expanded implant system (Table 16–18).[90] Pearl and Lippitt[318] and Collins and colleagues[99] have outlined many of the elements of modern arthroplasty technique.

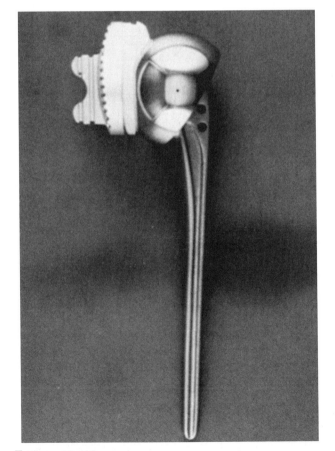

■ **Figure 16–125**
The monospherical total shoulder replacement. A slight amount of hooding has been incorporated into the design of the glenoid component. *(From Gristina AG, Romano RL, Kammire GC, and Webb LX: Total shoulder replacement. Orthop Clin North Am 18:445-453, 1987.)*

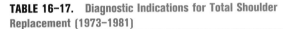

TABLE 16–17. Diagnostic Indications for Total Shoulder Replacement (1973–1981)

	No. of Shoulders
Rheumatoid arthritis	69
Osteoarthritis (primary and secondary)	62
Old trauma	60
Prosthetic revision	32
Arthritis of recurrent dislocation	26
Cuff tear arthropathy	16
Neoplasm	4
Congenital dysplasia	2
Glenohumeral fusion	2
Total	273

Adapted from Neer CS II, Watson KC, and Stanton FJ: Recent experience in total shoulder replacement. J Bone Joint Surg Am 64:319-337, 1982.

TABLE 16–18. Diagnoses in Patients Requiring Total Shoulder Arthroplasty*

	No. of Shoulders
Osteoarthritis	173
Rheumatoid arthritis	165
Traumatic arthritis	46
Cuff tear arthropathy	42
Failed surgery	
Total	34
Proximal humeral	21
Resection	3
Fusion	4
Osteonecrosis	15
Old sepsis	5
Other	8
Total	516

*December 1965 to June 1988.

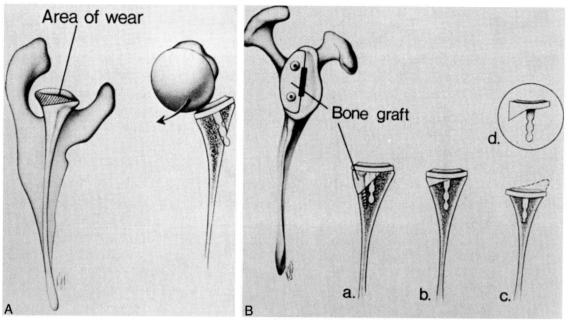

■ **Figure 16–126**

With arthritis of the shoulder, the glenoid may show uneven wear. If the glenoid component is cemented on the remaining subchondral bone surface, as illustrated in **A**, the prosthesis may subluxate in the direction of glenoid wear and the stem of the glenoid prosthetic component may perforate the scapular neck in the opposite direction. Neer and associates pointed out that as illustrated in **B**, this problem may be corrected by applying a bone graft to the area of wear as illustrated in **a**, by building up the worn area with methylmethacrylate as illustrated in **b**, by grinding away the prominent remaining bone in the area that has not been subject to wear as in **c**, or by using a custom-designed glenoid component as illustrated in **d**. *(From Neer CS II, Watson KC, and Stanton FJ: Recent experience in total shoulder replacement. J Bone Joint Surg Am 64:319-337, 1982.)*

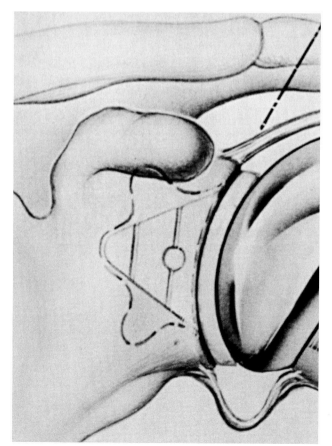

■ **Figure 16–127**

Demonstration of the cementing technique as used by Neer and associates. Subchondral bone is preserved, except for the slot for the keel portion of the component. Soft cancellous bone is removed from beneath a portion of the subchondral plate, from the base of the coracoid process, and to some degree, from the axillary border of the scapula. The remaining cancellous bony bed is carefully dried, and blood is removed. In this illustration, the *broken line* within the neck of the scapula shows the area of cancellous bone removal, which will be occupied by a prosthesis and polymethylmethacrylate. *(From Neer CS II, Watson KC, and Stanton FJ: Recent experience in total shoulder replacement. J Bone Joint Surg Am 64:319-337, 1982.)*

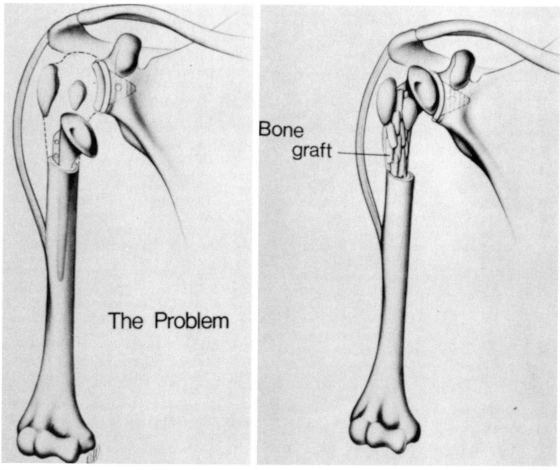

■ Figure 16–128

In certain shoulder arthritis problems, especially those associated with trauma, proximal humeral bone may be lost. If the prosthesis is set low to match the remaining bone, the prosthesis will subluxate inferiorly and the deltoid will be too long to develop any force. As illustrated on the *right,* Neer and associates proposed restoring humeral length, setting the prosthesis opposite the glenoid, and replacing the proximal humerus deficiency with bone graft. *(From Neer CS II, Watson KC, and Stanton FJ: Recent experience in total shoulder replacement. J Bone Joint Surg Am 64:319-337, 1982.)*

The 1980s saw the advent of a number of modular humeral component designs that tried to accommodate the variations in humeral anatomy and space available for the joint and humeral medullary canal diameters. On the glenoid side, some designs offered cementless fixation using screws and porous coatings on metal backing of the polyethylene (see Fig. 16–107). In the 1990s, increased emphasis was placed on restoring normal kinematics with anatomic location and orientation of the humeral and glenoid joint surfaces, advanced soft tissue balancing methods, and physiologic stabilization of the joint. Zuckerman and Cuomo provided a review of the indications and preoperative planning for glenohumeral arthroplasty,[449] Brems conducted a review of the evolution of the glenoid component,[52] and Rodosky and Bigliani reviewed the indications for glenoid resurfacing.[355]

Unfortunately, the results of most of the tens of thousands of surgeries performed for glenohumeral arthritis are not available, in large part because most "outcome" systems are too burdensome for the majority of surgeons carrying out shoulder reconstructions. During the 20 years since the advent of shoulder arthroplasty, the results of the procedure have been published for less than 2000

cases performed in the United States, an estimated 5% of the total. In that most of the published reports come from centers where relatively large numbers of these procedures are performed, it would be of immense interest to know to what degree the results of the other 95% were similar. Hasan and coworkers studied the distribution of shoulder replacements among surgeons and noted that the majority of shoulder replacement procedures are performed by surgeons who do 10 or fewer of these procedures per year. Thus, to the extent that most outcome data are derived from series performed by more experienced surgeons, it is impossible to know the results of shoulder arthroplasty in the context where it is used most often—community practice.[180,260]

Assessment of outcomes is further complicated by regional variation in the rates of shoulder replacement procedures. This variation suggests that appropriate indications for these procedures, as well as their clinical effectiveness, require further examination through well-designed clinical outcome studies. Vitale and associates[415] studied state-to-state variations in rates of total shoulder replacement and hemiarthroplasty. Rates for these procedures varied as much as 10-fold between states and were performed less often in states that were more densely populated. No significant relationship was established between the density of orthopaedic surgeons or shoulder specialists and the rates of either procedure.

An important advance is that simple and practical systems are now available by which surgeons can easily document the status of their patients before and sequentially after shoulder arthroplasty.[247,259,264,266,343] This documentation of treatment effectiveness will permit a comparison of different management approaches for defined groups of patients. If data on the more than 6000 shoulder arthroplasties being performed each year could be gathered, analyzed, and compared, shoulder surgeons would be in a powerful position to understand and progressively improve the effectiveness of the care that they offer their patients.

Milne and Gartsman[281] reviewed the cost of arthroplasty in 1992 and 1993 in a private practice in Houston, Texas. They found that the average cost for hemiarthroplasty was $15,656 and that for total shoulder arthroplasty was $16,606. Of this cost, 20% was for the surgeon, 75% for the hospital, 3% for the anesthesia, and 2% for consultations. Four percent of the patients were receiving workers' compensation, 43% were receiving private pay, and 53% were receiving Medicare. The average length of stay was 5 days with a range of 3 to 14 days.

Indications for Surgery

Glenohumeral arthroplasty is a technically demanding and powerful tool for reconstruction of an arthritic shoulder. Shoulder arthroplasty is considered when the following conditions are met:

1. *Substantial disability of the shoulder exists and is clearly related to loss of the normal glenohumeral articulation.* It is useful to document both the disability and the glenohumeral destruction with standardized tools such as the SST (see Table 16–4), the SF-36 (see Table 16–5), and defined radiographic views (see Figs. 16–41 and 16–42).
2. *The anatomy of the shoulder is amenable to reconstruction by shoulder arthroplasty* (i.e., there is sufficient bone stock, muscle strength, and tendon integrity to provide for a functional and robust reconstruction). In certain situations the presence of anatomic deficiencies may favor hemiarthroplasty over total shoulder arthroplasty, for example, when insufficient glenoid bone remains to support a glenoid component; when the humeral head is fixed in a superiorly displaced position relative to the glenoid (e.g., in cuff tear arthropathy), in patients with degenerative arthritis and an irreparable cuff,[431] in patients with rheumatoid arthritis and an irreparable cuff that is still concentric in shape,[24,383] and in patients with degenerative arthritis and a glenoid that has not eroded.[155,204]
3. *The patient is committed to the success of the procedure, has no contraindications, understands the limitations of a shoulder prosthesis, and has sufficient social support for the postoperative period.* The ideal patient for prosthetic arthroplasty has a positive attitude combined with the understanding that a shoulder arthroplasty is not meant to be used for heavy or jerky pushing, pulling, lifting, or overhead work. Active or recent infection, absent

deltoid function, and poor general health are considered contraindications. Patients with rheumatoid arthritis and other systemic diseases can be expected to have poorer general health and vitality than those with uncomplicated degenerative joint disease. Poor general health may lessen the desirability of shoulder reconstruction, even if the joint involvement is severe. Poor tissue quality, cuff deficiency, nonunion or malunion of the tuberosity, remote infection, previous shoulder surgery, previous trauma, alcoholism, smoking, narcotic use, significant parkinsonism, neuropathic arthropathy, obesity, crutch dependency, and unrealistic expectations all lessen the chance of a good result. Poor mental or emotional health may need management before shoulder reconstruction is undertaken; again, routine preoperative use of the SF-36 may alert the physician to such "red flags" (see Table 16-5).

4. *The surgeon is experienced and prepared to provide a technically excellent arthroplasty.* In that reconstruction of the shoulder is greater in complexity than that of the hip or knee, a similar type of learning curve and number of cases are necessary before mastery is achieved. According to the October 1993 to September 1994 National Inpatient Profile (HCIA Inc, 1995), the number of total knee reconstructions performed in 12 months in the United States was 211,872, whereas the number of total shoulder reconstructions was only 5895.* These data indicate that surgeons have only 3% of the opportunity to master total shoulder arthroplasty as they have to master total knee arthroplasty. Expressed another way, if the cases were distributed evenly, each of the 16,731 members of the American Association of Orthopaedic Surgeons would perform, on average, just over one total knee arthroplasty per month and one total shoulder arthroplasty every 3 years.

The shoulder arthroplasty surgeon must have a command of the anatomy as well as the techniques to safely manage the exposure, capsular contractures, abnormalities in glenoid version, cuff pathology, humeral deformities, and intraoperative problems. Although the approximate number of cases to achieve mastery has not been determined, it is recognized that for shoulder as well as for hip and knee reconstruction, "the surgeon is the method" and "experience is the great teacher."

Goals of Surgery

Shoulder arthroplasty provides the surgeon with the opportunity to restore the mechanics of glenohumeral motion, strength, stability, and smoothness.

Motion is re-established and obligate translation prevented by the following:

1. Releasing all adhesions and contractures at the humeroscapular motion interface (see Fig. 16-19).
2. Inserting a smooth humeral prosthesis whose articular surface area encompasses a substantial portion of the sphere (see Figs. 16-13 and 16-14).

---

*Similar data are presented by Madhok and associates,[252] who reviewed the trends in the use of upper limb replacements at the Mayo Clinic from 1972 to 1990.

3. Inserting a smooth glenoid prosthesis whose articular surface encompasses a relatively small portion of the sphere (see Fig. 16–14).
4. Removing blocking osteophytes (see Fig. 16–18).
5. Avoiding overstuffing of the joint (see Fig. 16–2).

Stability and **strength** are achieved by the following:

1. Normalizing glenoid and humeral joint surface location and orientation so that full surface contact occurs throughout the useful range of joint motion (see Fig. 16–20). Ballmer and associates[18] have studied in detail the effect of component articular surface geometry on the extent of glenohumeral joint surface contact. They found that for some commercially available prosthetic combinations, there was no position in which full surface contact occurred, whereas others offer a 117-degree range of positions of full surface contact. They pointed out that in the range of positions at which full surface contact takes place, there is no possibility for abutment of humeral bone or surrounding soft tissue against the glenoid edge. Furthermore, within this range, joint contact area is maximal, joint pressure is minimal, and the joint offers maximal stability. Conversely, outside the range of full surface contact, the edge of the glenoid may abut against humeral bone or soft tissue, joint contact pressure is increased, and instability may result.

   Pearl and associates[316] examined the ability of four commonly used shoulder replacement systems to replicate the articular geometry of the proximal end of the humerus and noted that this geometry may be extremely variable between patients. The investigators reported that despite attempts to optimize re-creation of the normal anatomy with different prosthetic combinations, the center of rotation was shifted superolaterally by an average of 14.7 mm. In addition, to reach this minimized shift in the center of rotation, optimal prosthetic combinations resulted in a diminution in the arc of the articular surface by an average of 26 degrees. In a related study of selected press-fit prosthetic systems, Pearl and colleagues determined that systems with the most geometric options were best able to match the normal three-dimensional geometry of the proximal end of the humerus.[317] The degree to which such alterations in normal proximal humeral geometry imposed by the prosthetic reconstruction are related to complications such as proximal migration and glenoid loosening has not been determined.
2. Selecting and positioning the new glenoid joint surface (see Figs. 16–26 and 16–27) so that effective arcs are available to balance the range of net humeral joint reaction forces usually encountered.
3. Re-establishing normal compressive muscle force (see Fig. 16–30) by releasing, repairing, balancing, and rehabilitating the cuff muscles (Figs. 16–129 and 16–130).

   The deltoid is the most important motor of the shoulder arthroplasty. The integrity of its origin, insertion, and nerve supply must be maintained. Maintenance of such integrity is most easily accomplished by gently approaching the joint through the deltopectoral interval and by identifying and protecting the axillary nerve both anteromedially as it crosses the

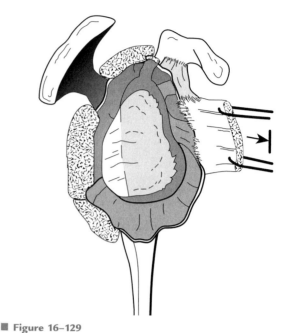

■ **Figure 16–129**
Contracted subscapularis tendon. *(Modified from Matsen FA III, Lippitt SB, Sidles JA, and Harryman DT II: Practical Evaluation and Management of the Shoulder. Philadelphia: WB Saunders, 1994.)*

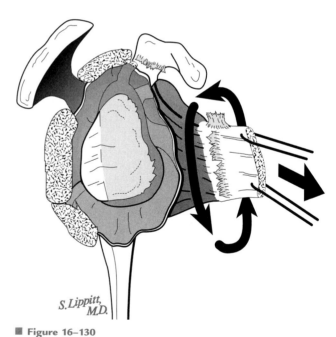

■ **Figure 16–130**
Three hundred sixty-degree subscapularis tendon release. *(Modified from Matsen FA III, Lippitt SB, Sidles JA, and Harryman DT II: Practical Evaluation and Management of the Shoulder. Philadelphia: WB Saunders, 1994.)*

subscapularis and the inferior capsule and laterally as it exits the quadrangular space and winds around the tuberosities on the deep surface of the deltoid. Rehabilitation of the deltoid is critical to achieve active motion after arthroplasty.

The rotator cuff mechanism is in jeopardy in shoulder arthroplasty for several reasons. The suprascapular nerve, which supplies the supraspinatus and

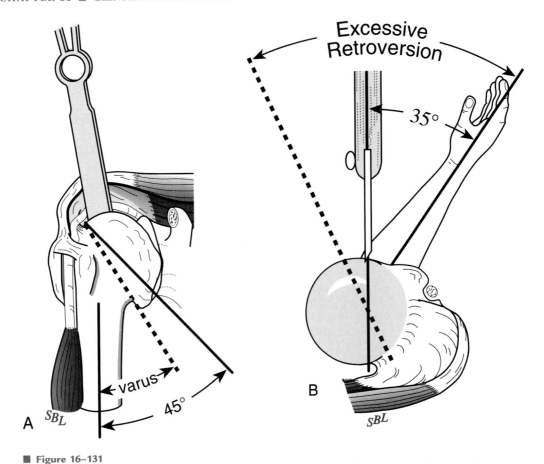

■ Figure 16–131

A, A cut that is too lateral risks detaching the cuff insertion superiorly. **B,** A humeral cut made in excessive retroversion risks detaching the cuff posteriorly. *(From Matsen FA III, Lippitt SB, Sidles JA, and Harryman DT II: Practical Evaluation and Management of the Shoulder. Philadelphia: WB Saunders, 1994.)*

infraspinatus, is at risk during surgical release as it courses medial to the coracoid and then down the back of the glenoid 1 cm medial to the glenoid lip. The cuff tendons are at risk during surgery because the humeral cut must come close to their insertion to the tuberosities superiorly and posteriorly. A humeral cut made in excessive retroversion is likely to detach the cuff posteriorly, and a cut made too low on the humerus is likely to detach the cuff superiorly (Fig. 16–131). Overstuffing the joint places the cuff under tension when the arm is adducted or rotated (see Fig. 16–40). Most shoulder arthroplasties are performed in older individuals, and the quality of the cuff tissue may be compromised not only by age-related changes but also by disuse imposed by chronic glenohumeral roughness. Shoulder arthroplasty may quickly restore motion and smoothness to the joint and place new and substantial demands on the poorer-quality cuff tissue. Thus, the rehabilitation program and the patient's activities after arthroplasty must *gradually* increase loads on the cuff to allow the tissue the opportunity to strengthen over time.

If a cuff defect exists at the time of arthroplasty, a cuff repair to bone can be carried out, provided that the quantity and quality of cuff tissue are sufficient to allow a secure repair under physiologic tension with the arm at the side. If these conditions are not met,

attempting cuff repair may not be worthwhile. If a cuff repair is carried out or if fixation of the tuberosities is performed, the rehabilitation after arthroplasty must be changed dramatically to allow for secure healing of the cuff mechanism to the humerus before active use is permitted. For these reasons, if the rotator cuff is deficient in quantity or quality, repair is not usually attempted. In these circumstances, hemiarthroplasty is often considered instead of total shoulder arthroplasty.

4. Ensuring that capsular ligaments are neither too short (in which case obligate translation may occur at the limits of motion) (see Fig. 16–7) nor too loose (in which case the joint may over-rotate beyond the positions at which the muscles can stabilize the head in the socket).

These considerations are critical. Reports suggest that almost one third of glenoid failures are associated with chronic glenohumeral instability after shoulder arthroplasty.[354-356]

Smoothness is provided by the following:

1. Inserting smooth prosthetic joint surfaces.
2. Managing all humeroscapular motion interface roughness.
3. Implementing immediate postoperative motion to prevent unwanted scar formation (Fig. 16–132). Early

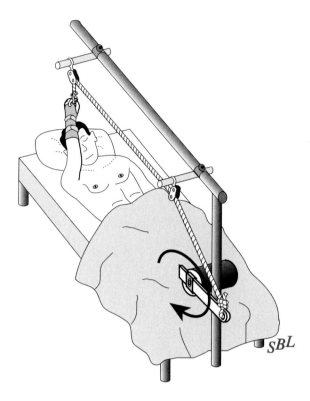

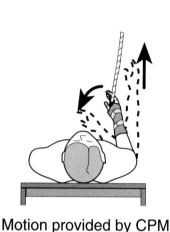

Motion provided by CPM

■ **Figure 16–132**
Continuous passive motion (CPM) is helpful for the first 24 to 48 hours after a procedure to mobilize the shoulder. Elevation to 90 degrees is easily achieved by using a simple pulley system with a motor-driven eccentric cam. *(From Matsen FA III, Lippitt SB, Sidles JA, and Harryman DT II: Practical Evaluation and Management of the Shoulder. Philadelphia: WB Saunders, 1994.)*

postoperative motion not only reduces the likelihood of adhesion formation but may also increase the strength of soft tissue repairs.[138]

Types of Arthroplasty

Three levels of glenohumeral arthroplasty are commonly used. The basic surgical approach, capsular balancing, and osteophyte removal are similar for all three:

Nonprosthetic arthroplasty is considered when osteophytes and capsular contractures block motion and function in the presence of congruent glenohumeral contact and reasonable cartilaginous space on radiographs. This option is particularly desirable in a young individual who plans to place continued heavy demands on the shoulder.

Prosthetic humeral hemiarthroplasty is considered in the following cases:

1. The humeral joint surface is rough, but the cartilaginous surface of the glenoid is intact* and sufficient glenoid arc is available to stabilize the humeral head.† In this situation, there is an even greater need to match the normal anatomy than in the case of total glenohumeral replacement.‡

2. Insufficient bone is available to support a glenoid component (e.g., after severe medial erosion of the glenoid in rheumatoid arthritis) (see Figs. 16–29 and 16–53).

3. The humeral head is upwardly displaced relative to the glenoid as in cuff tear arthropathy (see Fig. 16–34) or severe rheumatoid arthritis (see Fig. 16–58).

4. The patient has a history of remote joint infection.

5. Heavy demands will be placed on the joint (e.g., in motion disorders or anticipated heavy loading from occupation, sport, or lower extremity paresis).

Humeral hemiarthroplasty may be stabilized in cuff tear arthropathy, even though the superior lip of the glenoid is eroded away by superior humeral subluxation. In this situation, the prosthetic humeral head is captured by an acetabular-like socket consisting of the eroded upper glenoid, the coracoid, the coracoacromial ligament, and the acromion, provided that these structures have not been sacrificed by acromioplasty. It is vital that the surgeon not compromise this "socket" by sacrificing the anterior acromion or the coracoacromial ligament; otherwise, the humeral head is likely to be destabilized or "escape" in an anterosuperior direction.

In hemiarthroplasty for cuff tear arthropathy, the undersurface of the "acetabularized" coracoacromial arch

---

*Articular cartilage is assessed by preoperative radiographs, including CT scans, and at surgery by observation, palpation, and listening to the sound when the cartilage is struck with a small blunt elevator: thin cartilage or bare bone will cause the elevator to ring, whereas normal cartilage will yield only a dull "thunk."

†Frequently in degenerative joint disease and in capsulorrhaphy arthropathy, the posterior half of the glenoid concavity is eroded away and the shoulder is deprived of the effective glenoid arc (see Figs. 16–24 and 16–44). Thus, even if excellent articular cartilage exists on the anterior half of the glenoid, a humeral hemiarthroplasty cannot be stable without this posterior glenoid lip.

‡When performing hemiarthroplasty, the goal is to restore the humeral articular surface to its normal location and configuration. Because the glenoid is not replaced, the size, radius, and orientation of the prosthetic humeral joint surface must duplicate that of the original biologic humeral head. Information regarding the patient's normal humeral head anatomy may be obtained from radiographs of the opposite shoulder.

is found to be polished smooth with a consistent radius of curvature. The prosthetic humeral articular surface and the tuberosities must provide a smooth congruent surface to mate with this arch. Achieving this goal requires attention to selection and positioning of the humeral component and to sculpting the tuberosities. The best choice is a humeral prosthesis that duplicates the size and position of the humeral head that is excised. The large smooth joint contact area achieved in this procedure appears to be responsible for its success in restoring comfort and function in the difficult problem of cuff tear arthropathy. Care should be taken to avoid replacement of the head of the humerus with a "big head" that can overstuff the joint!

Total glenohumeral arthroplasty is considered when both joint surfaces are damaged and when both are reconstructible.

Rodosky and Bigliani[355] reviewed the indications for glenoid resurfacing. They pointed out that early in the history of shoulder arthroplasty it was recognized that when the glenoid was significantly diseased, problems with excessive excursion of the prosthetic head were noted. The goal of inserting a glenoid prosthesis was to provide a better fulcrum and therefore better strength and greater stability,[297] along with decreased friction and elimination of "glenoid socket pain."[355] Other potential benefits of the glenoid component include avoiding the progressive glenoid erosion seen when arthritis or fractures are treated with proximal humeral replacement alone.[35,100,283]

Comparison of Hemiarthroplasty and Total Shoulder Arthroplasty

At this point the literature comparing hemiarthroplasty and total shoulder arthroplasty seems to favor the former when arthritis and cuff deficiency are coexistent* and the latter in osteoarthritis and rheumatoid arthritis when the cuff is intact.† It is recognized that badly eroded glenoid bone cannot support a glenoid prosthesis.[297,298,304] Some studies have attempted to directly compare hemiarthroplasty and total shoulder arthroplasty for treatment of arthritic conditions of the glenohumeral joint. In a "similar," but unmatched series comparison, Boyd and associates[48] found that at 44-month follow-up, hemiarthroplasty and total shoulder arthroplasty produced similar results in terms of functional improvement. Pain relief, range of motion, and patient satisfaction were better with total shoulder arthroplasty than with hemiarthroplasty in the rheumatoid population. Progressive glenoid loosening was detected in 12% of total shoulder arthroplasties, but no correlation with pain relief or range of motion was noted. Gartsman and colleagues[152] randomized 51 shoulders undergoing shoulder replacement for osteoarthritis to receive either total shoulder arthroplasty (27 shoulders) or hemiarthroplasty (24 shoulders). At a mean follow-up of 35 months, total shoulder arthro-

plasty provided significantly greater pain relief than hemiarthroplasty did. In addition, total shoulder arthroplasty demonstrated a trend toward superior outcomes with respect to patient satisfaction, function, and strength, although statistical significance was not achieved by the numbers available for study. Three patients in the hemiarthroplasty group required revision for resurfacing the glenoid, whereas no patients in the total shoulder arthroplasty group required revision.

Prosthesis Selection

Many of the concepts guiding selection of a prosthesis have been presented earlier in the section of this chapter on mechanics. A few additional comments are offered here regarding selection of the prosthesis.

Desirable Characteristics of a Glenoid Prosthesis

1. The glenoid prosthesis should be as thin as structural properties allow to minimize joint stuffing (see Fig. 16-2). For this reason, all-polyethylene components have an advantage because metal backing takes up needed room in the joint.

2. The glenoid should be supported directly and intimately by bone (Fig. 16-133; see also Fig. 16-27) to avoid cracking away of a thin cement mantle. The high incidence of failure of metal-backed glenoid components has been recognized.[354-356] Preservation of subchondral bone and the use of all-polyethylene components result in loading patterns most similar to those found in a normal glenoid, whereas metal-backed components lead to high nonphysiologic stress.[144] Stone and associates[396] used finite element analysis to characterize and compare local stress at the bone-implant interface of a cemented all-polyethylene component and an uncemented metal-backed component. The all-polyethylene design demonstrated an overall stress pattern that was closer to the intact glenoid. Extremely high stress regions were found within the polyethylene near the metal interface in the metal-backed design.

3. The technique of fixation of the glenoid prosthesis should preserve bone stock and minimize the need for cement. Bone-prosthesis contact must be optimized by appropriate design, sizing, and bone preparation. Freehand bone preparation is too uncertain to routinely provide optimal stability without resorting to the interposition of cement (see Fig. 16-133). Drill guides can ensure that the fixation system achieves the desired relationship to the prepared glenoid face and minimizes the amount of bone removed.

4. The prosthesis selected must have an appropriate articular surface area[77] and diameter of curvature relative to the humeral prosthesis (Figs. 16-134 and 16-135; see also Figs. 16-14, 16-36, and 16-37).

   For the glenoid to stabilize the humeral head against transverse loads, it must be well supported by the bone beneath it. Clinical observations suggest that a primary mechanism of glenoid loosening is via the rocking horse mechanism when eccentric loads are

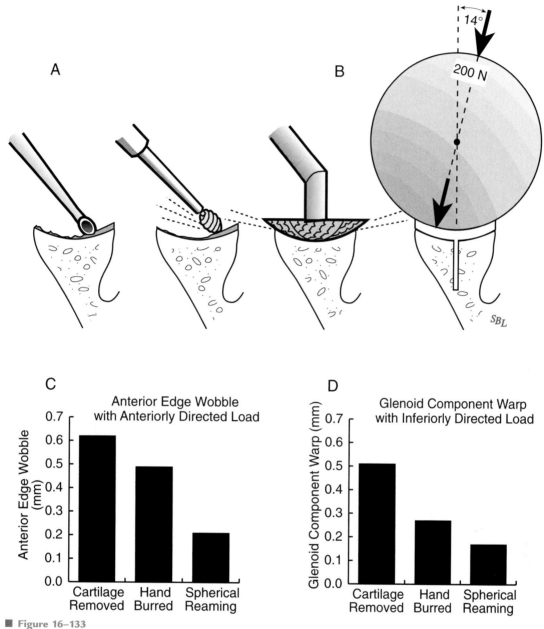

■ Figure 16–133

The effect of glenoid bone preparation on component stability. **A,** Three methods of bone preparation were compared: curettage, hand burring, and spherical reaming. **B,** Loads of 200 N were applied through a metal ball at an angle of 14 degrees with respect to the glenoid centerline. The glenoid was fixed only with a single uncemented flexible central peg. Displacement transducers measured the change in position of the edges of the glenoid component. **C** and **D,** Data on the stability of a glenoid component with three different types of glenoid surface preparation. Spherical reaming of the glenoid along the glenoid centerline significantly reduced the wobble (**C**) and warp (**D**) of the glenoid component and thus provided more glenoid component stability than did curettage or hand burring. *(From Matsen FA III, Lippitt SB, Sidles JA, and Harryman DT II: Practical Evaluation and Management of the Shoulder. Philadelphia: WB Saunders, 1994.)*

applied. In a series of 10 cadaver glenoids, the authors studied the effect of glenoid bone preparation on the stability of a 3-mm-thick, nonclinical glenoid component with a diameter of curvature of 60 mm on the surface apposed to bone.[262] To emphasize the effect of glenoid surface preparation, the component was secured to the bony glenoid with only a single, flexible, uncemented central peg. The component was loaded with an eccentric force of 200 N applied at an angle of 14 degrees to the glenoid centerline. While the compo-

nent was loaded, the wobble of the component with respect to bone and the warp or deformation of the component were measured with displacement transducers. The stability of the component was measured sequentially after three different glenoid preparations: (1) curettage of the articular cartilage, (2) meticulous burring of the bone by hand to fit the back of the component, and (3) preparation using a reamer with a diameter of curvature of 60 mm centered in a hole along the glenoid centerline. Spherical reaming

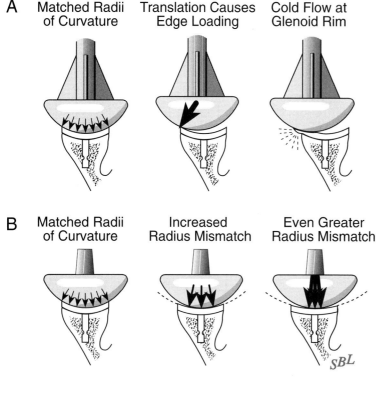

A   Matched Radii
of Curvature   Translation Causes
Edge Loading   Cold Flow at
Glenoid Rim

B   Matched Radii
of Curvature   Increased
Radius Mismatch   Even Greater
Radius Mismatch

■ **Figure 16–134**
A, When the joint surfaces of the glenoid and humeral components have identical radii of curvature, any amount of translation (however small) causes rim loading. Rim loading in turn results in high contact pressure, rim wear, and cold flow. **B,** When the radius of curvature of the surface of the glenoid component is larger than that of the humerus, joint pressure (load per unit area) is increased because of the degree of mismatch (see Figs. 16-38 and 16-39). *(Modified from Matsen FA III, Lippitt SB, Sidles JA, and Harryman DT II: Practical Evaluation and Management of the Shoulder. Philadelphia: WB Saunders, 1994.)*

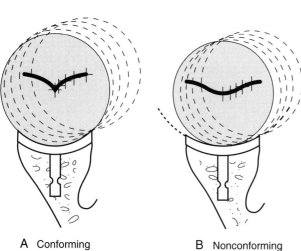

A   Conforming   B   Nonconforming

■ **Figure 16–135**
The path that the center of the humeral head takes during translation relative to the glenoid (the "glenoidogram" path). **A,** Conforming surfaces yield a tight V on the glenoidogram. **B,** When the glenoid diameter of curvature is slightly larger than that of the humerus, the glenoidogram yields a U shape. *(From Matsen FA III, Lippitt SB, Sidles JA, and Harryman DT II: Practical Evaluation and Management of the Shoulder. Philadelphia: WB Saunders, 1994.)*

dramatically diminished both the wobble and the warp of the glenoid component with eccentric loading when compared with the other two methods of bone preparation (see Fig. 16–133). It is likely that an even greater increment in stability would occur with concentric reaming of a deformed bony glenoid, such as that found in degenerative joint disease. This study demonstrates that precise contouring of the bone to fit the

back of the glenoid component provides excellent support of the prosthesis, even without the potential benefits of fixation with multiple pegs, keels, cement, screws, or tissue ingrowth. Spherical reaming along the anatomic glenoid centerline has two important advantages: (1) it normalizes glenoid version, and (2) it provides "bone back" support of the glenoid component with the opportunity for optimal stability and load transfer without the use of metal backing.

Fixation anterior and posterior to the meridian is used to prevent anterior and posterior rocking or "liftoff" during eccentric loading (see Fig. 16–35).

Glenohumeral arthroplasty provides the surgeon the opportunity to control the shape of the prosthetic glenoid concavity. The depth of the glenoid concavity is related to the dimensions of the face of the glenoid (superoinferior and anteroposterior breadth) and the radius of curvature (Fig. 16–136). For a given radius of joint surface curvature, larger components are deeper than smaller ones. For a given glenoid size, components with a smaller radius of curvature are deeper than those with larger radii of joint surface curvature.

If the glenoid and humeral radii of curvature are equal, the head will be held precisely in the center by concavity compression; no translation can occur unless the humeral head is allowed to lift out of the fossa (Fig. 16–137). Although this tight conformity provides excellent stability, it has the potential disadvantage that displacing loads applied to the humerus will be fully transmitted to the glenoid and thence to the glenoid-bone interface. In a biologic glenoid, compliance of the articular cartilage and glenoid labrum provides shock absorption for these transverse displacing loads. Because polyethylene is much stiffer than

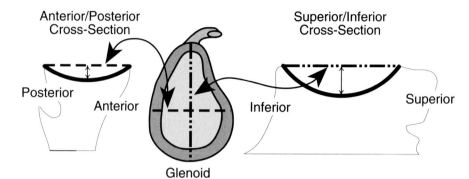

Glenoid

■ **Figure 16–136**
The width of the glenoid in the superoinferior direction is greater than the width of the glenoid in the anteroposterior direction. For a given radius of curvature, an increase in width results in an increase in depth. Thus, the depth of the glenoid as measured along the superoinferior direction is greater than the depth measured along the anteroposterior direction. *(From Matsen FA III, Lippitt SB, Sidles JA, and Harryman DT II: Practical Evaluation and Management of the Shoulder. Philadelphia: WB Saunders, 1994.)*

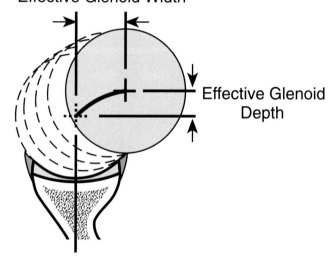

■ **Figure 16–137**
The glenoidogram is the path of the humeral head as it translates in a specified direction across the face of the glenoid away from the glenoid centerline under defined loads. The glenoidogram shows the effective glenoid depth and width for the specified direction of translation and loading conditions. *(Modified from Matsen FA III, Lippitt SB, Sidles JA, and Harryman DT II: Practical Evaluation and Management of the Shoulder. Philadelphia: WB Saunders, 1994.)*

cartilage and labrum, this shock absorption is not present in a prosthetic glenoid arthroplasty. Thus, glenoid fixation is at risk for substantial peak loads when the glenoid and humeral joint surfaces are totally conforming. Karduna and associates[214] demonstrated that prosthetically reconstructed shoulders developed higher peak force for a given translation as conformity increased. Rim loading also generated higher tensile strain in conforming joints than in nonconforming joints.

Some degree of shock absorption can be provided by a slight mismatch between the humeral and glenoid radii of curvature, that of the glenoid being slightly larger. This mismatch allows some translation before the humeral head must lift out of the fossa (the glenoidogram becomes more of a "U" than a tight "V"; see Fig. 16–135). This too is a compromise, however, in that the degree of mismatch decreases the contact area

and increases contact pressure with the potential risk of polyethylene failure. In a finite element model using conventional polyethylene, the surface area of contact with a typical 625-N (140-lb) body weight load was predicted to decrease dramatically with increasing degrees of radial mismatch (see Fig. 16–38). This drop in contact area gives rise to a corresponding increase in contact stress (see Fig. 16–39). For loads of 625 N, the contact stress exceeds the predicted yield stress for conventional polyethylene when the radial mismatch is greater than 3 mm.

Harryman and associates[175,262] demonstrated glenohumeral translation in normal shoulders with passive motion. Friedman[142] has used a radiographic technique to measure anteroposterior translation in 13 patients who underwent Neer or Cofield total shoulder arthroplasties (in each of which the diameters of curvature of the glenoid and humeral surfaces were equal). They measured an average of 4 mm (range, 0 to 12 mm) of posterior translation between horizontal elevation in the minus 30-degree (posterior) plane and horizontal elevation in the 60-degree (anterior) plane. Along with Matsen and associates[263] and Collins and coworkers,[98] they pointed out that this translation could contribute to loosening or to asymmetric wear (see Figs. 16–36, 16–37, and 16–134). Such a tendency for rim loading may be lessened if there is a slight diametric mismatch between the humerus and the glenoid (see Figs. 16–36, 16–37, and 16–135).

5. The mechanical properties of the glenoid prosthesis must have a sufficient yield stress for the anticipated loading conditions (see Figs. 16–38 and 16–39).
6. Glenoid preparation and component insertion must restore normal orientation with respect to the scapula.

A simple cadaver study demonstrated a practical method for normalizing orientation of the glenoid. The center of the face of the glenoid was located in each of 10 normal cadaveric scapulas. A drill was then inserted perpendicular to the face, starting at the glenoid center. In each case, the drill emerged from the anterior glenoid neck at the lateral aspect of the subscapularis fossa at a point midway between the upper and lower crura of the scapula (see Fig. 16–25). This spot is known as the "centering point." This point is easily palpated at arthroplasty surgery after an anterior capsular release has been performed (see Fig. 16–26). The line connecting it to the center of the glenoid face is the normalized glenoid centerline. Orienting the prosthetic glenoid to this normalized glenoid centerline enables the surgeon to correct pathologic glenoid version, which is frequently encountered in degenerative joint disease and other conditions that require shoulder arthroplasty (see Fig. 16–27).

Desirable Characteristics of the Humeral Prosthesis

1. The articular component must maximize the percentage of the sphere represented by the humeral articular surface area (see Figs. 16–9 and 16–13).[18]
2. The prosthesis design must allow replication of the anatomic location and orientation of the humeral articular surface (see Figs. 16–2 and 16–10).
3. The stem must provide secure humeral fixation in a way that preserves humeral bone stock.

If the component is press-fit in the medullary canal, the surgeon must recognize the restrictions that this fixation poses on positioning of the prosthesis. Ballmer and colleagues[19,262] pointed out that in a press-fit situation, the canal rather than the neck cut becomes the primary determinant of the mediolateral, anteroposterior, flexion-extension, and varus-valgus position of the component. In fact, with a snug canal fit, only 2 of the 6 potential degrees of freedom remain: component height and component version. Canal-fitting components are usually inserted after reaming the canal to the necessary depth and to a diameter judged to be safe and snug by the surgeon. The axis of this reamed proximal humeral canal is the "orthopaedic axis" of the humerus (Fig. 16–138). Again, the significance of this axis is that it defines much of the positional geometry of a humeral component press-fit into it. With this axis used as a reference, several geometric parameters were measured in 10 cadaveric humeri ranging in age from 37 to 78 years (mean of 60 years). The results are shown in Table 16–19. For components that fit snugly within the medullary canal, changes in humeral version must take place about the orthopaedic axis, which does not allow much latitude in version if the humeral

TABLE 16–19. Results of Several Geometric Parameters Measured in 10 Cadaveric Humeri Ranging in Age from 37 to 78 Years (Mean of 60 Years) with the "Orthopaedic Axis" of the Humerus Used as a Reference

	Range	Mean	Standard Deviation
Canal diameter (DC) (mm)	8–14	11	2
Head diameter (DH) (mm)	39–41	44	4
Neck length (ENL) (mm)	7–14	11	2
Joint surface angle (AH) (°)	104–120	113	5
Posterior head offset (OH) (mm)	(−3)–4	2	2

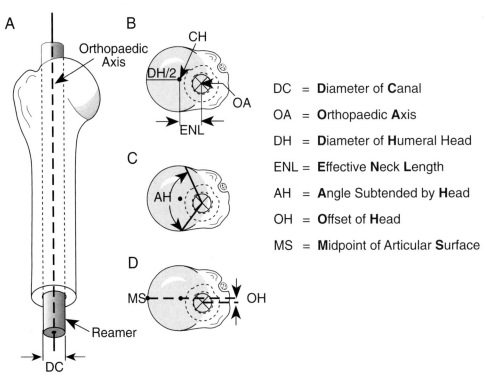

DC = **D**iameter of **C**anal

OA = **O**rthopaedic **A**xis

DH = **D**iameter of **H**umeral Head

ENL = **E**ffective **N**eck **L**ength

AH = **A**ngle Subtended by **H**ead

OH = **O**ffset of **H**ead

MS = **M**idpoint of Articular **S**urface

■ **Figure 16–138**

A, The humeral medullary canal is reamed to a diameter (DC) defining the orthopaedic axis (OA). **B,** The diameter of curvature of the humeral articular surface is DH (the radius is DH/2). The effective neck length (ENL) is the distance between the center of the humeral head (CH) and the orthopaedic axis (OA). **C,** The angle based at the orthopaedic axis and subtended by the humeral articular surface is AH. **D,** The offset of the center of the humeral head (OH) is defined as the perpendicular distance between the orthopaedic axis (OA) and a line connecting the midpoint of the articular surface (MS) and the center of the humeral head (CH). *(From Matsen FA III, Lippitt SB, Sidles JA, and Harryman DT II: Practical Evaluation and Management of the Shoulder. Philadelphia: WB Saunders, 1994.)*

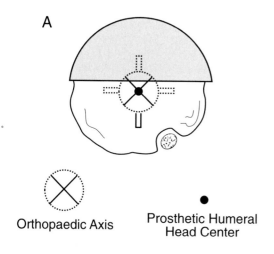

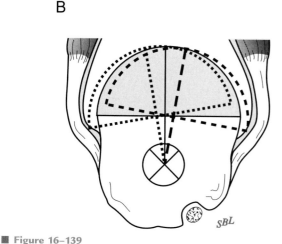

■ Figure 16–139

The effect of changing humeral version in a canal-fitting prosthesis is determined by the effective neck length of the prosthesis (the distance between the orthopaedic axis and the center of curvature of the head) and the amount of change in version. **A,** If the effective neck length is zero, no amount of change in version will affect the distance between the tuberosities and the glenoid that the soft tissues must span. **B,** For an anatomic humerus, the effective neck length is small (average, 11 mm). If the humeral neck cut is made just inside the cuff insertion to the tuberosities, little angular change of the humeral component can be accomplished without jeopardizing the integrity of the cuff insertion. Thus, in a canal-fitting humeral component, changes in version do not have a major effect on soft tissue balance. *(From Matsen FA III, Lippitt SB, Sidles JA, and Harryman DT II: Practical Evaluation and Management of the Shoulder. Philadelphia: WB Saunders, 1994.)*

articular surface is to be optimized (Fig. 16–139). For this reason and because the center of rotation of the head lies close to the orthopaedic axis, soft tissue tension is not substantially changed by alterations in humeral version (a very different situation from that encountered in the hip, where the center of rotation of the head is distant from the medullary axis of the shaft). Ballmer and colleagues[19] found that only a 2-mm change in combined head/neck length could be achieved by a change in the version of a prosthesis press-fit in the canal.

The strength of humeral fixation has been studied by experimental investigation. Harris and associates[174] compared rotational stability with three types of fixation, including press-fit, proximal cementation, and full cementation. Proximal cementation was noted to significantly reduce micromotion when compared with the press-fit technique, whereas full cementation did not increase rotational stability beyond that achieved with proximal cementation. Peppers and associates[321] similarly noted an inverse correlation between axial micromotion and canal fill when comparing these three types of fixation. Good fit and fill can often provide secure fixation without cement, but press-fitting does increase the risk of proximal humeral fracture.

Zuckerman[447] compared hospital reimbursement by Medicare for Diagnosis-Related Group (DRG) 491 (shoulder arthroplasty) and found an overall range of $4699 to $9856 with a mean of $6906 for urban locations and a mean of $5198 for rural locations. He found that the cost of humeral components ranged from $950 to $2250 whereas glenoid components ranged from $520 to $1250. Total shoulder systems ranged from $1470 to $2900. Thus, if the least costly implant system was used in a location with the greatest DRG reimbursement, it would account for $1470/$9856, or 15% of the hospital reimbursement. At the opposite extreme, if the most costly implant was used where DRG reimbursement was the least, it would account for $2900/$4699, or 62% of the total hospital reimbursement. In a prospective comparison of hemiarthroplasty versus total shoulder arthroplasty for treatment of glenohumeral osteoarthritis, Gartsman and colleagues[152] noted that placement of a glenoid component increased the cost per patient by $1177. In this series, however, three patients who had undergone hemiarthroplasty required revision glenoid resurfacing. The mean cost of this additional operation was $15,998.

■ MATSEN'S SURGICAL TECHNIQUE

Standardized preoperative radiographs are obtained to reveal the amount, quality, and orientation of the glenoid bone, as well as the size and configuration of the humerus down to where the tip of the humeral prosthesis will rest (see Figs. 16–41 and 16–42). Drawing the cuts and the implants on the preoperative radiographs with the manufacturer's templates helps the surgeon determine where the humeral and glenoid components should be positioned and whether any particular problems in their placement can be anticipated. **(V16-10)** Is there significant glenoid erosion or altered version? Are any potentially confusing glenoid osteophytes present? Is enough bone available to support a glenoid component? What is the radius of the humeral joint surface? Is the humeral canal straight? Is it cylindrical or funnel shaped? What size is it? What is the position of the tuberosities in relation to the canal and the joint surface? How much humeral bone will need to be excised? Are there other major abnormalities of bone structure that could change the procedure? In press-fit components, will the medullary space accommodate the size and shape of the stem and body of the prosthesis without a risk of fracture?

After a brachial plexus block or general anesthesia, the patient is placed in the beach chair position with the thorax up at an angle of 30 degrees. The shoulder is just off the edge of the operating table so that it can be moved freely through an entire range of motion. The anesthesiologist is positioned at the side of the neck on the opposite side from the shoulder being operated on. A careful double-skin preparation includes the entire arm and forequarter, anteriorly and posteriorly. Draping allows access to the entire scapula, clavicle, and humerus.

A *skin incision* is made over the deltopectoral groove along a line connecting the midpoint of the clavicle to the midpoint of the lateral aspect of the humerus and crossing over the coracoid process (Fig. 16–140). **(V16-11)** The deltopectoral interval is developed medial to the cephalic vein, with preservation of its major tributaries from the deltoid muscle (Fig. 16–141). No deltoid detachment is needed proximally or distally. Incising the clavipectoral fascia at the lateral edge of the conjoined tendon up to, but not through the coracoacromial ligament provides entry to the nonarticular humeroscapular motion interface (Fig. 16–142; see also Fig. 16–19). All adhesions in this interface are lysed from the axillary nerve medially to the point at which the axillary nerve exits the quadrilateral space posterolaterally. Burkhead and associates[66] have provided an excellent review of the surgical anatomy of this nerve.

The subscapularis is incised at its insertion to the lesser tuberosity along with the subjacent capsule (Fig. 16–143). **(V16-12)** This method of detachment maximizes the potential for a strong repair in that, as pointed out by Hinton and associates,[193] the inferior 40% of the belly of the

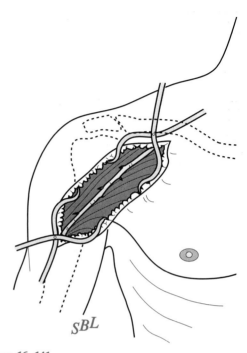

■ Figure 16–141

The cephalic vein identified in the deltopectoral groove. *(Modified from Pearl ML and Lippitt SB: Shoulder arthroplasty with a modular prosthesis. Tech Orthop 8:151-162, 1994. Original illustrator, S.B. Lippitt.)*

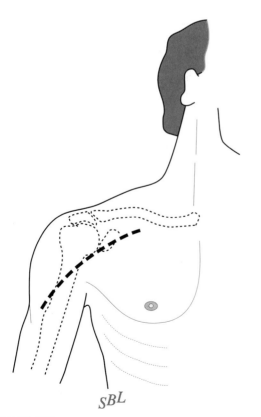

■ Figure 16–140

The skin incision for the extended deltopectoral approach uses the midclavicle, the tip of the coracoid process, and the deltoid tuberosity of the midhumerus as landmarks. *(Modified from Matsen FA III, Lippitt SB, Sidles JA, and Harryman DT II: Practical Evaluation and Management of the Shoulder. Philadelphia: WB Saunders, 1994.)*

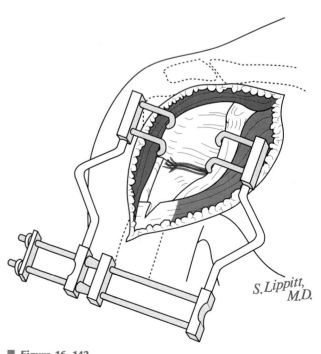

■ Figure 16–142

Self-retaining retractor below the conjoined tendon medially and the deltoid muscle laterally. *(From Pearl ML and Lippitt SB: Shoulder arthroplasty with a modular prosthesis. Tech Orthop 8:151-162, 1994. Original illustrator, S.B. Lippitt.)*

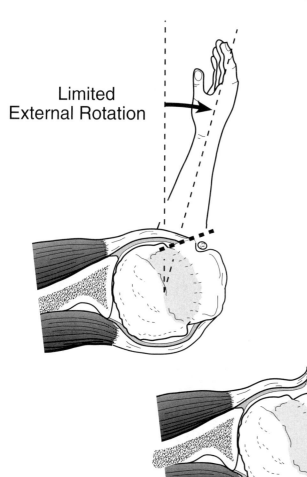

**Limited
External Rotation**

S. Lippitt,
M.D.

■ **Figure 16–143**
The subscapularis incision. The subscapularis and the subjacent
capsule are incised directly from the lesser tuberosity while
striving for maximal length of the tendon. *(Modified from Matsen
FA III, Lippitt SB, Sidles JA, and Harryman DT II: Practical Evaluation
and Management of the Shoulder. Philadelphia: WB Saunders, 1994.)*

**V16-13
V16-14**

subscapularis extends all the way to the bone rather than inserting as a tendon. A 360-degree release of the subscapularis tendon is then performed so that it moves freely with respect to the glenoid, the coracoid, the coracoid muscles, the axillary nerve, and the inferior capsule (see Figs. 16–129 and 16–130).

Humeral preparation is the next step in the arthroplasty. The humeral head is exposed anteriorly by *gentle* external rotation and slight extension. **(V16-13)** Special care is exercised in old patients and those with rheumatoid arthritis or other causes of fragile bone. Barriers to gentle external rotation may be an unreleased anterior capsule or posterior osteophytes (see Fig. 16–17).

The humeral osteotomy requires attention to detail. Although the degree of retroversion is often approximately 35 degrees, it may vary from 10 to 50 degrees. **(V16-14)** The ideal humeral cut is one that will allow positioning of the humeral prosthetic articular surface in the anatomic position. The cut plane must pass just inside the rotator cuff insertion to the tuberosity and resect the humeral articular surface without damaging the cuff insertion (Figs. 16–144 and 16–145). In degenerative joint disease, the apparent articular surface may not provide an accurate indication of the plane of humeral head resection. The angle of the cut with the humeral shaft must match that of the prosthesis being used—often about 45 degrees. The amount of humeral bone to be resected is compared for the different prosthetic options (see Fig. 16–2).

After the humeral osteotomy, the surgeon can get an idea of the joint volume remaining for the glenoid and humeral head components by pushing the humeral neck laterally with a finger. This step is helpful in determining the need for further soft tissue release. If the capsule is so tight that even the smallest head will not fit, more release is required (see Figs. 16–3 and 16–4). Cutting away more humerus is not an option because the humeral head has already been resected at the cuff insertion and further resection will jeopardize this essential attachment.

With the proximal end of the humerus displaced medially into the joint, the rotator cuff is palpated to establish its integrity. If a repairable defect through quality cuff tissue is identified, the retracted tendon is mobilized so that it will reach the tuberosity without undue tension when the arthroplasty components are in place and the arm is at the side (Fig. 16–146). However, two potential downsides of cuff repair in this circumstance are recognized: (1) in the presence of deficient tendon, cuff repair tightens the glenohumeral joint, and (2) cuff repair

V16-15

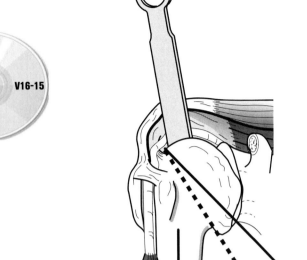

■ **Figure 16–144**
Humeral osteotomy planes. The preferred osteotomy plane starts just inside the insertion of the cuff to the greater tuberosity and proceeds medially at a 45-degree angle with respect to the long axis of the humeral shaft. If the osteotomy is incorrectly oriented such that it emerges at the margin of the osteophytes instead of the articular cartilage *(dotted line)*, the resulting cut will be in excessive varus. *(Modified from Matsen FA III, Lippitt SB, Sidles JA, and Harryman DT II: Practical Evaluation and Management of the Shoulder. Philadelphia: WB Saunders, 1994.)*

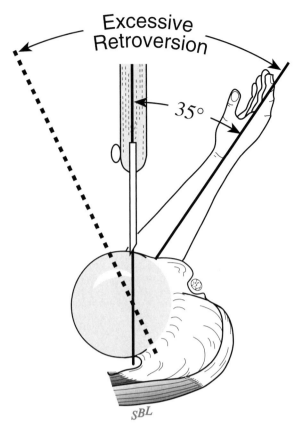

■ **Figure 16–145**
Humeral osteotomy planes. Humeral osteotomy also requires careful attention to version. An excessively retroverted cut *(dotted line)* will compromise the cuff insertion. *(Modified from Matsen FA III, Lippitt SB, Sidles JA, and Harryman DT II: Practical Evaluation and Management of the Shoulder. Philadelphia: WB Saunders, 1994.)*

changes the postoperative rehabilitation from active to passive motion until the tendon has healed.

The medullary canal of the humerus is reamed, beginning at a point lateral on the cut surface just behind the bicipital groove (Fig. 16–147). **(V16-15)** Starting with a small-diameter reamer, reaming is continued up to the diameter appropriate for the component. The reaming is performed in a slight valgus bias while protecting the biceps and cuff (Fig. 16–148). For prostheses that have press-fit stems, medullary reaming continues until a snug fit is achieved. This press-fit limits the degrees of freedom for placing the humeral component (see Fig. 16–139). If necessary, slots are made in the tuberosity to accommodate the fins and throat of the component (Fig. 16–149). The slot for the lateral fin should be just posterior to the bicipital groove. A trial component body is inserted so that the prosthetic neck is centered on the neck of the bony humerus. The trial component is used as a guide to excision of the osteophytes all around the humeral neck (see Fig. 16–18). Ideally, the horizontal and vertical distances between the tuberosity and the joint surface should be normalized (Fig. 16–150). It is particularly important that the superior aspect of the humeral articular surface

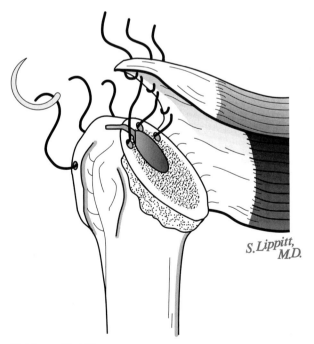

■ **Figure 16–146**
Repair of a rotator cuff tear. If tissue is of sufficient quantity and quality for a durable repair, drill holes are placed in the tuberosities for cuff attachment before insertion of the humeral component. *(Modified from Matsen FA III, Lippitt SB, Sidles JA, and Harryman DT II: Practical Evaluation and Management of the Shoulder. Philadelphia: WB Saunders, 1994.)*

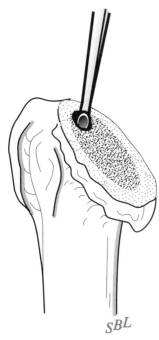

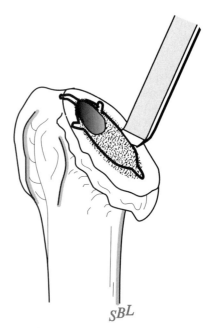

■ **Figure 16–147**
Making the pilot hole in the superior lateral cancellous surface just posterior to the bicipital groove to gain entrance to the humeral medullary canal. *(From Pearl ML and Lippitt SB: Shoulder arthroplasty with a modular prosthesis. Tech Orthop 8:151-162, 1994. Original illustrator, S.B. Lippitt.)*

■ **Figure 16–149**
A small curved osteotome is used to remove the cancellous bone outlined by the body-sizing osteotome. *(From Pearl ML and Lippitt SB: Shoulder arthroplasty with a modular prosthesis. Tech Orthop 8:151-162, 1994. Original illustrator, S.B. Lippitt.)*

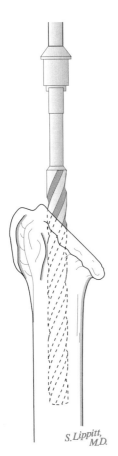

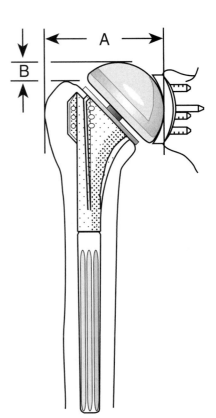

■ **Figure 16–148**
Reaming the humeral medullary canal. *(From Pearl ML and Lippitt SB: Shoulder arthroplasty with a modular prosthesis. Tech Orthop 8:151-162, 1994. Original illustrator, S.B. Lippitt.)*

■ **Figure 16–150**
The prosthesis in position, with reproduction of the normal tuberosity offset (A) and head height (B).

be no more than 5 mm above the top of the greater tuberosity.

By placing various trial humeral heads, the surgeon can select the size that allows 60 degrees of internal rotation of the abducted arm (the "scarecrow" test) and 15 mm of translation on the posterior drawer test (see Fig. 16–12). These two parameters are guides to the posterior capsular laxity usually necessary to achieve a satisfactory range of motion. A global periglenoid capsular release may be necessary to achieve this laxity (see Figs. 16–3 and 16–4). However, in degenerative joint disease, preoperative posterior subluxation usually obviates the need for posterior capsular release. An important interplay between position of the humeral component and capsular laxity is recognized (see Fig. 16–10).

PREPARATION OF THE GLENOID

Accurate preparation of the glenoid bone requires the excellent surgical exposure that results from excision of the humeral head and osteophytes and appropriate capsular release. (V16-16)

The goals of the glenoid part of the arthroplasty are (1) normalized glenoid orientation, (2) direct support of the component by precisely contoured bone, (3) secure fixation, and (4) avoidance of overstuffing (see Fig. 16–2).

Glenoid orientation is defined in terms of the glenoid centerline: the line perpendicular to the center of the normally oriented glenoid face. (V16-17) Shoulder arthroplasty surgeons should practice verifying the landmarks for a normal glenoid centerline by drilling holes perpendicular to the glenoid face of normal cadaveric scapulas and observing their exit in a consistent spot just medial to the anterior scapular neck: the "centering point" (see Fig. 16–25). This spot lies between the upper and lower crura of the body of the scapula as they approach the neck. After the capsular releases have been performed at surgery, this centering point can be palpated at the lateral extent of the subscapularis fossa. Because the location of this centering point is unaffected by arthritis, it is of great value in normalizing the orientation of a distorted glenoid face. It is particularly useful in correcting the increased retroversion of the glenoid face that commonly results from posterior erosion in degenerative joint disease.

An index finger identifies the centering point on the anterior scapular neck while a hole is drilled from the center of the glenoid face toward it (see Fig. 16–26). The orientation of the glenoid face is normalized by using a spherical reamer with a guiding peg inserted along the glenoid centerline drill hole (see Fig. 16–27). Appropriate positioning of retractors facilitates this reaming (Fig. 16–151). This technique is usually sufficient to manage posterior erosion; posterior glenoid bone grafting (Fig. 16–152) is rarely necessary. If there are reasons to not insert a glenoid component, this normalizing reaming provides an excellent nonprosthetic glenoplasty.

Once the reaming is completed, the glenoid centerline hole and the reamed glenoid surface can be used to precisely orient a drill guide for making additional fixation holes as required by the particular glenoid component design. Each hole is checked to determine whether it penetrates the scapula at its depth. Penetrating holes are cemented, but the cement is not pressurized.

A glenoid component is selected that covers the maximal amount of the prepared glenoid face with minimal overhang. The quality of the glenoid bone preparation is checked by inserting the glenoid trial component and ensuring that it does not rock even when the surgeon's finger applies an eccentric load to the rim.

After water spray irrigation, the holes are cleaned and dried with a spray of sterile CO_2 gas (Innovative Surgical Devices, Stillwater, MN 55082). A small amount of cement is injected into each of the holes with a large-tipped syringe. Holes that do not penetrate the scapula can be pressurized by the syringe. No cement is placed on the bony face of the glenoid; if the back of the glenoid component matches the prepared bony face, there is no advantage to an interposed layer of cement, which could fail and become displaced and consequently leave the glenoid component relatively unsupported. Contact between precisely contoured bone and polyethylene ("bone backing" as opposed to metal backing) provides an optimal load transfer mechanism (see Fig. 16–133). After the glenoid component is pressed into position, the absence of residual cement in the posterior of the shoulder is verified.

Insertion of the humeral body is the next step in the arthroplasty. Before insertion of the body, the surgeon places at least six No. 2 nonabsorbable sutures in secure bone at the anterior humeral neck for later attachment of the subscapularis tendon (Fig. 16–153). Final balancing of the soft tissues must be verified before the definitive humeral component is inserted. A shoulder arthroplasty with balanced soft tissues should allow (1) 60 degrees of internal rotation of the arm elevated in the coronal plane ("scarecrow" test), (2) 50% of posterior subluxation of the humeral head on the posterior drawer test, (3) 140 degrees of elevation, and (4) 40 degrees of external rotation of the adducted arm with the subscapularis approximated (see Fig. 16–12). (V16-18) A tighter shoulder will not only have limited range of motion but may also challenge the rotator cuff (see Fig. 16–40) and foster obligate translation at the extremes of motion with resultant rim loading, which risks glenoid loosening and component deformation (see Fig. 16–35). Some component systems are designed to allow a small amount of translation before rim loading occurs (see Figs. 16–36, 16–37, and 16–134).

The humeral component is then inserted into the prepared proximal end of the humerus. Height, version, and fixation are carefully checked. If sufficient stability of the prosthesis in the bone is not achieved with a press-fit,[263] autogenous cancellous graft harvested from the resected humeral head may be used. (V16-19) Selective placement of this graft can optimize the position as well as fixation of the component. Hacker and Matsen have shown that progressive impaction grafting can reduce the humeral void volume significantly.[44,169]

Before *closure,* the wound is thoroughly inspected for debris. The joint is put through a full range of motion to verify smoothness and lack of unwanted contact (e.g., between the medial aspect of the humerus and the inferior glenoid or the "Pooh Corner"). The wound is drained. The subscapularis is repaired securely to the humeral neck

V16-16 to V16-19

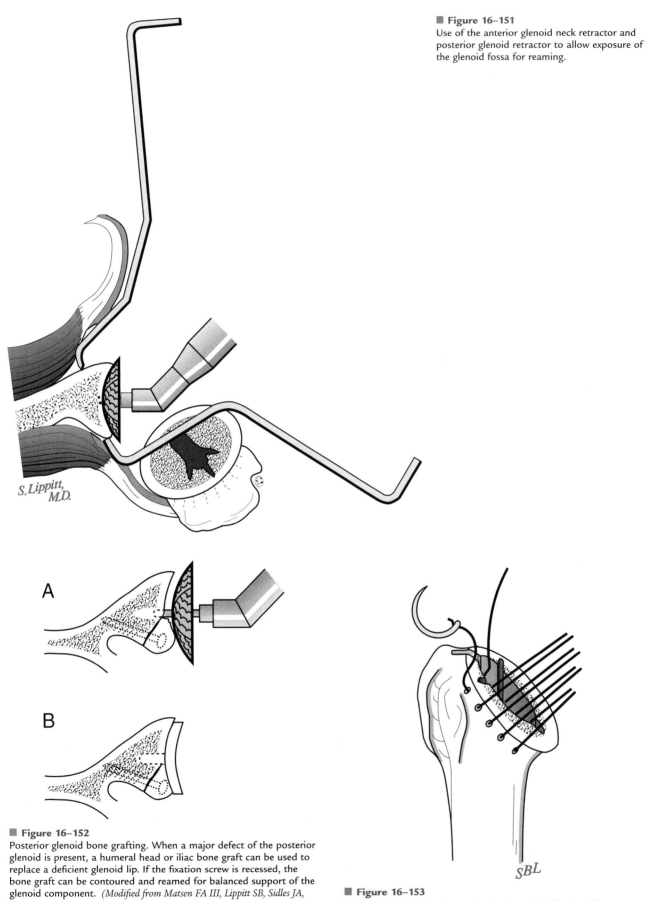

■ **Figure 16–151**
Use of the anterior glenoid neck retractor and posterior glenoid retractor to allow exposure of the glenoid fossa for reaming.

■ **Figure 16–152**
Posterior glenoid bone grafting. When a major defect of the posterior glenoid is present, a humeral head or iliac bone graft can be used to replace a deficient glenoid lip. If the fixation screw is recessed, the bone graft can be contoured and reamed for balanced support of the glenoid component. (*Modified from Matsen FA III, Lippitt SB, Sidles JA, and Harryman DT II: Practical Evaluation and Management of the Shoulder. Philadelphia: WB Saunders, 1994.*)

■ **Figure 16–153**
Placing sutures in the humeral neck through drill holes before insertion of the final humeral component.

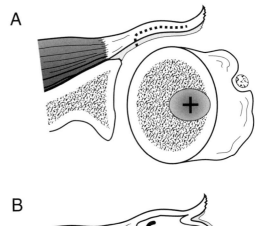

V16-20

■ **Figure 16–154**
Subscapularis tendon repair to drill holes in the anterior humeral neck medial to the lesser tuberosity. *(Modified from Matsen FA III, Lippitt SB, Sidles JA, and Harryman DT II: Practical Evaluation and Management of the Shoulder. Philadelphia: WB Saunders, 1994.)*

so that the adducted arm can be externally rotated by 40 degrees (Fig. 16-154). If additional subscapularis length is required, a "Z-plasty" can be performed (Fig. 16-155), although this technique compromises the strength of the tendon. The wound is closed in layers. Simple interrupted skin sutures are preferred when substantial drainage is anticipated or when wound healing may be impaired (e.g., in an individual taking corticosteroids or with thin rheumatoid skin). **(V16-20)**

Special Considerations

Degenerative Joint Disease

In this condition, the glenoid face is typically flattened and often eroded posteriorly as a result of chronic posterior subluxation (see Fig. 16–24). The glenoid may be distorted by peripheral osteophytes masking the location of the anatomic fossa. The humeral head may be flattened in a corresponding manner and effectively enlarged by the proliferation of "goat's beard" osteophytes from the anterior, inferior, and posterior articular rim. Intra-articular loose bodies may lie hidden in the subcoracoid or axillary recess. Anterior capsular and subscapularis contractures are common in degenerative joint disease and require release; however, posterior capsular release is not performed if posterior humeral subluxation is noted preoperatively.

Rheumatoid Arthritis

The basic principles of shoulder arthroplasty for rheumatoid arthritis are similar to those for degenerative

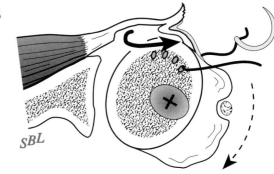

■ **Figure 16–155**
The inside-out Z-plasty. **A,** Additional length of the subscapularis tendon can be gained by splitting the capsule from the tendon medially and leaving their connection intact laterally. **B,** The medial end of the split capsule is reflected and attached to the humeral neck. *(Modified from Matsen FA III, Lippitt SB, Sidles JA, and Harryman DT II: Practical Evaluation and Management of the Shoulder. Philadelphia: WB Saunders, 1994.)*

arthritis, but some important differences exist. Rheumatoid tissue is much more fragile: the bone is more likely to fracture, and the muscle and tendons are more susceptible to tear. Thus, from the outset, extreme care must be taken to preserve bone and soft tissue integrity. We refer to these requirements for extraordinary gentleness as the "rheumatoid rules."

Because rheumatoid arthritis is an erosive and destructive disease, deficiencies of bone and the rotator cuff are more likely to occur than in degenerative joint disease. Thus, the soft tissues anteriorly may be insufficient to allow for lengthening of the subscapularis. The glenoid bone may be so eroded that insufficient stock is available to support a glenoid component. The rotator cuff may be partially or totally deficient. Thus, in the preoperative evaluation and in discussion with the patient concerning the possible outcomes of surgery, all these factors need to be considered.

The standard preoperative scapular anteroposterior and axillary radiographs are required to evaluate the humeral and glenoid bone stock. In rheumatoid arthritis, the glenoid erosion is usually medial (rather than posterior as in degenerative joint disease). For this reason, only minimal glenoid reaming may be necessary to achieve an excellent-quality fit to the back of the glenoid component. The potential fragility of the bone and soft tissues makes it particularly important that the joint not be overstuffed and that adequate soft tissue laxity be present for immediate postoperative motion. This is a particular challenge in diminutive patients with juvenile rheumatoid arthritis; such patients may also have a tiny humeral medullary canal. In addition, some patients may have insufficient joint volume to permit the insertion of a glenoid component despite complete soft tissue release.

Secondary Degenerative Joint Disease

In post-traumatic arthritis, the challenges may be even greater. The anatomy is likely to be distorted by previous fracture or surgery. The nonarticular humeroscapular motion interface is likely to be scarred, with important neurologic structures such as the axillary nerve being obscured. The tuberosities, the humeral shaft, and the glenoid may be ununited or malunited.

As a first step, the motion interface must be carefully freed, and the axillary nerve is identified both as it crosses the subscapularis and as it courses laterally on the deep surface of the deltoid. Case-by-case judgments must be made concerning the need for osteotomy in an attempt to restore more normal anatomic relationships while recognizing that additional healing and postoperative protection may be required. Again, the goal is restoration of anatomic relationships, firm fixation of components, soft tissue balance, stability, and smooth gliding in the humeroscapular motion interface.

Capsulorrhaphy Arthropathy

Shoulders affected by capsulorrhaphy arthropathy present additional challenges, such as neurovascular scarring from previous surgery, soft tissue contractures, bone deficiencies, implants from previous surgery, changes in glenoid version, and an increased potential for glenohumeral instability after the arthroplasty (see Fig. 16-8). Careful assessment of the preoperative axillary lateral film may alert the surgeon to the excessive posterior capsular laxity that results from chronic posterior humeral subluxation after anterior stabilization procedures. Such laxity may predispose the reconstructed shoulder to posterior instability. Thorough release of the subscapularis tendon is necessary to prevent obligate posterior translation from residual tight anterior structures. Excessive anterior soft tissue tension in combination with a lax posterior capsule may disrupt the normal balance of forces that keep the humeral head centered in the glenoid and result in rim loading of the posterior glenoid. Such loading renders the glenoid prosthesis susceptible to posterior wear and loosening. In addition, patients with capsulorrhaphy arthropathy are typically younger than those with primary degenerative or inflammatory arthritis conditions, and this factor must be weighed during consideration of the type of reconstruction planned.

Cuff Tear Arthropathy

This condition presents several unique challenges for regaining glenohumeral smoothness. The humeral head is subluxated in a superior position so that it articulates with the coracoacromial arch. The rotator cuff is almost never amenable to a strong repair, and the glenoid is eroded superiorly so that an acetabular-like structure is formed in continuity with the coracoacromial arch. Under these circumstances, normal glenohumeral relationships are very difficult to normalize and maintain by a durable cuff reconstruction. More often it is preferable to accept an altered joint relationship that adopts the "acetabulum" for secondary stability in the absence of primary stability from the rotator cuff. In this "special hemiarthroplasty," the articular surface of the proximal end of the humerus is resurfaced with a component matching the preoperative size and position of the humeral joint surface. The tuberosities are smoothed so that they are congruous with the humeral articular surface. Such smoothing allows for the proximal humeral convexity to match the "acetabulum" and to articulate smoothly within it. It is very important to avoid using "oversized" humeral components because they overstuff the joint, do not match the concavity of the "acetabulum," and restrict joint motion. In a special hemiarthroplasty, the patient is spared the necessity of protecting a rotator cuff repair, so immediate passive and active exercises can be instituted after surgery. The patient is also spared the risk of glenoid loosening from the rocking horse mechanism (see Fig. 16-35).

The ideal patient for this procedure has a normal deltoid muscle, a concentric coracoacromial "acetabulum" stabilizing the proximal end of the humerus (which is superiorly displaced with respect to the glenoid), concentric erosion of the upper glenoid fossa, a "femoralized" upper humerus with rounding off of the greater tuberosity, an irreparable rotator cuff defect, no previous surgical compromise of the acromion or coracoacromial ligament, favorable motivation, and realistic expectations.

In a series of 10 patients who underwent special hemiarthroplasty for rotator cuff tear arthropathy, the range of active motion and function were substantially

TABLE 16–20. Increment in Function after Special Hemiarthroplasty for Cuff Tear Arthropathy

	Preoperative	Postoperative
Active elevation	71° (range, 50–100)	115° (range, 50–160)
External rotation	30°	41°
Internal rotation	L5	L1
Perineal care	2/10 patients	9/10 patients
Reach opposite axilla	3/10 patients	10/10 patients
Comb hair	2/10 patients	8/10 patients
Sleep on side	2/10 patients	9/10 patients
Use above shoulder level	0/10 patients	6/10 patients

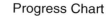

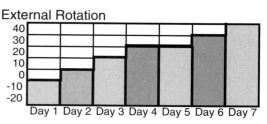

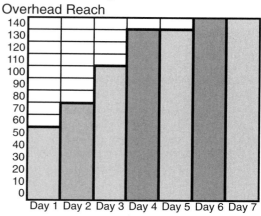

■ **Figure 16–156**

Typical wall charts showing the improvement in overhead reach and external rotation after surgery. *(From Matsen FA III, Lippitt SB, Sidles JA, and Harryman DT II: Practical Evaluation and Management of the Shoulder. Philadelphia: WB Saunders, 1994.)*

improved by this procedure (Table 16–20). These results are not as good as those for total glenohumeral arthroplasty because the patient lacks the benefit of both prosthetic glenoid smoothness and function of the rotator cuff.

Postoperative Rehabilitation

Rehabilitation is started immediately after surgery in the recovery room with the initiation of slow and gentle continuous passive motion (see Fig. 16–132).

For patients who have had an interscalene block before surgery, this early motion is pain free. Continuous passive motion should be stopped and the wrist brace removed every 2 to 3 hours for approximately 15 to 20 minutes to relieve any skin and nerve compression. A sling is worn between exercise sessions until active muscle control is regained.

The patient-conducted rehabilitation program is started on the day of surgery under instructions given by the surgeon or therapist. Although the program may vary with the details of the surgery performed, the following is a description of the basic program for shoulder arthroplasty. The stretching exercises include (1) elevation, (2) external rotation limited to 40 degrees, (3) internal rotation, (4) cross-body adduction, (5) grip strengthening, (6) elbow range of motion, (7) external rotator isometrics, and (8) anterior, middle, and posterior deltoid isometrics. The patient is instructed to perform a total of five exercise sessions spread evenly throughout the day both while in the hospital and at home after discharge.*

Charts are placed on the wall in full view of the patient's bed to graph the progress of elevation and external rotation (Fig. 16–156) as measured by the surgeon or therapist. Such charts provide positive feedback for rehabilitative progress.

For routine arthroplasty, the range-of-motion goals to be achieved before discharge are 140 degrees of elevation, 40 degrees of external rotation, and functional internal rotation and cross-body adduction. These goals may be modified according to the specific surgical procedure. Because the desired range has been achieved on the operating table, the patient's task is simplified: this range has to be maintained only during the postoperative period.

Elevation (overhead reach) is performed in the supine position (lying flat on the back) by grasping the wrist or elbow of the operative shoulder with the hand of the unoperated arm, pulling up toward the ceiling, and reaching overhead as high as possible to the goal of 140 degrees with the arm relaxed (see Fig. 16–75). A pulley or the forward lean (see Fig. 16–76) may also be useful in achieving elevation, especially if the opposite shoulder is involved in the arthritic process.

External rotation (rotation away from the body) is performed in the supine position (see Fig. 16–77) with the elbow on the operative side held against or close to the side of the body and flexed to 90 degrees. A stick is held in both hands so that the unaffected extremity pushes on the operative arm to externally rotate it to the goal of 40 degrees. Holding onto a door and turning away is another useful way to stretch external rotation (see Fig. 16–78).

Internal rotation is performed by grasping the wrist of the relaxed involved arm with the hand on the nonoperative side; the hands are lifted up the back as high as possible. A towel can also be used to assist with pulling the involved arm into internal rotation behind the back (see Fig. 16–79).

Cross-body adduction is performed while sitting or standing by grasping the elbow of the involved arm with the other hand. The involved arm is relaxed and the elbow is extended and pulled across the body until stretch is felt (see Fig. 16–80).

Active elbow motion is performed while standing to allow unimpeded or unrestricted flexion/extension and

---

*For example, if tuberosity or cuff fixation has been part of the procedure, external rotation isometrics and active elevation may be delayed.

supination/pronation. Grip strengthening is performed to maintain forearm tone and can be accomplished with a foam pad or tennis ball.

External rotator isometrics are performed with the forearm in neutral rotation. An attempt is made to move the wrist out to the side against the resistance of the other hand or a fixed object (see Fig. 16–82). Deltoid isometrics are also performed while standing or sitting. The arm is held in a neutral position and pushed forward, to the side, and to the back to exercise the anterior, middle, and posterior deltoids, respectively.

Supine presses are performed initially by holding a cloth or stick between both hands with the hands held close together (Fig. 16–157). From a starting position with the elbows bent and the hands lying across the chest, the stick is pushed straight to the ceiling with both hands in a slow and controlled manner and then slowly lowered back to the resting position at the chest. The space

between the two hands is progressively increased. As the shoulder becomes stronger, the hands are pushed to the ceiling in a slow and controlled manner independent of each other. With increasing strength, the exercise is conducted with a 1-lb weight that is held in the involved hand as it is pressed to the ceiling. When the patient is comfortable, the incline is gradually increased to eventually reach the upright position. All presses should be performed in a slow and controlled manner; the patient should progress to the next level only when 20 repetitions can be performed comfortably.

The patient is instructed in all these exercises on three occasions: (1) before surgery, (2) immediately after surgery, and (3) before leaving the hospital. Before discharge, the goals of assisted external rotation to 40 degrees and assisted elevation to 140 degrees must be accomplished.

Patients are placed in charge of their own rehabilitation and taught to progressively return to normal use of

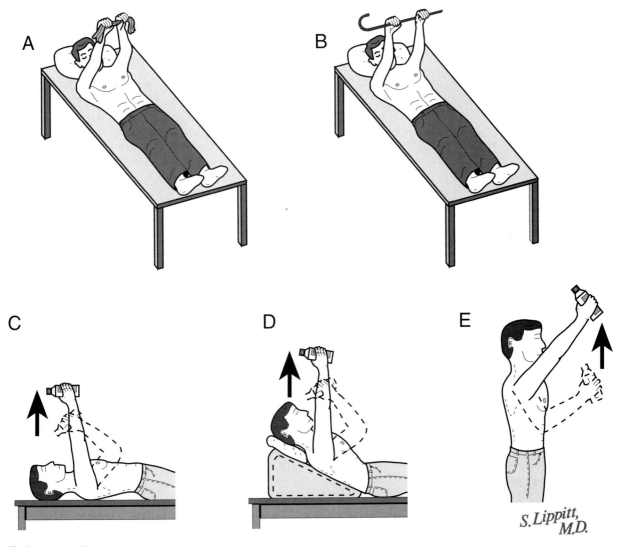

■ **Figure 16–157**
Progressive supine press exercises to strengthen flexion. The motion is always pushing up toward the ceiling and ends by lifting the shoulder blade off the bed. **A,** Start with two hands together holding a wash cloth; **B,** then two hands apart; **C,** then one hand with a 1-pint (i.e., 1-lb) weight; **D,** then one hand with a 1-pint weight with greater degrees of sitting up; and finally, **E,** one hand with a 1-pint weight while standing. *(Modified from Matsen FA III, Lippitt SB, Sidles JA, and Harryman DT II: Practical Evaluation and Management of the Shoulder. Philadelphia: WB Saunders, 1994.)*

the shoulder. Typically, keyboarding and driving are achieved at 2 weeks, swimming is initiated at 6 weeks, golf or tennis is started at 3 to 6 months, and chopping wood is precluded.

■ ROCKWOOD'S PREFERRED TECHNIQUE FOR SHOULDER ARTHROPLASTY

Although a number of surgical approaches for performing arthroplasty of the shoulder have been described, most procedures are performed through an anterior approach to the joint. The anterior, long deltopectoral approach without detaching the origin of the deltoid as described by Neer[303,304,353] is currently our preferred approach for shoulder arthroplasty. Two important principles of this approach are preservation of the anterior attachment of the deltoid to the clavicle and the acromion and protection of the axillary and musculocutaneous nerves.

The anterior portion of the deltoid must be preserved because no muscle can effectively compensate for loss of this powerful shoulder flexor.[66] Weakness of the posterior portion of the deltoid is less disabling because the latissimus dorsi is a strong synergistic muscle. Detachment of the anterior deltoid is problematic because secure reattachment of this muscle after shoulder arthroplasty is difficult and impairs postoperative rehabilitation for the patient.[95] Patients with a detached or denervated anterior deltoid after shoulder arthroplasty have a poor outcome in that they have limited motion and decreased strength, and they are extremely dissatisfied with the procedure.[164,436]

The relationship of the axillary and musculocutaneous nerves must always be of concern to the surgeon. Although positioning the arm in adduction and external rotation may make anterior approaches to the glenohumeral joint safer,[61,298,303,436] it is much better to identify the nerves and protect them during the entire surgical procedure. Burkhead and associates[64,66] have described in detail the tremendous variation in the course and position of these nerves from one specimen to another. Laceration of the axillary nerve denervates the entire deltoid muscle. Because all important shoulder function requires elevation in the scapular plane, injury to the axillary nerve is the most catastrophic neurogenic injury that can occur during shoulder arthroplasty. Disastrous consequences await surgeons who embark on a shoulder arthroplasty without exact knowledge of the location of the axillary nerve and fail to protect it.[164]

ANATOMIC LANDMARKS

Three anterior prominences—the clavicle, acromion, and coracoid—are excellent guides to placement of the incision and are intimately related to important structures when developing the exposure. The clavicle is just superior to the upper portion of the deltopectoral groove. Its position is readily palpable and marks the most superior aspect of the incision.

The acromion serves as a large surface area for attachment of the deltoid, and this large surface area increases the muscle's efficiency. If wide reflection of the deltoid becomes necessary, the deltoid should never be released from the acromion during arthroplasty; rather, the partial deltoid insertion can be released.[90,298,303] The interval between the acromion and the coracoid process is spanned by the tough, wide coracoacromial ligament. It is rarely necessary to divide or resect this ligament because it serves as a buttress to anterior displacement of the humeral head.

The coracoid serves as a "lighthouse" to the deltopectoral interval.[303] It lies within the deltopectoral groove, and palpation of it is a landmark for the position of the cephalic vein and the brachial plexus. The cephalic vein is intimately attached to the deltoid and directly overlies the coracoid. The brachial plexus and its terminal divisions lie medial to the base of the coracoid.

NERVES

The axillary nerve is one of the two terminal branches of the posterior cord of the brachial plexus. It arises posterior to the coracoid process and crosses the anteroinferior border and then the lateral border of the subscapularis muscle. At this point the nerve joins the posterior humeral circumflex artery, and together they exit posteriorly through the quadrangular space where the axillary nerve sends two branches to supply the capsule. The axillary nerve then splits into two major trunks. The posterior trunk gives off branches to the teres minor and posterior deltoid and terminates as the superior lateral cutaneous nerve. The anterior trunk passes forward around the humerus and supplies first the middle deltoid and then the anterior deltoid.[64,66,244]

The musculocutaneous nerve originates from the lateral cord of the brachial plexus and innervates the coracobrachialis muscle, as well as the biceps brachii and brachialis muscles. The coracobrachialis muscle is occasionally innervated directly from the lateral cord of the brachial plexus. Flatow and associates[136] noted that the lateral portion of the musculocutaneous nerve penetrates into the coracobrachialis muscle at a distance of 3.1 to 8.2 cm from the tip of the coracoid. However, we have seen cases in which the nerve comes from under the coracoid to then penetrate the conjoined tendon from the lateral side. The most common cause of damage to this nerve during shoulder arthroplasty is overzealous retraction. We prefer to not detach the conjoined tendons because they protect the neurovascular bundle during medial retraction of the pectoralis major muscle. Powerful retraction on the conjoined tendons, which are made up of the short head of the biceps and the coracobrachialis, may produce a traction injury to the musculocutaneous nerve. Careful attention to retraction should minimize this possibility.

SURGICAL APPROACH

Neer and associates[303,304,353] described the development of the currently preferred anterior deltopectoral surgical approach. Initially, a short deltopectoral approach with detachment of the anterior portion of the deltoid from the clavicle was used; however, this technique weakened the muscle and delayed postoperative rehabilitation. In 1976 and 1977, Neer used a superior approach with detachment of the middle section of the deltoid; however, this approach was found to weaken the middle part of the deltoid. In September 1977, Neer began to exclusively use the long deltopectoral approach, which has become the standard for shoulder arthroplasty because of greater ease of rehabilitation after surgery and is the technique described here.[298]

In 1977, the author (C.A.R.) recalls chatting with Neer about his approach, and it seemed incredible because I had trouble performing the arthroplasty procedure after detaching the majority of the anterior deltoid. I had to visit him and observe his technique before I could use it on my patients.

SURGICAL TECHNIQUE

The patient is positioned on the operating room table in the semi-Fowler position with the knees flexed to avoid

dependency (Fig. 16–158A). **(V16-21, 16-22)** The standard headrest from the operating table is removed and replaced with the McConnell headrest (McConnell Orthopaedic Equipment Co., Greenville, TX). This headrest allows the patient to be positioned at the top and edge of the table (see Fig. 16–158B and C), which is necessary to be able to extend the externally rotated arm off the side of the table down toward the floor and enable the surgeon to ream the intramedullary canal and insert the prosthesis. The patient's head should be secured to the headrest with tape, and tape can be used to secure the anesthesia tube to the headrest. Care should be taken to rest the head in a position that avoids hyperextension or tilting of the neck, which may cause compression of the cervical roots. We have found it best to position the table in the proper semi-Fowler position before securing the head to the headrest.

Plastic towel drapes are used to block out the area being prepared and to isolate the hair and anesthesia

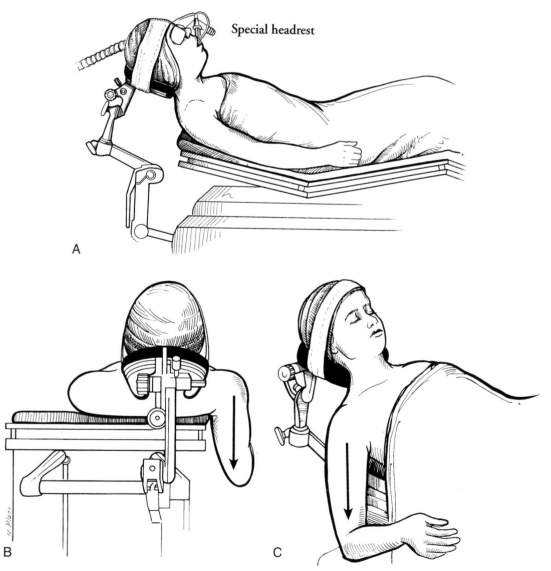

Special headrest

A

B

C

■ **Figure 16–158**
A, Proper positioning of the patient on the operating room table with the head supported by a McConnell headrest (**B**). **C**, The patient is on the top outer corner of the table so that the arm can be extended off the table down toward the floor.

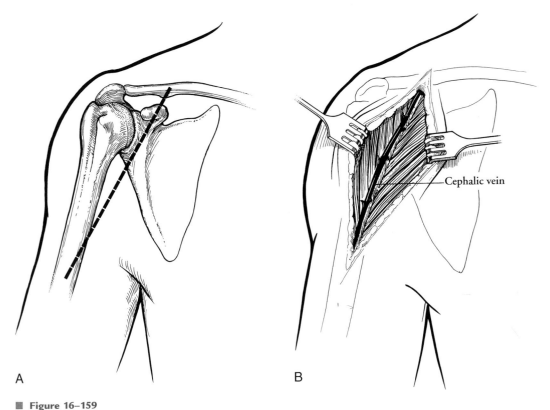

■ **Figure 16–159**

A, Placement of the surgical incision from the clavicle across the top of the coracoid down to the anterior aspect of the arm. **B,** The cephalic vein should be preserved and placed laterally with the deltoid muscle.

equipment from the operative field. The entire upper extremity is prepared, and the arm is draped free. The axilla is separated as much as possible from the sterile surgical field. After the skin incision is marked, the surgical site is covered with sterile adherent plastic drapes. A special shoulder drape pack is available that includes towel drapes, body drapes, gowns, gloves, and a marking pen (Shoulder Drape Pack, DePuy Co., Warsaw, IN). The skin incision is made in a straight line with the arm held in 30 degrees of abduction (Fig. 16–159A). The incision should begin from the superior aspect of the clavicle and then proceed over the top of the coracoid; the incision should extend down the anterior aspect of the arm. Once the incision has been made, the cephalic vein near the deltopectoral interval should be identified (see Fig. 16–159B) and protected because postoperative swelling and pain in the extremity will be decreased by preservation of this vein. The vein is usually intimately associated with the deltoid because of the many feeding vessels from the deltoid into the cephalic vein. It is for this reason that we recommend that the cephalic vein be taken laterally with the deltoid muscle. The feeding vessels coming into the vein from the region of the pectoralis major muscle should be clamped and tied to allow lateral retraction of the deltoid muscle with the vein. The deep surface of the deltoid is then freed from the underlying tissues by using a combination of blunt and sharp dissection all the way from its origin on the clavicle down to its insertion onto the humeral shaft. On occasion, as recommended by Neer, it may be necessary to partially free the insertion of the deltoid from the humeral shaft.

When the deep surface of the deltoid has been completely freed, abduct and externally rotate the arm. Protect the exposed surface of the deltoid with a moist laparotomy sponge, and retract the deltoid laterally with two Richardson retractors. We routinely use moist lap sponges during the procedure because they seem to be easier on the soft tissue. Next, retract the conjoined tendon medially with a Richardson retractor. It is rarely necessary to release a portion of the conjoined tendon or divide the coracoid process for additional exposure. The tendon of the upper portion of the pectoralis major is identified, and the upper portion of the tendon is released with an electrocautery cutting blade to aid in exposure of the inferior aspect of the joint (Fig. 16–160). Care must be taken to avoid injury to the long head of the biceps tendon during this maneuver. If the patient has a marked internal rotation contracture (i.e., −30 degrees or more), the entire pectoralis major tendon can be released from its insertion. This tendon release should not be repaired at the completion of the operation. The anterior humeral circumflex vessels are then identified on the lower third of the subscapularis tendon. The vessels are isolated, clamped, and ligated (Fig. 16–161). Because of the extensive anastomoses of blood supply in this area, other sources of bleeding should be expected and controlled with electrocautery during release of the subscapularis tendon.

It is now important to identify the musculocutaneous and axillary nerves. Palpate the musculocutaneous nerve as it comes from the brachial plexus into the medial aspect of the conjoined tendon (Fig. 16–162A). The nerve usually

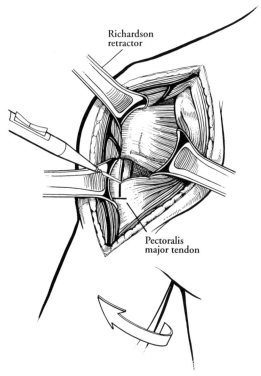

■ Figure 16–160
The deltoid and pectoralis major tendons are retracted and the upper portion of the pectoralis major tendon should be released. Care should be taken to not injure the underlying long head of the biceps tendon.

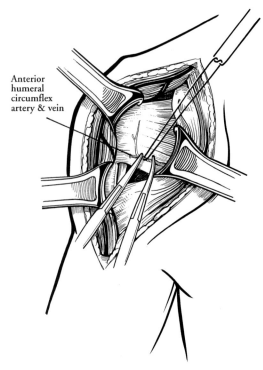

■ Figure 16–161
The anterior humeral circumflex vessels, which lie on the inferior portion of the subscapularis tendon, should be isolated and coagulated or ligated.

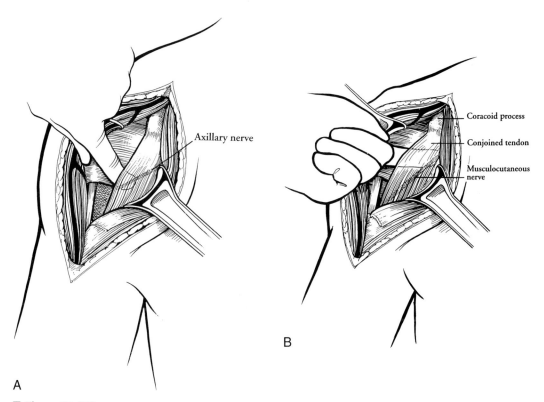

■ Figure 16–162
A and **B,** Identification of the musculocutaneous and axillary nerves.

penetrates the muscle about 4 to 5 cm inferior to the tip of the coracoid; however, as previously mentioned, the nerve may have a higher penetration into the conjoined muscle-tendon unit. The proximity of this nerve must be kept in mind during retraction of the conjoined tendon. The axillary nerve is then located by passing the volar surface of the index finger down along the anterior surface of the subscapularis muscle (see Fig. 16–162B). As the hand and wrist are supinated, the finger is rotated and hooked anteriorly to identify the axillary nerve (see Fig. 16–162A). Scarring and adhesions may result in the nerve being plastered onto the anterior surface of the subscapularis so that identification of the nerve is difficult. When this problem occurs, an elevator should be passed along the anterior surface of the subscapularis muscle to create an interval between the muscle and the nerve. Always identify the axillary nerve and carefully retract and hold it out of the way, especially during the critical steps of releasing and resecting the anteroinferior capsule. We have found that a Scoffield type of retractor works well to protect the axillary nerve.

The amount of passive external rotation present at this point in the procedure determines the specific technique for subscapularis tendon release. We currently release the tendon from its insertion into the lesser tuberosity, just medial to the long head of the biceps tendon (Fig. 16–163A). When a good stump of the subscapularis tendon has been freed up, heavy nonabsorbable 1-mm Dacron tape should be secured to the tendon with two or three "W" stitches or modified Kessler stitches. These sutures can then be used as traction sutures when freeing up the rest of the tendon from the underlying capsule and scar tissue. At the time of closure, the tendon is repaired back to the cut surface of the humerus with these sutures (see Fig. 16–163B). Release of the tendon from the lesser tuberosity and repair back to the cut surface of the neck of the humerus allow greater excursion of external rotation. If the patient's shoulder has marked limitation of external rotation, lengthen the tendon with a coronal Z-plasty technique (see Fig. 16–163C and D). Each centimeter of tendon lengthened will equal approximately 20 degrees of additional external rotation. When the coronal Z-plasty procedure is performed, include the capsule on the lateral stump of the tendon for additional strength. At the time of closure, the subscapularis tendon should be repaired with heavy nonabsorbable 1-mm surgical tape.

After the subscapularis tendon has been released, it must be completely freed up from the capsule and the anterior glenoid rim so that it once again becomes a dynamic muscle-tendon unit. This process requires that the subscapularis muscle-tendon unit be released 360 degrees around its circumference. Such release usually entails a fair amount of soft tissue dissection along the anterior aspect of the neck of the scapula. During this dissection, it is imperative to identify, protect, and retract the axillary nerve with a Scoffield-type retractor. It is important to have a free, dynamic, and functioning subscapularis muscle-tendon unit at the time of its repair.

On occasion, the capsule will be released at the time of subscapularis release. In this situation, the anterior capsule must be resected from the posterior surface of the subscapularis so that a free, dynamic subscapularis tendon can be achieved. If the capsule is just released from the glenoid and left in place, it will later scar back to the humerus and glenoid and once again limit external rotation. The anteroinferior capsule must then be released from the humerus all the way inferiorly to at least the 6

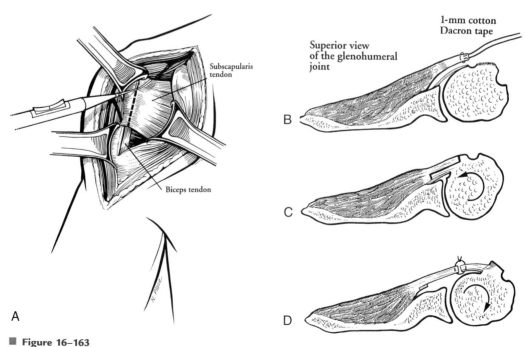

■ **Figure 16–163**

A, The subscapularis tendon should be released from its insertion into the lesser tuberosity. **B–D,** When the patient has –20 degrees or less of external rotation, the subscapularis tendon and capsule should be lengthened with a coronal Z-plasty technique.

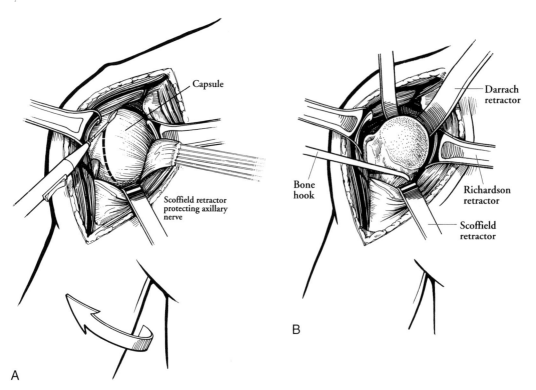

■ **Figure 16–164**
A, The capsule should be released from the neck of the humerus from the top to the bottom. Failure to release the capsule all the way inferiorly will lead to difficulty in displacing the head of the humerus up and out of the glenoid fossa. **B,** With Darrach retractors in the shoulder as a skid, a bone hook can be used to lift the head of the humerus out of the glenoid fossa while the arm is externally rotated and extended off the edge of the table.

o'clock position, even in the presence of a large inferior osteophyte (Fig. 16–164A). Failure to release the inferior capsule will make it very difficult to deliver the head up and out of the glenoid fossa. Later, the entire anteroinferior portion of the capsule will be released from the glenoid and discarded. Once the capsule has been released inferiorly, pass a small bone hook around and under the neck of the humerus. With a large Darrach retractor in the joint and a bone hook around the neck of the humerus, the arm is externally rotated, adducted, and extended off the edge of the table to deliver the head up and out of the glenoid fossa (see Fig. 16–164B). If the humeral head cannot be delivered in this fashion, the inferior capsule is probably still intact and must be further released. It is important to obtain this exposure with the arm extended off the side of the table in external rotation before proceeding with resection of the humeral head.

Technique for Nonconstrained Shoulder Arthroplasty*

Resection of the Humeral Head

Resection of the humeral head is a critical part of the procedure. When posterior glenoid erosion has not occurred, as determined by CT, the humeral head should be removed with the arm in 20 to 25 degrees of external rota-

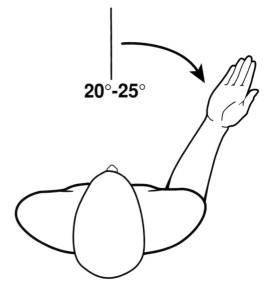

■ **Figure 16–165**
Before resection of the humeral head, the arm should be held parallel to the floor and externally rotated 20 to 25 degrees.

tion. This technique can be accomplished by flexing the elbow 90 degrees and then externally rotating the arm 20 to 25 degrees (Fig. 16–165). The varus-valgus angle of the head to be removed is determined with a humeral osteotomy template (Fig. 16–166A). **(V16-23)** Place the template along the anterior aspect of the arm parallel to the

---

*The surgical technique used in this chapter is adapted from the 1994 manual of DePuy, Inc., titled *Global Shoulder Arthroplasty System.*[352]

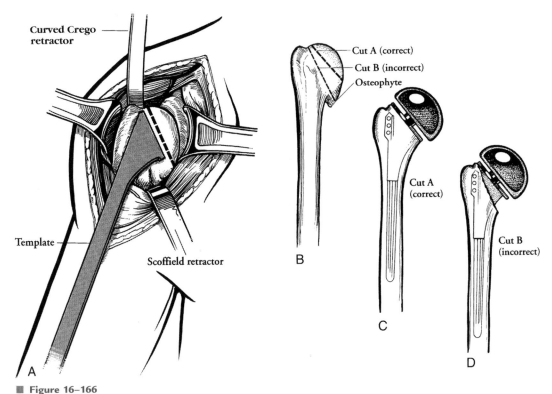

■ Figure 16–166
A, The template should be used to determine the proper angle of head resection. **B–D,** Failure to use the template when removing the head would lead to insufficient bone to support the neck of the prosthesis.

shaft of the humerus, and mark the angle at which the head will be removed with an electrocautery blade. The superolateral portion of the mark should be at the sulcus on the top of the shoulder (i.e., at the junction of the articular surface and the attachment of the rotator cuff on the greater tuberosity). In most cases, the inferior portion of the mark will be medial to the inferior osteophyte of the flattened and deformed humeral head (see Fig. 16–166B). Use of the osteotomy template will ensure that the prosthesis sits properly on the supporting medial neck of the humerus. If the resection is in too much of a varus position, support for the collar of the prosthesis will be compromised (see Fig. 16–166C and D).

If a preoperative axillary CT scan has shown posterior glenoid erosion, several options are available to the surgeon: removal of the anterior half of the glenoid with an air bur and glenoid reamer, placement of a bone graft on the posterior glenoid, or resection of the humeral head with the arm in less than 20 to 25 degrees of external rotation. For example, in shoulders with 10 degrees of posterior glenoid erosion, the head should be resected with the arm externally rotated only 10 to 15 degrees. With more than 25 degrees of posterior glenoid erosion, we generally use the air bur and special glenoid reamer to remove some of the anterior glenoid.

Before the oscillating saw is used to remove the head, the biceps tendon and insertions of the supraspinatus, infraspinatus, and teres minor into the proximal part of the humerus must be protected. Pass the large curved modified Crego retractor under the biceps, and curl it around to protect these structures during resection of the humeral head (Fig. 16–167). With the Darrach retractors

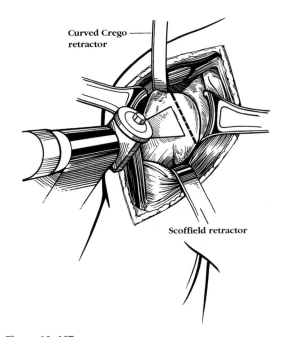

■ Figure 16–167
A modified Crego retractor should be passed under the biceps tendon and then curl around the back of the neck of the humerus to prevent the biceps and rotator cuff from being divided during removal of the head with an oscillating saw.

in the joint, a sagittal power saw is then used to remove the humeral head at the predetermined angle. During removal of the head, the arm must be parallel to the floor and the saw must be perpendicular to the floor.

Once the humeral head has been removed and with the Darrach retractors acting as a skid, use a bone hook in combination with extension and external rotation of the arm off the side of the table to deliver the cancellous bone surface of the proximal end of the humerus up and out of the incision (Fig. 16–168). Once again, positioning of the patient on the operating room table is extremely important because it is exceedingly difficult to insert the medullary canal reamers, as well as the prosthesis, unless the arm can be extended off the side of the table (see Fig. 16–158B and C). A 6-mm medullary canal reamer is used to make the pilot hole in the superolateral cancellous surface of the humerus. In this way, the reamer will pass directly down the intramedullary canal (Fig. 16–169A and B). The humeral reamer is inserted down the humerus until the top flute pattern is at the level of the cut surface of the bone. Once the initial reamer is seated, proceed with the 8-, 10-, and 12-mm reamers until one of the reamers begins to bite on the cortical bone of the intramedullary canal. The final reamer size that bites into the cortex will determine the stem size of the body-sizing osteotome and the implant. The reaming is done by hand and should not be performed with motorized equipment. Caution should be used to *not* over-ream the canal. Remember that the arm is being supported in external rotation and the reaming is being performed in an internal rotation direction. Over-reaming puts torque on the humerus and could create a stress riser or fracture. A body-sizing osteotome matching the size of the final reamer is selected; that is, if a 12-mm reamer was used, a 12-mm body-sizing osteotome and 12-mm intramedullary rod would be selected. The rod is then threaded into the osteotome body and inserted down the intramedullary

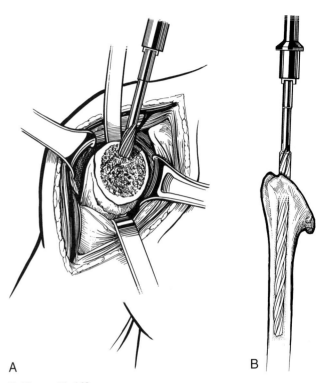

Figure 16–169
A, Initially, the 6-mm intramedullary reamer is placed eccentrically and as superior as possible into the proximal part of the humerus. B, Progressively larger reamers are used until the reamer begins to obtain purchase in cortical bone.

canal (Fig. 16–170A). Placing the rod down into the reamed canal prevents the sizing osteotome from drifting into a varus position. The collar on the body-sizing osteotome is used to determine proper rotation before cutting the bone. When the lateral fin of the osteotome touches the greater tuberosity, slide the collar down the osteotome until it touches cancellous bone. Then rotate the body-sizing osteotome until the collar lies flat on the cut bone surface. The body-sizing osteotome is tapped a few times with a mallet to drive the osteotome down into cancellous bone. Driving the body-sizing osteotome down into cancellous bone identifies the appropriate amount of bone to be removed to receive the body broach and creates the anterior, posterior, and inferior fin tracks. Before inserting the body broach, the cancellous bone can be removed with a small osteotome (see Fig. 16–170B).

Broaching with the trial body is an important step in the procedure. If a 12-mm reamer and 12-mm body-sizing osteotome have been used, a 12-mm broach should be used. With the broach locked into place (Fig. 16–171) in the driver-extractor tool, the fin tracks of the broach should be carefully lined up with the fin tracks previously established with the body-sizing osteotome. The broach should be carefully driven into place while being sure to maintain proper version of the broach by following the previously cut fin tracks. If the proximal part of the humerus is large in proportion to the intramedullary canal, a mismatched humeral body-stem combination is available. If the intramedullary canal was reamed to 12 mm and the proximal part of the humerus is quite large,

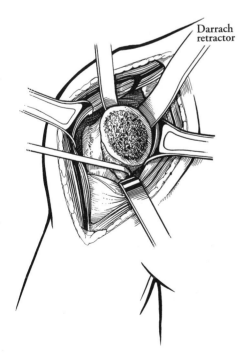

Figure 16–168
A Darrach retractor in the glenoid humeral joint will act as a skid. A bone hook can again be used to deliver the cut surface of the proximal end of the humerus up and out of the wound.

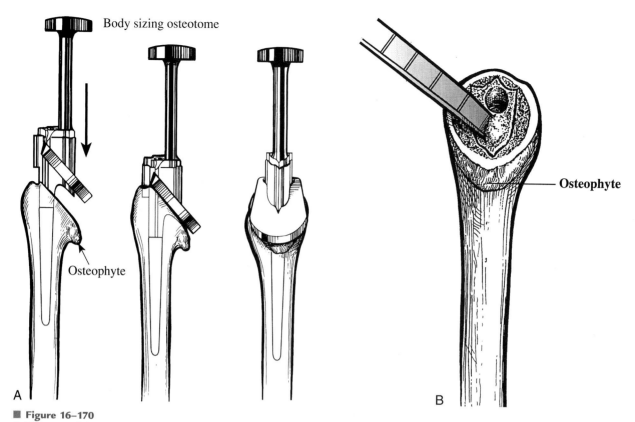

■ **Figure 16–170**

A, The stem of the body-sizing osteotome, which is the same size as the appropriate intramedullary canal reamer, is inserted down into the intramedullary canal of the humerus. **B,** The osteotome should be rotated until the collar lies flat on the cut surface of the bone to ensure that proper version for the prosthesis has been maintained.

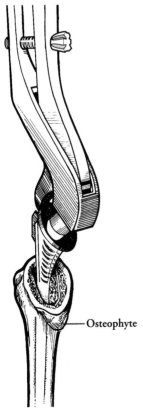

■ **Figure 16–171**

After insertion of the trial broach body with the driver extractor tool, the osteophytes should be removed with an osteotome and rongeur.

a 14/12 broach and prosthesis could be used. The final humeral prosthesis is approximately 1 mm larger than the corresponding broach size; thus, if the body broach is tight, a stable press-fit of the prosthesis can be achieved. Because the medullary canal is filled with the proper-sized stem and the body of the prosthesis fills the cancellous bone proximally, a press-fit of the prosthesis can usually be obtained. However, in the case of deficient cancellous bone proximally, as might be seen in patients with rheumatoid arthritis, cement may be required. If cement is required, we (C.A.R. and M.W.) do not use cement restricters or cement pressurization—we use just enough cement with finger pressure to prevent proximal rotation of the prosthesis. With the final broach in place, remove any osteophytes that extend inferiorly from the cut surface of the medial humeral neck with an osteotome or rongeurs (see Fig. 16–170B). While the glenoid fossa is being evaluated and prepared, the body broach should be left in place to protect the proximal end of the humerus from compression fractures or deformation by the humeral head retractors.

With the broach in place, use a humeral head retractor to displace the proximal end of the humerus posteriorly to expose the glenoid fossa (i.e., Carter Rowe, Fukuda, or DePuy retractor) (Fig. 16–172). The Scoffield retractor should again be used to protect the axillary nerve as the labrum and thickened anteroinferior capsule are removed. If the capsule is not excised and is left in place, it can become reattached to the glenoid and the humerus and once again restrict external rotation postoperatively.

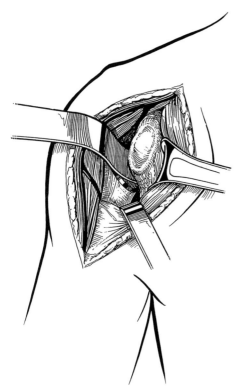

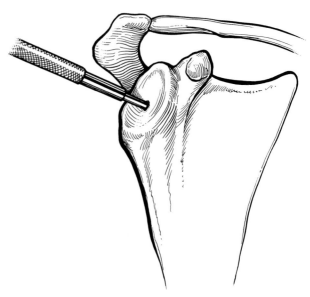

■ **Figure 16–173**
A central hole is placed in the glenoid fossa with a punch or an air bur.

■ **Figure 16–172**
When replacing the glenoid fossa with a prosthesis, various types of humeral head retractors can be used to expose the glenoid fossa.

Resection of the anteroinferior capsule has not led to any instability of the joint.

Hemiarthroplasty versus Total Shoulder Arthroplasty

If hemiarthroplasty is the procedure of choice, you are ready for final insertion of the prosthesis and reattachment of the subscapularis tendon. However, if a total shoulder replacement is planned, the following describes the steps for replacement of the glenoid.

Technique for Using the Five-Pegged Glenoid Prosthesis

A variety of glenoid sizer disks are used to determine the proper size of the glenoid. Select the one that best fits the size of the glenoid fossa. The disk that is used must be the same size or slightly smaller than the glenoid fossa. A larger disk and glenoid prosthesis could interfere with cuff function. Because the normal shoulder joint allows 6 mm of anteroposterior translation of the head in the glenoid fossa, glenoid prostheses have been developed with a diameter of curvature 6 mm larger than the corresponding humeral head.[175] Each of the glenoid sizer disks and trial prostheses are numbered—40xs, 40, 44, 48, 52, 56, or 56EL—and each has a different color. The numbers do not mean that the size is marked in millimeters; rather, each is 6 mm in diameter larger than the corresponding humeral head, which automatically allows for head translation in the glenoid prosthesis. If a No. 52 glenoid is selected, a 52-mm humeral head should be used, which allows for a 6-mm mismatch between the prosthetic head and the glenoid prosthesis.

With the humerus sufficiently displaced posteriorly, a hole is created in the center of the glenoid fossa with either a punch or an air bur (Fig. 16–173). Attach the gold-colored, anodized drill guide to the handle and place it into the glenoid fossa over the centering hole. Insert the gold-colored anodized drill bit into the guide, and drill until the guard hits the drill guide (Fig. 16–174). It is important that the drill bit be perfectly centered in the drill guide and that the power be engaged before the drill bit comes into contact with bone. If the drill bit is not properly aligned, the bit will bind in the guide, which can cause damage to the drill.

If the joint is so tight that the longer gold-colored, anodized drill bit cannot be inserted, the shorter silver bit may be used to create the central drill hole. After "bottoming out" the silver drill bit, the central drill guide should be removed and the drilling resumed until the silver drill bit bottoms out. The depth of the central drill hole achieved with the silver bit without using the central drill guide will be the same as though the longer gold anodized drill bit with the guide had been used. Next, attach to the drill the glenoid reamer that best fits the size of the glenoid fossa. Insert the hub of the reamer into the central hole and ream the glenoid until it has a smooth configuration that matches the size of the previously selected trial glenoid prosthesis (Fig. 16–175). Such reaming ensures a perfect fit between the back of the glenoid prosthesis and the face of the glenoid. The power to the glenoid reamer should be engaged while the tip of the reamer is in the pilot hole, but before it comes in contact with bone. If the reamer is held tightly against the glenoid before the power is started, the reamer may bind and cause damage to the power drill and bone.

The silver-colored peripheral drill guide is now attached to the handle. The central peg on the drill guide

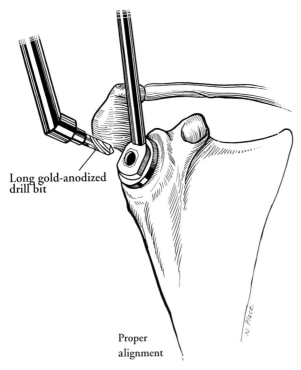

■ **Figure 16–174**

The long gold-anodized drill bit must be placed perfectly straight in the drill guide. If it is inserted at an angle, the drill bit can bind up in the drill guide and break the drill. A straight or 45-degree angled drill is available.

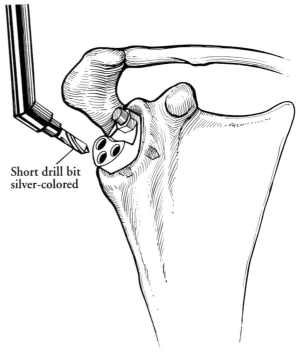

■ **Figure 16–176**

With the peripheral drill guide in place, the short silver drill bit should be used to drill the peripheral four holes in the glenoid fossa.

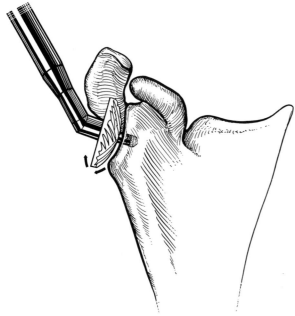

■ **Figure 16–175**

The hub of the glenoid reamer should be placed into the central hole. Reaming of the glenoid should be performed until the glenoid fossa is perfectly smooth and matches the back surface of the glenoid prosthesis.

slips into the hole previously drilled in the center of the glenoid fossa. Use the silver-colored drill bit, which is shorter than the gold anodized drill bit, to create four peripheral holes in the glenoid fossa (Fig. 16–176). Drill the superior hole first, and then place the antirotation peg to prevent any rotation of the guide while the other holes are being drilled.

Note that with the peripheral guide in place, it is a good idea to see whether sufficient room is available to drill the posterior hole. The shoulder joint is sometimes so tight that it is very difficult to displace the proximal part of the humerus enough posteriorly to be able to drill the posterior hole. If such is the case, you have several options; for example, release more of the posterior capsule, remove the posterior peg from the final prosthesis and use the remaining four pegs for fixation, or abandon use of the pegged glenoid and plan on using the keeled glenoid prosthesis.

Insert the previously selected, trial pegged glenoid prosthesis and keep it in place during sizing of the trial humeral head (Fig. 16–177). The final pegged glenoid prosthesis is slightly smaller than the trial prosthesis to allow room for cement.

Technique for Using the Keeled Glenoid Prosthesis

For application of the keeled component, use an air bur to partially create a slot in the glenoid fossa. Then insert the hub of the appropriate size of glenoid reamer into the slot and ream the glenoid until it has a smooth configuration that matches the size of the previously selected glenoid component. Continue to use the air bur with

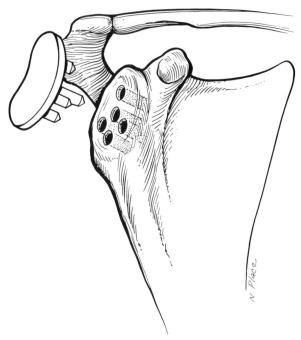

■ **Figure 16–177**

A trial pegged glenoid prosthesis is placed into position.

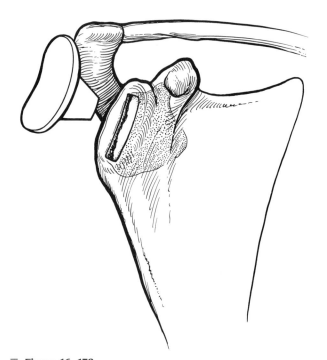

■ **Figure 16–178**

If a keeled glenoid prosthesis has been selected, the air bur is used to create a slot in the glenoid fossa. After the glenoid fossa has been reamed, a trial keel prosthesis is placed into position.

curets to remove enough bone to receive the keel (Fig. 16–178). Evacuate cancellous bone in the base of the coracoid and down the lateral border of the scapula to help lock in the keeled prosthesis with cement. The keel of the final prosthesis is slightly smaller than the trial prosthesis to accommodate the use of cement.

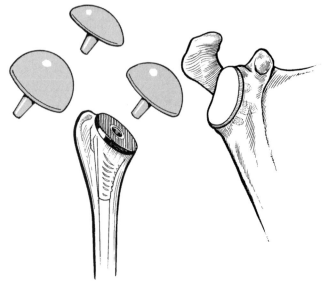

■ **Figure 16–179**

With the trial glenoid and broach body in place, an appropriately sized humeral head (i.e., short, medium, or long) is selected to balance the soft tissues.

Technique for Using the Anchor Peg Glenoid Prosthesis

The anchor peg glenoid is an all-polyethylene, minimally cemented, pegged glenoid prosthesis. It features a circumferentially fluted, central, interference-fit peg for tissue integration and three small, cemented peripheral pegs. This glenoid is designed to improve long-term fixation and was tested in a canine model. Radiographic, histologic, and mechanical tests were performed at three postoperative intervals (0, 3, and 6 months) in a canine survival study. The central, fluted peg of the anchor peg glenoid achieved bone ingrowth around the peg flanges in all cases. Results showed that the anchor peg design improved implant fixation, compared to conventional all-polyethylene, keeled glenoid designs. Also, the central fluted peg of the anchor peg glenoid was superior to a conventional cemented keeled design in achieving tissue integration and fixation in this weight-bearing animal model.[440a] **(V16-24)**

Selection of the Proper Head Size

(V16-25) With the trial body and glenoid prosthesis in place, select a suitable short, medium, or long humeral head (Fig. 16–179).

Note that the short head is **only** to be used with the 6- or 8-mm humeral prosthesis. If you use the short head with a size 10-mm or greater body, the collar of the humeral prosthesis will be larger than the humeral head, which could damage the surface of the glenoid. If the medium and long heads are too tight, you will have to remove more of the neck of the humerus and release more capsular tissue rather than using a short head.

The numeric size of the head is determined by the glenoid sizer disk selection. Selection of a humeral head of the appropriate length allows the soft tissues to be balanced with proper tension. With the correct head size in place, a stable configuration of the joint without gross anterior or posterior instability should be achieved. However, you should be able to displace the prosthesis posteriorly 50% out of the glenoid fossa. In addition, it should be possible to reapproximate the subscapularis tendon back to bone and have at least 30 to 50 degrees of external rotation, and you should be able to place the patient's hand on the opposite shoulder without any tension. If the fit of the humeral head is so tight that functional internal or external rotation cannot be achieved, more posterior capsule must be released or a shorter head should be used. Remember that the short head should be used only with a size 6 or 8 humeral body. If gross anterior or posterior instability exists, a longer head should be used.

Insertion of the Final Prosthesis

With the broach in place and the trial humeral head removed, displace the humerus posteriorly to prepare the glenoid fossa for insertion of the glenoid prosthesis. Insert a probe into each of the drilled holes to determine whether the holes have exited the anterior or posterior cortex of the glenoid. If exit holes are found, it is important to not put an excessive amount of cement in the holes, where it could extrude and possibly damage the surrounding soft tissues. **(V16-26)** Carefully irrigate or use pulsatile lavage to remove any clotted blood from the holes. For hemostasis, spray thrombin and insert Surgicel gauze into each of the holes. Mix half a package of methylmethacrylate, remove the gauze from the holes, and place a small amount of methylmethacrylate into each of the holes with your fingertip (Fig. 16–180). Only a small

amount of methylmethacrylate is necessary in each hole to create the proper cement mantle around each peg. Excessive cement extruding out of the holes and lying between the prosthesis and the glenoid fossa is undesirable for two reasons. First, it could create an uneven seat for the glenoid prosthesis, and second, the thin segments of cement from between the back of the glenoid prosthesis and the face of the glenoid may become fragmented and loose in the joint and cause damage to the polyethylene. Insert the glenoid prosthesis and hold it in position with finger pressure until the cement is cured and the prosthesis is secure (see Fig. 16–180).

If a keeled glenoid prosthesis is to be used, hemostasis in the keel hole must be achieved. The slot should be irrigated to remove any clots and then sprayed with thrombin and packed with Surgicel gauze and a lap sponge. When the methylmethacrylate is ready, remove the Surgicel gauze and the sponge and impact the cement into the slot with finger pressure. Firm finger pressure and several small batches of cement will ensure a good cement mantle in the slot to receive and secure the keeled prosthesis. As mentioned, cement between the glenoid fossa and the back of the prosthesis is undesirable. Insert the keeled prosthesis, and hold it in position with finger pressure until the cement has set and the prosthesis is secure (Fig. 16–181).

Repair of the Subscapularis Tendon

Before the humeral component is inserted, you must prepare for repair of the subscapularis back to the cut surface of the proximal end of the humerus. Because the tendon was released from its insertion onto the lesser tuberosity, we can gain length of the tendon and hence gain external rotation by reattaching it medially on the cut surface of the neck of the humerus. Three or four holes should be drilled into the anterior neck of the humerus with a small drill bit. Use a suture passer to pull loops of suture through these drill holes (Fig. 16–182).

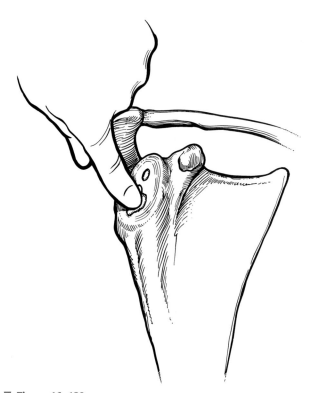

■ **Figure 16–180**
The drill holes are thoroughly irrigated, sprayed with thrombin, and packed with Surgicel gauze to dry up the drill holes. A small amount of bone cement is placed into each of the holes with fingertip pressure.

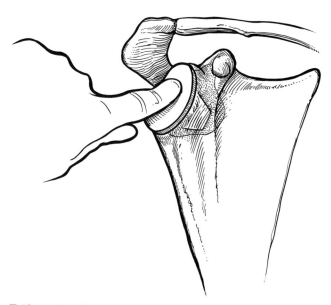

■ **Figure 16–181**
When a keeled prosthesis is used, the slot is cleaned, dried, and then packed with cement. The prosthesis is held in place with finger pressure until it has set up.

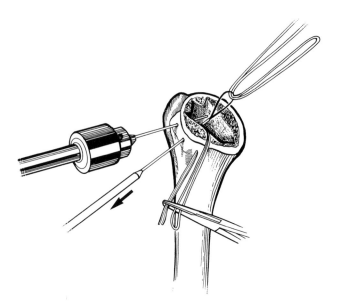

■ **Figure 16–182**
During preparation for repair of the subscapularis tendon, three or four drill holes are placed in the anterior neck of the humerus. With a suture passer, loops of sutures are placed through the drill holes. These loops of suture will be used later to pull the Dacron tape suture into the subscapularis tendon through the bone for secure fixation of the tendon to bone.

These loops of suture will be used later to pull the 1-mm nonabsorbable Dacron tape sutures in the subscapularis tendon out through the bone for secure fixation of the tendon back to bone.

Attach a humeral prosthesis that is the same size as the final broach size into the driver-extractor and insert the prosthesis down the humeral canal. The fins of the prosthesis must be aligned with the fin tracks previously created by the body broach. The final prosthesis is 1 mm larger overall than the broach so that a press-fit without cement can be obtained. Cancellous bone from the resected humeral head can be used as graft to help fill in any defects in the proximal part of the humerus or to ensure a good tight press-fit. The decision to use cement or a press-fit technique is up to the individual surgeon. In some cases, it may be necessary to use methylmethacrylate because of a previous surgical procedure, fractures, osteoporosis, rheumatoid arthritis, or degenerative cysts in the humerus. A set of long-stemmed humeral prostheses is available for revision cases or in the event of fractures of the shaft of the humerus.

Before the final humeral head is inserted, thoroughly clean the Morse taper socket in the humeral prosthesis with a dry sponge and insert the appropriate size of head. Use a plastic-tipped driver to secure the head in place by sharply striking it four to five times with a 2-lb mallet (Fig. 16–183). Make sure to impact the head down in the direction of the Morse taper. Grasp the head to ensure that it is securely attached to the humeral prosthesis. The pullout strength of a properly attached head into the body has been tested to be approximately 1400 lb. If for some reason the head needs to be removed, a special forked sled driver should be placed between the head and the body and tapped.

With gentle traction, internal rotation, and finger pressure on the humeral prosthesis, reduce the head into the

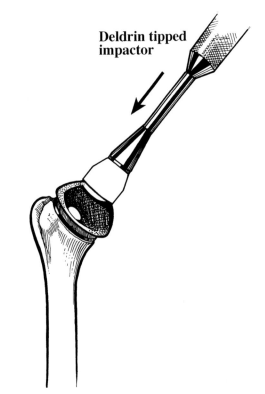

Deldrin tipped impactor

■ **Figure 16–183**
The head of the prosthesis is then impacted into the humeral body by using a Deldrin tipped impactor.

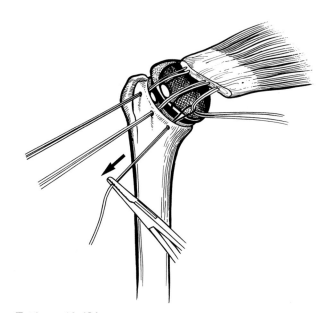

■ **Figure 16–184**
The loops of suture in the anterior surface of the neck of the humerus are used to pull the Dacron tape sutures previously placed in the subscapularis tendon out through the neck of the humerus, and then the Dacron tape sutures are tied.

glenoid fossa. A special plastic skid is available and should be used in place of the Darrach retractor to avoid scratching the humeral head. After joint irrigation, pass the previously placed Dacron tape sutures in the subscapularis tendon into the loop of sutures in the proximal part of the humerus, pull the loops and sutures through the bone, and secure the tendon back to bone (Fig. 16–184).

If the tendon was previously divided or was lengthened with a coronal Z-plasty technique, repair and secure it with heavy nonabsorbable sutures, such as 1-mm Dacron tape. The use of heavy 1-mm tape sutures allows immediate passive movement beginning the day of surgery without fear of detaching the subscapularis tendon.

Before wound closure, palpate the axillary nerve a final time to be sure that it is intact. Thoroughly irrigate the wound with antibiotic solution. Infiltrate the subcutaneous and muscle tissues with 0.25% bupivacaine solution to ease immediate postoperative pain. One or two portable wound evacuation units are used to prevent the formation of postoperative hematoma.

The wound may be closed according to the surgeon's preference. The deltopectoral fascia can be closed with a running 0 absorbable suture and the deep layer of fat with a 0 or 2-0 absorbable suture. Subcuticular fat is closed as a separate layer, and the skin is closed with a running subcuticular nylon suture. Careful attention to wound closure will result in a cosmetically acceptable incision.

If a humeral prosthesis needs to be removed, a special slap hammer extractor is available (Fig. 16–185). After the head has been removed, you should remove the Deldrin tip of the driver-extractor tool and replace it with a steel tip. The driver-extractor should be attached to the prosthesis. The slap hammer is screwed into the top of the driver-extractor, and then the handle is used to apply upward blows to remove the prosthesis. It may be necessary to use small osteotomes to loosen the prosthesis from bone or cement.

Results

Hemiarthroplasty Results

The results with the Neer design of hemiarthroplasty, or proximal humeral prosthetic replacement, are reported in Table 16-21. The results have been reported for osteonecrosis, osteoarthritis, rheumatoid arthritis, and the residuals of trauma. When this procedure is applied to the treatment of proximal humeral osteonecrosis, pain relief has been quite good, with rates ranging from 91% to

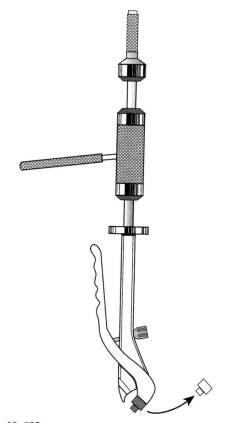

■ Figure 16–185
To remove a secure or cemented prosthesis, a special slap hammer is available. It requires that the driver-extractor tool be modified by tapping a hole in the top of the tool to receive the slap hammer.

100%, and the range of motion of the shoulder approaches normal. When this operation is applied to patients with rheumatoid arthritis, osteoarthritis, or the residuals of trauma, satisfactory pain relief is less consistently achieved but, with the exception of 3 of the 11 reported series, is still quite acceptable. Range of motion in these latter patients tends to be less and varies from one series to another; average active abduction ranged from one third to three quarters normal.

TABLE 16–21.   Results of Shoulder Hemiarthroplasty–Neer Design

Author, Year	Diagnosis	No. of Shoulders	No or Slight Pain (%)	Average Active Abduction (°) or Overall Rating
Neer, 1955[294]	Osteonecrosis	3	100	Excellent, good, good
Neer, 1974[296]	Osteoarthritis	47		20 excellent
				20 satisfactory
				6 unsatisfactory
Cruess, 1986[111]	Osteonecrosis	5	100	Approached normal
Bodey and Yeoman, 1983[40]	Osteoarthritis Rheumatoid arthritis	8	88	63°
Tanner and Cofield, 1983[404]	Old trauma	28	89	112°
Bell and Gschwend, 1986[30]	Mixed	17	59	91°
Petersson, 1986[323]	Rheumatoid arthritis	11	36	74°
Zuckerman and Cofield, 1986[448]	Osteoarthritis	39	82	134°
	Rheumatoid arthritis	44	91	112°
Hawkins et al, 1987[189]	Chronic dislocation	9	67	140°
Pritchett and Clark, 1987[335]	Chronic dislocation	7	100	5 good, 2 fair
Rutherford and Cofield, 1987[366]	Osteonecrosis	11	91	161°
Total		229	Weighted mean, 82%; median, 89%	Weighted mean of 8 series, 115°; median, 112°

In 1996, Williams and Rockwood[431] reported on treating 21 shoulders in 20 patients with glenohumeral arthritis and rotator cuff–deficient shoulders with a hemiarthroplasty procedure. After an average of 4 years of follow-up, 86% of the patients had achieved a satisfactory result according to the limited-goal criteria of Neer (i.e., pain was improved and deflection improved from an average of 70 degrees preoperatively to 120 degrees post-operatively). External rotation improved preoperatively from an average of 27 degrees to a postoperative average of 45 degrees. In none of the patients did postoperative instability of the shoulder develop.

In 1996, Bigliani, Glasson, and associates[155] treated 31 shoulders with osteoarthritis and an intact cuff with a hemiarthroplasty procedure. The patients were evaluated by the American Shoulder and Elbow Surgeons, Neer, and Constant end result scoring methods. They reported that the outcome varied with the amount of glenoid wear. However, in patients with a smooth concentric glenoid, they reported that 86% had excellent results and 7% had good results.

Sperling and Cofield[387] reported on the results of hemi-arthroplasty in 74 shoulders of 64 patients who were 50 years or younger. Significant pain relief and improvement in active abduction and external rotation were observed. Radiographic analysis revealed posterior glenoid erosion in 68% of cases. According to the Neer rating system, results were graded as excellent in 15 cases, satisfactory in 24 cases, and unsatisfactory in 35 cases. The estimated survivorship of the hemiarthroplasty prostheses was 92% at 5 years, 83% at 10 years, and 73% at 15 years. The risk of revision was highest in patients who underwent the treatment for sequelae of trauma. The authors concluded that although hemiarthroplasty successfully resulted in long-term pain relief in this subset of patients, the high rate of unsatisfactory results suggests that caution should be exercised when recommending this procedure for younger patients.

Total Shoulder Arthroplasty Results

The most commonly used total shoulder arthroplasty has been the Neer design. The results with this system are tabulated in Table 16–22. Most series contain a mixed diagnostic grouping and include patients with rheumatoid arthritis, osteoarthritis, old trauma, and a variety of less common diagnostic categories. As can be seen in Table 16–22, the percentage of patients who achieved satisfactory pain relief is quite high, and quite typically, slightly more than 90% of patients reported no or only slight pain after surgery. Motion data after surgery have not been as consistently reported as one might desire, but the amount of motion regained seems variable and dependent on the diagnostic category. For example, in the series reported by Cofield, mean active abduction after surgery for the entire group of patients reported was 120 degrees.[85] The average return of active abduction varied greatly according to the diagnosis: 141 degrees for patients with osteoarthritis, 109 degrees for those with post-traumatic arthritis, and 103 degrees for patients with rheumatoid arthritis. The return of movement in Cofield's series was not only dependent on the diagnosis but was also highly dependent on the condition of the rotator cuff and shoulder capsule and on avoidance of complications.[85]

The largest series of total shoulder arthroplasties of this category has been reported by Neer and colleagues.[304] They suggested two systems for grading results. Patients who received a full rehabilitation program were graded as excellent, satisfactory, or unsatisfactory. To achieve an excellent result, the patient had to be enthusiastic about the operation and have no significant pain, the patient could use the arm without limitations, strength approached normal, active elevation of the arm was within 35 degrees of the opposite normal side, and external rotation was 90% of the normal side. Patients with a satisfactory result had no more than occasional pain or aching with weather changes, good use of the shoulder for daily activities, elevation of at least 90 degrees, and rotation to 50% of the normal side. Muscle strength was at least 30% of the normal side, and patients expressed satisfaction with the operation. In an unsatisfactory result, the aforementioned criteria were not achieved. Neer has suggested a separate evaluation category for patients who undergo total shoulder replacement but whose muscles could be classified as detached and not capable of recovering function after repair because of fixed contracture or denervation. Patients with substantial bone loss, particularly bone loss in the proximal part of the humerus, might also be included within this evaluative category. In this setting, rehabilitation is aimed at achieving limited goals, the purpose being to gain a lesser range of motion but maintain stability. Neer has suggested that this limited-goals

TABLE 16–22.   Results of Total Shoulder Arthroplasty–Neer Design

Author, Year	Mean Follow-up (yr)	Diagnosis	No. of Shoulders	No or Slight Pain (%)	Average Active Elevation* (°)	Average External Rotation (°)
Neer et al, 1982[304]	3.1	Mixed	194			
Bade et al, 1984[15]	4.5	Mixed	38	93	118	
Cofield, 1984[85]	3.8	Mixed	73	92	120	48
Wilde et al, 1984[428]	3.0	Mixed	38	92		
Adams et al, 1986[1]	2.7	Mixed	33	91	96	
Hawkins et al, 1986[185]	3.0	Rheumatoid arthritis Osteoarthritis	70			
Barrett et al, 1987[21]	3.5	Mixed	50	88	100	54
Kelly et al, 1987[220]	3.0	Rheumatoid arthritis	40	88	75	40
Frich et al, 1988[140]	2.3	Mixed	50	92	58–78†	17–21†

*Elevation = abduction with 30 to 60 degrees of horizontal flexion.
†Range, depending on diagnosis.

TABLE 16–23. Follow-up on 194 Total Shoulder Arthroplasties (Clinical Ratings)

Diagnosis	No. of Shoulders	Excellent	Full Exercise Program		Limited-Goals Rehabilitation	
			Satisfactory	Unsatisfactory	Successful	Unsuccessful
Osteoarthritis (primary and secondary)	40	36	3	0	1	0
Arthritis of recurrent dislocation	18	13	3	1	1	0
Rheumatoid arthritis	50	28	12	3	7	0
Old trauma	41	16	7	12	6	0
Prosthetic revision	26	7	3	5	11	0
Cuff tear arthropathy	11	—	—	—	10	1
Miscellaneous (tumor, glenoid dysplasia, failed arthrodesis)	8	1	—	—	6	1
Total	194	101	28	21	42	2

Adapted from Neer CS II, Watson KC, and Stanton FJ: Recent experience in total shoulder replacement. J Bone Joint Surg Am 64:319–337, 1982.

TABLE 16–24. Results of Roentgenographic Analysis of Neer Total Shoulder Arthroplasty

Author, Year	No. of Shoulders	Glenoid Bone–Cement Junction Lucent Zones (%)			Shift in Position
		None	Any Area	Keel	
Neer et al, 1982[304]	194	70	30	12	
Bade et al, 1984[15]	38	33	67		
Cofield, 1984[85]	73	29	71	33	11
Wilde et al, 1984[428]	38	7	93	68	
Adams et al, 1986[1]	33			36	
Brems, 1993[52]	69	31	69		
Barrett et al, 1987[21]	50	26	74	36	10
Kelly et al, 1987[220]	40	17	83	63	

rehabilitation is successful when patients with these muscle or bone deficiencies achieve 90 degrees of elevation and 20 degrees of external rotation, maintain reasonable stability, and achieve satisfactory pain relief. The results achieved for Neer's large series of patients, including the numerous diagnostic categories, are displayed in Table 16–23. Other series of results with this type of prosthesis have been reported.[425]

Fehringer and associates[128] characterized shoulder-specific functional gains after total shoulder arthroplasty in relation to preoperative shoulder function in 102 shoulders with primary glenohumeral osteoarthritis. According to the SST, the average number of shoulder functions that could be performed improved from 4 of 12 preoperatively to 9 of 12 postoperatively. Ninety-four percent of shoulders demonstrated improvement in function, and postoperative function positively correlated with preoperative function. Significant improvement was noted in 11 of 12 shoulder functions that were examined. The chance of regaining a function that had been absent before surgery was 73%, whereas the chance of losing a function that had been present before surgery was 6%.

Goldberg and colleagues[157] studied the magnitude and durability of functional improvement after shoulder arthroplasty in 124 shoulders with primary osteoarthritis by using the SST, which was applied preoperatively and at sequential intervals postoperatively. Preoperatively, patients were able to perform 3.8 ± 0.3 of the 12 SST functions. Postoperatively, the number of functions that could be performed was consistent at different intervals: 8.0 ± 0.4 at 6 months, 9.5 ± 0.4 at 1 year, 10.0 ± 0.3 at 2 years, 9.2 ± 0.4 at 3 years, 9.6 ± 0.4 at 4 years, and 10.0 ± 0.4 at 5 years. The authors concluded that total shoulder arthro-

plasty can provide substantial improvement in shoulder function.

Godeneche and associates[156] performed a multicenter retrospective analysis of 268 shoulders that underwent anatomically designed shoulder arthroplasty for primary osteoarthritis at a mean follow-up of 30 months. The age- and gender-adjusted Constant score was 38% preoperatively and 97% postoperatively, and good or excellent results were observed in 77% of patients.

Roentgenographic analyses for a number of series of total shoulder arthroplasties using the Neer design are displayed in Table 16–24. All series report lucent lines or lucent zones at the glenoid bone-cement junction. These zones vary considerably in frequency among the different series, with ranges of 30% to 93% of shoulders reported. The keel portion of this implant serves as the significant means of attachment to the scapula, and the lucent zones seen at the cement-bone junction surrounding the keel are of great concern. The median percentage of the number of shoulders analyzed in which a lucent line was identified at the bone-cement junction of the keel part of the component is 36. The argument has been presented that when these lucent lines or zones are seen in patients, they are almost always present immediately postoperatively and clearly represent an error in surgical technique.[304] This may be the most common sequence of events associated with roentgenographic lucent zones at the glenoid bone-cement junction and emphasized the need for meticulous preparation of the bone bed and cementing at the time of surgery. However, it has also been reported that these lucent zones have not been present immediately after surgery but rather have developed over time.[85] Green and Norris[158] and Slawson and associates[381] provided a review of imaging techniques for evaluating glenohumeral arthroplasty.

Lazarus and associates[235] reviewed the initial postoperative radiographs of 328 patients with primary osteoarthritis who had been treated with total shoulder arthroplasty by 17 different surgeons. Of these cases, 39 patients had a keeled component and 289 had a pegged component. The radiographs were analyzed and graded according to the presence of radiolucent lines at the bone-cement interface and contact or seating of the base of the glenoid component on the glenoid surface. Only 20 of the 328 (6%) glenoids demonstrated no radiolucencies, including only 1 keeled component (2.5%). On a numeric scale with 0 indicating no radiolucency and 5 indicating gross loosening, the mean radiolucency score was 1.8 ± 0.9 for keeled components and 1.3 ± 0.9 for pegged components. Incomplete seating was also common, particularly in patients with keeled components. A wide range of seating grades was noted with a clear trend toward greater component seating with pegged components than with keeled components. A frequently observed pattern of incomplete seating was an unsupported posterior rim. Ninety-five of the 121 pegged components that had been inserted by the most experienced surgeon had better cementing than did the 85 of 168 pegged components that had been inserted by the remaining surgeons.

Franklin and coauthors have suggested a classification system for describing the radiographic appearance of the glenoid component.[139] Class 0 has no lucency; class 1 has lucency at the superior or inferior flange only; class 2 has incomplete lucency at the keel; in class 3, complete lucency is seen up to 2 mm around the component; class 4 is characterized by complete lucency greater than 2 mm around the component; in class 5A, the component has translated, tipped, or shifted in position; and in class 5B, the component has become dislocated from the bone.

In the series by Barrett and coworkers[21] and Cofield,[85] analyses have also included a shift in glenoid component position relative to the position achieved immediately after surgery. Analysis of component movement relative to the bone requires viewing of sequential radiograph over time because a lucent zone is often not seen. This finding implies component loosening, but it can easily be overlooked if serial radiographs are not studied.

Boorman and colleagues have demonstrated that the effect of total shoulder arthroplasty on self-assessed health status is comparable to that of hip and knee arthroplasty.[45]

Comparison of Hemiarthroplasty versus Total Shoulder Arthroplasty in Patients with Osteoarthritis

In 1996, Jensen and Rockwood[205] reported the end results of patients with osteoarthritis who were treated by hemiarthroplasty versus those who were treated by total shoulder arthroplasty. This retrospective review included 87 consecutive patients (117 shoulders). Forty-two patients were treated by hemiarthroplasty, and 75 patients were treated by total shoulder arthroplasty. A Neer prosthesis was used in 72 shoulders, and a modular global prosthesis was used in 45 shoulders. The average age was 63.5 years, and the average follow-up was 58 months. In 38

shoulders (25%), an irreparable rotator cuff was noted, and the majority of these patients were treated by hemiarthroplasty. At follow-up, which included comparing range of motion before and after the operative procedure, relief of pain, the ability to perform 15 different activities of daily living, and a review of radiographs, we did not find any statistical difference between patients treated by hemiarthroplasty and total shoulder arthroplasty.

Gartsman and associates[152] performed a prospective randomized analysis of 51 shoulders treated by arthroplasty for primary osteoarthritis, 37 of which underwent total shoulder arthroplasty and 24 underwent hemiarthroplasty. With the numbers available for study, no significant difference was found between the two groups with respect to the postoperative UCLA and American Shoulder and Elbow Surgeons outcome scores. Total shoulder arthroplasty provided significantly greater pain relief than hemiarthroplasty did and demonstrated a trend toward superior results in patient satisfaction, function, and strength. Three of the hemiarthroplasty patients required revision for resurfacing of the glenoid.

Norris and Iannotti[308,309] reported on a prospective multicenter outcome study comparing humeral head replacement and total shoulder arthroplasty for primary osteoarthritis. They evaluated the functional outcome, patient satisfaction, shoulder motion, strength, stability, and postoperative radiographs in this series of patients and compared the results of humeral head replacement and total shoulder arthroplasty. This series involved 19 surgeons using a single prosthetic design and enrolled 133 patients receiving total shoulder replacements and 43 receiving humeral head replacements. The authors concluded that prosthetic replacement for primary osteoarthritis yields excellent results with dramatic improvement in pain, function, and patient satisfaction. Patients were greatly improved by 3 months after the procedure and continued to improve over the first 12 months and have a stable functional outcome thereafter. The results of humeral head replacement for osteoarthritis with an intact rotator cuff and minimal glenoid wear were essentially equivalent to those of total shoulder arthroplasty. Full-thickness rotator cuff tears were uncommon with primary osteoarthritis; however, when present, such tears may result in less favorable results. Glenoid erosion was common in primary osteoarthritis and, when moderate or severe in degree, may adversely affect the functional outcome in humeral head replacement. In addition, glenoid erosion was associated with a higher degree of glenoid component lucent lines when a thick cement mantle was present beneath the base of the glenoid component in total shoulder arthroplasty. A thick cement mantle at the base of the component should be avoided in this situation because it adds to the increased incidence of glenoid lucent lines. Humeral lucent lines were uncommon but are more often seen with total shoulder arthroplasty, possibly because of polyethylene wear debris.

Comparison of Hemiarthroplasty versus Total Shoulder Arthroplasty in Patients with Rheumatoid Arthritis

Sneppen and associates[383] reported a prospective study of 62 shoulders with grade IV and V Larsen rheumatoid arthritis treated with a Neer total shoulder arthroplasty. At an average of 92 months, the authors reported that proximal migration had occurred in 55% of the patients and 40% showed radiographic loosening, translation, or displacement of the glenoid prosthesis. However, despite the glenoid loosening and displacement and loosening of the press-fit humeral components, 89% of the patients had good pain relief. The loosening did not influence range of motion or function. They concluded that a cemented hemiarthroplasty may be better treatment in the end stages of rheumatoid arthritis of the shoulder.

Basamania, Rockwood, and associates[24] reported that patients with rheumatoid arthritis who were treated by hemiarthroplasty had better results than did those treated by total shoulder arthroplasty. The patients consisted of 28 women and 9 men ranging in age from 22 to 77 years with an average age of 54 years. The average follow-up was 5.5 years (range, 2 to 14 years). In an effort to avoid loosening of the glenoid component secondary to proximal migration of the humeral prosthesis, 32 shoulders were treated by hemiarthroplasty and 13 shoulders were treated by total shoulder arthroplasty. Preoperatively, the average active flexion for all shoulders was 50 degrees, 21 degrees of external rotation and internal rotation to the lateral hip. Postoperatively, the average gain in motion for all shoulders was 42 degrees of active flexion, 10 degrees of external rotation, and six spinal levels for internal rotation. Twenty-four shoulders (53%) did not have the rotator cuff repaired because of massive irreparable effects that were associated with superior migration of the humeral head.

Patients treated by hemiarthroplasty had greater improvement in their postoperative range of motion. For these patients, the average gain in shoulder flexion was 53 degrees versus 38 degrees in shoulders treated by total shoulder arthroplasty. At latest follow-up, satisfaction was reported in 85% of the patients treated by total shoulder arthroplasty and in 94% of those treated by hemiarthroplasty.

Methods of Assessing Functional Outcome

Codman will be remembered in the annals of orthopaedic history as a pioneer in the study of shoulder disorders, but few except the most ardent of his followers are familiar with the role that he played as a visionary and champion of what is currently described as outcomes research.[82] Central to what Codman described in the early 1900s as an "end result" system was the admonition that every patient be monitored to determine whether the treatment was a success and, if not, to determine the reasons for failure so that such occurrences could be prevented in the future. Despite Codman's admonition almost 100 years ago, there continues to be a lack of standardized methods for measuring results and reporting complications associated with total shoulder implants. Unfortunately, the lack of a universally accepted outcome measurement system for shoulder arthroplasty increases methodologic flaws in structured literature reviews and often precludes meaningful retrospective or prospective comparisons between various arthroplasty series. The desirability of research methodologies that will improve the quality and

comparability of multicenter studies is underscored by our review of almost 50 total shoulder replacement series.* The results of this review revealed that only 33 of these reports assessed the outcome of treatment by applying a specific grading system. Moreover, there was a great lack of unanimity with regard to these evaluation schemes because 22 different grading systems were used. Other disconcerting factors were the variability in reported data, variations in terminology, and ill-defined standards of assessing complications; such factors make it difficult to systematically analyze many of these studies.

The necessity for improving study design, defining the important constituents of outcome measurement, and increasing the validity of orthopaedic clinical research has been emphasized by several authors.[107,113,150,364] It has been suggested that the current emphasis of orthopaedic clinical studies should be directed toward outcomes research that documents the effect of treatment on the health of those treated and the subsequent quality of their lives.[150] The American Shoulder and Elbow Surgeons proposed a standardized form for assessment of the shoulder that is applicable to all patients regardless of their diagnosis.[343] Such standardized forms represent assessment tools that will facilitate the analysis of multicenter studies, permit validity testing of measurement tools, and provide documentation of patient outcome in terms of economics and improved quality of life.

Hasan and associates[180] recently pointed out the importance of patient self-assessment in determining failure after shoulder arthroplasty. Failure has often been defined by the need for revision surgery, but the authors suggested that it may also be viewed as a result that does not meet the expectation of the patient. In 139 consecutive patients who were referred to the authors' institution for consultation because of dissatisfaction with the result of a previous shoulder arthroplasty, common characteristics of failure were characterized. The authors noted that the rate of revision underestimated the rate of failure as determined by a decline in patient self-assessed shoulder function. Almost three quarters of these patients complained of stiffness as a major functional problem after their shoulder arthroplasty, yet stiffness is rarely reported as a cause of failure after this procedure. These findings suggest the importance of documenting the clinical effectiveness of arthroplasty by using patient self-assessment of shoulder function, both before and after surgery.

Survivorship Analysis

The application of survivorship analysis to the evaluation of long-term clinical studies involving total hip replacement is well established.[103,116,117,206,315] Although nonparametric estimates of survivorship based on life tables and the Kaplan-Meier curve have proved useful in predicting the longevity of hip arthroplasties, the application of these instruments to total shoulder arthroplasty studies is limited to a few series.[54,91]

*See references 48, 54, 58, 60, 78, 94, 97, 105, 109, 123, 127, 129, 135, 140, 160, 161, 186, 220, 228, 234, 239, 245, 256, 270, 274-276, 301, 302, 313, 325, 329, 332-334, 357, 407, 422, 428.

In 1983, Cofield performed a nonparametric estimation of survivorship in 176 unconstrained total shoulder arthroplasties and predicted a 9.6% cumulative probability of failure at 5 years.[91] The criteria for failure were defined as the need for a major reoperation, which occurred in eight (4.5%) cases. Indications for reoperation included early dislocation in three shoulders, loosening of the glenoid component in three shoulders, and muscle transfer for axillary nerve paralysis and resectional arthroplasty for sepsis in one shoulder each. In a more recent article by the same author, this figure did not significantly change at an 11-year end point.[407] In 1989, Brenner and colleagues[54] used the Kaplan-Meier survivorship curve to analyze the results of 53 unconstrained total shoulder arthroplasties. Using a more rigid definition that considered failure as not only a need for reoperation but also patient dissatisfaction with the degree of pain relief, the authors reported an 11-year survival rate of only 73%.

In a large multicenter prospective study involving more than 470 unconstrained total shoulder arthroplasties, the 5-year survival rate was estimated at 97% (95% confidence interval).[349] A more rigid definition of failure, similar to the criteria proposed by Brenner and associates,[54] was applied to a subset of these patients whose diagnosis was restricted to osteoarthritis. For these patients, failure was defined by one of two parameters. The first parameter, as with the two previous studies, simply involved a need for reoperation after the index procedure. The second parameter was based on a patient self-assessment visual analog scale for pain. For this analysis, failure was defined as the point in time at which the patient reported shoulder pain that was equal or worse than the preoperative condition. For the osteoarthritis subgroup, the probability of 5-year survival was 92% when the more stringent criteria were used.

Sperling and Cofield[387] studied the survivorship of total shoulder arthroplasty and hemiarthroplasty in patients 50 years or younger. The estimated survival rate of total shoulder arthroplasty based on 36 patients for whom sufficient follow-up was available was 97% at 5 years, 97% at 10 years, and 84% at 15 years (95% confidence interval). The risk of revision surgery after total shoulder arthroplasty was higher when a rotator cuff tear was encountered during surgery. The estimated survival rate of hemiarthroplasty based on 78 patients was 92% at 5 years, 83% at 10 years, and 73% at 15 years. Hemiarthroplasty for sequelae of trauma was found to be a risk factor for revision. The variability in these results points to the inconsistency of the definition of "survival," including different criteria for revision surgery and the inclusion or exclusion of other parameters such as pain or function.

Patient Self-assessment

As a practical approach to measurement of effectiveness that can easily be applied in an active practice, one of us (F.A.M.) has used patient self-assessment methods (see earlier sections of this chapter). Since January 1992, all new patients with shoulder problems have been asked to complete the SST[247,262] to define their pretreatment shoulder function and the SF-36 to characterize their overall health status. The results from these pretreatment questionnaires serve as the baseline, or "ingo," for evaluating treatment effectiveness from the perspective of the patient. Follow-up questionnaires reveal the "outcome" of treatment from the patient's perspective. The difference between the outcome and the ingo is the effectiveness of the treatment. Table 16–25 presents some of these early data for the effectiveness of total arthroplasty or hemiarthroplasty for each of the indicated diagnoses. The preoperative scores are shown to the left of each arrow, and the follow-up score is shown to the right. The data include the SF-36 parameters for total body physical role function and comfort, as well as the 12 SST parameters that are specific to the shoulder. The SF-36 scores are the average of the scores of the patients. The SST scores are the percentage of the patients answering "yes" to the indicated question.

A convenient way to display these data is by using the Codman graph (Fig. 16–186), which shows the ingo and the outcome for each patient.

Matsen and colleagues[261] used these self-assessment methods to investigate factors contributing to the variability in improvement after shoulder arthroplasty. Patient demographics, preoperative health status, and preoperative shoulder function were compared with postoperative comfort, physical role function, and shoulder-specific function in 134 shoulders undergoing arthroplasty for degenerative joint disease. The strongest correlates with postoperative comfort included preoperative physical function, general health, and social function. The strongest correlates with postoperative physical role function included preoperative physical function and general health. The strongest correlates with postoperative shoulder function included male gender and preoperative physical function, shoulder function, social function, and mental health. The authors concluded that the overall well-being of the patient before surgery has a strong influence on the quality of the outcome after shoulder arthroplasty.

Although many approaches to the evaluation of shoulder arthroplasty have been proposed, simple functional self-assessments such as the SST and the SF-36 have several distinct advantages: (1) they are validated, (2) they reflect the status of the shoulder from the perspective of the patient, and (3) they lower the threshold for participation by patients and surgeons.

COMPLICATIONS

At the present time, complications associated with prosthetic devices or implants account for approximately 5% of the more than 3.5 million hospitalizations for musculoskeletal conditions.[292] This fact is interesting in light of the increasing patient population with permanent implants and the knowledge that the average age of patients undergoing total shoulder arthroplasty is the lowest of all major joint replacement groups.[277,293] Cofield and Edgerton have reviewed many of these complications in an instructional course lecture.[95]

Mirroring the increase in volume of total joint arthroplasties in general, the number of shoulder replacement

TABLE 16–25. Effectiveness of Total Arthroplasty or Hemiarthroplasty for Each of the Indicated Diagnoses

	DJD	2° DJD	RA	CTA	CA	AVN
Treatment	Total	Total	Total	Hemi	TSA	Hemi
Number of patients	87	20	11	14	6	4
Average follow-up (mo)	17	18	19	15	24	14
Physical role						
Preoperative average score	31	25	25	18	25	25
Postoperative average score	58	29	41	29	13	56
Comfort						
Preoperative average score	38	36	33	25	39	36
Postoperative average score	62	54	47	40	44	64
Sleep comfortably						
Preoperative average score	9	15	18	14	0	0
Postoperative average score	89	60	73	64	67	100
Comfort by side						
Preoperative average score	70	40	82	29	67	50
Postoperative average score	95	75	100	64	100	100
Wash opposite shoulder						
Preoperative average score	7	35	0	0	17	0
Postoperative average score	61	55	36	14	33	50
Hand behind head						
Preoperative average score	22	30	27	21	17	50
Postoperative average score	84	50	55	21	67	75
Tuck in shirt						
Preoperative average score	24	40	55	36	17	50
Postoperative average score	79	60	36	50	50	50
8 lb to shelf						
Preoperative average score	13	25	0	0	0	0
Postoperative average score	59	45	9	7	33	25
1 lb to shelf						
Preoperative average score	46	45	36	29	33	75
Postoperative average score	91	65	82	29	83	100
Coin to shelf						
Preoperative average score	55	50	27	36	33	75
Postoperative average score	92	70	91	29	83	75
Overhand toss						
Preoperative average score	5	15	0	7	0	0
Postoperative average score	44	25	18	14	33	0
Usual work						
Preoperative average score	36	45	36	21	67	25
Postoperative average score	71	40	64	14	67	75
Underhand toss						
Preoperative average score	52	45	27	36	33	25
Postoperative average score	72	55	55	29	50	75
Carry 20 lb						
Preoperative average score	62	60	45	43	33	50
Postoperative average score	82	60	73	36	67	75

AVN, avascular necrosis; CA, capsulorrhaphy arthropathy; CTA, cuff tear arthropathy; DJD, degenerative joint disease; RA, rheumatoid arthritis; TSA, total shoulder arthroplasty.

procedures has increased substantially in recent years. However, despite this growth, an annual average of less than 5000 total shoulder replacements was performed in the United States from 1990 to 1992, in contrast to 136,000 each for total hip and total knee arthroplasties over the same time period.[291] Although early and midrange follow-up studies of total shoulder arthroplasty have been encouraging, with good and excellent results in more than 90% of shoulders, widespread experience and long-term evaluations approaching that of lower extremity joint replacement are not presently available in the literature.*

A review of 43 series involving 1858 total shoulder arthroplasties reported over a 20-year period from 1975 to 1995 revealed a mean follow-up of only 3.5 years.† Additionally, less than 50% of these reports met the generally accepted, minimal 2-year follow-up criteria established by the peer review process. Of the 21 reports with a minimal follow-up of 2 years, only 5 studies (391 shoulders) had an average follow-up of 5 years or more.[22,54,58,234,407] It has been suggested that the duration of follow-up must be sufficient to allow assessment of all clinically relevant outcomes, including those that may occur long after the therapeutic intervention.[150] The use of an inappropriately short follow-up may fail to detect a potentially important difference in prosthetic survivorship or the long-term

*See references 6, 21, 22, 54, 85, 140, 186, 274, 275, 304.

†See references 14, 15, 21, 22, 48, 54, 58, 60, 78, 94, 97, 105, 109, 123, 127, 129, 135, 140, 160, 186, 220, 228, 234, 239, 245, 256, 270, 274-276, 301, 302, 313, 325, 329, 332-334, 357, 407, 422, 428.

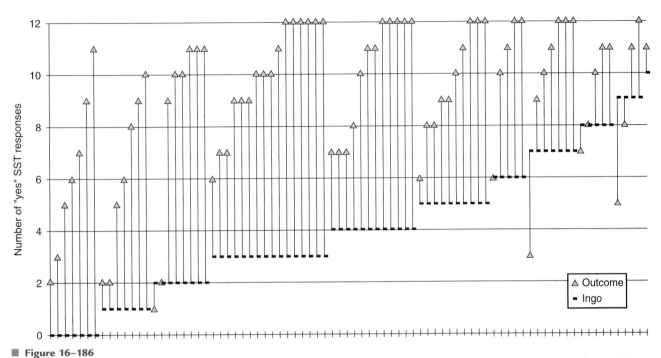

■ Figure 16–186
This Codman graph shows the efficacy of total shoulder arthroplasty (TSA) for 82 patients with glenohumeral degenerative joint disease (DJD) monitored for at least 1 year. The ordinate indicates the number of the 12 Simple Shoulder Test (SST) questions answered "yes." Each patient is represented by a *check mark* on the abscissa. The "ingo" for each patient is indicated by the *short horizontal line*. The outcome for each patient is indicated by the *arrow*. For each patient, efficacy is the height of the *vertical line* connecting the ingo to the outcome. The graph indicates that most but not all patients improved substantially after shoulder arthroplasty.

complication rate of various methods of treatments.[339] In the context of this concern, Neer and Kirby[301] stated in 1982 that an average follow-up of 3 years was not sufficient to assess many of the complications associated with total shoulder arthroplasty, and it is our opinion that this statement is just as relevant today. The fact that most shoulder arthroplasties are carried out by surgeons performing only one or two per year means that the results published are not indicative of the overall experience with this procedure and are likely to seriously underestimate the incidence of unsatisfactory results.[180]

Nonetheless, it is our purpose to review the most common problems associated with this procedure in the hope of providing a framework for understanding not only the rectifiable complications but also the failures in patients who have experienced an unfavorable outcome.

Complications of Constrained Total Shoulder Arthroplasty

Since the 1970s, several constrained total shoulder prostheses have been used for the treatment of various shoulder disorders. These implants include the Fenlin,[129,131] Bickel,[245] Stanmore,[97,105,239,313] Michael Reese,[329,332-334] Kölbel,[228] Kessel,[58] Laurence,[234] Zippel,[446] Liverpool,[40] trispherical,[161] and three different fixed-fulcrum prostheses designed by Neer and Averill.[298]

The development of these constrained shoulder prostheses resulted from the commonly held view that

glenohumeral instability would be a natural sequela of shoulders with ineffective, attenuated, or torn rotator cuffs. This incomplete understanding of shoulder kinematics led to a variety of nonanatomic shoulder arthroplasty devices that were designed with the twofold purpose of replacing the arthritic joint and restoring the joint stability that had presumably been lost as a result of rotator cuff pathology. It was also theorized that a prosthesis designed with an inherently stable fulcrum would permit the deltoid to elevate the humerus without assistance from the rotator cuff.[228,329,332-334]

The majority of constrained shoulder implants use a fixed-fulcrum or semifulcrum concentric ball-and-socket design. With the fixed-fulcrum implant, constraint is maximized by coupling of the humeral and scapular components, whereas the ball-and-socket prosthesis is somewhat less restricted. The basic structure of the latter design emulates a total hip prosthesis in that it provides simple static congruity and architectural stability. Unfortunately, the constrained nature of these devices in a joint that normally affords an almost unlimited range of motion results in a high incidence of complications. These complications occur as stress is transferred to the prosthesis-bone interface, and forces acting across the glenoid anchorage lead to loosening or mechanical failure.

Since their introduction, constrained total shoulder prostheses have met with limited success and have been associated with a uniformly high frequency of complications when compared with unconstrained implants. In a retrospective review of 314 constrained total shoulder arthroplasties reported in 10 series from 1975 through 1992, the overall incidence of complications was approximately 36% with limited follow-up in a number of reports (10-103).[58,97,105,129,228,234,239,245,313] In many cases, the length of follow-up was not specified or was less than 1 year. Only three reports established minimal 2-year follow-up criteria for inclusion in the respective study.[58,234,334] Over a similar study period, but with much longer follow-up, a review of 32 reports of unconstrained shoulder implants revealed a mean complication rate of only 16%.*

In an analysis of 296 constrained shoulder replacements described in seven reports, complications were numerous and included a 25% overall incidence of reoperations (range, 4% to 54%) that were mainly the result of the biomechanical considerations noted earlier.[58,105,228,234,239,245,333] More specifically, 82% of the complications were attributed to the following three factors in order of frequency: (1) mechanical loosening, (2) instability, and (3) implant failure secondary to plastic deformation, fracture, or dissociation of the components. Although these three factors were the most common problems noted in the literature, other complications such as sepsis,[105,239,313] neurovascular injury,[129,329] ankylosis,[234] and periprosthetic fracture[58,228,234,239,245,313,329,332,333] have also been described. In two studies, the number of failures was especially high, with a revision rate exceeding 50% of the total cases.[245,333] In 1979, Post and associates reported their early experience with a constrained shoulder prosthesis.[332] Eight years later in 1987, Post reported extended follow-up of the original series.[329] In this later report, 47 complications were noted in a series of 50 constrained total shoulder arthroplasties performed over a 13-year period. The majority of these complications were significant and included 10 broken or plastically deformed humeral components, 19 episodes of glenohumeral component instability, and 15 cases of mechanical loosening. Chronologically, implant failure was the most common initial complication, and the frequency of this problem increased from 33% to 48% with increasing follow-up (10-103). The problem of mechanical failure was addressed by altering two parameters: changing the implant material from stainless steel to a cobalt chrome alloy and improving the mechanical properties of the prosthesis by enlarging the humeral head and neck diameters. These implant modifications resulted in a substantial decrease in the rate of prosthetic failure, but at the cost of an increasing incidence of prosthetic dissociation and aseptic loosening. In fact, these two problems alone accounted for 85% of the complications reported by Post in a series and have also been noted by other investigators to be a frequent source of complications.[245,329]

Focusing briefly on these two problems, controlled dissociation of the glenoid and humeral components was actually part of the engineering rationale that was designed to protect the anchorage of the component by limiting the peak moments acting on the implant-bone interface. As the applied torque reaches a critical threshold (17 and 9 Nm for the Michael Reese and Kölbel pros-

theses, respectively), uncoupling of the glenoid and humeral components occurs. Unfortunately, this complication is rarely rectified without revision surgery to reduce the assembly. Regarding the other major complication, symptomatic aseptic loosening of the prosthesis posed difficulties at revision surgery because of loss of bone stock. Consequently, reoperations were often fraught with an even higher incidence of early loosening and ultimately resulted in resectional arthroplasty or arthrodesis of the glenohumeral joint. The generally poor results after reoperation for this complication led Post to conclude that a loose glenoid component could not be corrected by revision surgery.[329]

In conclusion, our review of the literature indicates that complications such as mechanical abutment, aseptic loosening, instability, and implant failure are disturbingly common in most constrained shoulder replacements and that reoperation rates are unacceptably high in many cases. An ever-expanding fundamental knowledge of shoulder anatomy and biomechanics suggests that these failures reflect not only an error in design rationale but also an underestimation of the forces involved in glenohumeral kinematics. Biomechanical studies by Inman and associates,[201] Poppen and Walker,[327,328] and Apreleva and colleagues[9] have determined that glenohumeral joint reactive forces approximate body weight during unrestricted active shoulder elevation. These compressive forces are greatly magnified with any additional load and increase linearly, with a maximum reached at 90 degrees of abduction. Clearly, the forces acting across the glenohumeral joint are impressive in magnitude and must be considered in the design of shoulder prostheses if untoward complications are to be avoided. To this end, further investigation of joint kinematics, prosthetic limitations, material properties, and survivorship data has influenced the evolution of constrained shoulder implants to more anatomically and physiologically unconstrained and semiconstrained prostheses. This same learning curve was observed with other joint replacement procedures in locations such as the knee and elbow, where constrained arthroplasties were similarly characterized by unacceptable failure rates.

At the present time, the indications for constrained total shoulder replacement surgery are exceedingly rare, and most investigators who have experience with this procedure reserve it strictly as a salvage operation. However, our analysis of the literature pertaining to constrained shoulder implants and the overwhelming number of complications associated with this type of prosthesis would lead us to question its efficacy even in this setting.

Complications of Unconstrained and Semiconstrained Total Shoulder Arthroplasty

Unconstrained and semiconstrained total shoulder arthroplasty has proved to be a highly successful procedure with good and excellent results in more than 90% of shoulders evaluated at early and midterm follow-up.†

---

*See references 48, 54, 58, 60, 78, 94, 109, 123, 127, 135, 140, 160, 161, 186, 220, 256, 270, 274-276, 301, 302, 313, 325, 357, 405, 407, 422, 428.

†See references 6, 21, 22, 54, 85, 140, 186, 274, 275, 304.

Despite this success, complications such as aseptic loosening, instability, limited implant longevity, sepsis, and periprosthetic fracture remain a concern, as it does for prosthetic arthroplasty in other major joints. According to Neer and associates,[304] four specific issues must be considered at the time of unconstrained shoulder replacement surgery if complications are to be minimized: (1) humeral head or glenoid bone deficiency, (2) a defective rotator cuff, (3) a deficient deltoid, and (4) chronic instability. Recognition of these variables along with careful patient selection, surgical precision, and a fundamental understanding of shoulder anatomy and kinematics will minimize the complications associated with this procedure.

Our review of the literature pertaining to total shoulder arthroplasty yielded 32 reports involving a total of 1615 shoulders.* These studies were published over a 19-year period from 1976 to 1995 and included at least 11 different unconstrained or semiconstrained prostheses. Even though various implants were used, the Neer prosthesis accounted for 70% of these devices.†

Although traditional unconstrained and semiconstrained shoulder replacement based on the Neer system has proved more than satisfactory, with numerous series reporting good and excellent results in most cases, the mean follow-up was only 42 months (range, 3 to 204 months), and 14 reports had less than a 2-year minimal follow-up. Furthermore, of the 18 reports that met the 2-year minimal evaluation period, only 8 series (432 shoulders) had a mean follow-up that exceeded 4 years.[15,22,78,97,135,186,301,302]

With that awareness of the potential shortcomings inherent in an analysis of complications associated with this duration of follow-up, our analysis revealed a mean overall complication rate of 16% (range, 0% to 62%) and included the following factors in order of frequency: component loosening, glenohumeral instability, rotator cuff tear, periprosthetic fracture, infection, implant failure including dissociation of modular prostheses, and deltoid weakness or dysfunction.[439]

Component Loosening

Although Péan is credited with performing the first artificial joint replacement of any type, it was not until after the independent pioneering work of McKee and Watson-Farrar[276] and Charnley[75] in the 1950s that total joint replacement was firmly established. Early complications associated with these devices centered around implant fixation. In 1960, Sir John Charnley suggested that the factors governing component loosening were by no means clearly understood.[74] Although problems related to component anchorage and progressive loosening were greatly improved by Charnley's introduction of polymethylmethacrylate, an incomplete understanding of aseptic loosening persists to the present day, and this complication remains a center of focus because of its ongoing threat to implant longevity.

Symptomatic loosening of glenoid and humeral components occurs with a combined incidence of 3.5% and is a major source of complications associated with total shoulder replacement surgery.‡ In fact, prosthetic loosening has the distinction of being the most common problem encountered in total shoulder arthroplasty, and it represents nearly a third of all complications.§ Most clinical and radiographic loosening involves failure of glenoid fixation, and this topic will occupy the central focus of the following discussion.

Kelleher and associates[217] pointed to the need for appropriate orientation of radiographs to evaluate the components in shoulder arthroplasty.

Glenoid Component Loosening

Glenoid component stability is determined by a complex interaction between intrinsic and extrinsic factors. Anatomic, biologic, and biomechanical factors are each critically important.

Multiple factors contribute to implant stability, including glenoid preparation, soft tissue balancing, wear debris, intercellular mediators of osteoclastic bone resorption, and the availability of glenoid bone stock for prosthetic fixation. Important extrinsic factors include prosthetic design considerations such as articular surface geometry, glenohumeral conformity, biomaterials, and the glenoid keel or peg morphology. In a report, Neer reviewed 46 total shoulder arthroplasties that had current radiographic evaluation and more than 10-year follow-up and found no evidence of clinical loosening.[298] Although clinical loosening of the glenoid is infrequent, radiolucent lines at the bone-cement interface of the glenoid component are common, with a frequency ranging from 30% to 96%.[21,22,58,85,186,220,304] As suggested by numerous authors,[94,98,139,298] this variation is partially attributed to nonstandardized methods of measurement, inconsistent definitions, and limitations of conventional radiography.

In 1982, Neer and associates[304] reported a 30% incidence of radiolucencies around the glenoid component in a series of 194 shoulders. More than 90% of these radiolucent lines were observed on the initial postoperative radiographs and were attributed to poor cementing technique. Six years later, an additional 214 implants were reviewed and found to have almost the same incidence of loosening, although the frequency of complete lines was much lower.[298] The authors emphasized that radiolucencies were not progressive during the period of follow-up and concluded that the clinical significance of these radiographic findings was unclear.

Offering a different perspective, other investigators have expressed concern that the appearance or progression of radiolucent zones may herald the onset of future problems related to symptomatic component loosening

---

*See references 14, 15, 21, 22, 48, 54, 58, 60, 78, 94, 109, 123, 127, 135, 140, 160, 186, 220, 256, 270, 274-276, 301, 302, 313, 325, 357, 405, 407, 422, 428.

†See references 14, 15, 21, 22, 48, 54, 60, 78, 123, 140, 186, 220, 274, 301, 302, 313, 325, 407, 428.

‡See references 8, 21, 54, 94, 140, 160, 186, 187, 270, 275, 276, 301, 313, 357, 387, 405, 407, 422, 428.

§See references 8, 14, 15, 21, 22, 48, 54, 58, 60, 78, 94, 109, 123, 127, 135, 140, 160, 186, 187, 220, 256, 270, 274-276, 301, 302, 313, 325, 357, 387, 405, 407, 422, 428.

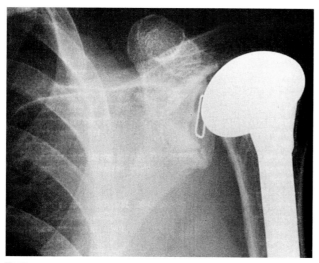

■ **Figure 16–187**

This anteroposterior radiograph shows a complete radiolucent line about the bone-cement interface of a glenoid component. This finding was present at the 6-month follow-up but showed no progression on several subsequent radiographic examinations. *(From Wirth MA and Rockwood CA: Complications of shoulder arthroplasty. Clin Orthop 307:47-69, 1994.)*

(Fig. 16–187).[12,21,58,85,94,186,216,407,430] A review of 350 shoulder replacements from five centers well known for their expertise in total shoulder arthroplasty revealed a 32% incidence (range, 10% to 96%) of progressive glenoid loosening.[21,48,58,85,186] One particular series from Sweden reported radiolucent zones around the glenoid component in 96% of 26 shoulders with a mean follow-up of 47 months.[58] Disconcertingly, no radiolucencies were observed around the glenoid component on immediate postoperative radiographs, but with increasing follow-up, this interval change had developed in 25 of 26 shoulders within 3 years after surgery. The development of these radiographic findings was associated with a slight decrease in function and a mild increase in pain.

In 1984, Cofield[85] reported improved shoulder motion and reliable pain relief in the majority of 73 Neer total shoulder arthroplasties with follow-up ranging from 2 to 6 years. Although the clinical results were excellent and compared favorably with other reports in the literature, 82% of the cases demonstrated radiolucencies at the bone-cement interface and 11% had radiographic evidence of component loosening. More recently, Torchia and associates[407] analyzed 89 total shoulder replacement arthroplasties that included extended evaluation of patients included in the original report. At a mean follow-up of 12 years (range, 5 to 17 years), 75 glenoid components (84%) had developed radiolucencies at the bone-cement interface and 39 glenoid implants (44%) demonstrated definite radiographic loosening as defined by a shift in component position or the presence of a complete bone-cement radiolucent line at least 1.5 mm in diameter. In a comparison of the original and recent reports, radiographic component loosening had increased fourfold according to established and consistently applied criteria over the extended study period. Even more concerning was the statistically significant association between radiographic glenoid

implant loosening and pain (P = .0001). With increasing duration of follow-up, the number of patients reporting satisfactory pain relief declined from 92% to 82%.

Concern about the prevalence of radiolucent lines around glenoid components and clinically apparent glenoid loosening has precipitated a host of recent investigations on the radiographic analysis of this problem. Lazarus and associates[235] reviewed the initial postoperative radiographs of 328 patients who underwent total shoulder arthroplasty for primary osteoarthritis. This series was composed of patients treated by 17 different surgeons and included 39 keeled components and 289 pegged components. A total of 308 glenoids (94%) demonstrated immediate postoperative radiolucencies. Incomplete seating of the glenoid was also common, particularly in patients with keeled components, and was frequently associated with an unsupported posterior rim. The most experienced surgeon had the best rate of optimal cementing and component seating.

Sperling and associates[388] reviewed 62 primary ingrowth total shoulder arthroplasties at a mean of 4.6 years after implantation to determine radiographic ingrowth of the prosthesis. A glenoid component was considered "at risk" when a complete lucent line, some part of which was at least 1.5 mm in width, surrounded the prosthesis or when migration or tilt of the prosthesis was detected. At-risk glenoids were present in 6.5% of cases and were not associated with any identifiable patient, disease, or surgical characteristics. Nagels and associates[289] examined radiolucencies around cemented glenoid components in 48 total shoulder arthroplasties with a mean follow-up of 5.3 years. Forty patients (83%) demonstrated radiolucencies in one or more areas. Progressive changes were observed predominantly at the inferior pole of the prosthesis. Thirteen glenoid components (27%) were loose, 5 of which showed progressive radiolucency and 8 demonstrated component shift. In five patients, additional analysis was performed with digital roentgen stereophotogrammetric analysis. After 3 years, loosening based on migration ranging from 1.2 to 5.5 mm developed in three of these five glenoids. In only one case of gross loosening did the standard radiographic signs of loosening corroborate the findings on stereophotogrammetric analysis. The authors concluded that traditional radiographs may underestimate the rate of early glenoid loosening because of the difficulty of obtaining standardized radiographs of the glenohumeral joint. Correlation of radiographic findings with clinical results was not undertaken in this study.

The present concerns of aseptic glenoid component loosening have led to a variety of new innovations, including cementless press-fitted, plasma-sprayed, and tissue ingrowth glenoid implants. The literature on this subject includes 150 cases from six series with an average follow-up of 3.5 years.[94,102,127,256,275,357] Deficiencies noted in many of these reports were incomplete radiographic review, insufficient follow-up, and inconsistent reporting methods; however, some of the preliminary data were encouraging and suggested a lower incidence of both radiolucencies and subsequent component loosening. Bonutti and associates[43] reported the use of arthroscopy to evaluate suspected glenoid loosening.

Wallace and associates[419] retrospectively compared the results of 58 total shoulder arthroplasties in which 32 cases involved a cemented glenoid component and 26 involved a cementless bone ingrowth prosthesis. The duration of follow-up ranged from 4 to 7 years. No significant differences could be detected between the groups with respect to pain, motion, shoulder function, or general health. Radiolucencies were noted in 41% of the cemented glenoids versus 23% of the uncemented glenoids. The proportion of glenoids classified as probably loose was three times greater in the cemented group. Eccentric wear of the posterior rim of the metal tray and focal osteolysis under the tray were seen in the bone ingrowth group, thus suggesting a potential for progression of radiographic loosening.

Boileau and associates[41] studied 40 shoulders with primary osteoarthritis that were prospectively randomized to receive either a cemented all-polyethylene glenoid component or a cementless metal-backed component. The presence of radiographic lucencies around the implants was significantly greater with polyethylene than with metal-backed glenoids (85% versus 25%, $P < 0.01$). Sixty percent of the radiolucent lines around cemented polyethylene components were present on immediate postoperative radiographs, and 25% were progressive but did not correlate with functional results. Periprosthetic radiolucencies were rare around metal-backed glenoids but, when present, were progressive. Loosening occurred in 20% of metal-backed cases and correlated with deteriorating functional results and increasing pain. Severe osteolysis was seen in these cases and was thought to stem from accelerated polyethylene wear caused by recurrent posterior humeral subluxation. Cavitary defects from this osteolysis precluded glenoid reimplantation at revision surgery. Based on this experience, the authors abandoned the use of metal-backed glenoids.

Although a number of different glenoid component designs were used in these studies, little published information specifically addresses the influence of glenoid morphology on implant stability. In 1988, Orr and colleagues used finite element analysis to examine several glenoid component design parameters.[311] The effect of keel geometry, metal backing, and superior constraints was assessed. The glenoid bone was modeled as a four-region homogeneous isotropic structure based on the material properties of the natural glenoid. For each of these regions, calculation of the yield strength, modulus of elasticity, and Poisson ratio was based on local bone density data from values in the literature. The authors concluded that keel geometry could be altered to approximate the stress distribution found in the natural glenoid to improve stability of the glenoid component. Anglin and associates[7] developed an experimental model to test glenoid loosening by cyclically subjecting components to superoinferior edge loading to mimic the rocking horse phenomenon thought to contribute to clinical glenoid loosening. Compression and distraction of the superior and inferior edges were measured with the humeral head displaced to each edge. The authors noted that a roughened fixation surface far outperformed a smooth fixation surface, curved backing showed almost half the distraction of flat backing, and

nonconstrained glenoids distracted less than more constrained glenoids.

Lacroix and associates[232] used finite element analysis to compare the cement layer stresses of keeled and pegged designs for modeled conditions of normal bone and rheumatoid arthritis bone. In normal bone, the 95% probability of cement survival was predicted to 94% of the cement mantle for the pegged prosthesis and 68% for the keeled prosthesis. In rheumatoid bone, however, the situation was reversed such that 86% of pegged prosthesis cement and 99% of keeled prosthesis cement had a greater than 95% survival probability. Bone stresses were affected little by the design. The authors concluded that a pegged glenoid is superior for normal bone whereas a keeled glenoid is superior for rheumatoid bone.

Murphy and colleagues[288] used finite element analysis to compare how cement stresses the effect of an anterior offset keel glenoid design and a conventional central keel design. The results predicted that the cement mantle in the offset keel design experiences less stress for the maximal joint load in abduction. The authors concluded that this design modification avoids contact between the keel and the cortical bone surface and that anterior placement of the keel situates it under the line of action of the resultant contact force in abduction.

Also in 1988, Fukuda and associates performed a biomechanical analysis of stability and fixation strength in four different glenoid designs: the Neer I, the Neer II (Kirschner Medical Corp, Fairlawn, NJ), the Cofield (Smith and Nephew Richards, Memphis, TN), and the Gristina (Howmedica, Inc., Rutherford, NJ) components.[146] The test results demonstrated less resistance to failure by pullout in a direction perpendicular to the face of the glenoid for the Neer-I high-density polyethylene glenoid that did not have a metal backing. The clinical significance of this finding is unclear, as suggested by Collins and associates, who proposed that glenoid component loosening resulted more often from eccentric or off-center compressive loads in contrast to a pullout mechanism of failure.[98] Furthermore, as suggested by Fukuda and colleagues, the fatigue testing did not consider the biologic stress shielding effect of metal-backed glenoid implants or the systemic response to metallic and polymeric wear debris.[146] Stone and associates[396] used finite element analysis to compare local stresses at the bone-implant interface of a cemented all-polyethylene glenoid and an uncemented metal-backed glenoid. The polyethylene component demonstrated a stress pattern that was closer to the intact glenoid. When the effects of concentric and eccentric loading conditions were compared, the subchondral bone stress magnitudes were substantially lower with the metal-backed component, thus suggesting that stress shielding may occur. High-stress regions were also found within the polyethylene near the interface with the metal backing.

In 1992, Friedman and associates studied the stress distributions of several glenoid component designs by two-dimensional finite element analysis.[144] It was hypothesized that adverse bone remodeling at the implant site would lead to aseptic loosening and that this loosening would be minimized by reproducing physiologic stress patterns across the natural glenoid. The analysis indicated that physiologic stresses were approximated when the subchondral bone was preserved.

The influence of fixation peg design on implant stability was evaluated by Giori and coworkers in a parametric study.[154] The parameters included the number and size of fixation pegs, as well as the aspect ratio (length/diameter). Five peg geometries of various shapes and sizes were tested for sheer stability. The results of the study suggested that components with multiple small pegs created a more uniform stress distribution in the anchoring material and provided more sheer stability per unit volume than did implants with fewer, but larger pegs.

Current concepts to enhance glenoid fixation and durability include preservation of the subchondral plate, concentric spherical reaming that ensures optimal bone support of the glenoid implant, diametral mismatching of the glenoid and humeral head to decrease eccentric loading, and the introduction of new glenoid designs and enhanced biomaterials.[98,200,379,441] Though theoretically and biomechanically sound, these concepts must remain as a focus of ongoing basic science and clinical research to determine whether this promising new technology will decrease the incidence of glenoid component failure.[437]

In addition to loosening, other mechanisms of glenoid failure also contribute to complications of total shoulder arthroplasty.[434] Gunther and associates[167] evaluated wear mechanisms contributing to failure of total shoulder glenoid components. Polyethylene glenoids were retrieved from 10 consecutive revision total shoulder replacements. The median time to revision was 4.3 years (range, 7 months to 16.5 years). Wear mechanisms were analyzed under low-power magnification, and a classification system was devised by grading the severity in four separate quadrants. The most prevalent damage modes were scratching (present in 90% of regions examined), abrasions (present in 68% of regions examined), pitting (present in 60% of regions examined), and delamination (present in 58% of regions examined). Component fracture was observed in four implants, and one component demonstrated complete wear through the polyethylene. The least prevalent modes of damage were deformation (present in 40% of regions examined), embedded debris (present in 28% of regions examined), and burnishing (present in 8% of regions examined). The inferior quadrant had the highest average damage score, but no significant differences were noted between any of the regions. The authors concluded that surface wear and subsurface fatigue were both contributory mechanisms of glenoid implant failure.

Scarlat and Matsen[374] reported on 39 retrieved glenoids. Among 19 cases with an available clinical history, the average time to retrieval was 2.5 years. Loosening was the most common cause for revision, and a history of instability was noted in more than a third of these cases. The articular surface contours of most of these components were altered by in vivo use, with obvious rim erosion in 28 glenoids, surface irregularities in 27 glenoids, fracture in 11 glenoids, and central wear in 9 glenoids. These observations suggest the potential for in vivo deformation of polyethylene, especially when the mechanics of arthroplasty are compromised. The authors concluded that the magnitude of contour alterations was sufficient to com-

promise the stability and smoothness of the prosthetic articulation.

Weldon and associates[426] investigated the effects of surface alterations on the intrinsic stability provided by the glenoid component. Intrinsic stability was determined by measuring the balance stability angles in 24 retrieved glenoids that demonstrated alterations in surface geometry from in vivo use. The balance stability angles of retrieved implants were often substantially reduced: 11 glenoids had diminished balance stability angles of 30% in at least one direction. The mean balance stability angle decrement in the most affected direction was 13.1 degrees (29.4%). In two thirds of retrieved components, the maximal decrement occurred along an oblique axis. The authors concluded that the changes in glenoid surface geometry from in vivo use may compromise the stability provided by the glenoid concavity.

Despite considerable success with total shoulder arthroplasty after the independent introduction of glenoid components by Kenmore,[221] Zippel,[445] and Neer[298] in the early 1970s, many problems remain unsolved (Fig. 16–188). An inability to resolve some of these issues and the apparent success with hemiarthroplasty have led some investigators to question the indications for glenoid resurfacing.[21,58,141,430]

In 1974, Neer[296] reviewed 47 shoulder hemiarthroplasties with an average follow-up of 6 years. Twelve patients were monitored for more than 10 years without evidence

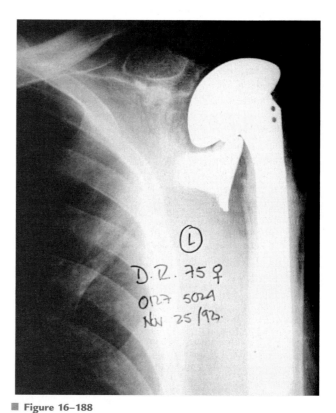

■ **Figure 16–188**

An anteroposterior radiograph made after the patient complained of acute worsening of symptoms that occurred when the shoulder "slipped out of place" while she was getting out of bed. Note the inferior dislocation of the metal-backed glenoid component. *(Adapted from Wirth MA and Rockwood CA: Complications of total shoulder replacement arthroplasty. J Bone Joint Surg Am 78:603-616, 1996.)*

of progressive degenerative changes or resorption of the glenoid fossae. Pain relief and functional recovery were the rule and led Neer to conclude that there was little reason to treat osteoarthritis with a more extensive replacement that might increase complications and jeopardize prosthetic longevity.

After Neer's report in 1974, several studies have documented good and excellent results with hemiprosthetic replacement of the shoulder, but only a few have compared the results of hemiarthroplasty with total shoulder arthroplasty in a similar patient population.[12,48,78,152,216,411] Interestingly, complications are less frequent with hemiarthroplasty of the shoulder, and statistically significant differences in overall pain relief, function, and patient satisfaction when compared with total shoulder arthroplasty have not been demonstrated.[12,22,48,78,84,216,220,411]

Several authors have described an association between symptomatic glenoid loosening, glenohumeral instability, and irreparable rotator cuff deficiencies.[21,98,141,186,325] These issues, in conjunction with the limited follow-up in most total shoulder arthroplasty series, the prevalence of osteolysis about the bone-cement interface of glenoid components, current knowledge pertaining to material properties in the pathogenesis of prosthetic loosening, and the association of symptomatic translation of the glenoid component with glenohumeral instability, lead us to conclude that the current indications for prosthetic glenoid arthroplasty need further refinement.

Glenoid Wear after Hemiarthroplasty

Cofield and Edgerton[95] pointed to the potential for medial migration and progressive glenoid wear after hemiarthroplasty. They pointed out that revision to total shoulder arthroplasty almost always resolved the process and symptoms. Levine and associates[241] reviewed glenoid surface wear in 31 hemiarthroplasties. Ten shoulders had primary osteoarthritis and 21 had secondary osteoarthritis. Glenoid surface wear was evaluated and classified as either type I, concentric (15 shoulders), or type II, nonconcentric (16 shoulders). Outcome correlated most significantly with the status of posterior glenoid wear. Patients with concentric, type I glenoids achieved 86% satisfactory results, whereas patients with nonconcentric, type II glenoids had only 63% satisfactory results. Although pain relief was similar in both groups, the unsatisfactory results were attributed to loss of forward elevation and external rotation in patients with type II glenoids. On the basis of these results, the authors concluded that hemiarthroplasty can be an effective treatment of both primary and secondary arthritis but should be reserved for patients with a concentric glenoid, which affords a better fulcrum for glenohumeral motion. Sperling and Cofield[387] noted glenoid erosion in 68% of 74 patients 50 years or younger who underwent hemiarthroplasty.

Rockwood and associates reported successful results with hemiarthroplasty in patients with osteoarthritis and rheumatoid arthritis.[24,204]

Humeral Component Loosening

Undeniably, difficulties with glenoid component fixation account for most complications related to aseptic loosening of total shoulder prostheses. In short- and mid-term follow-up studies, radiographic evaluation reveals a 5% incidence of implant subsidence or complete radiolucent lines measuring 2 mm or more about the humeral prosthesis.[21,48,54,85,91,304] Complete radiolucent lines were more frequently observed in uncemented humeral components, but clinical findings associated with loosening were rare and accounted for symptoms in less than 2% of patients.[21,22,48,54,58,91,304]

In a long-term series with a mean follow-up of 12 years, 49% of 81 press-fit humeral components had shifted in position.[407] Furthermore, 93% of the humeral prostheses that underwent a change in position also demonstrated radiolucent lines at the prosthesis-bone interface. In contrast, radiolucent lines were present in less than 50% of the 41 prostheses that did not reveal a change in position. Consistent with previous studies, only one of eight cemented humeral components developed a radiolucent line at the bone-cement interface, and none demonstrated a change in position.[21,54,94,140,160,276,357] As opposed to the statistically significant correlation between symptoms and loosening of the glenoid prosthesis, loosening of the humeral component was not associated with pain.

Sanchez-Sotelo and associates studied radiographic "at-risk" signs for humeral loosening in 43 cemented Neer II humeral components monitored for a mean of 6.6 years[372] and 72 press-fit Neer II humeral components monitored for a mean of 4.1 years.[373] A humeral component was judged to be radiographically at risk for clinical loosening when a radiolucent line 2 mm or greater was present in three or more zones or when tilt or subsidence was identified on sequential radiographs. Of the cemented components, none had undergone tilt or subsidence. Radiolucent lines greater than 2 mm were present in nine shoulders but were limited to two zones or less in all but one shoulder. The incidence, extent, and thickness of these radiolucent lines were significantly higher in total shoulder arthroplasty than hemiarthroplasty cases. Of the press-fit series, 40 components were judged to be at risk, and they tended to occur in patients with longer follow-up than in those without at-risk signs. Humeral components with at-risk lines had a higher rate of endosteal erosion and a greater number of zones with sclerosis. Subsidence and tilt occurred in 27 and 31 shoulders, respectively. The clinical outcomes in this series were not affected by the presence of at-risk radiographic lines.

Glenohumeral Instability

Glenohumeral instability after total shoulder arthroplasty is rarely discussed in the literature despite a frequency that varies between 0% and 35%* and the fact that it is the second leading cause of complications associated with prosthetic arthroplasty of this joint. From an extensive review of the literature, anterior, anterosuperior, or anteroinferior instability was found in 30 (43%) shoulders,† posterior instability in 14 (20%) shoulders,‡ inferior

---

*See references 22, 54, 78, 94, 160, 186, 270, 275, 276, 301, 313, 357, 407, 428.
†See references 22, 127, 160, 270, 275, 282, 301, 428, 440.
‡See references 12, 14, 21, 22, 54, 78, 94, 186, 301, 440.

instability in 3 (4%) shoulders,[140,301] multidirectional instability in 2 (4%) shoulders, and an unspecified direction of instability in 21 (30%) shoulders,[22,78,275,276,313,357,407] for an overall incidence of approximately 4%.

In normal glenohumeral joints, stability is provided by a hierarchy of mechanisms that labor in concert to ensure a virtually unlimited range of motion and uncompromised function. Small loads are offset by passive means such as joint surface architecture,[56,240,287] finite joint volume,[265] atmospheric pressure,[240,287,380] and the adhesion/cohesion of joint fluid.[381] Moderate loads are counterbalanced by the rotator cuff musculature, whose coordinated contractions resist displacing forces, and large loads are resisted by the capsulolabral structures and bone architecture.[265,375,380,409,421,440] Unfortunately, these complex interactions can become ineffective in shoulder arthroplasty, thus increasing the propensity for instability. This tendency increases the shoulder's dependence on precise soft tissue balancing and proper positioning of the prosthetic components to restore both the rotational and translational components of normal shoulder kinematics. Although the diagnosis of a fixed dislocation should be obvious when the triad of history, physical examination, and radiographic studies are properly applied, analysis of more subtle instability can be quite challenging when manifested as discomfort associated with a vague sense of shoulder dysfunction.

Anterior Instability

Anterior instability after shoulder replacement surgery is most commonly associated with subscapularis failure, glenoid anteversion, malrotation of the humeral component, or anterior deltoid dysfunction. Thirty shoulders with this complication were reported in the literature: 4 were managed expectantly with closed reduction and immobilization, 17 were treated by reoperation, and treatment was not specified for the remaining shoulders.[127,160,270,275,282,428,440]

In 1993, Moeckel and associates[282] described their findings and the results of reoperation in seven patients whose total shoulder arthroplasty had been complicated by anterior glenohumeral instability. At the time of surgery, all patients demonstrated disruption of the subscapularis tendon repair, and the tendon was mobilized and repaired. The anterior instability recurred in three shoulders (43%) but was successfully reconstructed with a secondary operative procedure in which a bone–Achilles tendon allograft was inserted as a static anterior restraint.

In our series, surgical exploration of three total shoulder arthroplasties with anterior instability revealed decreased retroversion of the humeral component (≤20 degrees) in all shoulders, disruption of the subscapularis in two shoulders, and erosion of the anterior glenoid in one shoulder.[440] One of these patients with a massive irreparable tear of the rotator cuff had previously undergone distal clavicle resection, coracoacromial ligament resection, and acromioplasty, which rendered the coracoacromial arch an incompetent restraint to anterior glenohumeral translation. Revision of these shoulders involved various techniques, including restoration of normal humeral component version, reconstruction of

the coracoacromial ligament, and transfer of the pectoralis major tendon.

Although inadequate retrotorsion of the humeral component may lead to increased anterior translation of the humeral head, clinically obvious anterior subluxation or dislocation will not usually occur unless the subscapularis is deficient or previous surgery has compromised the stabilizing effect of an intact coracoacromial arch. In our experience, disruption of the subscapularis repair is generally attributed to surgical technique, poor tissue quality, inappropriate physical therapy, or the use of oversized components. The use of thick metal-backed glenoid components or excessively large humeral head implants may dramatically increase the lateral humeral offset and thereby create an internal rotation contracture of the shoulder and stress the subscapularis repair during external rotation maneuvers.

Superior Instability

Progressive superior migration of the humeral head has been reported in association with dynamic muscle dysfunction, attenuation of the supraspinatus, failed rotator cuff repairs, and frank rupture of the rotator cuff.[21,48,50,85] In one series, major cuff tears were present in 20% of all patients and in 29% of patients with proximal migration. The amount of proximal humeral migration was independent of the size of the rotator cuff defect but correlated positively with the association of cuff deficiency and poor preoperative function.[50] Similarly, the series of Boyd and associates[48] noted proximal humeral migration in 29 (22%) of 131 total shoulder arthroplasties with an average follow-up of 44 months. Rotator cuff tears were present in only seven shoulders in this subgroup, thus suggesting that proximal migration may be secondary to an imbalance in the force couple between a strong deltoid and a weak, poorly rehabilitated rotator cuff.

Although superior migration of the humeral head is well recognized in the literature, it does not appear to be directly related to the development of shoulder discomfort or impending failure after hemiarthroplasty. In fact, Boyd and associates[48] noted no increased pain with proximal migration of the humeral head, and we have also made this observation. However, our concern is related to the loss of function and the potential complication of glenoid component loosening as a result of progressive superior humeral migration. In this setting, the humeral head articulates with the superior portion of the glenoid component and causes eccentric loading of the component and progressive loosening over time. This observation was reported by Barrett and colleagues,[21] who suggested that superior migration leads to eccentrically applied glenoid compressive forces, increased stress at the bone-cement interface, and eventual loosening of the glenoid component within the glenoid fossa. In 1988, Franklin and associates[139] reported an association between proximal humeral migration, incompletely reconstructible rotator cuff tears, and glenoid component loosening in seven cases of total shoulder arthroplasty. The amount of proximal humeral migration was closely correlated with the degree of glenoid loosening and superior tilting of the component. The translation of the glenoid component was referred to as a "rocking horse" glenoid, and the authors credited Gristina for first recognizing that eccentric loading would stress the glenoid anchorage.

From the preceding discussion of superior instability in conjunction with our experience during the past 20 years in performing humeral hemiarthroplasty for combined degenerative glenohumeral arthritis and irreparable rotator cuff tears, we can only conclude that humeral hemiarthroplasty is the procedure of choice for this condition.

Posterior Instability

Approximately 14 cases of posterior glenohumeral instability after total shoulder arthroplasty have been recorded in the literature.[14,21,54,78,94,186,301,304] This complication is frequently associated with increased retroversion of the glenoid component or excessive retroversion of the humeral prosthesis, posterior glenoid erosion, and soft tissue imbalance. Patients with long-standing arthritis of the glenohumeral joint usually demonstrate a characteristic wear pattern of the glenoid, and in most circumstances this wear pattern can be predicted by the disease process. For example, central glenoid erosion is the usual pattern of wear in rheumatoid arthritis, whereas posterior glenoid deficiency characterizes long-standing osteoarthritis. Failure to recognize posterior glenoid erosion may lead to placement of the glenoid component in excessive retroversion at the time of surgery, which can result in an increased propensity for posterior instability.[439] When the patient's physical examination demonstrates marked restriction of external rotation and the radiographic examination reveals posterior glenohumeral subluxation, the physician should be wary of uneven posterior glenoid wear. In this situation, CT of both shoulders will precisely define the degree of posterior glenoid deficiency and will greatly facilitate preoperative planning. In most situations, deficiencies of the posterior glenoid can be compensated by careful reaming of the anterior glenoid to normalize the glenoid version.[298,353] Occasionally, severe posterior glenoid deficiency will require bone grafting of the glenoid as described by Neer and Morrison.[302] However, glenoid grafting is technically difficult and the complication rate is high.

Patients who have posterior glenohumeral subluxation associated with long-standing osteoarthritis or a history of chronic posterior instability, whether recurrent or fixed, are at increased risk for posterior instability after shoulder replacement. Although proper placement of the humeral and glenoid components will minimize this tendency, avoidance of this complication is also critically dependent on soft tissue balancing. In most patients, the shoulder demonstrates restricted external rotation with a tight and contracted anterior soft tissue envelope. In contrast, the posterior capsule is stretched and its volume is greatly increased as a result of chronic and progressive posterior displacement of the humeral head. This combination of pathologic features is commonly seen in patients with capsulorrhaphy arthropathy, in whom surgically induced limitation in external rotation causes chronic posterior humeral subluxation. In such cases, the

posterior capsule may become attenuated and patulous. Careful inspection of the preoperative axillary lateral radiograph can alert the surgeon to the possibility of this pathologic constellation in patients with this diagnosis. Namba and Thornhill[290] described the use of posterior capsulorrhaphy for the management of intraoperative posterior instability.

The experience at the University of Texas Health Sciences Center at San Antonio regarding posterior glenohumeral instability after shoulder arthroplasty includes seven shoulders.[440,441] Objective findings in these shoulders included increased retroversion of the humeral component (≥80 degrees) in four shoulders, posterior glenoid erosion in four shoulders, and nonunion of the greater tuberosity (Fig. 16–189). These shoulders were revised by restoring normal retroversion of the humeral component, sculpting or reaming the glenoid to re-establish proper glenoid version, and performing posterior capsulorrhaphy to address the asymmetric soft tissue pathology.

Hill and Norris[192] reported on the results of bone grafting for restoration of glenoid volume and version at the time of shoulder arthroplasty. Posterior glenoid defects were treated by bone grafting in 12 patients, and the average correction in glenoid version amounted to 33 degrees. Failure to maintain correction was common and was associated with graft nonunion, dissolution, or shift. Steinmann and Cofield[394] reviewed 28 patients who underwent bone grafting for segmental glenoid wear as part of total shoulder arthroplasty. Autogenous humeral head grafts were used in 27 patients and fixed with 3.5-mm cortical lag screws in 25 patients. According to the Neer rating system, 13 shoulders were graded as excellent, 10 as satisfactory, and 5 as unsatisfactory. Symptomatic glenoid loosening developed in two patients and recurrent instability in two. Radiographic assessment revealed no glenoid lucencies in 13 patients, incomplete lucencies in 11, and complete lucencies in 4.

Inferior Instability

Inferior instability after shoulder arthroplasty usually occurs as a complication of treatment of acute proximal humeral fractures but has also been noted after total shoulder replacement in cases of prosthetic revision, chronic fractures, previous osteosynthesis, and uncomplicated rheumatoid arthritis or osteoarthritis.[127,140,141,304] Many of the patients with this complication demonstrate inadequate active motion and lack the ability to raise the arm above the horizontal plane because of shortening of the humerus, which renders the deltoid ineffective. Authors reporting this complication emphasize the importance of re-establishing anatomic humeral length, which in turn restores the resting tension of the deltoid and rotator cuff.[84,301,304] Such repair optimizes function by minimizing the tendency for inferior instability and subsequent weakness during elevation.

Rotator Cuff Tears

Postoperative tearing of the rotator cuff is the third most frequent complication of total shoulder arthroplasty,

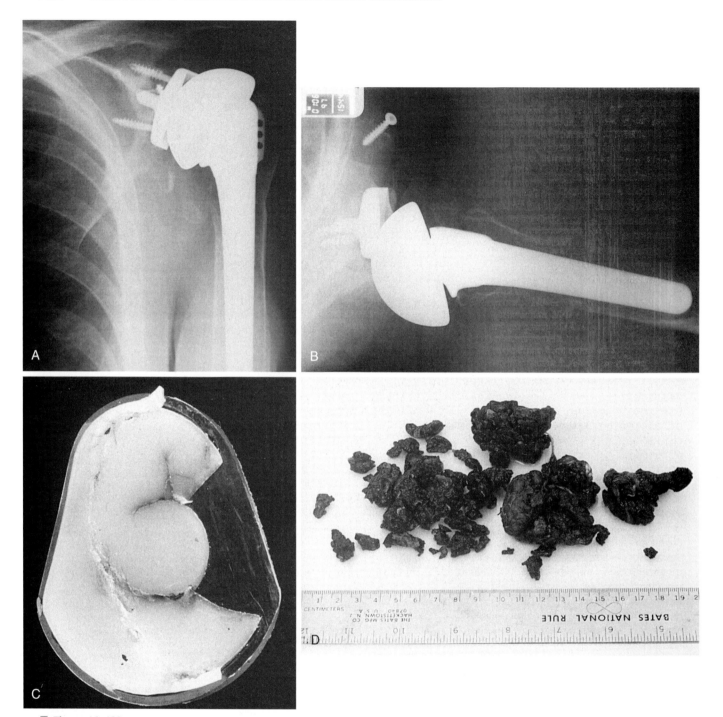

■ **Figure 16–189**
A, Anteroposterior radiograph of a 71-year-old man who had pain and a "mechanical clunk" with motion of the shoulder 2 years after surgery. Narrowing of the glenohumeral articulation suggests metal-on-metal contact. **B,** This axillary lateral radiograph shows posterior subluxation of the humeral head from the glenoid. **C,** At the time of revision surgery, performed 36 months after the primary arthroplasty, the glenoid component was loose. This photograph shows marked wear of the polyethylene insert, but the marked wear of the metal glenoid tray is not apparent. **D,** Metal-on-metal wear between the humeral head and the glenoid tray resulted in a proliferative metal synovial reaction. The volume of excised synovial tissue exceeded 240 cm³.

with an incidence of 2%. Although this entity is considered a common complication after shoulder replacement surgery, symptoms are usually minimal and reflect the natural history of cuff disease in the general population. A review of several large series suggests that both nonoperative and operative treatment has been used in the management of this complication; however, the benefits of

surgical intervention are somewhat unclear because recurrent tearing of the cuff and insignificant improvement in function and motion have been noted in several cases.[6,21,22,54,135,186,220,428]

In Neer and colleagues' 1982 report,[304] patients with massive rotator cuff deficiencies fared quite well after shoulder arthroplasty. This series included 2 paraplegic patients, 7 rheumatoid patients, and 10 patients with rotator cuff arthropathy whose shoulders were all graded as a successful result despite having massive rotator cuff tears. This experience led Neer to conclude that rotator cuff deficiency was not a contraindication to unconstrained total shoulder arthroplasty as advocates of constrained arthroplasty had suggested.

In our experience, most patients with symptoms suggesting a chronic rotator cuff tear will respond to expectant management consisting of an anti-inflammatory agent, moist heat, and a physician-directed rehabilitation program that emphasizes strengthening of the deltoid, the remaining rotator cuff, and the scapular stabilizing musculature. We reserve reoperation of postoperative rotator cuff tears for patients with persistent symptoms and for those with obvious functional deficits after acute trauma.

Sperling and associates[391] reviewed the use of specialized MRI to evaluate rotator cuff tears in patients with painful shoulder arthroplasties. Findings on imaging studies were correlated with those documented at the time of surgical revision. Full-thickness rotator cuff tears were present in 11 of 21 painful shoulder arthroplasties, 10 of which were predicted by MRI. Ten shoulders did not have a rotator cuff tear, and MRI correctly predicted its absence in 8 cases. The sensitivity in detecting a full-thickness rotator cuff tear based on this series was 91%, the specificity was 80%, the positive predictive value was 83% and the negative predictive value was 89%. The data from this preliminary study suggest that MRI may be a useful adjunct to clinical examination for determining the integrity of the rotator cuff when assessing and managing patients with a painful shoulder arthroplasty.

Periprosthetic Fractures

Although a prevalence of less than 2% might appear to be insignificant, periprosthetic shoulder fractures account for approximately 20% of all complications associated with total shoulder arthroplasty and often present difficult treatment challenges. We reviewed 14 reports describing 45 fractures of the glenoid or humerus associated with prosthetic replacement of the shoulder.* In several of these articles the mechanism of injury, subsequent management, and final outcome were either omitted or not discussed in detail, thus making analysis difficult. Nonetheless, we reviewed the results according to three parameters: the type of fracture, the temporal relationship of the fracture to surgery, and the clinical outcome. The clinical outcome was graded as satisfactory or unsatisfactory. A satisfactory rating was characterized by clinical and radiographic bony union, minimal to no symptoms, and the absence of associated complications such as component loosening. Our analysis revealed involvement of the humeral shaft or tuberosity in 86% of these injuries[14,21,48,139,186,220,275,313,407] and glenoid fractures in an additional 12% of cases.[186,220,274] The division of fracture complications into intraoperative and postoperative groups identified the former group as the most frequently

occurring, with an incidence of 62%. According to the clinical outcome parameters, 87% of the intraoperative fractures that were diagnosed and stabilized at the time of injury were graded as satisfactory. With regard to fractures occurring in the postoperative period, only 54% healed uneventfully with expectant management.

In 1989, Hawkins and associates[186] reported two humeral shaft fractures and two glenoid fractures in a series of 70 total shoulder arthroplasties, all of which were sustained intraoperatively. The humeral shaft fractures occurred in elderly patients with rheumatoid arthritis. Overzealous reaming, impaction of the humeral component, and excess torque placed on the humerus were all mentioned as mechanisms leading to fracture. The humeral shaft fractures were treated initially with cerclage wiring and postoperative immobilization, but both required reoperation. One was treated successfully with a long-stemmed revision humeral component, whereas the second was treated with compression plating. This last patient subsequently experienced a refracture distal to the plate, which was treated successfully with a humeral fracture brace.

Boyd and associates[49] reported seven patients who had a humeral fracture after either total shoulder arthroplasty or shoulder hemiarthroplasty. Trauma after a fall was the cause of fracture in six patients; and the final patient sustained the injury in a motor vehicle accident. Common to all injuries was a fracture pattern that involved the humeral shaft at the tip of the prosthesis. The initial treatment in four patients consisted of an Orthoplast or sugar tong splint, whereas two patients were initially immobilized with only a sling and swathe. Progressive loss of radial nerve function developed in both these patients and necessitated early operative intervention. Surgical management of the fractures consisted of open reduction and internal fixation with a dynamic compression plate in two patients and revision shoulder arthroplasty with a long-stemmed humeral component in three patients. All operatively treated fractures healed at an average of approximately 5 months after surgery. Of the two patients treated nonoperatively, nonunion developed in one, but further treatment was refused for medical reasons, and the other eventually required revision surgery unrelated to the humeral fracture. In the latter patient, the humeral fracture united with the tip of the prosthesis protruding outside the humeral shaft. Apparently, persistent symptoms were attributed to loosening of the glenoid component, and the humeral malunion was asymptomatic. In five of six patients the authors noted a decrease in shoulder motion from preinjury levels, but the extent of this decrease was unclear because information specifying the range of shoulder motion before injury was not available. In conclusion, Boyd and colleagues[49] emphasized several factors that influenced the natural history of fractures adjacent to humeral prostheses. These factors included the advanced age of many of the patients, osteopenia or poor bone quality, rheumatoid arthritis, and associated deficiencies of soft tissues. The authors also stressed that only one of seven fractures healed with immobilization alone, but the results of conservative fracture management could not be assessed in two patients because of the development of a radial nerve palsy that prompted subse-

*See references 6, 14, 21, 42, 48, 49, 127, 163, 186, 220, 274, 301, 313, 407.

quent operative intervention. Moreover, by admission of the investigators, these seven cases probably did not represent all of the periprosthetic fractures that occurred during the 15-year period of their study.

Wright and Cofield[444] presented a similar series of nine fractures that occurred at an average of 39 months after 499 arthroplasties with an average patient age of 70 years. The original indication for arthroplasty was either rheumatoid arthritis or old trauma. The authors concluded that long oblique and spiral fractures can be successfully treated nonoperatively if the alignment is acceptable. Operative treatment is considered for transverse or short oblique fractures at the level of the distal tip of the prosthesis or for those associated with a loose prosthesis. Autogenous bone grafting is recommended with all surgeries.

In 1994, we presented the results of treatment of fractures adjacent to humeral prostheses at the University of Texas Health Science Center at San Antonio.[163] The series consisted of 12 humeral fractures, 8 of which occurred as an intraoperative complication and 4 resulted from postoperative trauma. Of the eight intraoperative humeral fractures, six occurred during primary shoulder arthroplasty and two during revision procedures. In the primary arthroplasty group of six patients, fractures occurred during manipulation of the limb in two patients, reaming of the intramedullary canal in one patient, broaching of the canal in one patient, and insertion of the prosthesis in two patients. In the revision arthroplasty cases, both fractures occurred in areas of moderate to severe cortical thinning. Intraoperative fractures were managed by open reduction and internal fixation with simple cerclage wiring or by a long-stemmed prosthesis in conjunction with cerclage wiring (Fig. 16–190). All intraoperative fractures healed at an average of 8 weeks, with mean forward elevation of 122 degrees at final follow-up.

Four postoperative fractures occurred an average of 14 months after the index arthroplasty. All these injuries were managed with a fracture orthosis, and bone union was achieved at an average of 9 weeks after injury. At final evaluation, the average forward elevation was 121 degrees.

Treatment of periprosthetic shoulder fractures is divided into two seemingly divergent schools of thought. Bonutti and Hawkins[42] advocated aggressive treatment of these injuries, which included open reduction and internal fixation, bone grafting, and postoperative immobilization in a spica cast for a minimum of 6 weeks. Similarly, Boyd and associates[49] reported an increased likelihood of nonunion after nonoperative treatment and suggested that fractures treated operatively would fare better.

Campbell and coworkers[69] retrospectively reviewed 21 periprosthetic humeral fractures in 20 patients. Osteopenia was present in all patients and was graded as severe in 30%. For fractures proximal to the metaphysis, intramedullary fixation using the standard humeral stem and cerclage wiring provided superior results in terms of time to union, rehabilitation, and complication rate. Diaphyseal fractures that were treated by standard-stem arthroplasty with or without supplemental fixation had a longer time to union and a higher complication rate. Long-stem intramedullary fixation with cerclage wiring

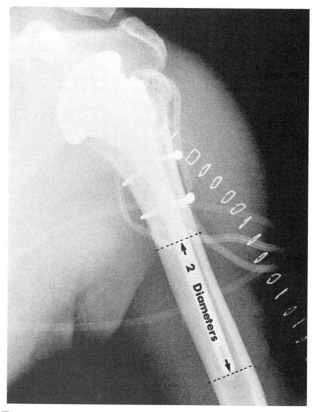

■ **Figure 16–190**

Anteroposterior radiograph demonstrating cerclage wire stabilization of a periprosthetic proximal humeral fracture. Note that the humeral stem bypasses the distal extent of the fracture by approximately two cortical diameters.

was thought to be the preferred treatment of unstable humeral shaft fractures. Cast or brace immobilization was effective for fractures distal to a stable prosthetic stem, but immobilization led to an increased risk of complications and prolonged rehabilitation.

Although one would expect uniform treatment guidelines based on the 11 patients in the reports of Bonutti and Hawkins[42] and Boyd and associates,[49] the results of the San Antonio experience involving 12 patients suggest an alternative and perhaps more conservative approach to the management of postoperative periprosthetic fractures. Of note, three patients in our series with fractures that extended distal to the tip of the prosthesis were managed with a fracture orthosis, and these fractures healed uneventfully. In all, five fractures that progressed to bone union were managed with an Orthoplast fracture brace, isometric exercises, and early range-of-motion rehabilitation. Our approach to intraoperative fractures was more aggressive because most of these injuries were treated by open reduction and internal fixation. Four intraoperative fractures were also managed by replacing the primary prosthesis with a long-stemmed revision component. Bone union was achieved in all cases without supplemental bone grafting or postoperative shoulder spica immobilization.

Although a meaningful comparison of various treatment modalities is difficult because of the few reported cases, we prefer to manage all intraoperative fractures by whatever means necessary to obtain a stable surgical construct. The purpose of this treatment is to restore stability to the limb, create an environment that is favorable to fracture healing, and allow unimpeded postoperative rehabilitation so that the functional result is not compromised by prolonged immobilization.

Intraoperative Periprosthetic Fractures

For the most part, intraoperative fractures of the humerus or glenoid arise from errors in surgical technique, many of which are avoidable. These surgical errors include inadvertent reaming, overzealous impaction, or manipulation of the upper extremity during exposure of the glenoid. Several points deserve emphasis.[42,49,163,186] First, spiral fractures of the humerus are usually observed when the shoulder is externally rotated by using the upper extremity as a lever arm. This maneuver places the humerus at risk for fracture because of the magnitude of torsional stress generated. The torsional force imparted to the humerus can be minimized by performing a complete anterior and inferior capsular release and by using a bone hook on the humeral neck to deliver the proximal end of the humerus out of the glenoid fossa. Occasionally, exposure is still less than optimal; however, it can be improved by continuing the inferior soft tissue release to the posteroinferior and posterior capsular structures. One must pay meticulous attention to detail while releasing the capsule from the glenoid in this region of the glenohumeral joint because of the close proximity of the axillary nerve as it passes through the quadrangular space. Second, if the arm is not extended off the side of the operating table, it is difficult to insert the trial prosthesis or medullary reamers, and perforation or complete fracture of the proximal part of the humerus may result. Third, after resection of the humeral head, the entry point of the trial stem or reamer should be superolateral in an eccentric location on the cancellous surface of the proximal end of the humerus. Such an entry point ensures that the trial stem or reamer will pass directly down into the medullary canal rather than medially, where it may perforate the humeral neck or medial cortex. Finally, hand reaming is preferred to power instrumentation because the latter may remove too much cancellous bone or increase the likelihood of perforating osteoporotic bone.

If an intraoperative fracture occurs, we have been pleased with the results of cerclage wiring and the use of a long-stemmed prosthesis if the situation warrants. For humeral fractures occurring proximal to the tip of the humeral prosthesis, simple cerclage wiring of the proximal end of the humerus and implantation of a standard-sized prosthesis is appropriate. Autogenous bone graft from the humeral head is used to make a slurry of cancellous bone, which is placed into the metaphyseal portion of the proximal end of the humerus after the stem of the prosthesis is inserted to the level of the metaphyseal-diaphyseal junction. The trial prosthesis is then used in a piston fashion to work the slurry of autogenous bone into the fracture site or other areas of bone deficiency before placing the final prosthesis. For fractures occurring entirely distal to the prosthesis or those occurring in the proximal portion of the humerus with distal extension beyond the tip of the prosthesis, we prefer to use a long-stemmed prosthesis that extends at least two humeral cortical diameters beyond the most distal extent of the fracture. Such treatment is accomplished by extending the deltopectoral incision into an extensile anterolateral approach to the humerus. The relatively straight, cylindrical anatomy of the humeral diaphysis is ideal for this method of intramedullary fracture fixation. This form of treatment has several advantages over dynamic compression plating or cerclage wiring alone. First, the need for secure screw purchase in bone, which is often of poor quality, is obviated. Second, bending and torsional loads are better tolerated and decrease the risk of implant failure. Third, a rigid and biomechanically sound surgical construct is usually ensured. Fourth, the extensile exposure and soft tissue dissection needed for plate fixation is avoided. Finally, the ever-present concern for stress shielding is minimized.

With regard to glenoid fractures, it is important to remember that stability of the glenoid component is affected by glenoid preparation, soft tissue balancing, and the availability of uncompromised glenoid bone stock for prosthetic fixation.[435] Scapular fractures adjacent to glenoid components may compromise implant stability and lead to symptomatic loosening. Bone grafting or revision glenoid components that are built up with a wedge to accommodate the defect can be used; however, if bone support cannot be ensured, resurfacing of the glenoid should not be performed. In this situation, the remaining glenoid is sculpted with a hand bur or glenoid reamer to match the radius of curvature of the head of the humeral component, and the glenoid component is omitted.

Postoperative Periprosthetic Fractures

As a rule of thumb, our initial approach to the management of postoperative periprosthetic fractures of the shoulder is more conservative than the usual methods of treatment recommended for similar fractures that occur during surgery. If a trial of expectant management is not contraindicated by the development of radial nerve palsy or another ominous complication, one can proceed with a simple regimen consisting of an Orthoplast fracture brace, isometric exercises for the entire upper extremity, and early motion as the pain and swelling subside. In our experience at the University of Texas Health Science Center at San Antonio, satisfactory results are often achieved with this simple form of initial treatment. However, it cannot be overemphasized that one must do what is necessary to ensure that early functional rehabilitation is not delayed because prolonged immobilization has been associated with poor results in our experience.

Infection

Infection after total shoulder arthroplasty is a rare, but potentially devastating complication with a prevalence of about 1%.[376] The unique predilection for bacterial seeding of endoprostheses is the result of several factors, including bacterial adhesion, glycoprotein encapsulation, bacterial resistance to antibiotics, physical properties of the implant such as chemical composition and surface texture, and inhibiting factors from ion elution. Of 39 cases reported in the literature, 18 had a mean interval of 17 months from the initial arthroplasty to the diagnosis of shoulder sepsis; 10 were classified as late infections and 6 as early infections, without specifying the exact time of occurrence.* In three shoulders the time of occurrence was not mentioned at all, thus making it impossible to determine the temporal relationship of the infection to the index arthroplasty.[94,276,357] In three reports,[81,108,243] the interval from the initial arthroplasty to the diagnosis of glenohumeral sepsis often exceeded a period of 12 months. An increased susceptibility to infection was correlated with host risk factors such as diabetes mellitus, rheumatoid arthritis, systemic lupus erythematosus, and remote sites of infection. Additionally, immunosuppressive chemotherapy, systemic corticosteroids, multiple steroid injections, and previous shoulder surgery were noted in 66% of patients from the combined series.[81,108,243] Though only speculation, the apparent increased risk of infection after local steroid injections may be attributed to the unique bursal anatomy of the shoulder. Inadvertent or purposeful injection of the subdeltoid, subscapular, or infraspinatus bursae or the sheath of the long head of the tendon of the biceps may provide an avenue for intra-articular bacterial invasion.

The value of preoperative laboratory tests (i.e., WBC count, erythrocyte sedimentation rate, and C-reactive protein), radioisotope scanning, and joint aspiration was difficult to ascertain because of rare and inconsistent reporting methods. Eighteen patients with infected shoulder arthroplasties from the series of Codd and associates[81] and 5 patients with septic shoulder arthroplasties treated at the University of Texas were combined for the purpose of analysis. Laboratory values for the preoperative erythrocyte sedimentation rate and WBC count averaged 55 mm/hr and 11,260/mm³, respectively. Radioisotope scans were interpreted as positive in 58% of shoulders, and positive joint aspiration cultures were found in only 38% of shoulders.

A review of 39 infected shoulder arthroplasties reported in the literature revealed *S. aureus* as the etiologic organism in 3 shoulders and *Candida parapsilosis* in 1 shoulder.* In the remaining shoulders, the infectious organism was not identified in the report. Our experience with five infected shoulder arthroplasties revealed *S. aureus* in three shoulders, *Staphylococcus epidermidis* in one shoulder, and a mixed infection in one shoulder.

As with other joint replacement surgery, infections can occur early or late, and optimal treatment depends on isolation of the pathogen through tissue or fluid specimens. Once the diagnosis has been made, several treatment options exist, including antibiotic suppression, irrigation and débridement, reimplantation, resectional arthroplasty, arthrodesis, and amputation. The type of treatment depends on a host of factors, including the time interval from arthroplasty to the diagnosis of sepsis, the feasibility of implant removal as dictated by anesthetic risk, the pathogen's virulence and susceptibility to antibiotics, and implant stability.

The differential diagnosis of a draining wound in the early postoperative period after shoulder replacement surgery must include early infection despite negative cultures and a lack of obvious constitutional symptoms. In this scenario, we advocate early wound exploration with irrigation, débridement, and the judicious use of parenteral antibiotics. The prosthesis is retained if the infection is secondary to a gram-positive organism and the components are stable. For early infections with gram-negative organisms or late deep wound infections, we are currently advising thorough débridement of granulation tissue and scar and removal of all biomaterials, including cement, followed by a 6-week course of parenteral antibiotics as advised by infectious disease consultation. The majority of infected shoulder implants that we have treated are managed with resectional arthroplasty; however, other modes of treatment can be used, such as glenohumeral arthrodesis or two-stage revision arthroplasty.

In one report, 18 infected shoulder arthroplasties were managed by resectional arthroplasty in 5 shoulders and endoprosthetic reimplantation with the use of antibiotic-impregnated cement in 13 shoulders.[81] In the latter group, eight components were revised with a one-stage reimplantation, and five were managed by reimplantation at a second operation. Pain decreased in most patients; however, interestingly, the degree of pain relief was not significantly different in patients undergoing reimplantation and those with resectional arthroplasty alone. Not surprisingly, functional results in terms of range of motion and the ability to perform activities of daily living were much better in the reimplantation group. For this reason, it is important to convey to patients that resectional arthroplasty of the shoulder is a salvage procedure that at best, allows patients to achieve acceptable pain relief, the ability to perform simple activities of daily living, and resolution of their infection.

Sperling and associates[390] reviewed 26 primary and 8 revision shoulder arthroplasties in which deep periprosthetic infection was diagnosed at an average of 3.5 years after arthroplasty. Twenty-one shoulders underwent resection arthroplasty, 6 of which had additional episodes of infection. Six shoulders were treated by extensive joint débridement and retention of the prosthesis, but reinfection developed in three, and resection arthroplasty was eventually required. Three shoulders underwent delayed reimplantation, with no recurrence of infection. The authors concluded that delayed reimplantation may offer the best hope of eradication of infection and maintenance of shoulder function. Seitz and Damacen[377] studied eight patients with shoulder sepsis who underwent staged exchange arthroplasty using antibiotic-impregnated methylmethacrylate spacers shaped and fitted to the patient's anatomy after extensive débridement of the joint. Intravenous antibiotic therapy followed for a minimum of 3 months. At the end of 6 months, patients were evaluated for clinical and laboratory signs of infection, and none were encountered. Exchange prosthetic reconstructions using standard implants fixed with antibiotic-impregnated cement were then performed. All patients experienced improvement in pain, but overhead function was limited. Based on the success

---

*See references 58, 81, 94, 127, 135, 160, 243, 270, 275, 301, 313, 357, 407.

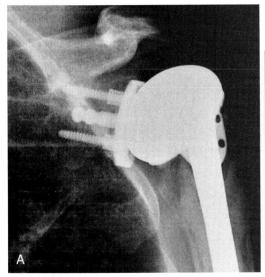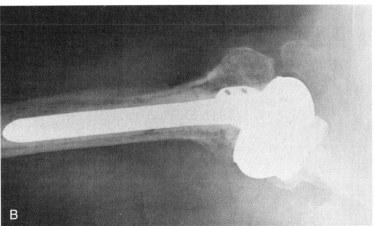

■ **Figure 16–191**

A and **B,** Radiographs of a patient who sustained a posterior shoulder dislocation that was complicated by dissociation of the polyethylene glenoid insert. Narrowing of the glenohumeral articulation suggests metal-on-metal contact.

of infection eradication, the authors concluded that the technique represented a satisfactory salvage option for managing glenohumeral sepsis after shoulder arthroplasty.

Although the literature is somewhat limited, several reports substantiate infection about a joint replacement from transient bacteremia secondary to dental manipulation, urinary tract infection, pneumonia, and genitourinary instrumentation.[1,305,395,397] Because of the variety of possibilities leading to secondary infection, we advocate prophylactic antimicrobial coverage individualized to each clinical situation.

Nerve Injuries

Approximately 14 cases of peripheral nerve or brachial plexus complications associated with total shoulder arthroplasty have been recorded in the literature.* Fortunately, most of these injuries involved neurapraxia and were managed expectantly with good results. However, in two cases, the mechanism of neural injury involved a laceration of the axillary nerve that occurred in heavily scarred surgical fields.[84] Although the majority of these complications involve the axillary nerve (six cases), injuries to the ulnar nerve (three cases), musculocutaneous nerve (two cases), median nerve (one case), and brachial plexus (two cases) have also been reported. Seven of these injuries resolved completely, two exhibited incomplete recovery, and one demonstrated no recovery. The recovery status of the remaining four neurologic injuries was not mentioned.

Lynch and associates[251] reported on 18 shoulders with neurologic deficits out of 417 arthroplasties. Thirteen shoulders had injuries involving the brachial plexus, usually the upper and middle trunks. Eleven shoulders

recovered well at 1 year. In most cases, traction was thought to be the cause of the injury.

Implant-Related Complications

Occasionally, shoulder replacement surgery is complicated by the development of implant-related failure. From our analysis of the literature we conclude that the prevalence of this complication is approximately 0.7%, and 80% of these failures have been observed in uncemented metal-backed glenoid components. Dissociation of the polyethylene glenoid insert from its metal tray,[94,120,275] fracture of the keel or metal glenoid backing,[94,120,256] fractured fixation screws,[256,275] and subluxation or dislocation of polyethylene subacromial spacers[54,78] have all been reported (Fig. 16–191).

Since their introduction in the late 1980s, modular total shoulder arthroplasty systems have been widely accepted for their ability to optimize soft tissue balancing, maximize proximal humeral metaphyseal and canal fit, facilitate glenoid revision, and permit conversion of hemiarthroplasty to total shoulder arthroplasty. Although some complications of total shoulder replacement surgery have been decreased by changes in prosthetic design, improved component fixation, and the evolution of biomaterials, new problems have arisen that are unique to modular shoulder implants. In 1991, Cooper and Brems[101] described a case report of a patient with recurrent dissociation of a modular humeral component that was ultimately revised to a Neer II humeral component. In addition to this case report and another case that was referred to our institution, we are aware of 11 cases of dissociation of the humeral component.[33] With the exception of one episode, all dissociations occurred within 6 weeks of the index arthroplasty procedure. Unlike previous case reports involving disassembly of modular femoral components used in the hip, none of the shoulder component dissociations were associated with joint

*See references 14, 21, 48, 135, 140, 160, 221, 274, 325, 407.

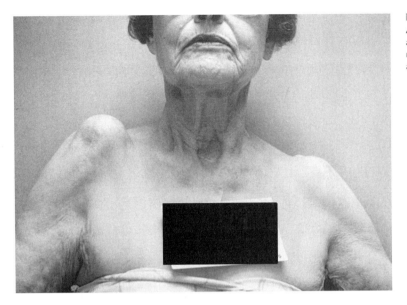

■ **Figure 16–192**

Appearance of the shoulder of a patient with loss of the anterior deltoid attachment after total shoulder replacement surgery. Note the anterior shoulder atrophy and the prominent humeral component.

dislocation or subsequent reduction maneuvers.[320,442] In fact, several of the patients in the report of Blevins and colleagues[38] were uncertain when the dissociation occurred. Similarly, our patient was unaware of a specific event that correlated with disassembly of the humeral prosthesis but had noted discomfort associated with shoulder dysfunction since the time of surgery. At the time of revision surgery, the posterior aspect of the humeral collar was subsided in the metaphyseal bone of the proximal end of the humerus and most likely precluded adequate seating of the Morse taper components during the initial arthroplasty procedure.

In the laboratory setting, biomechanical studies of Cooper and Brems[101] and Blevins and colleagues[38] have demonstrated that as little as 0.4 mL of water, saline, or blood may be enough to prevent locking of the Morse taper. To minimize such complications, the Morse taper socket of the modular prosthesis must be thoroughly free of tissue or fluids that would preclude an adequate weld of the Morse taper fixation. Additionally, it is imperative to recognize soft tissue or bone encroachment that might become interposed between the humeral head and the collar.

Deltoid Dysfunction

The technique of prosthetic replacement of the shoulder joint requires great familiarity with the anatomy and biomechanics of the shoulder. Critical to the final outcome of this procedure is maintenance of the deltoid origin and insertion because loss of the deltoid through a failed repair or injury to the axillary nerve results in a catastrophic loss of shoulder function.[15,108,165,301,304,428] Although optimal exposure is key to the ease at which total shoulder arthroplasty is accomplished, it is equally important to realize that the procedure can be performed through an extended deltopectoral approach without detaching the origin or insertion of the deltoid muscle.[350]

In Neer and colleagues' 1982 series of total shoulder replacements, three different surgical exposures were used.[304] Initially, a short deltopectoral approach was used that involved detachment of the anterior deltoid from the clavicle. The second approach was more superior and involved detachment of the middle deltoid, but both these exposures were discontinued because they were found to weaken the anterior and middle portions of the deltoid, respectively. The third approach, which Neer has advocated since 1977, entails a long deltopectoral interval and preserves the origin and insertion of the deltoid. Maintenance of the deltoid in this fashion facilitates early postoperative rehabilitation and minimizes the problems associated with the first two operative exposures. In 1982, Neer and Kirby included deltoid detachment as a major cause of failed unconstrained shoulder arthroplasty (Fig. 16–192).[301] These authors observed consistent weakening and atrophy of the deltoid in all except 3 of 37 patients. Fibrotic and ischemic changes in the anterior deltoid were presumably the result of overzealous retraction in most cases, whereas previous surgical approaches denervated the anterior deltoid in five patients. Overall, severe compromise of deltoid function was observed in 92% of failed unconstrained total shoulder and humeral head arthroplasties.

One of us (C.A.R.) has treated 36 patients who experienced postoperative loss of deltoid muscle function after shoulder operations, including endoprosthetic replacement procedures.[325] Nine of these replacement procedures were primary operations, and three were revision procedures. Of these 12 patients, 10 lost function of the anterior or anterior and middle deltoid secondary to a failed repair, and 2 lost complete function of the deltoid as a result of axillary nerve denervation. Patients were evaluated by using a standardized evaluation form proposed by the American Shoulder and Elbow Surgeons that independently documents the patient's pain, range of motion, strength, stability, and function. All patients were significantly disabled with a mean forward elevation of only 33 degrees (range of 0 to 75 degrees). Additionally, several patients demonstrated painful anterosuperior dislocation of the glenohumeral joint with attempted elevation of the upper extremity. Functional limitations were severe, with nine poor and three fair results based on 15 activities of daily living. Without question, loss of deltoid function because of denervation or detachment was poorly tolerated and resulted in pain and functional impairment.[165]

Revision Shoulder Arthroplasty

The number of shoulder replacement procedures performed in the United States has increased substantially in the past decade. Although widespread use of unconstrained total shoulder prosthetic designs has resulted in a marked decrease in complications, difficulties requiring reoperation are not uncommon. In a review of 22 shoulder arthroplasty series that reported this complication, the frequency of reoperation was 7%.* Although many of these operations consisted of soft tissue procedures for postoperative complications such as rotator cuff tears and glenohumeral instability, approximately 46% involved removal or revision of prosthetic components. A stratification of the latter two subgroups revealed revision of the glenoid, humeral, or both components in 16 shoulders, glenohumeral resectional arthroplasty in 10 shoulders, resection of the glenoid component in 7 shoulders, and glenohumeral arthrodesis in 4 shoulders. The treatment of several shoulders in these subgroups was not specified.

One of the greatest drawbacks in the surgical management of failed total shoulder prostheses is underestimating the technical demands and substantial complications that may occur with revision surgery of this magnitude. The literature reflects revision rates of 0% to 17% after shoulder arthroplasty, but publications that specifically address revision shoulder surgery are rare.

In 1982, Neer and Kirby[301] published a report on a series of 40 revision arthroplasties performed over a 9-year period. The index procedures included 31 hemiarthroplasties, 6 unconstrained total shoulder arthroplasties, and 3 constrained total shoulder replacements. The authors analyzed the index procedures and categorically assigned the causes of failure to one of three major groups: (1) general preoperative considerations such as neuromuscular problems, infection, or arthritis of adjacent joints; (2) surgical or prosthetic complications, including deltoid detachment, tuberosity nonunion, and component loosening or breakage; and (3) postoperative considerations such as residual or recurrent instability and inadequate rehabilitation. More than one cause of failure was noted in almost every case.

According to Neer and Kirby, the most common causes of failure included deltoid scarring and detachment, loss of external rotation as a result of contracture of the subscapularis, prominence or retraction of the greater tuberosity, glenoid insufficiency, and inadequate postoperative rehabilitation.[301] The common denominator in all failed hemiarthroplasties and unconstrained total shoulder replacements was adhesions of the rotator cuff and

deltoid that occurred as a result of prolonged immobilization. Revision surgery consisted of unconstrained total shoulder replacement in 32 shoulders, glenohumeral arthrodesis in 3 shoulders, a fixed-fulcrum constrained implant in 1 shoulder, and resectional arthroplasty and scar débridement in 2 shoulders each. It is important to emphasize that more than 80% of these revisions involved prostheses that had originally been inserted for displaced fractures and fracture-dislocations of the proximal end of the humerus. The degree of surgical difficulty in revision surgery was greatly magnified by contracture and muscle scarring, associated tuberosity malunion or nonunion, and bone loss with shortening of the humeral shaft. The results of the majority of these revisions were reported in another series and were found to be inferior to those of other diagnostic groups, thus prompting the authors to stress the importance of a successful primary procedure.[304]

In 1993, Caldwell and associates[68] reviewed 13 revision arthroplasties with an average follow-up of 36 months. Two total shoulder replacements and one hemiarthroplasty were revised for glenohumeral instability. Seven hemiarthroplasties were revised to total shoulder replacements secondary to glenoid arthropathy, and three total shoulder arthroplasties were revised because of loosening of the glenoid component. The results were considered satisfactory in only 62% of the cases, and five shoulders required seven reoperations. Glenoid loosening and incorrect version were regarded as the most frequent causes of revision surgery.

Wirth and Rockwood reviewed 38 failed unconstrained shoulder arthroplasties that were revised at the University of Texas Health Science Center at San Antonio between 1977 and 1993.[440] The initial indication for arthroplasty was acute trauma in 19 shoulders, osteoarthritis in 12 shoulders, post-reconstruction arthropathy in 5 shoulders, and rheumatoid arthritis in 2 shoulders. Five patients had undergone eight previous attempts at revision arthroplasty. Our analysis of these cases revealed findings that were similar to those of Neer and Kirby[301] in that failure was often multifactorial, thus making it difficult to associate failure with one specific factor in 70% of shoulders. Patients were divided into two groups, similar to those described by Neer and associates.[304] Shoulders in group I patients were characterized by infected prostheses, anterior deltoid dysfunction or axillary nerve injury, chronic intractable pain, severely limited range of motion, and poor function. These patients were treated by resectional arthroplasty, with the expectation that they would achieve only limited goals consisting of pain relief and the ability to perform simple activities of daily living (Fig. 16–193). Patients in group II were managed with a revision hemiarthroplasty or total shoulder replacement procedure. The most common complication leading to revision surgery was symptomatic glenohumeral instability (43%), including posterior instability in eight shoulders, anterosuperior instability in six shoulders, and inferior instability in four shoulders. The instability was correlated with inadequate humeral length and soft tissue balancing in 12 shoulders, component malpositioning or subsidence in 7 shoulders, asymmetric glenoid erosion in 5 shoulders, and failure of the sub-

---

*See references 15, 48, 54, 58, 84, 94, 109, 127, 135, 139, 160, 186, 220, 256, 275, 276, 301, 325, 357, 405, 422, 428.

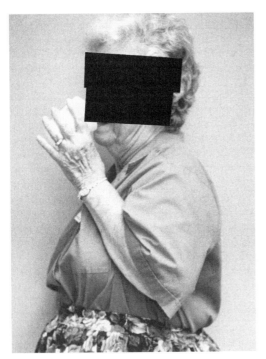

■ **Figure 16–193**

A 76-year-old patient demonstrating function of the upper extremity after resectional arthroplasty of a failed constrained total shoulder prosthesis. Although simple activities of daily living can be performed by adducting the arm to the body for stability, shortening of the humerus significantly limits deltoid effectiveness in elevation of the arm.

scapularis repair in 2 shoulders. Other causes of failure, listed in order of decreasing frequency, included anterior deltoid insufficiency, glenoid component loosening, glenoid erosion, humeral component loosening, tuberosity detachment or malunion, bony or fibrous ankylosis, glenohumeral infection, and dissociation of a modular humeral component.

Twenty-five shoulders were monitored between 2 and 9 years and included nine resectional arthroplasties. Seven of the nine shoulders (group I) obtained acceptable pain relief and were successful in achieving limited-goal activities; the other two shoulders required additional proximal humeral resection.[108] The remaining 16 shoulders (group II) were graded according to Neer's rating system, with five excellent, seven satisfactory, and four unsatisfactory results, which compared favorably with the findings of Caldwell and associates.[68] Of the four shoulders with an unsatisfactory result, all demonstrated marked anterior deltoid weakness and dysfunction.

Antuna and coworkers[8] retrospectively reviewed 48 shoulders that underwent glenoid revision surgery. Indications included loosening in 29 shoulders, implant failure in 14 shoulders, and malposition or wear leading to instability in 5 shoulders. Seventeen shoulders had associated instability. Reimplantation of a new glenoid was performed in 30 shoulders and removal of the glenoid implant followed by bone grafting in 18 shoulders. Patients without a glenoid component were significantly less satisfied with the procedure than were those who underwent reimplantation. Pain relief was

achieved in 86% of reimplanted patients versus 66% of patients who underwent glenoid removal. The authors concluded that patients who undergo glenoid reimplantation have more successful outcomes and that bone grafting may allow eventual reimplantation after graft consolidation.

Hawkins and associates[187] evaluated outcomes in 9 patients with symptomatic glenoid loosening who underwent surgical revision. In seven patients a prosthetic glenoid was replaced, and two patients had insufficient bone stock requiring hemiarthroplasty. The results demonstrated decreased pain and increased functional ability with overall patient satisfaction in seven patients. Two patients were considered failures as a result of recurrent glenoid loosening. The authors concluded that because of the risk of recurrent loosening, hemiarthroplasty may be an acceptable alternative to revision glenoid replacement.

Sperling and Cofield[387] reported 18 revision arthroplasties performed for the treatment of painful glenoid arthrosis in shoulders that had previously undergone hemiarthroplasty. The mean interval between hemiarthroplasty and revision to a total shoulder replacement was 4.4 years. Nearly 40% of the revised patients had an unsatisfactory outcome according to Neer's grading system, and such outcomes were most often due to limited motion and the need for a subsequent revision. The authors recommended the use of a modular prosthesis because many well-fixed prostheses had to be removed and revised for malposition.

In summary, there are many different causes of failure of primary shoulder arthroplasty, and the multifactorial nature of these problems makes analysis difficult. Revision shoulder arthroplasty represents a formidable challenge and requires careful preoperative evaluation if satisfactory management is to be expected. We agree with Neer and colleagues[304] that revision arthroplasty is the most technically challenging of shoulder replacement procedures and emphasize that although pain relief is usually achieved, a functioning deltoid is required if more than limited goals are to be expected.

Although major advances in total shoulder arthroplasty have been made in recent years, we would do well to remember that major complications can occur in shoulder arthroplasty and that these problems exert a substantial burden on the patient's health, function, and quality of life. It is with this in mind and in the spirit of Codman that we press on to carefully assess the failures with the purpose of preventing them in the future.

REFERENCES AND BIBLIOGRAPHY

1. Adams MA, Weiland AJ, and Moore JR: Nonconstrained total shoulder arthroplasty: An eight year experience. Orthop Trans 10:232-233, 1986.
2. Alasaarela EM and Alasaarela ELI: Ultrasound evaluation of painful rheumatoid shoulders. J Rheumatol 21:1642-1647, 1994.
3. Alasaarela E, Leppilahti J, and Hakala M: Ultrasound and operative evaluation of arthritic shoulder joints. Ann Rheum Dis 57:357-360, 1998.
4. Amstutz HC: The DANA Shoulder Replacement. Rutherford, NJ: Howmedica, 1982.
5. Amstutz HC, Sew Hoy AL, and Clarke IC: UCLA anatomic total shoulder. Clin Orthop 155:7-20, 1981.
6. Amstutz HC, Thomas BJ, Kabo JM, et al: The DANA total shoulder arthroplasty. J Bone Joint Surg Am 70:1174-1182, 1988.

7. Anglin C, Wyss UP, and Pichora DR: Mechanical testing of shoulder prostheses and recommendations for glenoid design. J Shoulder Elbow Surg 9:323-331, 2000.
8. Antuna SA, Sperling JW, Cofield RH, and Rowland CM: Glenoid revision surgery after total shoulder arthroplasty. J Shoulder Elbow Surg 10:217-224, 2001.
9. Apreleva M, Parsons IM, Warner JJ, et al: Experimental investigation of reaction forces at the glenohumeral joint during active abduction. J Shoulder Elbow Surg 9:409-417, 2000.
10. Armbuster TG, Slivka J, Resnick D, et al: Extraarticular manifestations of septic arthritis of the glenohumeral joint. AJR Am J Roentgenol 129:667-672, 1977.
11. Arntz CT, Jackins S, and Matsen FA III: Surgical management of complex irreparable rotator cuff deficiency. J Arthroplasty 6:363-370, 1991.
12. Arntz CT, Jackins S, and Matsen FA III: Prosthetic replacement of the shoulder for the treatment of defects in the rotator cuff and the surface of the glenohumeral joint. J Bone Joint Surg Am 75:485-491, 1993.
13. Arredondo J and Worland RL: Bipolar shoulder arthroplasty in patients with osteoarthritis: Short-term clinical results and evaluation of birotational head motion. J Shoulder Elbow Surg 8:425-429, 1999.
14. Averill RM, Sledge CB, and Thomas WH: Neer total shoulder arthroplasty [abstract]. Orthop Trans 4:287, 1980.
15. Bade HA III, Warren RF, Ranawat CS, and Englis AE: Long-term results of Neer total shoulder replacement. In Bateman JE and Welsh RP (eds): Surgery of the Shoulder. St Louis: BC Decker and CV Mosby, 1984, p 294.
16. Badet R, Walch G, and Boulahia A: Computed tomography in primary glenohumeral osteoarthritis without humeral head elevation. Rev Rheum Engl Ed 65:187-194, 1998.
17. Baker GL, Oddis CV, and Medsger TA Jr: Pasteurella multocida polyarticular septic arthritis. J Rheumatol 14:355-357, 1987.
18. Ballmer FT, Lippitt SB, Romeo AA, and Matsen FA III: Total shoulder arthroplasty: Some considerations related to glenoid surface contact. J Shoulder Elbow Surg 3:299-306, 1994.
19. Ballmer FT, Sidles JA, Lippitt SB, and Matsen FA III: Humeral head prosthetic arthroplasty: Surgically relevant geometric considerations. J Shoulder Elbow Surg 2:296-304, 1993.
20. Bankes MJ and Emery RJH: Pioneers of shoulder replacement: Themistocle Gluck and Jules Emile Pean. J Shoulder Elbow Surg 4:259-262, 1995.
21. Barrett WP, Franklin JL, Jackins SE, et al: Total shoulder arthroplasty. J Bone Joint Surg Am 69:865-872, 1987.
22. Barrett WP, Thornhill TS, Thomas WH, et al: Non-constrained total shoulder arthroplasty for patients with polyarticular rheumatoid arthritis. J Arthroplasty 4:91-96, 1989.
23. Barton NJ: Arthrodesis of the shoulder for degenerative conditions. J Bone Joint Surg 54:1759-1764, 1972.
24. Basamania CJ, Gonzales J, Kechele P, et al: Hemiarthroplasty vs total shoulder arthroplasty in patients with rheumatoid arthritis. Paper presented at the 10th Open Meeting of the American Shoulder and Elbow Surgeons, 1994, New Orleans.
25. Bateman JE: Arthritis of the glenohumeral joint. In The Shoulder and Neck. Philadelphia: WB Saunders, 1978, pp 343-362.
26. Bayley JIL and Kessel L: The Kessel total shoulder replacement. In Bayley I and Kessel L (eds): Shoulder Surgery. New York: Springer-Verlag, 1982, pp 160-164.
27. Bechtol CO: Bechtol Total Shoulder. Memphis, TN: Richards Manufacturing, 1976.
28. Becker W: Arthrodesis of the shoulder joint (review of 47 cases). In Chapchal G (ed): The Arthrodesis in the Restoration of Working Ability. Stuttgart, Germany: Georg Thieme, 1975, p 25.
29. Beddow FH and Elloy MA: The Liverpool total replacement for the glenohumeral joint. In Joint Replacement in the Upper Limb. London: Institution of Mechanical Engineering, 1977, pp 21-25.
30. Bell S and Gschwend N: Clinical experience with total arthroplasty and hemiarthroplasty of the shoulder using the Neer prosthesis. Int Orthop 10:217-222, 1986.
31. Beltran JE, Trilla JC, and Barjau R: A simplified compression arthrodesis of the shoulder. J Bone Joint Surg Am 57:538, 1975.
32. Benjamin A, Hirschowitz G, and Arden GP: The treatment of arthritis of the shoulder joint by double osteotomy. Int Orthop 3:211-216, 1979.
33. Benjamin A, Hirschowitz D, Arden GP, and Blackburn N: Double osteotomy of the shoulder. In Bayley I and Kessel L (eds): Shoulder Surgery. New York: Springer-Verlag, 1982, pp 170-175.
34. Bennett WF and Gerber C: Operative treatment of the rheumatoid shoulder [editorial]. Curr Opin Rheumatol 6:177-182, 1994.
35. Bigliani LU, Flatow EL, McCluskey GM, and Fisher RA: Failed prosthetic replacement in displaced proximal humerus fractures. Orthop Trans 15:747-748, 1991.
36. Bigliani LU, Weinstein DM, Glasgow MT, et al: Glenohumeral arthroplasty for arthritis after instability surgery. J Shoulder Elbow Surg 4:87-94, 1995.
37. Blauth W and Hepp WR: Arthrodesis of the shoulder joint by traction absorbing wiring. In Chapchal G (ed): The Arthrodesis in the Restoration of Working Ability. Stuttgart, Germany: Georg Thieme, 1975, p 30.
38. Blevins FT, Deng X, Torzilli PA, et al: Dissociation of humeral shoulder arthroplasty components. Paper presented at the 61st Annual Meeting of the American Academy of Orthopaedic Surgeons, 1994, New Orleans.
39. Blevins FT, Pollo FE, Torzilli PA, and Warren RF: Effect of humeral head component size on hemiarthroplasty translations and rotations. J Shoulder Elbow Surg 7:591-598, 1998.
40. Bodey WN and Yeoman PM: Prosthetic arthroplasty of the shoulder. Acta Orthop Scand 54:900-903, 1983.
41. Boileau P, Avidor C, Krishnan SG, et al: Cemented polyethylene versus uncemented metal-backed glenoid components in total shoulder arthroplasty: A prospective, double-blind, randomized study. J Shoulder Elbow Surg 11:351-359, 2002.
42. Bonutti PM and Hawkins RJ: Fracture of the humeral shaft associated with total replacement arthroplasty of the shoulder. J Bone Joint Surg Am 74:617-618, 1992.
43. Bonutti PM, Hawkins RJ, and Saddemi S: Arthroscopic assessment of glenoid component loosening after total shoulder arthroplasty. Arthroscopy 9:272-276, 1993.
44. Boorman R, Hacker S, Lippitt SB, and Matsen FA III: Impaction grafting technique for humeral component replacement and fixation in shoulder arthroplasty. Tech Shoulder Elbow Surg (in press).
45. Boorman R, Kopjar B, Fehringer E, Churchill RS, et al: The effect of total shoulder arthroplasty on self-assessed health status is comparable to that of total hip arthroplasty and coronary artery bypass grafting. J Shoulder Elbow Surg 12:158-163, 2003.
46. Bostrom C, Harms-Ringdahl K, and Nordemar R: Clinical reliability of shoulder function assessment in patients with rheumatoid arthritis. Scand J Rheumatol 20:36-48, 1991.
47. Boyd AD Jr, Aliabadi P, and Thornhill TS: Postoperative proximal migration in total shoulder arthroplasty. Incidence and significance. J Arthroplasty 6:31-37, 1991.
48. Boyd AD Jr, Thomas WH, Scott RD, et al: Total shoulder arthroplasty versus hemiarthroplasty. J Arthroplasty 5:329-336, 1990.
49. Boyd AD Jr, Thornhill TS, and Barnes CL: Fractures adjacent to humeral prostheses. J Bone Joint Surg Am 74:1498, 1992.
50. Boyd AD Jr, Thornhill TS, Thomas WH, et al: Post-operative proximal migration in total shoulder replacement: Incidence and significance. Paper presented at the Annual Meeting of the American Shoulder and Elbow Surgeons, 1989, New York.
51. Bradford DS, Szalapski EWJ, Sutherland DER, et al: Osteonecrosis in the transplant recipients. Surg Gynecol Obstet 159:328-334, 1984.
52. Brems J: The glenoid component in total shoulder arthroplasty. J Shoulder Elbow Surg 2:47-54, 1993.
53. Brems JJ: Rehabilitation following total shoulder arthroplasty. Clin Orthop 307:70-85, 1994.
54. Brenner BC, Ferlic DC, Clayton ML, and Dennis DA: Survivorship of unconstrained total shoulder arthroplasty. Paper presented at the Fourth International Conference on Surgery of the Shoulder, 1989, New York.
55. Brett AL: A new method of arthrodesis of the shoulder joint, incorporating the control of the scapula. J Bone Joint Surg 15:969, 1933.
56. Brewer BJ, Wubben RC, and Carrera GF: Excessive retroversion of the glenoid cavity: A cause of non-traumatic posterior instability of the shoulder. J Bone Joint Surg Am 68:724-731, 1986.
57. Brittain HA: Architectural Principles in Arthrodesis. Baltimore: Williams & Wilkins, 1942.
58. Brostrom LA, Kronberg M, and Wallensten R: Should the glenoid be replaced in shoulder arthroplasty with an unconstrained DANA or St. Georg prosthesis? Ann Chir Gynaecol 81:54-57, 1992.
59. Brownlee C and Cofield MD: Shoulder replacement in cuff tear arthropathy. Paper presented at the Open Meeting of the American Shoulder and Elbow Surgeons, 1986, New Orleans.
60. Brumfield RH Jr, Schilz J, and Flinders BW: Total shoulder replacement arthroplasty: A clinical review of 21 cases [abstract]. Orthop Trans 5:398, 1981.
61. Bryan JB, Schouder K, Tullos HS, et al: The axillary nerve and its relationships to common sports medicine shoulder procedure. Am J Sports Med 14:113-116, 1986.
62. Buechel FF, Pappas MJ, and DePalma AF: "Floating socket" total shoulder replacement: Anatomical, biomechanical, and surgical rationale. J Biomed Mater Res 12:89-114, 1978.
63. Burdge DR, Reid GD, Reeve CE, et al: Septic arthritis due to dual infection with Mycoplasma hominis and Ureaplasma urealyticum. J Rheumatol 15:366-368, 1988.
64. Burkhead WZ: Musculocutaneous and axillary nerve position after coracoid graft transfer. In Post M, Morrey BF, and Hawkins RJ (eds): Surgery of the Shoulder. St Louis: Mosby–Year Book, 1990, pp 152-155.
65. Burkhead WZ Jr and Hutton KS: Biologic resurfacing of the glenoid with hemiarthroplasty of the shoulder. J Shoulder Elbow Surg 4:263-270, 1995.
66. Burkhead WZ, Scheinberg RR, and Box G: Surgical anatomy of the axillary nerve. J Shoulder Elbow Surg 1:31-36, 1992.
67. Burri C: Indication, technique and results in prosthetic replacement of the shoulder joint. Acta Orthop Belg 51:606-615, 1985.
68. Caldwell GL Jr, Dines D, Warren R, et al: Revision shoulder arthroplasty [abstract]. Paper presented at the Annual Meeting of the American Shoulder and Elbow Surgeons, 1993, San Francisco.
69. Campbell JT, Moore RS, Iannotti JP, et al: Periprosthetic humeral fractures: Mechanisms of fracture and treatment options. J Shoulder Elbow Surg 7:406-413, 1998.

70. Campion GV, McCrae F, Alwan W, et al: Idiopathic destructive arthritis of the shoulder. Semin Arthritis Rheum 17:232-245, 1988.

71. Carroll RE: Wire loop in arthrodesis of the shoulder. Clin Orthop 9:185, 1957.

72. Chard MD and Hazleman BL: Shoulder disorders in the elderly (a hospital study). Ann Rheum Dis 46:684-687, 1987.

73. Charnley J: Compression arthrodesis of the ankle and shoulder. J Bone Joint Surg Br 33:180-191, 1951.

74. Charnley J: Anchorage of the femoral head prosthesis of the shaft of the femur. J Bone Joint Surg Br 42:28-30, 1960.

75. Charnley J: Low Friction Arthroplasty of the Hip. New York: Springer-Verlag, 1979.

76. Charnley J and Houston JK: Compression arthrodesis of the shoulder. J Bone Joint Surg Br 46:614-620, 1964.

77. Clare DJ, Wirth MA, Groh GI, and Rockwood CA Jr: Shoulder arthrodesis. J Bone Joint Surg Am 83:593-600, 2001.

78. Clayton ML, Ferlic DC, and Jeffers PD: Prosthetic arthroplasty of the shoulder. Clin Orthop 164:184, 1982.

79. Cockx E, Claes T, Hoogmartens M, and Mulier JC: The isoelastic prosthesis for the shoulder joint. Acta Orthop Belg 49:275-285, 1983.

80. Codd TP, Pollock RG, and Flatow EL: Prosthetic replacement in the rotator cuff–deficient shoulder. Tech Orthop 8:174-183, 1994.

81. Codd TP, Yamaguchi K, and Flatow EL: Infected shoulder arthroplasties: Treatment with staged reimplantations vs. resection arthroplasty. Paper presented at the 11th Open Meeting of the American Shoulder and Elbow Surgeons, 1995, Orlando, FL.

82. Codman EA: The Shoulder, Rupture of the Supraspinatus Tendon and Other Lesions in or about the Subacromial Bursa. Boston: Thomas Todd, 1934.

83. Cofield RH: Arthrodesis and resection arthroplasty of the shoulder. In McCollister EC (ed): Surgery of the Musculoskeletal System. New York: Churchill Livingstone, 1983, pp 109-124.

84. Cofield RH: Unconstrained total shoulder prostheses. Clin Orthop 173:97-108, 1983.

85. Cofield RH: Total shoulder arthroplasty with the Neer prosthesis. J Bone Joint Surg Am 66:899-906, 1984.

86. Cofield RH: Shoulder arthrodesis and resection arthroplasty. Instr Course Lect 34:268-277, 1985.

87. Cofield RH: Preliminary experience with bone ingrowth total shoulder arthroplasty. Orthop Trans 10:217, 1986.

88. Cofield RH: Total shoulder arthroplasty with bone ingrowth fixation. In Kolbel R, Helbig B, and Blauth W (eds): Shoulder Replacement. Berlin: Springer-Verlag, 1987, pp 209-212.

89. Cofield RH: Subscapularis tendon transposition for large rotator cuff tears. Tech Orthop 3:58, 1989.

90. Cofield RH: Degenerative and arthritic problems of the glenohumeral joint. In Rockwood CA and Matsen FA III (eds): The Shoulder. Philadelphia: WB Saunders, 1990, pp 678-749.

91. Cofield RH: Complications of shoulder arthroplasty. [ICL No. 317]. Paper presented at the Annual Meeting of the American Academy of Orthopaedic Surgeons, 1993, San Francisco.

92. Cofield RH: Uncemented total shoulder arthroplasty: A review. Clin Orthop 66:899-906, 1994.

93. Cofield RH and Briggs BT: Glenohumeral arthritis. J Bone Joint Surg Am 61:668-677, 1979.

94. Cofield RH and Daly PJ: Total shoulder arthroplasty with a tissue-ingrowth glenoid component. J Shoulder Elbow Surg 1:77-85, 1992.

95. Cofield RH and Edgerton BC: Total shoulder arthroplasty: Complications and revision surgery. Instr Course Lect 39:449-462, 1990.

96. Cofield RH, Frankle MA, and Zuckerman JD: Humeral head replacement in glenohumeral arthritis. J Shoulder Elbow Surg 2(suppl):S13, 1993.

97. Cofield RH and Stauffer RN: The Bickel glenohumeral arthroplasty. In Conference on Joint Replacement in the Upper Limb. London: Institute of Mechanical Engineering, 1977, pp 15-25.

98. Collins D, Tencer A, Sidles J, and Matsen FA III: Edge displacement and deformation of glenoid components in response to eccentric loading. J Bone Joint Surg Am 74:501-507, 1992.

99. Collins DN, Harryman DT II, Lippitt SB, et al: The technique of glenohumeral arthroplasty. Tech Orthop 6:43-59, 1991.

100. Compito CA, Self EB, and Bigliani LU: Arthroplasty and acute shoulder trauma: Reasons for success and failure. Clin Orthop 307:27-36, 1994.

101. Cooper RA and Brems JJ: Recurrent disassembly of a modular humeral prosthesis: A case report. J Arthroplasty 6:375-377, 1991.

102. Copeland S: Cementless total shoulder replacement. In Post M, Morrey BF, and Hawkins RJ (eds): Surgery of the Shoulder. St Louis: Mosby–Year Book, 1990, pp 289-293.

103. Cornell CN and Ranawat CS: Survivorship analysis of total hip replacements. Results in a series of active patients who were less than fifty-five years old. J Bone Joint Surg Am 68:1430-1432, 1986.

104. Cosendai A, Gerster JC, Vischer TL, et al: Destructive arthropathies associated with articular chondrocalcinosis. Clinical and metabolic study of 16 cases. Schweiz Med Wochenschr 106:8-14, 1976.

105. Coughlin MJ, Morris JM, and West WF: The semiconstrained total shoulder arthroplasty. J Bone Joint Surg Am 61:574-581, 1979.

106. Couteau B, Mansat P, Estivalezes E, et al: Finite element analysis of the mechanical behavior of a scapula implanted with a glenoid prosthesis. Clin Biomech (Bristol, Avon) 16:566-575, 2001.

107. Cowell HR and Curtiss PH Jr: The randomized clinical trial [editorial]. J Bone Joint Surg Am 67:1151-1152, 1985.

108. Craviotto DF, Seltzer DG, Wirth MA, and Rockwood CA Jr: Resection arthroplasty for salvage of failed shoulder arthroplasty. Paper presented at the Annual Meeting of the American Shoulder and Elbow Surgeons, 1994, New Orleans.

109. Cruess RL: Shoulder resurfacing according to the method of Neer. J Bone Joint Surg Br 62:116-117, 1980.

110. Cruess RL: Corticosteroid-induced osteonecrosis of the humeral head. Orthop Clin North Am 16:789-796, 1985.

111. Cruess RL: Osteonecrosis of bone: Current concepts as to etiology and pathogenesis. Clin Orthop 208:30-39, 1986.

112. Curran JF, Ellman MH, and Brown NL: Rheumatologic aspects of painful conditions affecting the shoulder. Clin Orthop 173:27-37, 1983.

113. Cutler SJ and Ederer F: Maximum utilization of the life table method in analyzing survival. J Chron Dis 8:699-712, 1958.

114. De Velasco Polo G and Cardoso Monterrubio A: Arthrodesis of the shoulder. Clin Orthop 90:178, 1973.

115. Dines DM, Warren RF, Altchek DW, and Moeckel B: Posttraumatic changes of the proximal humerus: Malunion, nonunion, and osteonecrosis. Treatment with modular hemiarthroplasty or total shoulder arthroplasty. J Shoulder Elbow Surg 2:121, 1993.

116. Dobbs HS: Survivorship of total hip replacements. J Bone Joint Surg Br 62:168-173, 1980.

117. Dorey F and Amstutz HC: Survivorship analysis in the evaluation of joint replacement. J Arthroplasty 1:63-69, 1986.

118. Dorwart RH, Genant HK, Johnston WH, and Morris JM: Pigmented villonodular synovitis of synovial joints: Clinical, pathologic, and radiologic features. AJR Am J Roentgenol 143:877-885, 1984.

119. Dorwart RH, Genant HK, Johnston WH, and Morris JM: Pigmented villonodular synovitis of the shoulder: Radiologic-pathologic assessment. AJR Am J Roentgenol 143:886-888, 1984.

120. Driessnack RP, Ferlic DC, and Wiedel JD: Dissociation of the glenoid component in the Macnab/English total shoulder arthroplasty. J Arthroplasty 5:15-18, 1990.

121. Ellman MH and Curran JJ: Causes and management of shoulder arthritis. Compr Ther 14:29-35, 1988.

122. Engelbrecht E and Heinert K: More than ten years' experience with unconstrained shoulder replacement. In Kolbel R, Helbig B, and Blauth W (eds): Shoulder Replacement. New York: Springer-Verlag, 1987, pp 85-91.

123. Engelbrecht E, Siegel A, Rottger J, and Heinert K: Erfahrungen mit der Anwendung von Schultergelenksendoprothesen. Chirurg 51:794, 1980.

124. Engelbrecht E and Stellbrink G: Total Schulterendoprosthese Modell (St. Georg). Chirurg 47:525-530, 1976.

125. Ennevaara K: Painful shoulder joint in rheumatoid arthritis: A clinical and radiological study of 200 cases with special reference to arthrography of the glenohumeral joint. Acta Rheum Scand Suppl 11:1-108, 1967.

126. Epps CH Jr: Painful hematologic conditions affecting the shoulder. Clin Orthop 173:38-43, 1983.

127. Faludi DD and Weiland AJ: Cementless total shoulder arthroplasty: Preliminary experience with thirteen cases. Orthopedics 6:431-438, 1983.

128. Fehringer EV, Kopjar B, Boorman RS, et al: Characterizing the functional improvement after total shoulder arthroplasty for osteoarthritis. J Bone Joint Surg Am 84:1349-1353, 2002.

129. Fenlin JM: Total glenohumeral joint replacement. Orthop Clin North Am 6:565-583, 1975.

130. Fenlin JM, Frieman BG, and Allardyce TJ: Hemiarthroplasty in rotator cuff tear arthropathy. J Shoulder Elbow Surg 4(suppl):S62, 1995.

131. Fenlin JM, Ramsey ML, Allardyce TJ, and Frieman BG: Modular total shoulder replacement. Design rationale, indications and results. Clin Orthop 307:37-46, 1994.

132. Fink B, Sallen V, Guderian H, et al: Resection interposition arthroplasty of the shoulder affected by inflammatory arthritis. J Shoulder Elbow Surg 10:365-371, 2001.

133. Field LD, Zabinski SJ, Dines DM, et al: Hemiarthroplasty of the shoulder for rotator cuff arthropathy. J Shoulder Elbow Surg 4(suppl):S62, 1995.

134. Figgie HE, Inglis AE, Goldberg VM, et al: An analysis of factors affecting the long-term results of total shoulder arthroplasty in inflammatory arthritis. J Arthroplasty 3:123-130, 1988.

135. Figgie MP, Inglis AE, Figgie HI, et al: Custom total shoulder arthroplasty for inflammatory arthritis. Paper presented at the Fourth International Conference on Surgery of the Shoulder, 1989, New York.

136. Flatow EL, Bigliani LU, and April EW: An anatomical study of the musculocutaneous nerve and its relationship to the coracoid process. Clin Orthop 244:166-171, 1989.

137. Fournie B, Railhac JJ, and Monod P: The enthesopathic shoulder. Rev Rhum Mal Osteoartic 54:447-451, 1987.

138. Frank CB: Ligament healing: Current knowledge and clinical applications. J Am Acad Orthop Surg 4:74-83, 1996.

139. Franklin JL, Barrett WP, Jackins SE, and Matsen FA III: Glenoid loosening in total shoulder arthroplasty; association with rotator cuff deficiency. J Arthroplasty 3:39-46, 1988.

140. Frich LH, Moller BN, and Sneppen O: Shoulder arthroplasty with the Neer Mark-II prosthesis. Arch Orthop Trauma Surg 107:110-113, 1988.

141. Frich LH, Sojbjerg JO, and Sneppen O: Shoulder arthroplasty in complex acute and chronic proximal humeral fractures. Orthopedics 14:949-954, 1991.

142. Friedman RJ: Glenohumeral translation after total shoulder arthroplasty. J Shoulder Elbow Surg 1:312-316, 1992.

143. Friedman RJ, Hawthorne KB, and Genez BM: The use of computerized tomography in the measurement of glenoid version. J Bone Joint Surg Am 74:1032-1037, 1992.

144. Friedman RJ, LaBerge M, Dooley RL, and O'Hara AL: Finite element modeling of the glenoid component: Effect of design parameters on stress distribution. J Shoulder Elbow Surg 1:261-270, 1992.

145. Friedman RJ, Thornhill TS, Thomas WH, and Sledge CB: Non-constrained total shoulder replacement in patients who have rheumatoid arthritis and class-IV function. J Bone Joint Surg Am 71:494-498, 1989.

146. Fukuda K, Chen C-M, Cofield RH, and Chao EYS: Biomechanical analysis of stability and fixation strength of total shoulder prostheses. Orthopedics 2:141-149, 1988.

147. Galinat BJ, Howell SM, and Kraft TA: The glenoid posterior acromion angle: An accurate method of evaluating glenoid version. Orthop Trans 12:727, 1988.

148. Garancis JC, Cheung HS, Halverson PB, and McCarty DJ: "Milwaukee shoulder"—association of microspheroids containing hydroxyapatite crystals, active collagenase, and neutral protease with rotator cuff defects. Arthritis Rheum 24:484-491, 1981.

149. Gariepy R: Glenoidectomy in the repair of the rheumatoid shoulder. J Bone Joint Surg Br 59:122, 1977.

150. Gartland JJ: Orthopaedic clinical research: Deficiencies in experimental design and determinations of outcome. J Bone Joint Surg Am 70:1357-1364, 1988.

151. Gartsman GM, Brinker MR, Khan M, and Karahan M: Self-assessment of general health status in patients with five common shoulder conditions. J Shoulder Elbow Surg 7:228-237, 1998.

152. Gartsman GM, Roddey TS, and Hammerman SM: Shoulder arthroplasty with or without resurfacing of the glenoid in patients who have osteoarthritis. J Bone Joint Surg Am 82:26-34, 2000.

153. Gerard P, Leblanc JP, and Rousseau B: Une prothèse totale d'épaule. Chirurgie 99:655-663, 1973.

154. Giori NJ, Beaupre GS, and Carter DR: The influence of fixation peg design on the shear stability of prosthetic implants. J Orthop Res 8:892-898, 1990.

155. Glasson JM, Pollock RG, Djurasovic M, et al: Hemiarthroplasty for glenohumeral osteoarthritis in a patient with an intact rotator cuff: Results correlated to degree of glenoid wear. Paper presented at the 12th Open Meeting of the American Shoulder and Elbow Surgeons, 1996, Atlanta.

156. Godeneche A, Boileau P, Favard L, et al: Prosthetic replacement in the treatment of osteoarthritis of the shoulder: early results of 268 cases. J Shoulder Elbow Surg 11:11-18, 2002.

157. Goldberg BA, Smith K, Jackins S, et al: The magnitude and durability of functional improvement after total shoulder arthroplasty for degenerative joint disease. J Shoulder Elbow Surg 10:464-469, 2001.

158. Green A and Norris TR: Imaging technique for glenohumeral arthritis and glenohumeral arthroplasty. Clin Orthop 307:7-17, 1994.

159. Green A and Norris TR: Shoulder arthroplasty for advanced glenohumeral arthritis after anterior instability repair. J Shoulder Elbow Surg 10:539-545, 2001.

160. Gristina AG, Romano RL, Kammire GC, and Webb LX: Total shoulder replacement. Orthop Clin North Am 18:444-453, 1987.

161. Gristina AG and Webb LX: The trispherical total shoulder replacement. In Bayley I and Kessel L (eds): Shoulder Surgery. New York: Springer-Verlag, 1982, pp 153-157.

162. Gristina AG, Webb LX, and Carter RE: The monospherical total shoulder. Orthop Trans 9:54, 1985.

163. Groh GI, Heckman MM, Curtis RJ, et al: Treatment of fractures adjacent to humeral prostheses. Orthop Trans 18:1072, 1994-1995.

164. Groh GI and Rockwood CA: Loss of Deltoid following Shoulder Operations: An Operative Disaster. Monterey, CA: Western Orthopaedic Association, 1992.

165. Groh GI, Simoni M, Rolla P, and Rockwood CA Jr: Loss of the deltoid after shoulder operations: An operative disaster. J Shoulder Elbow Surg 3:243, 1994.

166. Gschwend N: Is a glenoid component necessary for rheumatoid patients? Paper presented at the Second Congress of the European Shoulder and Elbow Society, 1988, Berne, Switzerland.

167. Gunther SB, Graham J, Norris TR, et al: Retrieved glenoid components: A classification system for surface damage analysis. J Arthroplasty 17:95-100, 2002.

168. Habermeyer P and Schweiberer L: Corrective interventions subsequent to humeral head fractures. Orthopade 21:148-157, 1992.

169. Hacker S, Boorman R, Lippitt SB, and Matsen FA III: Impaction grafting improves the fit of proximal humeral arthroplasty. J Shoulder Elbow Surg (in press).

170. Halverson PB, Cheung HS, and McCarty DJ: Enzymatic release of microspheroids containing hydroxyapatite crystals from synovium and of calcium pyrophosphate dihydrate crystals from cartilage. Ann Rheum Dis 41:527-531, 1982.

171. Halverson PB, Cheung HS, McCarty DJ, et al: "Milwaukee shoulder"—association of microspheroids containing hydroxyapatite crystals, active collagenase, and neutral protease with rotator cuff defects. II. Synovial fluid studies. Arthritis Rheum 24:474-483, 1981.

172. Halverson PB, Garancis JC, and McCarty DJ: Histopathological and ultrastructural studies of synovium in Milwaukee shoulder syndrome—basic calcium phosphate crystal arthropathy. Ann Rheum Dis 43:734-741, 1984.

173. Halverson PB, McCarty DJ, Cheung HS, and Ryan LM: Milwaukee shoulder syndrome: Eleven additional cases with involvement of the knee in seven (basic calcium phosphate crystal deposition disease). Semin Arthritis Rheum 14:36-44, 1984.

174. Harris TE, Jobe CM, and Dai QG: Fixation of proximal humeral prostheses and rotational micromotion. J Shoulder Elbow Surg 9:205-210, 2000.

175. Harryman DT II, Sidles JA, Clark JM, et al: Translation of the humeral head on the glenoid with passive glenohumeral motion. J Bone Joint Surg Am 72:1334-1343, 1990.

176. Harryman DT, Sidles JA, Harris SL, et al: The effect of articular conformity and the size of the humeral head component on laxity and motion after glenohumeral arthroplasty. J Bone Joint Surg Am 77:555-563, 1995.

177. Harryman DT II, Sidles JA, Harris SL, and Matsen FA III: Laxity of the normal glenohumeral joint: A quantitative in-vivo assessment. J Shoulder Elbow Surg 1:66-76, 1992.

178. Harryman DT II, Walker ED, Harris SL, et al: Residual motion and function after glenohumeral or scapulothoracic arthrodesis. J Shoulder Elbow Surg 2:275-285, 1993.

179. Hasan SS, Leith JM, Campbell B, et al: Characteristics of unsatisfactory shoulder arthroplasties. J Shoulder Elbow Surg 11:431-441, 2002.

180. Hasan S, Leith J, Smith KL, and Matsen FA III: The distribution of shoulder replacements among surgeons and hospitals is significantly different than that of hip or knee replacements. J Shoulder Elbow Surg 12:164-169, 2003.

181. Hattrup SJ and Cofield RH: Osteonecrosis of the humeral head: Relationship of disease stage, extent, and cause to natural history. J Shoulder Elbow Surg 8:559-564, 1999.

182. Hattrup SJ and Cofield RH: Osteonecrosis of the humeral head: Results of replacement. J Shoulder Elbow Surg 9:177-182, 2000.

183. Hauge MF: Arthrodesis of the shoulder: A simple elastic band appliance utilizing the compression principle. Acta Orthop Scand 31:272, 1961.

184. Hawkins RJ and Angelo RL: Glenohumeral arthrosis: A late complication of the Putti-Platt repair. J Bone Joint Surg Am 72:1193-1197, 1990.

185. Hawkins RJ, Bell RH, and Jallay B: Experience with the Neer total shoulder arthroplasty: A review of 70 cases. Orthop Trans 10:232, 1986.

186. Hawkins RJ, Bell RH, and Jallay B: Total shoulder arthroplasty. Clin Orthop 242:188-194, 1989.

187. Hawkins RJ, Greis PE, and Bonutti PM: Treatment of symptomatic glenoid loosening following unconstrained shoulder arthroplasty. Orthopedics 22:229-234, 1999.

188. Hawkins RJ and Neer CS II: A functional analysis of shoulder fusions. Clin Orthop 223:65-76, 1987.

189. Hawkins RJ, Neer CS II, Pianta RM, and Mendoza FX: Locked posterior dislocation of the shoulder. J Bone Joint Surg Am 69:9-18, 1987.

190. Hernigou P, Duparc F, and Filali C: Humeral retroversion and shoulder prosthesis. Rev Chir Orthop Reparatrice Appar Mot 81:419-427, 1995.

191. Hernigou P, Duparc F, and Hernigou A: Determining humeral retroversion with computed tomography. J Bone Joint Surg Am 84:1753-1762, 2002.

192. Hill JM and Norris TR: Long-term results of total shoulder arthroplasty following bone-grafting of the glenoid. J Bone Joint Surg Am 83:877-883, 2001.

193. Hinton MA, Parker AW, Drez DJ, and Altcheck D: An anatomic study of the subscapularis tendon and myotendinous junction. J Shoulder Elbow Surg 3:224-229, 1994.

194. Hjelkrem M and Stanish WD: Synovial chondrometaplasia of the shoulder. A case report of a young athlete presenting with shoulder pain. Am J Sports Med 16:84-86, 1988.

195. Hovelius LK, Sandstrom BC, Rosmark DL, et al: Long-term results with the Bankart and Bristow-Latarjet procedures: Recurrent shoulder instability and arthropathy. J Shoulder Elbow Surg 10:445-452, 2001.

196. Hsu HC, Wu JJ, Chen TH, et al: The influence of abductor lever-arm changes after shoulder arthroplasty. J Shoulder Elbow Surg 2:134-140, 1993.

197. Hucherson DC: Arthrodesis of the paralytic shoulder. Am Surg 25:430, 1959.

198. Hughes GM, Biundo JJJ, Scheib JS, and Kumar P: Pseudogout and pseudosepsis of the shoulder. Orthop Grand Rounds 13:1169-1172, 1990.

199. Huten D and Duparc J: L'arthroplastie prothetique dans les traumatismes complexes récents et anciens de l'épaule. Rev Chir Orthop 72:517-529, 1986.

200. Iannotti JP, Gabriel JP, Schneck SL, et al: The normal glenohumeral relationships: An anatomical study of one hundred and forty shoulders. J Bone Joint Surg Am 74:491-499, 1992.

201. Inman VT, Saunders JBDCM, and Abbott LC: Observations on the function of the shoulder joint. J Bone Joint Surg Am 26:1-30, 1944.

202. Jacobson SR and Mallon WJ: The glenohumeral offset ratio: A radiographic study. J Shoulder Elbow Surg 2:141-146, 1993.

203. Jenkinson ML, Bliss MR, Brain AT, and Scott DL: Peripheral arthritis in the elderly: A hospital study. Ann Rheum Dis 48:227-231, 1989.

204. Jensen K and Rockwood CA: Hemiarthroplasty vs total shoulder arthroplasty in patients with osteoarthritis of the shoulder. Orthop Trans 19:821, 1995-96.

205. Jensen K and Rockwood CA Jr: The value of preoperative computed tomography in shoulder arthroplasty. Paper presented at a combined meeting of the New Zealand and Australian Orthopaedic Associations, 1996, Perth, Australia.

206. Jinnah RH, Amstutz HC, Tooke SM, et al: The UCLA Charnley experience: A long-term follow-up study using survival analysis. Clin Orthop 221:164-172, 1986.

207. Johnson CA, Healy WL, Brooker AF Jr, and Krackow KA: External fixation shoulder arthrodesis. Clin Orthop 211:219-223, 1986.

208. Jones L: Reconstructive operation for nonreducible fractures of the head of the humerus. Ann Surg 97:217, 1933.

209. Jones L: The shoulder joint—observations on the anatomy and physiology: With an analysis of a reconstructive operation following extensive injury. Surg Gynecol Obstet 75:433, 1942.

210. Jónsson E: Surgery of the Rheumatoid Shoulder with Special Reference to Cup Hemiarthroplasty and Arthrodesis. Lund, Sweden: Infotryck, 1988.

211. Jónsson E, Egund N, Kelly I, et al: Cup arthroplasty of the rheumatoid shoulder. Acta Orthop Scand 57:542-546, 1986.

212. Jónsson E, Lidgren L, and Rydholm U: Position of shoulder arthrodesis measured with Moire photography. Clin Orthop 238:117-121, 1989.

213. Kalamchi A: Arthrodesis for paralytic shoulder: Review of ten patients. Orthopedics 1:204-208, 1978.

214. Karduna AR, Williams GR, Iannotti JP, and Williams JL: Total shoulder arthroplasty biomechanics. A study of the forces and strains at the glenoid component. J Biomech Eng 120:92-99, 1998.

215. Kechele P, Basmania C, Wirth MA, et al: Rheumatoid shoulder: Hemiarthroplasty vs. total shoulder arthroplasty. J Shoulder Elbow Surg 4(suppl):S13, 1995.

216. Kechele PR, Seltzer DG, Gonzalez JC, et al: Hemiarthroplasty vs. total shoulder arthroplasty for the rheumatoid shoulder. Paper presented at the 10th Open Meeting of the American Shoulder and Elbow Surgeons, 1994, New Orleans.

217. Kelleher IM, Cofield RH, Becker DA, and Beabout JW: Fluoroscopically positioned radiographs of total shoulder arthroplasty. J Shoulder Elbow Surg 1:306-311, 1992.

218. Kelly IG: Surgery of the rheumatoid shoulder. Ann Rheum Dis 49:824-829, 1990.

219. Kelly IG: Shoulder arthroplasty in rheumatoid arthritis. Clin Orthop 307:94-102, 1994.

220. Kelly IG, Foster RS, and Fischer WD: Neer total shoulder replacement in rheumatoid arthritis. J Bone Joint Surg Br 69:723-726, 1987.

221. Kenmore PI: A simple shoulder replacement. Paper presented at a Clemson University Biomaterials Symposium, 1973.

222. Kenmore PI, MacCartee C, and Vitek B: A simple shoulder replacement. J Biomed Mater Res 5:329-330, 1974.

223. Kessel L and Bayley JL: The Kessel total shoulder replacement. In Bayley I and Kessel L (eds): Shoulder Surgery. New York: Springer-Verlag, 1982, pp 160-164.

224. Kiss J, Mersich I, Perlaky GY, and Szollas L: The results of the Putti-Platt operation with particular reference to arthritis, pain, and limitation of external rotation. J Shoulder Elbow Surg 7:495-500, 1998.

225. Klimaitis A, Carroll G, and Owen E: Rapidly progressive destructive arthropathy of the shoulder—a viewpoint on pathogenesis. J Rheumatol 15:1859-1862, 1988.

226. Knight RA and Mayne JA: Comminuted fractures and fracture-dislocations involving the articular surface of the humeral head. J Bone Joint Surg Am 39:1343, 1957.

227. Kölbel R and Friedebold G: Schultergelenkersatz. Z Orthop 113:452-454, 1975.

228. Kölbel R, Rohlmann A, and Bergmann G: Biomechanical considerations in the design of a semi-constrained total shoulder replacement. In Bayley I and Kessel L (eds): Shoulder Surgery. New York: Springer-Verlag, 1982, pp 144-152.

229. Kraft SM, Panush RS, and Longley S: Unrecognized staphylococcal pyarthrosis with rheumatoid arthritis. Semin Arthritis Rheum 14:196-201, 1985.

230. Kronberg M, Brostrom LA, and Soderlund V: Retroversion of the humeral head in the normal shoulder and its relationship to the normal range of motion. Clin Orthop 253:113-117, 1990.

231. Krueger FJ: Vitallium replica arthroplasty on the shoulder: A case report of aseptic necrosis of the proximal end of the humerus. Surgery 30:1005-1011, 1951.

232. Lacroix D, Murphy LA, and Prendergast PJ: Three-dimensional finite element analysis of glenoid replacement prostheses: A comparison of keeled and pegged anchorage systems. J Biomech Eng 122:430-436, 2000.

233. Laumann U and Schilgen L: Varisierende subkapitale Osteotomie in Verbindung mit Schulterarthrodese und Oberarmamputation bei Plexusparese. Z Orthop 115:787, 1977.

234. Laurence M: Replacement arthroplasty of the rotator cuff deficient shoulder. J Bone Joint Surg Br 73:916-919, 1991.

235. Lazarus MD, Jensen KL, Southworth C, and Matsen FA III: The radiographic evaluation of keeled and pegged glenoid component insertion. J Bone Joint Surg Am 84:1174-1182, 2002.

236. Lee DH and Niemann KMW: Bipolar shoulder arthroplasty. Clin Orthop 304:97-107, 1994.

237. Lehtinen JT, Kaarela K, Belt EA, et al: Incidence of glenohumeral joint involvement in seropositive rheumatoid arthritis. A 15 year endpoint study. J Rheumatol 27:347-350, 2000.

238. Leslie BM, Harris JMI, and Driscoll D: Septic arthritis of the shoulder in adults. J Bone Joint Surg Am 71:1516-1522, 1989.

239. Lettin AWF, Copeland SA, and Scales JT: The Stanmore total shoulder replacement. J Bone Joint Surg Br 64:47-51, 1982.

240. Levick JR: Joint pressure-volume studies: Their importance, design and interpretation. J Rheumatol 10:353-357, 1983.

241. Levine WN, Djurasovic M, Glasson JM, et al: Hemiarthroplasty for glenohumeral osteoarthritis: Results correlated to degree of glenoid wear. J Shoulder Elbow Surg 6:449-454, 1997.

242. Levy O and Copeland SA: Cementless surface replacement arthroplasty of the shoulder. 5- to 10-year results with the Copeland mark-2 prosthesis. J Bone Joint Surg Br 83:213-221, 2001.

243. Lichtman EA: Candida infection of a prosthetic shoulder joint. Skeletal Radiol 10:176-177, 1983.

244. Linell EA: The distribution of nerves in the upper limb with reference to variabilities and their clinical significance. J Anat 55:79-112, 1921.

245. Linscheid RL and Cofield RH: Total shoulder arthroplasty: Experimental but promising. Geriatrics 31:64-69, 1976.

246. Lippitt SB, Harris SC, Harryman DT II, et al: In vivo quantification of the laxity of normal and unstable glenohumeral joints. J Shoulder Elbow Surg 3:215-223, 1994.

247. Lippitt SB, Harryman DT II, and Matsen FA III: A practical tool for evaluation function: The simple shoulder test. In Matsen FA III, Fu FH, and Hawkins RJ (eds): The Shoulder: A Balance of Mobility and Stability. Rosemont, IL: American Academy of Orthopaedic Surgeons, 1993, pp 510-518.

248. Louthrenoo W, Ostrov BE, Park YS, et al: Pseudoseptic arthritis: An unusual presentation of neuropathic arthropathy. Ann Rheum Dis 50:717-721, 1991.

249. Lugli T: Artificial shoulder joint by Péan (1893). The facts of an exceptional intervention and the prosthetic method. Clin Orthop 133:215-218, 1978.

250. Lusardi DA, Wirth MA, Wrutz D, and Rockwood CA Jr: Loss of external rotation after capsulorrhaphy of the shoulder. J Bone Joint Surg Am 75:1185-1192, 1993.

251. Lynch NM, Cofield RH, Silbert PL, and Hermann RC: Neurologic complications after total shoulder arthroplasty. J Shoulder Elbow Surg 5:53-61, 1996.

252. Madhok R, Lewallen DG, Wallrichs SL, et al: Utilization of upper limb replacements during 1972-90: The Mayo Clinic experience. Proc Inst Mech Eng [H] 207:239-244, 1993.

253. Mallon WJ, Brown HR, Vogler JB, and Martinez S: Radiographic and geometric anatomy of the scapula. Clin Orthop 277:142-154, 1992.

254. Marks SH, Barnett M, and Calin A: Ankylosing spondylitis in women and men: A case control study. J Rheumatol 10:624-628, 1983.

255. Marmor L: Hemiarthroplasty of the rheumatoid shoulder joint. Clin Orthop 122:201-203, 1977.

256. Martin SD, Sledge CB, Thomas WH, and Thornhill TS: Total shoulder arthroplasty with an uncemented glenoid component. Paper presented at the 11th Annual Meeting of the American Shoulder and Elbow Surgeons, 1995, Orlando, FL.

257. Marx RG, McCarty EC, Montemurno TD, et al: Development of arthrosis following dislocation of the shoulder: A case-control study. J Shoulder Elbow Surg 11:1-5, 2002.

258. Mason JM: The treatment of dislocation of the shoulder-joint complicated by fracture of the upper extremity of the humerus. Ann Surg 47:672, 1908.

259. Matsen FA III: Early effectiveness of shoulder arthroplasty for patients with primary glenohumeral degenerative joint disease. J Bone Joint Surg Am 78:260-264, 1996.

260. Matsen FA III: The relationship of surgical volume to quality of care: Scientific considerations and policy implications. J Bone Joint Surg Am 84:1482-1483, discussion 1483-1485, 2002.

261. Matsen FA III, Antoniou J, Rozencwaig R, et al: Correlates with comfort and function after total shoulder arthroplasty for degenerative joint disease. J Shoulder Elbow Surg 9:465-469, 2000.

262. Matsen FA III, Lippitt SB, Sidles JA, and Harryman DT II: Practical Evaluation and Management of the Shoulder. Philadelphia: WB Saunders, 1994, pp 1-242.

263. Matsen FA III, Rockwood CA Jr, and Iannotti J: Humeral fixation by press fit of a tapered metaphyseal stem. A prospective radiograph study. J Bone Joint Surg Am 85:304-308, 2003.

264. Matsen FA III, Smith KL, DeBartolo SE, and Von Oesen G: A comparison of patients with late-stage rheumatoid arthritis and osteoarthritis of the shoulder using self-assessed shoulder function and health status. Arthritis Care Res 10:43-47, 1997.

265. Matsen FA III, Thomas SC, and Rockwood CA Jr: Anterior glenohumeral instability. In Rockwood CA Jr and Matsen FA III (eds): The Shoulder. Philadelphia: WB Saunders, 1990, pp 534-540.

266. Matsen FA III, Ziegler DW, and DeBartolo SE: Patient self-assessment of health status and function in glenohumeral degenerative joint disease. J Shoulder Elbow Surg 4:345-351, 1995.

267. Matsunaga M: A new method of arthrodesis of the shoulder. Acta Orthop Scand 43:343, 1972.

268. Mau H and Nebinger G: Arthropathy of the shoulder joint in syringomyelia. Z Orthop 124:157-164, 1986.
269. May VR Jr: Shoulder fusion: A review of 14 cases. J Bone Joint Surg Am 44:65, 1962.
270. Mazas F and de la Caffiniére JY: Total arthroplasty of the shoulder: Experience with 38 cases [abstract]. Orthop Trans 5:57, 1981.
271. Mazas F and de la Caffiniére JY: Une prothèse totale d'épaule non rétentive: A propos de 38 cas. Rev Chir Orthop 68:161-170, 1982.
272. McCarty D: Crystals, joints, and consternation. Ann Rheum Dis 42:243-253, 1983.
273. McCarty DJ, Halverson PB, Carrera GF, et al: "Milwaukee shoulder"—association of microspheroids containing hydroxyapatite crystals, active collagenase, and neutral protease with rotator cuff defects. I. Clinical aspects. Arthritis Rheum 24:353-354, 1981.
274. McCoy SR, Warren RF, Bade HA, et al: Total shoulder arthroplasty in rheumatoid arthritis. J Arthroplasty 4:105-113, 1989.
275. McElwain JP and English E: The early results of porous-coated total shoulder arthroplasty. Clin Orthop 218:217-224, 1987.
276. McKee GK and Watson-Farrar J: Replacement of arthritis hips by the McKee-Farrar prosthesis. J Bone Joint Surg Br 48:245, 1966.
277. Medicare Hospital Utilization Data Bases: Consolidated Consulting Group, Fairfax, VA.
278. Medsger TA, Dixon JA, and Garwood VF: Palmar fasciitis and polyarthritis associated with ovarian carcinoma. Ann Intern Med 96:424-432, 1982.
279. Milbrink J and Wigren A: Resection arthroplasty of the shoulder. Scand J Rheumatol 19:432-436, 1990.
280. Mills KL: Severe injuries of the upper end of the humerus. Injury 6:13, 1974.
281. Milne JC and Gartsman GM: Cost of shoulder surgery. J Shoulder Elbow Surg 3:295-298, 1994.
282. Moeckel BH, Altchek DW, Warren RF, et al: Instability of the shoulder after arthroplasty. J Bone Joint Surg Am 75:492-497, 1993.
283. Moeckel BH, Dines DM, Warren RF, and Altcheck DW: Modular hemiarthroplasty for fractures of the proximal humerus. J Bone Joint Surg Am 74:884-889, 1992.
284. Mont MA, Payman RK, Laporte DM, Petri M, et al: Atraumatic osteonecrosis of the humeral head. J Rheumatol 27:1766-1773, 2000.
285. Mullaji AB, Beddow FH, and Lamb GHR: CT measurement of glenoid erosion in arthritis. J Bone Joint Surg Br 76:384-388, 1994.
286. Muller ME, Allgower M, Schneider R, and Willenegger H: Manual of Internal Fixation. New York: Springer-Verlag, 1979, pp 384-385.
287. Muller W: Uber den negativen Luftdruck im Gelenkraum. Dtsch A Chir 217:395-401, 1929.
288. Murphy LA, Prendergast PJ, and Resch H: Structural analysis of an offset-keel design glenoid component compared with a center-keel design. J Shoulder Elbow Surg 10:568-579, 2001.
289. Nagels J, Valstar ER, Stokdijk M, and Rozing PM: Patterns of loosening of the glenoid component. J Bone Joint Surg Br 84:83-87, 2002.
290. Namba RS and Thornhill TS: Posterior capsulorrhaphy in total shoulder arthroplasty: A case report. Clin Orthop 313:135-139, 1995.
291. National Health Interview: National Center for Health Statistics, 1988.
292. National Hospital Discharge Survey: National Center for Health Statistics, 1984-1990.
293. National Hospital Discharge Survey: National Center for Health Statistics, 1990-1992.
294. Neer CS II: Articular replacement for the humeral head. J Bone Joint Surg Am 37:215-228, 1955.
295. Neer CS II: The rheumatoid shoulder. In Cruess RR and Mitchell NS (eds): Surgery of Rheumatoid Arthritis. Philadelphia: JB Lippincott, 1971, pp 117-125.
296. Neer CS II: Replacement arthroplasty for glenohumeral arthritis. J Bone Joint Surg Am 56:1-13, 1974.
297. Neer CS II: Unconstrained shoulder arthroplasty. Instr Course Lect 34:278-286, 1985.
298. Neer CS II: Shoulder Reconstruction. Philadelphia: WB Saunders, 1990.
299. Neer CS II, Brown TH Jr, and McLaughlin HL: Fracture of the neck of the humerus with dislocation of the head fragment. Am J Surg 85:252-258, 1953.
300. Neer CS II, Craig EV, and Fukuda H: Cuff-tear arthropathy. J Bone Joint Surg Am 65:1232-1244, 1983.
301. Neer CS II and Kirby RM: Revision of humeral head and total shoulder arthroplasty. Clin Orthop 170:189-195, 1982.
302. Neer CS II and Morrison DS: Glenoid bone-grafting in total shoulder arthroplasty. J Bone Joint Surg Am 70:1154-1162, 1988.
303. Neer CS II and Rockwood CA: Fractures and dislocations of the shoulder. In Rockwood CA and Green DP (eds): Fractures in Adults. Philadelphia: JB Lippincott, 1984, pp 675-985.
304. Neer CS II, Watson KC, and Stanton FJ: Recent experience in total shoulder replacement. J Bone Joint Surg Am 64:319-337, 1982.
305. Nelson JP, Fitzgerald RH, Jaspers MT, and Little JW: Prophylactic antimicrobial coverage in arthroplasty patients [editorial]. J Bone Joint Surg Am 72:1, 1990.
306. Nguyen VD and Nguyen KD: "Idiopathic destructive arthritis" of the shoulder: A still fascinating enigma. Comput Med Imaging Graph 14:249-255, 1990.
307. Norris TR, Green A, and McGuigan FX: Late prosthetic shoulder arthroplasty for displaced proximal humerus fractures. J Shoulder Elbow Surg 4:271-280, 1995.
308. Norris T and Iannotti J: A Prospective Outcome Study Comparing Humeral Head Replacement and Total Shoulder Replacement for Primary Osteoarthritis of the Shoulder. Paper presented at the 12th Open Meeting of the American Shoulder and Elbow Surgeons, 1996, Atlanta.
309. Norris TR and Iannotti JP: Functional outcome after shoulder arthroplasty for primary osteoarthritis: A multicenter study. J Shoulder Elbow Surg 11:130-135, 2002.
310. Nussbaum AJ and Doppman JL: Shoulder arthroplasty in primary hyperparathyroidism. Skeletal Radiol 9:98-102, 1982.
311. Orr TE, Carter DR, and Schurman DJ: Stress analyses of glenoid component designs. Clin Orthop 232:217-224, 1988.
312. Pahle JA and Kvarnes L: Shoulder synovectomy. Ann Chirurg Gynaecol 198 (suppl 75):37-39, 1985.
313. Pahle JA and Kvarnes L: Shoulder replacement arthroplasty. Ann Chir Gynaecol 74(suppl 198):85-89, 1985.
314. Parikh JR, Houpt JB, Jacobs S, and Fernandes BJ: Charcot's arthropathy of the shoulder following intraarticular corticosteroid injections. J Rheumatol 20:885-887, 1993.
315. Pavlov PW: A fifteen year follow-up study of 512 consecutive Charnley-Müller total hip replacements. J Arthroplasty 2:151-156, 1987.
316. Pearl ML and Kurutz S: Geometric analysis of commonly used prosthetic systems for proximal humeral replacement. J Bone Joint Surg Am 81:660-671, 1999.
317. Pearl ML, Kurutz S, Robertson DD, and Yamaguchi K: Geometric analysis of selected press fit prosthetic systems for proximal humeral replacement. J Orthop Res 20:192-197, 2002.
318. Pearl ML and Lippitt SB: Shoulder arthroplasty with a modular prosthesis. Tech Orthop 8:151-162, 1994.
319. Pearl ML and Volk AG: Retroversion of the proximal humerus in relationship to prosthetic replacement arthroplasty. J Shoulder Elbow Surg 4:286-289, 1995.
320. Pellicci PM and Hass SB: Disassembly of a modular femoral component during closed reduction of the dislocated femoral component: A case report. J Bone Joint Surg Am 72:619-620, 1990.
321. Peppers TA, Jobe CM, Dai QG, et al: Fixation of humeral prostheses and axial micromotion. J Shoulder Elbow Surg 7:414-418, 1998.
322. Petersson CJ: Shoulder surgery in rheumatoid arthritis. Acta Orthop Scand 57:222-226, 1986.
323. Petersson CJ: Painful shoulders in patients with rheumatoid arthritis. Scand J Rheumatol 15:275-279, 1986.
324. Podgorski M, Robinson B, Weissberger A, et al: Articular manifestations of acromegaly. Aust N Z J Med 18:28-35, 1988.
325. Pollock RG, Deliz ED, McIlveen SJ, et al: Prosthetic replacement in rotator cuff-deficient shoulders. J Shoulder Elbow Surg 1:173-186, 1992.
326. Pollock RG, Higgis GB, Codd TP, et al: Total shoulder replacement for the treatment of primary glenohumeral osteoarthritis. J Shoulder Elbow Surg 4(suppl):S12, 1995.
327. Poppen N and Walker P: Normal and abnormal motion of the shoulder. J Bone Joint Surg Am 58:195-201, 1976.
328. Poppen N and Walker P: Forces at the glenohumeral joint in abduction. Clin Orthop 135:165-170, 1978.
329. Post M: Constrained arthroplasty of the shoulder. Orthop Clin North Am 18:455-462, 1987.
330. Post M: Shoulder arthroplasty and total shoulder replacement. In Post M (ed): The Shoulder. Philadelphia: Lea & Febiger, 1988, pp 221-278.
331. Post M and Haskell S: Michael Reese Total Shoulder. Memphis, TN: Richards Manufacturing, 1978.
332. Post M, Haskell SS, and Jablon M: Total shoulder replacement with a constrained prosthesis. J Bone Joint Surg Am 62:327, 1980.
333. Post M and Jablon M: Constrained total shoulder arthroplasty: Long-term follow-up observations. Clin Orthop 173:109-116, 1983.
334. Post M, Jablon M, Miller H, and Singh M: Constrained total shoulder joint replacement: A critical review. Clin Orthop 144:135-150, 1979.
335. Pritchett JW and Clark JM: Prosthetic replacement for chronic unreduced dislocations of the shoulder. Clin Orthop 216:89-93, 1987.
336. Putti V: Artrodesi nella tubercolosi del Ginocchio e della Spalla. Chir Organi Mov 18:217, 1933.
337. Radosevich DM, Wetzler H, and Wilson SM: Health Status Questionnaire (HSQ) 2.0: Scoring Comparisons and Reference Data. Bloomington, MN: Health Outcomes Institute, 1994.
338. Rand JA and Sim FH: Total shoulder arthroplasty for the arthroplasty of hemochromatosis: A case report. Orthopedics 4:658-660, 1981.
339. Raskob GE, Lofthouse RN, and Hull RD: Current concepts review: Methodological guidelines for clinical trials evaluating new therapeutic approaches in bone and joint surgery. J Bone Joint Surg Am 67:1294-1297, 1985.
340. Reeves B, Jobbins B, Dowson D, and Wright V: A total shoulder endo-prosthesis. N Engl J Med 1:64-67, 1974.
341. Rhoades CE, Neff JR, Rengachary SS, et al: Diagnosis of posttraumatic syringohydromyelia presenting as neuropathic joints. Clin Orthop 180:182-187, 1983.
342. Richard A, Judet R, and Reneá L: Acrylic prosthetic reconstruction of the upper end of the humerus for fracture-luxations. J Chir 68:537-547, 1952.

343. Richards RR, An K-N, Bigliani LU, et al: A standardized method for the assessment of shoulder function. J Shoulder Elbow Surg 3:347-352, 1994.

344. Richards RR, Beaton D, and Hudson AR: Shoulder arthrodesis with plate fixation: Function outcome analysis. J Shoulder Elbow Surg 2:225-239, 1993.

345. Richards RR, Sherman RMP, Hudson AR, and Waddell JP: Shoulder arthrodesis using a pelvic-reconstruction plate—a report of eleven cases. J Bone Joint Surg Am 70:416-421, 1988.

346. Richards RR, Waddell JP, and Hudson AR: Shoulder arthrodesis for the treatment of brachial plexus palsy. Clin Orthop 198:250-258, 1985.

347. Riggins RS: Shoulder fusion without external fixation: A preliminary report. J Bone Joint Surg Am 58:1007, 1976.

348. Roberts SNJ, Foley APJ, Swallow HM, et al: The geometry of the humeral head and the design of prostheses. J Bone Joint Surg Br 73:647-650, 1991.

349. Rockwood CA Jr: The technique of total shoulder arthroplasty. Instr Course Lect 39:437-447, 1990.

350. Rockwood CA Jr: Personal communication, 1995.

351. Rockwood CA Jr, Jarman RN, and Williams GR: Complications of shoulder arthrodesis using internal fixation. Orthop Trans 15:45, 1991.

352. Rockwood CA and Matsen RM: Global Shoulder Arthroplasty System. Warsaw, IN: DePuy Inc, 1994.

353. Rockwood CA Jr and Wirth MA: Global Total Shoulder Arthroplasty Video, Parts I and II. AAOS Individual Orthopaedic Instruction Video Award Winner, 1992.

354. Rodosky MW and Bigliani LU: Surgical treatment of nonconstrained glenoid component failure. Oper Tech Orthop 4:226-236, 1994.

355. Rodosky MW and Bigliani LU: Indications for glenoid resurfacing in shoulder arthroplasty. J Shoulder Elbow Surg 5:231-248, 1996.

356. Rodosky MW, Weinstein DM, Pollock RG, et al: On the rarity of glenoid failure. J Shoulder Elbow Surg 4(suppl):S13, 1995.

357. Roper BA, Paterson JMH, and Day WH: The Roper-Day total shoulder replacement. J Bone Joint Surg Br 72:694-697, 1990.

358. Rossleigh MA, Smith J, Straus DJ, and Engel IA: Osteonecrosis in patients with malignant lymphoma. Cancer 58:1112-1116, 1986.

359. Rountree CR and Rockwood CA Jr: Arthrodesis of the shoulder in children following infantile paralysis. South Med J 58:861, 1959.

360. Rowe CR: Re-evaluation of the position of the arm in arthrodesis of the shoulder in the adult. J Bone Joint Surg Am 56:913-922, 1974.

361. Rowe CR and Zarins B: Chronic unreduced dislocations of the shoulder. J Bone Joint Surg Am 64:494-505, 1982.

362. Rozencwaig R, van Noort A, Moskal MJ, et al: The correlation of comorbidity with function of the shoulder and health status of patients who have glenohumeral degenerative joint disease. J Bone Joint Surg Am 80:1146-1153, 1998.

363. Rozing PM and Brand R: Rotator cuff repair during shoulder arthroplasty in rheumatoid arthritis. J Arthroplasty 13:311-319, 1998.

364. Rudicel S and Esdiale J: The randomized clinical trial in orthopaedics: Obligation or option? J Bone Joint Surg Am 67:1284-1293, 1985.

365. Russe O: Schulterarthrodese nach der AO-methode. Unfallheilkunde 81:299, 1978.

366. Rutherford CS and Cofield RH: Osteonecrosis of the shoulder. Orthop Trans 11:239, 1987.

367. Rybka V, Raunio P, and Vainio K: Arthrodesis of the shoulder in rheumatoid arthritis: A review of 41 cases. J Bone Joint Surg Br 61:155, 1979.

368. Rydholm U and Sjogren J: Surface replacement of the humeral head in the rheumatoid shoulder. J Shoulder Elbow Surg 2:286-295, 1993.

369. Saha AK, Bhattacharyya D, Dutta SK: Total shoulder replacement: A preliminary report. Calcutta, India: SK Sitcar, 1975.

370. Samilson RL and Prieto V: Dislocation arthroplasty of the shoulder. J Bone Joint Surg Am 65:456-460, 1983.

371. Sanchez-Sotelo J, Cofield RH, and Rowland CM: Shoulder hemiarthroplasty for glenohumeral arthritis associated with severe rotator cuff deficiency. J Bone Joint Surg Am 83:1814-1822, 2001.

372. Sanchez-Sotelo J, O'Driscoll SW, Torchia ME, et al: Radiographic assessment of cemented humeral components in shoulder arthroplasty. J Shoulder Elbow Surg 10:526-531, 2001.

373. Sanchez-Sotelo J, Wright TW, O'Driscoll SW, et al: Radiographic assessment of uncemented humeral components in total shoulder arthroplasty. J Arthroplasty 16:180-187, 2001.

374. Scarlat MM and Matsen FA III: Observations on retrieved polyethylene glenoid components. J Arthroplasty 16:795-801, 2001.

375. Schwartz RR, O'Brien SJ, Warren RF, and Torzilli PA: Capsular restraints to anterior-posterior motion in the shoulder. Paper presented at the 4th Open Meeting of the American Shoulder and Elbow Surgeons, 1988, Atlanta.

376. Schwyzer HK, Simmen BR, and Gschwend N: Infection following shoulder and elbow arthroplasty: Diagnosis and therapy. Orthopade 24:367-375, 1995.

377. Seitz WH Jr and Damacen H: Staged exchange arthroplasty for shoulder sepsis. J Arthroplasty 17(4 suppl 1):36-40, 2002.

378. Sethi D, Naunton Morgan TC, et al: Dialysis arthropathy: A clinical, biochemical, radiological and histological study of 36 patients. Q J Med 77:1061-1082, 1990.

379. Severt R, Thomas BJ, Tsenter MJ, et al: The influence of conformity and constraint on translational forces and frictional torque in total shoulder arthroplasty. Clin Orthop 292:151-158, 1993.

380. Simkin PA: Structure and function of joints. In Schumacher HR (ed): Primer on the Rheumatic Diseases. Atlanta: Arthritis Foundation, 1988.

381. Slawson SH, Everson LI, and Craig EV: The radiology of total shoulder replacement. Radiol Clin North Am 33:305-318, 1995.

382. Smith-Peterson MN, Aufranc OE, and Larson CB: Useful surgical procedures for rheumatoid arthritis involving joints of the upper extremity. Arch Surg 46:764-770, 1943.

383. Sneppen O, Fruensgaard S, Johannsen HV, et al: Total shoulder replacement in rheumatoid arthritis: Proximal migration and loosening. J Shoulder Elbow Surg 5:47-52, 1996.

384. Sojbjerg JO, Frich LH, Johannsen HV, and Sneppen O: Late results of total shoulder replacement in patients with rheumatoid arthritis. Clin Orthop 366:39-45, 1999.

385. Spencer R and Skirving AP: Silastic interposition arthroplasty of the shoulder. J Bone Joint Surg Br 68:375-377, 1986.

386. Sperling JW, Antuna SA, Sanchez-Sotelo J, et al: Shoulder arthroplasty for arthritis after instability surgery. J Bone Joint Surg Am 84:1775-1781, 2002.

387. Sperling JW and Cofield RH: Revision total shoulder arthroplasty for the treatment of glenoid arthrosis. J Bone Joint Surg Am 80:860-867, 1998.

388. Sperling JW, Cofield RH, O'Driscoll SW, et al: Radiographic assessment of ingrowth total shoulder arthroplasty. J Shoulder Elbow Surg 9:507-513, 2000.

389. Sperling JW, Cofield RH, and Rowland CM: Neer hemiarthroplasty and Neer total shoulder arthroplasty in patients fifty years old or less. Long-term results. J Bone Joint Surg Am 80:464-473, 1998.

390. Sperling JW, Kozak TK, Hanssen AD, and Cofield RH: Infection after shoulder arthroplasty. Clin Orthop 382:206-216, 2001.

391. Sperling JW, Potter HG, Craig EV, et al: Magnetic resonance imaging of painful shoulder arthroplasty. J Shoulder Elbow Surg 11:315-321, 2002.

392. Steffee AD and Moore RW: Hemi-resurfacing arthroplasty of the shoulder. Contemp Orthop 9:51-59, 1984.

393. Steindler A: Orthopedic Operations: Indications, Technique, and End Results. Springfield, IL: Charles C Thomas, 1944, p 302.

394. Steinmann SP and Cofield RH: Bone grafting for glenoid deficiency in total shoulder replacement. J Shoulder Elbow Surg 9:361-367, 2000.

395. Stinchfield FE, Bigliani LU, Neu HC, et al: Late hematogenous infection of total joint replacement. J Bone Joint Surg Am 62:1345-1350, 1980.

396. Stone KD, Grabowski JJ, Cofield RH, et al: Stress analyses of glenoid components in total shoulder arthroplasty. J Shoulder Elbow Surg 8:151-158, 1999.

397. Sullivan PM, Johnston RC, and Kelley SS: Late infection after total hip replacement, caused by an oral organism after dental manipulation. J Bone Joint Surg Am 72:121-122, 1990.

398. Summers MN, Haley WE, Reveille JD, and Alarcon GS: Radiographic assessment and psychologic variables as predictors of pain and functional impairment in osteoarthritis of the knee or hip. Arthritis Rheum 31:204-209, 1988.

399. Svend-Hansen H: Displaced proximal humeral fractures: A review of 49 patients. Acta Orthop Scand 45:359, 1974.

400. Swanson AB: Implant resection arthroplasty of shoulder joint. In Swanson AB (ed): Flexible Resection Arthroplasty in the Hand and Extremities. St Louis: CV Mosby, 1973, pp 287-295.

401. Swanson AB: Bipolar implant shoulder arthroplasty. In Bateman JE and Welsh RP (eds): Surgery of the Shoulder. St Louis: CV Mosby, 1984, pp 211-223.

402. Swanson AB, deGroot G, Maupin BK, et al: Bipolar implant shoulder arthroplasty. Orthopedics 9:343-351, 1986.

403. Swanson AB, deGroot Swanson G, Sattel AB, et al: Bipolar implant shoulder arthroplasty: Long-term results. Clin Orthop 248:227-247, 1989.

404. Tanner MW and Cofield RH: Prosthetic arthroplasty for fractured and fracture-dislocations of the proximal humerus. Clin Orthop 179:116-128, 1983.

405. Thomas BJ, Amstutz HC, and Cracchiolo A: Shoulder arthroplasty for rheumatoid arthritis. Clin Orthop 265:125-128, 1991.

406. Tonino AJ and van de Werf GJIM: Hemiarthroplasty of the shoulder. Acta Orthop Belg 51:625-631, 1985.

407. Torchia ME, Cofield RH, and Settergren CR: Total shoulder arthroplasty with the Neer prosthesis: Long-term results. Orthop Trans 18:977, 1994-1995.

408. Tully JG Jr and Latteri A: Paraplegia, syringomyelia tarde and neuropathic arthrosis of the shoulder: A triad. Clin Orthop 134:244-248, 1978.

409. Turkel SJ, Panio MW, Marshall JL, and Girgis FG: Stabilizing mechanisms preventing anterior dislocation of the glenohumeral joint. J Bone Joint Surg Am 63:1208-1217, 1981.

410. Uematsu A: Arthrodesis of the shoulder: Posterior approach. Clin Orthop 139:169, 1979.

411. van Cappelle HGJ, and Visser JD: Hemiarthroplasty of the shoulder in rheumatoid arthritis. J Orthop Rheum 7:43-47, 1994.

412. van der Zwaag HM, Brand R, Obermann WR, and Rozing PM: Glenohumeral osteoarthrosis after Putti-Platt repair. J Shoulder Elbow Surg 8:252-258, 1999.

413. van Schaardenburg D, Van den Brande KJS, Ligthart GJ, et al: Musculoskeletal disorders and disability in persons aged 85 and over: A community survey. Ann Rheum Dis 53:807-811, 1994.

414. Varian JPW: Interposition Silastic cup arthroplasty of the shoulder. J Bone Joint Surg Br 62:116-117, 1980.
415. Vitale MG, Krant JJ, Gelijns AC, et al: Geographic variations in the rates of operative procedures involving rotator cuff repair. J Bone Joint Surg Am 81:763-772, 1999.
416. Wainwright D: Glenoidectomy in the treatment of the painful arthritic shoulder [abstract]. J Bone Joint Surg Br 58:377, 1976.
417. Wakitani S, Imoto K, Saito M, et al: Evaluation of surgeries for rheumatoid shoulder based on the destruction pattern. J Rheumatol 26:41-46, 1999.
418. Walch G, Badet R, Boulahia A, and Khoury A: Morphologic study of the glenoid in primary glenohumeral osteoarthritis. J Arthroplasty 14:756-760, 1999.
419. Wallace AL, Phillips RL, MacDougal GA, et al: Resurfacing of the glenoid in total shoulder arthroplasty. A comparison, at a mean of five years, of prostheses inserted with and without cement. J Bone Joint Surg Am 81:510-518, 1999.
420. Ware JE, Snow KK, Kosinski M, and Gandek B: SF 36 Health Survey Manual and Interpretation Guide. Boston: New England Medical Center, The Health Institute, 1993.
421. Warren RF, Kornblatt IB, and Marchand R: Static factors affecting posterior shoulder instability. Orthop Trans 8:1-89, 1984.
422. Warren RF, Ranawat CA, and Inglis AE: Total shoulder replacement indications and results of the Neer nonconstrained prosthesis. In Inglis AE (ed): The American Academy of Orthopaedic Surgeons Symposium on Total Joint Replacement of the Upper Extremity. St Louis: CV Mosby, 1982, pp 56-67.
423. Watson-Jones RW: Extra-articular arthrodesis of the shoulder. J Bone Joint Surg 15:862, 1933.
424. Weigert M and Gronert HJ: Zur Technik der Schultergelenksarthrodese. Z Orthop 112:1281, 1974.
425. Weiss APC, Adams MA, Moore JR, and Weiland AJ: Unconstrained shoulder arthroplasty. A five-year average follow up study. Clin Orthop 257:86-90, 1990.
426. Weldon EJ III, Scarlat MM, Lee SB, and Matsen FA III: Intrinsic stability of unused and retrieved polyethylene glenoid components. J Shoulder Elbow Surg 10:474-481, 2001.
427. Wheble VH and Skorecki J: The design of a metal-to-metal total shoulder joint prosthesis. In Joint Replacement in the Upper Limb. Conference Sponsored by the Medical Engineering Section of the Institution of Mechanical Engineers and the British Orthopaedic Association. London: Medical Engineering Institute, 1977, pp 7-13.
428. Wilde AH, Borden LS, and Brems JJ: Experience with the Neer total shoulder replacement. In Bateman JE and Welsh RP (eds): Surgery of the Shoulder. St Louis: BC Decker and CV Mosby, 1984, p 224.
429. Wilde AH, Brems JJ, and Boumphrey FRS: Arthrodesis of the shoulder: Current indications and operative technique. Orthop Clin North Am 18:463-472, 1987.
430. Williams GR and Rockwood CA Jr: Massive rotator cuff defects and glenohumeral arthritis. In Friedman RJ (ed): Arthroplasty of the Shoulder. New York: Thieme Medical, 1994, pp 204-214.
431. Williams GR and Rockwood CA Jr: Hemiarthroplasty in rotator cuff–deficient shoulders. J Shoulder Elbow Surg 5:362-367, 1996.
432. Williams GR Jr, Wong KL, Pepe MD, et al: The effect of articular malposition after total shoulder arthroplasty on glenohumeral translations, range of motion, and subacromial impingement. J Shoulder Elbow Surg 10:399-409, 2001.
433. Winalski CS and Shapiro AW: Computed tomography in the evaluation of arthritis. Rheum Dis Clin North Am 17:543-557, 1991.
434. Wirth MA, Agrawal CM, Mabrey JD, et al: Isolation and characterization of polyethylene wear debris associated with osteolysis following total shoulder arthroplasty. J Bone Joint Surg Am 81:29-37, 1999.
435. Wirth MA, Basamania C, and Rockwood CA Jr: Fixation of glenoid component: Keel vs. pegs. Oper Tech Orthop 4:218, 1994.
436. Wirth MA, Butters KP, and Rockwood CA Jr: The posterior deltoid-splitting approach to the shoulder. Clin Orthop 296:92-98, 1993.
437. Wirth MA, Korvick DL, Basamania CJ, et al: Radiologic, mechanical, and histologic evaluation of 2 glenoid prosthesis designs in a canine model. J Shoulder Elbow Surg 10:140-148, 2001.
438. Wirth MA and Rockwood CA Jr: Traumatic instability: Pathology and pathogenesis. In Matsen FA (ed): The Shoulder: A Balance of Mobility and Stability. Chicago: American Academy of Orthopaedic Surgeons, 1993.
439. Wirth MA and Rockwood CA Jr: Complications of shoulder arthroplasty. Clin Orthop 307:47-69, 1994.
440. Wirth MA and Rockwood CA Jr: Glenohumeral instability following shoulder arthroplasty. Paper presented at the 62nd Annual Meeting of the American Academy of Orthopaedic Surgeons, 1995, Orlando, FL.
440a. Wirth MA and Rockwood CA Jr, et al: Radiologic, mechanical, and histologic evaluation of two glenoid prosthesis designs in a canine model. J Shoulder Elbow Surg March/April:140-148, 2001.
441. Wirth MA, Seltzer DG, Senes HR, et al: An analysis of failed humeral head and total shoulder arthroplasty. Orthop Trans 18:977-978, 1994-1995.
442. Woolson ST and Potorff GT: Disassembly of a modular femoral prosthesis after dislocation of the femoral component: A case report. J Bone Joint Surg Am 72:624-625, 1990.
443. Worland RL and Arredondo J: Bipolar shoulder arthroplasty for painful conditions of the shoulder. J Arthroplasty 13:631-637, 1998.
444. Wright TW and Cofield RH: Humeral fractures after shoulder arthroplasty. J Bone Joint Surg Am 77:1340-1346, 1995.
445. Zippel J: Vollständiger Schultergelenkersatz aus Kunststoff und Metall. Biomed Technik 17:87, 1972.
446. Zippel J: Luxationssichere Schulterendoprothese Modell BME. Z Orthop 113:454-457, 1975.
447. Zuckerman JD: Shoulder arthroplasty—costs/results. Instructional Course Lecture No. 110 presented at the Annual Meeting of the American Academy of Orthopaedic Surgeons, 1996, Atlanta.
448. Zuckerman JD and Cofield RH: Proximal humeral prosthetic replacement in glenohumeral arthritis. Orthop Trans 10:231, 1986.
449. Zuckerman JD and Cuomo F: Glenohumeral arthroplasty: A critical review of indications and preoperative considerations. Bull Hosp Jt Dis 52:21-30, 1993.
450. Zuckerman JD and Matsen FA III: Complications about the glenohumeral joint related to the use of screws and staples. J Bone Joint Surg Am 66:175-180, 1984.
451. Zuckerman JD, Scott AJ, and Gallagher MA: Hemiarthroplasty for cuff tear arthropathy. J Shoulder Elbow Surg 9:169-172, 2000.

CHAPTER 17

NERVE PROBLEMS ABOUT THE SHOULDER

Scott P. Steinmann, M.D., and Robert J. Spinner, M.D.

• • • •

Patients with shoulder pain or injuries not infrequently have concomitant neurologic conditions, and orthopaedic surgeons caring for such patients must be aware of this potential complication. In addition, the practice of reconstructive shoulder surgery carries an inherent risk of iatrogenic injury to neighboring neurologic structures. Knowledge of the common nerve lesions about the shoulder will allow surgeons to recognize these entities when they see them, and familiarity with the relevant neural anatomy will help them avoid potential neural injuries when they operate. Surgeons must have a systematic approach to evaluating and treating these challenging patients with nerve-related disorders about the shoulder region.

CLINICAL EVALUATION

Patients with nerve injuries are often seen in situations involving significant trauma. Frequently, the patient may be confused, incoherent, sedated, or even unconscious, and it can be difficult to perform a satisfactory neurologic examination before initiating surgical care. Nonetheless, a good neurologic examination should be attempted in the emergency department. If an adequate examination cannot be performed for any reason, this fact should be noted in the patient's medical record. Specifically, if the function of a particular nerve cannot be assessed well preoperatively, the record should include such information. Too often in the emergency setting, the patient receives only a cursory evaluation and perhaps the most junior person on the orthopaedic surgical team writes in the clinical record that the extremity was "neurovascularly intact." These two words, if inaccurate, are sometimes the origin of unnecessary litigation. Such general terms should not be used when recording a patient's examination, but instead, individual muscle strength, sensory examination, and deep tendon reflexes should be carefully documented in the patient's record.

A neurologic evaluation of the upper extremity can be performed on a coherent patient in a relatively short time, even if the patient has a shoulder dislocation or proximal humeral fracture. It is often easiest to start at the hand and progress proximally during the examination. Radial, median, and ulnar nerve function can all be assessed by a thorough evaluation of the hand and wrist, which should take less than a minute. Elbow flexion and extension

strength are relatively simple to determine. One should be aware, however, that it is possible to flex the elbow strongly with the action of the brachioradialis without having any function of the biceps. Loss of motor or sensory function in the distal end of the extremity can help direct examination of the more proximal musculature. For example, loss of radial nerve function should make the examiner look closely at axillary nerve function because they are both derived from the posterior cord. Likewise, loss of median nerve function might also affect the musculocutaneous nerve if the lesion is in the lateral cord.

Progressing up the arm, the condition of the medial and lateral pectoral nerves can be assessed by individually testing the strength of each of the major portions of the pectoralis major. The deltoid and rotator cuff muscles are then examined. The deltoid can be assessed even in the case of a painful proximal humeral fracture or glenohumeral dislocation. With the arm at the side, the patient is instructed to push out or "elbow" the examiner's hand (one of which is placed at the lateral aspect of the elbow and the other over the deltoid region to feel for contracture). If the patient is in a great deal of pain and the examiner cannot adequately determine the condition of the axillary nerve, this information should be recorded in the clinical record. Do not assume that it "might" be okay.

Examining shoulder abduction is an important part of the examination both to record muscle strength and to visualize shoulder kinesis through the arc of motion. Two important points are relevant here. First, some patients can abduct the shoulder through a full arc of motion by using either just the supraspinatus or the deltoid in the face of complete paralysis of one or the other. Ensuring muscle contraction is a critical element in this part of the examination. Second, visualizing and palpating the scapula are a necessary part of the examination, especially when one is faced with dysfunction. For example, patients with winged scapulas from either serratus anterior or trapezius weakness may have difficulty abducting the arm fully without the scapula stabilized and may compensate with "trick motions." Physicians should recognize the clinical appearances and know the techniques to examine winging of the scapula, particularly with respect to distinguishing serratus anterior, trapezius, or rhomboid muscle dysfunction. In addition, a useful test for serratus anterior function, in which the inferior pole of the scapula is stabilized and the patient pushes the arm forward, can be applied even in a patient with a complete brachial plexus lesion; patients unable to push their arms forward could not otherwise perform the more "standard" pushoff test with the arms extended against the wall.

One needs to evaluate for other conditions causing lack of movement besides a neurologic etiology. Certainly, one needs to consider that the inability of a patient to externally rotate the arm or perform the "liftoff" test may represent either a neurologic lesion affecting the infraspinatus or subscapularis, a rotator cuff tear, or both. A patient who is feigning paralysis in the upper limb for secondary gain issues cannot "voluntarily" stop the latissimus dorsi from contracting while coughing.

Examination of the shoulder must include examination well above the shoulder and even above the neck, as well as the distal portion of the limb. Proximal and distal lesions must always be considered when one is examining a patient with shoulder pain or weakness and establishing a differential diagnosis. Cervical radiculopathy is a common cause of pain in the shoulder accompanied by motor weakness and sensory loss in the upper extremity. In this situation, flexion and extension of the cervical spine or Spurling's maneuver may reproduce or exacerbate the patient's symptoms. Upper motor neuron lesions can also result in shoulder weakness. In these cases, the deep tendon reflexes may be hyperreflexic, pathologic reflexes may be present, and tone may be increased. Referred pain should be excluded as a possibility during the clinical examination because cardiac or other intrathoracic complaints may be manifested as shoulder pain.

Finally, examination of the shoulder can be performed only with both shoulders exposed. Visualization is the first component of a physical examination, but this step is often neglected because of either time constraints or modesty issues. It is easy to "miss" atrophy of the spinatus muscles if one does not look at the bare scapula. Bilateral atrophy or weakness would certainly change the differential diagnosis and force the examiner to consider an underlying neurogenic or myopathic condition.

MUSCULOCUTANEOUS NERVE INJURY

Musculocutaneous nerve injury is most commonly associated with severe brachial plexus trauma. Although the nerve can be injured in glenohumeral dislocation, it is unusual to diagnose such injury as an isolated neuropathy.[38] If it is seen as an isolated nerve injury, it is most often associated with a form of penetrating trauma, open surgical reconstruction, or a direct blow to the chest (near the coracoid). Occasionally, musculocutaneous neuropathy can occur after strenuous physical activity such as rowing.[103]

The musculocutaneous nerve travels obliquely below the coracoid process and enters the coracobrachialis. The anatomy of this juncture has been investigated in several studies. Small branches of the nerve can be found inserting into the coracobrachialis as close as 17 mm below the coracoid.[60] The main trunk of the musculocutaneous nerve enters the coracobrachialis approximately 5 cm from the coracoid and exits at 7 cm.[53,60] The nerve then enters the biceps, typically more than 10 cm from the coracoid.[53] The nerve is at risk during anterior shoulder procedures that result in significant retraction medially or during medial surgical dissection. The Bristow procedure has been thought to be associated with injury to the nerve,[10] but such injury is probably related less to transfer and more to manipulation of the nerve.[28] The operating surgeon must recognize the protective value of maintaining the origins of the coracobrachialis and biceps. When these muscles are allowed to remain on the coracoid during surgery, they act as a tether to overzealous medial retraction. In fact, exposure of the posterior cord or the axillary nerve may lead to musculocutaneous nerve palsy as a result of retraction. Care must be taken to avoid excessive traction on the musculocutaneous nerve during dissection. Alternatively, detachment of the conjoint tendon allows excellent exposure and potentially decreased pressure in the entire brachial plexus. Actual detachment of these muscles from the coracoid and reattachment to the anterior glenoid (the Bristow procedure) will relax the musculocutaneous nerve. Nonetheless, the surgical manipulation required may result in damage to the nerve.

The nerve may also be damaged during arthroscopic surgery, although such injury is quite rare. Anterior portals straying medial to the coracoid put the musculocutaneous nerve and other branches of the brachial plexus at potential risk for injury. Low anterior portals such as the "5 o'clock portal" may bring instruments to within 10 mm of the nerve.[124] A patient with a musculocutaneous nerve lesion typically has a mixed sensory and motor lesion. Less commonly, a pure sensory lesion of the lateral antebrachial cutaneous nerve, the distal sensory termination of the musculocutaneous nerve, can occur. This injury can often have an atraumatic etiology. Patients may have numbness or paresthesia along the lateral elbow crease that extends distally along the anterolateral aspect of the forearm. Treatment involves splinting or corticosteroid injection and, possibly, surgical exploration.[157] Surgical exploration may on occasion reveal a thickened aponeurosis compressing the lateral antebrachial cutaneous nerve as it transits between the biceps and brachioradialis muscles. Patients may respond to surgical decompression of the nerve in this area.[42]

If a patient is seen after trauma or surgery with an injury to the musculocutaneous nerve, the patient should be observed for a period of 3 to 4 weeks. If at that time no improvement in function is noted, electromyography and nerve conduction studies (EMG/NCS) can be performed to assess the extent of nerve damage. Most postoperative musculocutaneous neuropathies are traction injuries that resolve over a period of weeks to months, depending on the extent of the injury.

If biceps function is not seen to improve either by clinical examination or by electrophysiologic studies, surgical exploration should be undertaken, ideally before 6 months has transpired from the injury. Surgical treatment options vary for persistent musculocutaneous neuropathy. If at surgical exploration the nerve appears intact but compressed by scar and demonstrates electrical conduction across the lesion, neurolysis may be the initial treatment. If a neuroma in continuity or transection of the nerve is discovered, additional treatment options may be considered.

In patients with an isolated musculocutaneous nerve injury, a standard approach would be to perform interpositional nerve grafting across the lesion. However, nerve transfers could also be used to shorten the distance (and time) for reinnervation or bypass a scarred or avascular segment. A new nerve transfer is the Oberlin transfer, a technique in which one or two fascicles of the ulnar nerve are transferred directly to the motor branch to the biceps.[92,119] The distance to achieve reinnervation is extremely short because the site of repair is in the proximal part of the arm (several centimeters from the biceps end-organ) rather than a more lengthy repair from the neck or shoulder region. This technique can be used in patients with upper plexus lesions. Grade 3 or 4 Medical Research Council (MRC) function was achieved in over 90% of patients treated with this technique in two large series (each with over 30 patients).[119,156] Reinnervation in the biceps was noted approximately 3 months after the procedure. Importantly, no patient suffered loss of distal ulnar nerve function or sensation.

If patients are seen longer than 1 year after musculocutaneous nerve injury, nerve repair or reconstruction is significantly less likely to be effective.[34,62,83,120,138,141,147]

Some of these patients still function extremely well solely by using their brachioradialis for elbow flexion. The majority of these patients, however, need augmentation. A number of tendon or muscle transfer procedures that achieve good results can be used. Popular options include Steindler's flexorplasty (proximal advancement of the flexor/pronator muscle group) and triceps, pectoralis major, pectoralis minor, and latissimus dorsi transfer. Free muscle transfer is also a possibility in patients without these other available potential donor muscles.

AXILLARY NERVE

The axillary nerve is one of the more commonly injured nerves about the shoulder. It is a terminal branch of the posterior cord and is derived from the fifth and sixth cranial nerves. The axillary nerve lies lateral to the radial nerve, posterior to the axillary artery, and anterior to the subscapularis muscle. It enters the quadrilateral space accompanied by the posterior humeral circumflex artery and is in close contact with the inferior shoulder capsule. It is easy to locate at surgery during an anterior exposure by sweeping an index finger inferiorly over the anterior subscapularis and gently hooking the axillary nerve while simultaneously palpating the nerve on the underside of the deltoid with the other index finger.[59] As it exits the space, the nerve continues to the posterior aspect of the humeral neck and divides into anterior and posterior branches. The position of the anterior branch is commonly reported as lying 4 to 7 cm inferior to the anterolateral corner of the acromion.[23] The posterior branch innervates both the teres minor and the posterior portion of the deltoid. The branch to the teres minor usually arises within or just distal to the quadrilateral space and enters the posteroinferior aspect of the teres minor muscle. The internal topography of the axillary nerve has been studied by Aszmann and Dellon.[8] As the nerve leaves the posterior cord, it is monofascicular, but as it enters the quadrilateral space, it has three distinct groups of fascicles: motor groups to the deltoid and teres minor and the sensory group of the superior lateral cutaneous nerve. The deltoid motor fascicles are found in a superolateral position; those of the teres minor and superior lateral cutaneous nerve are located inferomedially.

Most axillary nerve injuries occur as part of a combined brachial plexus injury; isolated axillary nerve injury occurs in only 0.3% to 6% of brachial plexus injuries.[153] Injury to the axillary nerve most frequently follows closed trauma involving traction on the shoulder. Axillary nerve paralysis is the most common neurologic complication of shoulder dislocations. Some patients with a proximal humeral fracture or shoulder dislocation may have a subclinical axillary nerve lesion evident by EMG/NCS but not clinically apparent because of the associated discomfort.[73,115,123,160,168] The vast majority of these patients recover from the nerve injury as they rehabilitate from the dislocation or fracture. Blunt trauma to the anterolateral aspect of the shoulder has also been noted to cause axillary nerve injury from compression of the nerve as it travels on the deep surface of the deltoid muscle.[128]

Open reconstructive surgery (Fig. 17–1) or newer arthroscopic techniques may put the axillary nerve at risk. For example, it has been demonstrated that capsular shrinkage procedures can create a local increase in temperature in the inferior capsule that can lead to nerve injury.[68,69] The nerve has been reported to be injured in 1% to 2% of thermal capsular shrinkage procedures, but fortunately, the vast majority of these injuries seem to be only temporary.[173] The axillary nerve is also at risk during capsular resection for adhesive capsulitis.[79] Because the nerve is in close proximity to the anteroinferior capsule, great care should be taken when resecting in this area. A safer method of inferior capsular resection in this area is to visualize the axillary nerve with the arthroscope during the procedure.

Young patients may be able to compensate for complete deltoid paralysis and can often perform activities of daily living with only partial disability. The shoulder can easily maintain a full range of motion with an intact rotator cuff. However, most patients will have early fatigue in the involved side if asked to perform repetitive activities. Although deltoid atrophy will be quite evident in a fit individual, in a less fit patient, the examiner may occasionally find it difficult to detect deltoid atrophy. Injury to the superior lateral cutaneous nerve of the arm may lead to sensory loss over the lateral aspect of the shoulder. It is possible for patients with a complete deltoid motor deficit to have only mild loss of sensation over the lateral part of the shoulder. The diagnosis of axillary neuropathy should not be determined by the presence or absence of lateral shoulder sensation. It is unclear whether the sensory branch is spared from injury or whether the sensory zone is supplied by overlapping innervation from other cutaneous branches.

The quadrilateral space syndrome has been described as another potential cause of posterior shoulder pain, and it presumably results from compression of the axillary nerve within the quadrilateral space. This syndrome is

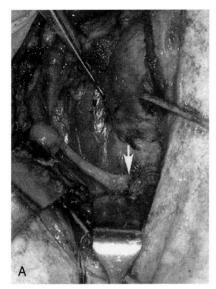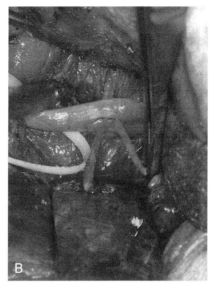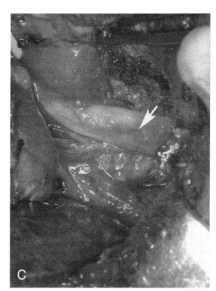

■ **Figure 17–1**

Axillary nerve palsy. This 21-year-old man underwent arthroscopic repair for recurrent left anterior shoulder dislocation. Postoperatively, new shoulder weakness and deltoid atrophy developed, and the patient was referred to our institution 6 months after the operation. He had 120 degrees of abduction and 160 degrees of forward flexion. Electromyography demonstrated dense fibrillations in the deltoid without voluntary activation. A severe axillary nerve lesion was diagnosed. **A,** At surgery, the conjoined tendon was taken down. The axillary nerve was encased in scar *(arrow)* and was decompressed. **B,** At the inferior portion of the glenoid, a suture anchor splitting the axillary nerve in half was noted. **C,** Stimulation across the lesion resulted in a deltoid response. The indentation within the nerve from which the suture anchor was removed can be seen *(arrow)*.

a controversial clinical entity; it may simply be a manifestation of Parsonage-Turner syndrome (brachial neuritis). Tenderness may be noted posteriorly along the shoulder joint; otherwise, the clinical examination is often normal. Deltoid atrophy or lateral sensory changes are uncommon, and EMG examination is usually normal. Magnetic resonance imaging (MRI) may demonstrate signal change indicative of denervation in the deltoid and teres minor muscles.[97] Observation is the usual treatment of quadrilateral space syndrome, with the vast majority of patients improving with time.[96] Surgical exploration of the quadrilateral space and release of scar or fibrous bands to achieve decompression of the axillary nerve are rarely needed.[25]

Patients with a history of blunt trauma to the axillary nerve should be observed over at least a 3-month period before operative treatment is considered. At 3 to 4 weeks, a baseline EMG/NCS examination should be obtained. Physical therapy, including active and passive exercises, should be initiated to preserve maximal range of motion and prevent joint contracture while awaiting return of function. Electrical stimulation of the deltoid has been used in an attempt to preserve muscle viability, although it is unclear whether this approach has any genuine effect.

The results of nonoperative treatment of a blunt traumatic lesion have generally been good. Leffert believes that axillary nerve injury after fracture or dislocation is more common than usually appreciated, yet the majority of patients progress to full recovery.[94] In a study of 73 patients with proximal humeral fracture or dislocation, 33% were noted on EMG to have an axillary nerve injury, with 9 complete and 15 partial lesions.[17] All patients

recovered with no objective loss of function, including those with complete nerve lesions. In a series of 108 elderly patients with anterior shoulder dislocation, 9.3% were found to have an axillary nerve injury, but all patients went on to full recovery by 12 months.[73] Nonetheless, some patients do not make the expected recovery. In these patients, surgical exploration with neurolysis or possibly nerve grafting can be undertaken if no clinical or EMG recovery is evident by 3 to 4 months.[5,36,117,133] If the patient has a history of a sharp penetrating wound or if a surgical injury has occurred, surgical exploration should be performed at an earlier date.

The proximal monofascicular structure of the axillary nerve with primarily motor fibers and its relatively short length from the posterior cord to the deltoid motor end plate are characteristics that lend themselves to surgical intervention. Alnot and Valenti reported on 37 axillary nerve surgeries, including 33 cases of sural nerve grafting, 3 neurolysis procedures, and 1 direct repair.[5] In 23 of the 25 isolated axillary nerve lesions, M4 or M5 strength was achieved. The fact that 33 of the 37 patients required sural nerve grafting illustrates the difficulty in adequately mobilizing the nerve for direct repair. The small number of patients undergoing neurolysis (3 of 37) is an indication that mild nerve compression by scar or fibrous bands is not common. Repair of the nerve with a short interposed, cabled sural nerve graft has been the most common method and has demonstrated the most consistent results.[4,21,36,126,129,134] We have found the use of intraoperative EMG techniques to be invaluable in evaluating neuromas and helping us decide whether to perform neurolysis alone or resect the neuroma and perform a graft. In all cases, we are also prepared to expose the axillary nerve posteriorly. In selected cases, such exposure is necessary to identify normal nerve more distally for grafting.

Other techniques for repair of the axillary nerve include nerve transfer. Direct neurotization with a donor nerve such as the medial pectoral, thoracodorsal, or radial has yielded satisfactory results in cases in which direct repair or short cable grafting of the axillary nerve itself is not possible or not preferable.[40,65,140] Nerve transfers using the spinal accessory nerve or upper intercostal nerves have been described but require an interpositional sural nerve graft[32,140] and have demonstrated less optimal results.[140,150]

Patients seen longer than 18 months after trauma usually do not benefit from surgical repair of the nerve because of the poor condition of the deltoid muscle and its motor end plates. In patients who have poor shoulder function limiting their activities of daily living but a normal rotator cuff, muscle transfer procedures can be considered. Potentially, if the posterior deltoid and middle deltoid are innervated and the anterior deltoid is not functioning, the posterior/middle deltoid can be rotated anteriorly on the clavicle. This procedure, however, has the potential to harm the remaining deltoid and is not strongly recommended.

Alternatively, the pectoralis major can be transposed laterally on the clavicle and acromion. Mobilization of the pectoralis major is limited somewhat by the relatively tight anatomic dimensions of the pectoral nerves. If complete deltoid paralysis is present, the trapezius can be mobilized off the clavicle and spine of the acromion, and the lateral acromion with attached trapezius can be inserted into the proximal end of the humerus. This procedure can restore some shoulder abduction to a patient who has none; however, it does create a change in the normal slope of the shoulder and therefore has a less than desirable cosmetic result. More advanced techniques such as free muscle transfer have been attempted, but the results have been less than uniform or satisfactory.

SPINAL ACCESSORY NERVE

Injury to the spinal accessory nerve can occur after penetrating trauma to the shoulder. Blunt trauma may also cause loss of trapezius function. Most commonly, surgical dissection in the posterior triangle of the neck, such as for lymph node biopsy, may expose the nerve to possible damage (Fig. 17–2).[88,104,112,163,172]

The spinal accessory nerve passes through the upper portion of the sternocleidomastoid muscle, which it innervates, and then crosses the posterior cervical triangle. The posterior cervical triangle is bordered anteriorly by the sternocleidomastoid muscle, posteriorly by the trapezius, and inferiorly by the clavicle. The nerve lies on the floor of the posterior triangle with only the overlying fascia as protection against injury.[41] It abuts the posterior cervical lymph nodes. The nerve enters the anterior surface of the trapezius and travels inferiorly, parallel to the medial border of the scapula.[80] The trapezius has a broad origin from the ligamentum nuchae to the 12th thoracic vertebra and inserts over the lateral part of the

clavicle, acromion, and spine of the scapula. The upper trapezius is the prime elevator of the scapula and acts to upwardly rotate the lateral aspect of the bone.

If the spinal accessory nerve is injured, the diagnosis is often missed and appropriate treatment may be delayed.[88] Patients usually have pain as their primary complaint. Loss of motion may be a secondary concern. Unless trapezius function is specifically tested, the diagnosis may not be recognized. Because of the common occurrence of anterior shoulder pain in these patients with occasionally only slight visible wasting of the trapezius muscle, the pain may be assumed to represent "postoperative pain" or be misinterpreted as resulting from another condition associated with shoulder pain, such as rotator cuff pathology. The trapezius receives some innervation from the upper cervical nerve roots, so complete atrophy of the muscle may not occur. The spinal accessory nerve supplies the sole innervation to the lateral portion of the muscle, which is critical in supporting abduction of the shoulder. If the patient is carefully observed, the scapula will appear to be rotated forward at the shoulder. The shoulder may hang lower or droop in comparison to the contralateral side. Winging of the scapula often occurs but is not as dramatic as that associated with injury to the long thoracic nerve. Usually, asking the patient to perform a shoulder shrug will produce the deformity, but a strong levator scapulae may compensate well and only minimal deformity may be noted. The patient may not be able to abduct the arm fully with the forearm either pronated or supinated.

Some of the pain that patients experience may come from strain of the other parascapular muscles as they attempt to compensate for the lack of trapezius function. Additionally, because the scapula cannot properly rotate the acromion away from the humerus as the arm is elevated, impingement of the rotator cuff may cause secondary rotator cuff tendinopathy. If attention is directed only at the rotator cuff, the underlying nerve pathology will be missed. In addition, the spinal accessory nerve, though mainly a motor nerve, still has sensory fibers. Injury to the nerve may also produce neuropathic pain. Finally, one should also examine for possible concomitant injury to other neighboring nerves such as the cervical plexus or great auricular nerve.

If the patient is seen within the first 6 months after injury, surgical exploration of the nerve can be performed. Although surgical repair of the nerve may be considered up to a year after injury, better results occur with treatment as soon after injury as possible.[88,104,163] We favor early exploration of these nerve injuries when they occur immediately after surgery, especially when the nerve was not identified and protected as part of the operation.

Surgical options include neurolysis, direct repair, or nerve grafting, depending on intraoperative observations and electrophysiologic testing. During surgical reconstruction, it is important to consider the acromion-mastoid distance in the anesthetized patient. If direct repair of the nerve is performed with the head tilted toward the operated shoulder, when the patient is awakened after surgery and transported to the recovery room, significant traction may occur and disrupt the repair. If the nerve ends are found to have retracted at surgery, it is

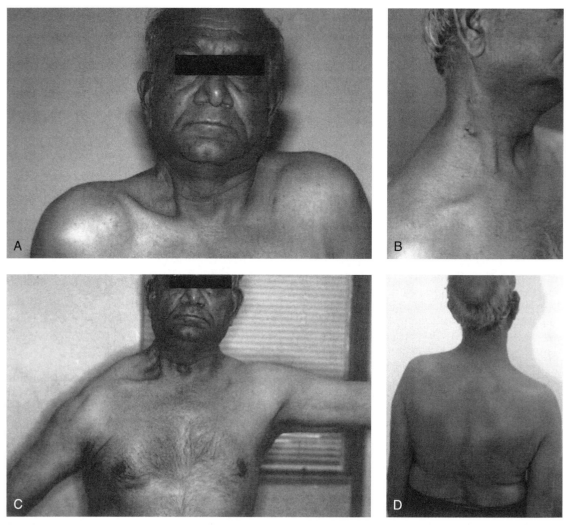

■ **Figure 17–2**

Spinal accessory nerve paralysis. This 53-year-old man underwent a cervical lymph node biopsy that was performed to exclude tuberculous lymphadenitis. The specimen was nondiagnostic. Severe pain and deformity developed in the affected shoulder after surgery. A postoperative pain syndrome was thought to have developed. The diagnosis of spinal accessory nerve paralysis was not made until several months later. **A,** An asymmetric shoulder shrug and trapezius atrophy are evident. **B,** A small transverse incision from the lymph node biopsy is seen directly posterior to the sternocleidomastoid muscle. This incision is directly over the oblique course of the accessory nerve. **C,** The patient had significant difficulty with shoulder abduction. **D,** Resultant shoulder droop can be seen from loss of the trapezius.

best to use an intervening graft such as a sural nerve or the great auricular nerve to allow for less tension on the repair (Fig. 17–3).

If more than 12 months has passed since injury to the spinal accessory nerve, nonoperative treatment may be considered if the patient has compensated reasonably well. The degree of disability varies from patient to patient. Some may have only a persistent ache in the shoulder, whereas others may feel and act completely disabled with respect to the upper extremity. Braces have been advocated as adjunctive treatment, but they are bulky and not used consistently by patients.[167] A patient symptomatic enough to attempt to use a brace is potentially a candidate for surgical reconstruction.

Modern surgical procedures currently involve dynamic muscle transfer techniques. Earlier historical procedures, however, initially involved mostly static repairs. Henry and others advocated static stabilization of the medial

aspect of the scapula to the vertebral spine with strips of fascia lata.[44,76,171] Dewar and Harris described lateral transfer of the levator scapulae to the lateral part of the scapula combined with a static fascial sling from the vertebral spine to the medial part of the scapula.[43] Static repairs with either fascia, tendon, or artificial materials, however, tend to stretch out or rupture over time.[91]

Dynamic transfer of the levator scapulae along with the rhomboid major and rhomboid minor was described in Germany by Eden and Lange.[51,89,90] Bigliani reported good results with this technique.[13,15,172]

The surgical approach for an Eden-Lange transfer involves a vertical incision midway between the vertebral spine and the medial edge of the scapula. The atrophied trapezius is divided, and the levator scapulae and rhomboids are released from the medial part of the scapula with a small piece of bone containing their insertions. This release can be accomplished with a small saw or an

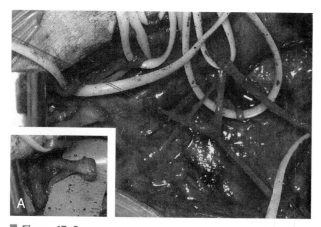
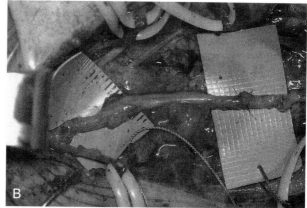

■ **Figure 17–3**

Spinal accessory nerve paralysis. **A,** The spinal accessory nerve was transected. A neuroma *(inset)* can be seen. A suture marks the distal stump. **B,** An interpositional graft repair (backgrounds) using the sural nerve was performed.

osteotome. The levator scapulae is passed subcutaneously to a horizontal incision over the lateral spine of the scapula, near the acromion. The levator should be placed as far laterally as possible on the spine of the scapula, usually 5 to 7 cm medial to the posterolateral edge of the acromion. The rhomboid major and minor can be elevated individually or together from the medial edge of the scapula. The dorsal scapular nerve is potentially at risk during this part of the procedure. The infraspinatus is partially elevated off of the scapula in a medial-to-lateral direction. The rhomboids are then placed as far lateral as possible, at least 4 cm, on the posterior aspect of the scapula and secured in place via suture and drill holes through the scapula. Alternatively, the rhomboid minor can be transferred cephalad to the spine of the scapula into the supraspinatus fossa. The infraspinatus is then sutured back in position over the transferred rhomboids. Postoperatively, patients are placed in a shoulder abduction brace that holds the arm at approximately 70 degrees of abduction for 4 weeks. This brace will relieve tension on the transferred muscles while healing takes place. At 4 weeks, a gradual strengthening program can begin.

This technique has shown good results, probably because it involves dynamic transfer of muscle rather than a static transfer, which might stretch or possibly wear out over time.[90] If an Eden-Lange procedure or a static transfer fails and a salvage situation exists, scapulothoracic fusion becomes a potential option. Scapulothoracic fusion should be reserved primarily for patients with fascioscapulohumeral dystrophy and global loss of shoulder muscle function. Different techniques have been used to perform scapulothoracic fusion, but most involve passing wires through the scapula and around several ribs with a broad iliac crest bone graft or metallic plate for support. The complication rate can be high with the potential for pneumothorax or hardware failure.

LONG THORACIC NERVE

Isolated injury to the long thoracic nerve is usually manifested as winging of the scapula. Velpeau first described injury to the long thoracic nerve causing paralysis of the serratus anterior in 1837.[166] However, winging of the scapula has multiple causes, with multidirectional instability probably being the most common cause of mild winging. Spinal accessory nerve injury can also cause winging, but this injury tends to be milder and results in more of a rotational deformity of the scapula. Additionally, some patients have volitional control over the scapula and can demonstrate significant winging on command.

The serratus anterior takes origin from the upper nine ribs and inserts on the anteromedial border of the scapula. This insertion is only a few millimeters wide at the mid-portion of the scapula, but it becomes more substantial at the inferior pole of the scapula. It is the inferior portion of the muscle that is important in maintaining protraction and upward rotation of the scapula during forward elevation of the shoulder. The long thoracic nerve has a relatively long course after taking origin from the C5, C6, and C7 nerve roots. After crossing over the first rib, it travels 10 to 20 cm to its motor end plate in the serratus anterior. It is vulnerable to blunt trauma over the first rib along the lateral chest wall and can be crushed by forceful displacement of the scapula.

The nerve is rarely injured as a result of penetrating trauma, but injury can occur from thoracic outlet surgery in the region of the first rib, breast surgery, or lateral chest wall procedures such as axillary node dissection.[164,175] Spontaneous cases of entrapment at the scalenus medius have been described. Probably, the most common cause of serratus anterior dysfunction is Parsonage-Turner syndrome. In fact, this condition is most likely the underlying cause of dysfunction attributed to overexertion, including athletic activities.

In idiopathic or nonpenetrating trauma cases, observation is the standard therapy. No specific physical therapy protocol has been found to be especially helpful other than continued use of the shoulder as tolerated. Braces have been advocated to help hold the scapula against the chest wall.[101] Though somewhat effective, braces are usually found to be awkward and are not well tolerated by patients. If monitored for 6 months to a year,

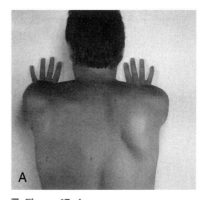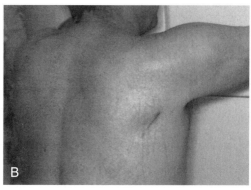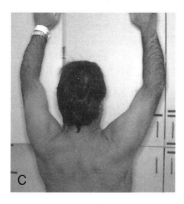

■ **Figure 17–4**

Long thoracic nerve palsy. A complete long thoracic nerve paralysis from Parsonage-Turner syndrome developed in this 36-year-old man. His winged scapula did not improve after 3 years. He had persistent pain in his shoulder and disability when performing overhead maneuvers. **A,** Prominent right scapula winging is noted preoperatively. **B,** Postoperatively, the winging has disappeared after pectoralis major transfer. The posterior incision has healed well. **C,** Postoperatively, his shoulder arc of motion has improved as well.

most patients with a nontraumatic or idiopathic cause tend to recover from the paralysis and regain serratus anterior function.[63]

Potential surgical options are available for treatment of injury to the long thoracic nerve in the early stages. If the patient is seen before 6 months, neurolysis of the nerve can be performed.[45] However, because of the length of the nerve, it is difficult to be certain where the lesion resides, and we do not recommend this approach for most patients. A more practical surgical procedure would be neurotization or nerve transfer from one or two intercostal nerves or the thoracodorsal nerve.[116,174] Because it is not usually clear where the damaged section is, the nerve can be connected with the donor nerve close to the motor end plate. This technique has been helpful in a small number of reported cases.[116,174] Many patients with atraumatic lesions recover spontaneously, so we do not routinely recommend surgery to the average patient before 6 or 9 months after development of the nerve deficit.

If a patient does not recover serratus anterior function and use of the shoulder is compromised, a number of reconstructive options are available (Fig. 17–4).* Scapulothoracic fusion has been performed when the scapula is fixed to the underlying ribs. Although this technique may eliminate winging of the scapula, it will decrease shoulder girdle motion by at least 30%, with mostly forward elevation and extension affected.[22] The technique involves the risk of pneumothorax, and the pseudarthrosis rate is not insignificant. For these reasons, it should be reserved for the salvage situation or for patients with symptomatic fascioscapulohumeral dystrophy.

Tendon transfers provide dynamic control of a winging scapula and are now our preferred method in patients who have had a neurologic deficit for 1 year or more. Tubby described transfer of the pectoralis major to the serratus anterior in 1904.[161] Although this transfer might offer initial relief of the winging, the paralyzed serratus anterior tends to stretch out with time, and this procedure is not recommended today. Other techniques described

include transfer of the pectoralis minor, rhomboids, or levator scapulae.[29,77,149]

The technique that seems to give the most consistent result is transfer of the pectoralis major to the scapula with tendon graft augmentation. Durman, Ober, and Marmor each described successful transfer of the pectoralis major with a fascial extension graft in a few cases.[49,102,118] More recent studies have demonstrated the excellent ability of this tendon transfer procedure to control winging of the scapula.[37,78,127,131,151,170] The pectoralis major is ideally suited as a transfer to substitute for the paralyzed serratus anterior. The direction of pull of the pectoralis major is similar to the path of the serratus anterior, and the bulk of the pectoralis major provides enough strength to resist winging of the scapula. The technique has been used with transfer of the entire pectoralis major or with only the sternal head (Fig. 17–5). Equally good results have been reported with both procedures. However, the sternal head of the pectoralis major is much more in line with the direction of pull of the serratus anterior than the clavicular head is, and it also provides for a less bulky transfer. Moreover, the sternal head is more substantial than the clavicular head and provides a stronger tendon transfer. Potential concerns of cosmesis or visible deformity of the anterior chest wall should be minimal. In most instances, regardless of whether the entire pectoralis major or the sternal head is transferred, there is little change in the normal contour of the anterior chest.

This procedure can be performed with a single large incision across the axilla or through two separate incisions. The two-incision technique is not technically harder than a single incision, is somewhat more cosmetic, and is the preferred procedure. The choice of tissue for augmentation of the transferred pectoralis major tendon depends on the surgeon's preference. The most common choice has been a large portion of fascia lata rolled into a tube. Other graft options include semitendinosus or gracilis autograft or allograft. Fascia lata can be rolled into a spiral tube and draped around the pectoralis major muscle and tendon to provide very strong proximal fixation. The native tendon of the pectoralis major is quite short, and it can be difficult to attach a long thin tendon

*See references 9, 29, 37, 67, 77, 78, 102, 127, 131, 132, 161, 164, 169.

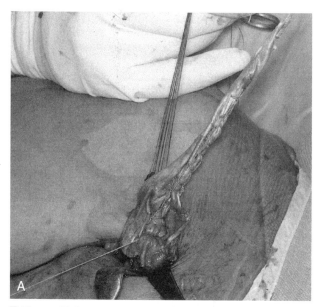
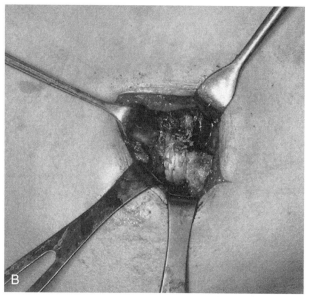

■ **Figure 17–5**
Long thoracic nerve palsy, operative photographs. **A,** Axillary exposure showing the sternal portion of the pectoralis tendon reinforced with a fascia lata graft before its transfer posteriorly to the scapula. **B,** The posterior approach shows the tendon secured to the scapula.

such as a semitendinosus or gracilis with the same degree of security. However, the use of hamstring tendons has not been associated with an increase in sudden failure of the graft.

At surgery, the patient should be positioned in the lateral decubitus position for easy access to the anterior and posterior aspects of the shoulder. The anterior approach is usually performed while a second surgical team is simultaneously harvesting fascia lata. This approach is made somewhat easier by the lateral position. The anterior incision (4 to 6 cm) is made almost entirely in the axillary crease and is extended only a centimeter superiorly. This technique results in a well-hidden, cosmetic incision. The sternal head of the pectoralis major is easily identified at the inferior margin of the muscle. The sternal head wraps posteriorly under the clavicular head and inserts more medial and superior to it. The sternal head is detached directly off the humerus, with care taken to avoid damage to the biceps tendon. The sternal head is then freed up medially onto the chest wall to allow greater excursion of the muscle. The harvested fascia lata graft should measure approximately 14 by 5 cm. At this point, the fascia lata is rolled into a spiral tube, draped around the pectoralis major tendon and muscle, and secured with multiple sutures. A heavy running locking suture is then placed through the fascia lata graft and tagged for transfer.

The posterior incision should be made at the junction of the middle and distal lateral edge of the scapula. It is important for an assistant to manually push the scapula as far anteriorly and laterally as possible. When this position is achieved, a 4-cm incision is made over the lateral edge of the scapula, and the muscles are cleared off the bone and retracted. An 8- to 10-mm hole is created in the scapula with a bur, just medial to the thick lateral mass of the scapula, to ensure a strong bony bridge during the healing period. A large bone hook is helpful at this stage to secure the scapula. Using a large, blunt clamp, a

subcutaneous path is created from the anterior incision along the chest wall to the posterior incision. Much of this dissection can be performed with digital palpation. This plane is safe because the brachial plexus is more superior and abducted with the arm. Once a clear path has been created for the pectoralis major/graft, the traction suture is passed posteriorly and the graft is pulled through the scapular fenestration in an anterior-to-posterior direction. The graft is then pulled tight in an attempt to abut the native pectoralis major tendon to the scapula. The tendon is then folded back and sutured to itself. It is important for the scapula to be held as far anterior on the chest wall as possible while these sutures are secured. No reports of "overtight" pectoralis major transfers have appeared in the literature. Any excess graft after suture fixation is excised. Drains are not usually needed at closure, and the arm is placed into a sling.

Postoperatively, the patient is told to use the sling full-time and to avoid any abduction of the shoulder. At 6 weeks after surgery, the sling can be discarded and the patient allowed to resume all normal daily activities with the arm. No lifting of objects heavier than a kilogram is permitted. A formal physical therapy program is not typically necessary. Patients tend to regain a normal range of motion quite readily. It is assumed that healing takes place during the initial 3- to 6-month period, and therefore return to manual labor or sporting activities is allowed after 6 months. Early failure has occasionally been reported after pectoralis major transfer, and such failure seems to be related to premature return to full function before complete healing.[37,78]

SUPRASCAPULAR NERVE

The suprascapular nerve originates from the C5 and C6 nerve roots at the junction of the upper trunk and its divisions. The nerve follows the omohyoid posteriorly and then runs inferiorly through the suprascapular notch, bridged by the superior transverse scapular ligament. The suprascapular artery and vein typically pass superior to the ligament. The suprascapular notch is a region where the nerve is relatively fixed in position. After exiting the suprascapular notch, the nerve gives off branches that innervate the supraspinatus. The nerve then continues medial to the superior edge of the glenoid and enters the spinoglenoid notch at the lateral margin of the scapular spine. As the nerve travels posteriorly, it may be less than 20 mm from the glenoid edge.[14] In the spinoglenoid notch, the spinoglenoid ligament can potentially impinge on the nerve. A spinoglenoid ligament, however, is not present in all patients.[82] After exiting the spinoglenoid notch, the nerve divides into two to four branches that enter the infraspinatus. Near the suprascapular notch, the suprascapular nerve also supplies articular branches to the shoulder joints. These fibers may explain the pain experienced by patients with suprascapular nerve lesions at the transverse scapular ligament. In contrast, more distal lesions such as at the spinoglenoid notch characteristically produce painless atrophy (of the infraspinatus). The cutaneous supply of the suprascapular nerve is still somewhat debatable. Some have described sensory fibers supplying the skin over the posterior of the shoulder; however, few patients are noted to have loss of sensation after nerve injury.

Patients with a suprascapular nerve injury typically complain of pain over the posterior and lateral aspects of the shoulder. Pain on deep palpation over the suprascapular notch may also be present. In addition, patients may have weakness of abduction, external rotation, or both and be noted to have atrophy of the supraspinatus and infraspinatus. In many individuals, the supraspinatus is difficult to visualize because a well-developed trapezius will cover the supraspinatus and make it difficult to see muscle wasting. Loss of muscle bulk in the infraspinatus, however, is fairly easy to see on clinical examination. Nonetheless, some patients will not demonstrate any atrophy on examination. Shoulder pain and mild weakness of abduction may be the only findings, thus making correct diagnosis difficult. An appropriate clinical examination with EMG/NCS will often detect suprascapular neuropathy. The diagnosis can easily be made if conduction velocity is delayed (in comparison to the contralateral side) and fibrillation potentials are noted in the supraspinatus or infraspinatus. In some patients, EMG/NCS may show only mild involvement. These patients should be examined carefully for other shoulder pathology that might have been missed during the clinical examination. Surgical treatment tends to not be as beneficial in these patients as those with substantial changes on EMG/NCS.[7] Because shoulder pain can be caused by several conditions, in these patients and especially those with only mild EMG/NCS findings, cervical disk disease, rotator cuff tear, impingement syndrome, and acromioclavicular joint degeneration should all be excluded.

Suprascapular neuropathy can occur from a variety of causes.[165] Direct blunt trauma to the shoulder or sudden twisting of the shoulder may acutely injure the nerve. A compressive injury may develop at the suprascapular or spinoglenoid notch. A common cause of nerve compression in this region is a ganglion cyst (Fig. 17–6).[6,7,16,56,109,135] The origin of a cyst in this region is presumed to be from the glenohumeral joint, and it is very often associated with degenerative tears of the glenoid labrum.[7,145] Repetitive rotatory motion of the shoulder, such as occurs during many sporting activities, may cause a chronic traction injury of the nerve. Neuropathy of the suprascapular nerve has been noted in participants of baseball, volleyball, tennis, and weightlifting.[1,6,16,20,35,39,52,143] Parsonage-Turner syndrome (acute brachial neuritis) may also result in an idiopathic etiology of suprascapular neuropathy. In rare instances, a fracture of the scapula that enters the suprascapular notch may also damage the nerve.[18,50,146]

Treatment of a patient with suprascapular neuropathy is based on the type of injury and the duration of dis-

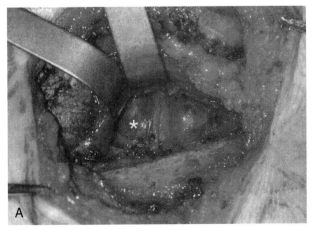
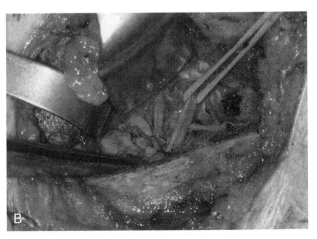

■ **Figure 17–6**
Suprascapular nerve compression. This 50-year-old man had left shoulder weakness over 6 months and was found to have moderate supraspinatus and infraspinatus weakness (grade 3/5) and atrophy. Electromyography showed denervation changes in both spinatus muscles. Magnetic resonance imaging demonstrated a large ganglion cyst near the suprascapular notch. **A,** At surgery, when the supraspinatus was retracted anteriorly, a large ganglion cyst *(asterisk)* was compressing the suprascapular nerve near the suprascapular notch. The nerve was splayed over the top of the cyst and flattened in appearance. **B,** The cyst was resected and the nerve decompressed.

ability, pain, and atrophy. A patient with a chronic neuropathy from repetitive shoulder motion, such as a baseball or volleyball player, should be placed in therapy and treated conservatively. Similarly, a patient with Parsonage-Turner syndrome should be observed for an extended period. Both groups, if monitored for 2 to 3 months, tend to demonstrate clinical improvement. The results of surgical intervention in these two groups are somewhat unpredictable.[7]

Patients with evidence of compressive neuropathy at either the suprascapular notch or the spinoglenoid notch should also be observed for improvement in function over a 2- to 3-month period. If they remain symptomatic after that time, surgical decompression can be performed.

Early surgical intervention (within a few weeks) is rarely needed, except in patients with an obvious ganglion cyst noted on MRI or the rare patient with intractable pain and significant compressive neuropathy noted on EMG/NCS. Patients with Parsonage-Turner syndrome will have considerable pain for the first few weeks of the neuropathy; they should not be operated on during this time because the pain will tend to dissipate in a few weeks.

The suprascapular nerve can be approached from an anterior, superior, or posterior direction. The anterior approach puts the remainder of the brachial plexus at risk and does not allow for exposure of the spinoglenoid notch.[144] A direct superior approach performed by splitting the trapezius in line with its fibers has been commonly recommended. This technique, however, results in a deep surgical wound in which the suprascapular notch and superior transverse scapular ligament can be visualized, but only a small distance of the suprascapular nerve itself can be exposed.

The posterior approach detaches the trapezius from the spine of the scapula 6 to 8 cm medial to the lateral edge of the acromion. The supraspinatus is then retracted posteriorly to visualize the suprascapular nerve and the notch. Careful exposure should be performed while in the area of the suprascapular notch because the artery and vein travel above it and, on occasion, a branch of the nerve may be above rather than below the superior transverse scapular ligament. If greater exposure of the nerve is needed with this approach, two additional steps can be performed. The trapezius can be detached laterally and anteriorly onto the acromioclavicular joint to allow wide exposure of the nerve. At closure, however, the trapezius will need to be accurately repaired back to the acromion.

If the nerve needs to be explored into the spinoglenoid notch, the posterior deltoid can be detached from the spine of the scapula, and exposure of the nerve from the infraspinatus to the suprascapular notch can then be achieved.

In cases involving a ganglion at the spinoglenoid notch, arthroscopic débridement of the cyst is an excellent technique. Arthroscopy also allows for visualization of the joint and the opportunity to débride any associated labral tears. Most of these posterosuperior labral tears are not amenable to surgical reattachment.

Good or better surgical results have been achieved in recovery of supraspinatus function. Infraspinatus recovery is more variable. The best results are seen in patients with nerve lesions from masses. The worst results are in

patients with neuropathy caused by fractures or severe trauma.

THORACIC OUTLET SYNDROME

Thoracic outlet syndrome is a difficult condition to accurately diagnose because of the lack of a gold standard for confirming the diagnosis. Some clinicians believe that it is overdiagnosed, and others think that it should be more commonly treated. The correct diagnosis is made more difficult because of the preponderance of subjective symptoms with few objective tests. Both radiographic and electrodiagnostic tests have been used to make the diagnosis, but no test is specific for thoracic outlet syndrome. The diagnosis is therefore primarily one of exclusion and is based on a patient's history and symptoms.

Despite any controversy about the prevalence of thoracic outlet syndrome, shoulder surgeons will undoubtedly encounter many patients with thoracic outlet symptoms (disputed thoracic outlet syndrome). These patients may complain of pain in the shoulder or neck region with radiation to the forearm or hand. Paresthesias may radiate along the upper part of the arm to the hand. Often, patients will perceive loss of sensation along the small and ring fingers. Bilateral symptoms are relatively common, with symptoms greater on the dominant side. A patient's pain typically begins gradually without a history of trauma. Trauma and impending lawsuits frequently becloud the clinical scenario. Frequently, patients complain of difficulty working overhead. Arm traction, such as carrying a heavy bag or luggage, can increase a patient's symptoms. Although the patient may complain of hand weakness and loss of sensation, the results of motor examination are typically normal. True neurogenic thoracic outlet syndrome may result from an anomalous relationship of the neurologic structures to a cervical rib or to fibrous bands and the like, and it typically produces lower trunk compression. These patients may have subtle ulnar-sided lumbrical weakness or display a Gilliatt-Sumner hand (more severe weakness in the hand intrinsic musculature beyond the ulnar nerve distribution). In addition, neurovascular compression may result from a reduced costoclavicular space (Figs. 17–7 to 17–9). A patient may on occasion have a vascular disorder (venous or arterial) responsible for the symptoms, although this type of vascular thoracic outlet syndrome is less common. In such cases, patients will often display objective findings such as a change in color of their hands or a chronically reduced pulse. Noninvasive vascular studies or an angiogram may demonstrate a compressed area in the vascular system of the upper extremity.

Several provocative tests have been described for thoracic outlet syndrome, most of which were originally proposed for vascular conditions. The Adson test was described for compression of the subclavian artery. The test is performed by having the patient turn the head to the affected side while inspiring deeply in a sitting position. The patient's radial artery is palpated and checked for loss of pulse. Loss of pulse is not indicative by itself of thoracic outlet syndrome because a large proportion of the population will demonstrate a variation in pulse

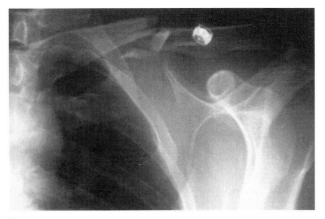

■ **Figure 17–7**
Clavicle fracture and upper trunk neurapraxia. This 48-year-old man sustained a midshaft clavicular fracture after a fall while snowboarding. Shortly after the injury he noted severe weakness in abduction and mild weakness in elbow flexion. An upper trunk lesion was diagnosed. Plain films demonstrate mild apical angulation of the clavicular fracture. The distal fragment was displaced 8 mm inferiorly. Small butterfly fragments were adjacent to the fracture. This neurologic deficit improved after 4 months.

during different upper extremity maneuvers. The Wright test involves hyperabduction of the shoulders with the elbows flexed more than 45 degrees. The Roos test involves elevation of the arm to 90 degrees of shoulder abduction and external rotation with 90 degree of elbow flexion accompanied by rapid opening and closing of the hands for up to 3 minutes. A modification of the Roos test is the elevated arm stress test (EAST), in which the hands are repetitively opened and closed with the shoulders elevated 180 degrees and the elbows extended. A positive test occurs when the patient reports a reproduction of the symptoms within 30 to 60 seconds. Percussion of the brachial plexus in the supraclavicular fossa may produce radiating paresthesias. None of these tests are universally accepted as a gold standard for thoracic outlet syndrome. An asymptomatic individual may not infrequently be found to have a falsely positive test when several of these tests are performed. The finding of a cervical rib on chest films must also be cautiously interpreted because it is a variation found in 1% of the population.

If a patient is believed to have thoracic outlet syndrome, conservative management is the usual initial treatment. Patients are taught to avoid activities that aggravate their symptoms. Poor posture is corrected and physical conditioning improved. An aerobic exercise plan will strengthen the accessory muscles of inspiration, help correct muscle imbalance, and lead to weight loss. Usually, patients are placed in a conservative management program for at least 9 to 12 months before considering operative options. If the patient is still unable to function after this period, decompression of the brachial plexus with or without rib resection may be considered. The most common surgical approaches are transaxillary,[136] supraclavicular, or combined. These procedures have advantages and disadvantages and advocates and critics. In general, however, the results of these techniques have been similar. Leffert and Perlmutter reported a high percentage of excellent results with the transaxillary

approach, and Sanders and colleagues reported similar results with a supraclavicular approach.[95,142] Surgery is performed earlier in patients with neurogenic thoracic outlet syndrome.

Thoracic outlet syndrome remains a diagnosis of exclusion because no diagnostic tests can accurately pinpoint the condition. All aspects of the history and physical examination must be examined carefully to make the diagnosis. Conservative measures are usually effective and should be the primary treatment. Surgical treatment may offer some benefit in selected individuals; however, the techniques are demanding and the potential for complications is high.

PARSONAGE-TURNER SYNDROME (BRACHIAL PLEXUS NEUROPATHY)

Brachial plexus neuropathy is also known as idiopathic brachial plexitis, brachial neuritis, neuralgic amyotrophy, brachial plexus neuropathy, serum neuritis, and shoulder-girdle neuritis, among others. It also is known as Parsonage-Turner syndrome after the two physicians who presented the first large series of patients in 1943.[121] The description dates back to 1887 when Dreschfeld[48] reported two siblings with nontraumatic brachial plexopathy and to 1889 when Feinberg[57] described a case of plexitis after influenza. It is a relatively uncommon condition overall with an annual incidence rate of 1 to 2 cases per 100,000 population.[11] Nevertheless, it is encountered several times per year by those treating shoulder or brachial plexus disorders.

Patients typically have an acute onset of periscapular pain that lasts several days to weeks. Motor weakness in the shoulder and arm associated with sensory loss ensues, usually when the pain is resolving. This triad of pain and motor and sensory disturbance is not always present, and painless neuropathy may occur on occasion. Certain peripheral nerves seem to be preferentially affected, including the long thoracic,[55,122] axillary, suprascapular, anterior interosseous, and radial nerves. The process frequently involves various components of the brachial plexus diffusely[54] and occurs bilaterally in over 10% of cases. In fact, other non–brachial plexus nerves, such as the phrenic nerve, or cranial nerves, such as the spinal accessory nerve, may be involved. It may also affect a single nerve (such as the anterior interosseous nerve). Men are affected slightly more often than women, generally between the third and sixth decades of life.[137] The disorder is typically monophasic, but recurrent attacks rarely occur.

The etiology of this nontraumatic condition remains unclear. It is thought to be immune mediated or inflammatory in nature. Its onset may follow a viral illness or other infection, immunization, pregnancy, trauma, extreme exercise, and surgery.[81,98,108,164] In some ways, it is thought to be similar to Bell's palsy affecting the facial nerve. Several pathologic specimens of affected brachial plexus elements have revealed inflammatory changes.[152] A familial component exists as well (hereditary neuralgic amyotrophy)[125,130]; these patients may have recurrent episodes and are affected at an earlier age than typical.

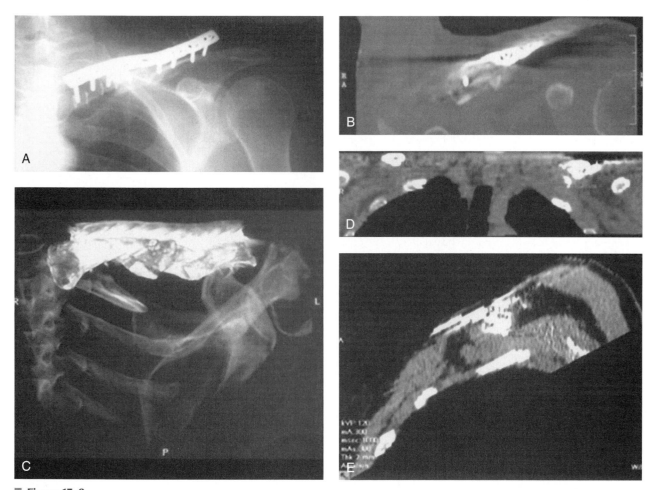

■ **Figure 17–8**

Neurogenic thoracic outlet caused by clavicular malunion. The clavicular fracture in this patient (illustrated in Fig. 17–7) progressed to nonunion. He also had pain near his acromioclavicular joint. He underwent a takedown of the nonunion, bone grafting, and internal fixation with a dynamic compression plate along with distal clavicular resection. The week after surgery he noted ulnar-sided hand paresthesias and then weakness in the hand. Over the next month, severe but incomplete lesions affecting the posterior cord, medial cord, and lateral contribution to the medial cord developed. The potential for iatrogenic compression of the brachial plexus in the thoracic outlet always exists for surgeons operating in or around the clavicle. **A,** Plain films showed the plate fixation and the inferior callus. **B** and **C,** Computed tomographic scans with reconstruction better characterized the inferior callus and showed the reduced costoclavicular space. **D,** On the left side, the shortest distance between the undersurface of the clavicle callus and the first rib was 10 to 11 mm versus 13 to 15 mm on the right in the coronal and sagittal planes (**E**). In addition, a well-defined fat plane beneath the clavicle seen on the right side was effaced by a soft tissue density on the left (**D**).

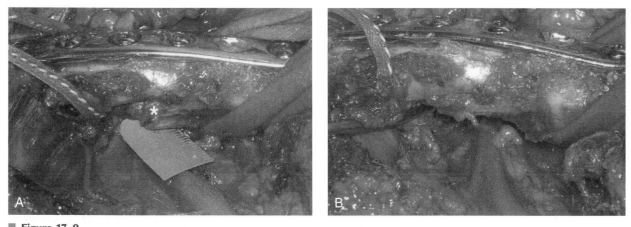

■ **Figure 17–9**

Neurogenic thoracic outlet syndrome caused by clavicular malunion (same patient as Figs. 17-7 and 17-8). **A,** Surgery was performed in view of the worsening deficit. A large hypertrophic portion of callus *(asterisk)* was seen compressing the lateral cord. **B,** The bony prominence was resected. Ample room was restored for the underlying neural elements. Passive range of motion did not alter the space, and a first rib resection was not deemed necessary. In the recovery room, his hand strength had improved one full grade. He made a full recovery by 3 months. Restoration of a normal costoclavicular space has been associated with favorable recovery of neural function in these types of cases.

The diagnosis of Parsonage-Turner syndrome can often be established by a good history and physical examination and exclusion of other disorders. Electrodiagnostic studies typically reveal a patchy, multifocal neurologic process that supports the diagnosis. Other serologic studies and cerebrospinal fluid are usually normal. Imaging studies reveal nonspecific changes (e.g., high signal intensity in affected muscles on T2-weighted MRI) but help eliminate other more common diagnoses of the neck and shoulder. Parsonage-Turner syndrome is frequently misdiagnosed and is a great masquerader of other diseases. It must be considered when establishing the differential diagnosis of shoulder pain or muscle weakness in the upper limb. It may mimic orthopaedic conditions, especially shoulder problems such as rotator cuff disease, impingement syndrome, adhesive capsulitis, bursitis, and others. Neurologic disorders, including cervical radiculopathy, other peripheral nerve conditions such as mononeuritis multiplex, chronic inflammatory demyelinating polyneuropathy or "entrapment syndromes," and transverse myelitis, must be excluded. Anterior interosseous nerve paralysis and long thoracic nerve lesions are examples of nerve lesions that are not uncommonly classified as entrapment because of the spontaneous onset that more accurately represents examples of Parsonage-Turner syndrome. As such, surgeons may take false credit for improving the clinical course by decompressing a nerve that might have recovered anyway based on its own natural history.

Overall, the prognosis is generally favorable, although recovery may take several years. However, not all patients recover, and many have residual deficits such as mild scapular winging. It is unknown whether these deficits predispose individuals to other shoulder pathology in the long term because of faulty shoulder mechanics. Despite the fact that this entity has been perceived as one producing largely reversible deficits, one series with late follow-up has demonstrated that patients may experience significant disability, limitations in activities of daily living, persistent pain, and difficulty returning to their original work.[66] Treatment is usually supportive and directed at decreasing pain with anti-inflammatory agents and other analgesics. Some physicians have tried steroids or intravenous immunoglobulin, although their efficacy has not been established. Maintaining range of motion and performing strengthening exercises are important, and a course of physical therapy is helpful. Residual deformities may be helped in certain cases with tendon transfers, which can provide improved stability or function and pain relief.

BRACHIAL PLEXUS INJURIES

Brachial plexus lesions (Fig. 17–10) can often lead to significant physical disability, psychological duress, and financial hardship. Complete loss of the use of one's limb or partial loss (e.g., one that does not allow positioning of a working hand in space) results in significant impairment with devastating consequences. Traumatic lesions typically affect young men and frequently result from motor vehicle or motorcycle accidents. Other mechanisms may

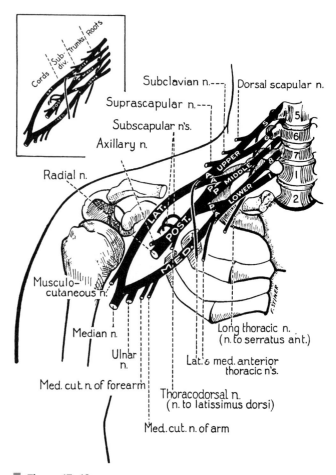

■ **Figure 17–10**
The brachial plexus. *(From Haymaker W and Woodhall B: Peripheral Nerve Injuries. Philadelphia: WB Saunders, 1953, p 210).*

be responsible for brachial plexus lesions, including obstetric birth palsy (occurring in approximately 1 in 2000 live births), penetrating injuries, radiation, compression (such as by a mass effect) (Fig. 17–11), tumors, entrapment, iatrogenic causes (e.g., after first rib resection, shoulder surgery), and inflammation.

Closed brachial plexus injuries are traction injuries. They result in distraction of the forequarter from the body. Narakas summarized the potential disrupting forces well: "The motorcyclist thrown in the air will have multiple impacts: the car, the roof, the road, each of which will have their own natural history and possible injury."[113] These forces may lead to supraclavicular, retroclavicular, infraclavicular, or combined patterns of injury affecting the brachial plexus from the rootlets to the terminal branches.

Supraclavicular injuries are the most common and the most severe. They are typically related to high-speed injuries. Such injuries most frequently lead to complete lesions (pan-plexal injuries), followed by upper pattern lesions (C5, C6, ± C7). Lower element (C8, T1) injuries are very rare. Downward traction on the arm or forcible widening of the shoulder-neck angle produces upper trunk injuries, whereas lower trunk injuries are produced by forcible upward traction of the arm. Depending on the duration and the amount of force, injuries may result in

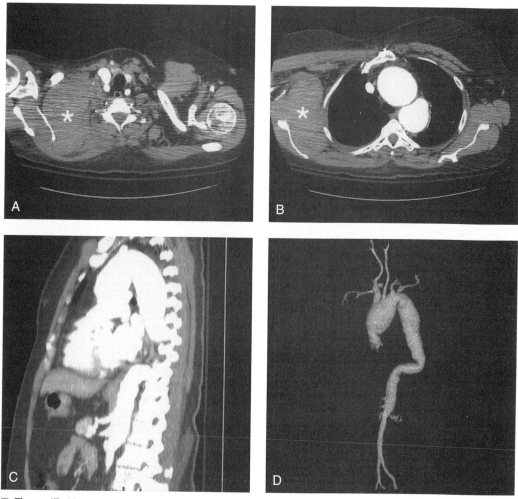

■ **Figure 17–11**

Brachial plexus compression by a large hematoma. A 55-year-old woman had a history of a previous ascending aortic aneurysm replacement with a composite graft. She was receiving chronic anticoagulation with warfarin (Coumadin) for her aortic valve replacement. She fell from a horse and sustained a tibial plateau fracture. She used crutches clumsily, and a neck hematoma developed "spontaneously" and painful paralysis in the right upper limb 1 week later. **A** and **B,** A large (12 × 9 cm) hematoma *(asterisk)* spanning from the supraclavicular portion to the scapula is compressing the brachial plexus. **C** and **D,** Three-dimensional reconstruction shows a 7-cm aortic aneurysm (seen in **B**). The aneurysm was an incidental finding and the hematoma was a result of crutch use and not from a ruptured aneurysm.

stretch lesions (neuromas), rupture, or avulsion. Stretch lesions are often longitudinal injuries. Nerve lesions that are in continuity have the best prognosis for recovery; rupture and avulsion have the poorest prognosis and require surgical intervention. Preganglionic injuries may lead to avulsion from the spinal cord (central avulsion) or rupture just distal to the spinal cord (intradural rupture). Preganglionic injuries may affect either the ventral or the dorsal roots individually or, more commonly, both. Avulsion is more common in the lower elements because of anatomic restraints in the upper levels. The upper elements have proximal branches (e.g., to the phrenic or serratus anterior) and transverse radicular ligaments that may be protective, whereas the lower elements do not have these branches or ligaments.

Infraclavicular injuries usually develop after a lower-energy impact and are often due to compression rather than traction. Many are incomplete lesions and recover spontaneously without surgery.[93] However, complete lesions do occur, sometimes with rupture and even avulsion. Infraclavicular lesions usually affect the cords and terminal branches and, occasionally, the roots. Injury to one or more terminal branches may occur as either a primary or a secondary site of injury (together with a supraclavicular or infraclavicular injury). These terminal branch injuries seem to occur at sites where the nerves are relatively fixed. For example, the musculocutaneous nerve may be predisposed to injury as it penetrates the coracobrachialis; the suprascapular nerve, at the transverse scapular notch; and the axillary nerve, at the quadrilateral space. Associated vascular injuries occur in 10% to 20% of infraclavicular brachial plexus cases. Coexisting bony injuries (e.g., clavicular, scapular, or humeral fractures or dislocations) may contribute to the neural injury acutely or in delayed fashion (such as with clavicular nonunion or malunion). Operative dissection of the infraclavicular brachial plexus may be extremely difficult because of the dense fibrosis.

The diagnosis of brachial plexus injuries is often elusive, and the resultant delay may have a negative impact on timely referral for specialized treatment. The diagnosis of brachial plexus injury can be suspected from a good history, supported by physical examination, and confirmed by electrodiagnostic or imaging studies. The mechanism of the injury, in particular, the position of the neck and arm in relation to the body after trauma, needs to be evaluated. A thorough primary and secondary assessment must be included to identify concomitant injuries to the head, chest, vessels, long bones, pelvis, and spine (associated symptoms and signs of myelopathy must also be sought). Multitrauma is common, and frequently other more critical injuries may receive attention while other (not minor) injuries may be missed. Detailed neurologic testing will reveal deficits affecting a discrete pattern. Ideally, the diagnosis of an injury to the brachial plexus should be made in the emergency department. Additional information that would be helpful is whether the injury is complete or incomplete, whether it involves the supraclavicular or infraclavicular region (or more than one injury), and whether it is a preganglionic or postganglionic injury. These localizations are helpful in planning treatment and predicting the prognosis.

Other diagnostic studies complement the physical examination. Plain radiographs of the chest may reveal an elevated diaphragm from a phrenic nerve injury. Radiographs of the cervical spine and other bones may demonstrate fractures. Angiography should be performed if vascular injury is suspected, especially when an acute brachial plexus injury is present in conjunction with an expanding hematoma, first rib fracture, widened mediastinum, or upper limb pulse abnormality. Electrodiagnostic studies are most useful about 3 weeks after the injury and can further localize the lesion and assess the degree of neural involvement. Computed tomography (CT)-myelography[110] should be performed when a supraclavicular lesion has been diagnosed and a preganglionic injury is being considered. We have used shoulder MRI to assess patients with nerve injuries associated with shoulder dislocations and proximal humeral fractures to ensure rotator cuff integrity, as well as in isolated suprascapular nerve lesions to identify ganglia. MRI of the brachial plexus is rapidly improving, but we have not yet found this imaging modality to be as helpful as CT-myelography in identifying root avulsions.

Features gleaned from a careful history, physical examination, and electrodiagnostic and imaging studies can suggest a preganglionic injury. Such features include the presence of deafferentiating pain; the finding of Horner's syndrome (miosis, ptosis, anhidrosis, enophthalmos), weak rhomboids or serratus anterior muscles, or an absent Tinel sign in the neck on physical examination; the presence of fibrillations in the paraspinal muscles or rhomboids or preserved sensory nerve action potentials in an anesthetic hand with absent motor nerve action potentials on electrical studies; and detection of an elevated hemidiaphragm or associated cervical fractures on radiographs and pseudomeningoceles (Fig. 17–12) or absent nerve rootlets on myelography.

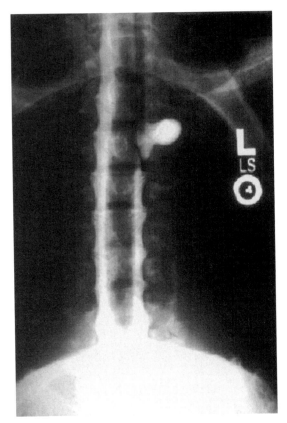

■ **Figure 17–12**
Large post-traumatic pseudomeningocele suggestive of a preganglionic lesion.

Timely diagnosis of a brachial plexus injury has therapeutic implications. For closed injuries, patients are typically observed for spontaneous improvement over the first several months. It is important to obtain a baseline examination and then monitor clinical and electrophysiologic examinations serially for improvement. Patients who demonstrate improvement in this time frame have sustained neurapractic injury. However, it is difficult to preoperatively determine which axonometric lesions (Sunderland grades II to IV) will recover spontaneously despite their differing prognoses. Grade II is associated with good spontaneous recovery, but grade IV has a poor prognosis. Patients should receive physical therapy for range of motion to prevent soft tissue contractures and to strengthen working muscles. Neuropathic pain should be managed by a specialist, especially when it is refractory to first-line medications, as is often the case with deafferentiated pain.

The decision to operate is complex. Surgery must balance the risks and benefits of waiting for potential spontaneous recovery with the realization that the window of opportunity for nerve recovery is finite. The timing of surgery is critical. Surgery is indicated for closed injuries when objective recovery has not been established on sequential examinations by 3 to 6 months. Clinical recovery, especially in the proximal muscles, is a favorable sign. However, one should be cautious and not unduly optimistic because of the potential for overinterpretation of an advancing Tinel sign, a positive squeeze test, or nascent potentials on EMG without additional signs of clinical recovery. If avulsion injury is suspected, one might perform surgery even earlier.

Nerve injuries from sharp (knife) objects should be explored early (within several days). Patients with an increasing deficit under observation should undergo early exploration. An increasing deficit often bespeaks a vascular injury such as from a pseudoaneurysm or an expanding hematoma. Nerve injuries associated with blunt trauma should be explored after several weeks when the ends of nerve have demarcated; nerve ends that may have been identified at the time of immediate vascular repair should be tacked down under tension, and then definitive treatment should be performed several weeks later. Nerve injuries associated with gunshot wounds should generally be treated nonoperatively; the majority are not associated with disruption of elements,[85] are neurapractic, and improve spontaneously. Fortunately, our experience with civilian injuries is limited, and we base our current approach on our vast experience from war injuries. Patients initially evaluated at a late stage (after 9 or 12 months) are better treated with reconstruction (e.g., functional free muscle transfer, tendon transfers, joint fusion) than with direct nerve surgery.

Before surgery, the surgical team should formulate a preoperative plan based on a careful review of all existing clinical and electrophysiologic examinations and studies. Surgeons need to consider many factors and tabulate a list of what is working (and what is not), what is available for transfer, and what is needed. Surgeons must balance realistic goals (based on injury patterns, timing of surgery, etc.) and expectations of the patient, the family, and themselves. Contingency plans should be established.

The brachial plexus is exposed through a supraclavicular and/or infraclavicular approach, depending on the level or levels of suspected injury. We favor exploration of both regions because we have been surprised by the frequency of double-level injuries. We use a transverse supraclavicular incision rather than a zigzag incision and a separate deltopectoral approach (with detachment of the pectoralis minor). Clavicular osteotomy is seldom necessary except in rare cases with predominantly retroclavicular pathology. If osteotomy is deemed necessary, predrilling and preplating should be performed with a low-contour compression plate (Fig. 17–13).

Exposure of the brachial plexus permits us to perform intraoperative electrophysiologic monitoring. It is well known that direct visualization or palpation of the external surface of a nerve does not accurately predict the nerve's histologic appearance or potential for recovery. We believe that a combination of intraoperative techniques is the most useful way to obtain additional data, define the nerve pathology, and prognosticate outcomes. Nerve action potentials (NAPs)[86,87,159] can help distinguish preganglionic and postganglionic injury and can differentiate between grades of axonometric injury. Somatosensory evoked potentials (SSEPs) may also be used to determine the presence or absence of nerve root avulsion. Although SSEPs test the sensory pathway per se, in most cases (but not all), one can draw inferences about the status of the ventral roots. Another shortcoming of SSEPs is that a positive response can be obtained with as few as 100 to 200

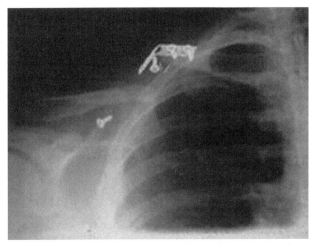

■ **Figure 17–13**

If clavicular osteotomy is necessary, it should be performed by a surgeon skilled in fixation. This case illustrates inadequate fixation of the clavicular osteotomy with a semitubular plate.

intact nerve fibers.[177] For example, avulsion may be diagnosed with an absent SSEP and a preganglionic NAP. A recovering neuroma will show a regenerative NAP (i.e., viable axons). A neuroma that does not conduct an NAP will exhibit a flat tracing and does not result in clinical recovery. The use of motor evoked potentials (MEPs) with transcranial electrical stimulation has recently been approved in the United States and allows the theoretical advantage of testing the integrity of motor root function.[24,162] All techniques require experience in interpretation. These types of recordings are better suited for detecting early regeneration in brachial plexus lesions than compound muscle action potential (CMAP) recordings. Given the distance to the end-organ, one would not anticipate that nerve reinnervation has reached the target muscle. However in partial lesions, CMAPs may also be helpful in determining the severity of the lesion (i.e., the number of functioning axons). We do not perform hemilaminectomy[27] or histochemical analysis with choline acetyltransferase[75] to identify avulsions, although we recognize the appeal afforded by these techniques.

Nerve repair is seldom possible except in instances of acute, sharp injury treated urgently. Standard approaches to brachial plexus surgery would be neurolysis of a recovering neuroma that shows a regenerative NAP and grafting of an advanced lesion that does not conduct an NAP or a rupture (direct repair is not generally practical).[106] Nerve stumps are sectioned back until good fascicular structure has been identified. Proximal dissection to a foraminal level is sometimes necessary to locate adequate quality in the proximal stump. Then, plexoplexal grafting is accomplished by interfascicular repair with microsurgical techniques. Interpositional grafts are placed to ensure adequate coverage of the proximal and distal faces of the nerve ends. Grafts should be sutured in place without tension. Typically, the repairs are performed with the arm abducted and externally rotated. Donor nerve grafts usually include the sural nerve (unilaterally or bilaterally), but other cutaneous nerves in the forearm or arm can also be used. We place several 9-0 sutures to coapt the nerve ends and then reinforce the repair with fibrin glue. After the repair is completed, the limb is gently mobilized through an arc of motion to test the tension. Although other groups have used intraoperative histology to identify the fascicular structure,[100] we have not. The limb is maintained in a shoulder immobilizer for 3 weeks to protect the suture lines. Thereafter, pendulum exercises are begun, and passive and active motion is instituted. Therapists also provide resting splints for immobile joints. We prescribe electrical stimulation, although we recognize that this technique has not been validated clinically. Patients are examined every 3 to 4 months for clinical signs of recovery.

Avulsions or preganglionic injuries can be treated by nerve transfer. Nerve transfer (neurotization) exchanges a nonfunctioning nerve with a dispensable or redundant working nerve. Nerve transfers are useful in the following situations: to treat avulsions, to achieve more rapid or predictable recovery of a distal target (i.e., an alternative to nerve grafting), and to power a free functioning muscle transfer. Nerve transfers provide a source of axons that permits surgeons to reconstruct additional targets with the intent of improving outcomes (Fig. 17–14). They should consist of a large number of "pure" motor or sensory axons (depending on the type of nerve transfer being performed) and preferably be synergistic. Patients should have the ability to relearn the new function independently, although induction exercises and re-education are necessary components of the postoperative program. Most importantly, when considering any nerve transfer, one needs to weigh the cost-benefit ratio, or the advantages and potential disadvantages of using a specific donor. Popular nerve transfers include the intercostals,[47,107,111] distal spinal accessory, cervical plexus, thoracodorsal, and pectoral branches.[19] With some of the newer transfers especially (e.g., phrenic[71,154,176] or contralateral C7[72,148] and fascicles of the ulnar or median nerves[155]), potential risks must be carefully considered before using them. Use of the phrenic nerve and contralateral C7 increases the number of donor nerves available and perhaps allows reconstructive strategies to be designed that will permit more distal reinnervation. Transfer of ulnar or median nerve fascicles to the biceps motor branch significantly shortens the time for reinnervation. Several large series have reported acceptable morbidity from all these techniques. Preliminary experience with the hypoglossal nerve[58,99] has been disappointing, however. Various combinations of nerve transfers are being used as part of brachial plexus reconstruction.

Historically, goals for a complete brachial plexus injury were limited. Surgery took on different paths, including "peak and shriek," above-elbow amputation with shoulder fusion, and elbow flexion with biceps neurotization with or without shoulder fusion. The main priorities of brachial reconstruction include restoration of elbow flexion, shoulder abduction, and stability; hand sensibility can be achieved in some cases. More distal motor function was considered unobtainable because of the length of regeneration needed.

Brachial plexus surgery is evolving, and older techniques are rarely performed. Amputation is not widely practiced because of poor compliance with use of an

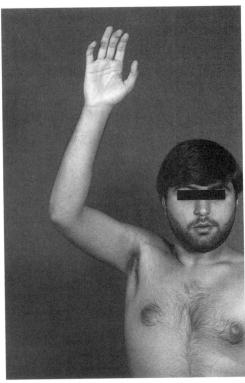

■ Figure 17–14
Brachial plexus reconstruction: nerve transfers for shoulder abduction. This 17-year-old sustained a high-speed motor vehicle accident 6 months previously. He had a spinal cord injury that was treated successfully with evacuation of a cervical epidural hematoma acutely. Initially he had a C5-C7 lesion but noted recovery in C6 and C7. Six months after injury, he had a flail shoulder, including weak rhomboids. Electromyography (EMG) showed fibrillations in the midcervical paraspinals. Myelography demonstrated a pseudomeningocele at C5. At surgery, nerve action potentials and somatosensory evoked potentials confirmed a preganglionic injury. He underwent nerve transfers involving the spinal accessory nerve to the suprascapular nerve and a triceps branch to the axillary nerve. By 1 year postoperatively, he had already regained more than 90 degrees of abduction and 45 degrees of external rotation. EMG confirmed nascent potentials in both the infraspinatus and deltoid muscles.

artificial limb and lack of pain resolution. Shoulder fusion is less often performed now for brachial plexus lesions. Voluntary control with neural reconstruction has been shown to be more preferable than a fused shoulder. Still, shoulder fusion (Fig. 17–15) is very reliable in cases of failed shoulder reconstruction or in patients with painful instability from paralysis of the deltoid and rotator cuff. Shoulder fusion is probably preferable to tendon transfers for adults with these lesions. One must remember that successful shoulder fusion requires a functioning trapezius, serratus anterior, levator scapulae, and rhomboids. The ideal position for shoulder fusion is controversial.

By adding other combinations of nerve transfers, brachial plexus surgeons have become more successful in achieving the major goals of restoring elbow flexion, shoulder abduction and stability, and hand sensibility than in the recent past. In the case of complete avulsion, conventional nerve transfers could include the accessory nerve to the suprascapular nerve, the intercostals to the

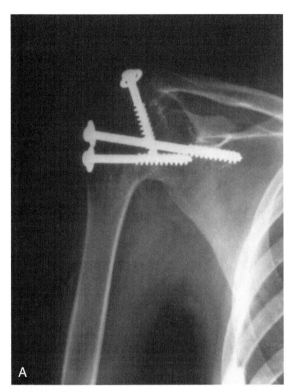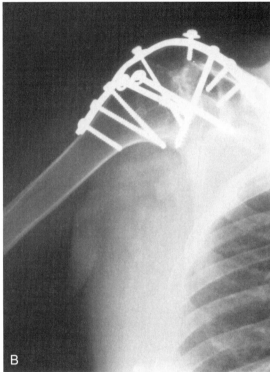

■ **Figure 17–15**
Shoulder fusion after brachial plexus injury. Two different techniques for shoulder fusion are illustrated: large cancellous screws (**A**) and a combination of plate and screw fixation (**B**).

biceps, and perhaps the intercostals to the median nerve to achieve these goals as part of the primary procedure.

With the emergence of newer techniques, some successful restoration of hand function (grasp and release) has been achieved, even in patients with a flail limb. These results, however, necessitate a more "aggressive" approach to reconstruction. Multiple nerve transfers for muscle and sensory function may be performed by themselves or together with free muscle transfer. For example, the same case of pan-plexus avulsion can be treated with a strategy of multiple neurotization, which might include the phrenic to the suprascapular nerve, the spinal accessory (via a sural nerve graft) to the musculocutaneous nerve, the contralateral C7 to the median nerve with a vascularized ulnar nerve graft, and the intercostals to the radial nerve and the long thoracic nerve.

Free muscle transfer can also be incorporated into the early reconstruction. Single-muscle transfer can restore elbow flexion with or without wrist dorsiflexion with reliable results. A muscle transfer that has been popular has been transfer of the gracilis muscle. A similar-size match between the gracilis and the biceps allows for ease of wound closure at the end of surgery, and the morbidity of gracilis harvest is minimal. Typically, the gracilis muscle origin is secured to the clavicle through drill holes, and the spinal accessory nerve and the gracilis motor nerve can be repaired under the clavicle. Alternatively, two or three intercostal nerves or a fascicle of the ulnar nerve[74] (when it is available) can be used in place of the spinal accessory nerve. The results of contralateral C7 neurotization of a free muscle have not been as successful.[33] The donor

vessels are repaired to ones from the thoracoacromial trunk. The tendon of the gracilis is then attached to the biceps tendon. Studies have shown improvement in elbow flexion strength, with 80% of patients achieving MRC grade 3 or better.[2,31] Free gracilis transfer allows early reinnervation of the free muscle by 3 to 6 months and maximal strength by 18 months. This free muscle technique can be modified to provide both elbow flexion and wrist extension by weaving the tendon beneath the mobile wad and into the extensor carpi radialis brevis. In one series, over half the patients obtained M3 or greater wrist extension.[2] In our experience, elbow flexion is slightly weakened when the free muscle is used for dual transfer rather than just a single function.

Double free muscle transfer for patients with four or five root avulsions has been successfully performed by Doi and colleagues.[46] The lofty goals of these two technically demanding procedures include independent voluntary elbow flexion and extension, independent voluntary finger flexion and extension, and protective sensation in the hand. Stage 1 includes exploration of the brachial plexus and free gracilis transfer with spinal accessory neurotization for elbow flexion and finger extension. Stage 2, performed several weeks later, consists of intercostal neurotization of another free gracilis muscle for finger flexion, combined with intercostal motor neurotization of the triceps and sensory neurotization of the median nerve. The gracilis muscle is attached to the second rib and secured into the tendons of the finger and thumb flexors. The donor vessels are repaired to the thoracodorsal vessels. Additional nerve transfers can also be added (using other available donors such as phrenic nerve or contralateral C7) to provide shoulder function/stabilization. Twenty-five of 26 patients obtained good or excellent elbow flexion and slightly more than half obtained satisfactory prehension (more than 30 degrees of total active motion of the fingers) and could position the hand in space.

Carlstedt and associates[26] and several other groups[12,61] have attempted reimplantation of avulsed spinal nerves into the spinal cord. Although regeneration across the central/peripheral nerve interface has been demonstrated in experimental animals and in humans, early experience with this technique in humans has been inferior to other more standard reconstructive procedures. As such, reimplantation is being performed only at several centers around the world, and its use in humans is still experimental.[158] It remains an exciting possibility for the future.

Another example of brachial plexus reconstruction in evolution can be seen with a typical C5-C6 pattern of functional loss as a result of avulsions. Such patients (Erb's palsy) would have absent shoulder abduction and external rotation and absent elbow flexion. In the past, the most common procedure would be transfer of two to three intercostal nerves. Studies have shown that direct transfer without a bridging nerve graft, performed before 6 months, will offer the best results.[33,64,83,138] Others have used the spinal accessory nerve with an intervening sural nerve graft with similar outcomes.[3,139,141] Other nerve transfers involving the medial pectoral, thoracodorsal,[40] phrenic, contralateral C7, and even the ipsilateral C7[72] could be performed. In the past decade, the Oberlin transfer (ulnar nerve fascicle) has been used with great success. Currently, this technique is becoming extremely popular and widespread. It has been performed via an end-to-side technique[62] and modified to transfer the median nerve fascicle or used to reinnervate both the biceps and the brachialis muscles.

The same clinical pattern of C5 and C6 loss can become more controversial if the surgeon finds C5 and C6 neuromas or ruptures rather than C5 and C6 avulsions. Should one perform a nerve graft from C5 or C6 if proximal stumps are available or should one perform a new transfer? Which of these techniques will produce better outcomes? If one were to perform nerve transfers, which ones would provide superior results?

Patients who are initially examined late after injury (after 9 months or 1 year) are probably best not treated with primary nerve surgery. Here, a combination of procedures, including muscle/tendon transfers, free muscle transfer, and bony procedures (shoulder fusion, other augmenting techniques), may be applied. Options may be limited because of the lack of available donors of sufficient strength.

Patients with brachial plexus surgery need careful and thoughtful long-term follow-up evaluation. Those who have made insufficient recovery from a primary nerve reconstruction may benefit greatly from a secondary (soft tissue or bony) procedure. In fact, a surgeon should consider leaving "something behind" should a salvage procedure need to be performed for which donor nerves might be needed. In addition, relatively minor operative procedures (such as flexor-to-extensor tendon transfers) can markedly improve function.

Treating neuropathic pain remains as difficult and challenging an issue as treating loss of function and may also require long-term patient follow-up. Neuropathic pain is best treated by a multidisciplinary approach within a pain clinic setting. Patients can be managed with a combination of various medications titrated to effect by experts in the field under close observation. Other modalities, including psychological support and physical therapy, should be admixed. Pain can improve over time, especially as reinnervation occurs. Primary nerve-related surgery can help relieve neuropathic pain, either with neurolysis or resection of neuromas or with nerve transfers. Patients with refractory pain from a root avulsion can also be treated by creating lesions at the dorsal entry zone (DREZ lesions)[114] or by spinal cord stimulators.

Despite the excitement that these new techniques have brought and the improved outcomes, the overall results are still sobering when we consider the magnitude of the problem. Great difficulty exists when analyzing outcomes. All to often we have insufficient data from a single surgeon using the same technique at the same time in the same matched set of individuals, without long-term follow-up. The definition of a good result or even a uniform classification has not been universally adopted. In the end, we are comparing apples, oranges, and lemons when we study operative outcomes.

Some generalizations can be made regarding outcomes. Ultimate recovery is dependent on many factors, including the extent and pattern of injury, the age of the patient, the patient's cooperation and rehabilitation, the surgeon's experience, and the time interval between injury and surgery. Outcomes are best for incomplete lesions or neuromas that conduct an NAP. Injuries to the upper plexal elements fare better than those to the lower elements (lower trunk, medial cord, etc); these latter elements do quite poorly with nerve surgery. Infraclavicular lesions and terminal branch injuries do better than supraclavicular injuries (note—the more distal the better). The best results can be achieved in those operated on before 6 months and in younger patients. Short grafts do better than long grafts. Nerve transfers offer the opportunity of speeding up the recovery process. The best results are seen when nerve transfers can be coapted directly without an interpositional graft. Standard nerve transfers to improve median nerve, ulnar nerve, and distal radial nerve function have not generally fared well. Double innervation of a joint is probably preferable to single innervation.[105] Nerve reconstruction, when at all achievable, seems to be more functional than tendon transfer or joint fusion.

Brachial plexus reconstruction has made great strides in the past few decades. Outcomes are better because of increased awareness and improved surgical techniques. In the past, few options were available other than amputation or benign neglect. Brachial plexus injuries have a lifelong impact on the quality of life of affected individuals. Most still have significant residual loss of function. Many have severe neuropathic pain and become dependent on narcotics.[30] Only about half these patients return to work. Continuing advancement in basic science, the development of new techniques, and refining of described procedures will ultimately improve outcomes and, one hopes, allow many more individuals to return to the workforce.

REFERENCES

1. Agre JC, Ash N, Cameron MC, and House J: Suprascapular neuropathy after intensive progressive resistive exercise: Case report. Arch Phys Med Rehabil 68:236-238, 1987.
2. Akasaka Y, Hara T, and Takahashi M: Restoration of elbow flexion and wrist extension in brachial plexus paralyses by means of free muscle transplantation innervated by intercostal nerve. Ann Chir Main Memb Super 9:341-350, 1990.
3. Allieu Y and Cenac P: Neurotization via the spinal accessory nerve in complete paralysis due to multiple avulsion injuries of the brachial plexus. Clin Orthop 237:67-74, 1988.
4. Alnot JY: L'epaule paralytique de l'adulte par lesions nerveuses peripheriques post-traumatiques. Acta Orthop Belg 65:10-22, 1999.
5. Alnot JY and Valenti P: Reparation chirurgicale du nerf axillaire. A propos de 37 cas. Int Orthop 15:7-11, 1991.
6. Antoniadis G, Richter HP, Rath S, et al: Suprascapular nerve entrapment: Experience with 28 cases. J Neurosurg 85:1020-1025, 1996.
7. Antoniou J, Tae SK, Williams GR, et al: Suprascapular neuropathy. Variability in the diagnosis, treatment, and outcome. Clin Orthop 386:131-138, 2001.
8. Aszmann OC and Dellon AL: The internal topography of the axillary nerve: An anatomic and histologic study as it relates to microsurgery. J Reconstr Microsurg 12:359-363, 1996.
9. Atasoy E and Majd M: Scapulothoracic stabilisation for winging of the scapula using strips of autogenous fascia lata. J Bone Joint Surg Br 82:813-817, 2000.
10. Bach BR Jr, O'Brien SJ, Warren RF, and Leighton M: An unusual neurological complication of the Bristow procedure. A case report. J Bone Joint Surg Am 70:458-460, 1988.
11. Beghi E, Kurland LT, Mulder DW, and Nicolosi A: Brachial plexus neuropathy in the population of Rochester, Minnesota, 1970-1981. Ann Neurol 18:320-323, 1985.
12. Bertelli JA and Ghizoni MF: Brachial plexus avulsion injury repairs with nerve transfers and nerve grafts directly implanted into the spinal cord yield partial recovery of shoulder and elbow movements. Neurosurgery 52:1385-1390, 2003.
13. Bigliani LU, Compito CA, Duralde XA, and Wolfe IN: Transfer of the levator scapulae, rhomboid major, and rhomboid minor for paralysis of the trapezius. J Bone Joint Surg Am 78:1534-1540, 1996.
14. Bigliani LU, Dalsey RM, McCann PD, and April EW: An anatomical study of the suprascapular nerve. Arthroscopy 6:301-305, 1990.
15. Bigliani LU, Perez-Sanz JR, and Wolfe IN: Treatment of trapezius paralysis. J Bone Joint Surg Am 67:871-877, 1985.
16. Black KP and Lombardo JA: Suprascapular nerve injuries with isolated paralysis of the infraspinatus. Am J Sports Med 18:225-228, 1990.
17. Blom S and Dahlback LO: Nerve injuries in dislocations of the shoulder joint and fractures of the neck of the humerus. Acta Chir Scand 136:461-466, 1970.
18. Boerger TO and Limb D: Suprascapular nerve injury at the spinoglenoid notch after glenoid neck fracture. J Shoulder Elbow Surg 9:236-237, 2000.
19. Brandt KE and Mackinnon SE: A technique for maximizing biceps recovery in brachial plexus reconstruction. J Hand Surg [Am] 18:726-733, 1993.
20. Briner WW Jr and Kacmar L: Common injuries in volleyball. Mechanisms of injury, prevention and rehabilitation. Sports Med 24:65-71, 1997.
21. Brown TD, Newton PM, Steinmann SP, et al: Rotator cuff tears and associated nerve injuries. Orthopedics 23:329-332, 2000.
22. Bunch WH and Siegel IM: Scapulothoracic arthrodesis in fascioscapulo-humeral muscular dystrophy. Review of seventeen procedures with three to twenty-one year follow-up. J Bone Joint Surg Am 75:372-376, 1993.
23. Burkhead WZ, Scheinberg RR, and Box G: Surgical anatomy of the axillary nerve. J Shoulder Elbow Surg 1:31-36, 1992.
24. Burkholder LM, Houlden DA, Midha R, et al: Neurogenic motor evoked potentials: Role in brachial plexus surgery. J Neurosurg 98:607-610, 2003.
25. Cahill BR, Palmer RE: Quadrilateral space syndrome. J Hand Surg [Am] 8:65-69, 1983.
26. Carlstedt T, Anand P, Hallin R, et al: Spinal nerve repair and reimplantation of avulsed ventral roots into the spinal cord after brachial plexus injury. J Neurosurg 93:237-247, 2000.
27. Carvalho GA, Nikkhah G, Matthies C, et al: Diagnosis of root avulsions in traumatic brachial plexus injuries. Value of computerized tomography, myelography, and magnetic resonance imaging. J Neurosurg 86:69-76, 1997.
28. Caspi I, Ezra E, Nerubay J, and Horoszovski H: Musculocutaneous nerve injury after coracoid process transfer for clavicle instability. Report of three cases. Acta Orthop Scand 58:294-295, 1987.
29. Chavez J: Pectoralis minor transplanted for paralysis of the serratus anterior. J Bone Joint Surg Br 33:21-28, 1951.
30. Choi PD, Novak CB, Mackinnon SE, and Kline DG: Quality of life and functional outcome following brachial plexus injury. J Hand Surg [Am] 22:605-612, 1997.
31. Chuang DC: Functioning free muscle transplantation for brachial plexus injury. Clin Orthop 314:104-111, 1995.
32. Chuang DC, Lee GW, Hashem F, and Wei FC: Restoration of shoulder abduction by nerve transfer in avulsed brachial plexus injury: Evaluation of 99 patients with various nerve transfers. Plast Reconstr Surg 96:122-128, 1995.
33. Chuang DCC, Wei FC, and Noordhoff MS: Cross-chest C7 nerve grafting followed by free muscle transplantations for the treatment of total avulsed brachial plexus injuries: A preliminary report. Plast Reconstr Surg 92:717-725, 1993.
34. Chuang DC, Yeh MC, and Wei FC: Intercostal nerve transfer of the musculocutaneous nerve in avulsed brachial plexus injuries: evaluation of 66 patients. J Hand Surg [Am] 17:822-828, 1992.
35. Coelho TD: Isolated and painless atrophy of the infraspinatus muscle. Left handed versus right handed volleyball players. Arq Neuropsiquiatr 52:539-544, 1994.
36. Coene LN and Narakas AO: Operative management of lesions of the axillary nerve, isolated or combined with other nerve lesions. Clin Neurol Neurosurg 94(suppl):S64-S66, 1992.
37. Connor PM, Yamaguchi K, Manifold SG, et al: Split pectoralis major transfer for serratus anterior palsy. Clin Orthop 341:134-142, 1997.
38. Corner NB, Milner SM, MacDonald R, and Jubb M: Isolated musculocutaneous nerve lesion after shoulder dislocation. J R Army Med Corps 136:107-108, 1990.
39. Cummins CA, Bowen M, Anderson K, and Messer T: Suprascapular nerve entrapment at the spinoglenoid notch in a professional baseball pitcher. Am J Sports Med 27:810-812, 1999.
40. Dai SY, Lin DX, Han Z, and Zhoug SZ: Transference of thoracodorsal nerve to musculocutaneous or axillary nerve in old traumatic injury. J Hand Surg [Am] 15:36-37, 1990.
41. Dailiana ZH, Mehdian H, and Gilbert A: Surgical anatomy of spinal accessory nerve: Is trapezius functional deficit inevitable after division of the nerve. J Hand Surg [Br] 26:137-141, 2001.
42. Davidson JJ, Bassett FH 3rd, and Nunley JA 2nd: Musculocutaneous nerve entrapment revisited. J Shoulder Elbow Surg 7:250-255, 1998.
43. Dewar FP and Harris RI: Restoration of function of the shoulder following paralysis of the trapezius by fascial sling fixation and transplantation of the levator scapulae. Ann Surg 132:1111-1115, 1950.
44. Dickson F: Fascial transplants in paralytic and other conditions. J Bone Joint Surg 19:405-412, 1937.
45. Disa JJ, Wang B, and Dellon AL: Correction of scapular winging by supraclavicular neurolysis of the long thoracic nerve. J Reconstr Microsurg 17:79-84, 2001.
46. Doi K, Muramatsu K, and Hattori Y: Restoration of prehension with the double free muscle technique following complete avulsion of the brachial plexus. Indications and long-term results. J Bone Joint Surg Am 82:652-666, 2000.
47. Dolenc VV: Intercostal neurotization of the peripheral nerves in avulsion plexus injuries. Clin Plast Surg 11:143-147, 1984.
48. Dreschfeld J: On some of the rarer forms of muscular atrophies. Brain 9:187-189, 1887.
49. Durman D: An operation for paralysis of the serratus anterior. J Bone Joint Surg 27:380-382, 1945.
50. Edeland HG and Zachrisson BE: Fracture of the scapular notch associated with lesion of the suprascapular nerve. Acta Orthop Scand 46:758-763, 1975.
51. Eden: Zur Behandlung der Trapeziuslaehmung mittels Muskelplastik. Dtsch Z Chir 184:387-397, 1924.
52. Eggert S and Holzgraefe M: Die Kompressionsneuropathic des Nervus suprascapularis bei Hochleistungsvolleyballern. Sportverletz Sportschaden 7:136-142, 1993.
53. Eglseder WA Jr and Goldman M: Anatomic variations of the musculocutaneous nerve in the arm. Am J Orthop 26:777-780, 1997.
54. England JD: The variations of neuralgic amyotrophy. Muscle Nerve 22:435-436, 1999.
55. England JD and Sumner AJ: Neuralgic amyotrophy: An increasingly diverse entity. Muscle Nerve 10:60-68, 1987.
56. Fehrman DA, Orwin JF, and Jennings RM: Suprascapular nerve entrapment by ganglion cysts: A report of six cases with arthroscopic findings and review of the literature. Arthroscopy 11:727-734, 1995.
57. Feinberg J: Fall von Erb-Klumpke Scher. Lahmung nach Influenza. Centralbl. 16:588-637, 1897.
58. Ferraresi S, Garozzo D, Ravenni R, et al: Hemihypoglossal nerve transfer in brachial plexus repair: Technique and results. Neurosurgery 50:332-335, 2002.
59. Flatow EL and Bigliani LU: Tips of the trade. Locating and protecting the axillary nerve in shoulder surgery: The tug test. Orthop Rev 21:503-505, 1992.
60. Flatow EL, Bigliani LU, and April EW: An anatomic study of the musculocutaneous nerve and its relationship to the coracoid process. Clin Orthop 244:166-171, 1989.
61. Fournier HD, Mercier PH, and Menei P: Lateral interscalenic multilevel oblique corpectomies to repair ventral root avulsions after brachial plexus

injury in humans; anatomical study and first clinical experience. J Neurosurg 95(suppl):202-207, 2001.

62. Franciosi LF, Modestti C, and Mueller SF: Neurotization of the biceps muscle by end-to-side neurorrhaphy between ulnar and musculocutaneous nerves. A series of five cases. Chir Main 17:362-367, 1998.

63. Friedenberg SM, Zimprich T, and Harper CM: The natural history of long thoracic and spinal accessory neuropathies. Muscle Nerve 25:535-539, 2002.

64. Friedman AH, Nunley JA 2nd, Goldner RD, et al: Nerve transposition for the restoration of elbow flexion following brachial plexus avulsion injuries. J Neurosurg 72:59-64, 1990.

65. Friedman AH, Nunley JA 2nd, Urbaniak JR, and Goldner RD: Repair of isolated axillary nerve lesions after infraclavicular brachial plexus injuries: Case reports. Neurosurgery 27:403-407, 1990.

66. Geertzen JH, Groothoff JW, Nicolai JP, and Rietman JS: Brachial plexus neuropathy. A long-term outcome study. J Hand Surg [Br] 25:461-464, 2000.

67. Gozna ER and Harris WR: Traumatic winging of the scapula. J Bone Joint Surg Am 61:1230-1233, 1979.

68. Greis PE, Burks RT, Schickendantz MS, and Sandmeier R: Axillary nerve injury after thermal capsular shrinkage of the shoulder. J Shoulder Elbow Surg 10:231-235, 2001.

69. Gryler EC, Greis PE, Burks RT, and West J: Axillary nerve temperatures during radiofrequency capsulorrhaphy of the shoulder. Arthroscopy 17:567-572, 2001.

70. Gu YD, Cai PQ, Xu F, et al: Clinical application of ipsilateral C7 nerve root transfer for treatment of C5 and C6 avulsion of brachial plexus. Microsurgery 23:105-108, 2003.

71. Gu YD and Ma MK: Use of the phrenic nerve for brachial plexus reconstruction. Clin Orthop 323:119-121, 1996.

72. Gu YD, Zhang GM, Chen DS, et al: Seventh cervical nerve transfer from the contralateral healthy side for treatment of brachial plexus root avulsion. J Hand Surg [Br] 17:518-521, 1992.

73. Gumina S and Postacchini F: Anterior dislocation of the shoulder in elderly patients. J Bone Joint Surg Br 79:540-543, 1997.

74. Hattori Y, Doi K, and Baliarsing AS: A part of the ulnar nerve as an alternative donor nerve for functioning free muscle transfer: A case report. J Hand Surg [Am] 27:150-153, 2002.

75. Hattori Y, Doi K, Fukushima S, and Kaneko K: The diagnostic value of intraoperative measurement of choline acetyltransferase activity during brachial plexus surgery. J Hand Surg [Br] 25:509-511, 2000.

76. Henry A: An operation for slinging a dropped shoulder. Br J Surg 15:95-98, 1927.

77. Herzmark M: Traumatic paralysis of the serratus anterior relieved by transplantation of the rhomboidei. J Bone Joint Surg Am 33:235-238, 1951.

78. Iceton J and Harris WR: Results of pectoralis major transfer for winged scapula. J Bone Joint Surg Br 69:108-110, 1987.

79. Jerosch J, Filler TJ, and Peuker ET: Which joint position puts the axillary nerve at lowest risk when performing arthroscopic capsular release in patients with adhesive capsulitis of the shoulder? Knee Surg Sports Traumatol Arthrosc 10:126-129, 2002.

80. Jobe C, Kropp WE, and Wood VE: The spinal accessory nerve in a trapezius splitting approach. J Shoulder Elbow Surg 5:206-208, 1996.

81. Johnson JK and Kendall HO: Isolated paralysis of the serratus anterior muscle. J Bone Joint Surg Am 37:567-574, 1955.

82. Kaspi A, Yanai J, and Pick CG: Entrapment of the distal suprascapular nerve. An anatomical study. Int Orthop 12:273-275, 1988.

83. Kawabata H, Shibata T, Matsui Y, and Yasui N: Use of intercostal nerves for neurotization of the musculocutaneous nerve in infants with birth-related brachial plexus palsy. J Neurosurg 94:386-391, 2001.

84. Ketenjian AY: Scapulocostal stabilization for scapular winging in fascioscapulohumeral muscular dystrophy. J Bone Joint Surg Am 60:476-480, 1978.

85. Kline DG: Civilian gunshot wounds to the brachial plexus. J Neurosurg 70:166-174, 1989.

86. Kline DG and Happel LT: A quarter century's experience with intraoperative nerve action potential recording. Can J Neurol Sci 20:3-10, 1992.

87. Kline DG and Hudson AR: Nerve Injuries: Operative Results for Major Nerve Injuries, Entrapments, and Tumors. Philadelphia: WB Saunders, 1995.

88. Kretschmer TAG, Braun V, Rath SA, and Richter HP: Evaluation of iatrogenic lesions in 722 surgically treated cases of peripheral nerve trauma. J Neurosurg 94:905-912, 2001.

89. Lange M: Die Behandlung der irreparablen Trapeziuslaehmung. Langenbecks Arch Klin Chir 270:437-439, 1953.

90. Lange M: Die operative Behandlung der irreparablen Trapeziuslaehmung. TIP Fakult Mecmuasi 22:137-141, 1959.

91. Langenskiold A and Ryoppy S: Treatment of paralysis of the trapezius muscle by the Eden-Lange operation. Acta Orthop Scand 44:383-388, 1973.

92. Leechavengvongs S, Witoonchart K, Uerpairojkit C, et al: Nerve transfer to biceps muscle using a part of the ulnar nerve in brachial plexus injury (upper arm type): A report of 32 cases. J Hand Surg [Am] 23:711-716, 1998.

93. Leffert RD: Brachial Plexus Injuries. New York, Churchill Livingstone, 1985.

94. Leffert RD: Neurological problems. In Rockwood CA and Matsen FA (eds): The Shoulder. Philadelphia: WB Saunders, 1990, pp 765-767.

95. Leffert RD and Perlmutter GS: Thoracic outlet syndrome. Results of 282 transaxillary first rib resections. Clin Orthop 368:66-79, 1999.

96. Lester B, Jeong GK, Weiland AJ, and Wickiewicz TL: Quadrilateral space syndrome: Diagnosis, pathology, and treatment. Am J Orthop 28:718-722, 1999.

97. Linker CS, Helms CA, and Fritz RC: Quadrilateral space syndrome: Findings at MR imaging. Radiology 188:675-676, 1993.

98. Malamut RI, Marques W, England JD, and Sumner AJ: Postsurgical idiopathic brachial neuritis. Muscle Nerve 17:320-325, 1994.

99. Malessy MJA, Hoffman CFE, and Thomeer RTWM: Initial report on the limited value of hypoglossal nerve transfer to treat brachial plexus avulsions. J Neurosurg 91:601-604, 1999.

100. Malessy MJA, van Duinen SG, Feirabend HKP, and Thomeer RT: Correlation between histopathological findings in C-5 and C-6 stumps and motor recovery following nerve grafting for repair of brachial plexus injury. J Neurosurg 91:636-644, 1999.

101. Marin R: Scapula winger's brace: A case series on the management of long thoracic nerve palsy. Arch Phys Med Rehabil 79:1226-1230, 1998.

102. Marmor L: Paralysis of the serratus anterior due to electric shock relieved by transplantation of the pectoralis major muscle. A case report. J Bone Joint Surg Am 45:156-160, 1983.

103. Mastaglia FL: Musculocutaneous neuropathy after strenuous physical activity. Med J Aust 145:153-154, 1986.

104. Matz PG and Barbaro NM: Diagnosis and treatment of iatrogenic spinal accessory nerve injury. Am Surg 62:682-685, 1996.

105. Merrell GA, Barrie KA, Katz DL, and Wolfe SW: Results of nerve transfer techniques for restoration of shoulder and elbow function in the context of a meta-analysis of the English literature. J Hand Surg [Am] 26:303-314, 2001.

106. Millessi H: Brachial plexus injuries: Nerve grafting. Clin Orthop 237:43-56, 1988.

107. Minami M and Ishii S: Satisfactory elbow flexion in complete (preganglionic) brachial plexus injuries: Produced by suture of third and fourth intercostals nerves to musculocutaneous nerve. J Hand Surg [Am] 12:1114-1118, 1987.

108. Misamore GW and Lehman DE: Parsonage-Turner syndrome (acute brachial neuritis). J Bone Joint Surg Am 78:1405-1408, 1996.

109. Moore TP, Fritts HM, Quick DC, and Buss DD: Suprascapular nerve entrapment caused by supraglenoid cyst compression. J Shoulder Elbow Surg 6:455-462, 1997.

110. Nagano A, Ochiai N, Sugioka H, et al: Usefulness of myelography in brachial plexus injuries. J Hand Surg [Br] 14:59-64, 1989.

111. Nagano A, Tsuyama N, Ochiai N, et al: Direct nerve crossing with the intercostals nerve to treat avulsion injuries of the brachial plexus. J Hand Surg [Am] 14:980-985, 1989.

112. Nakamichi K and Tachibana S: Iatrogenic injury of the spinal accessory nerve. Results of repair. J Bone Joint Surg Am 80:1616-1621, 1998.

113. Narakas AO: Traumatic brachial plexus lesions. In Dyck PJ, Thomas PK, Lambert EH, and Bunge R (eds): Peripheral Neuropathy, 2nd ed. Philadelphia: WB Saunders, 1984, pp 1394-1409.

114. Nashold BS Jr and Ostdahl RH: Dorsal root entry zone lesions for pain relief. A clinical and electrophysiological study. Brain Res 496:228-240, 1979.

115. Neviaser RJ, Neviaser TJ, and Neviaser JS: Concurrent rupture of the rotator cuff and anterior dislocation of the shoulder in the older patient. J Bone Joint Surg Am 70:1308-1311, 1988.

116. Novak CB and Mackinnon SE: Surgical treatment of a long thoracic nerve palsy. Ann Thoracic Surg 73:1643-1645, 2002.

117. Nunley JA and Gabel G: Axillary nerve. In Gelberman RH (ed): Operative Nerve Repair and Reconstruction. Philadelphia: JB Lippincott, 1991, pp 437-445.

118. Ober F: Transplantation to improve the function of the shoulder joint and extensor function of the elbow joint. In Lectures on Reconstruction Surgery of the Extremities, vol 2. 1944, pp 274-276.

119. Oberlin C, Beal D, Leechavengvongs S, et al: Nerve transfer to biceps muscle using part of ulnar nerve for C5-C6 avulsion of the brachial plexus: anatomical study and report of four cases. J Hand Surg [Am] 19:232-237, 1994.

120. Osborne AW, Birch RM, Munshi P, and Bonney G: The musculocutaneous nerve. J Bone Joint Surg Br 82:1140-1142, 2000.

121. Parsonage MJ and Turner JW: Neuralgic amyotrophy: The shoulder-girdle syndrome. Lancet 1:532-535, 1943.

122. Parsonage MJ and Turner JW: Neuralgic amyotrophy. Lancet 2:973-978, 1948.

123. Pasila M, Jaroma H, Kiviluoto O, and Sundholm A: Early complications of primary shoulder dislocations. Acta Orthop Scand 49:260-263, 1978.

124. Pearsall AWT, Holovacs TF, and Speer KP: The low anterior five-o'clock portal during arthroscopic shoulder surgery performed in the beach-chair position. Am J Sports Med 27:571-574, 1999.

125. Pellegrino JE, George RA, Biegel J, et al: Hereditary neuralgic amyotrophy: Evidence of genetic homogeneity and mapping to chromosome 17q25. Hum Genet 101:277-283, 1997.

126. Perlmutter GS: Axillary nerve injury. Clin Orthop 368:28-36, 1999.

127. Perlmutter GS and Leffert RD: Results of transfer of the pectoralis major tendon to treat paralysis of the serratus anterior muscle. J Bone Joint Surg Am 81:377-384, 1999.

128. Perlmutter GS, Leffert RD, and Zarins B: Direct injury to the axillary nerve in athletes playing contact sports. Am J Sports Med 25:65-68, 1997.

129. Petrucci FS, Morelli A, and Raimondi PL: Axillary nerve injuries—21 cases treated by nerve graft and neurolysis. J Hand Surg [Am] 7:271-278, 1982.

130. Phillips LH 2nd: Familial long thoracic nerve palsy: A manifestation of brachial plexus neuropathy. Neurology 36:1251-1253, 1986.

131. Post M: Pectoralis major transfer for winging of the scapula. J Shoulder Elbow Surg 4:1-9, 1995.
132. Rapp I: Serratus anterior paralysis treated by transplantation of the pectoralis minor. J Bone Joint Surg Am 36:852-854, 1954.
133. Richards RR, Hudson AR, Bertoia JT, et al: Injury to the brachial plexus during Putti-Platt and Bristow procedures. A report of eight cases. Am J Sports Med 15:374-380, 1987.
134. Rochwerger A, Benaim LJ, Toledano E, et al: Reparations chirurgicales du nerf axillaire. Resultats a cinq ans de recul. Chir Main 19:31-35, 2000.
135. Romeo AA, Rotenberg DD, and Bach BR Jr: Suprascapular neuropathy. J Am Acad Orthop Surg 7:358-367, 1999.
136. Roos D: Transaxillary approach for first rib resection to relieve thoracic outlet syndrome. Ann Surg 163:354-358, 1966.
137. Rubin DI: Neuralgic amyotrophy: Clinical features and diagnostic evaluation. Neurologist 7:350-356, 2001.
138. Ruch DS, Friedman A, and Nunley JA: The restoration of elbow flexion with intercostal nerve transfers. Clin Orthop 314:95-103, 1995.
139. Samardzic M, Grujicic D, Antunovic V, and Joksimovic M: Reinnervation of avulsed brachial plexus using the spinal accessory nerve. Surg Neurol 33:7-11, 1990.
140. Samardzic M, Rasulic L, Grujicic D, and Milicic B: Results of nerve transfers to the musculocutaneous and axillary nerves. Neurosurgery 46:93-101, discussion 101-103, 2000.
141. Samii M, Carvalho GA, Nikkhah G, and Penkert G: Surgical reconstruction of the musculocutaneous nerve in traumatic brachial plexus injuries. J Neurosurg 87:881-886, 1997.
142. Sanders RJ, Monsour JW, Gerber WF, et al: Scalenectomy versus first rib resection for treatment of the thoracic outlet syndrome. Surgery 85:109-121, 1979.
143. Sandow MJ and Ilic J: Suprascapular nerve rotator cuff compression syndrome in volleyball players. J Shoulder Elbow Surg 7:516-521, 1998.
144. Shupeck M and Onofrio BM: An anterior approach for decompression of the suprascapular nerve. J Neurosurg 73:53-56, 1990.
145. Skirving AP, Kozak TK, and Davis SJ: Infraspinatus paralysis due to spinoglenoid notch ganglion. J Bone Joint Surg Br 76:588-591, 1994.
146. Solheim LF and Roaas A: Compression of the suprascapular nerve after fracture of the scapular notch. Acta Orthop Scand 49:338-340, 1978.
147. Songcharoen P, Mahaisavariya B, and Chotigavanich C: Spinal accessory neurotization for restoration of elbow flexion in avulsion injuries of the brachial plexus. J Hand Surg [Am] 21:387-390, 1996.
148. Songcharoen P, Wongtrakul S, Mahaisavariya B, and Spinner RJ: Hemicontralateral C7 transfer to median nerve in the treatment of root avulsion brachial plexus injury. J Hand Surg [Am] 26:1058-1064, 2001.
149. Steindler A: Kinesiology of the Human Body under Normal and Pathological Conditions. Springfield, IL: Charles C Thomas, 1955, pp 476-478, 482-483.
150. Steinmann SP and Moran EA: Axillary nerve injury: Diagnosis and treatment. J Am Acad Orthop Surg 9:328-335, 2001.
151. Steinmann SP and Wood MB: Pectoralis major transfer for serratus anterior paralysis. J Shoulder Elbow Surg (in press).
152. Suarez GA, Giannini C, Bosch EP, et al: Immune brachial plexus neuropathy: Suggestive evidence for an inflammatory immune pathogenesis. Neurology 46:559-561, 1996.
153. Sunderland S: Nerve and Nerve Injuries. Edinburgh, Churchill Livingstone, 1978, pp 843-847.
154. Sungpet A, Suphachatwong C, and Kawinwonggowith V: Restoration of shoulder abduction in brachial plexus injury with phrenic nerve transfer. Aust N Z J Surg 70:783-785, 2000.
155. Sungpet A, Suphachatwong C, and Kawinwonggowit V: One-fascicle median nerve transfer to biceps muscle in C5 and C6 root avulsions of brachial plexus injury. Microsurgery 23:10-13, 2003.
156. Sungpet A, Suphachatwong C, Kawinwonggowit V, and Patradul A: Transfer of a single fascicle from the ulnar nerve to the biceps muscle after avulsions of upper roots of the brachial plexus. J Hand Surg [Br] 25:325-328, 2000.
157. Swain R: Musculocutaneous nerve entrapment: A case report. Clin J Sport Med 5:196-198, 1995.
158. Thomeer RT, Malessy MJ, and Marani E: Nerve root repair [comment]. J Neurosurg 96:138-139, 2002.
159. Tiel RL, Happel LT, and Kline DG: Nerve action potential recording, method and equipment. Neurosurgery 31:103-109, 1996.
160. Travlos J, Goldberg I, and Boome RS: Brachial plexus lesions associated with dislocated shoulders. J Bone Joint Surg Br 72:68-71, 1990.
161. Tubby A: A case illustrating the operative treatment of paralysis of the serratus magnus by muscle grafting. BMJ 2:1159-1160, 1904.
162. Turkof E, Millesi H, and Turkof R: Intraoperative electroneurodiagnostics (transcranial electrical motor evoked potentials) to evaluate the functional status of anterior spinal roots and spinal nerves during brachial plexus surgery. Plast Reconstr Surg 99:1632-1641, 1997.
163. Vandeweyer EGD and de Fontaine S: Traumatic spinal accessory nerve palsy. J Reconstr Microsurg 14:259-261, 1998.
164. Vastamaki M: Pectoralis minor transfer in serratus anterior paralysis. Acta Orthop Scand 55:293-295, 1984.
165. Vastamaki M and Goransson H: Suprascapular nerve entrapment. Clin Orthop 297:135-143, 1993.
166. Velpeau A: Luxations de L'epaule. Arch Gen Med 14(suppl 2):269-305, 1837.
167. Villanueva R: Orthosis to correct shoulder pain and deformity after trapezius palsy. Arch Phys Med Rehabil 58:30-34, 1977.
168. Visser CP, Coene LN, Brand R, and Tavy DL: Nerve lesions in proximal humeral fractures. J Shoulder Elbow Surg 10:421-427, 2001.
169. Vukov B, Ukropina D, Bumbasirevic M, et al: Isolated serratus anterior paralysis: A simple surgical procedure to reestablish scapulo-humeral dynamics. J Orthop Trauma 10:341-347, 1996.
170. Warner JJ and Navarro RA: Serratus anterior dysfunction. Recognition and treatment. Clin Orthop 349:139-148, 1998.
171. Whitman A: Congenital elevation of the scapula and paralysis of the serratus magnus muscle. JAMA 9:1332-1334, 1932.
172. Wiater JM and Bigliani LU: Spinal accessory nerve injury. Clin Orthop 368:5-16, 1999.
173. Wong KL and Williams GR: Complications of thermal capsulorrhaphy of the shoulder. J Bone Joint Surg Am 83(suppl 2):151-155, 2001.
174. Wood MB: Personal communication, 2002.
175. Wood V and Frykman G: Winging of the scapula as a complication of first rib resection: A report of six cases. Clin Orthop 149:160-163, 1980.
176. Xu W-D, Gu Y-D, Xu J-G, and Tan LJ: Full-length phrenic nerve transfer by means of video-assisted thoracic surgery in treating brachial plexus avulsion injury. Plast Reconstr Surg 110:104-111, 2003.
177. Zhao S, Kim D, and Kline DG: Somatosensory evoked potentials induced by stimulating a variable number of nerve fibers in rat. Muscle Nerve 16:1220-1227, 1993.

CHAPTER 18

CALCIFYING TENDINITIS*

Hans K. Uhthoff, M.D.,   Geoffrey F. Dervin, M.D.,   and Joachim F. Loehr, M.D.

• • • •

Calcifying tendinitis of the rotator cuff is a common disorder of unknown etiology in which reactive calcification usually undergoes spontaneous resorption in the course of time with subsequent healing of the tendon. During the deposition of calcium, the patient may be either free of pain or suffer only a mild to moderate degree of discomfort, but the disease becomes acutely painful when the calcium is being resorbed.

HISTORICAL REVIEW

The subacromial-subdeltoid bursa was recognized as a source of painful shoulders by Duplay[44] as early as 1872, and he described the condition as scapulohumeral periarthritis, later also called Duplay's disease.[157,158] Numerous other nomenclature has since been used. A bursal localization of calcific deposits was first assumed by Painter,[123] who was also the first to demonstrate the radiologic appearance of the disease, and by Stieda and colleagues.[12,172] However, surgical exploration soon established that the calcification was primarily in the rotator cuff tendons.[30,198] In his classic textbook on the shoulder, Codman[31] stated definitively: "The deposits do not arise in the bursa itself, but in the tendons beneath it." Wrede[198] gave a masterly description of the disease, including the pathologic changes in the tendon: "The cells resemble more and more chondrocytes, meanwhile the fiber arrangement of the tendon is lost."

The intratendinous localization of calcification has been repeatedly confirmed by later authors.[153,154,158] Nonetheless, such confirmation did not stop the proliferation of newer nomenclature, and terms such as peritendinitis calcarea,[154] periarthropathy,[131] and calcified peritendinitis[43] are well known. In the English literature, calcific or calcified tendinitis is more generally accepted. We, however, prefer *calcifying tendinitis,* a term that to our knowledge was first used by Plenk[135] and later by De Sèze and Welfling ("tendinite calcifiante").[41] This term denotes the evolutionary process that is directed at spontaneous healing, contrary to the other terms, which imply progressive deterioration. Whereas mainly in Europe the term *tendinosis* is most often used,[195] in North America the terms *tendinitis* or *tendonitis* are given preference.

ANATOMY

The anatomy of the shoulder has been dealt with in earlier chapters. A few aspects of the rotator cuff tendons relevant to calcifying tendinitis are discussed briefly in this section. The cuff tendons that blend with the capsule of the glenohumeral joint before insertion into bone consist of the supraspinatus in its most superior portion, the infraspinatus and teres minor posteriorly and posteroinferiorly, and the subscapularis anterior to the supraspinatus. The first three tendons insert into the greater tuberosity, whereas the subscapularis attaches to the lesser tuberosity. At the zone of the tendon where calcification takes place, we were unable to histologically distinguish between the deeper, more collagenous tendon and the joint capsule, a fact already noted by Codman.[31] Cells of the synovial layer were often inconspicuous.

The supraspinatus tendon is the most frequent site of cuff tendinopathy. It is 2 to 3 cm long and traverses the subacromial compartment, which is rigidly limited by the coracoacromial arch above and the humeral head below. Codman[31] pointed out that diseases in the supraspinatus tendon tend to occur in a specific area of the tendon: "about half an inch proximal to the insertion." He called this area the "critical portion," which was later renamed by Moseley and Goldie[112] as the "critical zone." The vascularity of this area has been repeatedly investigated because hypoperfusion is believed to possibly initiate the degenerative changes that subsequently result in calcification or tear.

The rotator cuff tendons are regularly supplied by the suprascapular, anterior circumflex humeral, and posterior circumflex humeral arteries. In addition, contributions are received from the thoracoacromial, suprahumeral, and subscapular arteries in descending order of frequency.[147] The vascularity of the cuff tendons, especially that of the supraspinatus, has been studied in many cadaver shoulders by microangiography simultaneously with histology. Moseley and Goldie[112] found that the supraspinatus was well supplied by a network of vessels coming from both the muscular and the osseous ends of the tendon that

---

*The first edition of this chapter was written with Dr. Kiriti Sarkar, who unfortunately is now deceased.

anastomosed in the area of the "critical zone." They stated that there is "no evidence that the critical zone is much less vascularized than any other part of the tendinous cuff." On the other hand, microangiographic studies by Rothman and Parke[148] showed that the "critical zone" was markedly "undervascularized," and their histologic examinations corroborated this view. Although the supraspinatus tendon was most frequently involved, the infraspinatus and subscapularis tendons showed zones of hypovascularity as well. Brooks and associates[21] performed a quantitative histologic study of the cuff and concluded that the supraspinatus and infraspinatus are equally hypovascular in their distal 15 mm and that the diameter of vessels decreases toward the bony insertion.

Rathbun and Macnab[136] documented in their cadaver study a zone of avascularity in the supraspinatus tendon near its bony insertion. This avascularity was dependent on the position of the arm. They showed that when Micropaque (barium sulfate) was injected into the vessels with the arm of the cadaver in the position of adduction, the "critical zone" did not fill. The nonfilling area sometimes extended up to the point of insertion. If the vessels of the contralateral shoulder of the same cadaver were injected after passive abduction, they filled completely throughout the tendon. Therefore, the authors postulated that the zone of avascularity was a "wring-out" effect resulting from pressure of the head of the humerus on the tendon. In a more recent study, Tillmann[176] documented that the zone of insertion of the supraspinatus is avascular because of pressure/compression.

Our histologic findings have been similar to those of previous authors.[89] There is hardly an area in the supraspinatus tendon that is conspicuously devoid of vascular channels. However, we have observed that vascular channels, especially the larger ones, are abundant in the loose connective tissue underneath the bursa but are relatively scarce in the dense collagenous portion close to the joint. Interestingly, this pattern of vascularity is already evident in the supraspinatus tendon of the fetus (Fig. 18–1), even before the fascicular arrangement of the tendon fibers has occurred.

Our histologic studies of cadaver tendons were supplemented by microangiographic studies that consistently showed an area of underfilling at the articular aspect of the tendon near its insertion, regardless of the position of the arm.[89]

It is obvious, then, that the question of reduced or lack of vascular perfusion in certain areas of the cuff tendons is not entirely settled. Maneuvering the cadaveric arm to obtain optimal results with microangiography is not easy. Furthermore, it is doubtful that microangiography can reveal the entire vasculature up to capillary levels. However, it seems safe to assume that an anatomic as well as transient hypoperfusion exists in cuff tendons, particularly in the deeper portion of the supraspinatus.

INCIDENCE

Reports on the overall incidence of tendon calcification vary tremendously. The variation depends not only on the clinical material used but also on the radiographic

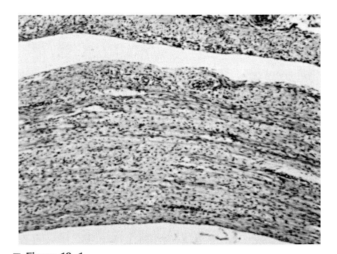

■ Figure 18–1

The supraspinatus tendon close to the bony insertion in a 20-week-old human fetus. Note the rather rich vascular supply in the part of the tendon close to the bursa. On the other hand, vessels are scarce in the articular part. (Goldner; original magnification, ×100).

technique. Bosworth examined both shoulders of 6061 office workers and found an incidence of calcification of 2.7%.[16,17] Welfling and colleagues[191] radiographed 200 shoulders of persons without any complaints and found calcifications in 15 (7.5%). Rüttimann[152] radiographed 100 individuals without symptoms and found a 20% incidence of calcification.

The incidence of calcification in 925 painful shoulders reported by Welfling and collaborators[191] was 6.8%. When broken down by age groups, patients between 31 and 40 years had a 19.5% incidence of calcification. Evidently, the peak at this age did not correspond with the peak seen in patients with rotator cuff tears. They therefore concluded that the diseases represent different entities. Friedman radiographed the shoulders of 228 patients with a painful rotator cuff and found calcific deposits in 75.[52] Fifty-four of the 75 individuals with calcification were between 30 and 49 years of age. Bosworth estimated that 35% to 45% of patients with calcareous deposits will eventually become symptomatic.[16,17]

Plenk[135] found that 82% of the calcifications were located in the supraspinatus tendon. Bosworth[16,17] found 90% in the supraspinatus and infraspinatus. DePalma and Kruper[40] reported an incidence of 74% when assessing the supraspinatus alone, whereas the incidence of simultaneous calcific deposits in the supraspinatus and other short rotators was 90%. In Bosworth's series,[16,17] calcifications in the supraspinatus occurred in 51%, in the infraspinatus in 44.5%, in the teres minor in 23.3%, and in the subscapularis in 3%. Obviously, deposits were sometimes seen in more than one tendon.

In general, authors agree that women are affected more often than men. Bosworth[16,17] reported an incidence of 76.7% in women; DePalma and Kruper[40] reported an incidence of 60.3%; Welfling and collaborators[191] reported an incidence of 62%; Lippmann[87] as well as Hartig and Huth[68] reported 64%; and in our series of 127 patients, the incidence was 57%. A higher incidence in men (56%) was reported by Friedman.[52] An even higher incidence was seen by Hsu and coworkers.[73] Of 82 patients, 61 men suffered from calcifying tendinitis (74%).

The age distribution varies slightly among authors. Welfling and collaborators[191] reported the highest incidence in persons between 31 and 40 years of age, whereas DePalma and Kruper[40] found calcifying tendinitis in 36% of patients in the 40- to 50-year-old group. In our series, 53 patients (42%) were in the 40- to 49-year-old group. Welfling and coworkers[191] state that in their group of 925 individuals, no calcification was seen in patients older than 71 years, and McLaughlin[101] reported that no calcification was detected in about 1000 older cadavers in an anatomy laboratory. It seems that men peak slightly later than women do. Lippmann[87] had similar results: the average age of women was 47 years and that of men was 51 years. Hsu and associates[73] reported that 56 of 82 patients were older than 60 years. They concluded that the sex and age of patients with calcifying tendinitis are different in Asians. Nutton and Stothard[118] reported the presence of calcifying tendinitis in a 3-year-old child.

Occupation seems to play a role in calcifying tendinitis. In DePalma and Kruper's group,[40] 41% were housewives and 27% were professionals, executives, and salespersons. In our series, 43% were housewives, and 44% were persons who had a clerical job.

The right shoulder is usually affected more often than the left. This difference amounted to 64% in Hartig and Huth's study,[68] 57% in DePalma and Kruper's series,[40] and 51% in our series. Bilateral involvement was found in 24.3% by Welfling and coworkers.[191] In DePalma and Kruper's series,[40] the difference was 13%. Of our patients, 17% came back with calcification of the opposite shoulder; this incidence increases with increasing length of the follow-up period.

The incidence of simultaneous calcifications around the hip in 23 patients radiographed in Welfling and associates' series[191] amounted to 62.5%, whereas the incidence was only 4% in control subjects.

All authors agree that calcifying tendinitis is not related to any generalized disease process, and Welfling and colleagues[191] rightly conclude that tendon calcification constitutes a disease entity on its own. Neither McLaughlin[101] nor Rüttimann[152] could find a correlation between tendon tear and calcific tendinitis. Partial tears occur mostly on the bursal side when the deposit ruptures into the bursa. Ruptures into the glenohumeral joint are said to occur extremely seldom.[63] Patte and Goutallier[125] observed two cases. Hsu and collaborators[73] found arthrographic evidence of rotator cuff tearing in 28% (23 patients). We did not record a single instance of a complete cuff tear. Morimoto and colleagues[107] observed calcification of the coracoacromial ligament in one patient.

Most authors agree that no relationship exists between calcifying tendinitis and trauma.

CLASSIFICATION

Several classifications of calcifying tendinitis have been proposed. Bosworth[16,17] divided the deposits into three categories according to their size and corresponding clinical significance: (1) small (up to 0.5 mm), (2) medium (0.5 to 1.5 mm), and (3) large (>1.5 mm). He believed that small deposits have little clinical significance, whereas deposits larger than 1.5 mm are likely to give rise to symptoms. DePalma[39] classified calcifying tendinitis into acute, subacute, and chronic, according to the degree and duration of symptoms. It has been suggested that some patients with the chronic form who have acute exacerbations should be classified in a separate category because they have a better prognosis. Patte and Goutallier[125] classified the deposits into localized and diffuse forms. Radiologically, the localized form is round or oval, dense, and homogeneous and lies close to the bursal wall; it tends to heal spontaneously. In contrast, the diffuse form is situated much deeper in the tendon, close to the bony insertion, and radiologically has a heterogeneous appearance. The diffuse form produces more symptoms and takes longer to disappear.

We have not used these classifications in the clinical management of our patients with calcifying tendinitis because they do not take into account the cyclic nature of the disease. It is, however, important to remember that radiologically visible calcifications in the cuff tendons may occur with diseases other than calcifying tendinitis. Dystrophic calcifications can be seen around the torn edges of the tendon after a complete tear.[196] Massive calcification, as seen in the Milwaukee shoulder or in cuff arthropathy with a complete tear, is associated with severe osteoarthritic changes in the glenohumeral joint and, to some extent, the acromioclavicular joint.[2,65,99,116] Dystrophic calcification associated with a tear has a poor prognosis and is indicative of progressive degenerative changes; it is not comparable with the spontaneous healing of the tendon in calcifying tendinitis. Moreover, dystrophic calcifications, contrary to reactive calcifications, do not occur in the midtendon but arise much closer to the bony insertion.

PATHOLOGY

Four key histologic findings are found in calcifying tendinitis:

1. Fibrocartilaginous metaplasia during the precalcific stage
2. Deposition of calcium crystals in the fibrocartilaginous matrix during the formative phase of the calcific stage
3. Cell-mediated resorption of the calcific deposit during the resorptive phase of the calcific stage
4. Tendon restitution during the postcalcific stage

Because the etiology of calcifying tendinitis is still a matter of speculation, we believe that a careful study of its pathology is necessary before any logical assumptions can be made about the pathogenetic mechanism.

Under the light microscope, the calcific deposits appear multifocal, separated by fibrocollagenous tissue or fibrocartilage (Fig. 18-2). The latter consists of easily distinguishable chondrocytes, described by Archer and collaborators[7] as chondrocyte-like cells, within a matrix showing varying degrees of metachromasia (Fig. 18-3).

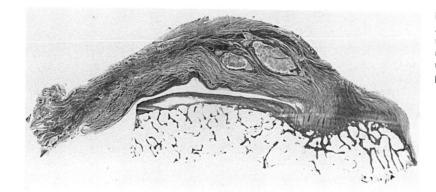

■ **Figure 18–2**
Autopsy specimen of a 45-year-old woman showing the typical location of multiple calcific deposits in the more superficial (bursal) part of the supraspinatus tendon. The bursal reaction is minimal. The deeper part is spared (azan; original magnification, ×3).

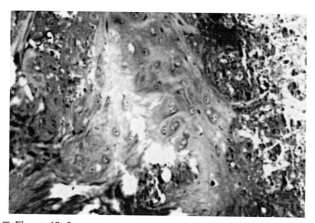

■ **Figure 18–3**
A fibrocartilaginous area between calcific deposits (C) shows typical chondrocytes surrounded by a metachromatic matrix. The appearance characterizes the formative phase. The deposits are partly in clumps and partly granular (toluidine blue, ×100).

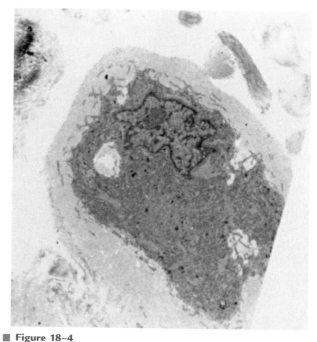

■ **Figure 18–4**
The ultrastructure of a chondrocyte surrounded by a pericellular matrix shows a nucleus with an indented margin and the cytoplasm containing a fairly extensive rough endoplasmic reticulum and vacuoles (uranyl acetate and lead citrate, ×6500).

The appearance of chondrocytes within the tendon substance near calcifications was noted by Wrede[198] in 1912, by Harbin[66] in 1929, by Sandström and Wahlgren[154] in 1937, by Howorth[72] in 1945, and by Pedersen and Key in 1951.[127] The ultrastructure of these chondrocytes shows that the cells often have a fair amount of cytoplasm containing a well-developed endoplasmic reticulum, a moderate number of mitochondria, one or more vacuoles, and numerous cell processes (Fig. 18–4). The margin of the nucleus is indented. The cells are surrounded by a distinct band of pericellular matrix with or without an intervening lacuna.

The fibrocartilaginous areas are generally avascular. The intercellular substance is metachromatic, and glycosaminoglycan-rich pericellular halos are prominent around rounded cells.[7] Surprisingly, monoclonal collagen staining by Archer and colleagues[7] did not reveal the presence of type II collagen. In our studies using type II collagen monoclonal antibodies, we occasionally documented its presence. The difference in outcome may be due to differences in tissue preparation, source of monoclonal antibodies, and staining technique. In contrast to the fibrocartilage, the fibrocollagenous tissue abutting against the calcification may appear compressed, with formation of a pseudocapsule around the deposits. The neighboring tendon fibers may show thinning and fibrillation.

The calcium deposits may be loosely granular or appear in clumps. With the transmission electron microscope, aggregates of rounded structures containing crystalline material are found in a matrix of amorphous debris or irregularly fragmented collagen fibers (Fig. 18–5). When examined by scanning electron microscopy, calcific deposits appear as rocky bulks engulfed in mortar.[51] The irregularly rectangular crystals are sometimes found within membrane-bound structures resembling matrix vesicles, also called calcifying globules.[4,6,14] Infrequently, crystalline densities seem to be embedded between collagen fibers.

Examination by chemical methods, x-ray diffraction, and infrared spectrometry, as well as thermogravimetry, has shown that the crystals are carbonated apatite.[50] However, high-resolution transmission electron microscopy revealed that the crystals are much larger than the classic apatite crystals and have a different configuration.[185]

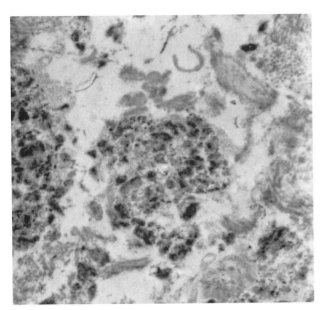

■ Figure 18–5
Rounded structures resembling matrix vesicles contain electron-dense crystalline structures (uranyl acetate and lead citrate, ×23,200).

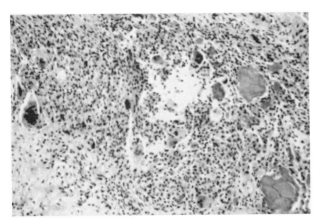

■ Figure 18–6
A "calcium granuloma" contains scattered small deposits of calcium, macrophages, and multinucleated giant cells (hematoxylin and eosin, ×100).

In 1915, Moschkowitz[108] identified deposits within the tendon but stated that they failed to evoke a cellular reaction. A few years before, however, Wrede[198] had already written that although inflammation or vessels were notably absent around some deposits, "young mesenchymal cells, epithelioid cells, leukocytes, a certain number of lymphocytes and occasionally giant cells" were present at other sites of calcification. The presence of these cells is compatible with resorptive activity at that stage. Indeed, the marked cellular reaction around calcific deposits—the "calcium granuloma"—was considered by Pedersen and Key[127] to be the characteristic lesion of calcifying tendinitis. The granulomatous appearance is imparted by the presence of multinucleated giant cells (Fig. 18–6) and macrophages. Archer and coauthors[7] interpreted the presence of the latter two cell types as a resorption phenomenon. The cellular reaction is often

accompanied by capillary or thin-walled vascular channels around the deposits (Fig. 18–7). The margin and the interior of the deposits are infiltrated by macrophages and a few leukocytes, including polymorphonuclear cells and fibroblasts. Phagocytosed substance within macrophages or multinucleated giant cells can easily be discerned (Fig. 18–8). The ultrastructure of these cells shows electron-dense crystalline particles in cytoplasmic vacuoles (Fig. 18–9), but the crystals are slightly different in appearance from those in the extracellular deposits.[155] Some of the intracellular accumulations have a rounded aspect and are known as microspheroliths or psammomas (Fig. 18–10).

Small areas representing the process of repair can be found in the general vicinity of calcification, and these areas show considerable variation in appearance. Granulation tissue with young fibroblasts and newly formed capillaries contrasts with well-formed scars with vascular channels and maturing fibroblasts that are in the process of alignment along the long axis of the tendon fibers (Figs. 18–11 and 18–12). Using monoclonal antibodies against collagen type III, we were able to confirm collagen neoformation, most pronounced around vascular channels.

Calcific deposits in the wall of the subacromial bursa also tend to be multifocal (Fig. 18–13). A cellular reaction is seldom seen around the bursal deposits.[156]

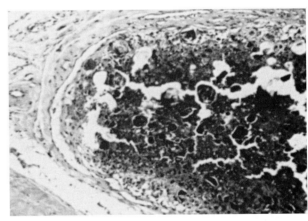

■ Figure 18–7
Capillary channels surround a calcific deposit (toluidine blue, ×100).

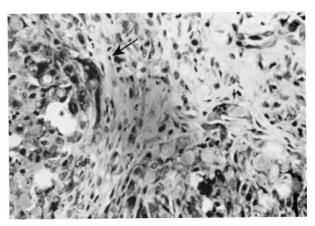

■ Figure 18–8
Macrophages and multinucleated giant cells contain a phagocytosed substance *(arrow)* (toluidine blue, ×250).

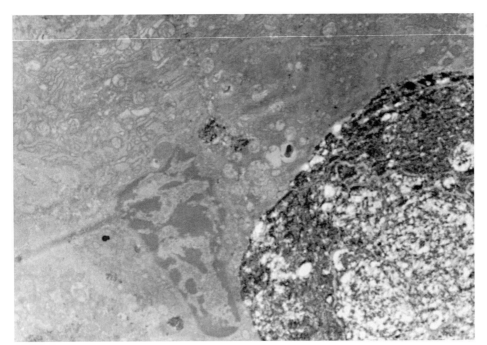

■ **Figure 18–9**
The ultrastructure of a macrophage shows apparently phagocytosed electron-dense material in the cytoplasm (uranyl acetate and lead citrate, ×11,500).

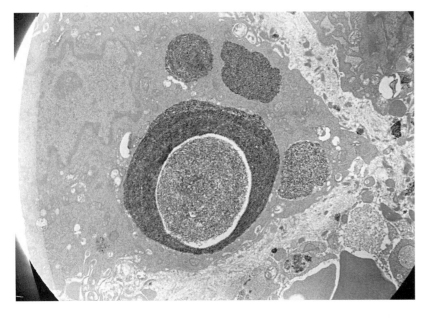

■ **Figure 18–10**
This electron microphotograph shows a psammoma inside a macrophage beside three smaller accumulations of electron-dense material. The multilayered structure of the psammoma is quite evident (uranyl acetate and lead citrate, ×14,500).

PATHOGENESIS

Codman[31] proposed that degeneration of the tendon fibers precedes calcification. The fibers become necrotic, and dystrophic calcification follows. Degeneration of fibers of the rotator cuff tendons because of a "wear-and-tear" effect and aging has been postulated or demonstrated by many investigators. Obviously, these two causes are interrelated. It is reasonable to assume that the rotator cuff tendons suffer a "wear-and-tear" effect because the glenohumeral joint is not only a universal but probably also the most used joint in the body. Studies performed in Sweden seem to indicate that stress and strain induced by work involving the arm can lead to supraspinatus tendinitis.[70] However, there are no indications that calcifying

tendinitis would develop in time in even a worker engaged in heavy manual labor, and Olsson[120] has shown that the cuff tendons from the dominant arm show no more evidence of degeneration than those from the contralateral arm.

Aging is considered to be the foremost cause of degeneration in cuff tendons. Brewer[19] believes that with aging comes a general diminution in the vascularity of the supraspinatus tendon along with fiber changes. The well-delineated bundles of collagen or the fascicles that constitute the distinctive architecture of the tendon show the most conspicuous age-related changes, beginning at the end of the fourth or fifth decade.[120] The majority of the fascicles undergo thinning and fibrillation, which is defined as a degenerative process characterized by

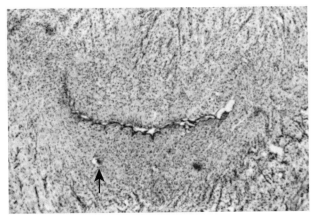

■ Figure 18–11
Granulation tissue is almost completely replacing the area that was occupied previously by calcific deposits. A speck of calcium is still visible *(arrow)*. The central portion shows amorphous precipitate (hematoxylin and eosin, ×40).

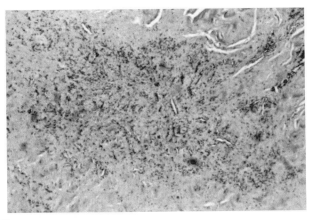

■ Figure 18–12
A scar composed of collagenous tissue represents the area of healing in the tendon (hematoxylin and eosin, ×40).

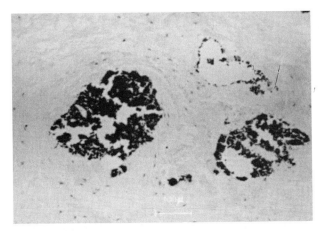

■ Figure 18–13
Multiple foci of calcific deposits in the wall of the subacromial bursa do not show any cellular reactions (hematoxylin and eosin, ×40).

splitting and fraying of the fibers. The thinned fascicles show irregular cellular arrangement, and the fragmented fibers are often hypocellular. The intervening connective tissue that carries the blood vessels between the fascicles may appear to be increased when contrasted with the volume of the fascicles. In our experience, it is difficult to ascertain the numerical decrease in vessels, but more vessels with thicker walls are consistently found in the cuff tendons of aged individuals.

Because calcifying tendinitis seldom affects persons before the fourth decade, it can be argued that primary degeneration of tendon fibers is responsible for the subsequent deposition of calcium. Following Codman's suggestion of the degenerative nature of calcifying tendinitis,[31] subsequent investigators have found ample histologic evidence for the sequence of degeneration, necrosis, and calcification.[56,58,103] According to McLaughlin,[101] the earliest lesion is focal hyalinization of fibers that eventually become fibrillated and get detached from the surrounding normal tendon. Continued motion of the tendon grinds the detached, curled-up fibers into a "wen-like substance" consisting of necrotic debris on which calcification occurs. This sequence of events was demonstrated experimentally by Macnab[96] in the course of investigations on the effects of interruption of the vascular supply to the Achilles tendon of rabbits. Pedersen and Key,[127] who are also in favor of the concept of degenerative calcification, state that "calcium is deposited in the necrotic collagenic tissue."

Mohr and Bilger[105] believe that the process of calcification starts with necrosis of tenocytes along with a concomitant intracellular accumulation of calcium, often in the form of microspheroliths, also known as psammomas. Contrary to Mohr and Bilger,[105] we never observed psammomas during the early phases of formation, but we did observe them regularly during the phase of resorption (see Fig. 18–10). Our electron microscopic examinations leave no doubt that the electron-dense material is situated intracellularly and not extracellularly, as seen in the pathologic conditions cited by these authors. Moreover, it is unfortunate that these authors do not distinguish between calcifications at the insertion and intratendinous calcifications (i.e., the site of calcifying tendinitis). The biochemical aspects of soft tissue calcifications have been published by Seifert.[161]

Authors' Opinion

The aforementioned investigators failed to distinguish between fundamentally different histologic aspects of calcifying tendinitis and dystrophic calcification. Lippmann[87] observed that "the early deposit, located in a totally avascular bed, provokes no tissue reaction." He contrasted this statement with "the mechanism of absorption that primarily is dependent upon vascularity and inflammation." Moreover, Jones[78] deplored the fact that "proper assessment of the natural repair process in acute cases has not been made."

We would like to add that neither the self-healing nature of calcifying tendinitis nor the various aspects of its pathology are characteristic of a degenerative disease.

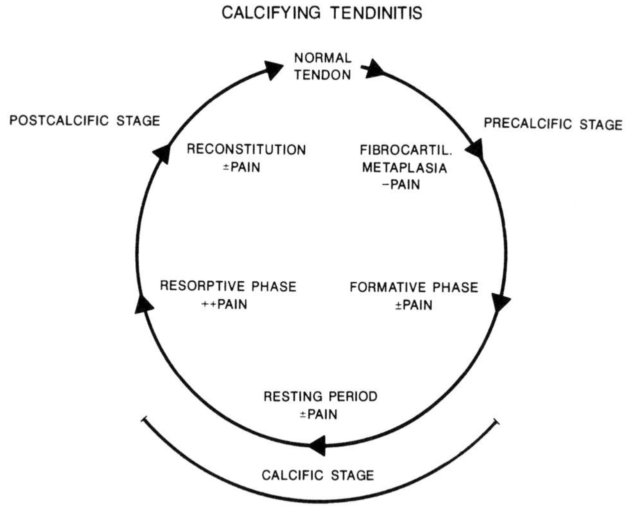

CALCIFYING TENDINITIS

■ Figure 18–14
Evolution of calcifying tendinitis.

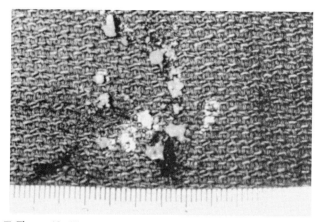

■ Figure 18–15
The calcium removed from a patient during the formative phase has a granular aspect.

We believe that the process of calcification is actively mediated by cells in a viable environment.[130,138,155,178,180-183,185] Moreover, there cannot be the slightest doubt that formation of the calcium deposit must precede its resorption.

Calcifying tendinitis has three distinct stages:

1. Precalcific (metaplasia of matrix)
2. Calcific (calcification of matrix and resorption of calcific deposits)
3. Postcalcific (reconstitution of matrix) (Fig. 18–14)

Precalcific Stage

In the precalcific stage, the site of predilection for calcification undergoes fibrocartilaginous transformation. This metaplasia of tenocytes into chondrocytes is accompanied by metachromasia, which is indicative of the elaboration of proteoglycan.

Calcific Stage

This stage is subdivided into the formative phase and the resorptive phase.

Formative Phase

In the ensuing calcific stage, calcium crystals are deposited primarily in matrix vesicles that coalesce to form large areas of deposits.[155] For convenience of description, we have used the term "formative phase" to describe the initial period of the calcific stage.[185] If the patient undergoes surgery at this stage, the deposit appears chalk-like (Fig. 18–15) and has to be scooped out for removal. At this time, the area of fibrocartilage with the foci of calcification is generally devoid of vascular channels. Septa of fibrocartilage separating the foci of calcification stain positively metachromatic. They do not consistently stain positively for collagen type II, which is known to be a component of fibrocartilage. These fibrocartilaginous septa are gradually eroded by the enlarging deposits.

Resorptive Phase

After a variable period of inactivity of the disease process ("resting period" in the schema), the spontaneous resorption of calcium is heralded by the appearance of thin-walled vascular channels at the periphery of the deposit. Soon thereafter, the deposit is surrounded by macrophages and multinucleated giant cells that phagocytose and remove the calcium. This step is the last one in the calcific stage, which we have called the "resorptive phase." If an operation is performed at this stage, the calcific deposit is a thick, white, cream-like or toothpaste-like material (Fig. 18–16).

Postcalcific Stage

Simultaneously with the resorption of calcium, granulation tissue containing young fibroblasts and new vascular channels begins to remodel the space occupied by calcium. These sites stain positively for collagen type III. As the scar matures, fibroblasts and collagen eventually align along the longitudinal axis of the tendon. During this remodeling process, type III collagen is replaced by type I. We have called this stage of tendon reconstitution "postcalcific." Figure 18–17 outlines the correlation

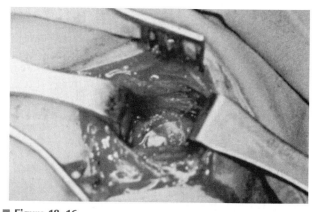

■ Figure 18–16
After opening a deposit that was in the resorptive phase, a cream-like fluid spurted out under pressure; it can be seen in the wound margins.

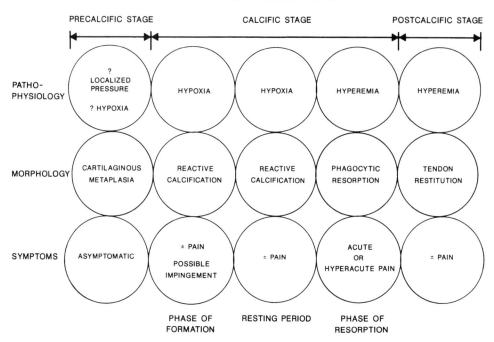

THE PATHOPHYSIOLOGY, MORPHOLOGICAL ALTERATIONS AND SYMPTOMS DURING VARIOUS PHASES

■ **Figure 18–17**
The pathophysiology, morphologic alterations, and symptoms are shown during various stages of calcifying tendinitis. In the course of evolution of the disease, the stages are likely to overlap each other.

between pathogenesis, morphologic findings, and symptoms during the various stages of calcifying tendinitis.

Although the pathogenesis of the calcifying process can be reasonably constructed from morphologic studies, it is difficult to determine what triggers the fibrocartilaginous transformation in the first place. Codman[31] suggested tissue hypoxia as the primary etiologic factor. This hypothesis still remains attractive because of the peculiarity of the tendon vasculature and shoulder mechanics. We have found an increased frequency of HLA-A1 in patients with calcifying tendinitis, thus indicating that these individuals may be genetically susceptible to the condition.[164] Factors that trigger the onset of resorption also remain unknown. Our phase of formation seems to be identical to Lippmann's early phase of increment,[87] whereas his late phase of increment is analogous to our phase of resorption.

CLINICAL FINDINGS

Clinical keys identifying calcifying tendinitis are as follows:

1. Pain, most pronounced during the resorptive phase
2. Reduced range of motion, mostly secondary to pain
3. Radiologic evidence of intratendinous calcification
4. Positive sonographic findings

Pain is the cardinal symptom of calcifying tendinitis.[15,79,84,170,174]

We would like to strongly emphasize that an understanding of the pathogenetic mechanism of calcifying tendinitis is essential for clinical evaluation and management of this disease entity. There is a tendency to assume that calcifying tendinitis, as most diseases, begins with

acute symptoms and progresses to a chronic state. Others maintain that we are dealing with two separate disease entities. Our understanding of the disease is entirely to the contrary. We believe that the initial stage of formation of the deposit, which lacks a vascular and cellular reaction, is likely to cause few symptoms or just nondebilitating discomfort because the intratendinous tissue tension is hardly raised by the deposit. Thus, the disease generally begins with chronic symptoms, if any at all. Larger deposits can lead to impingement against the coracoacromial ligament (see Fig. 18-2), a fact already observed by Baer[9] in 1907 during surgery. During the later phase of calcium resorption, on the other hand, exudation of cells along with vascular proliferation must enlarge the tissue space considerably and thus produce raised intratendinous pressure, which causes pain. The pain is probably further exacerbated as the increased volume of the tendon impinges on the unyielding structures that limit the subacromial compartment.

In fact, the subclinical nature of the formative phase of calcification has been recognized by many authors. Codman[31] stated that "the usual history is not acute pain at the beginning." Wilson[193] noted that many patients might know about a calcium deposit in one or both shoulders for months or years before an acute attack. Lippmann[87] stressed the well-known fact that early deposits are usually symptomless and that acute pain signals "the onset of 'break-up' of the deposit." Pinals and Short[134] wrote: "... calcium deposition precedes rather than follows the development of an acute attack of calcific periarthritis and the attack is accompanied by disintegration and gradual disappearance of the deposit." Similarly, Gschwend and associates[63] believed that the calcification is often symptomless at the beginning, whereas its disappearance is associated with pain.

It is therefore evident that we are not dealing with two unrelated disease processes, an acute and a chronic calcific tendinitis, but a disease cycle. Lippmann[87] described a phase of increment followed by a short, self-limited phase of disruption. Each phase has its characteristics. During the phase of increment, the symptoms were described as being mild, the consistency of the deposit was said to be hard and chalky, and no inflammation was noted. During the phase of disruption, the pain was severe, the consistency allowed tapping, and radiographs showed a fluffy deposit. Lippmann[87] concluded that failure to identify the phase of the cycle resulted in crediting "useless therapeutic measures with magical healing power and, on the other hand, led to the performance of needless surgical procedures."

Clinical findings depend on the acuteness of the symptoms. Simon[165] believed that a definite relationship exists between the intensity of symptoms and their duration. The symptoms can last up to 2 weeks when they are acute, 3 to 8 weeks when they are subacute, and 3 months or more when they are chronic. Pendergrass and Hodes[128] observed that the acute symptoms subside in 1 to 2 weeks, even in the absence of treatment. It is also known that symptoms may change rapidly.

During the subacute and chronic phases, patients complain of pain or tenderness. They are usually able to localize the point of maximal tenderness. Radiation of pain is the rule, the insertion of the deltoid being the most frequent site of pain referral. Referred pain was seen in 42.5% of the patients of De Sèze and Welfling.[41] Radiation of pain occurred more often in the arm than toward the neck. Wrede[198] and many authors after him found that clinical symptoms are often absent. Usually, range of motion is decreased by pain, patients cannot sleep on the affected shoulder, and they often complain of an increase in pain during the night. A painful arc of motion between 70 and 110 degrees has been described by Kessel and Watson,[82] but these authors were unable to classify these patients into any of their three types of the painful arc syndrome (posterior, anterior, and superior). In 97 patients with this syndrome, they found 12 cases of calcification. Patients often have the sensation of catching when going through the arc of motion. This sensation is most probably due to localized impingement, which in turn leads to loss of scapulohumeral rhythm. Impingement between the calcium deposit and the coracoacromial ligament during abduction had already been noted by Baer[9] and by Wrede.[198] A further sign of the long-standing symptoms of calcifying tendinitis is atrophy of both spinatus muscles. Although some authors have reported the presence of swelling and redness on clinical examination, we were never able to find these signs.

During the acute phase, the pain is so intense and excruciating that patients refuse to move their shoulders. De Sèze and Welfling[41] believe that this severe pain leads to locking. Any attempt at mobilization of the glenohumeral joint will be resisted by the patient. Patients hold their arms close to their bodies in internal rotation.

Although we have described involvement of the bursa in painful shoulder syndromes,[155] its involvement in various phases of calcifying tendinitis has not been documented in detail.

During the formative phase, the subacromial bursa is not the site of widespread reaction. Only in the presence of impingement[115] is a zone of hyperemia observed around the calcium deposit (Fig. 18-18). Carnett[24] noted that bursitis is a minor and infrequent feature.

During the resorptive phase, bursitis is said to be a source of pain. However, during surgery, the bursal reaction is minimal and often limited to localized hyperemia (Fig. 18-19). This reaction is not usually severe enough to cause bursal thickening; in fact, the calcific deposit often shines through the deep or visceral layer of the bursa. Litchman and colleagues[88] also noted the absence of bursal inflammation. Many authors state that rupture of the deposit into the bursa causes a crystalline type of bursitis and, consequently, pain. We would like to emphasize again that only during the resorptive phase does the consistency of the deposit allow rupture into the bursa. DePalma and Kruper[40] noted that deposits rupturing into the bursa are encountered in acute cases. De Sèze and Welfling[41] monitored 12 patients with rupture of the deposit into the bursa. Only eight patients had symptoms. In our histologic specimens we could observe synovial cells resorbing calcium. No inflammatory reaction, in

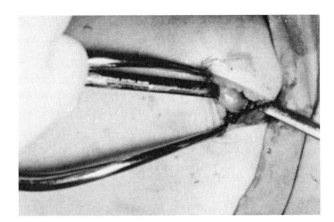

■ **Figure 18–18**
Intraoperative photograph after opening the bursal cavity. The whitish area of a deposit during the formation phase is surrounded by slight bursal hyperemia.

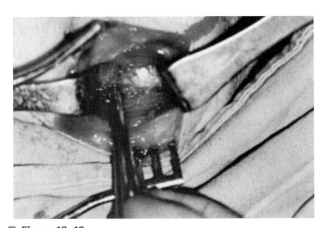

■ **Figure 18–19**
Intraoperative photograph of a patient during the resorptive phase. The whitish deposit shines through the bursal wall, which is locally hyperemic.

particular, no leukocytes or lymphocytes, accompanied this resorptive process. It therefore seems probable that the edema and proliferation of cells and vessels cause an increase in intratendinous pressure that evokes pain rather than a localized bursal reaction. This impression seems to be confirmed by intraoperative observations during the acute phase. Key[83] reported: "In some hyperacute cases of short duration, the calcific material is thin or milk-like in consistency and may be under such pressure that when the surface of the tendon is incised, the contents of the deposit may spurt out into the air." An identical observation has been made by Friedman.[52]

In 41 operated patients, we correlated symptoms with radiologic findings and with consistency of the deposit.[180] Of 31 patients with chronic symptoms, 24 had radiographic signs compatible with formation and 29 had chalk-like granular calcium deposits. Of 10 patients with acute symptoms, 8 had radiographic signs typical of resorption and 9 exhibited a toothpaste-like consistency of their deposit.

Should calcifying tendinitis be considered a systemic disease as Pinals and Short[134] have speculated? There is no good evidence despite the high incidence of calcifications occurring in other sites. With the exception of an increased incidence of HLA-A1 in patients with calcifying tendinitis, all other laboratory test results are normal.[164] An associated illness was never reported,[88] and Gschwend and associates[63] were unable to prove an association with diabetes or gout, although this association had been repeatedly suspected by various authors but never documented. A relationship to occupation must be suspected, given the high incidence of clerical workers observed by us and other investigators. Litchman and colleagues,[88] on the other hand, stated that no relationship to occupation could be found. A possible correlation between stiff and painful shoulders and calcifying tendinitis has been suspected for approximately 90 years.[20,29] We could observe only a single case of this syndrome. Lundberg[95] reported 24 patients with calcification among 232 with a frozen shoulder. This finding does not point toward a strong correlation between calcifying tendinitis and frozen shoulder.

RADIOLOGY

The calcium deposits in calcifying tendinitis are localized inside a tendon. They are not usually in continuity with bone, nor do they extend into bone. DePalma and Kruper[40] observed extensions into bone in 8 of 136 patients. The only other occurrence has been reported by Toriyama and associates.[177] Calcium deposits close to bone must be clearly distinguished from the stippled calcifications seen at the tendon insertion in patients with dystrophic calcification.

In all cases of suspected calcification of tendons, a radiograph must be taken. Radiologic assessment is also important during follow-up examinations because it permits assessment of changes in density and extent.

Initial radiographs should include anteroposterior films in neutral rotation as well as internal and external rotation. Deposits in the supraspinatus are readily visible on films in neutral rotation, whereas deposits in the infraspinatus and teres minor are best seen in internal rotation. Calcifications in the subscapularis occur only in rare cases, and a radiograph in external rotation will show them well. Axillary views are rarely indicated. Scapular views, however, will help determine whether a calcification is causing impingement. Ruptures into the bursa will appear as a crescent-like shadow overlying the actual calcification and extending over the greater tuberosity, with the extent of the bursa outlined well (Fig. 18-20).

The presence of calcium deposits, particularly in the acute or resorptive phase, is often barely visible on radiographs (Fig. 18-21). In these cases, xerography (see Fig. 18-20) or sonography is helpful.[33,49,68] We suspect that computerized radiography may give similar results. Loew and colleagues[94] reported their experience with magnetic resonance imaging (MRI) in 75 patients. Calcifications appear on T1-weighted images as areas of decreased signal intensity (Fig. 18-22), whereas T2-weighted images frequently show a perifocal band of increased signal intensity compatible with edema.

Bursograms have not been shown to be of great value in our experience.[179] When arthrograms are performed, they show a distinct delineation between the deposit and the joint cavity. We believe that they are indicated only in exceptional cases, especially when a tear is suspected.

Not only do radiographs allow confirmation of the absence or presence of calcium deposits, they also permit proper localization. Furthermore, the extent, delineation, and density can be well appreciated.[184] Moreover, serial radiographs are helpful in assessment of the evolution of the disease (Fig. 18-23).

DePalma and Kruper[40] described two radiologic types. Type I has a fluffy, fleecy appearance, and its periphery is poorly defined. This type is usually encountered in acute cases. An overlying crescent-like streak indicates a rupture

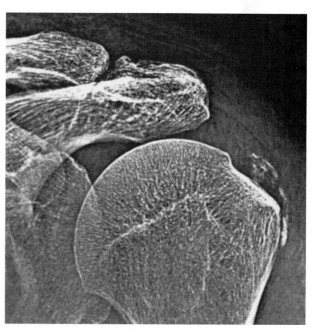

■ **Figure 18–20**
Xerogram of a calcium deposit in the resorptive phase. Note the presence of calcific material in the bursa.

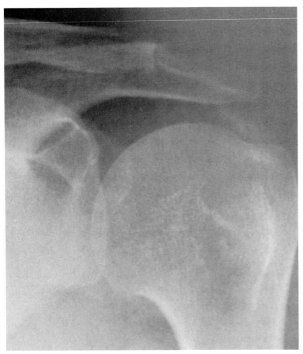

■ Figure 18–21
Calcifying tendinitis during the resorptive phase. The deposit is fluffy and ill defined.

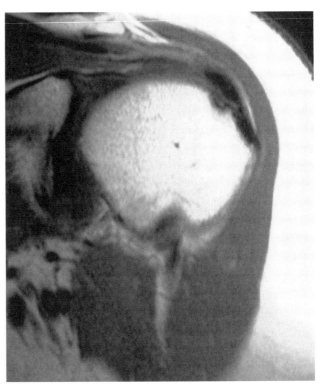

■ Figure 18–22
T1-weighted magnetic resonance image in the frontal plane of a calcific deposit (dark area).

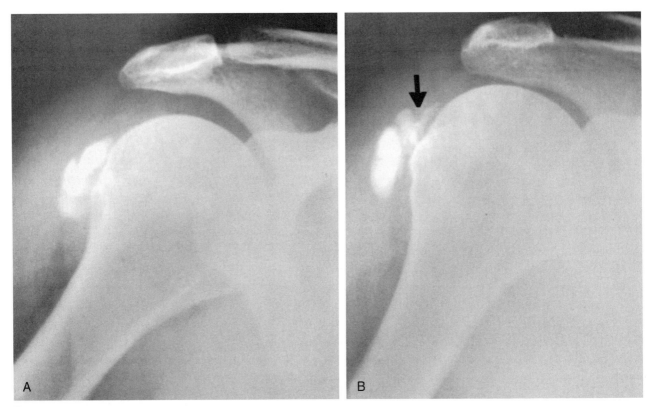

■ Figure 18–23
Calcifying tendinitis of the infraspinatus. At the time of the first consultation, symptoms were chronic. **A,** At that time the deposit was dense, homogeneous, and well defined. This pattern is typical of the formative phase. **B,** Four months later, the patient reported the spontaneous onset of acute pain. Note the beginning of resorption. The *arrow* points to an area of decreased density with irregular margins that is typical of the resorptive phase.

of the deposit into the bursa, which occurs only in this type. Type II is more or less discrete and homogeneous. Its density is uniform, and the periphery is well defined. This type is seen in subacute and chronic cases. Moreover, DePalma and Kruper[40] reported that in 52% of their patients, the calcification was seen as a single lesion.

De Sèze and Welfling[41] observed that in the presence of acute pain, the deposit was less dense and the margins were not well defined. In chronic cases, on the other hand, the margins were well defined and the calcification was dense. They described the following radiologic sequence in acute cases. First, a fluffy, ill-defined intratendinous deposit is followed in time by calcific material in the bursa only, and finally, no calcific material can be seen at all. We believe, however, that calcific material can often be seen in both the bursa and the tendon, that the calcific material disappears rather rapidly from the bursa, and that a faintly visible shadow often remains in the tendon for some time.

Our observations confirm those made by DePalma and Kruper[40] and by De Sèze and Welfling.[41] During the formative or chronic phase, the deposit is dense and well defined and of homogeneous density (see Fig. 18–23A). During the resorptive or acute phase, the deposit is fluffy, cloud-like, and ill defined, and its density is irregular (see Fig. 18–21). Communications with the bursa have been observed only during the latter phase.

Most authors agree that radiologic evidence of degenerative joint disease is usually lacking. This absence of such evidence, of course, holds true mostly for patients in the fourth and fifth decades of life. It is therefore not surprising that in the group of patients reported by Hsu and collaborators,[73] the incidence of degenerative joint changes was higher. In three of our patients in the sixth decade, we observed acromioclavicular osteophytes. We agree with Ozaki and coworkers[122] that these changes are secondary in nature and that they occur in response to rotator cuff pathology.

Bony changes at the insertion of the supraspinatus into the greater tuberosity can sometimes be seen after resorption of the deposit. Whether these alterations occur more often after intraosseous extension of the calcium deposit into bone is difficult to confirm.

The calcifications seen in arthropathies have a quite different appearance. They are stippled and overlie the bony insertion. They are always accompanied by degenerative bony or articular changes. Moreover, the acromiohumeral compartment or interval is always narrowed. These calcium deposits constitute dystrophic calcifications; they must be clearly distinguished from reactive intratendinous calcifications.

According to Hartig and Huth,[68] sonography is more sensitive than radiography in detecting calcium deposits (Figs. 18–24A and B and 18–25A and B). Deposits could be visualized in 90% of their 217 patients radiologically and in 100% sonographically (as well as histologically). The role of high-resolution ultrasonography in the management of calcifying tendinitis has also been stressed by Chiu.[28]

LABORATORY INVESTIGATIONS

Calcifying tendinitis is not associated with any abnormalities in calcium and phosphorus metabolism. Therefore, serum values are within normal limits. Alkaline phosphatase is also normal. No increase is seen in the number of white blood cells, and the erythrocyte sedimentation rate is normal.

In our attempts to further distinguish between degenerative and reactive tendinopathies, we proceeded with tissue typing in 50 patients with calcifying tendinitis and compared the results with those of 36 patients with a tear of the rotator cuff and with 982 control patients.[164] HLA-A1 was present in 50% of the patients with calcifications, 27.8% of the patients with tears, and 26.7% of controls. There is a statistically significant difference between patients suffering from calcifying tendinitis and those with a tear, the P value being .0025.

Nakase and colleagues[114] described the presence of multinucleated giant cells synthesizing cathepsin K. Obviously, this activity is related to the resorptive phase. Localization and expression of osteopontin in patients

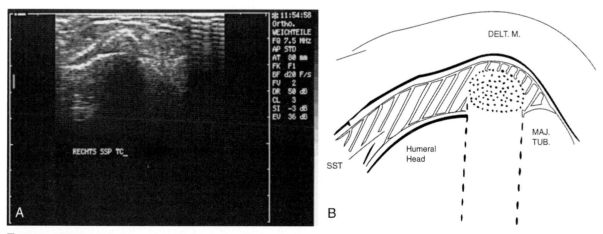

■ **Figure 18–24**
A, Ultrasonography of a calcific deposit in the supraspinatus tendon (coronal section, Siemens SI-400). **B,** Drawing of the ultrasonographic picture. DELT. M., deltoid muscle; MAJ. TUB., greater tuberosity; SST, supraspinatus tendon.

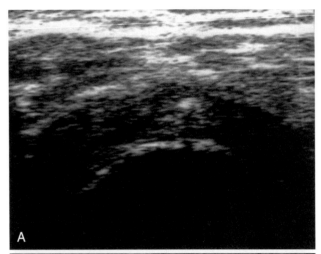

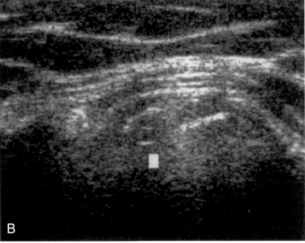

■ **Figure 18–25**
Sonographic (7.5 MHz) depiction of a calcific deposit.
A, Anteroposterior plane. **B,** Lateral plane.

with calcifying tendinitis have been described by Takeuchi and Sugamoto.[173]

During screening of patients with calcifications, serum glucose values and the level of uric acid and iron should be determined.

COMPLICATIONS

Although calcification starts inside the tendon, it may occasionally extend into muscle or bone. DePalma and Kruper[40] noted that in cases of osseous penetration, the point of entry was to be found at the sulcus, the interval between the articular cartilage and insertion of the tendon. They observed that intraosseous deposits were always in continuity with intratendinous calcifications. In their experience, bone involvement led to protracted symptoms; deposits in these patients were resistant to conservative measures, and they advocated surgical removal.

Bicipital tendinitis may complicate calcifying tendinitis. It occurred in 16 of 136 patients reported by DePalma and Kruper.[40]

As stated earlier, frozen shoulder may occur in association with calcification. It was seen by DePalma and Kruper[40] in 7 of 94 patients. They believed that frozen shoulder was caused by an inflammatory process whereby adhesions occur between the cuff and the humeral head.

Rupture of the deposit into the bursa cannot be regarded as a complication. Complete tears, however, must be included, and to our knowledge, they have been reported only by Patte and Goutallier,[125] who observed rupture of the deposit into the glenohumeral joint, seen only in the type that they call diffuse calcification.

Complications from surgery must be of little importance because they have not been reported. Careful attention must be paid to spare the axillary nerve during splitting of the deltoid. Postoperative wound infection has not been seen by us, and all wounds healed without undue delay.

Recurrence of calcification after surgical removal has been observed by us in 1 of 127 operated patients. In other patients in whom the deposit was not completely removed, spontaneous disappearance of the deposit was rather slow.

DIFFERENTIAL DIAGNOSIS

Here again we wish to insist on a proper distinction between reactive and dystrophic calcification. In calcifying tendinitis, the major portion of the deposit is situated inside the tendon without being either in continuity or in contact with bone. Dystrophic calcifications, on the other hand, are part of a degenerative process at the enthesis with concomitant radiologic evidence of osteoarthritis and a rotator cuff tear leading to narrowing of the interval between the humeral head and the acromion. These calcifications are small and stippled and sit just over the greater tuberosity.

O'Leary and collaborators observed tophaceous deposits in the supraspinatus and crystals in the synovial fluid in a patient with anterior shoulder pain and a strongly positive impingement sign.[119a]

TREATMENT

Clinical keys for treatment are as follows:

1. The first line of treatment is conservative.
2. For dense, well-circumscribed deposits refractory to conservative care: surgery, preferably arthroscopic.
3. For ill-defined, cloudy deposits: needling, aspiration, lavage; immediately in patients with excruciating pain. Surgery is rarely indicated.

Treatment varies according to the training and expertise of the treating physician. In general, rheumatologists seem to favor a conservative approach more often than surgeons do. The approach also depends on the acuteness of symptoms and on the patience of the physician and patient. Some impatience is understandable because no one knows how long the disease will last in its chronic phase or when the calcification will spontaneously disappear. In 1963 Moseley[111] reported on a comparison of results of nonoperative and operative treatment; he could not find a significant difference. Broad outlines of treatments have also been reported.[137,194]

Nonoperative

The natural evolution of the deposit has been followed by Gärtner[54] in 235 patients over a 3-year period. Radiologically dense deposits disappeared in 33%, in contrast to 85% of fluffy accumulations.

Gschwend and coworkers[63] estimate that at least 90% of patients are treated conservatively. In a series of 100 patients reported by Litchman and colleagues,[88] only 1 patient underwent surgery.

All authors agree about the need for adequate physiotherapy.[11,102] Range-of-motion and pendulum exercises and, later on, muscle-strengthening exercises are recommended. In acute cases, gentle attempts at mobilization are preceded by the local application of ice, whereas local heat is recommended in chronic cases. Infrared treatment should be understood as the local application of heat. Ultrasonography is said to be able to mobilize the calcium crystals, but no randomized study proving its value could be found by Griffin and Karselis.[61] These authors observed pain relief, which is thought to result from a physiologic rise in tissue temperature. The main aim of physiotherapy is a decrease in muscle spasm and prevention of stiffness. Relief of pain can sometimes be obtained by placing the arm on a pillow in abduction.[24] The treatment regimen outlined is indicated mainly for chronic cases. Whether pulsed ultrasound will have a positive effect on dissolution of the calcium deposit remains to be seen.

Extracorporeal Shock Wave Therapy

"The role of ESWT as a physical treatment has yet to be established by further, large, well-designed trials."

A.G. White[192]

Several points should be taken into consideration when contemplating the use of extracorporeal shock wave therapy (ESWT):

1. No randomized multicenter study has been published.
2. Clear indications related to the phase of calcification (formation, resorption) exist.
3. No general agreement has been reached regarding the optimal energy/frequency.
4. Cost of the equipment may be a factor.

ESWT had its beginning with success in the lithotripsy of various types of kidney stones. The technique gained interest among orthopaedic surgeons when it became evident that bone could be microfractured by the application of shock waves.[23] Initial studies focused on the possible effect of ESWT on fracture healing, as well as the treatment of pseudarthrosis.[60] Valchanou and Michailov[186] were among the first to evaluate shock wave therapy for pseudarthroses, and it became evident that in some cases, particularly in atrophic pseudarthroses, shock wave therapy could stimulate healing and resolution of nonunion in more than 50% of patients.[188] The effects of ESWT in sports orthopaedics were published by Steinacker and Steuer.[169]

Loew and Jurgowski,[91] Dahmen and colleagues,[37] Fritze,[53] and Rompe and associates[142,146] directed their interest to the possible effects of ESWT on the dissolution of calcific deposits within shoulder tendons. Loew and Jurgowski[91] reported a better outcome in patients treated by ESWT than by a 3-month trial of conservative therapy. Similar numbers have since been reported by Brunner and colleagues[22] and Wang and coworkers.[189] The mechanical effects of shock waves were investigated by Perlick and associates.[129]

Daecke and collaborators[36] reviewed 115 patients examined at 3 and 6 months and reported that in 50% of the patients, radiographic changes within the calcium deposit were seen 3 months after ESWT whereas at 6 months, 70% had morphologic changes when compared with the initial deposits, specifically, breakup of single deposits and diminution in particle size. Rompe and coauthors[144] published an initial study of 40 patients who received 1500 impulses under regional anesthesia during a single session; the patients were monitored for 24 weeks. Twenty-five patients had complete or partial disappearance of the calcific deposit after 24 weeks. This study was expanded to 100 patients and reported again in 1997[143]; similar numbers showing radiographic changes (75%) were found, with 90% having complete dissolution. Loew and coworkers[92] studied 20 patients with "chronic, symptomatic calcifying tendinitis" and reported an improvement in symptoms, but the 12-week follow-up period was rather short. Their controls were patients in whom MRI did not show any secondary changes in the rotator cuff or underlying bone, although local hematomas developed in 14 of 20 patients after treatment. Thirty percent of their patients had an improvement in the Constant score,[32] and in 7 the deposit disappeared completely.

When one compares the various treatment options, one has to be aware that no real consensus has yet been reached between the various author groups regarding how to compare their results. One should also be aware that the treatment can be applied either with a low-, medium-, or high-energy delivery system, depending on the amount of energy desired in the focus. The frequency of the shock waves may be modulated as well. A further variable is whether one session or multiple sessions of ESWT are used.[92] Some authors[93,143] suggested a grading scale from 1 to 5 between low- and high-energy applications. The amount of energy considered to be low is less than $0.08 \, mJ/mm^2$, medium energy is considered to be $0.28 \, mJ/mm^2$, and high energy is anything above $0.6 \, mJ/mm^2$. Energies and the frequency of treatment used by various authors are listed in Table 18–1.

Technical Points

Electromagnetic, piezoelectric, or electrohydraulic systems are used for shock wave generation. The action of extracorporeal shock waves can either be directly destructive, with the applied energy of the shock wave being converted into local kinetic energy and direct transfer of the energy into the calcific deposit, or indirectly destructive, with the shock wave producing cavitations leading to breakup of the calcific deposit.[143]

TABLE 18-1. Energy and Frequency of Application of Extracorporeal Shock Wave Therapy by Various Authors

Study	Energy/Frequency	Follow-up Time	n	Results*
Loew et al. (1995)[93]	2000, 22 kV, repeat after 14 days	6 wk, 12 wk	20	6 excellent, 8 much improved, 1 better, 4 unchanged, 1 poor
Loew et al. (1995)[92]	2 × 2000 14 days, 21 kV	6 wk, 12 wk	20	70% subject. improvement, 60% rad. calcific depot changes
	1 × 2000, 21 kV		20	60% subject. improvement, 50% rad. calcific depot changes
	1 × 2000, 18 kV		20	30% subject. improvement, 10% rad. calcific depot changes
Daecke et al. (1997)[36]	1 × 2000, 22 kV	3 mo, 6 mo	115/2	3 mo, 32% rad. calcific depot changes
	2 × 2000 (7 days), 22 kV	3 mo, 6 mo	115/2	3 mo, 50%; 6 mo, 70% rad. calcific depot changes
Rompe (1997)[143]	0.28 mJ/mm	3, 6, 12, 24 wk	100	67% (24 wk) subject. improvement, 75% rad. calcific depot changes
Brunner et al. (1997)[22]	1534 (3 × 14 days)	12 wk	70	64.4% (def. 50% much improved)
Dahmen et al. (1995)[37]	0.08 mJ/mm	6, 12, 18 mo	76	67% better, 3 mo conservative treatment

*The results refer to the subjective improvement as a percentage of the radiographic changes in the deposit at the moment of follow-up.

The initial studies involving therapy for pseudarthrosis demonstrated a dose-dependent action on cortical bone healing, as well as an increase in bone formation with the application of higher doses.[188] Another study could not demonstrate a dose-dependent action on the vitality of osteoblasts in cell cultures.[93] Delius and Draenert[38] tried to explain the action of ESWT as local secondary tissue warming as a result of energy transfer, which would lead locally to edema formation and secondary cell membrane disruption. This action would then cause local petechial bleeding as a side effect.

The main action of ESWT on the shoulder seems to consist of a transfer of physical energy that causes disintegration of the calcific deposit or initiates changes in its consistency. Cell-mediated resorption must obviously follow the disintegration because no natural pathways exist as in the case after breakup of gallstones or kidney stones. A further effect might be an increase in vascularization in the area of the tendon, close to the focus of energy application.

Charrin[27] described the role of high-resolution ultrasonographic guidance during shock wave therapy.

From a review of the literature with a meta-analysis,[69] it becomes evident that in approximately 50%, high-energy ESWT is not successful (four studies[36,133,142,151] were used). The reason for these failures is thought to be the different types of calcific composition, the variability in the size and structure of the deposits, and their location (see Fig. 18–23). Single calcific deposits seem to have the best prognosis for successful dissolution, whereas those with a fluid or paste-like consistency would yield the least success.[143] This difference in prognosis is also known from the results of arthroscopic treatment.[75,106,141] The results reported give an approximately 80% success rate for patients treated by arthroscopy, with those having complete removal of radiographically visible deposits enjoying the best outcomes. In contrast, Tillander and Norlin[175] found good results after subacromial decompression only, without touching the deposits at the time of surgery. Seventy-nine percent of the deposits had decreased or disappeared at follow-up.

Loew and colleagues[93] demonstrated that the results of ESWT were dependent on the energy dose and not related to the size and type of the calcific deposit found at the beginning of treatment. They believed that a single session with approximately 2000 shock impulses of medium to high energy would give the best results in most cases. They compared their results with needling and found that it had a similar rate of success in treating calcifying tendinitis. Ebenbichler and coauthors[45] reported that with their ESWT therapy, 47% of patients had improved at 6 weeks versus only 10% in a sham group. At 6 months, 65% had improved versus only 20% in the sham group. Forty-two percent of their patients had no residual calcific deposit at 6 months on control radiographs.

Maier and co-workers treated 52 patients with calcific deposits. The patients received an average density flow of 0.15 mJ/mm² and were followed for 18 months. Twenty-one deposits disappeared, and 31 persisted. The clinical and radiologic outcome was independent of the size of the deposit.[97a]

Schmitt and coworkers[160] used low-energy ESWT for tendinitis of the supraspinatus tendon, but they could not report any better results than with standard conservative measures. They concluded that symptomatic tendinitis was not a good indication for ESWT. In a clinical double-blind study, Speed and associates[168] compared the effect of ESWT with that of sham treatment in patients with rotator cuff tendinitis. They failed to find an added benefit of ESWT. It must be noted, however, that these authors did not distinguish between noncalcific and calcific tendinitis.

Haake and coworkers[64] compared their results with those of radiotherapy for calcifying tendinitis and could not find a significant difference in outcome. They used six applications of radiation at 0.5 Gy and compared it with ESWT at 0.33 mJ/mm² applied in three sessions.

Only one controlled prospective study on ESWT has been performed, that by Daecke and coworkers.[35] These authors examined the effect of high-energy ESWT and its complications over a 4-year period. They evaluated two groups totaling 115 patients (67 men and 48 women) with a mean age of 49 years who received either one or two sessions of ESWT. The inclusion criteria consisted of the presence of painful calcifying tendinitis for more than 12 months that was unresponsive to conservative therapy, including subacromial steroid infiltration. They included only deposits that had a homogeneous structure and were sharply outlined with a minimal diameter of 15 mm. None of the patients had a rotator cuff tear, and no arthritis or any other related problem was present. Patients in group A received a single 2000-impulse, high-energy shock wave therapy, whereas group B received two sessions of the same dose 1 week apart. All patients were given local anesthesia before the shock wave therapy.

Patients were asked to not accept any further therapy for at least 6 months after the treatment and were encouraged to use the arm in daily activities. The results were assessed at 3-month and 6-month intervals and 4 years after the initial therapy. Besides the clinical assessment, standard radiographs were obtained at follow-up, and the Constant score was used to evaluate the patients.[32] The percentage of patients seen at follow-up was 87% at 3 months and 72% at 6 months. Ninety-two percent of the initial population could be re-interviewed at 4 years. At this point, 20% elected to undergo surgery on the affected shoulder. Comparison of both groups shows that only 23 patients receiving the single session of high-dose ESWT (A) and 37% of the patients receiving two sessions of ESWT (B) had received no further therapy between the 6-month follow-up and the examination at 4 years. The radiographic changes were found to be most profound at the first follow-up (67% within the first 3 months); the number then decreased over time, with further changes noted in only 17% of the patients after 6 months and complete dissolution in 16% during the last 3 years at the 4-year final follow-up examination. The frequency of subjective success, as asked for in the patient questionnaire, was found to be higher in group B (two sessions) than in group A (one session) but was not statistically significant; however, when compared with the preoperative assessment, it was significantly improved for both groups. The radiographic findings were graded as partial or complete resorption and amounted to 30% (A) and 52% (B) at 3 months, 47% (A) and 77% (B) at 6 months, and 93% for both groups after 4 years. The differences were significant only at the 6-month interval ($P < .046$). The Constant score increased in both groups from 49 and 44 points before ESWT to 88 and 85 points at the 4-year mark. No significant difference was found between the two groups. No evidence of humeral head necrosis or bone infarct was detected, and no rotator cuff tear after 4 years was thought to possibly have been induced by ESWT. In patients who had undergone further surgical therapy (22), no cartilage damage was found in the shoulder joint at the time of surgery that could be related to ESWT. Three patients were found to have hypertrophic bursal tissue. This study showed that ESWT applied in doses of 1000 to 2000 impulses at $0.4\ mJ/mm^2$ did not have any detrimental long-term effect on the shoulder joint such as secondary rotator cuff degeneration or cartilage damage. The authors thought that the results of ESWT were only slightly inferior to those of any surgical techniques, but that anesthetic and surgical risks could be avoided completely. These authors[34] published the same study with the same results in 2002.

Complications, Risks, and Contraindications to ESWT

It should be noted that shock wave therapy does have its own risks, which depending on the type of energy used, will lead to a localized pain sensation after therapy, a petechial type of bleeding, and possibly, subcutaneous hematoma. Most patients undergoing high-energy shock wave therapy will require local anesthesia.

The risk of avascular necrosis and tendon degeneration seems to be low. Maier and colleagues[97] used MRI to review the results of ESWT at energies of up to $0.12\ mJ/mm^2$; they could not detect any changes within the tendon or bone in 24 patients after the procedure. Daecke and associates[35] did not find any instances of avascular necrosis 4 years after treatment.

Contraindications to ESWT are divided into general and local. General contraindications are any type of infection, pacemaker use, pregnancy, and local tumors. Local contraindications are avascular necrosis of the humeral head, heterotopic ossification, osteomyelitis, and open growth plates, thus excluding patients younger than 18 years from consideration for this treatment.

Summary

When comparing the differing results of various treatment modalities, one should keep in mind that as other studies have demonstrated, during the natural course of calcifying tendinitis the calcific deposits may spontaneously disappear in 9% of patients over a 37-month period.[55] Bosworth[17] reported a yearly resolution rate of approximately 3% in a population of 138 patients. Therefore, it seems difficult to assess the long-term outcome of any study because of the natural course of the calcific deposits.[167] Wolk and Wittenberg[197] thought that in their collective experience, 70% of patients could be successfully treated with conservative measures only. A more invasive therapy must therefore give either better or faster success.

ESWT is believed to produce dose-dependent changes in the calcific deposit within the first 6 months after initial treatment, whereas in longer follow-up, no significant changes can be found.[35] One should be aware that only one prospective follow-up study has been conducted thus far; it did not demonstrate any adverse effects on rotator cuff tissues or the cartilage and bone of the involved shoulder joints. One should also be aware of a possible bias in the results because concomitant physiotherapy is often administered to patients after any procedure, be it ESWT, surgery, needling, or subacromial injections. Therefore, the results can easily be modified as a result of the attentive care that is directed to the shoulders involved, as well as the natural outcome of the disease.[57] In Daecke and coworkers' study,[35] the number of patients with partial or complete resorption of the calcification was higher than the number with subjective improvement at the 6-month examination. This result seems to indicate that persistent calcific deposits might very well be responsible for persistent discomfort. Only in two cases in their study was resorption not complete at the 4-year mark. Of interest is that no recurrences of any calcific deposits were noted in this study.

ESWT seems to be an effective therapeutic tool for the appropriate type of calcific deposit in the correct phase of calcifying tendinitis.[90,145] One should be aware that the cost incurred is high in comparison to conservative measures, not only for the apparatus required but also for preparation of the patient in the clinical setting and for the follow-up needed. This disadvantage is also true for any minimally invasive procedures such as arthroscopy. A persistent calcific deposit with persisting pain might become an indication for a surgical procedure such as arthroscopic removal.

The paucity of experimental investigations on the effect of ESWT on tissues is surprising. Only one study could be found.[121] Studies comparing different treatment protocols are also needed, as stated by Seil and coworkers.[162]

We consider this technique as still being under trial, and one will have to wait for longer follow-up studies, a larger patient population, and reports from other centers before being able to comment on the strict indications and details of the technique.

Authors' Opinion

ESWT has been advocated as conservative therapy for calcifying tendinitis. The variables of this therapy include the frequency of the shock waves, the amount of energy applied, and the number of sessions. Additional variables are the size and location of the deposit, as well as the radiologic appearance. Most of the published studies come from Europe. Besides, controversy still exists regarding its effectiveness in the light of the natural course of the disease.

We believe that ESWT may be indicated in patients with a solitary and compact deposit when other conservative regimens lasting at least 3 months have failed. At a minimum, a local anesthetic should be applied. The patient must be informed of the possible side effects and risks, such as local pain, subcutaneous petechial bleeding, hematoma, and incomplete disappearance of calcification. There does not seem to be a need to include avascular necrosis and permanent soft tissue injury because none of these complications have been reported in the literature.

Needling and Lavage

In acute cases, easing pain becomes a priority. Patterson and Darrach[126] and later Lapidus[85] recommended needling and injection of local anesthetics. Gärtner[54] monitored 33 patients for 1 year after needling and observed resorption of the deposit in 23 patients. Repeated perforations seem to decrease intratendinous pressure. An additional lavage may also help remove part of the deposit. Its effect on symptoms was studied by Pfister and Gerber[132] in 149 of 212 patients after 5 years. Sixty percent were free of pain, 34% had marked relief, and 6% were unchanged. Lavage can be effective only in the presence of radiologic evidence of resorption. The site of needle insertion is based on the site of maximal tenderness and radiographic localization. To better locate the deposits, Aina and colleagues[1] described a modified ultrasonic-guided fine-needle technique. Although these injections had to be repeated in some patients twice or three times, Harmon[67] reported that they led to excellent results in 78.9% of more than 400 patients. DePalma and Kruper's results were less good; they obtained 61% good, 22% fair, and 17% poor results.[40]

Some authors suggest the addition of a corticosteroid preparation to local treatment. Gschwend and colleagues[63] note that its action is short and its effect is exclusively symptomatic. Dhuly and associates[42] showed that corticosteroids inhibit vascular proliferation, local hyperemia, and macrophage activity. Lippmann[87] warned that

corticosteroids abort the activity that leads to disruption and return the deposit to a static phase. Harmon[67] believed that the addition of corticosteroids did not accelerate the process of resorption but did reduce muscle spasms. Murnaghan and McIntosh[113] treated 27 patients with lidocaine (Xylocaine) injections alone and 24 with hydrocortisone and found no difference in results. During the acute phase, analgesics are absolutely necessary to calm the often excruciating pain. Nonsteroidal anti-inflammatory drugs are often recommended. No randomized study, however, could be found to document their salutary effect on the process of resorption.

Radiation

In the past, radiotherapy enjoyed an important place in the treatment of calcifying tendinitis.[10,18] Milone and Copeland[104] treated 136 patients with radiotherapy. They concluded that "patients with the acute syndrome experience the most favorable response." Of 54 patients in the acute phase, 49 had excellent and good results, whereas only 15 of 24 patients with chronic pain obtained the same degree of relief. The percentage of patients with chronic symptoms who had similar results fell to 33% in Young's[199] and Chapman's[26] series. Of 609 patients reported by Harmon,[67] 79 received radiotherapy. Of these patients, 28 needed surgical excision at a later date. Plenk[135] concluded that radiotherapy was ineffective. In a series of 38 patients, Plenk irradiated 21 patients and interposed a lead shield between the source of radiation and the shoulder in 17 patients. The calcium deposit disappeared in 67% of the shielded patients and 44% of the irradiated patients. Plenk gained the impression that in acute cases, irradiation delayed resorption in five of nine patients, whereas in shielded patients, the deposit persisted in only one of eight patients. In this context, Gschwend and colleagues' sarcastic remark that in acute cases any form of treatment is successful[63] is noteworthy. "Therapy cannot hinder the success," they conclude. Although radiotherapy is not an acceptable mode of treatment in North America any more, a recent report from France recommends the use of "anti-inflammatory radiotherapy." Ollagnier and colleagues[119] reported good results in 68% of 47 patients. It seems that their assessment has been based mainly on pain relief.

Surgery

Bosworth[16,17] expressed the opinion of many surgeons when he wrote that the quickest and most dependable way of relieving patients of large and troublesome deposits is by open surgery. Vebostad[187] obtained excellent and good results with surgery in 34 of 43 patients. Litchman and colleagues[88] believe that prolonged waiting in the chronic group leads to adhesive capsulitis and frozen shoulder. This view is not commonly shared. Gschwend and associates[63] formulated the following indications for surgery:

1. Progression of symptoms
2. Constant pain interfering with activities of daily living
3. Absence of improvement in symptoms after conservative therapy

They reported excellent and good results in 25 of 28 subjects. Moseley[109,110] restricts the indication to recommending surgery for large deposits in the mechanical phase. He, like most other authors, is in favor of conservative treatment for acute cases. DePalma and Kruper[40] reported 96% good results and only 4% fair results after surgery. The time of recovery after surgery is surprisingly long. In DePalma and Kruper's series,[40] 53% recovered in 2 to 6 weeks, and in an additional 30%, recovery took 5 to 10 weeks. DePalma and Kruper gained the impression that the period of convalescence was longer in patients treated surgically than in those managed conservatively. The observation of Carnett[24] is of equal interest: the postoperative pain clears up less rapidly in chronic than in acute cases. Our investigations have shown that postoperative symptoms persist for much longer than anticipated.[100]

Surgical Techniques

Arthroscopy

Arthroscopy has become a common tool for dealing with pathology in the shoulder. The main indication is not for a purely diagnostic evaluation any more, but rather as a surgical procedure for correcting intra-articular changes or subacromial pathology.*

Significant experience is accumulating with arthroscopic treatment of calcifying tendinitis in patients refractory to conservative and nonoperative measures. The potential advantages are obvious: less dissection, the ability to examine for additional pathology, and shorter recovery periods. The major questions revolve around the efficacy of the technique and whether the time to final recovery can be shortened.

Technical Considerations

Preoperative external rotation and neutral anteroposterior views appear to localize the calcific deposit best.[8] Rupp and coworkers[150] used preoperative ultrasonography to help localize the deposit and identify the distance between it and the biceps tendon in the transverse plane and the greater tuberosity in the longitudinal plane. The use of a graduated probe introduced through the anterior portal during glenohumeral arthroscopy allows for targeted outside-in insertion of a 14-gauge spinal needle referenced to the biceps tendon (Fig. 18-26); the appearance of a calcific deposit at the tip of the needle confirms the correct location. A nonabsorbable dark suture can be fed through the lumen of the needle to establish a landmark to aid in identification of the deposit on the bursal side, where definitive management will occur. Needling of the deposit will optimally result in a snowstorm appearance, but such is not always the case and depends on the consistency of the calcific deposit. Ark and colleagues[8] found that the use of two lateral portals facilitates visualization and surgical access. Confirmatory localization with needling can be followed by two to three longitudinal slits if calcific egress is not consistent with the amount of

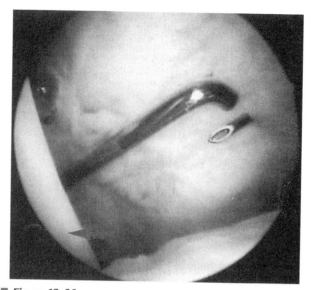

■ **Figure 18–26**

Graduated probe inserted into the subacromial space referenced to the biceps tendon and greater tuberosity to aid in localization of the spinal needle at calcific deposits. *(From Rupp S, Seil R, and Kohn D: Preoperative ultrasonic mapping of calcium deposits facilitates localization during arthroscopic surgery for calcifying tendinitis of the rotator cuff. Arthroscopy 14:540-542, 1998.)*

deposit on radiographs. Jerosch and associates[76] could identify the deposit by bursoscopy alone in 10 patients and relied on needling the cuff to locate it successfully in 40 of 48 patients. Despite meticulous preoperative evaluation and careful intraoperative visualization, one should not expect to find all deposits. Molé and colleagues[106] could not locate the lesion in 12% of their arthroscopic cases. Even in open series, the deposit is not always identified despite serial longitudinal slits in the tendon—as Rochwerger and coworkers[141] found in 15% of their patients.

Arthroscopic Technique

The patient is placed in a beach chair position for surgery under general endotracheal anesthesia, with interscalene regional anesthesia in place for postoperative relief of pain. The portals used are placed in the posterior, anterolateral, and if needed, the anterolateral and posterolateral positions.

Initially, the glenohumeral joint is explored through the posterior portal with a 4.5-mm, 30-degree-tilt arthroscope. A vascular injection pattern of the rotator cuff tendons indicative of an inflammatory response to the calcific deposit can occasionally be seen on the articular surface of the tendon,[141] and this site may then be marked with a suture.

After drainage of the joint, the scope is removed and introduced into the subacromial space, where a working cannula is inserted through the anterolateral portal, and the surface of the rotator cuff is palpated. In many cases a bursal leaf might be present and require partial resection with a full-radius resector. The acromion is then inspected, as well as the coracoacromial ligament and the border of the acromioclavicular joint. The rotator cuff is examined methodically by palpating the cuff for any hard-

---

*See references 3, 13, 25, 46-48, 74, 77, 81, 117, 124, 139, 159, 166, 171.

ening indicative of a calcific deposit. Needling can be performed, and usually an 18-gauge spinal needle will fill with calcific material when withdrawn from the tendon. Such filling can be observed through the scope in the subacromial space. Depending on the consistency of the deposit, the calcium might extrude as a paste but is generally seen as small flakes in sharply demarcated deposits, which is the ideal indication for arthroscopic therapy. In some cases, the so-called snowstorm appearance might occur. Once the deposit is identified, we prefer to make a longitudinal incision in line with the direction of the fibers with the needle in the superficial part of the rotator cuff to avoid any deep penetrating cuts. Palpation with the hook will then usually allow one to liberate the calcific deposit, but care must be taken to not create a rotator cuff defect by using large curets or possibly knives and tissue cutters.

Careful irrigation of the subacromial space is then performed because the calcific debris can act as an irritating agent in the subacromial bursa. Subacromial decompression is performed only if associated pathology is present, such as an obvious acromial beak or signs of subacromial impingement; the same is true for associated acromioclavicular joint pathology such as osteophytes.

Once the subacromial space has been drained, one may consider reinspection of the glenohumeral joint to ensure that no rotator cuff rupture has occurred. Otherwise, the instruments are removed and the portal holes are closed with a skin suture.

Postoperative management consists of range-of-motion exercises 24 hours after arthroscopy. The exercises start with pendulum exercises, and then active assisted exercises are begun after the third day and progress to active exercises as tolerated by the patient. Usually, no arm sling is necessary, except for patient comfort at night.

Results

Jerosch and coauthors[75] reported the results of arthroscopic treatment of persistent shoulder pain and calcific tendinitis in a retrospective analysis of 48 patients. The calcific deposit was removed whenever possible (40 patients) by needling and resection with a sharp spoon or synovial resector. All patients were treated by arthroscopic subacromial decompression, but acromioplasty was reserved for those with type III acromia on the supraspinatus outlet view[13] or intraoperative findings of cuff impingement (33 patients). At a mean follow-up of 21 months, the Constant score[32] significantly improved from 38 to 86. Patients with disappearance of the calcific deposit postoperatively had significantly better outcomes than did those without radiographic changes. The addition of acromioplasty did not improve the results, and the authors do not recommend its inclusion. The presence of an os acromiale could justify acromioplasty.[74] In a related 3- to 6-year follow-up study, Hoe-Hanson and associates[71] examined the influence of cuff pathology on shoulder function after subacromial decompression. They could not find any long-term deterioration of the cuff tendons.

Ark and coworkers[8] reviewed a cohort of 23 patients (53% were women, and the mean age was 49 years [range, 33 to 60]) with chronic calcifying tendinitis of the shoulder after a brief trial of conservative therapy. Subacromial bursectomy was performed in all patients, nine underwent coracoacromial ligament release for hypertrophy, and acromioplasty was performed on three for bony overhang and suspected soft tissue impingement. At a mean follow-up of 26 months (range, 12 to 47) in 22 patients, 11 had full motion and complete pain relief and 9 had full motion and occasional episodes of pain. Two patients complained of persistent pain and required repeat surgery, with acceptable results. Follow-up radiographs demonstrated that 13 patients had partial removal of calcium whereas 9 had complete removal of calcium, but these findings did not correlate with the clinical results.

Molé and colleagues[106] retrospectively evaluated the results of arthroscopic treatment of chronic calcifying tendinitis in 112 patients (64% women) within a multicenter study of the French Society of Arthroscopy. The patients had a mean age of 45 years (range, 28 to 67) with an average duration of symptoms of 40 months, and 80% received an average of five subacromial corticosteroid infiltrations. Several subacromial procedures were used: 107 acromioplasties were performed, 18 of which included coracoacromial ligament release, and 5 patients had bursectomies only. The calcific deposit was resected in most cases but was not directly addressed in 37% of the patients, intentionally in 25% and through an inability to localize the deposit in the other 12%. At a mean follow-up of 21 months (range, 12 to 53), this study found an objective success rate of 89% and a patient subjective satisfaction rate of 82% as determined by the Constant score.[32] Based on follow-up radiographs, 88% of patients had complete disappearance of the calcific deposit. No recurrences and no secondary rotator cuff tears were noted. Patients returned to work at a mean of 3 months, and full functional recovery occurred by 6 months, quite similar to their results with open surgery. The results were not associated with patient age or with the radiographic features (type, size, localization) of the calcification. The results, however, did correlate with the arthroscopic procedure: a trend toward a better outcome was observed when the calcification had been removed. Acromioplasty did not improve the results of resection but was considered necessary when the calcification could not be found or was intentionally ignored.

Re and Karzel[137] thought that arthroscopic surgery was ideal for patients who failed to improve with conservative measures. They reported a good success rate with arthroscopic removal of the calcific deposit. Kempf[80] presented a classification of calcifications into four groups and stated that calcifications that are heterogeneous, type D, are rather difficult to deal with because they might have multiple deposits that are very hard to find during either open or arthroscopic surgery.

The answer to the question of whether acromioplasty should always be performed at the time of surgical excision of a calcific deposit remains controversial.[59] Molé and collaborators,[106] as well as Re and Karzel,[137] reviewed their respective patients and could not demonstrate an improvement in results when surgical excision was combined with acromioplasty. Johnson[77] believed that acromioplasty was indicated only in patients in whom an associated pathology of the subacromial space was present, such as a hooked or beaked acromion. The same applies to exclusive resection of the coracoacromial ligament. His finding confirms the experience gained in subacromial impingement surgery, in which no benefit of simple ligament resection has been seen unless performed in association with acromioplasty. In patients with diffuse type D calcification, however, the French group[80,86] suggests that acromioplasty be considered because it seems unlikely to them that removal of the deposit alone would be successful. It is interesting to note that Goutallier and coworkers[59] recommend a simple anterior acromioplasty without any attempt at removal of the calcific deposit; they report good results. A concomitant tear of the rotator cuff is a very rare finding.[75,140] Nevertheless, proper exploration is always indicated, and if a tear is found, a mini-open or conventional repair might be indicated.

In summary, most authors were able to show similar results with arthroscopic and open techniques for removal of calcium deposits. The use of preoperative ultrasound should help localize the deposits with a frequency similar to that of open techniques. Whereas short-term morbidity can be expected to be decreased with arthroscopy, no study has definitively shown faster resolution of symptoms postoperatively or a quicker return to work, probably because the studies referenced have all been retrospective and not designed to look at speed of recovery. A multicenter randomized study would be required to definitively prove this aspect of treatment given the relative infrequency with which most of these patients come to surgery. Similarly, a comparison with ESWT would also be enlightening to better select which patients are best treated with either modality.

Complications seem to be rare and are mainly reported as insufficient pain relief, often secondary to unsuccessful removal of the calcific deposit.[59,80] Rupture of the rotator cuff may be a sequela.

Authors' Preferred Technique

We consider patients who complain about persistent pain and have an obvious calcific deposit candidates for arthroscopic surgery. All these patients should have undergone a trial of physical therapy, possibly combined with non-steroidal anti-inflammatory medication and rarely with more than one subacromial steroid injection.[149] The chief complaint of these patients is a chronic aching type of pain that is accentuated by activity and occurs at night.

On radiographs, most of the calcific deposits are located in the supraspinatus tendon (70%), and a shoulder series consisting of anteroposterior views in neutral, internal, and external rotation and an axial view, as well as a view in the plane of the scapula, are obtained. Because ultrasonography (see Figs. 18-24A and B and 18-25A and B) often permits determination of the site of the deposit, we have reduced this series to two anteroposterior views in internal and external rotation and one view in the plane of the scapula. We consider calcific deposits that are dense and sharply demarcated as ideal for arthroscopic removal; these deposits should preferably be monolocular and not heterogeneous.

Open Procedures (Fig. 18-27)

In discussing the surgical technique, Gschwend and colleagues[62,63] recommend a muscle-splitting approach but

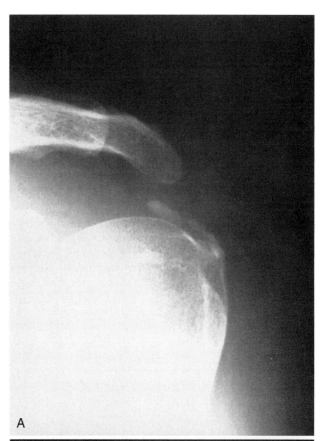

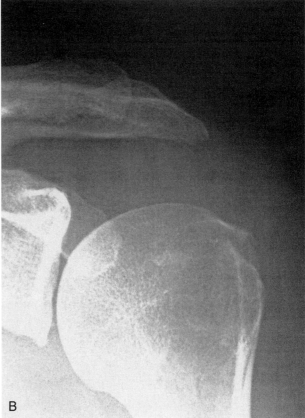

■ Figure 18–27
A, Preoperative radiograph of a multilobulated dense calcific deposit in a patient with a concomitant impingement syndrome secondary to an acromial spur. B, State after acromioplasty and removal of deposit.

warn against detachment of the deltoid. They are in favor of resection of the coracoacromial ligament. Vebostad[187] could not find an improvement in results when he added partial resection of the acromion, which according to his description, seems to have consisted of an anterior acromioplasty. Occasionally, serial vertical tendon incisions become necessary when the deposit is not readily identifiable. Resch[139] recommends that an acromioplasty be performed in those with radiologic or arthroscopic changes only. This recommendation is based on a series of 43 patients. In 1975, Vebostad[187] reported the results of an isolated subtotal acromionectomy performed in five patients in whom the deposit could not easily be found during surgery. He obtained good and excellent relief of symptoms in four patients. Goutallier and colleagues[59] recommended an isolated anterior acromioplasty without removal of the calcium deposit in instances of "heterogeneous calcifications which infiltrate the tendon." Most of the 19 calcifications disappeared during the first postoperative year.

After surgery, early mobilization is recommended. If a sling is worn, it must be removed at regular intervals for exercise.

■ AUTHORS' PREFERRED METHOD OF TREATMENT

Our therapeutic approach is based mainly on the severity of symptoms. Of course, the radiologic features of the deposit will also be taken into consideration (Table 18-2).

Because it is our firm belief that symptoms during the formative phase are chronic or even absent and that acute symptoms accompany the process of resorption, we will first present our management during the formative phase. Patients with subacute symptoms are classified as belonging to the formative phase unless radiographs show evident signs of resorption.

FORMATIVE PHASE

During the formative phase, we favor a conservative approach. Surgical removal is the exception and is performed only when an adequate conservative approach has failed and the symptoms interfere with either work or activity of daily living.

CONSERVATIVE MEASURES

The patient is instructed to perform a daily program of exercises to maintain full mobility of the glenohumeral joint. We also instruct the patient to position the arm in abduction as often as possible, which can be achieved by placing the arm on the backrest of a chair or on a seat beside the patient. While lying down, a pillow should be placed in the axilla. Application of moist heat is also suggested if the symptoms are subacute. Diathermy may be included. Although ultrasound is used occasionally in our physiotherapy department and some patients have commented on its beneficial effect, we have seen no evidence that this treatment modality accelerates the disappearance of calcium deposits.

Local intrabursal corticosteroid injections are never used in patients with chronic symptoms. Only in the presence of impingement causing subacute symptoms do we give one intrabursal corticosteroid injection mixed with lidocaine. Needling of dense, homogeneous deposits has never been attempted. Attempts at lavage have not been successful in our hands, which is not surprising given the chalk-like consistency of the deposit.

Nonsteroidal anti-inflammatory drugs are not prescribed when the symptoms are chronic, but they are prescribed for 1 week to 10 days when subacute symptoms are present. Analgesics are rarely indicated.

Patients are assessed clinically and radiologically every 4 weeks. In cases in which the outcome of conservative treatment is not satisfactory and the patient meets our criteria for surgical intervention, the indication is discussed with the patient. If the patient consents, removal of the calcium deposit is done on a short-stay basis in the hospital. A history and physical examination as well as all laboratory tests and radiographs (chest and affected shoulder) are completed 1 week before surgery. On the day of surgery, the patient is admitted to our short-stay unit and discharged the same day after surgery. Before being discharged, the patient will be seen by the physiotherapist to ensure that a proper postoperative exercise program is followed.

SURGICAL TECHNIQUE

Removal of calcium deposits is performed under general anesthesia. The patient is in a supine position, and a sandbag is placed under the affected shoulder. We make

TABLE 18–2.   Outline of the Treatment Approach

Symptom	Therapy	Effects
Chronic pain	Conservative	Maintenance of ROM and strength
	Avoid cortisone	
	Surgery, if unsuccessful and if interference with work and ADL	
Acute pain	Needling and lavage	Decompression
		Hyperemia↓
	Single cortisone injection	Phagocytosis↓
	Pendulum and ROM exercises	Avoidance of frozen shoulder
Subsiding pain	Rest in abduction	Relieve stretch pressure↓
		Blood flow↑
	ROM and strengthening exercises	Avoidance of frozen shoulder and muscle weakness
	Avoid cortisone	

ADL, activities of daily living; ROM, range of motion.

sure that the side of the patient to be operated on is as close to the edge of the table as possible. The arm is draped free to ensure full mobilization of the arm during surgery. Depending on the choice and training of the surgeon, the operation is performed arthroscopically or by open means. The arthroscopic technique has been well described in the foregoing pages. For open procedures, we make a skin incision from the acromion to the coracoid process, as recommended by Neer.[116] The deltoid fibers are bluntly separated. A stitch to protect the axillary nerve in the distal portion near the deltoid split has not been found necessary. The deltoid muscle is not detached from the acromion. The bursa is then opened, and the edges are retracted with army-navy retractors. The bursal wall is inspected. The coracoacromial ligament is then identified and cleaned of all overlying soft tissue. Care is taken to visualize the posterior edge of the ligament. The state of the ligament is recorded. We have never observed a thickening, although it was described by Watson.[190] The narrowness of the interval between the rotator cuff and the ligament is then tested, generally with the little finger. Introduction of this finger is made easier with longitudinal traction of the arm. While the finger is in place, the arm is rotated and lifted in position between flexion and abduction. The undersurface of the acromion is also palpated. If the space between the ligament and the rotator cuff is "tight," it is usually necessary to proceed with an anterior acromioplasty, although this procedure is definitely an exception. Even though anterior acromioplasty makes inspection of the rotator cuff and its covering bursal wall easier, we recommend against regular use of this procedure. External and internal rotation of the arm will permit inspection of the entire rotator cuff. If a bursal reaction is present, its location and extent are recorded. It is generally limited to a hyperemic reaction around the calcific deposit that shines through the bursal wall. We do not perform a bursectomy. The tendon is then incised in the direction of its fibers, and the calcific mass is treated by curettage. We then proceed with limited resection of the frayed tendon edges, which are usually sites of calcium encrustation. Sometimes more than one deposit is present, and separate tendon incisions are required. A proper preoperative radiograph is very important to determine not only the location but also the number of deposits. If no calcium can be seen during inspection, small incisions are made at the site of suspected calcifications as determined by radiography.

After the deposit has been removed, copious lavage is performed. The shoulder is moved through its full range of motion, the tendon edges are approximated if necessary, and the wound is closed in layers. A sling is applied after surgery. We again hasten to add that this sling must be removed at least four times a day for pendulum and gentle passive or active assisted range-of-motion exercises. The sling is removed completely after 3 days, and active exercises are started. We encourage patients to keep the arm in abduction as often as possible. If postoperative pain is severe, local ice packs should be applied. We have never resorted to postoperative corticosteroid injections.

RESORPTIVE PHASE

TECHNIQUE OF LAVAGE

During the phase of resorption when the symptoms are acute or in the presence of subacute symptoms when radiographs indicate ongoing resorption, we attempt lavage of the deposit with two 18-gauge needles. A local anesthetic (2% lidocaine without epinephrine) is used to freeze the sites of needle placement, and 5 mL is injected into the bursa. The site of lavage is based on the location of tenderness and radiographic localization. Two percent lidocaine is also used for lavage. Calcium particles can easily be recognized in the outflow. If lavage is not successful, needling usually helps decrease intratendinous pressure. At the end of lavage or needling, we proceed with an intrabursal corticosteroid injection only if the pain is excruciating. This injection will not be repeated.

The patient is instructed to apply ice and perform pendulum exercises. Analgesics are prescribed. Although we always instruct the patient to take nonsteroidal anti-inflammatory drugs for 1 week, we have no absolute proof of their beneficial effect. After the first treatment, the patient will be asked to report back 3 or 4 days later. As soon as the symptoms decrease, usually after 1 week, the patient is referred to physiotherapy for range-of-motion and strengthening exercises. Radiographs are taken 4 weeks after the first visit. They almost always show a considerable decrease, if not disappearance of the deposit. Ultrasound has not been used by us during the resorptive phase.

We have not observed a single case of frozen shoulder or adhesive capsulitis in patients treated in this fashion. One patient with this syndrome, however, was seen in consultation. This patient had been treated with systemic corticosteroid medication and a sling for 6 weeks.

INDICATIONS FOR SURGERY

Although at the beginning of our intensive involvement with calcifying tendinitis we operated during the acute phase, we now believe that surgery is not indicated at a time when nature is attempting and usually succeeding in removing the calcific deposit. This approach was advocated in 1970 by De Sèze and Welfling,[41] who stated that in the hyperalgic phase, the disease generally heals easily with supportive measures only. In patients who meet the indications for arthroscopic surgery, this approach may be chosen.

CONCLUSION

The success of management of patients with calcifying tendinitis depends on a thorough understanding of the disease process. Obviously, formation of the deposit must precede its resorption. Moreover, clinical observations leave no doubt that spontaneous resorption usually takes place, the moment of the onset of resorption being the only question.

Factors responsible for the fibrocartilaginous metaplasia and ensuing calcification, as well as those triggering the resorptive process, are far from being known. Their elucidation should be the goal of future research.

Experimental reproduction of localized tendon calcification has not been too successful. Attempts were made at the level of the rotator cuff with the use of a plastic mold under the supraspinatus. This foreign body as well as the surgical trauma never led to changes compatible with calcifying tendinitis. Selye[163] published the results obtained with his calciphylaxis model, which led to tendon calcification in only one strain of mice. However, there is no question that calciphylaxis is a systemic metabolic disease and not a localized disease process. We have had the opportunity to examine specimens of tendon and ligament calcification in inbred tiptoe-walking Yoshimura (TWY) mice from the Japanese Research Council. The sections showed multiple sites of cartilaginous metaplasia in ligaments and tendons, followed by calcification around chondrocytes.

REFERENCES AND BIBLIOGRAPHY

1. Aina R, Cardinal E, Bureau NJ, et al: Calcific shoulder tendinitis: Treatment with modified US-guided fine-needle technique. Radiology 221:455-461, 2001.
2. Ali SY: Crystal induced arthropathy. In Verbruggen G and Veys EM (eds): Degenerative Joints, vol 2. New York: Elsevier, 1985.
3. Altcheck DW, Warren RF, Wickiewicz TL, et al: Arthroscopic acromioplasty. J Bone Joint Surg 72:1198-1207, 1990.
4. Anderson HC: Electron microscopic studies of induced cartilage development and calcification. J Cell Biol 35:81-101, 1967.
5. Anderson HC: Vesicles associated with calcification in the matrix of epiphyseal cartilage. J Cell Biol 41:59-72, 1969.
6. Anderson HC: Calcific diseases. Arch Pathol Lab Med 107:341-348, 1983.
7. Archer RS, Bayley JI, Archer CW, and Ali SY: Cell and matrix changes associated with pathological calcification of the human rotator cuff tendons. J Anat 182:1-11, 1993.
8. Ark JW, Flock TJ, Flatow EL, and Bigliani LU: Arthroscopic treatment of calcific tendinitis of the shoulder. Arthroscopy 8:183-188, 1992.
9. Baer WS: The operative treatment of subdeltoid bursitis. Johns Hopkins Hosp Bull 18:282-284, 1907.
10. Baird LW: Roentgen irradiation of calcareous deposits about the shoulder. Radiology 37:316-324, 1941.
11. Bateman JE: The Shoulder and Neck. Philadelphia: WB Saunders, 1978.
12. Bergemann D and Stieda A: Über die mit Kalkablagerungen einhergehende Entzündung der Schulterschleimbeutel. Munch Med Wochenschr 52:2699-2702, 1908.
13. Bigliani LU, Morrison DS, and April EW: The morphology of the acromion and its relationship to rotator cuff tears. Orthop Trans 10:228, 1986.
14. Bonucci E: Fine structure and histochemistry of "calcifying globules" in epiphyseal cartilage. Z Zellforsch 103:192-217, 1970.
15. Booth RE Jr and Marvel JP Jr: Differential diagnosis of shoulder pain. Orthop Clin North Am 6:353-379, 1975.
16. Bosworth BM: Examination of the shoulder for calcium deposits. J Bone Joint Surg 23:567-577, 1941.
17. Bosworth BM: Calcium deposits in the shoulder and subacromial bursitis: A survey of 12,122 shoulders. JAMA 116:2477-2482, 1941.
18. Brenckmann E and Nadaud P: Le traitement des calcifications périarticulaires de l'épaule par radiothérapie. Arch d'Electric Med 40:27-29, 1932.
19. Brewer BJ: Aging of the rotator cuff. Am J Sports Med 7:102-110, 1979.
20. Brickner WM: Shoulder disability: Stiff and painful shoulder. Am J Surg 26:196-204, 1912.
21. Brooks CH, Revell WJ, and Heatley FW: A quantitative histological study of the vascularity of the rotator cuff tendon. J Bone Joint Surg Br 74:151-153, 1992.
22. Brunner W, Thüringer R, Ascher G, et al: Die extrakorporelle Stosswellentherapie in der Orthopaedie—Drei-Monatsergebnisse in 443 Faellen. Orthop Praxis 33:461-464, 1997.
23. Buerger RA, Witzsch U, Haist J, et al: Extracorporeal shockwave therapy of pseudo-arthrosis. J Urol 147:26-29, 1992.
24. Carnett JB: The calcareous deposits of so-called calcifying subacromial bursitis. Surg Gynecol Obstet 41:404-421, 1925.
25. Caspari RB and Thal R: A technique for arthroscopic subacromial decompression. Arthroscopy 8:23, 1992.
26. Chapman JF: Subacromial bursitis and supraspinatus tendinitis: Its roentgen treatment. Calif Med 56:248-251, 1942.
27. Charrin N: Shockwave therapy under US guidance in rotator cuff calcific tendinitis. Rev Rhum Engl Ed 68:241-244, 2001.
28. Chiu CH: The role of high resolution of ultrasonography in the management of calcific tendinitis of the rotator cuff. Ultrasound Med Biol 27:735-743, 2001.
29. Codman EA: On stiff and painful shoulders. Boston Med Surg J 154:613-620, 1906.
30. Codman EA: Bursitis subacromialis, or periarthritis of the shoulder joint. Publications of the Mass Gen Hospital in Boston 2:521-591, 1909.
31. Codman EA: The Shoulder. Boston: Thomas Todd, 1934.
32. Constant CR and Murley AHG: A clinical method of functional assessment of the shoulder. Clin Orthop 214:160-164, 1987.
33. Crass JR: Current concepts in the radiographic evaluation of the rotator cuff. Crit Rev Diagn Imaging 28:23-73, 1988.
34. Daecke W, Kusnierczak D, and Loew M: Long-term effects of extracorporeal shockwave therapy in chronic calcific tendonitis of the shoulder. J Shoulder Elbow Surg 11:476-480, 2002.
35. Daecke W, Kusnierczak D, and Loew M: Extracorporale Stosswellentherapie (ESWT) bei der Tendinosis calcarea der Rotatorenmanschette. Orthopade 31:645-651, 2002.
36. Daecke W, Loew M, Schuhknecht B, and Kusnierczak D: Der Einfluss der Applikationsdosis auf die Wirksamkeit der ESWA bei der Tendinosis calcarea der Schulter. Orthop Praxis 33:119-123, 1997.
37. Dahmen GP, Meiss L, Nam VC, and Skroudies B: Extracorporale Stosswellentherapie (ESWT) zur Behandlung von knochennahem Weichteilbereich an der Schulter. Extracta Orthop 11:25-27, 1992.
38. Delius M and Draenert K: Einfluss hochenergetischer Stosswellen auf Knochen. In Siebert W (ed): Stosswellenanwendungen an Knochen. Hamburg, Germany: Dr. Kovac Verlag, 1997, pp 10-11.
39. DePalma A: Surgery of the Shoulder, 2nd ed. Philadelphia: JB Lippincott, 1973.
40. DePalma AF and Kruper JS: Long term study of shoulder joints afflicted with and treated for calcific tendinitis. Clin Orthop 20:61-72, 1961.
41. De Sèze S and Welfling J: Tendinites calcifiantes. Rhumatologie 22:5-14, 1970.
42. Dhuly RG, Lauler DP, and Thorn GW: Pharmacology and chemistry of adrenal glucocorticosteroids. Med Clin North Am 57:1155-1165, 1973.
43. Dieppe P: Crystal deposition disease and the soft tissues. Clin Rheum Dis 5:807-822, 1979.
44. Duplay S: De la périarthrite scapulohumérale et des raideurs de l'épaule qui en sont la conséquence. Arch Gen Med 513:542, 1872.
45. Ebenbichler GR, Erdogmus CB, Resch KL, et al: Ultrasound therapy for calcific tendonitis of the shoulder. N Engl J Med 340:1533-1538, 1999.
46. Ellman H: Arthroscopic subacromial decompression: Analysis of one- to three year results. Arthroscopy 3:173-181, 1987.
47. Ellman H: Shoulder arthroscopy: Current indications and techniques. Orthopedics 11:45-51, 1988.
48. Ellman H: The controversy of arthroscopic vs. open approaches to shoulder instability and rotator cuff disease. Paper presented at the Fourth Open Meeting of the American Society of Shoulder and Elbow Surgeons, 1988, Atlanta.
49. Farin PU and Jaroma H: Sonographic findings of rotator cuff calcifications. J Ultrasound Med 14:7-14, 1995.
50. Faure G and Daculsi G: Calcified tendinitis: A review. Ann Rheum Dis 42(suppl):49-53, 1983.
51. Faure G, Netter P, Malaman B, et al: Scanning electron microscopic study of microcrystals implicated in human rheumatic diseases. Scanning Electron Microsc 3:163-176, 1980.
52. Friedman MS: Calcified tendinitis of the shoulder. Am J Surg 94:56-61, 1957.
53. Fritze J: Extracorporeal shockwave therapy (ESWT) in orthopedic indications: A selective review. Versicherungsmedizin 50(5):180-185, 1998.
54. Gärtner J: Tendinosis calcarea—Behandlungsergebnisse mit dem Needling. Z Orthop Ihre Grenzgeb 131:461-469, 1993.
55. Gärtner J, Heyer A: Calcific tendonitis of the shoulder. Orthopade 24:284-302, 1995.
56. Ghormley JW: Calcareous tendinitis. Surg Clin North Am 4:1721-1728, 1961.
57. Gimblett PA, Saville J, and Eball P: A conservative management protocol for calcific tendinitis of the shoulder. J Manipulative Physiol Ther 22:622-627, 1999.
58. Glatthaar E: Zur Pathologie der Periarthritis humeroscapularis. Dtsch Z Chir 251:414-434, 1938.
59. Goutallier D, Duparc F, and Allain J: Treatment of calcific tendinopathies through a simple acromioplasty. Paper presented at the European Symposium of the Shoulder, April 26-28, 1996, St Etienne, France, pp 205-206.
60. Graff J, Richter KD, Pastor J: Wirkung hochenergetischer Stosswellen auf Knochengewebe. Verh Ges Urol 39:76, 1989.
61. Griffin EJ and Karselis TC: Physical agents for physical therapists. In Ultrasonic Energy, 2nd ed. Springfield, IL: Charles C Thomas, 1982.
62. Gschwend N, Patte D, and Zippel J: Die Therapie der Tendinitis calcarea des Schultergelenkes. Arch Orthop Unfallchir 73:120-135, 1972.
63. Gschwend N, Scherer M, and Löhr J: Die Tendinitis calcarea des Schultergelenkes. Orthopade 10:196-205, 1981.
64. Haake M, Sattler A, Gross MW, et al: [Comparison of extracorporeal shockwave therapy (ESWT) with roentgen irradiation in supraspinatus tendon syndrome—a prospective randomised single-blind parallel group comparison.] Z Orthop Ihre Grenzgeb 139:397-402, 2001.
65. Halverson PB, McCarty DJ, Cheung HS, and Ryan LM: Milwaukee shoulder syndrome. Ann Rheum Dis 43:734-741, 1984.

66. Harbin M: Deposition of calcium salts in tendon of supraspinatus muscle. Arch Surg 18:1491-1512, 1929.
67. Harmon HP: Methods and results in the treatment of 2580 painful shoulders. With special reference to calcific tendinitis and the frozen shoulder. Am J Surg 95:527-544, 1958.
68. Hartig A and Huth F: Neue Aspekte zur Morphologie und Therapie der Tendinosis calcarea der Schultergelenke. Arthroskopie 8:117-122, 1995.
69. Heller KD, Niethard FU: Der Einsatz der extracorporalen Stosswellentherapie in der Orthopaedie—eine Metanalyse. Z Orthop Ihre Grenzgeb 136:390-401, 1998.
70. Herberts P, Kadefors R, Hogfors C, and Sigholm G: Shoulder pain and heavy manual labor. Clin Orthop 191:166-178, 1984.
71. Hoe-Hansen CE, Palm L, and Norlin R: The influence of cuff pathology on shoulder function after arthroscopic subacromial decompression: A 3- and 6-year follow-up study. J Shoulder Elbow Surg 8:585-589, 1999.
72. Howorth MB: Calcification of the tendon cuff of the shoulder. Surg Gynecol Obstet 80:337-345, 1945.
73. Hsu HC, Wu JJ, Jim YF, et al: Calcific tendinitis and rotator cuff tearing: A clinical and radiographic study. J Shoulder Elbow Surg 3:159-164, 1994.
74. Hutchinson MR and Veenstra MA: Arthroscopic decompression of shoulder impingement secondary to os acromiale. Arthroscopy 9:28-32, 1993.
75. Jerosch J, Strauss JM, and Schmiel S: Arthroscopic therapy of tendinitis calcarea—acromioplasty or removal of calcium? Unfallchirurg 99:946-952, 1996.
76. Jerosch J, Strauss JM, and Schmiel S: Arthroscopic treatment of calcific tendinitis of the shoulder. J Shoulder Elbow Surg 7:30-37, 1998.
77. Johnson LL: The subacromial space and rotator cuff lesions. In Johnson LL (ed): Diagnostic and Surgical Arthroscopy of the Shoulder. St Louis: CV Mosby, 1993, pp 377-380.
78. Jones GB: Calcification of the supraspinatus tendon. J Bone Joint Surg Br 31:433-435, 1949.
79. Jozsa L, Baliut BJ, and Reffy A: Calcifying tendinopathy. Arch Orthop Trauma Surg 97:305-307, 1980.
80. Kempf JF: Arthroscopie de l'épaule. J Chir (Paris) 129:271-275, 1992.
81. Kempf JF: Arthroscopic treatment of rotator cuff calcifications by isolated excision. Paper presented at the European Symposium of the Shoulder, April 26-28, 1996, St Etienne, France, pp 206-209.
82. Kessel L and Watson M: The painful arc syndrome. J Bone Joint Surg Br 59:166-172, 1977.
83. Key LA: Calcium deposits in the vicinity of the shoulder and other joints. Ann Surg 129:737-753, 1949.
84. Kozin F: Painful shoulder and the reflex sympathetic dystrophy syndrome. In McCarty DJ (ed): Arthritis and Allied Conditions, 10th ed. Philadelphia: Lea & Febiger, 1985.
85. Lapidus PW: Infiltration therapy of acute tendinitis with calcification. Surg Gynecol Obstet 76:715-725, 1943.
86. Levigne C: Are there indications for adjunct acromioplasty in the arthroscopic treatment of rotator cuff calcifications? Paper presented at the European Symposium of the Shoulder, April 26-28, 1996, St Etienne, France, pp 206-209.
87. Lippmann RK: Observations concerning the calcific cuff deposit. Clin Orthop 20:49-60, 1961.
88. Litchman HM, Silver CM, Simon SD, and Eshragi A: The surgical management of calcific tendinitis of the shoulder. Int Surg 50:474-482, 1968.
89. Loehr JF and Uhthoff HK: The microvascular pattern of the supraspinatus tendon. Clin Orthop 254:35-38, 1990.
90. Loew M, Daecke W, Kusnierczak D, et al: Shock-wave therapy is effective for chronic calcifying tendinitis of the shoulder. J Bone Joint Surg Br 81:863-867, 1999.
91. Loew M and Jurgowski W: Initial experiences with extracorporeal shockwave lithotripsy (ESWL) in treatment of tendinosis calcarea of the shoulder. Z Orthop Ihre Grenzgeb 131:470-473, 1993.
92. Loew M, Jurgowski W, Mau HC, and Thomsen M: Treatment of calcifying tendinitis of the rotator cuff with extracorporeal shock waves: A preliminary report. J Shoulder Elbow Surg 4:101-106, 1995.
93. Loew M, Jurgowski W, and Thomsen M: Die Wirkung extracorporaler Stosswellen auf die Tendinosis calcarea der Schulter—Ein vorlaeufiger Bericht. Urologe A 34:49-53, 1995.
94. Loew M, Sabo D, Mau H, et al: MR imaging of the rotator cuff with calcifying tendinitis [abstract FH 060]. Paper presented at the 6th International Congress on Surgery of the Shoulder (ICSS), June 1995, Helsinki, Finland.
95. Lundberg J: The frozen shoulder. Acta Orthop Scand 119(suppl):1-59, 1969.
96. Macnab I: Rotator cuff tendinitis. Ann R Coll Surg 53:271-287, 1973.
97. Maier M, Durr HR, Kohler S, et al: Analgesic effect of low energy extracorporeal shock waves in tendinosis calcarea, epicondylitis humeri radialis and plantar fasciitis. Z Orthop Ihre Grenzgeb 138:34-38, 2000.
97a. Maier M, Lieb A, Köhler S, and Refoir HJ: Stosswellenbehandlung bei Tendinosis calcarea der Schulter—das Therapieergebnis ist unabhängig von der Grösse der Verkalkung. Orthopadische Praxis 39:290-293, 2003.
98. Maier M, Stabler A, Schmitz C, et al: On the impact of calcified deposits within the rotator cuff tendons in shoulders of patients with shoulder pain and dysfunction. Arch Orthop Trauma Surg 121:371-378, 2001.
99. McCarty DJ, Halverson PB, Carrera GF, et al: "Milwaukee shoulder": Association of microspheroids containing hydroxyapatite crystals, active collagenase, and neutral protease with rotator cuff defects. I. Clinical aspects. Arthritis Rheum 24:464-473, 1981.

100. McKendry RJR, Uhthoff HK, Sarkar K, and St George-Hyslop P: Calcifying tendinitis of the shoulder: Prognostic value of clinical, histologic and radiologic features in 57 surgically treated cases. Rheumatology 9:75-80, 1982.
101. McLaughlin HL: Lesions of the musculotendinous cuff of the shoulder. III. Observations on the pathology, course and treatment of calcific deposits. Ann Surg 124:354-362, 1946.
102. McLaughlin HL: Selection of calcium deposits for operation—the technique and results of operation. Surg Clin North Am 43:1501-1504, 1963.
103. Meyer AW: Chronic functional lesions of the shoulder. Arch Surg 35:646-674, 1937.
104. Milone FP and Copeland MM: Calcific tendinitis of the shoulder joint. AJR Am J Roentgenol 85:901-913, 1961.
105. Mohr W and Bilger S: Morphologische Grundstrukturen der kalzifizierten Tendopathie und ihre Bedeutung für die Pathogenese. Z Rheumatol 49:346-355, 1990.
106. Molé D, Kempf JF, Gleyze P, et al: Résultats du traitement arthroscopique des tendinopathies non-rompues de la coiffe des rotateurs. 2. Calcifications de la coiffe. Rev Chir Orthop Reparative Appar Mot 79:532-541, 1993.
107. Morimoto K, Mori E, Nakagawa Y: Calcification of the coracoacromial ligament. A case report of the shoulder impingement syndrome. Am J Sports Med 16:80-81, 1988.
108. Moschkowitz E: Histopathology of calcification of the spinatus tendons associated with subacromial bursitis. Am J Med Sci 149:351-361, 1915.
109. Moseley HF: Shoulder Lesions, 3rd ed. Edinburgh: Churchill Livingstone, 1960.
110. Moseley HF: The natural history and clinical syndromes produced by calcified deposits in the rotator cuff. Surg Clin North Am 43:1489-1494, 1963.
111. Moseley HF: The results of nonoperative and operative treatment of calcified deposits. Surg Clin North Am 43:1505-1506, 1963.
112. Moseley HF and Goldie I: The arterial pattern of the rotator cuff of the shoulder. J Bone Joint Surg Br 45:780-789, 1963.
113. Murnaghan GF and McIntosh D: Hydrocortisone in painful shoulder. Controlled trial. Lancet 21:798-800, 1955.
114. Nakase T, Takeuchi E, Sugamoto K: Involvement of multinucleated giant cells synthesizing cathepsin K in calcified tendinitis of the rotator cuff tendons. Rheumatology 39:1074-1077, 2000.
115. Neer CS II: Impingement lesions. Clin Orthop 173:70-77, 1983.
116. Neer CS II, Craig EV, and Fukuda H: Cuff-tear arthropathy. J Bone Joint Surg Am 65:1232-1244, 1983.
117. Nutton RW, McBirnie JM, and Phillips C: Treatment of chronic rotator-cuff impingement by arthroscopic subacromial decompression. J Bone Joint Surg Br 79:73-76, 1997.
118. Nutton RW and Stothard J: Acute calcific supraspinatus tendinitis in a three year old child. J Bone Joint Surg Br 69:148, 1987.
119. Ollagnier E, Bruyère G, Gazielly DF, and Thomas TH: Medical treatment of calcifying tendinopathies of the rotator cuff. Paper presented at the European Symposium of the Shoulder, April 26-28, 1996, St Etienne, France, p 202.
119a. O'Leary ST, Goldberg JA, and Walsh WR: Tophaceous gout of the rotator cuff: A case report. J Shoulder Elbow Surg 12:200-201, 2003.
120. Olsson O: Degenerative changes of the shoulder and their connection with shoulder pain. Acta Chir Scand 181(suppl):1-110, 1953.
121. Orhan Z, Alper M, Akman Y, et al: An experimental study on the application of extracorporeal shock waves in the treatment of tendon injuries: Preliminary report. J Orthop Sci 6:566-570, 2001.
122. Ozaki J, Fuijimoto S, Nakagawa Y, et al: Tears of the rotator cuff of the shoulder associated with pathological changes in the acromion. J Bone Joint Surg Am 70:1224-1230, 1988.
123. Painter CF: Subdeltoid bursitis. Boston Med Surg J 156:345-349, 1907.
124. Patel VR, Singh D, Calvert PT, and Bayley JI: Arthroscopic subacromial decompression: Results and factors affecting outcome. J Shoulder Elbow Surg 8:231-237, 1999.
125. Patte D and Goutallier D: Calcifications. Rev Chir Orthop 74:277-278, 1988.
126. Patterson RL and Darrach W: Treatment of acute bursitis by needle irrigation. J Bone Joint Surg 19:993-1002, 1937.
127. Pedersen HE and Key JA: Pathology of calcareous tendinitis and subdeltoid bursitis. Arch Surg 62:50-63, 1951.
128. Pendergrass EP and Hodes PJ: Roentgen irradiation in treatment of inflammations. AJR Am J Roentgenol 45:74-106, 1941.
129. Perlick L, Korth O, Wallny T, et al: [The mechanical effects of shock waves in extracorporeal shock wave treatment of calcific tendinitis—an in-vitro model.] Z Orthop Ihre Grenzgeb 137:10-16, 1999.
130. Perugia L and Postacchini F: The pathology of the rotator cuff of the shoulder. Ital J Orthop Haematol 11:93-105, 1985.
131. Pfister J and Gerber H: Behandlung der Periarthropathia humeroscapularis calcarea mittels Schulterkalkspülung: Retrospektive Fragebogenanalyse. Z Orthop Ihre Grenzgeb 132:300-305, 1994.
132. Pfister J, Gerber HJ: Chronic calcifying tendinitis of the shoulder—therapy by percutaneous needle aspiration and lavage: A prospective open study of 62 shoulders. Clin Rheumatol 16:269-274, 1997.
133. Pigozzi F, Giombini A, Parisi A, et al: The application of shock-waves therapy in the treatment of resistant chronic painful shoulder. A clinical experience. J Sports Med Phys Fitness 40:356-361, 2000.
134. Pinals RS and Short CL: Calcific periarthritis involving multiple sites. Arthritis Rheum 9:566-574, 1966.

135. Plenk HP: Calcifying tendinitis of the shoulder. Radiology 59:384-389, 1952.
136. Rathbun JB and Macnab J: The microvascular pattern of the rotator cuff. J Bone Joint Surg Br 52:540-553, 1970.
137. Re LP Jr and Karzel RP: Management of rotator cuff calcifications. Orthop Clin North Am 24:125-132, 1993.
138. Remberger K, Faust H, and Keyl W: Tendinitis calcarea. Klinik, Morphologie, Pathogenese und Differentialdiagnose. Pathologe 6:196-203, 1985.
139. Resch H: Calcific Tendinitis. Paper presented at the European Symposium of the Shoulder, April 26-28, 1996, St Etienne, France, p 210.
140. Resch H and Beck E: Arthroskopie der Schulter. Berlin, Springer-Verlag, 1991, pp 147-152.
141. Rochwerger A, Franceschi JP, Viton JM, et al: Surgical management of calcific tendinitis of the shoulder: An analysis of 26 cases. Clin Rheumatol 18:313-316, 1999.
142. Rompe JD, Burger R, Hopf C, and Eysel P: Shoulder function after extracorporeal shock wave therapy for calcific tendinitis. J Shoulder Elbow Surg 7:505-509, 1998.
143. Rompe JD, Kuellmer K, Vogel J, et al: Extracorporale Stossswellentherapie—Experimentelle Grundlagen, klinischer Einsatz. Orthopade 26:215-228, 1997.
144. Rompe JD, Rummler F, Hopf C, et al: Extracorporeal shock wave therapy for calcifying tendinitis of the shoulder. Clin Orthop 321:196-201, 1995.
145. Rompe JD, Zoellner J, and Nafe B; Shockwave therapy versus conventional surgery in the treatment of calcifying tendinitis of the shoulder. Clin Orthop 387:72-82, 2001.
146. Rompe JD, Zollner J, Nafe B, and Freitag C: [Significance of calcium deposit elimination in tendinosis calcarea of the shoulder.] Z Orthop Ihre Grenzgeb 138:335-339, 2000.
147. Rothman RH, Marvel JP Jr, and Heppenstall RB: Anatomic considerations in the glenohumeral joint. Orthop Clin North Am 6:341-352, 1975.
148. Rothman RH and Parke WW: The vascular anatomy of the rotator cuff. Clin Orthop 41:176-186, 1965.
149. Rowe CR: Injection technique for the shoulder and elbow. Orthop Clin North Am 19:773-777, 1988.
150. Rupp S, Seil R, and Kohn D: Preoperative ultrasonic mapping of calcium deposits facilitates localization during arthroscopic surgery for calcifying tendinitis of the rotator cuff. Arthroscopy 14:540-542, 1998.
151. Rupp S, Seil R, and Kohn D: Tendinosis calcarea of the rotator cuff. Orthopade 29:852-867, 2000.
152. Rüttimann G: Uber die Häufigkeit röntgenologischer Veränderungen bei Patienten mit typischer Periarthritis humeroscapularis und Schultergesunden. Inaugural Dissertation, Zurich, 1959.
153. Sandström C: Peritendinitis calcarea: Common disease of middle life: Its diagnosis, pathology and treatment. AJR Am J Roentgenol 40:1-21, 1938.
154. Sandström C and Wahlgren F: Beitrag zur Kenntnis der "Peritendinitis calcarea" (sog. "Bursitis calculosa") speziell vom pathologisch-histologischen Gesichtspunkt. Acta Radiol (Stockh) 18:263-296, 1937.
155. Sarkar K and Uthoff HK: Ultrastructural localization of calcium in calcifying tendinitis. Arch Pathol Lab Med 102:266-269, 1978.
156. Sarkar K and Uthoff HK: Ultrastructure of the subacromial bursa in painful shoulder syndromes. Virchows Arch 400:107-117, 1983.
157. Schaer H: Die Periarthritis humeroscapularis. Ergebn Chir Orthop 29:211-309, 1936.
158. Schaer H: Die Duplay'sche Krankheit. Med Klin 35:413-415, 1939.
159. Schiepers P, Pauwels P, Penders W, et al: The role of arthroscopy in subacromial pathology. Retrospective study of a series of arthroscopic acromioplasties. Acta Orthop Belg 66:438-448, 2000.
160. Schmitt J, Haake M, Tosch A, et al: Low-energy extracorporeal shock-wave treatment (ESWT) for tendinitis of the supraspinatus. A prospective, randomised study. J Bone Joint Surg Br 83:873-876, 2001.
161. Seifert G: Morphologic and biochemical aspects of experimental extraosseous tissue calcification. Clin Orthop 69:146, 1970.
162. Seil R, Rupp S, Hammer DS, et al: [Extracorporeal shockwave therapy in tendinosis calcarea of the rotator cuff: Comparison of different treatment protocols.] Z Orthop Ihre Grenzgeb 137:310-315, 1999.
163. Selye H: The experimental production of calcific deposits in the rotator cuff. Surg Clin North Am 43:1483-1488, 1963.
164. Sengar DPS, McKendry RJ, and Uthoff HK: Increased frequency of HLA-A1 in calcifying tendinitis. Tissue Antigens 29:173-174, 1987.
165. Simon WH: Soft tissue disorders of the shoulder. Frozen shoulder, calcific tendinitis, and bicipital tendinitis. Orthop Clin North Am 6:521-539, 1975.
166. Snyder SJ: Arthroscopic evaluation and treatment of the rotator cuff. In Snyder SJ (ed): Shoulder Arthroscopy. New York: McGraw-Hill, 1993.
167. Speed CA and Hazleman BL: Calcific tendinitis of the shoulder. N Engl J Med 340:1582-1584, 1999.
168. Speed CA, Richards C, Nichols D, et al: Extracorporeal shock-wave therapy for tendonitis of the rotator cuff. J Bone Joint Surg Br 84:509-512, 2001.

169. Steinacker T and Steuer M: Use of extracorporeal shockwave therapy (ESWT) in sports orthopedics. Sportverletz Sportschaden 15:45-49, 2001.
170. Steinbrocker O: The painful shoulder. In Hollander JE (ed): Arthritis and Allied Conditions, 8th ed. Philadelphia: Lea & Febiger, 1972.
171. Stephens SR, Warren RF, Payne LZ, et al: Arthroscopic acromioplasty: A 6- to 10-year follow-up. Arthroscopy 14:382-388, 1998.
172. Stieda A: Zur Pathologie der Schultergelenkschleimbeutel. Arch Klin Chir 85:910-924, 1908.
173. Takeuchi E and Sugamoto K: Localization and expression of osteopontin in the rotator cuff tendon in patients with calcifying tendinitis. Virchows Arch 438:612-617, 2001.
174. Thornhill TS: The painful shoulder. In Kelley WN, Harris ED, Shaun R, and Sledge CB (eds): Textbook of Rheumatology, 2nd ed. Philadelphia: WB Saunders, 1985.
175. Tillander BM and Norlin RO: Change of calcifications after arthroscopic subacromial decompression. J Shoulder Elbow Surg 7:213-217, 1998.
176. Tillmann B: Rotatorenmanschettenrupturen. Operative Orthop Traumatol 4:181-184, 1992.
177. Toriyama K, Fukuda H, Hamada K, and Noguchi T: Calcifying tendinitis of the infraspinatus tendon simulating a bone tumor. J Shoulder Elbow Surg 3:165-168, 1994.
178. Uthoff HK: Calcifying tendinitis, an active cell-mediated calcification. Virchows Arch 366:51-58, 1975.
179. Uthoff HK, Hammond DI, Sarkar K, et al: The role of the coracoacromial ligament in the impingement syndrome: A clinical, radiological and histological study. Int Orthop 12:97-104, 1988.
180. Uthoff HK and Loehr J: Calcifying tendinitis. In Rockwood CA and Matsen FA (eds): The Shoulder, 2nd ed. Philadelphia: WB Saunders, 1998, pp 989-1008.
181. Uthoff HK, Loehr J, Hammond I, and Sarkar K: Aetiologie und Pathogenese von Rupturen der Rotatorenmanschette. In Helbig B and Blauth W (eds): Schulterschmerzen und Rupturen der Rotatorenmanschette. Berlin: Springer-Verlag, 1986, pp 3-9.
182. Uthoff HK, Loehr J, and Sarkar K: The pathogenesis of rotator cuff tears. In Takagishi N (ed): The Shoulder. Tokyo: Professional Postgraduate Services, 1986, pp 211-212.
183. Uthoff HK and Sarkar K: Tendopathia calcificans. Beitr Orthop Traumatol 28:269-277, 1981.
184. Uthoff HK, Sarkar K, and Hammond I: Die Bedeutung der Dichte und der Schärfe der Abgrenzung des Kalkschattens bei der Tendinopathia calcificans. Radiologe 22:170-174, 1982.
185. Uthoff HK, Sarkar K, and Maynard JA: Calcifying tendinitis. Clin Orthop 118:164-168, 1976.
186. Valchanou VD and Michailov P: High energy shock waves in the treatment of delayed and non union of fractures. Int Orthop 15:181-184, 1991.
187. Vebostad A: Calcific tendinitis in the shoulder region: A review of 43 operated shoulders. Acta Orthop Scand 46:205-210, 1975.
188. Vogel J, Hopf C, Eysel P, and Rompe JD: Application of extracorporeal shock-waves in the treatment of pseudarthrosis of the lower extremity—Preliminary results. Arch Orthop Trauma Surg 116:480-483, 1997.
189. Wang CJ, Ko JY, and Chen HS: Treatment of calcifying tendinitis of the shoulder with shock wave therapy. Clin Orthop 387:83-89, 2001.
190. Watson M: The impingement syndrome in sportsmen. In Bateman JE and Welsh RP (eds): Surgery of the Shoulder. Philadelphia: BC Decker, 1984, pp 140-142.
191. Welfling J, Kahn MF, Desroy M, et al: Les calcifications de l'épaule. II. La maladie des calcifications tendineuses multiples. Rev Rheum 32:325-334, 1965.
192. White AG: Book reviews. J Bone Joint Surg Br 84:1208, 2002.
193. Wilson CL: Lesions of the supraspinatus tendon: Degeneration, rupture and calcification. Arch Surg 46:307-325, 1943.
194. Wittenberg RH, Rubenthaler F, Wolk T, et al: Surgical or conservative treatment for chronic rotator cuff calcifying tendinitis—a matched-pair analysis of 100 patients. Arch Orthop Trauma Surg 121:56-59, 2001.
195. Wolf WB: Shoulder tendinoses. Clin Sports Med 11:871-890, 1992.
196. Wolfgang GL: Surgical repairs of the rotator cuff of the shoulder. J Bone Joint Surg Am 56:14-26, 1974.
197. Wolk T and Wittenberg RH: [Calcifying subacromial syndrome—clinical and ultrasound outcome of non-surgical therapy.] Z Orthop Ihre Grenzgeb 135:451-457, 1997.
198. Wrede L: Über Kalkablagerungen in der Umgebung des Schultergelenkes und ihre Beziehungen zur Periarthritis humeroscapularis. Langenbecks Arch Chir 99:259-272, 1912.
199. Young BR: Roentgen treatment for bursitis of shoulder. AJR Am J Roentgenol 56:626-630, 1946.

CHAPTER 19

THE BICEPS TENDON

W. Z. (Biceps Buzzy) Burkhead, Jr., M.D.,   Michel A. Arcand, M.D.,   Craig Zeman, M.D.,
Peter Habermeyer, M.D.,   and Gilles Walch, M.D.

• • • •

"Charlie Neer's never seen biceps tendinitis. Frank Jobe's never seen biceps tendinitis. I've never seen biceps tendinitis. You've been here from Dallas for 24 hours and you've seen a case of biceps tendinitis?" I'm going to find you a dermatology residency at Duke and send you there on a bus!!!

- C.A.R. to W.Z.B.
July 2, 1983, 1:15 p.m.
Audie Murphy VA
The day I thought my career ended.

In 1983 it was not uncommon to see patients who had undergone isolated biceps tenodesis when in reality their symptoms emanated from rotator cuff disease and impingement syndrome, thus Dr. Rockwood's above admonition. It is quixotic to think, however, that the biceps escapes the degenerative process or is unable to produce symptoms on its own or in conjunction with other pathologic entities of the shoulder.

The long head of the biceps brachii is the proverbial stepchild of the shoulder. It has been blamed for numerous painful conditions of the shoulder from arthritis to adhesive capsulitis. Kessell and Watson[144] described the tendon as "somewhat of a maverick, easy to inculpate but difficult to condemn." Lippman[158] likened the long head of the biceps to the appendix: "An unimportant vestigial structure unless something goes wrong with it." Throughout time this tendon has been tenodesed, translocated, pulled through drill holes in the humeral head, débrided with an arthroscope, and tenotomized, sometimes with marginal results.

Exposure of the biceps by the French surgeon Patte,[113] as well as arthroscopy, has shed new light on the pathophysiology of the long biceps tendon. The advent of magnetic resonance imaging (MRI) used for diagnostic purposes around the shoulder has allowed clinicians to visualize this tendon through a noninvasive imaging modality. These new techniques have provided fundamental insight into shoulder pathology, which in turn has yielded important implications in the treatment of lesions of the long head of the biceps tendon.

This chapter will present a historical perspective of treatment of lesions of the biceps tendon, review the pertinent anatomy, attempt to explain the function of this tendon, and present a review of current concepts on the etiology, diagnosis, and management of these lesions.

HISTORICAL REVIEW

Hippocrates[123] was the first to call attention to the possibility of pathologic displacement of muscle and tendons in dislocations. Accurate depictions of the anatomy of the biceps region and intertubercular groove appeared in the 1400s (Fig. 19-1A). Traumatic injuries to the bicipital region are depicted in a German wound manikin in the 1500s (Fig. 19-1B).

The first reported case of dislocation of the tendon of the long head of the biceps brachii muscle was in 1694 by William Cowper in a book titled *Myotoma Reformata.*[59] In his case, a woman who was wringing clothes felt something displace in her shoulder. Three days after the injury he examined her and noticed a depression of the external part of the deltoid, accompanied by rigidity in the lower biceps and an inability to extend the forearm. The tendon was reduced by manipulation and the patient immediately recovered use of the arm. This miraculous recovery is seldom seen in our practice. Recognition of this injury was accepted by Boerhaave and Bromfield.[33] Cowper's observation became subject to suspicion, though, because of his plagiarism of the Dutch anatomist Godfried Bidloo.[27] Before Cowper's description, most reported cases of biceps injury were undoubtedly a result of direct trauma, most likely as depicted in Figure 19-1B.

In 1803, Monteggia[199] reported a second case resembling that of Cowper's, except that the dislocation was habitual. From that time until 1910, numerous additional clinical reports appeared.[110,114,235,248,249] It was not until 1841 that Soden[271] reported a case of biceps dislocation that was clinically proven at necropsy. Hueter[130] clearly described the signs and symptoms of lesions of this tendon.

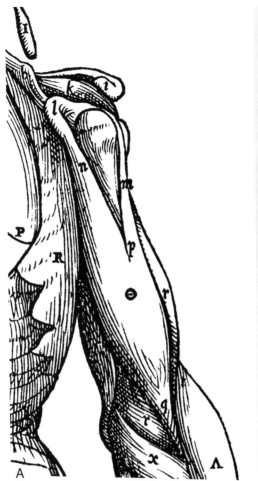

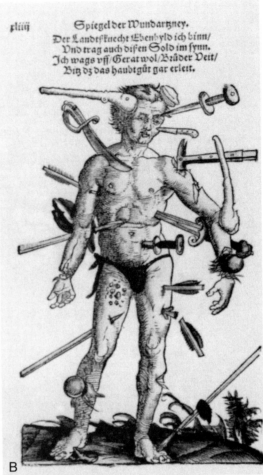

■ Figure 19–1
A, Close-up of the three tendons of the biceps brachii: short head (N), long head (M), distal tendon (Q). *(From the Sixth Plate of Muscles. Possibly by Jan Stevenz van Calcar [Flemish ca. 1499-1550]. From Andreas Vesalius: DeHumani Corporis Fabrica. Basel: Johannes Oporinus, 1543).* **B,** Probable mechanism of injury to the biceps before Cowper's description. Notice the saber-type incision in the opposite shoulder. *(Anonymous wound manikin, 1517. From von Gersdorff H: Feldthbuch der Wundartzney. Strasbourg: Hans Schotten, 1540.) (Reprinted with permission from Karp D: ARS Medica: Art, Medicine, and the Human Condition. Philadelphia, Copyright © 1985, the University of Pennsylvania Press.)*

However, there was controversy. Jarjavey,[136] discussing cases in 1867, believed that most of the symptoms were related to subacromial bursitis and that simple luxation did not exist. Some authors[12,33] believed that the lesion was secondary to arthritis or concomitant problems. Callender[36] mentioned one case of recurring dislocation in which the tendon could not be retained in the groove because of fibrous tissue. Duplay[73-75] described "periarthrite scapulo-humerale." It is evident from his work that this condition included tendinitis of the biceps.

McClellan[175] discussed the function of the biceps tendon:

Furthermore, the long tendon of the biceps muscle which is lodged below the tuberosities pierces the capsular ligament and passes over the head of the humerus to the top of the glenoid cavity, strengthens the upper anterior part of the joint and prevents the head of the humerus from being brought against the acromion, processing the normal upward movements of the arm. In fact it is mainly by the normal position of this tendon, assisted somewhat by atmos-

pheric pressure, that the head of the humerus is retained in its natural position.

Bera[25] in 1910 believed that osteitis reduced the height of the lesser tuberosity and thus led to instability. In the 1920s, valuable contributions were made by Meyer.[183-190] He discussed his observations based on a total of 59 cases of spontaneous dislocation of the long head of the tendon and 20 cases of complete rupture. He was the first to describe the supratubercular ridge (Fig. 19–2), degenerative changes on the undersurface of the acromion, the acromioclavicular joint, and the coracoacromial ligament. Meyer concluded that attrition, particularly after use of the extremity in abduction and external rotation, led to gradual destruction of the capsule proximal to and in the region of the lesser tuberosity. Dislocation ensued as a consequence of weakness of the capsule in this region.

According to Schrager,[262] F. Pasteur,[236] then medical colonel of the military hospital at Val de Gras, recognized the condition of bicipital tendinitis in all its aspects, described it fully, and raised it to the status of a distinct

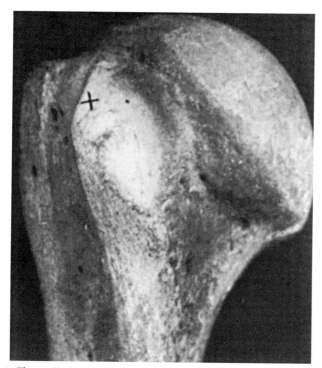

■ **Figure 19–2**
Original photograph of the supratubercular ridge taken by Meyer.
(From Gilcreest EL: Dislocation and elongation of the long head of the biceps brachii. Analysis of six cases. Ann Surg 104:118-138, 1936.)

clinical entity. In 1934, the specificity of the diagnosis of biceps tendinitis was questioned by Codman,[50] who wrote, "Personally, I believe that the sheath of the biceps is less apt to be involved than are other structures. I have never proved its involvement in a single case. I think that the substance of the tendon of the supraspinatus is most often involved." In the 1940s, Lippmann,[157,158] Tarsy,[279] and Hitchcock and Bechtol[124] all believed that bicipital tendinitis was an important cause of shoulder pain and individually described operations for the relief of symptoms. In 1950, DePalma[66] described degenerative changes in the biceps tendon that occurred with aging and reported on both operative and conservative management. Although he was grateful that more surgeons were recognizing the disorder (bicipital tendinitis), he thought that many were still reluctant to give this disorder the importance it deserved. Based on gross and microscopic examination in 78 cases, he concluded that bicipital groove tenosynovitis is the most common cause of a painful and stiff shoulder.

In 1972, Neer[207] described the anterior impingement syndrome, in which anterior acromial spurring with thickening and fibrosis of the coracoacromial ligament causes impingement wear on the rotator cuff and biceps tendon. He pointed out a close association between rupture of the biceps tendon and rotator cuff tears.

Although the pendulum had swung away from primary bicipital tendinitis and isolated biceps tendon instability over the past 30 years, it now appears to be swinging back. Several authors have published results of the diagnosis and treatment of isolated biceps tendinitis and dislocation. O'Donohue[222] reported on surgical techniques for treating the subluxating biceps tendon in

athletes. Neviaser and colleagues[219] recommended tenodesis of the biceps at the time of acromioplasty and excision of the distal part of the clavicle as part of the four-in-one arthroplasty, and in 1987, Post[244] presented a series of patients with primary bicipital tenosynovitis.

In the late 1980s and early 1990s, the frequent use of MRI and arthroscopy to visualize the long head of the biceps tendon has provided valuable insight into biceps pathology. In 1985, Andrews and coauthors[9] described tears in the superior labrum of the glenohumeral joint at its attachment to the biceps tendon. In 1990, Snyder and colleagues[270] first described the superolabral anterior-to-posterior (SLAP) lesion. They classified this lesion of the superior glenoid labrum and biceps anchor into four types.

Walch[294,295] classified both subluxations and dislocations of the biceps tendon in the early 1990s. Since then, he has gone on to identify pulley lesions. Pulley lesions involve the rotator interval and cuff. These "hidden" lesions[297] affect the stabilizers of the long head of the biceps tendon. He stated that they are not always visible on arthroscopic examination and may sometimes require open exploration of the rotator interval to identify them. Study of these lesions has directly incriminated the superior glenohumeral and coracohumeral ligaments and the subscapularis and supraspinatus in the process of biceps subluxation and dislocation. Bennet[23] has shown that good visualization of the rotator interval, including the coracohumeral and superior glenohumeral ligaments, is possible with the arthroscope. Placement of the arm in flexion and internal rotation improves the arthroscopist's ability to see these structures and even allows probing of the area. It has been over 300 years since Cowper[59] described his first case, and despite an increasing amount of research, controversy over the importance of this lesion still exists.

ANATOMY

The long head of the biceps brachii originates, in most cases, at the supraglenoid tubercle and glenoid labrum in the superior-most portion of the glenoid (Fig. 19–3). Some authors[168,224] have described absence of the intra-articular portion of the long head of the biceps or an extra-articular structure. The tendon itself is approximately 9 cm long. At its origin the tendon presents a variable insertion type. It may be bifurcated, trifurcated, or present with a single insertion point.

In a study by Habermeyer and associates,[112] the biceps was found to originate off the supraglenoid tubercle in 20% of specimens studied. Its origin was off the superior posterior aspect of the labrum in 48% of specimens studied, and 28% of specimens had origins from both the tubercle and the labrum.

In a different study, Pal and coworkers[232] showed that in 70% of specimens examined, the biceps tendon origin was mostly off the posterosuperior portion of the glenoid labrum. Usually, only a small part of the tendon was attached to the supraglenoid tubercle in these specimens. However, in 25% of specimens, a major portion of the biceps tendon was attached to the supraglenoid tubercle.

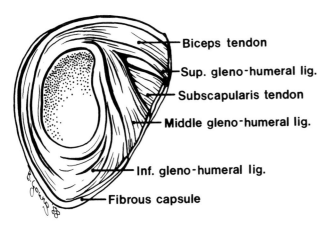

■ **Figure 19–3**
The biceps tendon is seen inserting on the superior-most portion of the glenoid labrum. Its origin may be simple, bifurcated, or trifurcated.

A close association was noted between the glenoid labrum and the biceps tendon, both grossly and histologically by Cooper and collaborators.[56] Primary attachment of the biceps tendon to the superior portion of the labrum was noted before it inserted onto the supraglenoid tubercle. Collagen fibers of the labrum and biceps tendon were found to be intimately blended in this area.

In a study by Vangsness and colleagues,[287] 105 cadaveric shoulders were dissected to investigate the origin of the biceps tendon from the labrum and its relationship to the supratubercular groove. They classified insertions into four types (Fig. 19–4). Type I, which occurred in 22% of specimens, had a labral attachment that was entirely posterior with no contribution to the anterior labrum. In type II, the labral contribution was mostly posterior with a small anterior band present; this type occurred in 33% of their specimens. Type III insertion had an equal contribution to both the anterior and posterior labrum and was found in 37% of their specimens. Type IV origins occurred in 8% of specimens and showed a mostly anterior labral contribution to the biceps origin.

The cross-sectional characteristics of the long head of the biceps change during its course from the supraglenoid tubercle down to the musculotendinous junction. At its origin, the tendon measures 8.5 × 7.8 mm. In the area of strongest demand, the entrance to the bicipital sulcus, the tendon measures 4.7 × 2.6 mm. Finally, at its musculotendinous junction, the tendon measures 4.5 × 2.8 mm.[121]

McGough and associates tested the tensile properties of the long head of the biceps tendon in specimens without demonstrable pathology.[177,178] They measured the cross-sectional area of the biceps tendon in three areas—proximal, middle, and distal. The tendon was found to be 22.7 ± 9.3 mm², 22.7 ± 3.5 mm², and 10.8 ± 2.8 mm², respectively. There was no statistically significant difference between the three regions. A difference in shape of the tendon was found between the proximal and middle portions of the long head of the biceps tendon. The proximal part of the tendon was flatter and tended to become more circular as it entered the bicipital groove. Cyclic stress relaxation was 18% ± 4% for the specimens. The ultimate tensile strength and ultimate strain and strain energy density were measured for all the specimens, and the results of these tests were 32.5 ± 5.3 MPa, 10.1% ± 2.7%, and 1.9 ± 0.4 MPa, respectively. The modulus of elasticity was calculated to be 421 ± 212 MPa. The mode of failure of the tendons was complete rupture within the midpoint of the tendon substance in all cases.

The course of the long head of the biceps tendon is oblique over the top of the humeral head and down into the bicipital (intertubercular) groove. Once out of the groove, the tendon continues down the ventral portion of the humerus and becomes musculotendinous near the insertion of the deltoid and the pectoralis major.

The angle formed by a line from the bottom of the groove to a central point on the humeral head is constant and corresponds to the retrotorsion angle measured from the epicondyles (Fig. 19–5).[104] This angle is important and can be used as a guide when placing a humeral head prosthesis. The bicipital tendon, though intra-articular, is extrasynovial. The synovial sheath reflects on itself to form a visceral sheath that encases the biceps tendon (Fig. 19–6). The sheath is open, communicates directly with the glenohumeral joint, and ends in a blind pouch at the level of the bicipital groove.

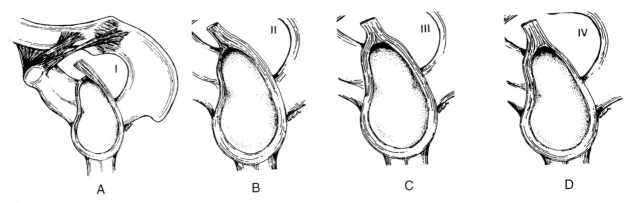

■ **Figure 19–4**
A, Type I: The labral attachment is entirely posterior, with no contribution to the anterior labrum (22%). **B,** Type II: Most of the labral contribution is posterior (33%). **C,** Type III: There are equal contributions to both the anterior and the posterior parts of the labrum (37%). **D,** Type IV: Most of the labral contribution is anterior, with a small contribution to the posterior labrum (8%). *(From Vangsness CT Jr, Jorgenson SS, Watson T, and Johnson DL: The origin of the long head of the biceps from the scapula and glenoid labrum. An anatomical study of 100 shoulders. J Bone Joint Surg Br 76:951-954, 1994.)*

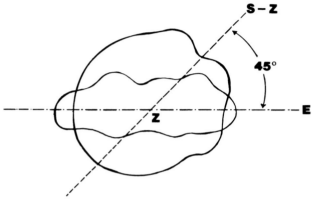

■ **Figure 19–5**

A line (S-Z) drawn through the center of the bottom of the bicipital groove and intersecting with a line drawn across the humeral condyles (E) accurately depicts retroversion of the humeral head. *(Redrawn from Habermeyer P, Kaiser E, Knappe M, et al: Functional anatomy and biomechanics of the long biceps tendon. Unfallchirurg 90:319–329, 1987.)*

The long head of the biceps muscle receives its blood supply from the brachial artery. Three arteries supply blood to the bicipital tendon. The distal portion of the tendon receives branches from the deep brachial artery. The proximal part of the tendon also receives branches from the anterior circumflex humeral artery. In the intertubercular sulcus, a branch of the anterior circumflex humeral artery gives rise to two small branches running in cranial and caudad directions.

The tendon of the long head of the biceps can be divided into two zones. The first is the traction zone, in which the tendon of the biceps closely resembles a normal tendon, and the second is the sliding zone, which is the fibrocartilaginous portion of the tendon that is in contact with the bony groove. The density of intratendinous vessels in the traction zone is comparable to the vascularization of other tendons. In the sliding zone, vascularization of the biceps tendons is markedly decreased. No vessels are present in the part of the tendon on which the humerus slides. This area has also been shown to be composed of fibrocartilage.[149] The portion of the long head of the biceps inside the bicipital groove possesses a mesotendon that arises from the posterolateral portion of its groove.[112] Vascularization appears to play a minor role in the pathogenesis of biceps tendon rupture.

The biceps tendon has classically been described as having an intra-articular portion and a grooved portion. Experimental studies have shown that this type of classification is not 100% accurate. Because of the humeral head sliding on the biceps tendon, the position of the arm dictates the amount of intra-articular tendon present. The maximal amount of intra-articular tendon occurs with the arm in adduction and extension, whereas in extremes of abduction, very little tendon is actually residing inside the joint.

The long head of the biceps and the short head of the biceps form a common tendon before inserting onto the radial tubercle (Fig. 19–7). A third muscle belly has been described in some specimens. Mercer[182] and Gilcreest[95] measured the tensile strength of the biceps tendon and found it to range from 150 to 200 lb. The blood supply of the muscle belly attached to the long head of the biceps is via the brachial artery.[112] The nerve supply to this muscle is via the musculocutaneous nerves stemming from C5-C7.

Soft Tissue Restraint

As the long biceps tendon courses from its origin on the superior aspect of the glenoid labrum and supraglenoid tubercle to its muscular insertion, it is kept in its anatomic position by several structures. Among the most important

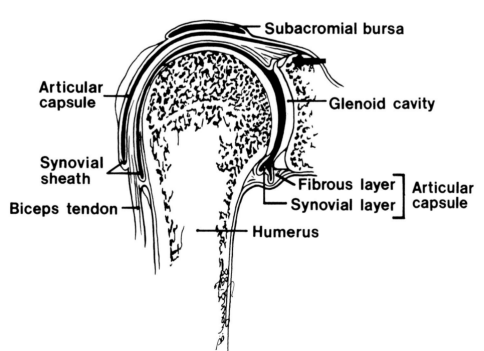

■ **Figure 19–6**

This figure illustrates both the insertion of the biceps onto the superior glenoid labrum as well as the supraglenoid tubercle *(black arrow)* and the reflection of the synovial sheath, which maintains the tendon as an extracapsular structure while it is on its intra-articular course.

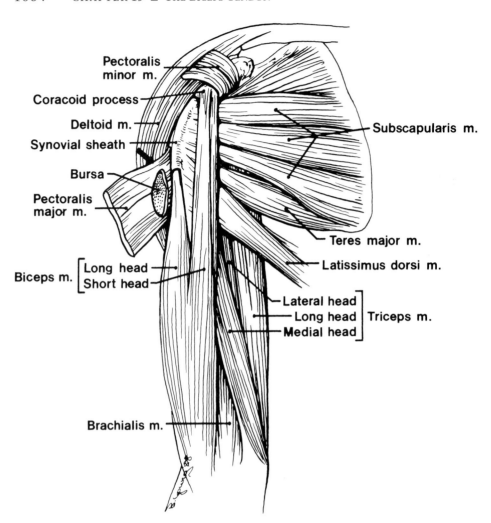

Pectoralis minor m.

Coracoid process

Deltoid m.

Synovial sheath

Bursa

Pectoralis major m.

Biceps m. [Long head / Short head]

Brachialis m.

Subscapularis m.

Teres major m.

Latissimus dorsi m.

Lateral head / Long head / Medial head] Triceps m.

■ **Figure 19–7**
General anatomic relationships of the long head of the biceps. Note how the pectoralis major and falciform ligament *(large black arrow)* cross over the tendon and help stabilize it after it exits the groove.

of these structures are the capsuloligamentous tissues. These structures play a major role in retaining and stabilizing the long head of the biceps tendon in its groove. The supraspinatus, subscapularis, coracohumeral ligament, and superior glenohumeral ligament all play a vital role in stabilizing the biceps.

Rotator Interval

The rotator interval is the area between the supraspinatus and subscapularis tendons. This triangular area, which contains both the coracohumeral and the superior glenohumeral ligaments, has as its medial boundary the coracoid process.

In its anatomic position, the intra-articular portion of the biceps tendon runs underneath the coracohumeral ligament, which lies between and strengthens the interval between the subscapularis and supraspinatus.

The rotator interval is an integral part of the cuff and capsule and can be distinguished only by sharp dissection.[205] The most important retaining structure in this area is the portion of the shoulder capsule thickened by the coracohumeral ligament and the edges of the subscapularis and supraspinatus tendons; this part of the capsule bridges the tuberosities in the uppermost portion

of the sulcus (Figs. 19–8 and 19–9). *This portion of the capsule is the first and chief obstacle to medial dislocation of the tendon, and Meyer*[183,188] *found that in all of his cases of dislocation it had been torn or stretched.* Codman,[50] in commenting on Meyer's work, stated that in his opinion, "displacement of the tendon is a result of rupture at that portion of the musculotendinous cuff, which is inserted into the inner edge of the intratubercular notch." These results were confirmed by Sakurai and colleagues,[261] who observed an intact transverse humeral ligament in 25 specimens with medial displacement of the biceps.

The rotator interval contains two structures that are important in stabilization of the biceps tendon in the groove. The coracohumeral ligament has a broad thin origin on the coracoid. This origin is along the lateral border of the coracoid, and as the ligament passes laterally, it divides into two main bands. One band inserts onto the anterior edge of the supraspinatus tendon and the greater tuberosity. The other inserts onto the superior border of the subscapularis, the transverse humeral ligament, and the lesser tuberosity (Figs. 19–10 and 19–11). The coracohumeral ligament has extensions that envelope the cuff tendons and blend into the superficial and deep layers of the supraspinatus and subscapularis tendons and the articular capsule. These extensions reinforce the capsule in the rotator interval at the border of the tendinous cuff.[51]

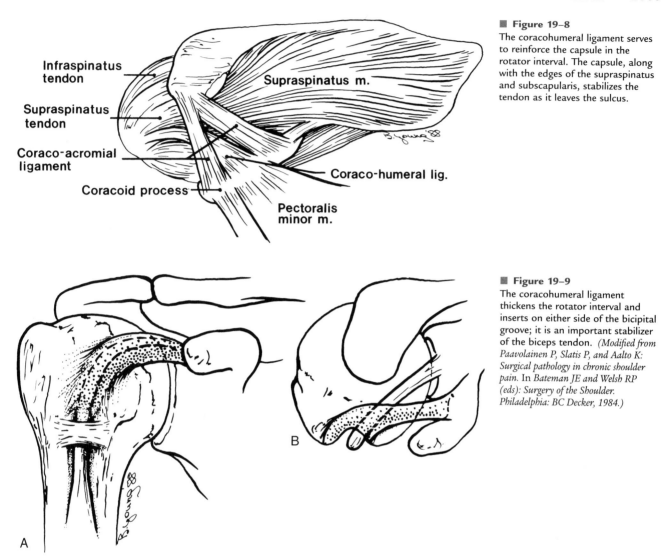

■ **Figure 19–8**
The coracohumeral ligament serves to reinforce the capsule in the rotator interval. The capsule, along with the edges of the supraspinatus and subscapularis, stabilizes the tendon as it leaves the sulcus.

Infraspinatus tendon

Supraspinatus m.

Supraspinatus tendon

Coraco-acromial ligament

Coracoid process

Coraco-humeral lig.

Pectoralis minor m.

■ **Figure 19–9**
The coracohumeral ligament thickens the rotator interval and inserts on either side of the bicipital groove; it is an important stabilizer of the biceps tendon. *(Modified from Paavolainen P, Slatis P, and Aalto K: Surgical pathology in chronic shoulder pain. In Bateman JE and Welsh RP (eds): Surgery of the Shoulder. Philadelphia: BC Decker, 1984.)*

A   B

The coracohumeral ligament is superficial to the shoulder capsule and overlies the biceps tendon.

The superior glenohumeral ligament is the second structure that adds stability to the biceps in the rotator interval. It arises from the labrum adjacent to the supraglenoid tubercle, inserts onto the superior lateral portion of the lesser tuberosity, and is united to the medial aspect of the coracohumeral ligament. This structure crosses the floor of the rotator interval.[221] Along with the coracohumeral ligament, the superior glenohumeral ligament forms a reflection pulley for the biceps tendon. This pulley is also in direct contact with the insertion of the subscapularis tendon. As can be seen by descriptions of the superior glenohumeral and coracohumeral ligaments, these structures blend together to form a sleeve above the entrance to the bicipital groove. This circular sleeve is comparable to the pulleys on the finger flexor tendons.[294] These structures prevent medial dislocation of the long biceps tendon. Although the superior glenohumeral ligament was previously considered insignificant, it appears to be an important stabilizer for the biceps tendon.

Cole and coauthors[52] described the anatomy of the rotator interval in adults and fetuses. They classified rotator intervals into two types. Type I intervals had a contiguous layer of capsule in the region of the superior and middle glenohumeral ligaments. A type II interval had a defect in the capsule between the superior and middle glenohumeral ligaments. The most frequent type of configuration was the type II interval, which occurred in 28 of 37 specimens. This study suggests that interval defects may be a congenital phenomenon. In Werner and colleagues' study[305] of the rotator interval, the superior glenohumeral ligament was found to make a U-shaped sling to stabilize the biceps tendon in the groove. They described two types of superior glenohumeral ligaments. Type I ligaments had fibers that covered more of the inferior aspect of the long head of the biceps tendon than was the case with type II ligaments. The fasciculus obliquus also had a significant role in investing the biceps tendon when examined microscopically. The subscapularis was not found to be involved in this suspensory sling. This suspensory mechanism protects the biceps against anterior shearing stresses. The authors concluded that the superior glenohumeral ligament is the most important stabilizing structure for the biceps tendon and that injury to this sling might lead to anterior bicipital instability.

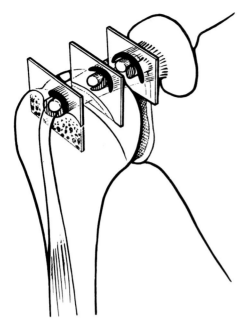

■ Figure 19–10

Schematic diagram showing the interrelationship of the coracohumeral ligament, superior glenohumeral ligament, and long biceps tendon at several planes in the rotator interval. The long biceps tendon (white) is positioned centrally. The coracoacromial ligament (black) forms a crescent-shaped roof above it, and the superior glenohumeral ligament (hatched area) forms a U-shaped trough. (From Habermeyer P and Walch G: The biceps tendon and rotator cuff disease. In Burkhead WZ Jr [ed]: Rotator Cuff Disorders. Media, PA: Williams & Wilkins, 1996, pp 142-159.)

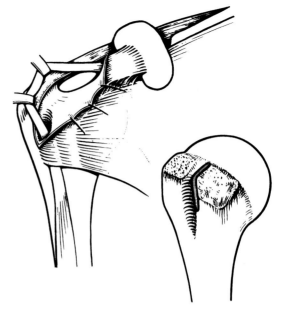

■ Figure 19–11

The rotator interval has been opened to demonstrate the common attachment of the coracohumeral ligament and superior glenohumeral ligament on the humeral head. (From Habermeyer P and Walch G: The biceps tendon and rotator cuff disease. In Burkhead WZ Jr [ed]: Rotator Cuff Disorders. Media, PA: Williams & Wilkins, 1996, pp 142-159.)

The Groove

The supraspinatus and subscapularis tendons fuse to form a sheath that surrounds the biceps tendon at the proximal end of the groove. Fibers from the subscapularis tendon pass below the biceps tendon and join with fibers from the supraspinatus to form the floor of the sheath (Fig. 19-12). The floor of the sheath is formed by the superior portion of the subscapularis and supraspinatus tendons. A slip from the supraspinatus forms the roof of the sheath along with the superior glenohumeral and coracohumeral ligaments. The deep portion of the sheath runs adjacent to the bone and forms a fibrocartilaginous lining in the groove that extends approximately 7 mm distal to the entrance of the groove.[54]

The transverse humeral ligament's role in providing stability of the biceps in its sulcus has been disputed by several authors.[183,227,261] Traditional teaching showed that the biceps was kept in the sulcus by action of the transverse ligament (Fig 19-13). Meyer[183] found that this structure was either too weak or often entirely absent. Paavolainen[227] and coworkers were unable to dislocate the biceps, even after sectioning the intertubercular transverse ligament, as long as the rotator cuff was intact.[205]

Once the tendon has entered the groove, the principal structure containing the tendon is the falciform ligament, a tendinous expansion from the sternocostal portion of the pectoralis major. It forms a margin with the deep aspect of the main tendon that stabilizes the biceps. The falciform ligament is attached to both lips of the groove and blends with the capsule at the shoulder joint.

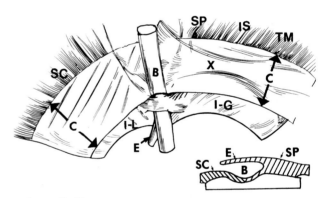

■ Figure 19–12

Drawing of the deep surface of the rotator cuff–capsule complex after it has been detached from the humerus. The diagram in the inset is a cross section of the bicipital groove and related structures. Note the relationships of the capsule (C), subscapularis (SC), supraspinatus (SP), infraspinatus (IS), and teres minor (TM) tendons, as well as the confluence of the supraspinatus and subscapularis tendons proximal to their insertions on the lesser (I-L) and greater (I-G) tuberosities. In the inset, the complex sheath surrounding the biceps tendon (B) is shown diagrammatically in cross section. The deep portion of this sheath is formed by the subscapularis tendon, and a slip (E) from the supraspinatus tendon forms a roof over the biceps tendon. Also shown is the pericapsular band (X). (From Clark JM and Harryman DT II: Tendons, ligaments, and capsule of the rotator cuff. Gross and microscopic anatomy. J Bone Joint Surg Am 74:713-725, 1992.)

Osseous Anatomy

The bicipital groove (Fig. 19-14) is formed between the lesser and greater tuberosities. The medial wall is made up of the lesser tuberosity, whereas the lateral wall is the edge of the greater tuberosity. Cone and colleagues[53] have studied the bicipital groove. They measured the medial wall angle and the width and depth of the intertubercular

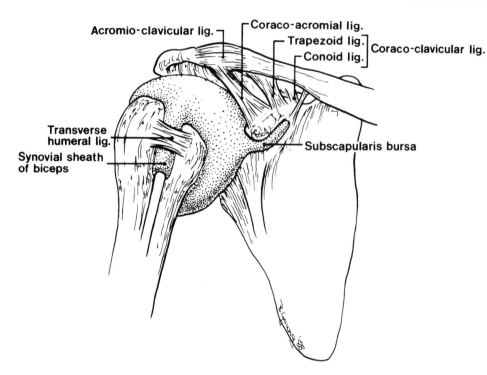

Acromio-clavicular lig.
Coraco-acromial lig.
Trapezoid lig.
Conoid lig.
Coraco-clavicular lig.
Transverse humeral lig.
Synovial sheath of biceps
Subscapularis bursa

■ **Figure 19–13**
The ligaments around the shoulder. Meyer[183] found the transverse ligament to be too weak or entirely absent.

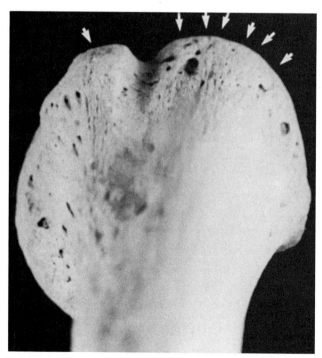

■ **Figure 19–14**
The bicipital groove is made up of the walls of the lesser tuberosity *(small arrow)* and greater tuberosity *(multiple arrows)*. *(From Cone RO, Danzig L, Resnick D, and Goldman AB: The bicipital groove: Radiographic, anatomic, and pathologic study. AJR Am J Roentgenol 41:781-788, 1983. Copyright © 1983, American Roentgen Ray Society.)*

lips of the intertubercular sulcus. The middle width was measured between the walls of the intertubercular sulcus, a point equal to half the depth of the sulcus. The difference between measurements was wide, but the ratio of the width was constant at 1.6 from the top to the middle distances. The average depth of the groove was found to be 4.3 mm (range, 4 to 6 mm).

In a separate study, Ueberham and Le Floch-Prigent[284] measured the intertubercular sulcus in dry bones. They found the total length of the groove to be 27.5 mm. On average, the proximal part of the intertubercular sulcus was 12.4 mm and the distal part was 15.1 mm. They noted that the groove was deepest in the middle and shallower at both its proximal and distal ends. They measured the angle between the proximal segment of the groove and its distal part and found it to be 142 degrees and quite variable. A supratubercular ridge was present in 45% of specimens and was thought to force the biceps anteriorly, thereby increasing the risk of dislocation. This abnormality was found in isolation in 17% of specimens or in association with one other lesion in 18%.

Variability in the medial wall angle was confirmed in studies by Hitchcock and Bechtol,[124] Habermeyer and associates,[112] and Cone and colleagues.[53] Hitchcock and Bechtol[124] found that the medial wall angle was 90 degrees in 10% of specimens, 75 degrees in 35%, 60 degrees in 34%, 45 degrees in 13%, 30 degrees in 6%, and 15 degrees in 2% (Fig. 19–16). In Habermeyer and coworkers' study,[112] as well as Hitchcock and Bechtol's study,[124] the medial wall angle was found to correlate with the probability of subluxation of the long head of the biceps tendon. Cone and colleagues,[53] on the other hand, did not find any correlation between the incidence of subluxation and low medial wall angles.

Vettivel and associates[291] found that the intertubercular sulcus of the humerus was related to handedness. In

groove (Fig. 19–15). The mean value of the medial wall angle was 56 degrees (range, 40 to 70 degrees). The width of the intertubercular sulcus was measured in two locations on the bicipital groove view. The top width was determined as the distance between the medial and lateral

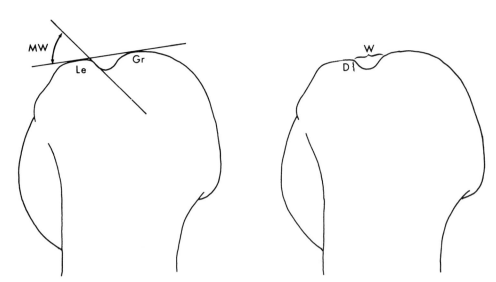

■ **Figure 19–15**
Measurements taken by Cone and associates, including the medial wall angle and the width and depth of the bicipital groove. D, depth of groove; Gr, greater tuberosity; Le, lesser tuberosity; MW, medial wall angle; W, width of groove. *(From Cone RO, Danzig L, Resnick D, and Goldman AB: The bicipital groove: Radiographic, anatomic, and pathologic study. AJR Am J Roentgenol 41:781-788, 1983. Copyright © 1983, American Roentgen Ray Society.)*

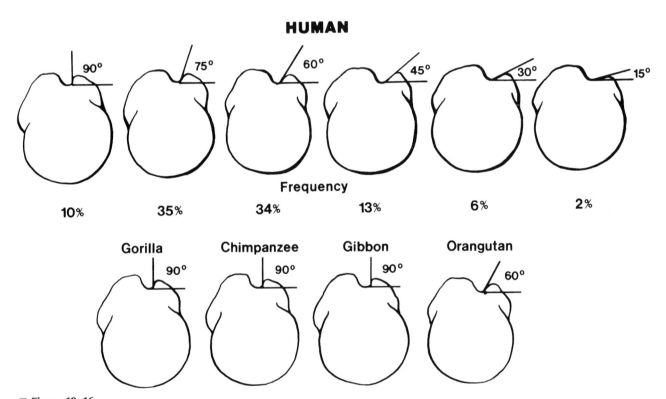

■ **Figure 19–16**
A, Humans are unique in having variations in the bicipital groove. **B,** The groove of the biceps in primates is constant within species.
(Modified and redrawn from Hitchcock HH and Bechtol CO: Painful shoulder. Observations on the role of the tendon of the long head of the biceps brachii in its causation. J Bone Joint Surg Am 30:263-273, 1948.)

their study, the intertubercular sulcus was wider and had an acute medial wall angle on the side of the specimen's dominant arm. They believe that this difference was due to greater stress passing through the tendon in the dominant extremity, especially during manual activities.

Comparative Anatomy

Hitchcock and Bechtol,[124] using specimens from the Museum of Natural History in Chicago, outlined changes in the relationship of the scapula and bicipital groove from the quadruped to the erect biped (Fig. 19–17). They described a progressive anteroposterior flattening of the thorax resulting in an increased angle that the scapula forms with the thorax and a relative lateral displacement of the scapula. Humans have a relatively short forearm and lateral part of the scapula. Such anatomy necessitates greater medial rotation of the humerus to enable the hand to reach the midline. The anteroposterior flattening of the thorax and the short forearm were compensated for, but only incompletely, by torsion of the humerus. In the

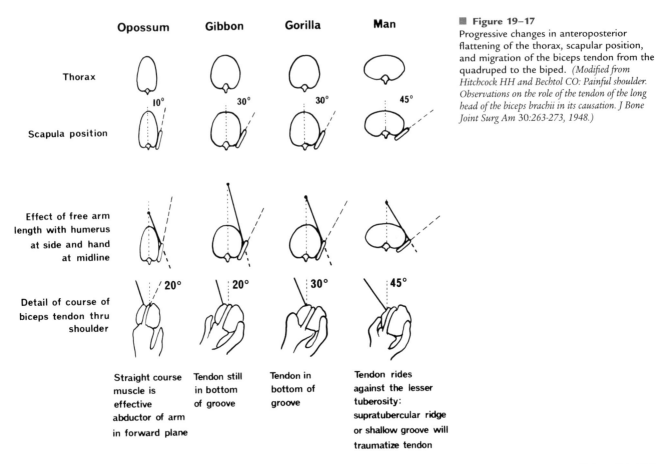

| Opossum | Gibbon | Gorilla | Man |

Thorax

Scapula position

10°   30°   30°   45°

Effect of free arm length with humerus at side and hand at midline

Detail of course of biceps tendon thru shoulder

20°   20°   30°   45°

Straight course muscle is effective abductor of arm in forward plane

Tendon still in bottom of groove

Tendon in bottom of groove

Tendon rides against the lesser tuberosity: supratubercular ridge or shallow groove will traumatize tendon

■ **Figure 19–17**
Progressive changes in anteroposterior flattening of the thorax, scapular position, and migration of the biceps tendon from the quadruped to the biped. *(Modified from Hitchcock HH and Bechtol CO: Painful shoulder. Observations on the role of the tendon of the long head of the biceps brachii in its causation. J Bone Joint Surg Am 30:263-273, 1948.)*

quadruped opossum, the biceps tendon takes a straight course through the bicipital groove and is an effective abductor of the forelimb in the forward plane. However, in humans, the tendon is lodged against the lesser tuberosity, where a supratubercular ridge or shallow groove can traumatize the tendon. Humans are unique among the primates in having marked variations (see Fig. 19–18) in configuration of the bicipital groove.

The human arm was derived from the foreleg of the quadruped. Whereas the forelimb was devised to bear weight in the quadruped, in humans the upper limb has moved away from the body. For effective use of the limb, it must move not only against its own weight but also against the weight of other objects. This short power arm has to act against a long lever arm, a situation that produces unfavorable mechanical conditions leading to tendinitis of the rotator cuff and biceps.

Developmental Anatomy

During the ninth week of gestation, the limbs undergo rotation. The upper limb rotates dorsally at the elbow. This rotation is reflected in the shoulder as humeral retroversion, which averages 35 degrees. This rotation, in essence, leaves the biceps tendon behind on the anterior aspect of the shoulder in the groove and requires that the biceps cross the joint obliquely at a 30- to 45-degree angle rather than proceeding in a straight line laterally as in quadrupeds.

The development of the glenohumeral joint is similar to that of other synovial joints in the human body.

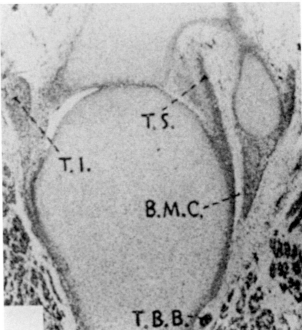

■ **Figure 19–18**
At approximately 7 weeks' gestation, the joint is well formed and the humeral head is spherical. The biceps tendon (T.B.B.) is seen clearly in the groove. This picture is taken before rotation occurs; the biceps tendon will eventually assume a position less lateral than shown here. The other structures in this picture are the tendons of the infraspinatus (T.I.) and subscapularis (T.S.) and the bursa of the coracobrachialis (B.M.C.). *(From Gardner E and Gray DJ: Prenatal development of the human shoulder and acromioclavicular joint. Am J Anat 92:219, 1953.)*

According to Gardner and Gray,[89] it involves two basic processes. Initially, an inner zone forms between the two developing bones of the joint, followed by the creation of cavities by enzymatic action. The inner zone often comprises three layers: a chondrogenic layer on either side of a looser layer of cells. The joint capsule and many of the intra-articular structures, such as the synovial membrane, the ligaments, the labrum, and the biceps tendon, are formed from this inner zone of tissue. Giuliani and associates[101] confirmed that the tendon of the long head of the biceps brachii arises in continuity with the anlage of the glenoid labrum. At approximately 7 weeks of gestation, the joint is well formed, the humeral head is spherical, and the tendons of the infraspinatus, subscapularis, and biceps, as well as the glenoid labrum, can be seen (Fig. 19–18).

Pathologic Anatomy

Some authors[66-68,70] believe that tenosynovitis is the chief cause of pain in bicipital tendinitis and that it leads to an altered gliding mechanism of the tendon sheath. They describe gradual pathologic changes in the area of the biceps tendon, initially including capillary dilation and edema of the tendon with progressive cellular infiltration of the sheath and synovium and the development of filmy adhesions between the tendon and the tendon sheath. In the chronic stage, fraying and narrowing of the biceps tendon occur along with minimal to moderate synovial proliferation and fibrosis and, ultimately, replacement of the tendon fibers by fibrous tissue and organization of dense fibrous adhesions between the tendon passing through the bicipital groove and across the joint. The biceps tendon passes directly under the critical zone of the supraspinatus tendon. Claessens and Snoek[44] described microscopic changes consistent with a relatively avascular state, including atrophic irregular collagen fiber,

fissurization and shredding of tendon fibers, fibrinoid necrosis, and a productive inflammatory reaction with an increase in fibrocytes (Fig. 19–19). Refior and Sowa found that the origin of the tendon and the portion of the tendon that exits the sulcus were sites of predilection for microscopic degeneration of the tendon (Fig. 19–20).[253] They believed that these areas are at the highest risk for rupture of the tendon. Macroscopic changes noted in cadaver studies by DePalma[66-70] and by Claessens and colleagues[42,44] included tendinitis with shredding of the tendon fibers by osteophytes, adhesions between the synovial sheaths and between the tendon and its osteofibrous compartment, subluxation or dislocation of the tendon, and rupture of the tendon with retraction of the distal portion or adhesion of the distal portion to the sulcus. Although it was common belief that the tendon, when it dislocates, always displaced medial to the lesser tuberosity riding over the subscapularis tendon (Fig. 19–21B), Petersson[238] in his study found only one such case. In the majority of cases in his series, internal degeneration of the subscapularis in the region of the lesser tuberosity had occurred and allowed the tendon to dislocate medially under the subscapularis (Fig. 19–21C). Similar pathologic findings were described by DePalma (Fig. 19–22). Sakurai and coworkers[261] studied three groups of patients with chronic shoulder pathology. Patients with an intact rotator cuff, group 1, did not have any flattening of the tendon in the intertubercular region. Half the patients with partial-thickness tearing or small rotator cuff tears, group 2, had flattening of the tendon in the intertubercular groove. Patients with massive rotator cuff tears, group 3, had tendon flattening in 66% of the specimens. Bicipital fraying was seen in 16% of these cases. Medial displacement was noted in 12% of group 2 and 38% of group 3. Rupture of the biceps tendon was seen in 16% of group 3 specimens. In their study these authors measured bicipital height, which included the height of the soft tissues. They demonstrated a significant difference in height of

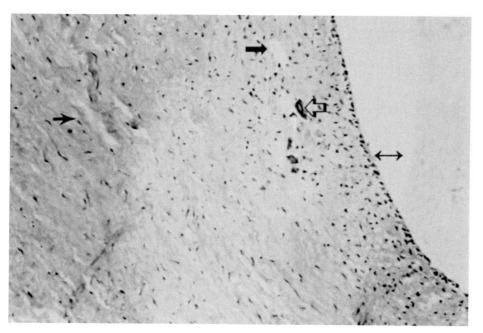

■ **Figure 19–19**
Pathology in a degenerative biceps tendon. The *double arrow* indicates the synovial membrane, the *open arrow* points to dystrophic calcification, the *closed arrow* marks total loss of fibers, and the *arrowhead* indicates fissuring in the collagen with a disorderly collagen pattern. A productive inflammatory reaction with an increase in fibrocytes is seen in the lower right corner.

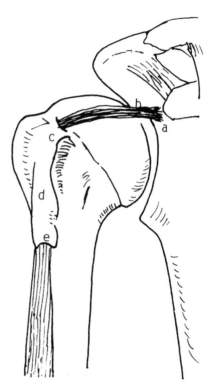

■ **Figure 19–20**
Areas of the long tendon of the biceps examined histologically.
a, Glenoid origin of the tendon; b, proximal intra-articular region;
c, entrance to the bicipital groove; d, bicipital groove; and e, exit
of the bicipital groove. Sites b and c are the most common sites of
degeneration. *(From Refior HJ and Sowa D: Long tendon of the biceps
brachii: Sites of predilection for degenerative lesions. J Shoulder Elbow Surg
4:436-440, 1995.)*

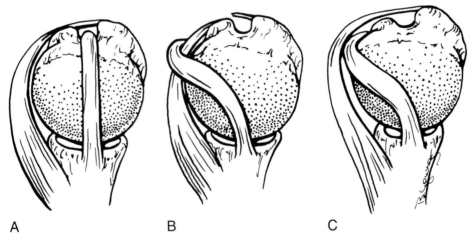

A   B   C

■ **Figure 19–21**
A, The normal relationship of the biceps tendon in the groove covered by the transverse ligament.
B, Rupture of the transverse ligament and subluxation of the biceps tendon out of the groove, with
the tendon lying anterior to the subscapularis muscle. **C,** Intratendinous disruption of the
subscapularis found in the majority of cases by Petersson, in which the subscapularis insertion
degenerates and the tendon subluxates beneath the muscle tendon belly. The subscapularis tendon
may have an attachment to the greater tuberosity through the coracohumeral and transverse
ligaments. *(Modified from Petersson CJ: Degeneration of the gleno-humeral joint: An anatomical study. Acta
Orthop Scand 54:277-283, 1983.)*

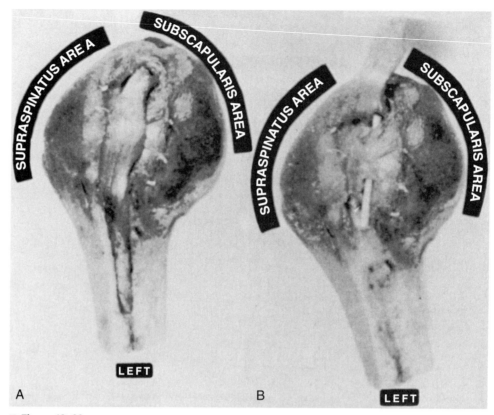

■ **Figure 19–22**
Obliteration of the bicipital groove by inflammation, with subluxation of the tendon lying in a fascial sling made by the insertion of the subscapularis. *(From DePalma A: Surgery of the Shoulder, 2nd ed. Philadelphia: JB Lippincott, 1983.)*

the medial wall in patients with medial displacement of the biceps and those without instability. They were unable to show a difference between the three groups in height of the medial wall of the groove. After analyzing these functions, the authors concluded that the long head of the biceps could potentially compensate for deficient rotator cuff function. The result of this compensation is relative stenosis of the tendon in the groove. Other gliding disorders can also result from this mismatch between the enlarged tendon size and the noncompliant bony groove. This mismatch may be responsible for degeneration of the soft tissue along the medial wall of the sulcus causing a pulley lesion and resulting instability.

The biceps tendon and its enveloping synovial sheath can be affected by inflammatory or infectious processes of the glenohumeral joint as a result of their anatomic location and course. Tumorous conditions affecting the synovium of the shoulder may also involve the sheath of the tendon.[58] Therefore, tenosynovitis of the biceps accompanies septic arthritis of the shoulder, as well as rheumatic inflammation, osteoarthritis, hemodialysis arthropathy,[278] and crystalline arthritis. The clinical syndrome in these cases is dominated by the articular pathology. In the past, biceps rupture has been reported to occur in conjunction with tuberculous and luetic infection.

Osteochondromatosis has also been reported in the shoulder and bicipital sheath.[62] This disorder causes pain and loose body formation in the shoulder. Detection of loose bodies in the bicipital sheath on radiography or MRI should arouse suspicion of this pathologic process. Treatment by synovectomy has been successful.

OSSEOUS PATHOANATOMY

The shape of the groove has been implicated frequently in the pathogenesis of biceps tendon rupture.[66-68,70,104,124] A shallow flattened groove (Fig. 19–23) is commonly associated with subluxation or dislocation of the biceps tendon, and a narrow groove with a sharp medial wall and an osteophyte at the aperture is associated with bicipital tendinitis and rupture (Fig. 19–24). Spurs on the floor of the groove may erode the tendon (Fig. 19–25). Although these groove abnormalities may contribute to bicipital tendon problems, it is more likely that some are changes in response to pathology of the soft tissues around the shoulder. In all degenerative conditions about the shoulder, soft tissue changes precede bony changes; for instance, rotator cuff disorders, fibrosis, bursitis, and tendinosis or enesthopathy precede the formation of spurring in the anterior acromion. Synovitis and cartilage degeneration precede spur formation in the acromioclavicular joint. It seems logical that changes in the bicipital groove and its opening follow changes in the tendon, capsule, ligaments, and synovium around it.

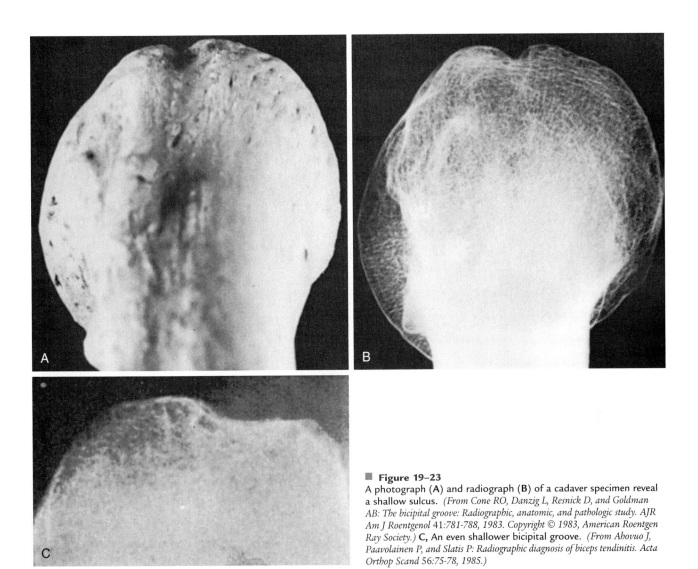

Figure 19–23

A photograph (**A**) and radiograph (**B**) of a cadaver specimen reveal a shallow sulcus. *(From Cone RO, Danzig L, Resnick D, and Goldman AB: The bicipital groove: Radiographic, anatomic, and pathologic study. AJR Am J Roentgenol 41:781-788, 1983. Copyright © 1983, American Roentgen Ray Society.)* **C,** An even shallower bicipital groove. *(From Ahovuo J, Paavolainen P, and Slatis P: Radiographic diagnosis of biceps tendinitis. Acta Orthop Scand 56:75-78, 1985.)*

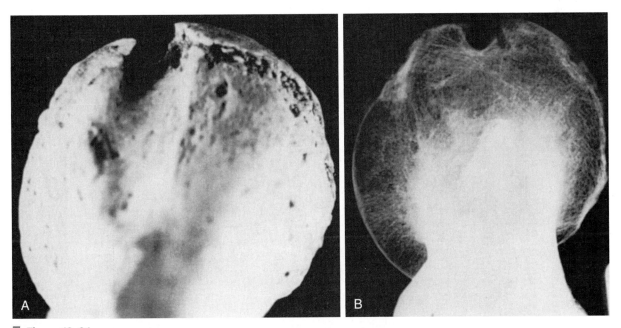

Figure 19–24

Pathologic specimen (**A**) and groove radiograph (**B**) of the bicipital groove with a 90-degree medial wall angle and medial osteophyte at the aperture, seen commonly with bicipital tendinitis and rupture. *(From Cone RO, Danzig L, Resnick D, and Goldman AB: The bicipital groove: Radiographic, anatomic, and pathologic study. AJR Am J Roentgenol 41:781-788, 1983. Copyright © 1983, American Roentgen Ray Society.)*

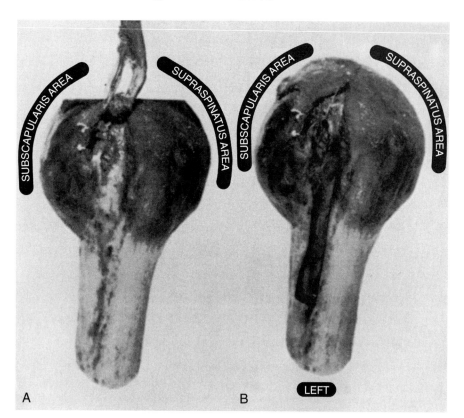

■ **Figure 19–25**

A, A large bony spur is seen in the floor of the groove. A corresponding defect is present in the biceps tendon. **B,** The tendon has been replaced in the groove. *(From DePalma A: Surgery of the Shoulder, 2nd ed. Philadelphia: JB Lippincott, 1983.)*

Bony Anomalies

Bony anomalies and variations have been proposed as a cause of subluxation and tendinitis of the biceps tendon. The supratubercular ridge has been described by Meyer[183] as a ridge that extends forward and downward from the region of the articular cartilage to the upper and dorsal portions of the lesser tuberosity (Fig. 19–26). Its incidence, according to Cilley,[39] was 17.5% in 200 humeri examined. The ridge, when present, decreases the depth of the sulcus and diminishes the effectiveness of the tuberosity as a trochlea. Meyer believed that the ridge pushes the biceps tendon against the transverse ligament, thereby favoring dislocation.

In Hitchcock and Bechtol's series,[124] the supratubercular ridge was found to be markedly developed in 8% and moderately developed in 59%. Hitchcock and Bechtol[124] found a direct correlation between the presence of a supratubercular ridge and spurs on the lesser tuberosity (medial wall spurs). In their series, medial wall spurs were found in approximately 45% of patients with a supratubercular ridge. When no supratubercular ridge was present, only 3% of the humeri had spurs on the lesser tuberosity (Fig. 19–26C). They concluded that spurs on the lesser tuberosity developed in response to pressure from the biceps tendon being pressed up against the tuberosity by the supratubercular ridge.

A supratubercular ridge was found in approximately 50% of patients by Cone and colleagues[53] but did not correlate very well with the presence of bicipital groove spurs. They thought that the medial wall spur was related more to a traction enostosis, or reactive bone formation at the site of a tendon or ligament insertion of the transverse humeral ligament. In one specimen, the transverse humeral ligament was completely ossified and the bicipital groove was converted into a bony tunnel. They agree with DePalma that the presence of bony spurs on the floor of the bicipital groove is related to chronic bicipital tenosynovitis (Fig. 19–27).

Some authors believe that primary bicipital tendinitis is more common than usually described. Pfahler and colleagues[241] compared the ultrasound and radiographic findings of patients with chronic shoulder pain and normal controls. Forty-three percent of their subjects with degenerative changes in the bicipital groove had sonographic evidence of inflammation of the biceps tendon. Ultrasound findings of bicipital tendinitis correlated with a small total opening angle of less than 80 degrees on radiographs in 65% of their cases. Patients with a flat medial angle had signs of bicipital tendinitis 47% of the time. In patients with bicipital rupture, 61% had a shallow medial angle. They concluded that 65% of their patients with anterior shoulder pain had changes in the anatomy of their bicipital groove. They believed that these patients represented cases of primary bicipital tendinitis.

FUNCTION OF THE BICEPS TENDON

Basmajian and Latif[16] characterized the actions of the biceps brachii muscle as flexion of the elbow joint when the forearm is in the neutral or supinated position. They found that it contributed very little to flexion at the elbow with the forearm in a pronated position. The biceps was also important in decelerating the rapidly moving arm, such as occurs during forceful overhand throwing.

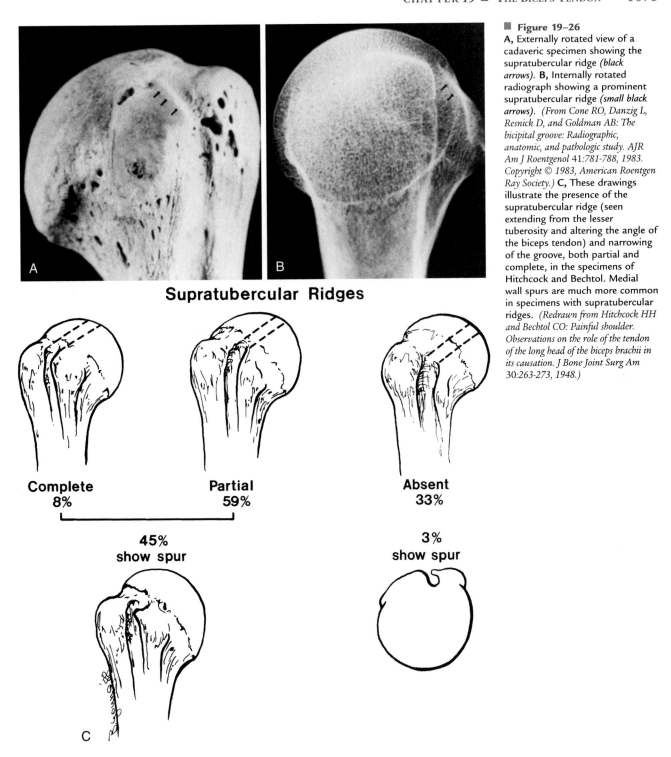

Supratubercular Ridges

Complete
8%

Partial
59%

Absent
33%

45%
show spur

3%
show spur

■ **Figure 19–26**

A, Externally rotated view of a cadaveric specimen showing the supratubercular ridge *(black arrows)*. **B,** Internally rotated radiograph showing a prominent supratubercular ridge *(small black arrows)*. *(From Cone RO, Danzig L, Resnick D, and Goldman AB: The bicipital groove: Radiographic, anatomic, and pathologic study. AJR Am J Roentgenol 41:781-788, 1983. Copyright © 1983, American Roentgen Ray Society.)* **C,** These drawings illustrate the presence of the supratubercular ridge (seen extending from the lesser tuberosity and altering the angle of the biceps tendon) and narrowing of the groove, both partial and complete, in the specimens of Hitchcock and Bechtol. Medial wall spurs are much more common in specimens with supratubercular ridges. *(Redrawn from Hitchcock HH and Bechtol CO: Painful shoulder. Observations on the role of the tendon of the long head of the biceps brachii in its causation. J Bone Joint Surg Am 30:263-273, 1948.)*

The function of the biceps at the elbow has been well worked out, and it is generally agreed that the biceps brachii is a strong supinator of the forearm and a weak flexor at the elbow. Debate continues, however, on the exact function of the biceps at the shoulder level. Most anatomy texts regard the biceps as a weak flexor of the shoulder.[126] Studies on function of the biceps tendon can be divided into three broad categories: direct observation, electromyographic (EMG) studies, and biomechanical cadaver studies.

Direct Observation

Multiple investigators[124,157,158,160] have observed that the biceps tendon does not slide in the groove but, rather, the humerus moves on a fixed passive biceps tendon during shoulder motion. From adduction to complete elevation of the arm, the groove moves along the tendon for a distance of as much as 2 to 5 cm. To facilitate this motion, the synovial pouch (see Figs. 19–2 and 19–6) extends from the shoulder joint to line the intertubercular groove for a

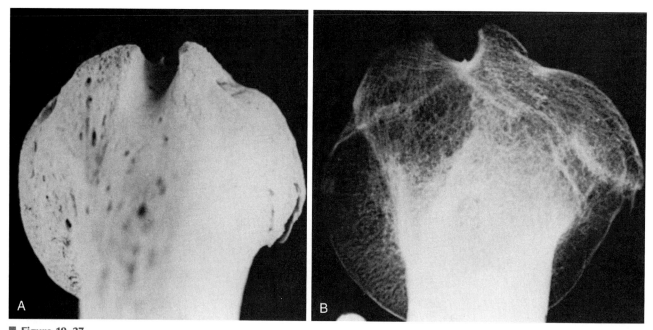

■ **Figure 19–27**

A, A spur in the floor of the bicipital groove thought by Cone and colleagues to be significant in biceps tendinitis, as opposed to a medial wall spur, which was seen in a number of normal specimens. **B,** Groove radiograph of the same structure. *(From Cone RO, Danzig L, Resnick D, and Goldman AB: The bicipital groove: Radiographic, anatomic, and pathologic study. AJR Am J Roentgenol 41:781-788, 1983. Copyright © 1983, American Roentgen Ray Society.)*

greater part of its extent. Below this bursa, the tendon glides through its peritendineum.

When the arm is in full external rotation, the tendon occupies the floor of the groove, and its more proximal portion exercises pressure on the humeral head. Therefore, it was originally believed that only in external rotation did the long head act directly on the shoulder as a head depressor and somewhat enhance the power of abduction of this joint. A vector diagram has been used by Lucas[162] to establish the resultant force of the biceps as that of depressing the head (Fig. 19–28). Figure 19–29 illustrates how the biceps acts as a static head depressor to prevent migration of the humeral head into the acromion by the pull of the deltoid.

Elevation of the arm in internal rotation causes minimal excursion of the tendon, whereas in external rotation, maximal excursion occurs. With the arm in the position of full abduction, 1.3 cm of tendon remained in the shoulder joint. When the arm is depressed and externally rotated, 5 cm of tendon is in the shoulder joint, for an overall excursion of 3.7 cm. Therefore, Lippmann[158] believed that the tendon should not be considered as two part, an intracapsular and a groove portion, because of this movement of the humeral head along the tendon (Fig. 19–30).

Rowe[259] states that in chronic rupture of the rotator cuff, the head depressor responsibility of the biceps tendon increases, and the tendon is often found to be hypertrophied. Bush[35] noted an increased depressor effect of the tendon when it was transplanted laterally for repairing cuff defects.

Andrews and colleagues[9] observed the biceps tendon and the superior glenoid–labrum complex arthroscopically during electrical stimulation of the biceps. They noted definite superior lifting of the labrum and compression of the glenohumeral joint. They observed that in this respect the biceps is a "shunt muscle of the shoulder" and does help stabilize the glenohumeral joint during throwing. Its primary role during throwing, they agree, is still deceleration of the elbow, and it is this sudden deceleration that leads to tearing of the superior glenoid–labrum complex by the biceps tendon.

In a study by Itoi and colleagues,[134] the long head and short head of the biceps were shown to have similar function as anterior stabilizers of the glenohumeral joint with the arm in abduction and external rotation. It was further demonstrated that as shoulder stability decreases as a result of sectioning of the inferior glenohumeral ligament, such as occurs during development of a Bankart lesion, both heads of the biceps were shown to have increased stabilizing function to resist anterior displacement of the head. They concluded that during rehabilitation of patients with chronic anterior instability, strengthening of the biceps should be included in nonoperative treatment of these lesions.

Kumar and associates[150] also studied the stabilizing role of the biceps tendon. They were able to show that severing the long head of the biceps tendon while both heads were tensed caused significant upward migration of the humeral head. In this manner, the long head of the biceps is important in stabilizing the humeral head in the glenoid during powerful elbow flexion and forearm supination. They warned against sacrifice of the intra-articular portion of the long head of the biceps tendon because of the danger of producing instability during forced elbow flexion and supination.

Continued support for the role of the long head of the biceps tendon in glenohumeral stability has recently been

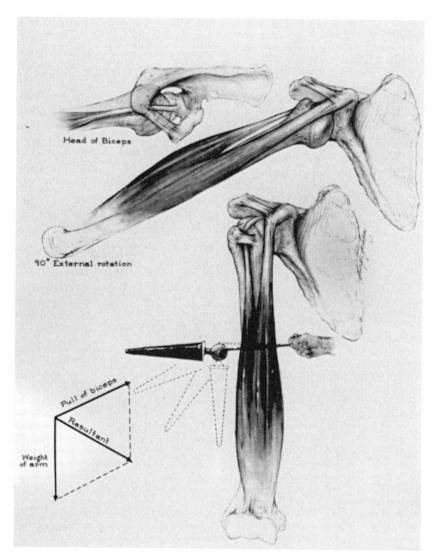

Head of Biceps

90° External rotation

Pull of biceps

Resultant

Weight of arm

■ **Figure 19–28**
Artist's conception and vector diagram of the resultant force of the biceps tendon. *(From Lucas DB: Biomechanics of the shoulder joint. Arch Surg 107:425-432, 1973. Copyright 1973, American Medical Association.)*

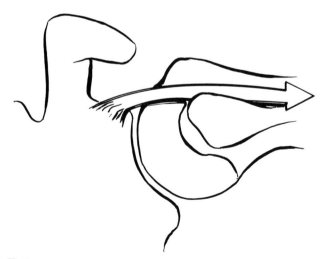

■ **Figure 19–29**
From this illustration it is evident that the biceps tendon is at least a static head depressor. Given the line of pull and the resultant vector, it is an active head depressor, though undoubtedly a weak one as shown by the percentage of recruitment on electromyographic analysis. *(Redrawn from Habermeyer P, Kaiser E, Knappe M, et al: Functional anatomy and biomechanics of the long biceps tendon. Unfallchirurg 90:319–329, 1987.)*

published.[171,230] In Pagnani and colleagues' study,[230] cadaveric shoulders were subjected to anterior, posterior, and inferior force at varying arm angles. The amount of translation that occurred was measured with and without a force applied to the biceps. The results showed decreased translation of the glenohumeral joint in all directions when a 55-N force was applied to the biceps. The effect was greatest at middle and lower elevations. Rotation of the shoulder joint also influenced the results. External rotation decreased posterior translation, whereas internal rotation decreased anterior translation. This force also decreased superior and inferior translation of the glenohumeral joint. They concluded that the biceps centers the humeral head on the glenoid and thus stabilizes the fulcrum and allows motion to occur.

Malicky and coworkers[171] showed that the biceps provides 30 N of force for translation of the humeral head when the arm is in neutral rotation. Its effect was smallest when the arm was in external rotation. The force required to subluxate the joint may be modulated by the position of the groove. In neutral rotation, the biceps may add concavity compression as well as a posterior force of the head on the glenoid. In external rotation, the biceps

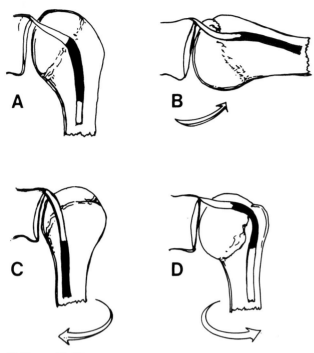

■ **Figure 19–30**
Lippmann found by direct observation under local anesthesia that the biceps tendon slid freely in its sheath on motion of the shoulder. Motion of the tendon in its groove appears only with motion of the shoulder joint. At any given position, a different amount of the biceps tendon can be found within the joint. *(Modified from Lippmann RK: Bicipital tenosynovitis. N Y State J Med 90:2235-2241, 1944.)*

applies an anterior force on the humeral head and may actually destabilize the joint in the anterior direction.

Warner and McMahon[301] studied seven patients with isolated rupture of the long head of the biceps tendon. This lesion was documented surgically or with MRI. They showed an increase in superior translation of the humeral head at all degrees of humeral abduction when compared with the contralateral control. This phenomenon was not seen at zero degrees of elevation. They concluded that isolated loss of the biceps could lead to impingement syndrome in patients with a type II or III acromion.

Electromyographic Evaluation

Basmajian[16] was a pioneer in evaluating the musculoskeletal system, including the shoulder, with integrated-function and dynamic-spectrum EMG analysis. He reported both heads of the biceps to be active during shoulder flexion, with the long head being most active.[15] Habermeyer and associates[112] performed EMG analysis, whereas Cybex testing was performed on normal individuals. Clear EMG activity was seen in the biceps during abduction, its peak being found at 132 degrees of abduction. Interestingly, they found the muscle to be active even with the arm in neutral rotation; that is, the biceps is active in abduction even when the arm is not externally rotated. In flexion, they found that the main activity was recorded during the first 90 degrees. The biceps was active in external but not internal rotation. The effectiveness of the long head of the biceps is greater in external rotation

when its tension is maximal. In arm adduction and internal rotation, the long head was always inactive, whereas the short head was active in half the cases of adduction and only seldom active in internal rotation. The biceps was totally inactive in extension.

Laumann[153,154] has divided the contribution of various muscles around the shoulder to shoulder flexion by percentage. Based on his work, he estimated that the biceps contributes approximately 7% of the power of flexion.

Furlani[87] studied EMG participation of the biceps in movements of the glenohumeral joint. He found that in flexion of the shoulder with an extended elbow, both the long and short heads of the biceps brachii were active in the majority of cases, regardless of the presence or absence of resistance. In abduction without resistance, the biceps was inactive. The addition of resistance increased the activity of the biceps to 10%.

Ting and coworkers[281] performed EMG analysis on the long head of the biceps in patients with rotator cuff tears. In all their patients, the EMG record was expressed as a percentage of the activity recorded during maximal effort. They correlated their data with operative findings. During both shoulder abduction and flexion, four of five subjects tested demonstrated a significantly greater degree of EMG activity in the biceps tendon in the extremity with a torn cuff than in the contralateral uninjured shoulder. In addition, all shoulders with compromised rotator cuffs proved to have a significantly larger tendon at the time of surgery than noted in controls, thus confirming the observations of Rowe.[259] Ting and colleagues[281] suggested that the lateral head of the biceps may be a greater contributor to abduction and flexion in the compromised shoulder than in the normal shoulder and that the concomitant enlargement of the tendon may represent use-induced hypertrophy. They therefore recommended not sacrificing the intracapsular portion of the tendon for graft material or tenodesing the tendon indiscriminately in the groove as a routine part of rotator cuff repair and acromioplasty.

The biceps' contribution to the shoulder during throwing has been evaluated by Jobe and associates[138] and by Perry.[237] In these studies, biceps function correlated with motion occurring at the elbow and not in the shoulder. A relatively stable elbow position during acceleration was accompanied by a marked reduction in the muscle's intensity. During follow-through, the need for deceleration of the rapidly extending elbow and pronating forearm was accompanied by peak biceps action. They showed no activity in the biceps muscle during the act of throwing, except when the elbow was active. Peak activity was only 36% of its maximal capacity. With a 9-cm² cross section and only half of the muscle related to the long head, the humeral force is small. In Perry's words: "It seems doubtful that the long head (biceps tendon) is a significant stabilizing force at the glenohumeral joint." Glousman and associates,[102] on the other hand, reported increased activity in the biceps during throwing in patients with unstable shoulders. Therefore, it seems that the biceps takes on more importance if the primary stabilizers are injured.

EMG activity in patients with a less than 5-cm rotator cuff tear was found to be increased in comparison to healthy subjects by Ozaki.[225] This increased activity could be compensating for decreased function of the torn cuff. Ozaki, like Ting and coworkers,[281] postulates that this increasing activity could be responsible for the hypertrophy of the long head of the biceps that is often seen accompanying small and medium rotator cuff tears.[226] Patients with massive tears and dislocated biceps tendons had no similar increase in activity.

Biceps and rotator cuff EMG activity was found to precede motion of the glenohumeral joint in a study by David and colleagues.[61] They found that EMG activity in these muscles occurs 0.092 ± 0.038 to 0.215 ± 0.045 seconds before actual internal or external rotation movement. The deltoid and pectoralis major muscles were also activated before glenohumeral motion, but at a significantly later time, 0.030 ± 0.047 to 0.12 ± 0.053 seconds. They postulated that the biceps and rotator cuff muscles were stiffening the joint to provide stability before initiating movement. Once movement initiated, the activity of the biceps was dependent on the direction of the movement. Little activity was found in the biceps during internal rotation, but more activity was seen during external rotation.

Sakurai and associates[260] studied EMG activity in the biceps while maintaining the elbow in a brace in neutral rotation. Surface electrodes were used to measure EMG activity of the deltoid and biceps muscles. Their results showed EMG activity in both the long and short heads of the biceps with all motions of the shoulder independent of elbow position. In their study, the biceps acted as an active flexor and abductor of the shoulder. It also showed activity with rotation. External rotation induced a larger amount of activity than internal rotation did. They also demonstrated greater fatigability of the biceps in relation to the deltoid. Accordingly, they thought that the biceps was at higher risk for injury than the deltoid was.

On the other hand, two other studies found no significant active role for the biceps in glenohumeral stability. In their study, Yamaguchi and colleagues[312,313] kept the elbow fixed at 100 degrees of flexion with the forearm in neutral rotation in an attempt to relax the elbow flexors. They also used EMG activity of the brachioradialis as a control for biceps EMG activity. Their results showed little to no activity in the biceps tendon, even in the group of patients in whom the head depressor effect of the cuff musculature was compromised. Furthermore, no difference was noted between the EMG activity of the brachioradialis and the biceps. They concluded that the biceps' role in stability is probably a passive one. In this relaxed position, the long head of the biceps did not actively contribute to stability of the humeral head.

Using a similar experimental design, Levy and coworkers[156] studied the EMG activity of the biceps and rotator cuff muscles with intramuscular electrodes during motion of the shoulder. A brace was used to control elbow motion. Three different elbow positions were tested. The shoulders were moved in flexion, external rotation, and internal rotation at two different speeds and with a 5-lb weight. The results showed no activity in the biceps tendon when elbow motion was controlled. The authors point out that many activities performed by the arm require both elbow and shoulder motion. In their experimental design they purposely removed elbow motion. The lack of bicipital activity seems to reflect this control of the elbow. They state that the EMG activity in the biceps in other studies may have occurred because of active motion or stabilization of the elbow by the biceps. They conclude that the biceps is not active in isolated motion of the shoulder.

Summary

It appears from a review of the literature that based on the finding of consistent EMG activity with shoulder flexion and abduction independent of elbow flexion and given the resultant force of the biceps muscle, the biceps tendon does have a weak active head depressor or stabilizing effect. Because of its anatomic position, it serves as a superior checkrein to humeral head excursion and therefore at the very least acts as a static head depressor. As long as the tendon is located in its groove, the humeral head will slide up and down on the tendon and on the glenoid face in the normal fashion. With tears of the rotator cuff and medial subluxation of the biceps tendon, this checkrein effect is lost. The lack of EMG activity with disassociation of shoulder and elbow motion may not be clinically relevant.

The tendon's activity seems to increase in pathologic states of the shoulder such as rotator cuff tears and shoulder instability, as evidenced by increased EMG activity as well as observation of hypertrophy and resistance to translation. The observation of increased superior translation of the humeral head in patients with confirmed bicipital rupture reinforces these findings. Based on this evidence, one cannot recommend that tenodesis of the long head of the biceps tendon be routinely performed at the time of acromioplasty or that the tendon be used as a free graft for performing rotator cuff repairs if it is otherwise normal. On the other hand, if during the preoperative workup or at the time of surgery pathologic changes are found that implicate the biceps in pain production, the downside of decreased shoulder function is small in comparison to the risk of continued pain.

CLASSIFICATION OF BICIPITAL LESIONS

Biceps lesions have historically been divided into biceps tendinitis and biceps instability. Biceps tendinitis was further divided into primary tendinitis, which was due to pathology of the biceps tendon sheath, and secondary biceps tendinitis, which had an associated lesion causing the tendinitis. An example is rheumatoid arthritis, osteoarthritis, or impingement causing bicipital tendinitis. More recently, a classification by anatomic locale has been offered by Walch.[296]

Primary biceps tendinitis has been likened to de Quervain's tenosynovitis by Lapidus and Guidotti.[152] The presence of thickening and stenosis of the transverse ligament and sheath and narrowing of the tendon underneath the sheath was demonstrated by these authors. DePalma[66-70] showed that the severity of the process is governed by the duration of the condition and the age of the patient. Post and colleagues[245] found consistent inflammation within

the intertubercular portion of the tendon with proliferative tenosynovitis, as well as irregularity of the walls of the
groove. There seems to be no reports of inflammation of
the intra-articular portion of the biceps. Codman[50]
believed that primary biceps tendinitis was a rare entity,
whereas DePalma[66-70] thought that it was a common cause
of stiff and painful shoulders. In DePalma's series, 39% of
cases had associated disorders. Crenshaw and Kilgore[60]
were also proponents of primary biceps tendinitis,
although 40% of their patients had an associated lesion.
They concluded that whether the biceps tendon or its
sheath is involved primarily or secondarily is not important, but that tenosynovitis was the chief cause of pain
and limitation of motion in pericapsulitis.

Many authors[67,68,207-210,244,245] believe that the pathology
seen in the biceps is directly related to its intimate relationship with the rotator cuff. As they pass under the
coracoacromial arch, both are involved in the impingement syndrome.

"Isolated" rupture of the biceps tendon has been
described by several authors.[55,126,188,229] Neer believed that
most biceps tendon ruptures were associated with
supraspinatus tendon tears. Some studies have shown isolated rupture of the biceps tendon occurring in 25% of
patients.[64] When computed tomographic (CT) arthrograms are performed on patients who have the clinical criteria for isolated rupture of the long head of the biceps,
the incidence of isolated lesions decreases to 6%.[64] In an
arthroscopically controlled study of isolated biceps
tendon lesions, a 2.2% rate of isolated biceps rupture was
documented. These studies show the rarity of isolated
rupture of the long head of the biceps. Many authors have
described bicipital groove osteophytes that were thought
to cause rupture of the long head of the biceps.[55,133,188,228]
Studies using CT scans have shown that the depth and
width of the bicipital groove do not have pathognomonic
significance.[64]

Although primary bicipital tendinitis was recognized
as a frequent cause of shoulder pain in the 1940s and
1950s, today it is a diagnosis that is made much less frequently. Even though we do not doubt the existence of

TABLE 19-1.   Slatis and Aalto Classification

Type A	Impingement tendinitis
Type B	Subluxation of the biceps
Type C	Attrition is primary

this lesion, it is very uncommon. It should be considered
a diagnosis of exclusion.

Slatis and Aalto[268] have offered what appears to be a
useful clinical classification of biceps lesions (Table 19-1).
It is based on pathoanatomy and appears to have
prognostic significance according to their review. It is as
follows:

Slatis and Aalto Classification

Type A: Impingement Tendinitis

Type A was tendinitis secondary to impingement syndrome and rotator cuff disease. The torn cuff exposes the
biceps to the rigid coracoacromial arch, and such exposure results in tendinitis (Figs. 19-31 and 19-32). This
type is the most frequent cause of biceps tendinitis.

Type B: Subluxation of the Biceps Tendon

Type B was called subluxation pathology. In this category,
all pathologies of the biceps that included subluxation
and dislocation of the tendon were included (Fig. 19-33).
In this group, lesions of the coracohumeral ligament
allow the biceps tendon to gradually become displaced
medially. This lesion can occur in an isolated fashion or it
can be associated with tears of the supraspinatus and subscapularis. As the tendon slips in and out of its sulcus,
inflammation and fraying develop. The tendon can finally
fully displace into a sling of ruptured cuff in early cases.
In more severe and later cases, the tendon may actually
dislocate intra-articularly. The groove becomes shallower
during this process as it fills with scar.

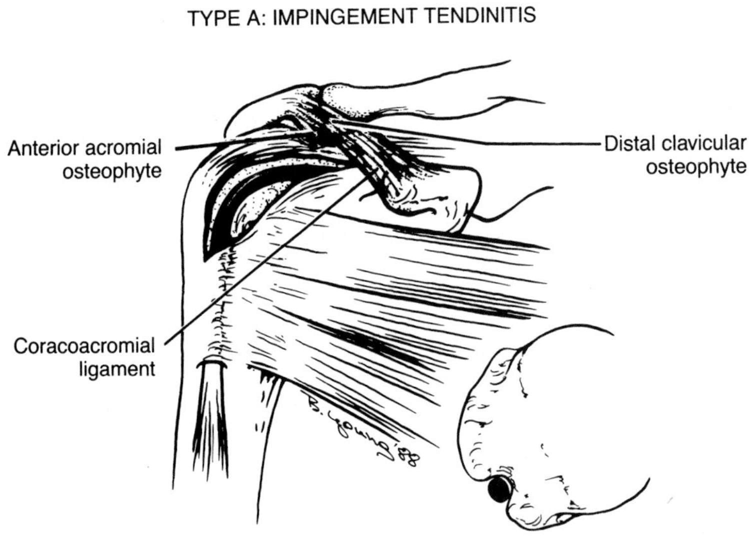

TYPE A: IMPINGEMENT TENDINITIS

Anterior acromial osteophyte

Distal clavicular osteophyte

Coracoacromial ligament

■ **Figure 19-31**
Type A impingement tendinitis. Rupture of the rotator
cuff exposes the tendon to compression between the
acromion above and the humeral head below. The
tendon normally lies in its groove. (*Modified from
Paavolainen P, Slatis P, and Aalto K: Surgical pathology in
chronic shoulder pain. In Bateman JE and Welsh RP [eds]:
Surgery of the Shoulder. Philadelphia: BC Decker, 1984.*)

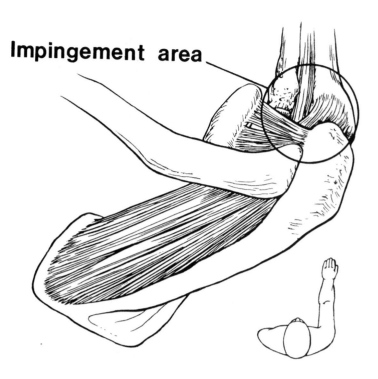

Impingement area

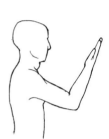

■ **Figure 19–32**
When the arm is forward-flexed, the impingement area (i.e., the groove, biceps tendon, and anterior cuff) comes in contact with the coracoacromial arch. The longer the acromial process, the more likely the biceps will be involved. (*Courtesy of Charles A. Rockwood, Jr., M.D.*)

TYPE B: SUBLUXATION

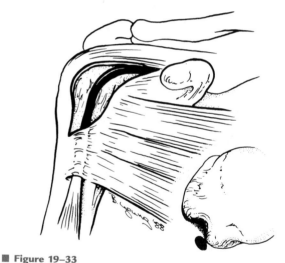

TYPE C: ATTRITION TENDINITIS

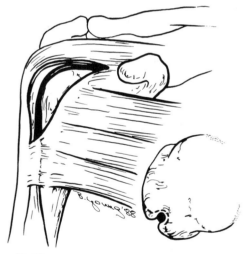

■ **Figure 19–33**
Type B subluxation of the biceps. A tear in the medial portion of the coracohumeral ligament causes subluxation and medial displacement of the tendon from the bicipital groove. Note the filling of the groove with fibrous tissue. (*Modified from Paavolainen P, Slatis P, and Aalto K: Surgical pathology in chronic shoulder pain. In Bateman JE and Welsh RP [eds]: Surgery of the Shoulder. Philadelphia: BC Decker, 1984.*)

■ **Figure 19–34**
The cuff is exposed to show the pathology of constriction of the biceps tendon within the groove. Local formation of new bone and connective tissue causes stenosis of the bicipital groove and subsequent attrition of the tendon of the long head of the biceps.

Type C: Attrition Tendinitis

Attrition tendinitis was the third category. These types of lesions were primary lesions of the biceps tendon that occurred inside the canal. In this type of tendinitis, inflammation in the tight canal causes pain and degeneration of the biceps tendon (Fig. 19–34). These changes are associated with spurring and fraying of the tendon. Inflammation of the sheath causes the formation of spurs and stenosis of the groove. This condition was thought to be extremely painful and rare.

Habermeyer and Walch's Classification

Habermeyer and Walch[113] classified lesions of the biceps tendon in a different manner (Table 19-2). They noted that the biceps tendon could be involved in pathology in different anatomic locations. In their classification, lesions of the biceps are found either (1) at the origin, (2) in the rotator interval, or (3) in association with rotator cuff tears.

TABLE 19-2. Habermeyer and Walch's Classification of Biceps Lesions

I. Origin	II. Interval Lesions	III. Associated with RCT
	A. Biceps tendinitis B. Isolated ruptures C. Subluxation 　　Type I: Superior 　　Type II: At the groove 　　Type III: Malunion or nonunion of the lesser tuberosity	A. Tendinitis B. Dislocation 　　Type IA: Extra-articular with a partial subscapularis tear 　　Type IB: Extra-articular with an intact subscapularis 　　Type II: Intra-articular C. Subluxation with RCT D. LHB rupture with RCT

LHB, long head of the biceps; RCT, rotator cuff tear.

Origin Lesions

Origin lesions are described as lesions affecting the attachment of the biceps tendon to the supraglenoid tubercle and to the superior glenoid labrum. These lesions can involve the biceps origin from the superior labrum and spare the fibers coming off the supraglenoid tubercle, or they can include lesions in which the superior glenoid rim is avulsed off the glenoid and pulled away with the biceps tendon. These lesions have been observed to occur with the use of muscle stimulation. Biomechanical data by Grauer and coworkers[108] have shown that strain on the labrum from the working biceps is greatest when the arm is in overhead abduction.

Lesions that affect the origin of the biceps tendon can occur in many different ways. These lesions have been described by Andrews and colleagues[9] as lesions of the anterior superior labrum in throwing athletes. These lesions are usually due to traction injuries in throwing athletes, especially during the release phase of throwing. They are associated with biceps tendon tears in 10% of cases.[9] These lesions can also be caused by falls on the outstretched arm with the shoulder in abduction and slight forward flexion.[270] In addition, acute inferior traction as well as abduction–external rotation injuries can cause these lesions.[111]

Snyder and colleagues[270] introduced the term SLAP (superior labrum, anteroposterior) lesion in 1990. These authors classified SLAP lesions into four basic types. Type I is a lesion of the superior labrum. It shows marked fraying of the edges of the labrum, but the labral attachment to the glenoid is solid. This lesion does not really involve the biceps tendon. In a type II lesion, the superior labral–biceps complex is stripped from the underlying glenoid. This stripping causes the labral-biceps anchor to be unstable in that portion of the biceps origin that is not inserted onto the supraglenoid tubercle. Type III lesions involve a bucket handle tear of the superior labrum in which the biceps tendon is not involved. Type IV lesions, on the other hand, have a bucket handle tear with splitting that extends into the biceps tendon.

Variations of SLAP lesions have also been described in association with complete rupture of the long head of the biceps.[34,111] SLAP lesions are covered more completely elsewhere in this text.

Interval Lesions

Habermeyer and Walch[113] divided interval lesions into three types: biceps tendinitis, subluxation of the long head of the biceps tendon, and isolated rupture.

Biceps Tendinitis

Biceps tendinitis is clinically characterized by chronic shoulder pain with tenderness over the bicipital groove and a positive Speed test. When these criteria are used, 90% of all painful shoulders could be considered to have biceps tendinitis. Pathologic examination of biceps tendons in these shoulders rarely shows degenerative or microtraumatic lesions. Such changes of the biceps tendon have been reported in only 5% of cases.

Primary Bicipital Tendinitis

This lesion, according to Walch and Habermeyer,[113] can be diagnosed only by arthroscopy. Findings of erythema and a vascular reaction around the long head of the biceps and in the groove are usually observed. For this diagnosis to be made, the shoulder must have a complete passive range of motion. The tendon should not be subluxated or dislocated out of its groove. Mechanical fraying of the bicipital tendon caused by osteophytes or narrowing of the groove from fracture is considered secondary. In their experience of over 3 years of arthroscopy of the shoulder looking specifically for isolated biceps tendinitis, they have been unsuccessful in finding one case. Isolated biceps tendinitis remains a diagnosis of exception.[294]

Subluxation of the Long Head of the Biceps Tendon

The definition of instability of the long head of the biceps tendon is poorly standardized and controversial.[72,172,222,228,238]

Walch[294] defines subluxation of the long head of the biceps tendon as partial or incomplete loss of contact between the tendon and its bony groove. He defined dislocation as complete loss of contact between the tendon and its bony groove. Subluxation has been divided into three types by Walch.[294]

Superior Subluxation—Type I

This lesion occurs when the superior glenohumeral and the coracohumeral ligaments are partially or completely torn. The result of this tearing is that the long head of the biceps tendon above the entrance of the groove is subluxated superiorly. The subscapularis tendon is intact. The subscapularis tendon prevents true dislocation of the tendon. A type I lesion is a discontinuity of the tendoligamentous rotator interval sling surrounding the long head of the biceps tendon that allows the tendon to migrate superiorly.

Subluxation in the Groove—Type II

The lesion responsible for this type of subluxation is located inside the bony groove. The tendon slips over the medial rim of the bone of the groove and rides on the border of the lesser tuberosity. This lesion is caused by tearing of the outermost fibers of the subscapularis tendon, as well as some fibers that align the floor. The principle criterion for type II biceps tendon subluxation is partial rupture of the outer superficial tendinous portion of the subscapularis muscle. This lesion can involve the whole groove or only a portion of it.

Malunion and Nonunion of the Lesser Tuberosity—Type III

Fracture-dislocation of the lesser tuberosity with malunion or nonunion can allow the biceps tendon to slip in and out of its groove. This lesion is seen after proximal humeral fractures. Affected patients complain of pain with internal rotation of the humerus.

Isolated Rupture of the Biceps Tendon Occurring in the Rotator Interval

Severe primary tendinitis of the tendon in the interval can cause weakening of the tendon and its eventual rupture in this area.

Biceps Tendinitis Associated with Rotator Cuff Tears

Patients in this subgroup have tendinitis of the biceps secondary to exposure of the biceps to the rigid coracoacromial arch. These patients have a rotator cuff tear but no dislocation or subluxation of the biceps tendon. The biceps is inflamed and painful and may appear hypertrophic when viewed through the arthroscope.

Dislocation Associated with Rotator Cuff Tears

Extra-articular Dislocation Associated with Subscapularis Lesions (Type IA)

Extra-articular dislocation combined with a partial tear of the subscapularis tendon occurs when the biceps tendon is completely dislocated over the lesser tuberosity. Despite superficial tearing of the subscapularis tendon, the deep portion of the subscapularis is intact. This intact portion allows the biceps tendon to line up over the lesser tuberosity and prevents the biceps from entering the joint. In this type of dislocation, the outer layer of the subscapularis tendon is always torn. This injury is an evolutional type II subluxation.

Extra-articular Dislocation of the Long Head of the Biceps Tendon Associated with an Intact Subscapularis (Type IB)

The biceps tendon can dislocate over an intact subscapularis tendon. This condition is extremely rare. The long head of the biceps tendon is found lying superficial to the intact subscapularis tendon. An associated tear of the supraspinatus tendon is always seen. This type was found in 3% of 70 patients with biceps dislocations.[220]

Intra-articular Dislocation of the Long Head of the Biceps Tendon (Type II)

Intra-articular dislocation of the long biceps tendon combined with a complete tear of the subscapularis tendon is type II. In this category, complete dislocation of the biceps is found in the intra-articular location. It usually occurs in conjunction with extensive tearing of the rotator cuff. The subscapularis tendon is torn completely from its attachment on the lesser tuberosity, and the biceps tendon can become interposed into the joint. The biceps tendon is then opposed to the glenoid labrum and can be entrapped in the anterior joint space during rotational movements of the humerus. Subluxation of the biceps can also be associated with rotator cuff tearing.

Ruptures of the Biceps Associated with Rotator Cuff Tears

The biceps can also rupture as a consequence of rotator cuff tears. Walch[295] has shown the frequency with which these lesions are associated. As has been stated earlier, an isolated rupture of the biceps tendon is extremely rare. Most biceps tendon ruptures are associated with rotator cuff tears, usually as a result of impingement of the biceps and supraspinatus tendons in the area of the biceps sulcus.

TLC Classification

In an attempt to somehow simplify how to think about these complex lesions, the senior one of us has developed the simple pneumonic TLC. The TLC system (Table 19-3) takes into account three distinct factors: the status of the biceps tendon (T), the anatomic location (L) of the pathologic process, and associated pathologic conditions of the rotator cuff (C). With this classification, subtypes such as I, IIA, IIB, IIC, III, or IV do not need to be memorized; there are merely three things to remember when thinking about the biceps. TLC should be easy to recall because that is how the biceps should be handled.

TABLE 19-3.   TLC Classification

TENDON	Stable	Unstable	Tendinitis	Rupture
LOCATION	Origin	Interval	Groove	Musculotendinous junction
CUFF	Intact	Partial tear	Complete tear	Tendinosis

INCIDENCE

In 1934, DePalma[66-70] stated that tenosynovitis of the long head of the biceps brachii tendon is the most common antecedent of painful and stiff shoulders. He believed that this was true in both younger and older individuals. In his 1954 series,[70] the lesion was encountered in 77 men and 98 women ranging in age from 16 to 69 years. The highest incidence was between the ages of 45 and 55. Bilateral involvement was observed in 8% of cases. More severe lesions were found in the older decades of life, where more severe degenerative changes prevail. In 61.2% of cases, the bicipital tenosynovitis was a localized pathologic process. In 38.8% of cases, inflammation in the biceps tendon and sheath was part of a generalized and chronic inflammatory process. DePalma[66-70] believed that bicipital tenosynovitis was the initiating agent in 80% of cases of frozen shoulder. Regardless of the cause, bicipital tenosynovitis was always a concomitant of a frozen shoulder.

Calcific tendinitis of the long head of the biceps brachii is uncommon.[255] This lesion has been described in two places. The first is the insertion of the biceps tendon into the supraglenoid tubercle and superior labrum. The second is in the distal portion of the groove near the musculotendinous junction. Calcific tendinitis occurred more frequently in a series by Goldman.[104] Nine cases of insertion tendinitis were seen in 119 cases of calcific tendinitis of the shoulder, as opposed to 11 of 19 for the more distal location.

Injuries to the superior labrum and biceps tendon complex occur infrequently. In a series by Andrews and colleagues,[9] 10% of 73 throwing athletes had associated partial tears of the biceps tendon and labral pathology. Burkhart and Fox[34] described two cases of complete tears of the biceps associated with SLAP lesions.

According to McCue and coworkers[176] and O'Donohue,[222] biceps tendinitis and subluxation are common causes of anterior shoulder pain in throwing athletes. It is more common in football quarterbacks because of the weight of the ball and the need for additional pushing action and in softball pitchers because of forceful supinator strain with arm and forearm flexion.

Lapidus and Guidotti[152] identified 89 patients with tendinitis of the long head of the biceps in a total of 493 patients treated for shoulder pain, for an incidence of 18%. Paavolainen and colleagues[228] reported on patients who failed to respond to conservative care and were referred to a shoulder center. A preoperative diagnosis of bicipital tendinitis was made before arthrotomy in 38 of 126, or 30%. Postoperatively with direct inspection of the biceps tendon, the incidence was much higher; 54% of the operative specimens showed some evidence of biceps tendinitis. In patients with cuff ruptures, the incidence was 31 of 51, or 60%. If the rotator cuff was intact (no full-thickness tear), the incidence was approximately 50%. Although the cuff was "intact" at surgery, most of these cuffs did show some evidence of degeneration, edema, and signs of stage I and II impingement. Medial dislocation of the biceps tendon occurred in 12 of 51 cases with the cuff ruptured and in 9 of 75 cases when the cuff was intact, for an overall incidence of dislocation of 17%. Frank rupture of the biceps tendon was seen in 8 of the 126 patients, or 6%.

Because bicipital tenosynovitis occasionally accompanies impingement syndrome, it remains a relatively common cause of anterior shoulder pain. However, as an isolated entity (i.e., primary bicipital tenosynovitis), it is much less common.

ETIOLOGY

Although the majority of biceps tendon dislocations occur secondarily as a result of degeneration and attrition of the anterior cuff and coracohumeral ligament,[85-89,183-190,207,208,210,211] acute traumatic dislocation of the tendon of the biceps has been described. Abbott and Saunders[2] in 1939 presented six cases with operative findings. Four were caused by a fall with a direct blow to the shoulder or from an indirect force after a fall on the outstretched hands. Two occurred during heavy lifting. All but one of these patients had a concomitant injury to the rotator cuff as well.

DePalma[66-70] and later Michele[191] divided the etiology of biceps tendinitis by the age group of the patient. In the younger age group, anomalies of the bicipital groove together with repeated trauma are the major factors in initiating the syndrome. In the older age group, degenerative changes in the tendon are the predominant etiologic factor.

Like most other musculoskeletal problems, the etiology of biceps pathology is most likely multifactorial. Chief among the causes is the anatomic location of the tendon. The blood supply of the tendon has been studied by Rathbun and Macnab[252] and shown to be diminished, with a critical zone similar to that seen in the supraspinatus (Fig. 19–35). In abduction, there is a zone of avascularity in the intracapsular portion of the tendon that is thought to be caused by pressure from the head of the humerus, the so-called wringing-out phenomenon. Occupational causes also exist because patients who perform repetitive overhead lifting and throwing are more prone to rupture, elongation, and dislocation of the biceps. Meyer[183-190] reasoned that capsular defects leading to problems with the biceps resulted from repeated and continual use of the arm in a position of marked abduction and external rotation. Borchers[30] and later DePalma[66-70] explained spontaneous rupture within the groove on the basis of osteophytic excrescences, which eventually wear away the tendon. Etiologic factors based on variations in the groove have been discussed previously.

The etiology of calcific deposits in the biceps may be active or passive. Hydroxyapatite deposition disease has been described and can occur in varied tendons throughout the body. The reader is referred to Chapter 18 for a detailed description of active calcification. In a study by Refior and Sowa,[253] histologic analysis of the biceps tendon was performed and showed degeneration at the biceps origin and in the region in which the biceps tendon exits the groove. They noted kinking and destruction of the collagen fibers in both these areas. Whether this degeneration is responsible for inducing calcification in some susceptible patients is debatable.

Intra-articular lesions of the biceps and superior labrum can be caused by several mechanisms. The first is

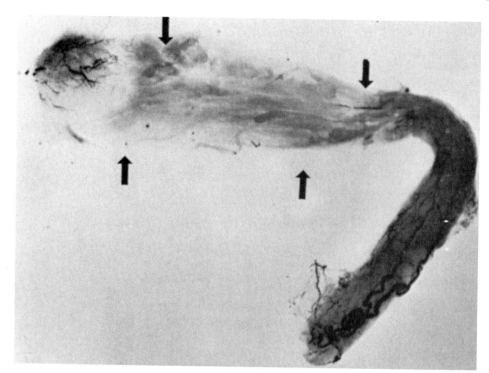

■ **Figure 19–35**
Zone of relative avascularity seen in the biceps. *(From Rathbun JB and Macnab I: The microvascular pattern of the rotator cuff. J Bone Joint Surg Br 52:540-553, 1970.)*

a fall on the outstretched hand that drives the humeral head up into the labrum and the tendon.[270] Andrews and colleagues[9] noted that excessive and forceful contraction of the biceps in throwing athletes, especially baseball pitchers and quarterbacks, can induce traction and avulsion of the biceps and superior labral complex in the deceleration phase of throwing. Finally, SLAP lesions can also be created by traction on an adducted arm.

Recently, Gerber and Sebesta[91] described an anterior internal impingement syndrome similar to the posterior internal impingement syndrome described by Walch and colleagues.[297] In their study, contact between the superior glenohumeral ligament and the anterior rim of the glenoid occurred while performing the Hawkins modified impingement test at 120 degrees of anterior elevation. The undersurface of the subscapularis tendon came into contact with the anterior glenoid rim when the arm was placed between 80 and 100 degrees of flexion. Contact of the superior glenohumeral ligaments and subscapularis on the anterior glenoid rim could explain fraying of these deep structures that do not come into contact with the anterior acromion. These findings were found most commonly in the dominant arm of manual laborers.

Patients maintained on dialysis with long-standing kidney failure can have shoulder pain and may have symptoms similar to biceps tendinitis. Often, the etiology of this syndrome is a synovitis caused by the deposition of amyloid-like substances. This entity is a rare cause of shoulder pain.[278] Another rare cause of bicipital pain and degeneration is a tumoral condition such as osteochondromatosis of the bicipital sheath.[63]

PREVENTION

Prevention of biceps injuries in workers and athletes entails the same type of preventive rehabilitation that is used in athletes for their rotator cuff, including warm-up passive stretching, strengthening, and avoidance of painful activities during the time of symptoms. Strengthening should include all the muscles of the rotator cuff to improve the force couple and decrease impingement. The parascapular muscles should also be rehabilitated. A better balanced shoulder musculature will prevent or at least decrease the vicious circle of impingement tendinitis, irritation, and muscle weakness, followed by altered biomechanics, subluxation, and further impingement. Persons who do manual labor involving heavy lifting or repetitive overhead work, such as carpenters, should probably spend as much time stretching before undertaking their jobs as football and baseball players spend before undertaking theirs. Stretching of the biceps tendon is maximal when the shoulder is fully extended and externally rotated and the elbow is fully extended as well.

Careful pre-employment screening and testing, including muscular strength, can help identify shoulder problems before employees begin working. Deficits noted could be corrected with exercise before beginning a job that requires heavy lifting or overhead use of the arm. The scapular lateral outlet view and the 30-degree caudal tilt x-ray view may possibly be used to prevent people at risk for impingement from taking jobs that would put their shoulders at risk for injury.

Overhand athletes, especially pitchers and quarterbacks, should warm up and stretch their rotator cuff as well as their paraspinal and arm muscles before training sessions and competition. They should be encouraged to strengthen the muscles of their upper extremity, especially the rotator cuff. Athletes should also be monitored closely to prevent overuse syndromes from developing. The use of a pitching rotation in young baseball pitchers can allow some of these players to rest adequately.

CLINICAL FEATURES OF BICIPITAL LESIONS

There is no substitute in any medical condition for an accurate history and physical examination. This statement is especially true for subtle lesions of the shoulder such as biceps tendinitis and instability.

Patients with bicipital tendinitis usually have chronic pain in the proximal anterior area of the shoulder. The pain sometimes extends down the arm into the region of the biceps muscle belly. It can, like pain from impingement syndrome, radiate to the deltoid insertion. Usually, the pain from bicipital tendinitis does not radiate into the neck or distally beyond the biceps. In most cases, patients have no history of major trauma, although as has been stated previously, acute trauma can predispose to bicipital tendinitis, rupture, or dislocation. Typically, the patient is young or middle aged with a history of repetitive use of the arm in overhead activity. The pain is less intense at rest and worse with use. Neviaser[212] states that there is no significant night pain, whereas Simon[267] believes that nocturnal exacerbation is common. In our experience, all painful conditions of the shoulder are worse at night because of compression loading and because the supine position places the shoulder at or below the level of the heart. Rolling over on the involved shoulder further increases the problem by decreasing the venous return from the upper extremity. The pain from calcific tendinitis of the biceps is of such great intensity that the patient often walks the floor at night.

Bicipital symptoms are frequently seen in patients who participate in sports. Any activity at or above the horizontal level that brings the tuberosities, the intervening groove, the biceps tendon, and the rotator cuff in direct contact with the anterior acromion, coracoacromial ligament, or the anterior edge of the glenoid can either as a single event or through repetitive trauma produce pathology in the biceps.

Biceps instability is seen most commonly in throwing athletes. Motion is often accompanied by a palpable snap or pop at a certain position in the arc of rotation. The patient indicates pain in the front of the shoulder, usually reproduced by raising the arm up to 90 degrees. Biceps rupture appears frequently with acute pain and sometimes with an audible pop in the shoulder. Over the next several days, the patient will notice a change in contour of the arm and ecchymosis.

Calcific tendinitis in the distal part of the long head of the biceps tendon is clinically manifested as anterior shoulder pain in young and middle-aged adults. The pain of distal tendon involvement is usually referred to the anterior region of the shoulder. The duration and severity of this pain can vary.

Physical Examination

Physical examination reveals point tenderness in the biceps groove, which is best localized with the arm in about 10 degrees of internal rotation.[174] With the arm in this position, the biceps tendon should be facing directly anteriorly and located 3 inches below the acromion (Fig. 19–36).[208] Point tenderness in this area (i.e., 7 cm below

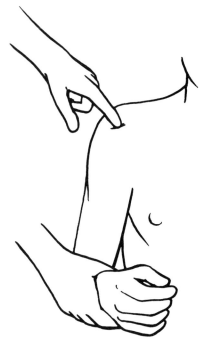

■ **Figure 19–36**
Matsen and Kirby[174] found that the biceps tendon can be palpated directly anteriorly with the arm in 10 degrees of internal rotation. This position is the same as that used before performing the deAnquin and Lippmann tests (described in the text).

the anterior acromion) should move with rotation of the arm. It often disappears as the lesser tuberosity and groove rotate internally under the short head of the biceps and coracoid. The tenderness of subdeltoid bursitis is generally more diffuse and should not move with arm rotation. The tenderness seen with impingement is often diffuse and accompanied by tenderness in the arm, acromion, coracoacromial ligament, and coracoid process. However, it does not move with rotation. This "tenderness in motion" sign is, in our opinion, the most specific for bicipital lesions. It does not, however, differentiate biceps instability from tendinitis. Many authors have stated that the biceps can be felt subluxating out of the groove. It is difficult to discern whether what one is feeling is actually a subluxating tendon or the muscle bundles of the deltoid rolling up underneath one's finger as it is pressed against the humerus. Anyone who has looked at the biceps surgically should have trouble thinking that he is actually palpating the tendon, especially in a well-muscled individual.

Slight restriction of abduction and internal rotation may be noted. This loss of motion is usually due to pain and not to capsular constriction and should improve with local anesthetic injection. Pain is felt with abduction and internal rotation, abduction and external rotation, and resisted forward flexion of the shoulder.

Several tests have been reported to aid in the diagnosis of biceps pathology. Few data, however, have been reported regarding the sensitivity or specificity of any of these tests in patients with shoulder pain. The most important question when performing provocative tests on any part of the musculoskeletal system is "Does this

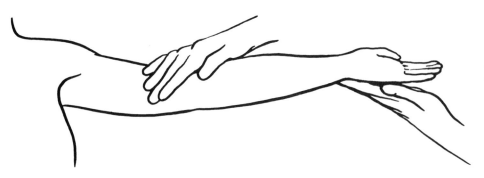

Speed's test. The biceps resistance test is performed with the patient flexing the shoulder against resistance with the elbow extended and the forearm supinated. Pain referred to the biceps tendon area constitutes a positive test.

maneuver specifically reproduce the patient's pain?" Selective injection with obliteration of pain is an extremely important part of clinical evaluation of the shoulder. There is no substitute for clinical experience, repeated examination, selective injection, and a cautious approach to anterior shoulder pain. Many poor results from surgery in this region come from a surgical procedure being performed too early or directed only at the biceps lesion. Repeated examination may show evolution of an impingement syndrome, adhesive capsulitis, or evidence of glenohumeral instability. The following tests have been described by authors in the past for isolating lesions in the biceps tendon:

1. Speed's test (Fig. 19–37).[90] The patient flexes the shoulder against resistance while the elbow is extended and the forearm supinated. The pain is localized in the bicipital groove.

   Recently, Bennett[22] has tested the sensitivity and specificity of the Speed test. He correctly remarked that we have a lot of data about the positive and negative predictive value of expensive diagnostic studies, but validation of our clinical examination is often lacking. He compared the results of Speed's test with pathology seen during arthroscopy. Speed's test was considered to be correctly positive only when a macroscopic lesion was found on the biceps or superior labrum. Speed's test was determined to be 90% sensitive for shoulder pain, but it was only 13% specific for bicipital pathology. The positive predictive value was 23% and the negative predictive value was 83%. This study showed that although the Speed test was developed and identified as a test for bicipital tendinitis, it is not very useful for diagnosing this pathology. On the other hand, a positive Speed test was sensitive enough to suggest that anterior shoulder pathology was present.

2. Yergason's sign (Fig. 19–38).[315] This test is performed with the patient's elbow flexed. The patient is asked to forcibly supinate against resistance. Pain referred to the front and inner aspect of the shoulder in the bicipital groove constitutes a positive sign. Post[244] found an incidence of 50% positivity with this sign in patients with primary bicipital tendinitis. The advantage of Yergason's test is that the shoulder is not moving and a more pure biceps examination is performed.

3. Biceps instability test (Fig. 19–39).[1] Dislocation of the tendon, complete or incomplete, may be differentiated from peritendinitis by the test of Abbott and Saunders.[2] After full abduction of the shoulder, the arm, which is held in complete external rotation, is slowly

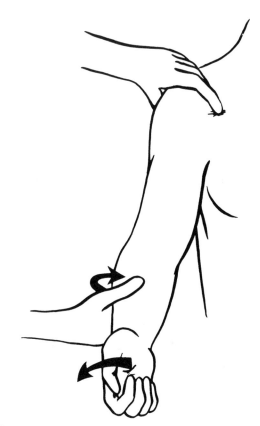

■ **Figure 19–38**
Yergason's sign. With the arm flexed, the patient is asked to forcefully supinate against resistance from the examiner's hand. Pain referred to the anterior aspect of the shoulder in the region of the bicipital groove constitutes a positive test.

brought down to the side in the plane of the scapula. A palpable and even audible and sometimes painful click is noted as the biceps tendon, now forced against the lesser tuberosity, becomes subluxated or dislocated from the groove.

4. Ludington's test (Fig. 19–40).[164] In Ludington's test, patients are asked to put their hands behind their head. In this position of abduction and external rotation, patients are asked to flex their biceps isometrically, and pain is felt in the region of the bicipital groove in those with tendinitis. If the examiner's finger is in the groove at the time of the contraction, subluxation can sometimes be felt. Subtle differences in the contour of the biceps in cases of elongation are best noted in this fashion.

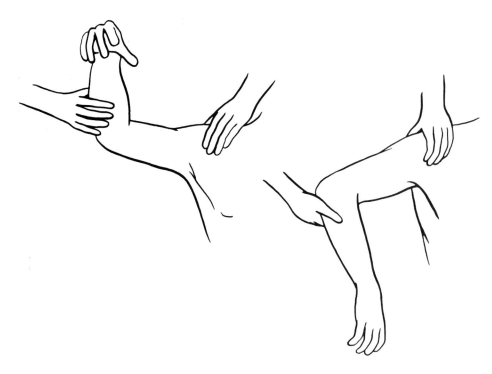

■ **Figure 19–39**
Biceps instability test (described by Abbott and Saunders). During palpation of the biceps in the groove while taking the arm from an abducted, externally rotated position to a position of internal rotation, a palpable or audible painful click is noted as the biceps tendon is forced against or over the lesser tuberosity.

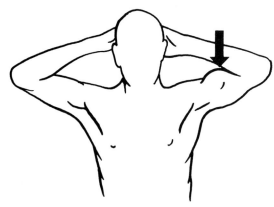

■ **Figure 19–40**
Ludington's test. The patient is asked to put his hands behind his head and flex his biceps. The examiner's finger can be in the bicipital groove at the time of the test. Subtle differences in the contour of the biceps are best noted with this maneuver. In this illustration the patient has a ruptured biceps at the left shoulder.

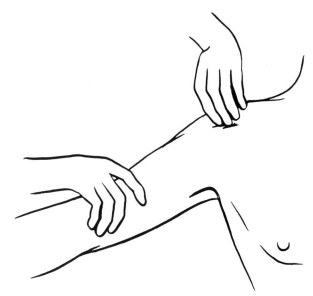

■ **Figure 19–41**
DeAnquin's test. The patient's arm is rotated while the examiner has his finger in the most tender spot in the bicipital groove. A positive test occurs in biceps tendinitis when the patient feels pain as the tendon glides beneath the finger.

5. deAnquin's test (Fig. 19–41).[276] The arm is rotated with the examiner's finger on the most tender spot. Pain is felt immediately as the tendon glides beneath the finger.
6. Lippmann's test.[157] Lippmann's test produces pain when the tendon is displaced from one side to the other by the probing finger and released. The probing is done about 3 inches from the shoulder joint, with the elbow flexed at a right angle. I think that we are more often rolling the deltoid muscle up with this test and the biceps is not being palpated.
7. Hueter's sign.[130] Hueter's sign is positive when flexion of the supinated forearm (primarily a biceps function) is less forceful than flexion of the pronated forearm.

Physical examination in patients with a complete biceps rupture is much less subtle (Fig. 19–42) because of the obvious deformity that develops. A hollowness is evident in the anterior portion of the shoulder, accompanied by balling up of the biceps below the midbrachium. In these patients it is important to look specifically for cuff atrophy because tears of the biceps in the older population are frequently associated with attrition-type tears in the rotator cuff preceding the biceps rupture. These tears may or may not have been symptomatic before the

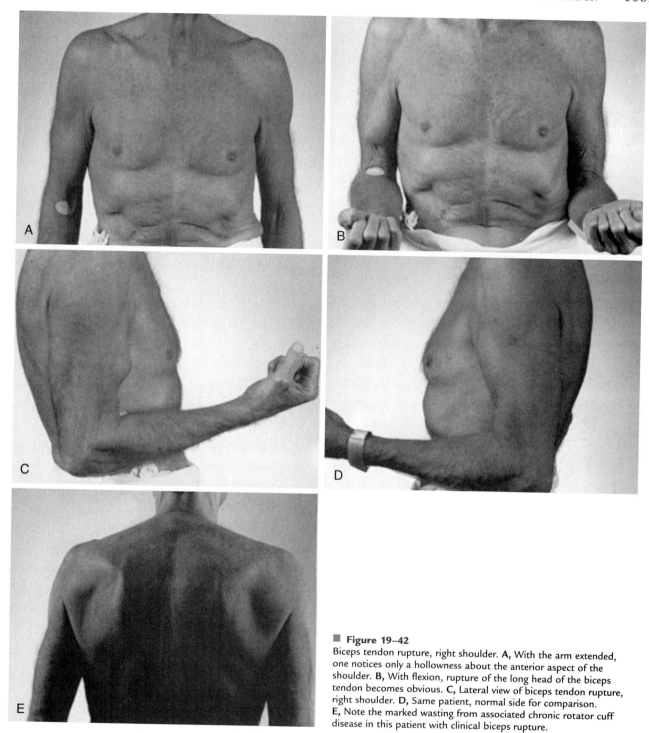

■ **Figure 19–42**
Biceps tendon rupture, right shoulder. **A,** With the arm extended, one notices only a hollowness about the anterior aspect of the shoulder. **B,** With flexion, rupture of the long head of the biceps tendon becomes obvious. **C,** Lateral view of biceps tendon rupture, right shoulder. **D,** Same patient, normal side for comparison. **E,** Note the marked wasting from associated chronic rotator cuff disease in this patient with clinical biceps rupture.

bicipital rupture, but it is not uncommon for the patient to have a history of being treated in the remote past for "bursitis." Some patients report an improvement in their shoulder pain after complete rupture of the long head of the biceps tendon. These patients often seek care for pain in the contralateral shoulder. The rupture usually occurred several years before the onset of pain in the currently symptomatic shoulder. The patient often fails to remember or mention the incident until the "Popeye" biceps is discovered on physical examination.

ASSOCIATED CONDITIONS

The following are associated conditions and are discussed under "Differential Diagnosis":

1. Impingement syndrome
2. Adhesive capsulitis
3. Rheumatoid arthritis and osteoarthritis
4. Glenohumeral instability
5. Coracoid impingement syndrome
6. Thoracic outlet/brachial plexopathy/plexitis

7. Peripheral nerve entrapment, cervical radiculopathy
8. Dialysis patients
9. Rare tumors

Concomitant Injuries

One should remain alert for a wide range of lesions when evaluating a biceps rupture. Such lesions include extensive damage to the rotator cuff and variable degrees of brachial plexus stretch, which are occasionally seen in association with biceps rupture and almost invariably occur as the result of a fall on a posteriorly outstretched arm in an elderly patient. Occasionally, anterior dislocation of the shoulder accompanies the injury. Humeral fractures and fracture-dislocations can occur. The biceps can become interposed and block reduction of both fractures and dislocations.[129,135,179] An extensive area of ecchymosis of the chest associated with the injury should tip off the examiner that the biceps tendon rupture is not an isolated injury. In isolated biceps rupture, the swelling and ecchymoses should be limited to the brachium.

DIAGNOSTIC TESTS

Plain Film Radiology

Frequently, routine plain films of the shoulder are normal in biceps tendinitis. Consequently, special views have been developed for the bicipital groove, and other imaging techniques have been used to evaluate this tendon.

Fisk's Method

In the Fisk method[84] (Fig. 19-43), the patient holds the cassette and leans over the table. The biceps groove is marked, and the central beam is perpendicular to the groove.

Bicipital Groove View

In the bicipital groove view described by Cone and colleagues (Fig. 19-43B),[53] the patient is supine with the arm in external rotation. The central beam is directed parallel

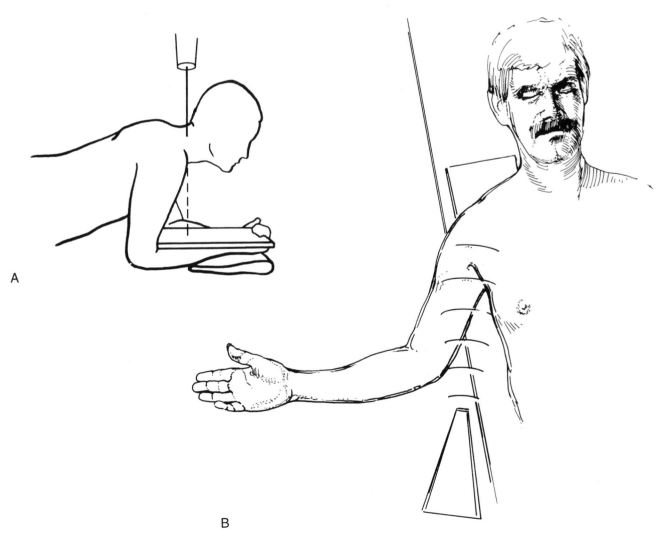

■ **Figure 19–43**
A, Fisk's method. The patient holds the cassette while leaning over the table to bring the bicipital groove perpendicular to the central beam of the x-ray. **B,** Bicipital groove view. The central beam is directed parallel to the coronal axis of the humerus and angled 15 degrees medially. The patient is supine with the arm in the externally rotated position.

to the coronal axis of the humerus and angled 15 degrees medially. The film cassette is held perpendicular to the superior aspect of the shoulder. From the radiographs, the medial wall angle, the width, and the presence or absence of bicipital groove spurs, coexisting degenerative changes in the greater or lesser tuberosity, and a supratubercular ridge can be determined (Fig. 19–44). In a study by Ahovuo[4] in which radiographic findings were correlated with surgical findings, half the patients with surgically proven bicipital tendinitis had degenerative changes in the walls of the groove. In patients with attrition tendinitis, the depth of the groove was 4.8 mm or more and its inclination was 58 degrees or more. A shallow groove was seen more frequently with bicipital dislocation.

Two additional views that are helpful in the differential diagnosis of biceps tendinitis are the caudal tilt view[256] radiograph and the outlet view of Neer and Poppen.[211] The caudal tilt radiograph is a standing anteroposterior view of the shoulder with a 30-degree caudal tilt of the x-ray beam (Fig. 19–45). With this technique, the degree of anterior acromial prominence or spurring can be appreciated. The outlet view is a trans-scapular radiograph performed with a 10-degree caudal tilt. The easiest way to take this radiograph is to have the patient stand with the spine of the scapula perpendicular to the cassette. The x-ray beam should be parallel to the spine, but with a 10-degree caudal tilt (Fig. 19–45B).

Arthrography

Shoulder arthrography can provide information on the state of the biceps tendon. Many shallow grooves contain a normal tendon.[4] Whether a shallow groove on plain films is associated with dislocation of the biceps can be determined by an arthrogram. Sometimes the dislocation

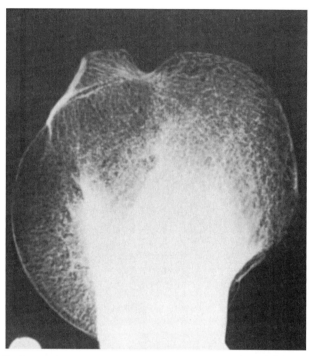

■ **Figure 19–44**
Normal bicipital groove projection. *(From Cone RO, Danzig L, Resnick D, and Goldman AB: The bicipital groove: Radiographic, anatomic, and pathologic study. AJR Am J Roentgenol 41:781-788, 1983. Copyright © 1983, American Roentgen Ray Society.)*

is obvious in the anteroposterior view (Fig. 19–46). In other patients, a groove view must be performed with contrast instilled to make the diagnosis.[117,119,120] In biceps tendinitis, the sharp delineation of the tendon may be lost.[117] In rheumatoid arthritis, irregularities in the sheath of the biceps tendon may be caused by synovitis. However, in the

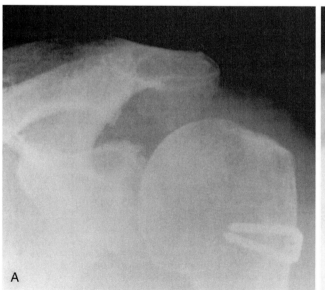

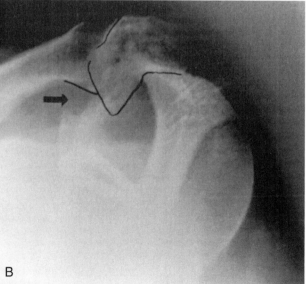

■ **Figure 19–45**
A, A 30-degree caudal tilt radiograph reveals anterior acromial spurring with a "shark's tooth" appearance. The patient had undergone biceps tenodesis but continued to have pain after surgery. His pain was completely relieved and function was greatly improved by acromioplasty and rotator cuff repair. **B,** An outlet view of the same patient demonstrating a type III acromion with marked inferior spurring and narrowing in the supraspinatus outlet. *(The film is somewhat underexposed; the lines were added to aid in reproduction.)*

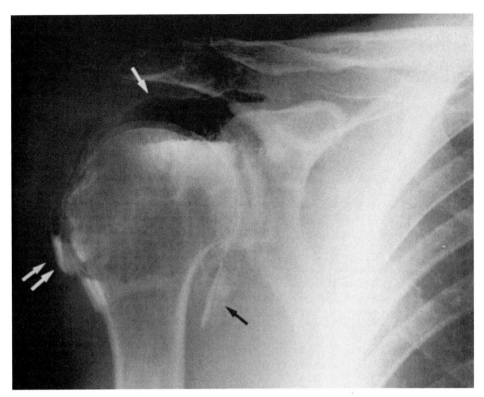

■ Figure 19–46
Anteroposterior arthrogram revealing medial dislocation of the biceps tendon, as indicated by the medial position of the biceps sheath *(black arrow)*. This patient also sustained a massive rupture of the rotator cuff at the time of the injury. Note the presence of air in the subacromial bursa *(single white arrow)* and contrast medium *(double white arrow)* in the subdeltoid bursa. *(Courtesy of Guerdon Greenway, M.D., and Robert Chapman, M.D.)*

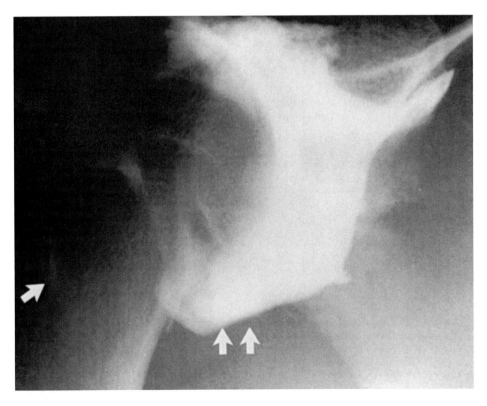

■ Figure 19–47
The arthrogram in adhesive capsulitis will frequently show nonfilling of the bicipital groove because of constriction in the bicipital sheath *(arrow)*. This finding is similar to the restriction that occurs in the axillary recess *(double arrows)*.

study by Ahovuo,[4] the arthrogram showed no difference in filling of the tendon sheath in patients with surgically verified biceps tendinitis and those with a normal tendon. Arthrography in patients with biceps tendinitis may show that the cuff is intact and that the biceps is poorly outlined, has a thickened sheath, or is elevated at its origin.[214,216] In patients with adhesive capsulitis, the biceps sheath, like the subscapularis recess and dependent axillary fold, contracts (Fig. 19–47). The tendon and bicipital groove can also be assessed with CT arthrography (Fig. 19–48).

MRI with gadolinium-enhanced arthrography is oftentimes used to evaluate the shoulder. This test can be used

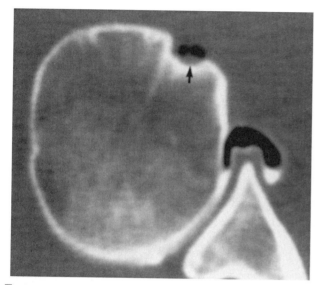

Figure 19–48

The bicipital tendon is seen *(black arrow)* seated in the groove on a computed tomographic arthrogram.

in much the same way as a CT arthrogram but provides better imaging and contrast of soft tissues in the area. MRI can also be used to evaluate the superior labral–biceps complex. A gadolinium arthrogram in this case is used to help identify superior labral avulsions and tearing of the bicipital attachment to the supraglenoid tubercle and the labrum.

Reflection pulley lesions can also be diagnosed with MRI arthrography. Weishaupt and colleagues[304] evaluated three criteria to diagnose these disorders in patients with a surgically proven pulley lesion. The signs that they evaluated were a thickened superior border of the subscapularis tendon three to five sections below the humeral head on axial gradient echo images, poorly defined superior border of the subscapularis tendon at its insertion site on the lesser tuberosity, and the pulley lesion, which was a collection of contrast material anterior to the superior border of the subscapularis above the level of the coracoid process on axial images in the expected area of the rotator interval. They found these signs to be valuable in the diagnosis of pulley lesions. The thickened border of the subscapularis tendon was the most sensitive and specific sign.

Ultrasonography

When comparing arthrography with sonography of the biceps, Middleton and colleagues[193] found that although sonography and arthrography were equally successful in facilitating evaluation of the bony anatomy of the bicipital groove, sonography gave a superior image of the biceps tendon within the groove (Fig. 19–49). Not only can the tendon be visualized in the groove, but the intra-articular portion and that portion just distal to the groove can also be visualized (Fig. 19–49B and C). In Middleton and associates' study, 16 patients were found to have biceps tendon sheath effusions or swelling detected by sonography (Fig.

19–49D); 15 of these patients had associated pathologic conditions elsewhere in the joint, the majority being rotator cuff tears.

It has previously been documented that the biceps tendon sheath often does not fill when a rotator cuff tear is present,[212-219] either because of associated tendinitis and contracture of the capsule or because of the fact that dye leaks out of the joint through the tear in the supraspinatus before enough pressure is generated to force the dye into the bicipital groove. Inasmuch as arthrograms often do not disclose a biceps tendon or sheath abnormality in many of the patients in which ultrasound was positive, Middleton and colleagues[192] concluded that sonography is the imaging method of choice in patients with suspected biceps tendon lesions.

An ultrasound subluxation test was able to detect subluxation in 12 of 14 (86%) patients who had surgically verified subluxation of the biceps tendon. The test was performed by placing the transducer over the bicipital groove and maximally externally rotating the humerus.[80] This test can be done with the transducer in the transverse and longitudinal planes. On transverse images, subluxation of the tendon is seen by the to-and-fro motion of the biceps as it rides over the lesser tuberosity. On longitudinal images, the biceps tendon moves away from the humerus in its extra-articular position. In the two cases missed at ultrasonography, external rotation was not possible because of pain or adhesive capsulitis. Static scanning produced a similar percentage (86%) of dislocation diagnoses. The ultrasound examination failed or could not be performed in 6% of their patients. No false-positive results occurred.[80]

AUTHORS' COMMENT

The sonogram is an excellent noninvasive test for biceps and cuff lesions. It is, however, very examiner dependent, and if equivocal, arthrography should be performed. A positive sonogram, like the clinical entity of biceps rupture itself, should also make one suspicious that rotator cuff pathology coexists.

Magnetic Resonance Imaging

MRI can be used to visualize the normal biceps tendon, both intra-articularly and in its groove. For optimal MRI evaluation, images should be obtained in the axial, oblique, and sagittal planes. The oblique and sagittal planes provide the best visualization of the intra-articular portion of the biceps tendon in the rotator interval.[283] The axial plane is best for showing the descending portion of the biceps in the groove. MRI is also useful for imaging rotator cuff pathology, which is frequently found in association with biceps lesions.[143,188]

Subluxations or dislocations can be visualized with MRI. With dislocation, the tendon is usually shown as being displaced out of its groove and is seen lying medial to the lesser tuberosity (Fig. 19–50A and B). Subluxation can be identified when the tendon is noted to overlie the lesser tuberosity on some images. This test can also be used to visualize an intra-articular dislocation of the biceps. Care must be taken because osteophytes and scar tissue can resemble the presence of a tendon in the groove.[288]

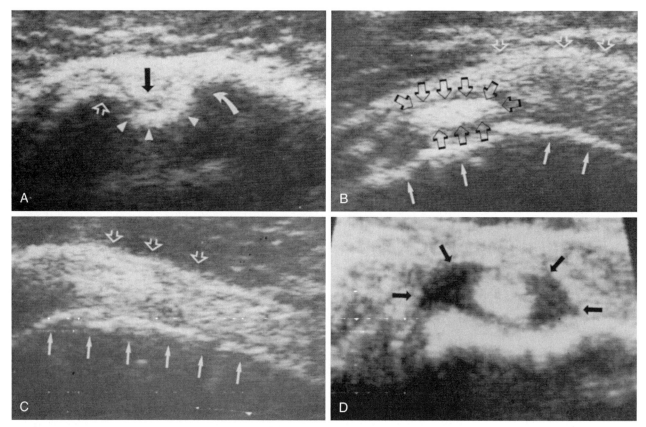

■ **Figure 19–49**

A, Transverse sonogram of the anterior aspect of the shoulder showing the bicipital groove *(arrowheads)* as a semicircular depression in the proximal part of the humerus formed by the lesser tuberosity medially *(open arrow)* and the greater tuberosity laterally *(curved arrow)*. The biceps tendon is seen as an echogenic ellipse within the groove *(black arrow)*. **B,** Sonogram perpendicular to the long axis of the intra-articular portion of the biceps tendon *(open black arrowheads)*, seen between the subscapularis anteriorly and the supraspinatus posteriorly. The deep surface of the deltoid muscle is shown by *open white arrowheads* and the humeral head by *solid white arrows*. **C,** On longitudinal scans, the biceps tendon appears as an echogenic band sandwiched between the upper portion of the humeral head *(solid arrows)* and the lower portion of the deltoid *(open white arrows)*. **D,** Transverse sonogram of the distal part of the biceps tendon showing biceps sheath effusion *(arrows)* surrounding the biceps tendon. *(From Middleton WD, Reinus WR, Tetty WG, et al: Ultrasonographic evaluation of the rotator cuff and biceps tendon. J Bone Joint Surg Am 68:440-450, 1986.)*

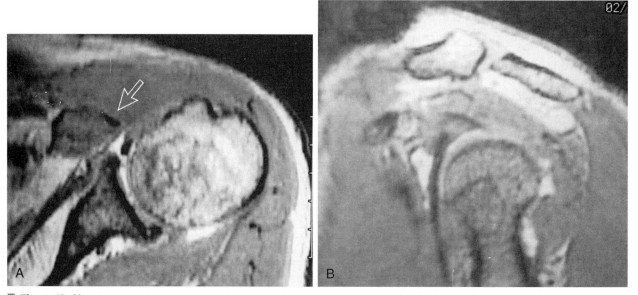

■ **Figure 19–50**

A, The biceps tendon *(open arrow)* is seen in an intra-articular position. Note the absent groove and change in signal intensity of the subscapularis. **B,** A sagittal oblique magnetic resonance image reveals the biceps anterior to the humeral head.

Biceps tendinitis is a much more difficult diagnosis to make on MRI, but it can be suggested by certain criteria. One criterion is fluid out of proportion to the intra-articular fluid in the shoulder. In shoulders with a large joint effusion, fluid surrounding the tendon can be a normal finding, but the presence of little intra-articular fluid and a lot of fluid in the biceps sulcus may be indicative of tendinitis (Fig. 19–51A and B). Thickening of the tendon and increased intensity on T1- and T2-weighted images can suggest degenerative changes in the tendon. This degeneration may be diffuse or occur in segmental areas.[283]

SLAP lesions can be diagnosed with the use of MRI. Studies have shown that SLAP lesions can be evaluated with gadolinium-enhanced as well as plain MRI.[46] In gadolinium-enhanced scans, contrast can help delineate lesions of the superior labrum and biceps anchor. Gadolinium can be seen infiltrating under the labrum in type II SLAP lesions. Even with non–gadolinium-enhanced scans, changes in the superior labrum and subluxated bucket handle tears can be seen in the joint.

MRI is also useful in diagnosing biceps ruptures (Fig. 19–52A and B). A rupture is easier to diagnose than a

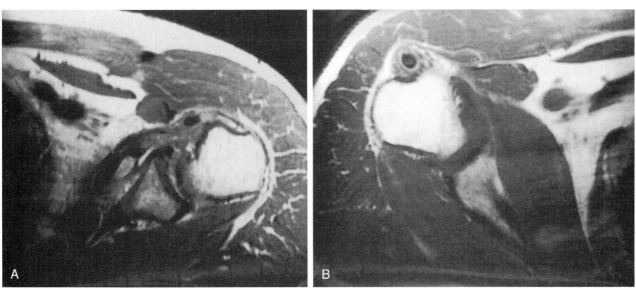

■ Figure 19–51
A, A coronal plane T2-weighted magnetic resonance image reveals increased fluid in the biceps sheath in comparison to the glenohumeral joint in an individual with surgically confirmed biceps tendinitis. **B,** An axial T1-weighted image in the same patient reveals tenosynovitis of the biceps.

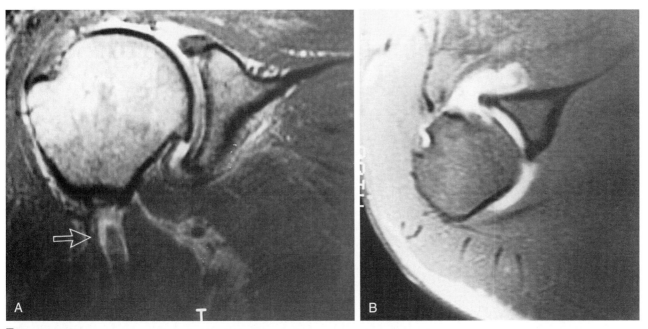

■ Figure 19–52
A, A coronal view magnetic resonance image (MRI) shows the location of the proximal biceps stump *(open white arrow)* to be at the distal end of the biceps groove. **B,** An axial view MRI of same patient reveals the biceps absent from the groove. Note the medial osteophytic ridge.

partial tear, clinically and with MRI. Ruptures are diagnosed by nonvisualization of the tendon at any point along its anatomic course. Klug and Moore[147] refer to such nonvisualization as the empty groove sign. Sometimes, an intra-articular stump can be seen. Obviously, one must be careful to make sure that the biceps tendon is not dislocated in the groove before making the diagnosis of a biceps rupture. Other useful signs that can be seen on MRI that may help diagnose ruptures are atrophy and retraction of the distal portion of the proximal part of the tendon. Tears are more difficult to diagnose. Tearing may alter the morphology and result in an irregular or notched appearance of the tendon. Tears can also be inferred by sudden changes in cross-sectional diameter of the tendon.[283] Longitudinal tears may be easier to see than transverse tears because they are visualized on several coronal and sagittal cuts. Signal change in the tendon itself can also represent partial tearing of the tendon. Focal lines and globular zones of high signal on long transient echo sequences are two types of signal change that can represent tears in the tendon.[147] Focal transverse partial lesions of the tendon can be difficult to see because they can be missed by the wide cuts or be dismissed as artifact because they show up on only one cut. MRI has been used to identify osteochondromatosis of the biceps sheath.[69]

Zanetti and coworkers[316] evaluated the sensitivity and specificity of several MRI findings on MRI arthrography to determine their usefulness. They found that caliber changes of the biceps, contour irregularities, and signal intensity changes in both the axial and parasagittal planes were all useful in attempting to diagnose tendinitis in the biceps tendon. These authors assigned sensitivity and specificity values to each finding for each observer, with only slight interobserver agreement for each of these signs. They concluded that using several criteria in two imaging planes allows a reasonably accurate diagnosis of biceps pathology.

Spritzer and colleagues[273] evaluated the use of several diagnostic criteria to diagnose bicipital pathology. They found that a tendon perched on the lesser tuberosity was both specific and sensitive for bicipital instability. Moderate interobserver agreement was noted for this criterion. Tendon shape and an obtuse intertubercular angle were found to be useful criteria. The reader's impression of the presence of instability of the biceps was also helpful in determining bicipital pathology. Abnormal signal and fluid around the biceps tendon was not a sensitive or specific criterion for the evaluation of bicipital pathology in their study. Kappa scores for this criterion were fair to poor. They concluded that the presence of a flat or degenerated tendon perched on the lesser tuberosity with an obtuse angle was highly suggestive of bicipital instability.

MRI is often ordered before consultation with a specialist. These images are sometimes read by radiologists who do not have a lot of experience in musculoskeletal pathology. Errors and omissions can sometimes occur on these readings. These errors can at times change the treatment required. For example, in a patient in whom arthroscopic treatment of impingement is planned, the intraoperative finding of bicipital tearing will change the plan significantly. The special instrument sets required for biceps tenodesis may require special ordering in some institutions. The surgeon's ability to diagnose tearing in the biceps on MRI can drastically alter the planned treatment or allow the proper equipment to be available. Relying on an inexperienced radiologist may not be the preferred method of imaging in this situation, and some interpretive pressure is therefore placed on the surgeon. Our personal preference is to procure the images on all studies performed on our patients at the time of consultation and surgery. In this way, interpretive skills can be improved so that the surgeon can detect bicipital and other hard-to-identify lesions and not have to rely on the interpretive skills of an inexperienced radiologist. If consultation with a musculoskeletal radiologist is available, it is used to help interpret difficult studies.

Arthroscopy

Arthroscopy remains the best method for visualizing the biceps tendon in its intra-articular location (Fig. 19–53). It is also very useful for imaging other lesions that may be causing chronic anterior shoulder pain.[8,9,223,308] Lesions of the biceps anchor and superior labrum can be visualized and repaired with arthroscopy. Arthroscopy provides the examiner with both static and dynamic visualization of the biceps, thereby helping to diagnose subtle cases of instability.

This technique can be used to evaluate numerous conditions that can cause anterior shoulder pain. Small bursal-side tears can be seen along with lesions related to anterior instability, impingement syndrome, labral tears without instability, and bicipital tendinitis. With the arthroscope, subtle anterior and posterior glenoid labral tears and cartilaginous head defects can be visualized; these lesions are not always seen on CT scans or MRI. A disadvantage of arthroscopy is that it is an invasive procedure that normally requires general anesthesia. As in all surgical procedures, insertion of the arthroscope poses a risk of infection and cartilage damage. Extra-articular lesions of the biceps may not be appreciated with the arthroscope. Arm position can help relax the biceps tendon to allow better visualization. Placing the elbow in flexion and supination and the shoulder in flexion and external rotation can accomplish this goal. Using a probe to pull the biceps tendon into the joint can also help the surgeon see a part of the tendon that may not be visualized during routine examination.[81] By using this method, an extra 3 to 5 cm of tendon can be visualized. Sometimes, fraying of the tendon in the intertubercular region can be brought into the joint and detected.

Visualization of the rotator interval is also important when performing arthroscopy of the shoulder. Pulley lesions can be visualized and probed to see whether damage has occurred.[22] The use of a 70-degree scope can sometimes be of assistance when performing this examination. Flexing the shoulder 60 to 90 degrees with the scope placed anteriorly in the joint allows the surgeon to see the interval structures. Internal rotation of the arm relaxes the subscapularis and allows the interval ligaments, rotator cuff tendons, and bicipital pulley to be probed. Identification of injury to these structures should

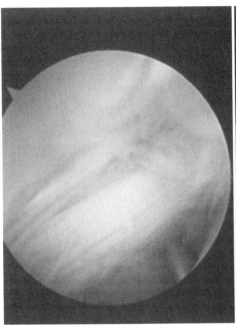 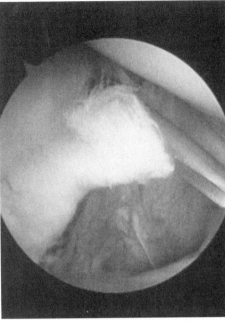

■ **Figure 19–53**
An arthroscopic view of the right shoulder reveals an intra-articular biceps with shredding of fibers secondary to loss of the sling and chronic subluxation out of the proximal part of the groove.

allow the surgeon to determine treatment of the lesion. A careful and systematic examination is the best tool available to identify and treat shoulder lesions. The examiner should not be afraid of using anterior and posterior portals to complete this examination.

COMPLICATIONS

The most common complication of biceps tendon rupture or dislocation is, as has been emphasized previously, failure to recognize disruption of the rotator cuff. The majority of rotator cuff tears are secondary to chronic impingement wear and tendinitis. Some patients will sustain an acute massive cuff avulsion as a result of trauma. Although the results of cuff débridement and decompression are impressive in terms of pain relief and restoration of range of motion, if the patient is young (younger than 60 years) and wants to maintain a strong shoulder for use above the horizontal, an approach involving early diagnostic workup and aggressive surgery is preferred.

Adhesive capsulitis can follow a number of painful conditions about the shoulder. Because biceps tendinitis has previously been associated with adhesive capsulitis, early recognition of this condition and treatment with anti-inflammatory agents, moist heat, and early, gentle patient-directed range-of-motion exercises may aid in preventing or shortening this often painful, long process.

Nontreatment of biceps ruptures, especially in the elderly, is accepted by many patients and physicians. Very few of these individuals note any dysfunction related to the biceps rupture itself. Predictably, patients with a bicipital rupture who have an intact brachialis muscle will have no decrease in flexion strength at the elbow. Loss of supination strength has been estimated by Warren and associates to be between 10% and 20% with Cybex testing.[302,303]

Phillips and coworkers[242] could not find a significant difference in patients who had operatively treated proximal biceps tendon ruptures and those who had nonoperative treatment. All the patients in this study were middle aged and older. Some patients in this study who had objective weakness did not feel functionally impaired.

DIFFERENTIAL DIAGNOSIS

Because tendinitis of the long head of the biceps usually accompanies other conditions and primary bicipital tendinitis is a diagnosis of exclusion, the other clinical entities that can mimic or be associated with this entity must be remembered. They are impingement syndrome, adhesive capsulitis, rheumatoid arthritis and osteoarthritis, glenohumeral instability, coracoid impingement syndrome, thoracic outlet syndrome or brachial plexopathy/plexitis, peripheral nerve entrapment, and cervical radiculopathy.

One pertinent historical feature is the mechanism of injury. Information about the injury should include the amount and direction of force applied, whether it was direct or indirect, and the position that the arm was in during application of the force. Was the onset insidious? Has the patient had gradual loss of motion over a period of several months? Had the patient engaged in any unusual overhead activity before the onset of symptoms? Did the patient have an injury to the shoulder before or been treated for "bursitis"? Has the patient engaged in activities that require overhead use of the arm, such as swimming, throwing, or tennis? What makes the pain better; what makes the pain worse? Where does the patient feel the pain most in his shoulder? Does activity improve or exacerbate the painful phenomenon? The shoulder should be inspected for atrophy of the deltoid, infraspinatus, supraspinatus, and trapezius; swelling; and obvious biceps ruptures. The patient should be examined from the front, the side, and the back and a comparison with the other side made. Physical examination should include cervical spine range of motion and detailed neurovascular examination, including deep tendon reflexes, sensation, strength testing, and specific physical tests for thoracic outlet syndrome. Range of motion of the shoulder should be examined. Both active and passive range of forward flexion, abduction, external rotation, internal rotation, and extension should be noted. The relative contribution of glenohumeral and scapulothoracic joint motion should be assessed. Anterior apprehension testing as well as anterior, posterior, and inferior drawer tests should be performed. The examiner should look for the impingement sign[207] and the impingement reinforcement sign of Hawkins.[120] The acromioclavicular joint is palpated, and a compression test, or a hug test, specific for acromioclavicular joint arthritis is performed. Specific areas of point tenderness over the anterior acromion, coracoacromial ligament, and coracoid are noted. The biceps tendon is palpated in the groove, anteriorly at a position of approximately 10 degrees of internal rotation, 4 to 6 cm distal to the acromion (see Fig. 19–36). A helpful point in determining whether this is the tendon and groove area is to see whether the point of tenderness moves with rotation of the humerus. In diffuse bursitis, the tenderness will not move, whereas it will with an inflamed biceps. The point of tenderness of bicipital tendinitis may completely disappear underneath the coracoid on marked internal rotation. The diagnosis of primary bicipital tendinitis must be arrived at by exclusion of the other, more common causes of anterior shoulder pain.

MRI is a useful tool to differentiate between primary bicipital tendinitis and impingement syndrome. Along with plain radiographs that include a trauma series, a supraspinatus outlet view and a 30-degree caudal tilt view can be used to help diagnose impingement-type syndrome. MRI can be used to demonstrate changes in the rotator cuff tendons, or it may show normal tendons and increased signal in and around the biceps tendon, which would confirm primary bicipital tendinitis and more than likely exclude impingement-type lesions.

Biceps Tendinitis versus Impingement Syndrome

To differentiate primary bicipital tendinitis from impingement tendinitis, selective injection with a local anesthetic is helpful. In patients with impingement syndrome without bicipital involvement, the pain is located more proximally, with tenderness primarily over the anterior acromion, coracoacromial ligament, and supraspinatus tendon insertion. The impingement and impingement reinforcement signs are positive. In patients with an impingement syndrome, injection of lidocaine (Xylocaine) into the subacromial space usually relieves all the patient's pain. In patients who have associated bicipital tendinitis, pain is located distally in the groove, subacromial injection does not relieve all of their pain, and they continue to have pain over the bicipital groove. Further injection of lidocaine into the sheath with obliteration of pain confirms the associated bicipital tendinitis. It is important to remember that the subdeltoid bursa, which covers the groove, is continuous with the subacromial bursa and that inadvertent injection into this area will anesthetize the subacromial bursa. Therefore, we recommend injecting the subacromial bursa first, doing so from the midlateral acromion to avoid inadvertent injection of lidocaine into the groove. Only if subacromial injection has absolutely no effect on the patient's pain and isolated biceps injection relieves all pain and restores 100% of motion will I make a clinical diagnosis of primary bicipital tendinitis. A positive response to injection has been found to be a predictor of good long-term results.[26]

A bicipital injection technique has been described by Kerlan.[143] The patient is placed supine with the arm over the table. The elbow is bent and the shoulder extended with the arm in external rotation to decrease the distance from the groove to the surface. The biceps tendon is located anteriorly, and a mark is made on the skin. The area is prepared in sterile fashion and injected. It is extremely important, especially if corticosteroids are used, that the injection be into the sheath and not into the tendon proper. Direction of the needle superiorly tangential to the tendon should eliminate this complication. The fluid must flow easily; if any resistance is felt, the needle should be repositioned. Because of the anatomy of the sheath and its communication with the joint, I use a very low volume of local anesthetic, only 2 to 3 mL of 1% Xylocaine, during the biceps ablation test.

Claessens and Snoek[44] thought that intra-articular injection of an anesthetic is important in differentiating rotator cuff tendinitis from bicipital tendinitis. Although this is true of bursal-side lesions, undersurface tears of the rotator cuff or labral lesions will be anesthetized with this technique as well. Radiography, sonography, and arthrography should be used to confirm one's clinical impression.

Anterior Shoulder Instability

The pain associated with anterior subluxation of the glenohumeral joint can be noted in the anterior portion of the shoulder. At the same time, patients may often have pain posteriorly from capsular stretching. The pain is episodic in nature and associated with a palpable and audible clunk, such as has been described previously with medial dislocation of the biceps. The pain generally lasts for several days after a major subluxation episode. If the brachial plexus is inflamed and stretched, pain and paresthesias can be experienced transiently or in varying degrees for several weeks or months. The mechanism of injury described for both these conditions is similar in that they both occur with forced external rotation. However, biceps lesions are more apt to occur with forced external rotation of the adducted arm. When differentiating shoulder instability from subluxation of the biceps tendon, provocative tests are helpful. In anterior shoulder instability, the maximal point of apprehension and clicking should be in 90 degrees of abduction and maximal external rotation (i.e., a positive apprehension sign). Pain in the anterior part of the shoulder occurs as the humeral head translates across the torn glenoid labrum. Pain can also be felt posteriorly at this time secondary to cuff stretching. In a patient with a subluxating biceps tendon, the pain is not maximal until the arm is brought down from the position of maximal abduction and external rotation, and the click occurs as the examiner begins to internally rotate the arm (i.e., biceps instability test). Yergason's and Speed's signs should be negative in patients with anterior shoulder instability, but positive if the biceps is inflamed. Special roentgenographic views for shoulder instability should be obtained (see Chapter 5 on radiology of the shoulder). The CT arthrogram can be extremely helpful in demonstrating lesions of the anterior cartilaginous labrum in patients with instability. The biceps tendon can be visualized within its groove on CT arthrography.

MRI with gadolinium contrast can also be helpful in cases of instability, much in the same way as CT arthrography. Although this study is not as useful in demonstrating Bankart-type lesions, it can show findings similar to those seen on CT arthrography with this lesion. The disadvantage of using MRI is that bony lesions are not seen as well as they are on CT arthrograms. MRI can also be used to visualize the biceps tendon and evaluate its position and whether it is inflamed.

If the diagnosis remains unclear after the aforementioned studies, examination under anesthesia, arthroscopy, or both can be performed. Examination under anesthesia combined with glenohumeral arthroscopy allows the surgeon to directly visualize the anterior labrum as well as the intra-articular portion of the biceps tendon. The aperture of the sulcus and the surrounding cuff tissue can be seen during arthroscopy. A Bankart lesion and a positive drive-through sign are both suggestive of glenohumeral instability as a cause of pain, especially if no lesion can be noted on the intra-articular portion of the biceps tendon during arthroscopy. The biceps tendon can be pulled into the joint with a probe during arthroscopy so that a greater length of the tendon can be examined. The bicipital sling can be examined arthroscopically by abducting and externally rotating the shoulder. Internal rotation of the arm will relax the subscapularis tendon and interval ligaments and thus allow these anterior structures to be probed.[22]

Glenoid Labrum Tears without Instability

Glenoid labrum tears without instability, such as those that occur in the superior third of the labrum in close proximity to the biceps, can cause symptoms similar to those of subluxation of the biceps tendon. These superior labrum tears can occur in baseball players and other throwing athletes and frequently cause symptoms very similar to those of a subluxating bicipital tendon or a rotator cuff tear (see Chapter 25 on shoulder injuries in athletes). An audible or palpable clunk occurs as the tear flips in and out of the joint and impinges on the humeral head during rotation above the horizontal. A high index of suspicion for this lesion should be present if one is dealing with shoulder pain in a throwing athlete. These patients sometimes have more pain with release because of the deceleration effect of the biceps pulling on the torn labrum. CT arthrography will occasionally miss this

lesion, and the best way to differentiate this problem from a subluxating biceps tendon is by glenohumeral arthroscopy.

MRI is useful in imaging this type of lesion. Studies using gadolinium-enhanced as well as plain MRI are helpful in making this diagnosis. Arthroscopy can evaluate this lesion well.

Adhesive Capsulitis

Patients with adhesive capsulitis frequently have tenderness in the anterior aspect of the shoulder in the region of the bicipital groove and anterior portion of the subdeltoid bursa.

In evaluating patients with painful and stiff shoulders who have direct areas of point tenderness over the bicipital groove, I will inject this area with lidocaine, initially without cortisone, to see what effect this agent has on motion. If one injects and infiltrates the tendon sheath with 2 to 3 mL of lidocaine and the patient's pain is obliterated but no appreciable change in motion has occurred, one can be sure that one is dealing with adhesive capsulitis or frozen shoulder and not just a painful stiff shoulder from biceps tendinitis. If injection into the biceps region eliminates pain and motion returns in full, bicipital tendinitis is present. Whether it is part of the impingement syndrome can be determined by clinical examination and subacromial injection.

Glenohumeral Arthritis

Early arthritis of the glenohumeral joint is frequently manifested as anterior shoulder pain with limited range of motion. Because the biceps tendon is an intra-articular structure, it will be involved in any process within the joint. Inflammatory changes occur in the visceral layer of the synovium of the biceps recess, just as they do in the subscapular and axillary recess. Plain radiography may show spurring of the proximal end of the humerus with a ring osteophyte and flattening of the glenoid. Before the development of obvious osseous spur formation, double-contrast arthrography can reveal thinning of the articular cartilage.

Coracoid Impingement Syndrome

Warren and colleagues[302,303] and Gerber and associates[92] described the role of the coracoid process in coracoid impingement syndrome. They have noted symptoms similar to those of biceps tendinitis and instability. Based on CT scan data, Gerber and coworkers[92] calculated the normal coracoid-to-humeral distance (8.6 mm) and noted that it is decreased in those with coracoid impingement (average, 6.7 mm). The syndrome has been described in patients with an excessively long or laterally placed coracoid process and in those who have undergone bone block and osteotomy procedures for instability. Symptoms of coracoid impingement are dull pain in the front of the shoulder referred to the anterior, upper part of the arm and occasionally extending down into the forearm. The pain is consistently brought about by forward flexion and internal rotation or by adduction and internal rotation. In contrast to the more common type of impingement, forward flexion was most often painful between 120 and 130 degrees rather than 60 to 120 degrees. The diagnosis is established clinically by obliteration of the patient's pain by subcoracoid injection. The importance of considering this entity before performing surgery on the biceps tendon has been pointed out by Dines and associates[72]; they reported a series in which a third of their failures from biceps tenodesis were related to undiagnosed coracoid impingement syndrome.

Thoracic Outlet Syndrome

Thoracic outlet syndrome is frequently manifested as some anterior shoulder pain. It is generally associated with paresthesias in the distribution of the lower trunk of the brachial plexus (i.e., the ulnar two fingers). Neck pain, parascapular pain, and radiation into the pectorals are not uncommon. The body habitus may be asthenic, with a long neck and round back, or endomorphic, with pendulous breasts. The shoulders slope forward and downward because of rhomboid, levator, and trapezius weakness. Provocative tests for thoracic outlet syndrome, such as Wright's maneuver, Adson's test, or Roos' overhead grip test, will be positive whereas Yergason's, Speed's, and the impingement tests will be negative or equivocal. Subacromial and bicipital injections should not alleviate the pain completely. Cervical spine series looking specifically for cervical ribs, as well as Doppler examination and EMG, are useful adjuncts to clinical testing. However, the diagnosis remains a clinical one.

Brachial Neuritis

Viral brachial plexitis (syndrome of Parsonage and Turner) is an extremely painful condition that is frequently manifested as anterior shoulder pain. Early in the course of this condition, which usually follows a viral illness, pain exceeds the neurologic findings, and one may be fooled into thinking that acute calcific tendinitis is present. Later, numbness and weakness with obvious atrophy become prominent. The course is variable.

Peripheral Nerve Entrapment/Cervical Radiculopathy

The common syndromes of peripheral nerve entrapment—carpal tunnel syndrome, ulnar neuritis, and posterior interosseous nerve entrapment—may all cause anterior shoulder pain that is referred and can potentially be confused with bicipital tendinitis. Cervical radiculopathy, especially involving C5-C6, can also mimic primary shoulder lesions. Careful and repeated neurologic examination followed by EMG and nerve conduction velocity tests can help distinguish among these entities. In patients with persistent anterior shoulder pain, especially if typical neurogenic pain is present, the workup for primary shoulder pathology is negative, and neurologic

examination is unrevealing, one must consider the possibility of a tumor in the apex, mediastinum, or diaphragm region.

Tumors

Osteochondromatosis has been described in the bicipital sheath. This lesion can cause chronic anterior shoulder pain in patients. The classic symptoms of catching may not be present when just the bicipital sheath is involved. If the rest of the shoulder joint is involved, classic symptoms may be present.

Dialysis Arthropathy

Arthropathy secondary to dialysis is a painful chronic shoulder condition found in patients maintained on long-term dialysis. These patients have degeneration of their joint as a result of synovial inflammation and amyloid deposition. This condition is easily diagnosed because the patient is on dialysis and has radiologic signs of degeneration. This condition seems to also affect the biceps tendon and sheath, as well as the joint itself.

TREATMENT OF BICIPITAL LESIONS: REVIEW OF CONSERVATIVE TREATMENT

Bromfield[33] in 1773 discussed the technical aspects of reducing dislocations of the biceps tendon. Treatment of tendinitis was initially discussed by Schrager[262] in the 1920s. Recommendations during the 1920s and 1930s included morphine, sudden traction, diathermy, massage, faradization, and light and x-ray treatment. Milgram[194-197] and later Lapidus[151] were proponents of procaine hydrochloride (Novocain) infiltration and aspiration of the calcific deposits in cases of acute calcific tendinitis.

DePalma[67] initially treated bicipital tenosynovitis conservatively with hydrocortisone injections directly into the tendon, under the transverse ligament, and noted improvement in 10 of 18 cases. He recommended, as a rule, three or four 1-mL injections into the tendon under the transverse ligament at weekly intervals. It is now apparent from data by Kennedy and Willis[142] that this interval is too frequent. The injection should be made only in the tendon sheath, and the tendon itself should not be directly injected. In conservatively treated patients, they noted excellent results in 29%, good in 45%, fair in 9%, and poor in 16%.

Habermeyer and Walch[113] prefer nonoperative therapy for isolated tendinitis of the long head of the biceps tendon. They recommend a single intra-articular injection of cortisone and oral anti-inflammatory drugs in the acute stages of the disease. These authors recommend immobilization and local ice therapy combined with a conservative regimen of physical therapy. Physical therapy, including isometric and isokinetic strengthening of the rotator cuff, is the key in rehabilitating these patients.

Bicipital tendinitis secondary to impingement syndrome may respond to conservative treatment of the rotator cuff pathology. Subacromial injections of corticosteroids may be of assistance in a patient with a large rotator cuff tear who refuses surgery. Because the intra-articular and subacromial spaces communicate, there is less need to inject the area of the biceps tendon specifically in these cases.

RESULTS OF NONOPERATIVE TREATMENT OF BICEPS RUPTURE

A slight functional deficit occurs after disruption of the long head of the biceps tendon. After a period of conservative care, including range-of-motion exercises, moist heat, and strengthening, most patients have relatively normal strength and flexion and only minimal loss of supination power.[128-131,133] Carroll and Hamilton[37] studied 100 patients who sustained a rupture of the biceps brachii as a result of forced extension. Follow-up function was ascertained by the patient's ability to lift weights. They believed that a patient could return to work earlier and suffered no residual disability with conservative treatment. Treated conservatively, the patients in their series returned to work at an average of 4 weeks. It therefore was thought that a conservative approach should be adopted in treating this type of injury.

Warren and colleagues,[303] using Cybex testing in 10 patients with chronic biceps rupture, failed to find any statistically significant loss of elbow flexion strength and only a 10% loss of elbow supination strength. Phillips and coworkers[242] confirmed some of Warren and colleagues' findings. Cybex testing was used to assess the objective outcome of patients treated with long-term nonoperative therapy versus operative therapy. In 19 patients, no significant difference in supination or elbow flexion strength was found.

REVIEW OF OPERATIVE TREATMENT

Surgical treatment of the biceps tendon received little attention before Gilcreest[96] in 1926. He was the first to suggest suturing the stump of the tendon to the coracoid process, and he described intracapsular, intertubercular, and labral junction ruptures of the tendon. In 1939, Abbott and Saunders[2] reviewed six cases of surgical treatment of biceps dislocations. Their procedure involved stabilizing the biceps tendon, with half the tendon affixed through drill holes and the intracapsular portion left intact. In their review, four of the six patients required a reoperation for pain, and all patients had some pain, weakness, and limited range of motion, even after a second operation. Poor results from their procedure stemmed from two problem areas: (1) the procedure as described prevents the normal upward and downward motion of the humerus on the bicipital tendon, and (2) too much attention was paid to the biceps lesion and not enough attention was placed on the cuff rupture and impingement-producing area. The one patient in their series who did have a good result had the biceps replaced into the groove and the fibrous roof reconstructed.

Lippmann[157,158] recommended tenodesis of the long head of the biceps to the lesser tuberosity (Fig. 19–54) to

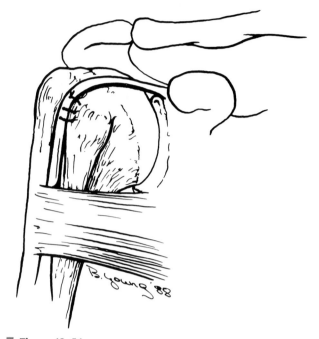

■ Figure 19–54
Lippmann's technique of suturing the biceps tendon to the lesser tuberosity for adhesive capsulitis.

shorten the course of frozen shoulder. He strongly believed, based on 12 operated cases, that periarthritis, or frozen shoulder, was caused by tenosynovitis of the long head of the biceps.

Hitchcock and Bechtol[124] in 1948 described tenodesis of the biceps tendon within the groove with an osteal periosteal flap (Fig. 19–55). Hitchcock's name has become synonymous with tenodesis of the biceps tendon in the bicipital groove. According to the authors, extensive fixation of the long head of the biceps tendon to the floor of the intertubercular groove in the manner they described greatly expedites convalescence, promotes loss of pain, and facilitates rapid functional recovery. However, they supplied no objective data to support this statement; they described primarily case results and stated that in 26 such cases, the results have been most satisfactory. The authors recognized the association of other lesions, such as rupture of the rotator cuff. Their main concern was that peritendinitis of the biceps tendon not be overlooked and not the converse (i.e., overlooking rotator cuff pathology when biceps symptoms predominate).

In 1954, DePalma and Callery[70] reported on 86 cases of bicipital tenosynovitis managed operatively, the bulk of which were treated by suturing the long head of the biceps tendon into the coracoid process (Fig. 19–56). Shortly before publication, several patients underwent tenodesis of the tendon in the groove, with a staple for fixation. The rationale cited for this change was that the three-prong staple provided firm fixation of the tendon and that tenodesis in the groove eliminated much of the dissection on the anterior aspect of the shoulder joint necessary to expose the coracoid process. Of the 86 cases, only 59 were available for follow-up (average, 27 months). Twenty-three were complicated by frozen shoulder. Excellent results were achieved in 64%, good results in 16%, fair results in

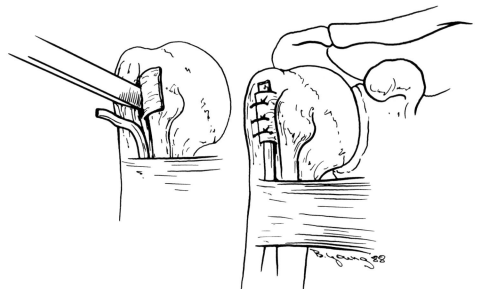

■ **Figure 19–55**
Hitchcock's procedure. With an osteotome, a bed is made in the intertubercular groove by elevating a portion of the floor from the outside inward. The tendon is roughened and then sutured beneath this osteal periosteal flap with heavy nonabsorbable sutures. The transverse humeral ligament is laid down over the tendon and the osteal periosteal flap.

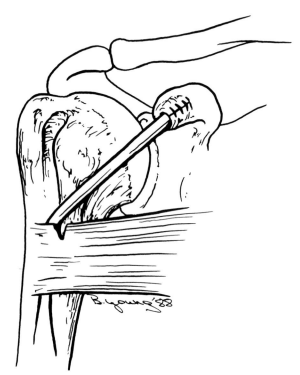

■ **Figure 19–56**
Tenodesis of the long head of the biceps to the coracoid process. This procedure was initially described by Gilcreest and popularized by DePalma. It involves medial dissection and potential denervation of the deltoid if done through a deltoid-splitting approach. It also theoretically changes the long head from a static head depressor to an active head elevator. *(Modified from Crenshaw AH and Kilgore WE: Surgical treatment of bicipital tenosynovitis. J Bone Joint Surg 45:1496-1502, 1966.)*

8%, and poor results in 10%; thus, 80% of their patients overall achieved an excellent or good result. Analysis of the poor results revealed errors in diagnosis and technique and reflex sympathetic dystrophy.

Michele[191] in 1960 described the keystone tenodesis. In this technique, a rectangular block of bone, including the bicipital groove, is removed. The bone is decorticated. The bony trough is prepared for insertion and exit of the tendon by placing two semilunar holes at the central poles at the sites of the remaining portion of the intertubercular sulcus. The tendon and sheath of the biceps are replaced into the defect and the bone block returned to its original position. The periosteum is then sutured back to secure the bony block in place. Michele reported on 16 cases in which roentgenograms demonstrated persistence of the entrance and exit holes and "smooth gliding of the biceps through the holes." Maneuverability was complete in all directions and asymptomatic. The patients had no recurrence of symptoms.

In 1966, Crenshaw and Kilgore[60] reported on the surgical treatment of bicipital tendinitis. They used the Hitchcock procedure in most of their cases and performed a total of 65 Hitchcock, 5 DePalma, and 3 Lippmann procedures. Relief of moderate to severe pain was good in 90% of patients, but 2% continued to complain of "mild, nagging pain." Restoration of motion in their series was often disappointing, with only 85% of normal motion noted at follow-up. Interestingly, half the patients who had good motion before surgery actually lost motion after the Hitchcock procedure. One has to wonder what the addition of an acromioplasty would have done to these results.

Keyhole tenodesis (Fig. 19–57) of the biceps origin was described in 1974 by Froimson and Oh[86] for the treatment of rupture, instability, and tendinitis of the biceps. They reported on 12 shoulders in 11 patients, with an average follow-up of 24 months. The results were satisfactory in all their patients, but they stated that patients with tenosynovitis enjoyed less than excellent results because of associated pericapsulitis. The authors cited several advantages of keyhole tenodesis: (1) the procedure avoids hardware and undue medial dissection; (2) the procedure removes the remnant of the biceps tendon, thereby allowing motion of the humeral head and avoiding intra-articular derangement; and (3) the inherent stability of their method gives one confidence to begin early, gentle

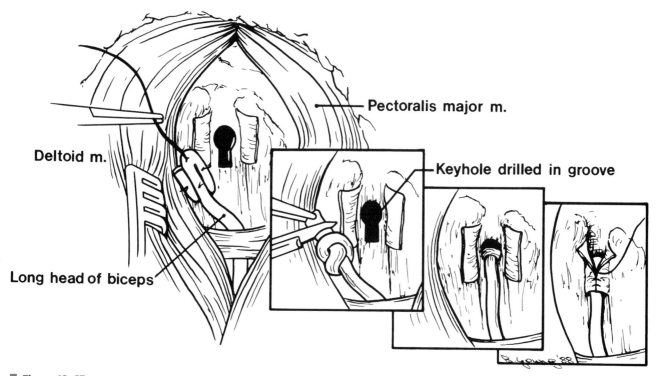

■ Figure 19–57

Keyhole tenodesis as described by Froimson and Oh. The biceps tendon is rolled into a thick ball in the proximal stump and then sutured together into a knot. A keyhole is made in the groove with a dental bur. The tendon is then inserted into the keyhole and the transverse ligament repaired over the tendon with nonabsorbable suture. Post has recommended marking the groove and the tendon with methylene blue before incision of the tendon to determine the normal tension of the tendon postoperatively. *(Modified from Froimson AI and Oh I: Keyhole tenodesis of biceps origin at the shoulder. Clin Orthop 112:245-249, 1974.)*

range of motion of both the shoulder and elbow. It should be noted that humeral fractures have been reported without keyhole tenodesis.[317]

Dines and coauthors[72] commented on surgical treatment of lesions of the long head of the biceps in 1982. Seventeen patients underwent tenodesis of the long head of the biceps into the humeral head via the keyhole technique, and 3 were treated by transfixion of the tendon into the coracoid. In addition, excision of the coracoacromial ligament was performed in 14 of their 20 patients. They had 6 failures out of 20 patients (30%). Revision surgery was required in four of six patients. In four failures in the tendinitis group, three were found to have an impingement syndrome. One patient had typical anterior impingement, and two had coracoid impingement. The other patient was later noted to have glenohumeral instability. The patients who did well in their series were older patients averaging 41 years of age. In these patients, excision of the coracoacromial ligament was part of the operation. However, it is their recommendation now that acromioplasty and coracoacromial ligament release be performed. In patients who were found to have coracoid impingement, coracoid osteotomy later relieved their pain. The most salient recommendation and lesson from this review is that at the time of surgical exposure, if biceps tenodesis is planned, the subacromial space and the interrelationship of the coracoacromial arch and the tendon must be observed. Careful preoperative evaluation as well as examination under anesthesia will reveal concomitant anterior instability. It was their impression that

isolated inflammation of the long head of the biceps is an infrequent finding unless injury to the biceps tendon in the groove has occurred. The entity of a subluxating biceps tendon is still questionable in their opinion. They state, "The role of the biceps tendon in the production of shoulder pain is difficult to assess and easily overestimated. Biceps tendon inflammation may be a secondary manifestation of an impingement syndrome. Unless treated, surgery for impingement syndrome will not be successful."

O'Donohue[222] presented a series of 56 cases of biceps instability treated with the Hitchcock procedure; 71% reported excellent progress, 77% said that they could throw satisfactorily, and 77% resumed their sport. They concluded that in a young, motivated athlete for whom throwing is important, this procedure is a very worthwhile operation.

Neviaser and colleagues[219] reported on the four-in-one arthroplasty for relief of chronic subacromial impingement. In this procedure all elements of the coracoacromial arch are addressed. The four-in-one arthroplasty includes anterior acromioplasty, excision of the coracoacromial ligament, excision of the distal end of the clavicle, and biceps tenodesis. Eighty-six percent of their 89 patients had no pain whatsoever, whereas 13% had pain only with excessive exercise. Motion was improved in 81%.

Most of the early studies showing good results of biceps tenodesis had very scant and short follow-up. Cofield and Becker[51] reviewed the long-term results of 51 patients (54 shoulders) with isolated biceps tenodesis. At 6 months, 94% thought that they had benefited from the procedure; however, satisfactory results fell to 52% at an average of 7 years. Fifteen percent underwent subsequent surgery, primarily cuff repairs and acromioplasty, and 33% continued to have moderate to severe pain. In another long-term study, Berleman and Bayley[26] obtained approximately 70% good and excellent results without deterioration in the longer term. Ogilvie-Harris and Wiley[223] reported on the arthroscopic findings and treatment of biceps tendon lesions. The usual lesion consisted of fraying of the tendon, with loose fronds hanging down into the joint. The fraying appeared to be greatest at the point where the biceps tendon entered the groove. The arthroscopic procedure consisted of débridement of the tendon and, in some cases, attempts at dilation of the orifice. Their series included 46 patients with lesions of the biceps tendon, some of whom had previously undergone rotator cuff repairs. The biceps tendon appeared to be adherent to the undersurface of the rotator cuff in these individuals. These adhesions were freed arthroscopically. Of patients with isolated lesions of the biceps tendon, "Three fourths of them did well with simple débridement." However, they admit that the follow-up was short, only 24 months. Only four of nine patients who had the biceps tendon released from the undersurface of the rotator cuff had "relief of symptoms."

In 1987, Post[244] presented 21 patients in whom the diagnosis of primary tendinitis of the long head of the biceps was made. In his cases, he excluded any with associated impingement syndrome, rotator cuff pathology, recurrent anterior shoulder instability, and repeated biceps tendon subluxation. All patients in his series had marked tenderness over the long head of the biceps, a negative impingement sign, and little or no relief of pain with subacromial injection. Fifty percent of the cases had a positive Yergason sign. Seventeen patients in his series underwent biceps tenodesis via the keyhole technique; four had a transfer to the coracoid process. In the transfer group, two excellent and two good results were achieved. One patient required manipulation under anesthesia. Of 17 patients who had a keyhole tenodesis, 13 results were excellent and 2 were good, with 1 failure. Two of these patients did require manipulation. In the one patient who was considered a failure in this group, symptoms and findings of impingement syndrome developed postoperatively and eventually required a partial anterior acromioplasty. In the tenodesis group, 88.3% good and excellent results were achieved. On the basis of his experience, it is Post's conviction that primary biceps tendinitis does occur as an isolated entity. Moreover, when it does occur, it is observed in the intertubercular groove alone.

Habermeyer and Walch[113] believe that chronic bicipital tendinitis combined with chronic subacromial impingement syndrome is best treated by subacromial decompression. They recommend biceps tenodesis only in patients younger than 40 years with isolated biceps tendinitis refractory to conservative treatment. For subluxating or dislocating bicipital lesions, they recommend two types of reconstruction. If patients have underlying subacromial impingement, a procedure to address this disease is also performed.

The first technique to operatively repair instability is reconstruction of the rotator interval sling and repair of the subscapularis tendon. The extensions of the supraspinatus and subscapularis tendons are formed into a lasso at the entrance of the groove to prevent it from re-subluxating. The second technique is either a biceps tenodesis using some of the various previously mentioned techniques or the Walch tubularization technique (Fig. 19-58). In this technique, the widened and damaged tendon is formed and fixed into a tube with a running suture. The groove is then deepened with an impactor, and the tendon is relocated into the groove. The damaged rotator interval and subscapularis and supraspinatus tendons are repaired. Berlemann and Bayley have recently reviewed biceps tenodesis with the keyhole technique and found approximately 65% good and excellent results. Multiple pathologies were encountered in most shoulders.[26] Walch[299] and colleagues recently reviewed their cases of bicipital instability in 445 patients who underwent rotator cuff repair. The incidence of bicipital instability in patients who had rotator cuff repairs was 16%. In 80% of these cases, a fibrous fascia extending from the subscapularis to the bicipital groove was present. This fascia gave the impression of normal anatomy. Once opened, the subscapular lesions and dislocation of the biceps could be seen. Bicipital subluxations were associated with limited lesions of the subscapularis and supraspinatus tendons. Dislocations, on the other hand, were found in conjunction with massive tears of the subscapularis, supraspinatus, and infraspinatus. Clinically, these patients had pseudoparalysis of their arm. In their experience, dislocation of the biceps tendon over an intact subscapularis tendon was rare. They suggested that opening the rotator interval is an essential part of open rotator cuff repairs to avoid missing bicipital subluxation.

The senior one of us has investigated the biomechanical strength of four different forms of biceps tenodesis.[318] Simple techniques such as anchor fixation or suture to soft tissue alone are stronger than the more complex keyhole or Hitchcock techniques. The authors found that the tendon was the weakest link in the chain. Doubling the biceps at the time of tenodesis improves the pullout strength of the surgical construct.[317]

ARTHROSCOPIC TREATMENT

Current treatment of bicipital tendinitis focuses on arthroscopic tenotomy and tenodesis. The use of arthroscopic biceps tenotomy for the treatment of bicipital tendinitis originated with Walch as an associated technique during repair of massive rotator cuff tears. The technique is simple and involves release of the tendon at its origin on the superior glenoid labrum. The distal end of the tendon is allowed to retract into the bicipital groove. In a study by Kempf and colleagues,[141] biceps tenotomy resulted in an improved level of physical activity, active mobility, and pain parameters. In contrast, their results also showed a prolonged and complicated postoperative course with more postoperative painful reactions and limitation of passive motion. Statistical analysis of their results showed that the benefits of bicipital tenotomy

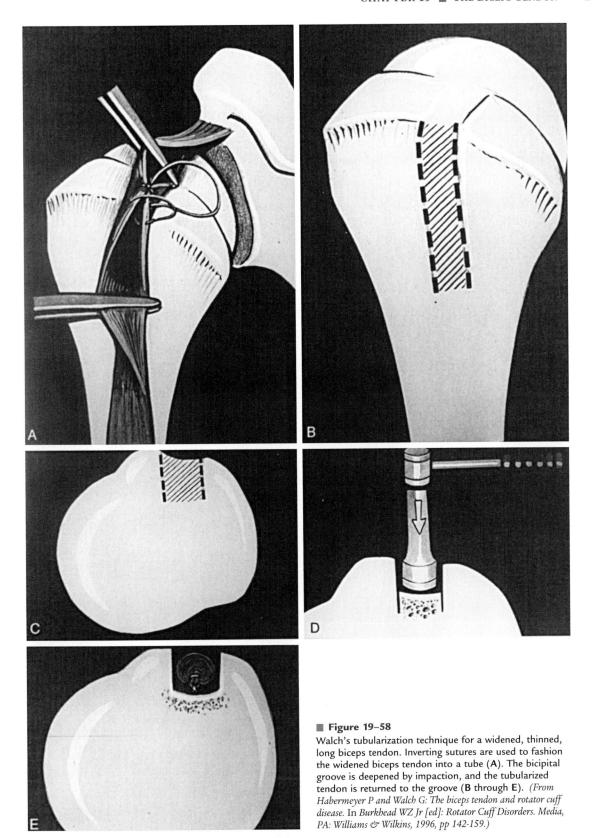

■ **Figure 19–58**
Walch's tubularization technique for a widened, thinned, long biceps tendon. Inverting sutures are used to fashion the widened biceps tendon into a tube (**A**). The bicipital groove is deepened by impaction, and the tubularized tendon is returned to the groove (**B through E**). *(From Habermeyer P and Walch G: The biceps tendon and rotator cuff disease. In Burkhead WZ Jr [ed]: Rotator Cuff Disorders. Media, PA: Williams & Wilkins, 1996, pp 142-159.)*

were especially evident in patients with a two-tendon tear of the rotator cuff.

Gill and coworkers[100] showed good results with use of the American Shoulder and Elbow Surgeons scoring system to evaluate the outcome of bicipital tenotomy. A significant improvement in pain and function was noted after the procedure, as well as a 13% complication rate. One patient did not like the cosmetic result and had a biceps tenodesis performed, and impingement developed in two patients after the procedure. The authors believed that tenotomy was a good treatment option that provided good results. Thomazeau and associates[280] also showed good results in their study when tenotomy was used to treat bicipital pathology found during the treatment of rotator cuff tears. Walch and colleagues used biceps tenotomy as a palliative treatment in patients with massive cuff tears. They reported decreased pain at rest and no loss of function after biceps tenotomy in patients with the following preoperative criteria. The patients were older than 50 years and had a humeral head–to–acromion distance of less than 7 mm. No tenotomy was performed if antero-superior subluxation was present. No cosmetic problems occurred in their patients, which they attributed to the normal atrophy present at this age.[300]

The use of arthroscopic bicipital tenodesis has evolved more recently as a result of improved arthroscopic instruments and techniques. The three techniques that we have experience with involve the use of acromioclavicular ligament (ACL) fixation screws to fix the tendon and an anchor technique as described by Gartsman and Hammerman.[90] Peter Habermeyer's technique involves the use of sutures to perform tenodesis to the capsule. These techniques have no long-term follow-up because they have only recently been developed. Most are performed with currently used methods of fixation in both open and arthroscopic surgery. The use of screws for holding ACL grafts is well documented, and many surgeons currently use suture anchors to perform their open biceps tenodesis. Placement of the tendon in the groove as the location for the tenodesis has been shown to give good results, as we have just discussed. Surgeons are using arthroscopic techniques to decrease the morbidity associated with shoulder surgery and speed recovery. Because of these facts, we think that these techniques should be discussed in this section.

The first arthroscopic technique, described by Boileau and coauthors,[28] uses a suture or needle to mark the biceps tendon as it enters the groove. The biceps is then released from its origin. Once it is in the subacromial space, the surgeon isolates the suture and opens the transverse ligament over the bicipital groove arthroscopically. The biceps tendon is delivered out through the wound or a cannula placed directly over the groove. At least 25 mm of tendon is retained to ensure good fixation. A guide pin from an ACL set is then driven into the humeral head while staying parallel to the acromion and chest wall with the arm kept in approximately 10 degrees of external rotation so that the bicipital groove is facing forward. The pin is tapped out through the deltoid and skin once it has pierced the posterior cortex of the humerus. An absorbable stitch is placed through the biceps tendon to allow the tendon to be pulled into

the hole. The tendon is then measured to make sure that an appropriately sized hole is made in the bone. The bone is drilled up to, but not beyond the posterior cortex with a cannulated drill of proper size. The guidewire is kept in place and the proximal end of the pin used as a suture passer to pull the tendon into the bone tunnel. An appropriately sized screw is then placed over a second guide pin placed in the tunnel. The screw is driven in until it is completely buried, and the holding suture is pulled out (Fig. 19-59).

The second variation of this technique of biceps tenodesis uses a similar approach but specific instruments to place the screw. The advantage of this technique is that it does not require the use of a pin that passes out of the humerus. By not having a pin pass out of the humerus, the frequency of injury to the axillary nerve, chest wall, and blood vessels is decreased.

The second technique uses two suture anchors placed in the groove approximately 1 cm apart to fix the tendon in the groove.[90] A mattress-type suture is used in conjunction with the anchors to secure the biceps in the groove. The advantage of the suture anchor technique is that it poses little risk to the nerves and blood vessels of the arm. No special instruments are required other than the instruments used to perform arthroscopic rotator cuff repairs. The open variation of this technique is performed by a large number of surgeons and seems to give good results (Fig 19-60).

Biceps tenodesis can also be performed in situ by using sutures to fix the tendon to the capsule. The biceps is inspected with an arthroscope through the posterior portal. A needle is placed through the bicipital tendon distal to the pathology. Suture is passed through the needle and brought out through the anterior portal. A second suture is placed through the biceps in the same manner. Scissors are then used to cut the biceps. The proximal suture ends are retrieved with a clamp through a tunnel in the subcutaneous tissue. The sutures are tied and the tenodesis is complete. Any remaining biceps anchor is removed and smoothed to a stable base (Fig 19-61).

Arthroscopic bicipital tenodesis is technically demanding and may not be a technique to be used by surgeons who do not perform a lot of operative shoulder arthroscopy. Because of the increased use of arthroscopy in resident training programs and fellowships, these techniques may become more widespread in the future.

Treatment of SLAP lesions is dependent on their type. Type I SLAP lesions are usually degenerative lesions that are often associated with rotator cuff or intra-articular pathology. Treatment of this lesion, as recommended by Field and Savoie,[83] Grauer and colleagues,[108] and Snyder and coworkers,[270] is correction of the underlying abnormality and possibly shaving of the degenerated labrum. Type II SLAP lesions have been repaired with suture techniques as well as a tacking technique to re-establish the biceps anchor onto the glenoid edge.[111,269] Type III lesions usually require débridement of the bucket handle tear.[270] The surgeon should also assess the patient for other associated pathology. Type IV lesions generally require stabilization of the biceps anchor with either suturing techniques or a tacking technique similar to that used for

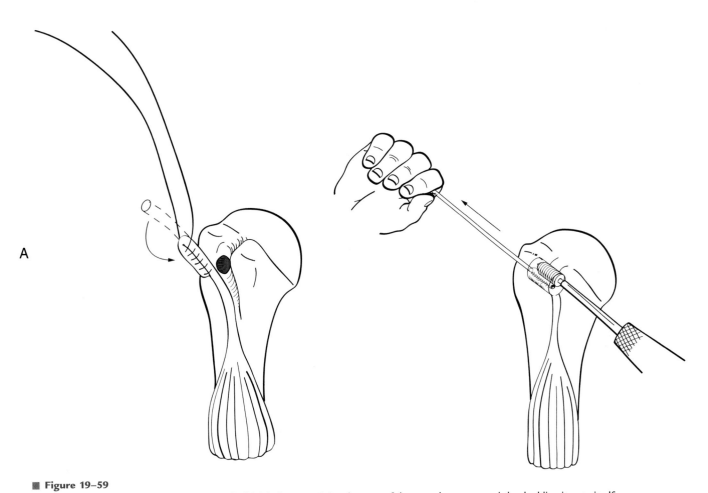

■ **Figure 19–59**

A, The biceps tendon is located and fixed in the bicipital groove. It is taken out of the cannula to prepare it by doubling it onto itself.

Continued

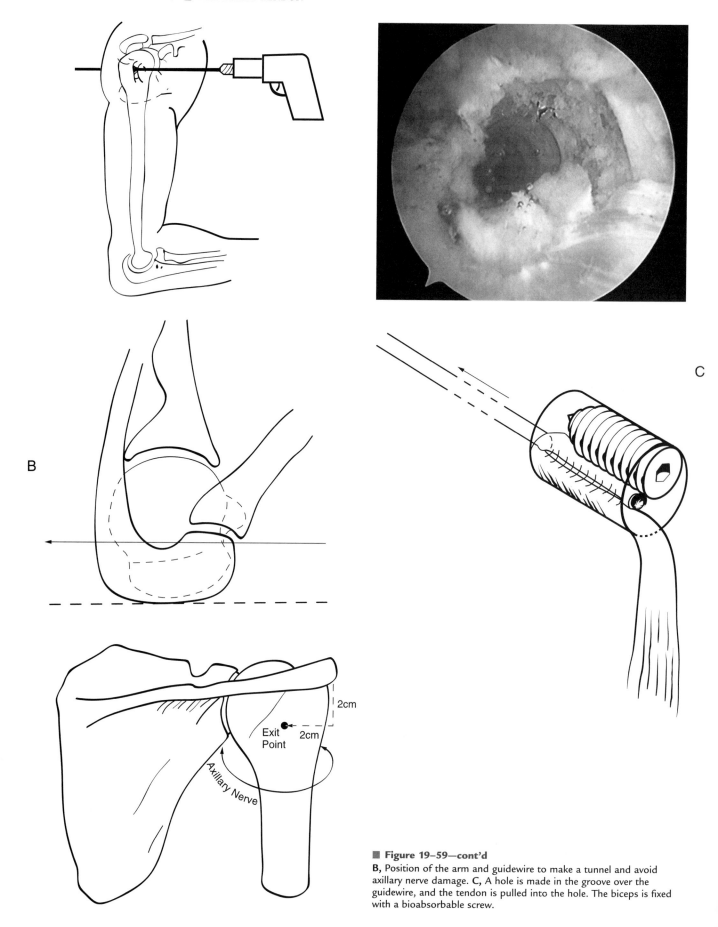

Figure 19–59—cont'd
B, Position of the arm and guidewire to make a tunnel and avoid axillary nerve damage. C, A hole is made in the groove over the guidewire, and the tendon is pulled into the hole. The biceps is fixed with a bioabsorbable screw.

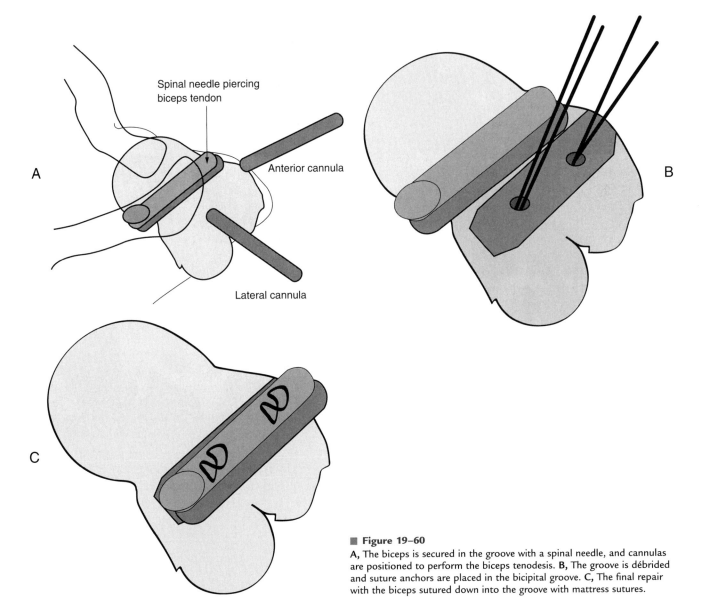

Spinal needle piercing
biceps tendon

A

Anterior cannula

Lateral cannula

B

C

■ **Figure 19–60**
A, The biceps is secured in the groove with a spinal needle, and cannulas
are positioned to perform the biceps tenodesis. **B,** The groove is débrided
and suture anchors are placed in the bicipital groove. **C,** The final repair
with the biceps sutured down into the groove with mattress sutures.

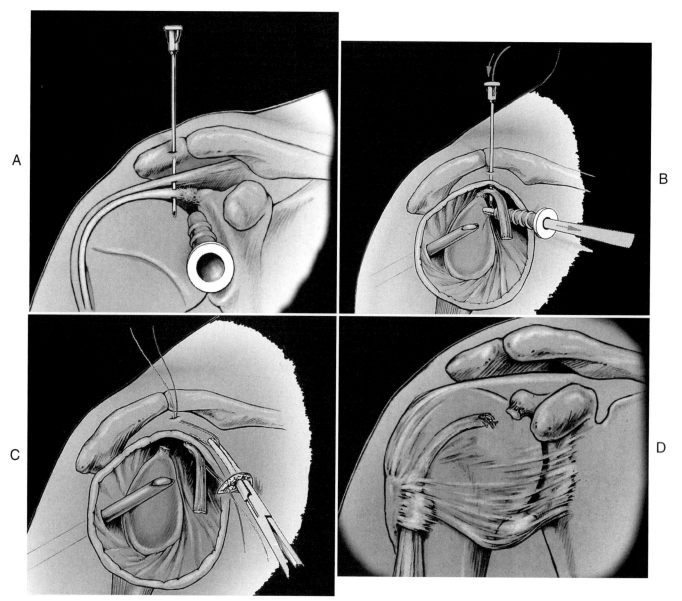

■ **Figure 19–61**

A, A needle is placed into the biceps tendon distal to the pathology on the biceps from a separate stab hole anterior to the acromion.
B, A suture is passed into the needle and retrieved from the lateral or anterior portal. A second suture is also placed via the same method.
C, Resection of the proximal part of the biceps is performed. The proximal suture limbs are retrieved subcutaneously and tied. **D,** The sutures are cut and the tenodesis is complete. *(Courtesy of Dr. Peter Habermeyer.)*

type II lesions. Resection of the bucket handle tear may be necessary.

Open operative treatment of synovial osteochondromatosis of the biceps tendon gave good results in a case report presented by Covall and Fowble.[57,58] Débridement of the diseased synovium in hemodialysis-related shoulder arthropathy has produced some good results according to Takenaka and associates.[278]

■ AUTHORS' PREFERRED METHODS OF TREATMENT

Treatment of lesions of the biceps tendon and associated pathology must be individualized to the patient. With the

exception of acute traumatic rupture of the tendon in a young patient or in association with a massive cuff tear in an active patient, management should be viewed as a continuum with prolonged (several months) conservative care and repeated evaluation. As long as the patient is making slow, gradual improvement, surgical intervention is not recommended. Surgical treatment is indicated only after a minimum of 6 months of conservative care. We have divided the treatment of chronic lesions according to the classification of Paavolainen and associates.[227]

■ IMPINGEMENT TENDINITIS

Treatment of bicipital tendinitis, when associated with coracoacromial arch impingement (enthesopathy), closely follows the treatment outlined by Neer in his original and follow-up articles. The stages and treatment of this clinical entity are well described in Chapter 15.

Glenohumeral arthroscopy is used to visualize the intra-articular portion of the biceps and glenoid labrum and the undersurface of the rotator cuff. The biceps tendon can be pulled into the joint with a probe and synovitis demonstrated if present. If an open approach seems more appropriate, the deltotrapezial fascia is taken down from the posterior corner of the acromioclavicular joint out to the anterolateral corner of the acromion. The distal end of the clavicle is resected with a saw. A Rockwood two-step acromioplasty is then performed with a straight osteotome (Fig. 19–62). The advantages of this double-cut approach are that (1) it ensures adequate removal of anterior bone, (2) it allows the surgeon to better appreciate the thickness of the acromion, and (3) it avoids leaving residual anteromedial and anterolateral acromion that can still cause impingement (Fig. 19–63).

Based on the previously mentioned study, the biceps is tenodesed into the groove with screw-type anchors and permanent sutures. The proximal end is sutured into the rotator interval. If significant tendinosis has occurred, the tendon is doubled back on itself to increase the pullout strength of the reconstruction.

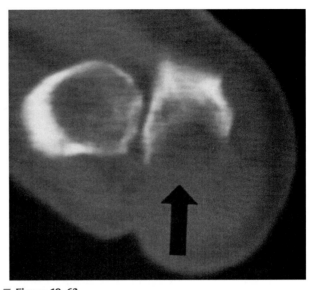

■ Figure 19–63

An anterior acromioplasty has been performed by using a curved osteotome in a single oblique acromioplasty. This procedure, unfortunately, left residual anterior acromion with residual coracoacromial ligament attached to the medial aspect *(arrow)*, as seen on this computed tomographic scan. For this reason, initially I recommend an anterior acromionectomy performed with a straight osteotome (as taught by Rockwood).

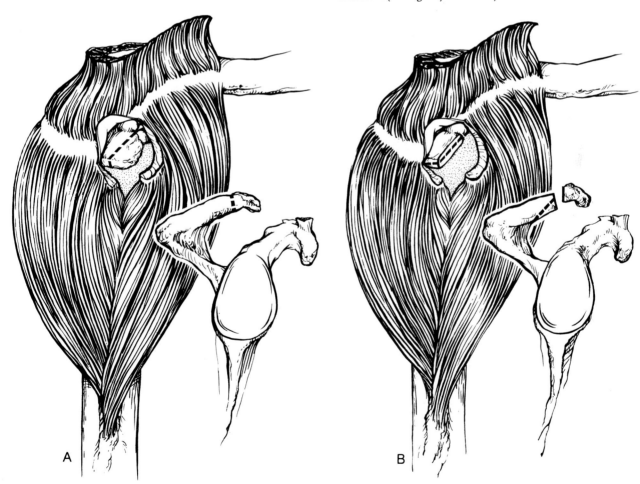

■ Figure 19–62

A, The anterior acromionectomy is shown by the *dashed line*. It is accomplished by making a vertical cut with an osteotome. The amount of acromion removed is all bone anterior to the anterior border of the clavicle. **B,** The *dashed line* indicates the anteroinferior acromioplasty. *(Courtesy of Charles A. Rockwood, Jr., M.D.)*

Post and colleagues[245] recommend marking the biceps tendon and intertubercular groove with methylene blue after the bicipital groove is opened but before the intertubercular portion is cut so that after the tendon is cut, these adjacent areas can be matched again at the time of tenodesis. We try to tension the repair such that the arm can be fully extended without placing undo pressure on the surgical construct.

When we use arthroscopic subacromial decompression for the treatment of impingement, we prefer an arthroscopic biceps tenodesis technique to fix the tendon in the groove. Our experience has been that patients are very satisfied with use of arthroscopic techniques, and takedown of the deltoid is not required. This technique also avoids violating the rotator interval. When performing arthroscopic tenodesis we try to pass our marking suture or a needle through the tendon as far down the groove as we can. The needle often penetrates the tendon at the level of the cuff insertion. Knowledge of this position helps us determine arthroscopically where the tendon should be fixed, in much the same way as Post's methylene blue technique. After release of the biceps proximally, the tendon retracts if a suture is used, and it becomes located distally in the groove. Driving a spinal needle into the bone prevents retraction of the biceps after release. After delivery of the tendon into the cannula in the bone tunnel technique, we can use the suture to measure the distance between our tendon, the point where we want the tendon to be fixed, and the position at which we will make our bone tunnel. If our point of fixation is 1 cm distal to the suture, we must make our tunnel 1 cm distal to the entry point of the bicipital groove. When the biceps tendon is held in position by a needle, the biceps can be fixed in situ because it has not retracted once the release is performed.

In stage III impingement, by definition, the rotator cuff has a full-thickness tear. These patients generally have severe spurring in the anterior acromial and distal clavicular areas. Frequently, if the anterior cuff is involved, subluxation, hypertrophy, degenerative changes, or frank rupture of the biceps tendon may be present. In these patients, a formal open anterior acromioplasty and cuff repair are performed with reconstruction of the rotator cuff. If the biceps is dislocated, but perfectly normal, it is replaced in the groove, and after suturing the supraspinatus via either a tendon-to-tendon or tendon-to-bone technique, the rotator interval is closed and the edges of the subscapularis and coracohumeral ligament complex are sutured to the repaired supraspinatus to re-create the stabilizing effect at the aperture of the tuberosities (Fig. 19-64). On the other hand, if the biceps tendon is tenodesed or any attritional wear is noted, seldom is an attempt made to repair chronic ruptures (longer than 6 weeks). Patients are informed preoperatively that they will continue to have a bulge in the lower portion of the brachium. The intra-articular stump is removed to prevent possible impingement in the joint.

When arthroscopic repair is used to treat full-thickness defects in the rotator cuff, the aforementioned bicipital tenodesing techniques can be used. We are very careful to avoid destabilizing the coracoacromial arch when decompressing the subacromial space. Even when using arthroscopic techniques we must remain vigilant of the superior stabilization afforded by an intact long head of the biceps

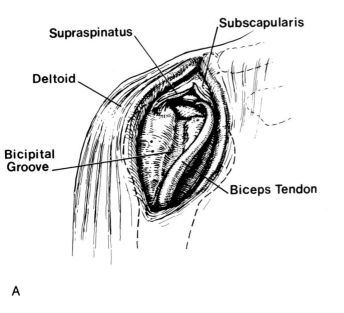

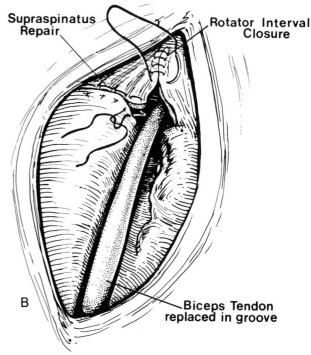

■ **Figure 19–64**

A, Rotator cuff tear and dislocated biceps tendon. B, The rotator cuff has been repaired into a bony trough and the rotator interval closed with the tendon replaced in the groove.

tendon. The larger the rotator cuff tear, the more likely we are to preserve the biceps.

BICEPS INSTABILITY

In our experience, surgically proven biceps instability is always related to a degenerative process in the cuff, restraining capsule, and coracohumeral ligament in the proximal portion of the groove. As with impingement tendinitis, primary attention should be placed on repair of the rotator cuff, as well as careful decompression of the coracoacromial arch. It has been well established that the main stabilizer of the biceps tendon is the musculotendinous cuff and the coracohumeral ligament. These structures can be injured acutely or by the mechanisms previously described, and fixed or recurrent subluxation of the biceps tendon can occur. If the injury is acute and the patient is younger than 65 years, MRI is recommended to diagnose this condition and evaluate the status of the rotator cuff. If the biceps is dislocated, we recommend early open reduction of the tendon with reconstruction of the fibrous roof, supraspinatus, and subscapularis, combined with an acromioplasty procedure, if indicated (see Fig. 19–64). It is important to remember that once the diagnosis of a dislocated biceps tendon is made, a rotator cuff tear is also diagnosed. Whereas in the older (over 65) age group this injury can be accepted and treated nonoperatively, younger (less than 50) patients will fare better if the tendon is replaced and the fibrous roof reconstructed; alternatively, if significant tenderness is present, biceps tenodesis can be performed. Because of the increasing activity in the older population, we are not using age as an absolute indication to guide our operative intervention as much as we did a few years ago. Older active patients with a dislocated biceps tendon may benefit from relocation of the tendon and rotator cuff repair just as much as younger patients do. In older, less active patients, we continue to try to treat biceps instability nonoperatively if possible.

ISOLATED BICEPS LESIONS

In patients with isolated biceps lesions, subacromial injection offers absolutely no improvement in pain, but pain and motion consistently respond to local anesthetic injections into the bicipital groove region. These patients generally respond to the judicious use of rest, aspirin or nonsteroidal anti-inflammatory agents, moist heat, and gentle patient-directed exercises. The judicious use of corticosteroids by injection can also be helpful. The injection should be into the bicipital sheath and should require only minimal pressure on the syringe and a low volume of fluid; specifically, 2 to 3 mL of lidocaine and 1 mL of water-soluble steroid should be used. The technique of injection has been described previously under "Differential Diagnosis." Numerous case reports have described tendon ruptures that are temporally and causally related to corticosteroid injections. Such ruptures have involved the patellar and Achilles tendons, the flexor and extensor tendons of the hand, and the long head of the biceps tendon. Although some tendons, especially those in an older patient with systemic disease or attrition tendinitis, may rupture as a result of the disease process, there is a

strong suggestion that injection into the tendon contributes to tendon degradation. Kennedy and Willis[142] have shown collagen necrosis as well as disorganization and loss of the normal parallel collagen arrangement in Achilles tendons injected with corticosteroids, in addition to a 35% loss of failure strength at approximately 48 hours after injection. The failure strength of the tendon returns at approximately 2 weeks; however, ultrastructural changes in the tendon persist for 6 weeks. Consequently, patients are asked to avoid any strenuous activity for 3 weeks. In our experience, patients are injected at a minimum of 6-week intervals and then only one to two or, perhaps in unusual cases, three times. Injections have been shown to be more efficacious than placebo or naproxen (Naprosyn) in the treatment of chronic shoulder pain and are equivalent to the use of indomethacin (Indocin).[285,286] Unfortunately, some patients with this problem cannot tolerate nonsteroidal anti-inflammatory agents in the doses required.

If the patient fails to respond to nonoperative care over a 6- to 12-month period, surgery is recommended. Because the results of isolated biceps tenodesis have not been spectacular in the long term and impingement syndrome has developed after biceps tenodesis, subacromial decompression is routinely performed.

ISOLATED BICEPS RUPTURE IN PATIENTS YOUNGER THAN 50 YEARS

In younger, active patients, particularly those involved in overhead sports or weightlifting or jobs requiring forceful supination, a sudden overload can result in an isolated biceps rupture. The rupture may be within the muscle-tendon junction rather than the long head tendon. Physical examination and ultrasonography of the biceps should be able to isolate the point of rupture. Sonography or MRI of the rotator cuff should be used to determine the status of the rotator cuff. If physical examination is consistent with an acute rupture and the sonogram is equivocal or negative, an arthrogram can be obtained. In these patients with high functional expectations, early repair is the best alternative. If the rupture is musculotendinous or at the transverse ligament and sonography is negative for a cuff tear, early repair using a Bunnell-type weave suture through a deltopectoral incision is performed. This group of patients is the only one in which use of the deltopectoral approach is recommended.

ACUTE BICIPITAL RUPTURE IN PATIENTS OLDER THAN 50 YEARS

If the patient is physically inactive, a graduated, leave-alone method (GLAM) technique of rest, anti-inflammatory medications, and moist heat is used. During this period the patient is instructed in how to keep shoulder movement free by passive motions. If the patient is physically active, an early aggressive diagnostic workup should be performed. Such workup usually consists of an MRI scan; however, arthrography or sonography can be performed. One will generally find an "acute" cuff tear as well as the biceps tendon rupture. Many of these patients will in reality have an acute extension of a chronic tear or no

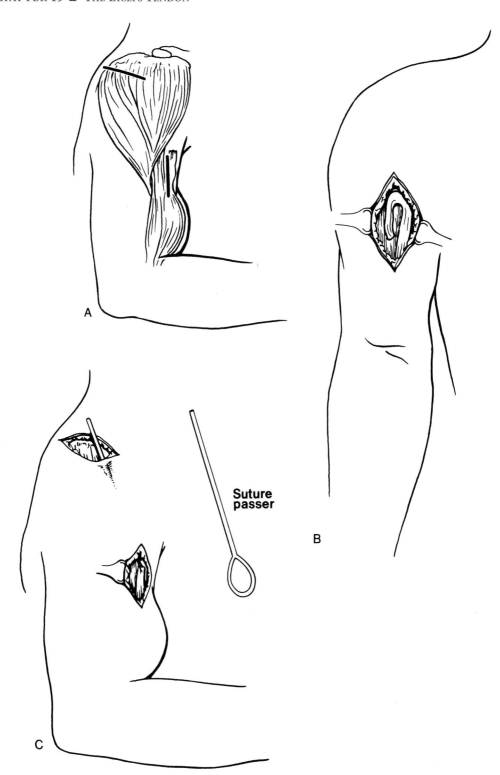

■ Figure 19–65
A, Two-incision approach to bicipital tendon rupture. The proximal incision is exactly the same as used for an anterior acromioplasty. The distal incision allows one to pick up the tendon of the biceps in the sulcus created by the defect in the biceps. The incision does not have to be very long, and only subcutaneous tissue and fascia need to be incised; a suture passer can then be used. B, Exposure of the ruptured biceps tendon through the counterincision in the sulcus, magnified in this view. A 3-cm incision is all that is required to pick up the end of the tendon in this region. C, A suture passer is used to bring the tendon into the proximal wound for tenodesis or repair.

extension at all. The two-incision approach in these cases is used if the rupture is less than 6 weeks old (Fig. 19–65A). If a tear is present in the rotator cuff, anterior acromioplasty with cuff repair and bicipital tenodesis is performed. The biceps tendon is exposed through a separate incision in the brachium (Fig. 19–65B). The subcutaneous tissue is incised and edema and old hemorrhage evacuated. The tendon can be curled up in this area or stuck proximal to the pectoralis insertion. With the use of a suture passer inserted down from above through the bicipital groove and into the lower wound, the tendon is advanced into the superior wound (Fig. 19–65C). A biceps tenodesis in the groove is then performed.

SLAP LESIONS

Treatment of SLAP lesions is covered fully in Chapter 8.

CALCIFIC TENDINITIS

Calcific tendinitis is treated as described in Chapter 18.

POSTOPERATIVE CARE

Unless there is some tension on the cuff repair with the arm at the side, a Velcro elastic immobilizer is used postoperatively for 3 weeks. The patient is encouraged to take the elbow out and gently flex and extend it passively with the opposite hand the night of the surgery. Gentle pendulum exercises are initiated on the first postoperative day. Passive flexion performed by the patient (with the other arm), nurse, or therapist is begun on the second postoperative day. Because holding onto a pulley handle requires some active contraction of the biceps, we generally instruct a family member in gentle, passive forward flexion and external rotation. At 1 month, the pulley can safely be used and gentle, active elbow flexion begun. Strengthening of the repaired cuff, deltoid, and biceps generally begins at 2 months and becomes more vigorous at 3 months. Patients usually return to work at jobs that require moderate lifting at approximately 6 months.

SUMMARY

Inflammation and degeneration of the biceps tendon often accompany rotator cuff pathology. Because of its unique anatomic position and close relationship to the coracoacromial arch, this tendon is susceptible to secondary injury and inflammation.

Biomechanically, the biceps tendon appears to function as a weak dynamic and static head depressor. In a normal shoulder it contributes little to humeral head depression, whereas in a shoulder with a rotator cuff tear, in vitro studies suggest an increase in the depressor role of the biceps. Accordingly, routine tenodesis of the biceps tendon or its use as a free graft in rotator cuff repair is not recommended.

The biceps tendon's primary restraints against dislocation are the coracohumeral ligament, superior glenohumeral ligament, and the rotator cuff, proximal to the groove. Because of its intimate relationship to the coracoacromial arch, whenever one considers a diagnosis of biceps pathology, one should also consider rotator cuff

pathology. When possible, subluxation of the biceps can be treated by replacement of the tendon into the groove and reconstruction of the rotator cuff combined with subacromial decompression.

Isolated biceps tenodesis or tenotomy is not recommended unless one is treating a massive cuff tear. The addition of anterior acromioplasty with excision of the coracoacromial ligament adds little morbidity to surgery on the biceps tendon in patients with an intact cuff and improves the results. Recognition that the diagnosis of isolated biceps tendon pathology is a diagnosis of exclusion, coupled with long-term conservative care for painful conditions about the shoulder, can often obviate the need for surgery and improve the results if surgical procedures are required.

Finally, a note of caution is in order. Although biceps tenotomy has gained popularity recently, patients must be prepared to live with the attendant deformity, and some will have significant pain at the site of tendon relocation for several months. Others may complain of chronic pain, fatigue, and cramping if their activities of daily living require repetitive forceful supination. Careful informed consent and patient selection are necessary to avoid medicolegal entanglements.

ACKNOWLEDGMENTS

(1) The senior author would like to thank Karen Lozano very much for her valuable help and tremendous patience in preparing this manuscript. She is a jewel of a human being who makes me look much better than I really am. (2) I still think that guy at the VA needs an arthroscopic biceps tenodesis!

REFERENCES

1. Abbott LC and Lucas DB: The function of the clavicle: Its surgical significance. Ann Surg 140:583-597, 1954.
2. Abbott LC and Saunders LB de CM: Acute traumatic dislocation of the tendon of the long head of biceps brachii; report of 6 cases with operative findings. Surgery 6:817-840, 1939.
3. Adams R: Abnormal conditions of the shoulder-joint. In Cyclopaedia of Anatomy and Physiology, vol. 4. London: Longman, 1847-1849, p 595.
4. Ahovuo J: The radiographic anatomy of the intratubercular groove of the humerus. Eur J Radiol 2:83, 1985.
5. Ahovuo J, Paavolainen P, and Slatis P: Radiographic diagnosis of biceps tendinitis. Acta Orthop Scand 56:75-78, 1985.
6. Ahovuo J, Paavolainen P, and Slatis P: Diagnostic value of sonography in lesions of the biceps tendon. Clin Orthop 202:184-188, 1986.
7. Anciaux-Ruyssen A and Claessens H: L'arthrographic de l'epaule. J Belg Radiol 39:837, 1956.
8. Andrews J and Carson W: Shoulder joint arthroscopy. Orthopedics 6:1157-1162, 1983.
9. Andrews J, Carson W, and McLeod W: Glenoid labrum tears related to the long head of the biceps. Am J Sports Med 13:337-341, 1985.
10. Anglesio B: Osteotomia per omero varo. Arch Orthop 46:417-428, 1930.
11. Ashurst J: The Principles and Practice of Surgery. Philadelphia: HC Lea, 1871, p 287.
12. Baer WS: Operative treatment of subdeltoid bursitis. Bull Johns Hopkins Hosp 18:282-284, 1907.
13. Baker BE and Bierwagen D: Rupture of the distal tendon of the biceps brachii. Operative versus non-operative treatment. J Bone Joint Surg Am 67:414-417, 1985.
14. Basmajian JV: Muscles Alive, 4th ed. Baltimore: Williams & Wilkins, 1978.
15. Basmajian JV: Muscles Alive, 5th ed. Baltimore: Williams & Wilkins, 1985.
16. Basmajian JV, Latif MA: Integrated actions and function of the chief flexors of the elbow. J Bone Joint Surg Am 39:1106-1118, 1957.
17. Bateman JE: The Shoulder and Environs. St Louis: CV Mosby, 1944.

18. Bateman JE: The Shoulder and Neck. Toronto: WB Saunders, 1978.
19. Bateman JE: The Shoulder and Neck, 2nd ed. Philadelphia: WB Saunders, 1978.
20. Becker DA and Cofield RH: Biceps brachii tenodesis for chronic tendinitis. Long term follow-up. Orthop Trans 210:447, 1986.
21. Bedi SS and Ellis W: Spontaneous rupture of the calcaneal tendon in rheumatoid arthritis after local steroid injection. Ann Rheum Dis 29:494-495, 1970.
22. Bennett WF: Specificity of the Speed's test: Arthroscopic technique. Arthroscopy 14:789-796, 1998.
23. Bennett WF: Visualization of the anatomy of the rotator interval and bicipital sheath. Arthroscopy 17:107-111, 2001.
24. Bennett GE: Shoulder and elbow lesions of professional baseball pitcher. JAMA 117:510-514, 1941.
25. Bera A: Syndrome Commun, Rupture, Elongation, Luxation du Tendon du Long Biceps. Paris: These, 1910-1911.
26. Berlemann U, Bayley I: Tenodesis of the long head of biceps brachii in the painful shoulder: Improving results in the long term. J Shoulder Elbow Surg 4:429-435, 1995.
27. Bidloo G: Anatomia Humani Corporis. Amstelodami, 1685.
28. Boileau P, Krishnan SG, Coste JS, and Walch G: Arthroscopic biceps tenodesis: A new technique using bioabsorbable interference screw fixation. Arthroscopy 18:1002-1012, 2002.
29. Booth RE and Marvel JP: Differential diagnosis of shoulder pain. Orthop Clin North Am 6:353-379, 1975.
30. Borchers E: Die ruptur der sehne des langen biceps kopfes. Beitr Klin Chir 90:635-648, 1914.
31. Bossuet: Two cas de luxation du tendon de la longue portion du biceps brachii. Bull Soc Anat Phys 28:154, 1907.
32. Brickner WM: JAMA 69:1237-1243, 1918.
33. Bromfield W: Chirgical Observations and Cases. London: 1773, p 76.
34. Burkhart SS and Fox DL: SLAP lesions in association with complete tears of the long head of the biceps tendon: A report of two cases. J Arthrop Rel Surg 8:31-35, 1992.
35. Bush LF: The torn shoulder capsule. J Bone Joint Surg Am 57:256, 1975.
36. Callender GW: Dislocation of muscles and their treatment. BMJ, July 13, 1878.
37. Carroll RE and Hamilton LR: Rupture of biceps brachii—a conservative method of treatment. J Bone Joint Surg Am 49:1016, 1967.
38. Cartland JP, Crues JV III, Stauffer A, et al: MR imaging in the evaluation of SLAP injuries of the shoulder. Findings in 10 patients. AJR Am J Roentgenol 159:787-792, 1992.
39. Cilley: Quoted by Meyer AW. Arch Surg 17:493-506, 1928.
40. Claessens H: De pijnlijke schouder. Belg T Geneesk, p 1050, 1956.
41. Claessens H and Anciauz-Ruyssen A: L'arthrographie de l'epaule. Acta Orthop Belg 3-4:289, 1956.
42. Claessens H and Biltris R: Diagnostic differentiel entre les lesions de la coiffe musculotendineuse et celles de la longue portion du biceps. J Belg Rheumatol Med Phys 20:53, 1965.
43. Claessens H and Brosgol M: Rapport: Les lesions traumatiques des parties molles de l'epaule. Acta Orthop Belg 2:97, 1957.
44. Claessens H and Snoek H: Tendinitis of the long head of the biceps brachii. Acta Orthop Belg 38:1, 1972.
45. Claessens H and Veys E: Les arthrites et l'arthrose de l'articulation scapulo-humerale. J Belg Rheumatol Med Phys 72:73, 1965.
46. Clark DD, Ricker JH, and MacCollum MS: The efficacy of local steroid injection in the treatment of stenosing tenovaginitis. Plast Reconstr Surg 51:179-180, 1973.
47. Clark JM and Harryman DT: Tendons, ligaments and capsule of the rotator cuff. J Bone Joint Surg Am 74:713-725, 1992.
48. Clark KC: Positioning in Radiography, vol 1, 9th ed. London: William Heinemann, 1973.
49. Codman EA: The supraspinatus syndrome. Boston Med Surg J 150:371-374, 1904.
50. Codman EA: The Shoulder. Boston: Thomas Todd, 1934.
51. Cofield RH and Becker D: Surgical tenodesis of the long head of the biceps brachii for chronic tendinitis. Paper presented at the 53rd Annual Meeting of the American Academy of Orthopaedic Surgeons, February 21, 1986, New Orleans.
52. Cole BJ, Rodeo SA, O'Brien SJ, et al: The anatomy and histology of the rotator interval capsule of the shoulder. Clin Orthop 390:129-137, 2001.
53. Cone RO, Danzig L, Resnick D, and Goldman AB: The bicipital groove: Radiographic, anatomic, and pathologic study. AJR Am J Roentgenol 41:781-788, 1983.
54. Conti V: Arthroscopy in rehabilitation. Orthop Clin North Am 10:709-711, 1979.
55. Cooper A: A Treatise on Dislocations and Fractures of the Joints. Boston: Lilly, Wait, Carter & Hendee, 1832, p 407.
56. Cooper DE, Arnoczky SP, O'Brien SJ, et al: Anatomy, histology and vascularity of the glenoid labrum. An anatomical study. J Bone Joint Surg Am 74:46-52, 1992.
57. Covall DJ and Fowble CD: Arthroscopic treatment of synovial chondromatosis of the shoulder and biceps tendon sheath. J Arthrop Rel Surg 9:602-604, 1993.
58. Covall DJ and Fowble CD: Synovial chondromatosis of the biceps tendon sheath. Orthop Rev 23:902-905, 1994.
59. Cowper W: Myotomia Reformata. London: 1694, p 75.
60. Crenshaw AH and Kilgore WE: Surgical treatment of bicipital tenosynovitis. J Bone Joint Surg Am 48:1496-1502, 1966.
61. David G, Magarey ME, Jones MA, et al: EMG and strength correlates of selected shoulder muscles during rotations of the glenohumeral joint. Clin Biomech 15:95-102, 2000.
62. David T and Drez DJ: Synovial chondromatosis of the shoulder and biceps. Orthopedics 23:611-613, 2000.
63. Day BH, Govindasamy N, and Patnaik R: Corticosteroid injections in the treatment of tennis elbow. Practitioner 220:459-462, 1978.
64. Dejour D and Tayot O: La rupture isolee de la longue portion du biceps. Journees Lyonnaise de l'Epaule. Lyon, France: 1993.
65. Demuynck M and Zuker RM: Biceps tendon rupture after successful reinnervation: A case report. Acta Orthop Belg 61:55-58, 1995.
66. DePalma AF: Surgery of the Shoulder. Philadelphia: JB Lippincott, 1950.
67. DePalma AF: The painful shoulder. Postgrad Med 21:368-376, 1957.
68. DePalma AF: Surgical anatomy of the rotator cuff and the natural history of degenerative periarthritis. Surg Clin North Am 43:1507-1520, 1963.
69. DePalma AF: Surgery of the Shoulder, 2nd ed. Philadelphia: JB Lippincott, 1983.
70. DePalma AF and Callery GE: Bicipital tenosynovitis. Clin Orthop 3:69-85, 1954.
71. Despates H: Gaz Hebd 15:374-378, 1878.
72. Dines D, Warren RF, and Inglis AE: Surgical treatment of lesions of the long head of the biceps. Clin Orthop 164:165-171, 1982.
73. Duplay S: Arch Gen Med 2:513-542, 1872.
74. Duplay S: On scapulo-humeral periarthritis (Paris Clinical Lectures). Med Presse 69:571-573, 1900.
75. Duplay S and Reclus P: Traite de Chirurgie, vol 1. Paris: G Masson, 1880-1882, p 825.
76. Dupont L, Gamet D, and Perot C: Motor unit recruitment and EMG power spectra during ramp contractions of a bifunctional muscle. J Electromyogr Kinesiol 10:217-224, 1927.
77. Ellman H: Arthroscopic subacromial decompression. Paper presented at a meeting of the Society of American Shoulder and Elbow Surgeons, 1986, New Orleans.
78. Ennevaara K: Painful shoulder joint in rheumatoid arthritis: Clinical and radiologic study of 200 cases with special reference to arthrography of the glenohumeral joint. Acta Rheumatol Scand Suppl 2:11-116, 1967.
79. Ewald: Traumatic ruptures usually due to arthritis deformans or other diseases of shoulder. Munch Med Wochnschr 74:2214-2215, 1927.
80. Farin PU, Jaroma H, Harju A, and Soimakallio S: Medial displacement of the biceps brachii tendon: Evaluation with dynamic sonography during maximal external shoulder rotation. Radiology 195:845-848, 1995.
81. Favorito PJ, Harding WG 3rd, and Heidt RS Jr: Complete arthroscopic examination of the long head of the biceps tendon. Arthroscopy 17:430-432, 2001.
82. Fenlin JM Jr and McShane RB: Conservative open anterior acromioplasty. Orthop Trans 11:229-230, 1987.
83. Field LD and Savoie FH: Arthroscopic suture repair of superior labral detachment lesions of the shoulder. Am J Sports Med 21:783-790, 1993.
84. Fisk C: Adaptation of the technique for radiography of the bicipital groove. Radiol Technol 37:47-50, 1965.
85. Freeland AE and Higgins RW: Anterior shoulder dislocation with posterior displacement of the long head of the biceps tendon. Arthrographic findings. A case report. Orthopedics 8:468-469, 1985.
86. Froimson AI and Oh I: Keyhole tenodesis of biceps origin at the shoulder. Clin Orthop 112:245-249, 1974.
87. Furlani J: Electromyographic study of the m. biceps brachii in movements at the glenohumeral joint. Acta Anat (Basel) 96:270-284, 1976.
88. Gainer BJ, Piotrowski G, Truhl J, et al: The throw: Biomechanics and acute injury. Am Sports Med 8:114-118, 1980.
89. Gardner E and Gray DJ: Prenatal development of the human shoulder and acromioclavicular joint. Am J Anat 92:219-276, 1953.
90. Gartsman GM and Hammerman SM: Arthroscopic biceps tenodesis: Operative technique. Arthroscopy 16:550-552, 2000.
91. Gerber C and Sebesta A: Impingement of the deep surface of the subscapularis tendon and the reflection pulley on the anterosuperior glenoid rim: A preliminary report. J Shoulder Elbow Surg 9:483-490, 2000.
92. Gerber C, Terrier F, and Ganz R: The role of the coracoid process in the chronic impingement syndrome. J Bone Joint Surg Br 67:703-708, 1985.
93. Gerster AG: Subcutaneous injuries of the biceps brachii, with two new cases and some historical notes. N Y Med J 27:487-502, 1878.
94. Gigis P, Natsis C, and Polyzonis M: New aspects on the topography of the long head of the biceps brachii muscle. One more stabilizer factor of the shoulder joint. Bull Assoc Anat 79: 9-11, 1995.
95. Gilcreest EL: Rupture of muscles and tendons, particularly subcutaneous rupture of the biceps flexor cubiti. JAMA 84:1819-1822, 1925.
96. Gilcreest EL: Two cases of spontaneous rupture of the long head of the biceps flexor cubiti. Surg Clin North Am 6:539-554, 1926.
97. Gilcreest EL: The common syndrome of rupture, dislocation and elongation of the long head of the biceps brachii. An analysis of one hundred cases. Surg Gynecol Obstet 58:322-339, 1934.
98. Gilcreest EL: Dislocation and elongation of the long head of the biceps brachii. Analysis of six cases. Ann Surg 104:118-138, 1936.

99. Gilcreest EL and Albi P: Unusual lesions of muscles and tendons of the shoulder girdle and upper arm. Surg Gynecol Obstet 68:903-917, 1939.

100. Gill TJ, McIrvin E, Mair SD, and Hawkins RJ: Results of biceps teneotomy for the treatment of pathology of the long head of the biceps brachii. J Shoulder Elbow Surg 10:247-249, 2001.

101. Giuliani P, Scarpa G, Marchini M, and Nicoletti P: Development of scapulohumeral articulation in man, with special reference to its relation to the tendon of the long head of the biceps muscle of the arm. Arch Ital Anat Embriol 82:85-98, 1977.

102. Glousman R, Jobe F, Tibone J, et al: Dynamic electromyographic analysis of the throwing shoulder with glenohumeral instability. J Bone Joint Surg Am 70:220-226, 1988.

103. Godsil RD Jr and Linschied RL: Intratendinous defects of the rotator cuff. Clin Orthop 69:181-188, 1970.

104. Goldman AB: Shoulder Arthrography. Boston: Little, Brown, 1981, pp 239-257.

105. Goldman AB: Calcific tendinitis of the long head of the biceps brachii distal to the glenohumeral joint: Plain film radiographic findings. Am J Radiol 153:1011-1016, 1989.

106. Goldman AB and Ghelman B: The double contrast shoulder arthrogram. A review of 158 studies. Radiology 127:658-663, 1978.

107. Goldthwait JE: An anatomic and mechanical study of the shoulder joint, explaining many of the cases of painful shoulder, many of the recurrent dislocations and many of the cases of brachial neuralgias or neuritis. Am J Orthop Surg 6:579-606, 1909.

108. Grauer JD, Paulos LE, and Smutz WP: Biceps tendon and superior labral injuries. Arthroscopy 8:488-497, 1992.

109. Green JS: Dislocation of the long head of the biceps flexor cubiti muscle. Virginia Med Monthly 4:106, 1877-1878.

110. Guermonprez MA: Posterior luxation of shoulder. Rupture of lesser tuberosity, rupture and luxation of tendon of long head of biceps. Recovery. Bull Soc Anat Paris 4:1890.

111. Habermeyer P, Brunner U, Treptow U, and Wiedemann E: Arthroskopische over-the top-naht bei der Behandlung von S.L.A.P. Lasionen der Schulter. Arthroskopie 6:253-271, 1993.

112. Habermeyer P, Kaiser E, Knappe M, et al: Functional anatomy and biomechanics of the long biceps tendon. Unfallchirurg 90:319-329, 1987.

113. Habermeyer P and Walch G: The biceps tendon and rotator cuff disease. In Burkhead WZ Jr (ed): Rotator Cuff Disorders. Media, PA: Williams & Wilkins, 1996, p 142.

114. Haenisch GF: Fortsch Rontgenstr 15:293-300, 1910.

115. Ha'eri GB and Maitland A: Arthroscopic findings in the frozen shoulder. J Rheumatol 8:149-152, 1981.

116. Ha'eri GB and Wiley AM: Advancement of the supraspinatus muscle in the repair of ruptures of the rotator cuff. J Bone Joint Surg Am 63:232-238, 1981.

117. Haggart GE and Allen HA: Painful shoulder: Diagnosis and treatment with particular reference to subacromial bursitis. Surg Clin North Am 15:1537-1560, 1935.

118. Hall-Craggs EC: Anatomy as a Basis for Clinical Medicine. Baltimore: Urban & Schwartzberg, 1985, p 111.

119. Hammond G, Torgerson W, Dotter W, and Leach R: The painful shoulder. American Academy of Orthopaedic Surgeons Instructional Course Lectures. St Louis: CV Mosby, 1971, pp 83-90.

120. Hawkins RJ and Kennedy JC: Impingement syndrome in athletes. Am J Sports Med 8:151-158, 1980.

121. Heikel HVA: Rupture of the rotator cuff of the shoulder. Acta Orthop Scand 39:477-492, 1968.

122. Herberts P, Kadefors R, Andersson G, and Petersen I: Shoulder pain in industry: An epidemiological study on welders. Acta Orthop Scand 52:299-306, 1981.

123. Hippocrates: Quoted by Duplay, Reclus and Garrison.

124. Hitchcock HH and Bechtol CO: Painful shoulder. Observations on the role of the tendon of the long head of the biceps brachii in its causation. J Bone Joint Surg Am 30:263-273, 1948.

125. Ho CP: MR imaging of the rotator interval, long head of the biceps and associated injuries in the overhead throwing athlete. Magn Reson Imaging Clin N Am 7:23-37, 1999.

126. Hollinshead WH: Anatomy For Surgeons, vol 3. New York: Harper & Row, 1969, p 325.

127. Hollinsworth GR, Ellis RM, and Hattersley TS: Comparison of injection techniques for shoulder pain: Results of a double blind, randomized study. BMJ 287:1339-1341, 1983.

128. Horowitz MT: Lesions of the supraspinatus tendon and associated structures. Investigation of comparable lesions in the hip joint. Arch Surg 38:990-1003, 1939.

129. Howard HJ and Eloesser L: Treatment of fractures of the upper end of the humerus: An experimental and clinical study. J Bone Joint Surg 16:1-29, 1934.

130. Hueter C: Zur Diagnose der Verletzungen des M. Biceps Brachii. Arch Klin Chir 5:321-323, 1864; and also Grundriss der Chirurgie, vol 2, p 735.

131. Ingelbrecht: Arch Franco-Belges Chir 29:922-923, 1926.

132. Inman VT and Saunders JB de CM: Observations on the function of the clavicle. Calif Med 65:158-166, 1946.

133. Inman VT, Saunders JB de CM, and Abbott LC: Observations on the function of the shoulder joint. J Bone Joint Surg 26:1-30, 1944.

134. Itoi E, Kuechle DK, Newman SR, et al: Stabilizing function of the biceps in stable and unstable shoulders. J Bone Joint Surg Br 75:546-550, 1993.

135. Janecki CJ and Barnett DC: Fracture dislocation of the shoulder with biceps interposition. J Bone Joint Surg Am 61:1-143, 1979.

136. Jarjavey JF: Luxation du tendon du biceps humeral et des tendons des peroniers lateraux. Gaz Hebd Med (Paris) 4:325-327, 357-359, 387-391, 1867.

137. Jobe FW and Jobe CM: Painful athletic injuries of the shoulder. Clin Orthop 173:117-124, 1983.

138. Jobe FW, Moines DR, Tibone JE, et al: An EMG analysis of the shoulder in pitching. A second report. Am J Sports Med 12:218-220, 1984.

139. Jobe FW, Tibone JE, Perry J, et al: An EMG analysis of the shoulder in throwing and pitching. A preliminary report. Am J Sports Med 11:3-5, 1983.

140. Jungmichel D, Winzer J, and Lippoldt G: Tendon rupture of the biceps muscle of the arm and its treatment with special reference to the key hole operation. Beitr Orthop Traumatol 33:226-232, 1986.

141. Kempf JF, Gleyze P, Bonnomet F, et al: A multicenter study of 210 rotator cuff tears treated by arthroscopic acromioplasty. Arthroscopy 15:56-66, 1999.

142. Kennedy JC and Willis RB: The effects of local steroid injections on tendons: A biomechanical and microscopic correlative study. Am J Sports Med 4:11-21, 1976.

143. Kerlan RK: Throwing injuries to the shoulder. In Zarins B, Andrews JR, and Carson WG (eds): Injuries to the Throwing Arm. Philadelphia: WB Saunders, 1985, p 114.

144. Kessel L and Watson M: The painful arc syndrome. Clinical classification as a guide to management. J Bone Joint Surg Br 59:166-172, 1977.

145. Kieft GJ, Bloem JL, Rozing PM, and Obermann WR: Rotator cuff impingement syndrome: MR imaging. Radiology 166:211-214, 1988.

146. Killoran PJ, Marcove RL, and Freiberger RH: Shoulder arthography. AJR Am J Roentgenol 103:658-668, 1968.

147. Klug JD and Moore SL: MR imaging of the biceps muscle-tendon complex. Magn Reson Imaging Clin N Am 5:755-765, 1997.

148. Kneeland JB, Middleton WD, Carrera GF, et al: MR imaging of the shoulder: Diagnosis of rotator cuff tears. AJR Am J Roentgenol 149:333-337, 1987.

149. Koltz I, Tillman B, and Lullmann-Rauch R: The structure and vascularization of the biceps brachii long head tendon. Ann Anat 176:75-80, 1994.

150. Kumar VP, Satku K, and Balasubramaniam P: The role of the long head of biceps brachii in the stabilization of the head of the humerus. Clin Orthop 244:172-175, 1989.

151. Lapidus PW: Infiltration therapy of acute tendinitis with calcification. Surg Gynecol Obstet 76:715-725, 1943.

152. Lapidus PW and Guidotti FP: Local injection of hydrocortisone in 495 orthopedic patients. Ind Med Surg 26:234-244, 1957.

153. Laumann U: Decompression of the subacromial space: An anatomical study. In Bayley I and Kellel L (eds): Shoulder Surgery. Berlin: Springer-Verlag, 1982, pp 14-21.

154. Laumann U: Kinesiology of the shoulder joint. In Kolbel R, Bodo H, and Blauth W (eds): Shoulder Replacement. New York: Springer-Verlag, 1987.

155. Levitskii FA and Nochevkin VA: Plastic repair of the tendon of the long head of the biceps muscle. Vestn Khir 130:92-94, 1983.

156. Levy AS, Kelley BT, Lintner SA, et al: Function of the long head of the biceps at the shoulder: Electromyographic analysis. J Shoulder Elbow Surg 10:250-255, 2001.

157. Lippmann RK: Frozen shoulder, periarthritis, bicipital tenosynovitis. Arch Surg 47:283-296, 1943.

158. Lippmann RK: Bicipital tenosynovitis. N Y State J Med 90:2235-2241, 1944.

159. Lloyd-Roberts GC: Humerus varus. Report of a case treated by excision of the acromion. J Bone Joint Surg Br 35:268-269, 1953.

160. Logal R: Rupture of the long tendon of the biceps brachii muscle. Clin Orthop 2:217-221, 1976.

161. Loyd JA and Loyd HA: Adhesive capsulitis of the shoulder: Arthrographic diagnosis and treatment. South Med J 76:879-883, 1983.

162. Lucas DB: Biomechanics of the shoulder joint. Arch Surg 107:425-432, 1973.

163. Lucas LS and Gill JH: Humerus varus following birth injury to the proximal humeral epiphysis. J Bone Joint Surg 29:367-369, 1947.

164. Ludington NA: Am J Surg 77:358, 1923.

165. Lundberg BJ: The frozen shoulder: Clinical and radiographical observations, the effect of manipulation under general anesthesia, structure and glycosaminoglycans content of the joint capsule. Local bone metabolism. Acta Orthop Scand 119:1-49, 1969.

166. Lundberg BJ: Glycosaminoglycans of the normal and frozen shoulder joint capsule. Clin Orthop 69:279-284, 1970.

167. Lundberg BJ and Nilsson BE: Osteopenia in the frozen shoulder. Clin Orthop 60:187-191, 1968.

168. MacDonald PB: Case report: Congenital anomaly of the biceps tendon and anatomy within the shoulder joint. Arthroscopy 14:741-742, 1998.

169. Macnab I: Rotator cuff tendinitis. Ann R Coll Surg Engl 53:271-287, 1973.

170. Makin M: Translocation of the biceps humeri for flail shoulder. J Bone Joint Surg Am 59:490-491, 1977.

171. Malicky DM, Soslowsky LJ, Blasier RB, and Shyr Y: Anterior glenohumeral stabilization factors: Progressive effects in a biomechanical model. J Orthop Res 14:282-288.

172. Mariani EM and Cofield RA: The tendon of the long head of the biceps brachii: Instability, tendinitis and rupture. Advances in Orthopaedic Surgery. Baltimore: Williams & Wilkins, 1988, pp 262-268.

173. Mariani PP, Bellelli A, and Botticella C: Case report: Arthroscopic absence of the long head of the biceps tendon. Arthroscopy 13:499-501, 1997.
174. Matsen F and Kirby R: Office evaluation and management of shoulder pain. Orthop Clin North Am 13:45, 1982.
175. McClellan: Textbook of Surgery, 1892.
176. McCue FC III, Zarins B, Andrews JR, and Carson WG: Throwing injuries to the shoulder. In Zarins B, Andrews JR, and Carson WG (eds): Injuries to the Throwing Arm. Philadelphia: WB Saunders, 1985, p 98.
177. McGough R, Debski RE, Taskiran E, et al: Tensile properties of the long head of the biceps tendon. Paper presented at a closed meeting of the American Shoulder and Elbow Surgeons, 1995.
178. McGough R, Debski RE, Taskiran E, et al: Tensile properties of the long head of the biceps tendon. Knee Surg Sports Traumatol Arthrosc 3:226-229, 1996.
179. McLaughlin HL: Lesions of musculotendinous cuff of shoulder; observations on pathology, course and treatment of calcific deposits. Ann Surg 124:354, 1946.
180. McLaughlin HL: Dislocation of the shoulder with tuberosity fracture. Surg Clin North Am 43:1615-1620, 1963.
181. Meagher DM, Pool R, and Brown M: Bilateral ossification of the tendon of the biceps brachii muscle in the horse. J Am Vet Med Assoc 174:283-285, 1979.
182. Mercer A: Partial dislocations: Consecutive and muscular affections of the shoulder joint. Buffalo Med Surg J 4:645-652, 1859.
183. Meyer AW: Spolia anatomica. Absence of the tendon of the long head of the biceps. J Anat 48:133-135, 1913-1914.
184. Meyer AW: Anatomical specimens of the unusual clinical interest. II. The effect of arthritis deformans on the tendon of the long head of the biceps brachii. Am J Orthop Surg 13:86-95, 1915.
185. Meyer AW: Unrecognized occupational destruction of the tendon of the long head of the biceps brachii. Arch Surg 2:130-144, 1921.
186. Meyer AW: Further observations upon use destruction in joints. J Bone Joint Surg 4:491-511, 1922.
187. Meyer AW: Further evidences of attrition in the human body. Am J Anat 34:241-267, 1924.
188. Meyer AW: Spontaneous dislocation of the tendon of the long head of the biceps brachii. Arch Surg 13:109-119, 1926.
189. Meyer AW: Spontaneous dislocation and destruction of the tendon of the long head of the biceps brachii. Arch Surg 17:493-506, 1928.
190. Meyer AW: Chronic functional lesions of the shoulder. Arch Surg 35:646-674, 1937.
191. Michele AA: Bicipital tenosynovitis. Clin Orthop 18:261, 1960.
192. Middleton WD, Reinus WR, Totty WG, et al: Ultrasonographic evaluation of the rotator cuff and biceps tendon. J Bone Joint Surg Am 68:440-450, 1986.
193. Middleton WD, Kneeland JB, Carrera GF, et al: High resolution MR imaging of the normal rotator cuff. AJR Am J Roentgenol 148:559-564, 1987.
194. Milgram JE: Pathology and treatment of calcific tendinitis and bursitis of the shoulder. Scientific exhibit presented at the 1939 Meeting of the American Academy of Orthopaedic Surgeons.
195. Milgram JE: Bursitis—pathology and treatment of calcific tendinitis and bursitis by aspiration and vascularization. Med Rev Mex 125:283-305, 1945.
196. Milgram JE: Shoulder anatomy. Instructional Courses Volume. American Academy of Orthopedic Surgeons, Chicago, January 1946, pp 55-68.
197. Milgram JE: Aspiration of bursal deposits (quoted by Crowe, Harold). Bull Am Acad Orthop Surg, p 11, April 1963.
198. Minami M, Ishii S, Usui M, and Ogino T: A case of idiopathic humerus varus. J Orthop Trauma Surg 20:175-178, 1975.
199. Monteggia GB: Instituzioni Chirurgiche. Milan: G Truffi, 1829-1830, p 179; also Part II, 1803, p 334.
200. Monu JUV, Pope TL Jr, Chabon SJ, and Vanarthos WJ: MR diagnosis of superior labral anterior posterior (SLAP) injuries of the glenoid labrum: Value of routine imaging without intra-articular injection of contrast material. AJR Am J Roentgenol 163:1425-1429, 1994.
201. Moseley HF: Rupture of supraspinatus tendon. Can Med Assoc J 41:280-282, 1939.
202. Moseley HF: Shoulder Lesions. Springfield, IL: Charles C Thomas, 1945, pp 58-65.
203. Moseley HF and Goldie I: The arterial pattern of the rotator cuff of the shoulder. J Bone Joint Surg Br 45:780-789, 1963.
204. Moseley HF and Overgaard B: The anterior capsular mechanism in recurrent anterior dislocation of the shoulder: Morphological and clinical studies with special reference to the glenoid labrum and the glenohumeral ligaments. J Bone Joint Surg Br 44:913-927, 1962.
205. Muller TH and Gohlke F: Synovial chondromatosis of the biceps tendon. Paper presented at the 6th International Congress on Surgery of the Shoulder, June 27-July 4, 1995, Helsinki and Stockholm.
206. Murthi AM, Vosburg CL, and Neviaser TJ: The incidence of pathologic changes of the long head of the biceps tendon. J Shoulder Elbow Surg 9:382-385, 2000.
207. Neer CS II: Anterior acromioplasty for the chronic impingement syndrome in the shoulder. J Bone Joint Surg Am 54:41-50, 1972.
208. Neer CS II: Impingement lesions. Clin Orthop 173:70-77, 1983.
209. Neer CS: Less frequent procedures. In Neer CS II (ed): Shoulder Reconstruction. Philadelphia: WB Saunders, 1990, pp 426-427.
210. Neer CS and Marberry TA: On the disadvantages of radical acromionectomy. J Bone Joint Surg Am 63:416-419, 1981.
211. Neer CS II and Poppen NK: Supraspinatus outlet. Orthop Trans 11:234, 1987.
212. Neviaser JS: Adhesive capsulitis of the shoulder. A study of the pathological findings in periarthritis of the shoulder. J Bone Joint Surg 27:211-222, 1945.
213. Neviaser JS: Surgical approaches to the shoulder. Clin Orthop 91:34, 1973.
214. Neviaser JS: Arthrography of the Shoulder. Springfield, IL: Charles C Thomas, 1975.
215. Neviaser JS, Neviaser RJ, and Neviaser TJ: The repair of chronic massive ruptures of the rotator cuff of the shoulder by use of a freeze-dried rotator cuff. J Bone Joint Surg Am 60:681, 1978.
216. Neviaser RJ: Lesions of the biceps and tendinitis of the shoulder. Orthop Clin North Am 11:343-348, 1980.
217. Neviaser RJ and Nevaiser TJ: Lesions of the musculotendinous cuff of the shoulder: diagnosis and management. Instr Course Lect 30:239-257, 1981.
218. Neviaser TJ and Neviaser RJ: Lesions of the long head of the biceps tendon. Instr Course Lect 30:250-257, 1981.
219. Neviaser TJ, Neviaser RJ, and Neviaser JS: The four in one arthroplasty for the painful arc syndrome. Clin Orthop 163:107, 1982.
220. Nove-Josserand L: Subluxation et luxation du tendon du long biceps. Journees Lyonnaise de l'Epaule. Lyon, France: 1993.
221. O'Brien SJ, Arnoczky SP, Warren REF, and Rozbruch RS: Developmental anatomy of the shoulder and anatomy of the glenohumeral joint. In Rockwood CA and Matsen FA III (eds): The Shoulder. Philadelphia: WB Saunders, 1990, pp 15-17.
222. O'Donohue D: Subluxating biceps tendon in the athlete. Clin Orthop 164:26, 1982.
223. Ogilvie-Harris DJ and Wiley AM: Arthroscopic surgery of the shoulder: A general appraisal. J Bone Joint Surg Br 68:201-207, 1986.
224. Ogowa K and Naniwa T: A rare variation of the biceps: A possible cause of degeneration of the rotator cuff. J Shoulder Elbow Surg 7:295-297, 1998.
225. Ozaki J: Repair of chronic massive rotator cuff tears with Teflon felt. In Burkhead WZ Jr (ed): Rotator Cuff Disorders. Media, PA: Williams & Wilkins, 1996, p 385.
226. Ozaki J: Personal communication, 1996.
227. Paavolainen P, Bjorkenheim JM, Slatis P, and Paukku P: Operative treatment of severe proximal humeral fractures. Acta Orthop Scand 54:374-379, 1983.
228. Paavolainen P, Slatis P, and Aalto K: Surgical pathology in chronic shoulder pain. In Bateman JE and Welsh RP (eds): Surgery of the Shoulder. Philadelphia: BC Decker, 1984.
229. Packer NP, Calvert PT, Bayley JIL, and Kessel L: Operative treatment of chronic ruptures of the rotator cuff of the shoulder. J Bone Joint Surg Br 65:171-175, 1983.
230. Pagnani MJ, Deng XH, Warren RF, et al: Role of the long head of the biceps brachii in the glenohumeral stability: A biomechanical study in cadavera. J Shoulder Elbow Surg 5:255-262, 1996.
231. Painter CF: Subdeltoid bursitis. Boston Med Surg J 156:345-349, 1907.
232. Pal GP, Bhatt RH, and Patel VS: Relationship between the tendon of the long head of biceps brachii and the glenoid labrum in humans. Anat Rec 229:278-280, 1991.
233. Pappas AM, Goss TP, and Kleinman PK: Symptomatic shoulder instability due to lesions of the glenoid labrum. Am J Sports Med 11:279-288, 1983.
234. Parkhill CS: Dislocation of the long head of the biceps. Int J Surg 10:132, 1897.
235. Partridge R: The case of Mr. John Soden. Communication to the Royal and Chirurgical Society of London, July 6, 1841.
236. Pasteur F: Les algies de L'epaule et la physiotherapie. La teno-bursite bicipitale. J Radiol Electrol 16:419-429, 1932.
237. Perry J: Muscle control of the shoulder. In Rowe C (ed): The Shoulder. New York: Churchill Livingstone, 1988, p 26.
238. Petersson CJ: Degeneration of the gleno-humeral joint: An anatomical study. Acta Orthop Scand 54:277-283, 1983.
239. Petersson CJ: Spontaneous medial dislocation of the tendon of the long biceps brachii. Clin Orthop 211:224-227, 1986.
240. Petri M, Dobrow R, Neiman R, et al: Randomized, double-blind, placebo-controlled study of the treatment of the painful shoulder. Arthritis Rheum 30:1040-1045, 1987.
241. Pfahler M, Branner S, and Refior HJ: The role of the bicipital groove in tendinopathy of the long biceps tendon. J Shoulder Elbow Surg 8:419-424, 1999.
242. Phillips BB, Canale ST, Sisk TD, et al: Ruptures of the proximal biceps tendon in middle-aged patients. Orthop Rev 22:349-353, 1993.
243. Pinzur M and Hopkins G: Biceps tenodesis for painful inferior subluxation of the shoulder in adult acquired hemiplegia. Clin Orthop 206:100-103, 1986.
244. Post M: Primary tendinitis of the long head of the biceps. Paper presented at a Closed Meeting of the Society of American Shoulder and Elbow Surgeons, 1987, Orlando, FL.
245. Post M, Silver R, and Singh M: Rotator cuff tear. Diagnosis and treatment. Clin Orthop 173:78-91, 1983.
246. Postacchini F: Rupture of the rotator cuff of the shoulder associated with rupture of the tendon of the long head of the biceps. Ital J Orthop Traumatol 12:137-149, 1986.
247. Postacchini F and Ricciardi-Pollini T: Rupture of the short head tendon of the biceps brachii. Clin Orthop 124:229-232, 1977.
248. Postgate J: Displacement of long tendon of biceps. Med 3:615, 1851.

249. Pouteau C: Melanges de Chirurgie. Lyons, France: G Regnault, 1760, p 433.
250. Ptasznik R and Hennessey O: Abnormalities of the biceps tendon of the shoulder: Sonographic findings. AJR Am J Roentgenol 164:409-414, 1995.
251. Quinn CE: Humeral scapular periarthritis. Observations on the effects of x-ray therapy and ultrasound therapy in cases of "frozen shoulder." Ann Phys Med 10:64-69, 1967.
252. Rathbun JB and Macnab I: The microvascular pattern of the rotator cuff. J Bone Joint Surg Br 52:540-553, 1970.
253. Refior HJ and Sowa D: Long tendon of the biceps brachii: Sites of predilection for degenerative lesions. J Shoulder Elbow Surg 4:436-440, 1995.
254. Resnick D: Shoulder arthrography. Radiol Clin North Am 19:243-253, 1981.
255. Resnick D and Niwayama G: The Shoulder. In Diagnosis of Bone and Joint Disorders, 2nd ed. Philadelphia: WB Saunders, 1988, pp 1733-1764.
256. Rockwood C, Burkhead W, and Brna J: Anterior acromial morphology in relation to the caudal tilt radiograph. Unpublished manuscript.
257. Rokito AS, Bilgen OF, Zuckerman JD, and Cuomo F: Medial dislocation of the long head of the biceps tendon: Magnetic resonance imaging evaluation. Am J Orthop 25:314-323, 1996.
258. Rothman RH and Parke WW: The vascular anatomy of the rotator cuff. Clin Orthop 41:176-182, 1965.
259. Rowe CR (ed): The Shoulder. New York: Churchill Livingstone, 1988, p 145.
260. Sakurai G, Ozaki J, Tomita Y, et al: Electromyographic analysis of shoulder joint function of the biceps brachii muscle during isometric contraction. Clin Orthop 345:123-131, 1998.
261. Sakurai G, Ozaki J, Tomita Y, et al: Morphologic changes in the long head of biceps brachii in rotator cuff dysfunction. J Orthop Sci 3:137-142, 1998.
262. Schrager VL: Tenosynovitis of the long head of the biceps humeri. Surg Gynecol Obstet 66:785-790, 1938.
263. Schutte JP and Hawkins RJ: Advances in Shoulder Surgery. Orthopedics 10:1725-1728, 1987.
264. Seeger LL, Ruszkowski JT, Bassett LW, et al: MR imaging of the normal shoulder: Anatomic correlation. AJR Am J Roentgenol 148:83-91, 1987.
265. Sheldon PJH: A retrospective survey of 102 cases of shoulder pain. Rheum Phys Med 11:422-427, 1972.
266. Simmonds FA: Shoulder pain: With particular reference to the "frozen" shoulder. J Bone Joint Surg Br 31:426-432, 1949.
267. Simon WH: Soft tissue disorders of the shoulder. Frozen shoulder, calcific tendinitis, and bicipital tendinitis. Orthop Clin North Am 6:521-538, 1975.
268. Slatis P and Aalto K: Medial dislocation of the tendon of the long head of the biceps brachii. Acta Orthop Scand 50:73-77, 1979.
269. Snyder SJ: Repair of type II SLAP lesion using suture anchors and permanent mattress sutures. Paper presented at the Ninth Annual Meeting of the San Diego Shoulder Association, 1992, San Diego, CA.
270. Snyder SJ, Karzel RP, Del Pizzo W, et al: SLAP lesions of the shoulder. Arthroscopy 6:274-279, 1990.
271. Soden J: Two cases of dislocation of the tendon of the long head of the biceps. Med Chir 24:212, 1841.
272. Soto-Hall R and Haldeman KO: Muscles and tendon injuries in the shoulder region. Calif West Med 41:318-321, 1934.
273. Spritzer CE, Collins AJ, Cooperman A, and Speer KP: Assessment of instability of the long head of the biceps tendon by MRI. Skeletal Radiol 30:199-207, 2001.
274. Stanley E: Observations relative to the rupture of the tendon of the biceps at its attachment to the edge of the glenoid cavity. Med Gaz 3:12-14, 1828-1829.
275. Stanley E: Rupture of the tendon of the biceps at its attachment to the edge of the glenoid cavity. Med Gaz 3:12, 1829.
276. Steindler A: Interpretation of pain in the shoulder. AAOS Instructional Course Lecture. Ann Arbor, MI: JW Edwards, 1958, p 159.
277. Stevens HH: The action of short rotators on normal abduction of arm, with a consideration of their action on some cases of subacromial bursitis and allied conditions. Am J Med 138:870, 1909.
278. Takenaka R, Fukatsu A, Matsuo S, et al: Surgical treatment of hemodialysis-related shoulder arthropathy. Clin Nephrol 38:224-230, 1992.
279. Tarsy JM: Bicipital syndromes and their treatment. N Y State J Med 46:996-1001, 1946.
280. Thomazeau H, Gleyze P, Frank A, et al: Le débridement endoscopic des ruptures transfixantes de la coiffe des rotateurs: Étude rétrospective multicentrique de 283 cas a plus de 3 ans de recul. Rev Chir Orthop 86:136-142, 2000.
281. Ting A, Jobe FW, Barto P, et al: An EMG analysis of the lateral biceps in shoulders with rotator cuff tears. Paper presented at the Third Open Meeting of the Society of American Shoulder and Elbow Surgeons, 1987, California.
282. Treves F: Surgical Applied Anatomy. Philadelphia: HC Lea's Son & Co., 1883.
283. Tuckman GA: Abnormalities of the long head of the biceps tendon of the shoulder: MR imaging findings. Am J Radiol 163:1183-1188, 1994.
284. Ueberham K and Le Floch-Prigent P: Intertubercular sulcus of the humerus: Biometry and morphology of 100 dry bones. Surg Radiol Anat 20:351-354, 1998.
285. Valtonen EJ: Subacromial triamcinolone, hexacetonide and methylprednisolone injections in treatment of supraspinatus tendinitis. A comparative trial. Scand J Rheumatol Suppl 16:1-13, 1976.

286. Valtonen EJ: Double acting betamethasone (celestone chronodose) in the treatment of supraspinatus tendinitis: A comparison of subacromial and gluteal single injections with placebo. J Intern Med Res 6:463-467, 1978.
287. Vangsness CT Jr, Jorgenson SS, Watson T, and Johnson DL: The origin of the long head of the biceps from the scapula and glenoid labrum. J Bone Joint Surg Br 76:951-954, 1994.
288. van Leersum M and Schweitzer ME: Magnetic resonance imaging of the biceps complex. Magn Reson Imaging Clin N Am 1:77-86, 1993.
289. Veisman IA: Radiodiagnosis of subcutaneous ruptures of the biceps tendons. Ortop Traumatol Protez 31(7):25-29, 1970.
290. Verbrugge J, Claessens H, and Maex L: L'arthrographie de l'epaule. Acta Orthop Belg 3-4:289, 1956.
291. Vettivel S, Indrasingh I, Chandi G, and Chandi SM: Variations in the intertubercular sulcus of the humerus related to handedness. J Anat 180:321-326, 1992.
292. Vigerio GD and Keats TE: Localization of calcific deposits in the shoulder. AJR Am J Roentgenol 108:806-811, 1970.
293. Volkmann R: Luxationen der Muskeln und Sehnen. Billroth Pitha's Handb Allgemeinen Speciellen Chir 2:873, 1882.
294. Walch G: La pathologie de la longue portion du biceps. Conference d'enseignement de la SOFCOT, 1993, Paris.
295. Walch G: Synthese sur l'epidemiologie et l'ethiologie des ruptures de la coiffe des rotateurs. Journees Lyonnaise de l'Epaule. Lyon, France: 1993.
296. Walch G: Posterosuperior glenoid impingement. In Burkhead WZ Jr (ed): Rotator Cuff Disorders. Media, PA: Williams & Wilkins, 1996, pp 193-198.
297. Walch G, Boileau P, Noel E, and Donell ST: Impingement of the deep surface of the supraspinatus tendon on the posterosuperior glenoid rim: An anatomical study. J Shoulder Elbow Surg 1:238-245, 1992.
298. Walch G, Madonia G, Pozzi I, et al: Arthroscopic tenotomy of the long head of the biceps in rotator cuff ruptures. In Gazielly DF, Gleyze P, and Thomas T (eds): The Cuff. New York: Elsevier, 1998, pp 350-356.
299. Walch G, Nove-Josserand L, Boileau P, and Levigne C: Subluxations and dislocations of the tendon of the long head of the biceps. J Shoulder Elbow Surg 7:100-108, 1998.
300. Walch G, Nove-Josserand L, Levigne C, and Renaud E: Tears of the supraspinatus tendon with "hidden" lesions of the rotator interval. J Shoulder Elbow Surg 3:353-360, 1994.
301. Warner JJP and McMahon PJ: The role of the long head of the biceps brachii in superior stability of the glenohumeral joint. J Bone Joint Surg Am 77:336-372, 1995.
302. Warren RF: Lesions of the long head of the biceps tendon. Instr Course Lect 34:204-209, 1985.
303. Warren RF, Dines DM, Inglis AE, and Pavlos H: The coracoid impingement syndrome. Paper presented at the Second Meeting of the Society of American Shoulder and Elbow Surgeons, American Academy of Orthopaedic Surgery, February 19-20, 1986, New Orleans.
304. Weishaupt D, Zanetti M, Tanner A, et al: Lesions of the reflection pulley of the long biceps tendon: MR arthrographic findings. Invest Radiol 34:463-469, 1999.
305. Werner A, Mueller T, Boehm D, and Gohlke F: The stabilizing sling for the long head of the biceps tendon in the rotator cuff interval: A histoanatomic study. Am J Sports Med 28:28-31, 2000.
306. White JW: A case of supposed dislocation of the tendon of the long head of the biceps muscle. Am J Med Soc 87:17-57, 1884.
307. White RH, Paull DM, and Fleming KW: Rotator cuff tendinitis: Comparison of subacromial injection of a long acting corticosteroid versus oral indomethacin therapy. J Rheumatol 13:608-613, 1986.
308. Wiley AM and Older MW: Shoulder arthroscopy: Investigations with a fiberoptic instrument. Am J Sports Med 8:31-38, 1980.
309. Winterstein O: On the periarthritis humero-scapularis and on the rupture of the long biceps tendon. Arch Orthop Unfallchir 63:19-22, 1968.
310. Withrington RH, Girgis FL, and Seifert MH: A placebo-controlled trial of steroid injections in the treatment of supraspinatus tendinitis. Scand J Rheumatol 14:76-78, 1985.
311. Wolfgang GL: Surgical repair of tears of the rotator cuff of the shoulder. J Bone Joint Surg Am 56:14-26, 1974.
312. Yamaguchi K, Riew KD, Galatz LM, et al: Biceps function in normal and rotator cuff deficient shoulders: An electromyographic analysis. Orthop Trans 18:191, 1994.
313. Yamaguchi K, Riew KD, Galatz LM, et al: Biceps during shoulder motion. Clin Orthop 336:122-129, 1997.
314. Yeh L, Pedowitz R, Kwak S, et al: Intracapsular origin of the long head of the biceps tendon. Skeletal Radiol 2:178-181, 1999.
315. Yergason RM: Rupture of biceps. J Bone Joint Surg 13:160, 1931.
316. Zanetti M, Weishaupt D, Gerber C, and Hodler J: Tendinopathy and rupture of the tendon of the long head of the biceps brachii muscle: Evaluation with MR arthrography. AJR Am J Roentgenol 170:1557-1561, 1998.
317. Zimmerman JA, Arcand MA, Doane R, and Burkhead WZ Jr: Biomechanical evaluation of four different methods of biceps tenodesis.

CHAPTER 20

THE STIFF SHOULDER

Douglas T. Harryman II, M.D.,* and Mark D. Lazarus, M.D.

• • • •

Y ou slowly reach toward your alarm clock after yet another restless night. You use your all-too-familiar maneuver to contort your body to turn it off. After remembering to put your shirt on your painful sleeve first, your wife helps tuck it in. Thankfully, she also remembers to place the breakfast cereal on the bottom shelf, within your range. As you drive to work, the car in front of you suddenly stops. Instinctively, you grip the wheel and the sudden jolt results in a searing pain. Once at work, that guilty feeling returns as coworkers assist in many of your tasks. After work, you decline your son's offer for a game of catch because of your inability to throw. Feeling exhausted and irritated, you lie down early and await another sleep-deprived night. Such is a day in the life of a patient with a stiff and painful shoulder.

To attain the complete range of shoulder motion, four articulations and two bursal-lined interfaces of the shoulder girdle must have stable alignment, smooth articular and motion plane surfaces, and an absence of periarticular soft tissue contractures. The musculotendinous units that interconnect the bones and joints of the shoulder girdle must retain flexibility and freedom of excursion to fully mobilize the extremity through its entire arc of motion. When joint surfaces are normal, are stably aligned, and have no skeletal block, a restriction in range is classified as stiffness. Stiffness may result from pathologic connections between motion interfaces, contracture of periarticular soft tissues, shortened muscle-tendon unit excursion, or a combination of causes. When a person with shoulder stiffness seeks medical assistance from a practitioner, the challenge remains to determine the pathophysiology of the stiffness and, more importantly, the remedy.

CLASSIFICATION OF SHOULDER STIFFNESS

In 1923, Jones and Lovett distinguished two principal types of shoulder stiffness based on clinical examination.[159] In the latter half of the 20th century, five different investigators proposed a dichotomous nomenclature to classify clinical shoulder stiffness, each according to his own diagnostic criteria.[161,188,216,261,330] The two main

clinical themes lending themselves to subgroup typing were the severity of the stiffness and the presence or absence of an associated etiology. In their classification scheme, Reeves and Neviaser relied primarily on arthrographic criteria,[216,261] Kay and Withers divided stiffness according to the severity of restricted motion,[161,330] and Lundberg sought the etiology.[188]

A loosely woven common thread among these classifications is the presence or absence of trauma. Reeves used the subgrouping "idiopathic frozen shoulder" and "post-traumatic stiff shoulder" and related his arthrographic findings to the clinical descriptions provided by Jones and Lovett.[159,261] Lundberg based the definition of primary and secondary frozen shoulders on the presence or absence of a significant initiating traumatic event.[188] As Reeves and Matsen and associates have indicated, these categories of shoulder stiffness clearly have independent historical and clinical examination findings.[195,261]

Definition of Shoulder Stiffness

In the late 19th century, Duplay in France and, soon after, Putnam in North America described "scapulohumeral periarthritis," which encompassed a broad spectrum of pathologic conditions causing similar symptoms of painful shoulder stiffness and dysfunction.[88,256] Rotator cuff tendinitis and tears, biceps tendinitis or tears, calcific deposits, acromioclavicular arthritis, and other painful conditions causing shoulder stiffness were often combined together under the term "periarthritis." Unfortunately, this term is still in usage today and has become synonymous with a wide range of afflictions of the shoulder.[14,37,60,80,174,260,264,335,336] Because of the lack of specific diagnostic criteria and persistent confusion surrounding use of the term "periarthritis," some have recommended discarding it.[130,264]

In 1934, Codman recognized a pattern of muscle spasm and glenohumeral stiffness and coined the term "frozen shoulder."[65] He said that this entity was "difficult to define, difficult to treat and difficult to explain from the point of view of pathology." He also "presumed" that the symptoms were related to tendinitis of the rotator cuff. Although this term fails to describe the pathologic process, it does provide a great description of the clinical picture. Like "periarthritis," Codman's "frozen shoulder" terminology is also a general descriptive term referring to shoulders that are stiff and painful.[58,228,343]

In 1945, Neviaser proposed the term "adhesive capsulitis,"[213] which he believed better described the underlying pathology. Neviaser identified a "chronic inflammatory process involving the capsule of the shoulder causing a thickening and contracture of this structure which secondarily becomes adherent to the humeral head." Today, this term is often used synonymously with frozen shoulder and, unfortunately, is also commonly used as an incorrect synonym for stiffness occurring secondary to an inciting event.

Zuckerman polled members of the American Shoulder and Elbow Surgeons (ASES) to ensure the best consensus on the definition of frozen shoulder syndrome after having defined it summarily as "a condition of uncertain etiology characterized by significant restriction of both active and passive shoulder motion that occurs in the absence of a known intrinsic shoulder disorder." That definition was accepted by the workshop committee at the 1992 symposium "The Shoulder: A Balance of Mobility and Stability" and published by the American Academy of Orthopaedic Surgeons.[343]

Authors' Preferred Classification

Matsen and associates combined Codman's original clinical observation of global motion restriction, Reeves's consideration of the implication of the presence or absence of a significant traumatic event, and contemporary understanding of the findings present in a stiff shoulder and classified stiffness as either a "frozen shoulder" or a "post-traumatic stiff shoulder." A frozen shoulder is defined as having

An idiopathic global limitation of humeroscapular motion resulting from contracture and loss of compliance of the glenohumeral joint capsule.[195]

Although this definition is stated in one sentence, three important criteria are included within it:

1. Idiopathic—there should be no history of a significant traumatic event that preceded the onset.
2. Global limitation—motion is restricted in all directions.
3. Glenohumeral—the process is recognized as a capsular one.

To avoid the risk of introducing additional categories for shoulder stiffness, the authors have instead simply assigned stiff shoulders that are not idiopathic frozen shoulders to the "post-traumatic stiff shoulder" category. The authors define this group as having

A limitation in humeroscapular motion after an injury, low-level repetitive trauma, or part of an accompanying condition that results in a contracture of structures participating in the glenohumeral or humeroscapular motion interfaces.

As will be discussed later, the "post-traumatic" group easily can be subdivided according to the type of injury

(for instance, trauma or surgery) or disease process. This system also nicely corresponds to the distinction suggested by Lundberg in which stiffness is separated into "primary" and "secondary" frozen shoulder syndrome.[188] Lundberg's secondary frozen shoulders were defined as those with a known intrinsic or extrinsic precursor typically causative of shoulder pain and dysfunction that ultimately leads to global stiffness.

PATHOPHYSIOLOGY

Although the etiology of stiffness remains elusive, our understanding of its pathogenesis is increasing. Recent investigations have focused on the inflammatory cellular morphology and immunologic response, humoral mediators, and immunologic predisposition as possible initiators of the process that results in capsular fibrosis. Many plausible pathogenic mechanisms have been proposed during the last 60 years, yet none of the factors occasionally isolated and associated with the pathogenesis of frozen shoulder has been consistently found (Table 20–1).[141]

Early investigators localized the "freezing" of frozen shoulder to the interface of the rotator cuff and subacromial space, hence the term "periarthritis."[65,88,256] Little to no basic science supports involvement of this interface in the pathology of a primary frozen shoulder.

Riedel was the first to suggest that the basic pathology of shoulder stiffness may be localized to the joint capsule.[270] In 1945, Neviaser described the surgical, arthrographic, and histologic findings occurring in the synovium and subsynovial capsular regions of patients with painful shoulder stiffness.[213] On biopsy and histologic examination, he identified perivascular infiltration and capsular thickening, contracture, and fibrosis. He also identified a normal synovial layer.

Later in the same decade, Simmonds took biopsy samples of the hypervascular "tight inelastic tissue" around the joint and identified some focal necrosis that he attributed to tendon degeneration.[293] He postulated that this process led to chronic inflammation, especially around the biceps tendon, contracture, and tears of the rotator cuff.

Lundberg also did not find pathologic changes in the synovial cells lining the joint, but he identified an increase in the density of capsular collagen and a pattern of glycosaminoglycan distribution that he likened to a repair reaction.[188] These observations pointed to inflammation of the capsule as an essential precursor of the process leading to capsular fibrosis. McLaughlin, however, noted an "obvious inflammatory reaction involving the entire synovial lining of the shoulder joint and the biceps tendon sheath" in only 10% of his cases, and in the "great majority of cases neither clinical nor histologic evidences of inflammation were observed."[199] He concluded that perhaps "acute synovitis represents one phase in the life cycle of this condition."

Macnab studied the association between rotator cuff degeneration and painful stiffness.[190] At open capsular release and biopsy, he identified round and lymphoid cell infiltrates and attributed them to an autoimmune

TABLE 20-1. Proposed Pathogenic Mechanisms for Primary Frozen Shoulder

Mechanism	Disorder	Pathology	Etiology Excluded by
Autoimmune	Collagen-vascular disorders	Type IV reaction (to infarcted cuff tendon)	Absence of immune complexes and autoantibodies, no other affected joints
Inflammatory	Infectious arthritis	Viral, bacterial, or fungal infection	Absence of prodromal illness and systemic symptoms
Crystal arthropathy	CPPD disease and gout	Crystal deposition	Absence of recurrences, crystals, and inflammatory phases
Reactive arthropathy	Spondyloarthritides and ankylosing spondylitis	Seronegative arthritis	No systemic manifestations; normal joint fluid, no blood markers
Hemarthrosis	Hemoglobinopathies and trauma	Chemical irritation (hemosiderin)	No capsulitis or fibrositis with hemoglobinopathies
Paralytic	Suprascapular nerve palsy	Compression neuropathy	Absence of EMG or conduction abnormalities
Algodystrophy	Autonomic neuropathy	Neuropathic disturbance and hypervascularity	No sensory or vascular deficiency, stellate ganglion block not helpful
Degenerative	Rotator cuff tendon and degeneration/infarction	Microvascular infarction	Absence of tendon inflammation or infarction
Traumatic	Trauma and immobilization	Injury synovitis and tissue contracture	Brief shoulder stiffness after prolonged casting in the majority
Psychogenic	Hysteria and hypochondriasis	Depression, dependence, and chronic pain disorder	Similar MMPI between patients and controls
Fibrogenic	Cytokine induction of fibroplasia	Tissue contracture in response to cytokines, inflammatory cell products, and platelet-derived growth factor	No exclusion, current theory in text

CPPD, calcium pyrophosphate dihydrate; EMG, electromyogram; MMPI, Minnesota Multiphasic Personality Inventory.
From Harryman DT II: Shoulders: Frozen and stiff. Instr Course Lect 42:247–257, 1993.

response against degenerative collagen particles from a hypovascular supraspinatus tendon.

The inflammatory reaction histologically observed by Neviaser, Lundberg, and McLaughlin could represent a response to injury, an infectious agent, chemical mediation, or an autoimmune reaction with cellular and humoral components. In an attempt to find immunologic clues, a study of 40 patients with frozen shoulder was undertaken by Bulgen and colleagues. They found that pretreatment increased circulating immune complex levels and C-reactive protein and decreased lymphocyte transformation as a result of stimulation by phyto-hemagglutinin and concanavalin A relative to a control group.[44] The implications of these findings were impaired cell-mediated immunity and increased circulating immune complexes associated with an autoimmune process. Repeat testing after time and treatment showed that values tended to approach control levels. Bulgen and associates also analyzed serum immunoglobulin levels in 25 patients with frozen shoulder and age- and sex-matched controls.[46,48] Serum IgA levels were reduced significantly in patients with a frozen shoulder, and this decrease persisted after clinical recovery. Lymphocyte transformation in response to phytohemagglutinin in 21 patients also showed significant depression. Despite early findings that indicated the presence of an immunologic basis for the disease, recent reports have failed to support these findings or identify immunologic tests useful in diagnosis, treatment, or prediction of outcome.[338]

Investigation has also centered on identifying a predisposition to stiffness by the use of immunologic cellular markers. Initial research focused on the presence of certain histocompatibility antigens. For instance, the presence of HLA-B27 was reported as being more common in patients with frozen shoulder (42%) than in controls (10%).[47] This result, however, was later refuted by the same authors.[46] As with other diseases, identifying a predisposition may be resolved only after genotypic analysis.[1,309]

An association between clinical frozen shoulder and Dupuytren's contracture has been identified by multiple authors dating back to 1936.[296] These reports identify rates of association ranging from 18% to as high as 52%. More recent investigators likened the histologic changes in the glenohumeral capsule to Dupuytren's contracture in the palm and further noted that in the shoulder capsule, the inflammatory component was absent or localized to the synovial and subsynovial layers.[49,126] Bunker and Anthony performed manipulation and open excisional biopsy of the coracohumeral ligament and rotator interval capsule in patients who failed to improve with conservative treatment of frozen shoulder.[49] Tissue specimens revealed active fibroblastic proliferation amidst thick nodular bands of collagen accompanied by some transformation to a smooth muscle phenotype (myofibroblasts). These fibroblastic histologic features were very similar to those in Dupuytren's disease of the hand, with no inflammation and no synovial involvement. Fibrotic accumulation is most evident in later phases of the inflammatory response, with collagen and matrix synthesis taking place after chemotactic and cellular responses have occurred. These findings, therefore, may reflect only one phase of the disease.[199]

A proliferative pathologic repair by active fibroblasts occurs in response to inflammatory infiltration of connective tissue by mononuclear cells that produce polypeptide growth factors. Rodeo and associates compared capsular tissue samples from patients undergoing arthroscopy who had adhesive capsulitis, nonspecific synovitis, or a normal capsule to determine specific cytokines involved in the inflammatory and fibroblastic response.[277] Their results indicate that cytokines such as transforming growth factor-β (TGF-β), platelet-derived growth factor (PDGF), and hepatocyte growth factor (HGF) are involved in the early inflammatory stages of adhesive capsulitis. PDGF is a mitogenic agent that causes fibroblastic cell proliferation, and TGF-β increases extracellular matrix, both being potential precursors of capsular fibrosis. A more recent study by Suzuki and associates further demonstrated that specific growth factors stimulate capsular fibroblasts in a canine model. They found that PDGF-AB, HGF, and insulin-like growth factor type I all stimulated the migration of fibroblasts from three different parts of a canine shoulder model: the upper and lower parts of the medial glenohumeral ligament and the posterior capsule.[302]

In a related study, Hannafin and colleagues attempted to correlate the three histopathologic phases of fibroplasia detected in biopsy samples of shoulders with adhesive capsulitis with the clinical examination and arthroscopic findings in the capsule. They hypothesized that the hypervascular synovitis provokes a progressive fibroblastic response in the adjacent capsule that results in diffuse capsular fibroplasia, thickening, and contracture (Fig. 20–1).[126] Based on these immunohistochemical and histologic findings, these investigators proposed an algorithm of pathology leading to capsular fibrosis (Fig. 20–2). With the use of this model, they believe that investigators are poised to devise agents that may interrupt the cytokinetic connection and cellular-mediated response leading to capsular fibroplasia.

Matrix metalloproteinases (MMPs), a family of naturally occurring proteinases that control collagen matrix remodeling, have been implicated as a contributing factor in the pathogenesis of frozen shoulder.[51,152] Hutchinson and coworkers reported frozen shoulder developing in 12 patients after treatment with the MMP inhibitor marimastat for gastric carcinoma.[152] Bunker and colleagues examined capsular tissue from patients with frozen shoulder and Dupuytren's contracture and from normal individuals.[51] The tissue was analyzed for various factors, one of which was MMPs and their inhibitors. When compared with normal capsule or capsule derived from patients with Dupuytren's contracture, the capsule of patients with frozen shoulder demonstrated an increase in mRNA for MMPs, as well as a natural MMP inhibitor. These results suggest that abnormalities in MMP expression are a factor in frozen shoulder, although a causal relationship has not been established.

NORMAL MOTION AND PATHOMECHANICS OF SHOULDER STIFFNESS

What determines the functional limit of shoulder range? The answer depends on our skeletal morphology, our articular surface area, and the flexibility of the connecting capsule, ligaments, musculotendinous units, and integument. If a sphere were mapped about the shoulder to describe its range of motion, we could reach approximately a third of its inner surface with the tip of our elbow using humerothoracic range and a quarter using humeroscapular motion alone (Fig. 20–3). The sum of humerothoracic elevation is achieved from motion at two articulations in a ratio of glenohumeral-to-scapulothoracic range of approximately 2 : 1.[103,153,255]

Defined further, humerothoracic motion occurs between the articular surfaces of the glenohumeral ball-and-socket joint and two major bursal-lined surfaces defined as the humeroscapular motion interface (HSMI) and the scapulothoracic motion interface (STMI).[195] In a glenohumeral joint with smooth articular surfaces, clinical shoulder stiffness occurs as a result of (1) contractures shortening the length of the intra-articular capsule, ligaments, or muscle-tendon units; (2) adhesions along gliding surfaces such as the rotator cuff or biceps tendons;

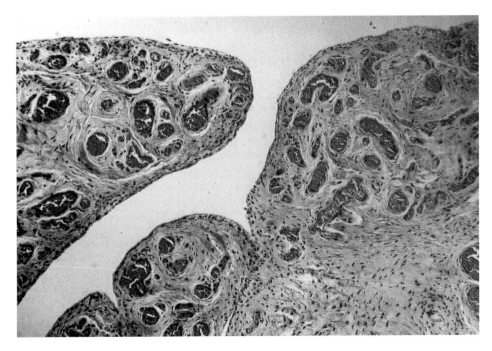

■ **Figure 20–1**

This capsular biopsy specimen shows proliferation of synovial cells at the surface with underlying capsular fibroplasia. The capsular matrix is densely collagenous. Evidence of neovascularization (red cell–filled capillaries) is present (hematoxylin and eosin stain, 40×). *(Courtesy of S. Rodeo, M.D.[277])*

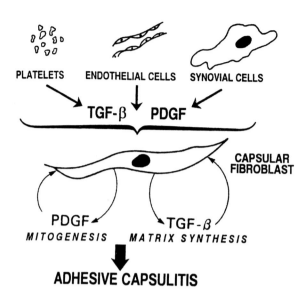

■ Figure 20–2

Theoretical algorithm leading to fibroplasia.[277] Transforming growth factor-β (TGF-β) and platelet-derived growth factor (PDGF), produced locally by synovial cells, platelets, and endothelial cells, stimulate capsular fibroblasts by a paracrine mechanism. Production of these cytokines by capsular fibroblasts, in the setting of upregulation of TGF-β and PDGF receptors on these capsular fibroblasts, suggests that an autocrine mechanism may amplify the paracrine stimulation of these cells. *(Courtesy of S. Rodeo, M.D.[277])*

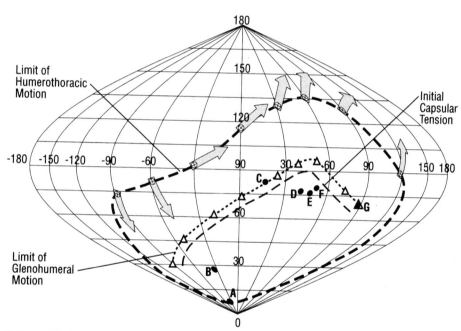

■ Figure 20–3

Global graphic diagram of shoulder motion. The *outer dashed line* is the limit of humerothoracic motion (in vivo glenohumeral plus scapulothoracic). The *dotted line* is the boundary of glenohumeral motion alone (in vivo after scapulothoracic fusion). The area between the *outer dashed line* and the *dotted line* represents the contribution of scapulothoracic motion. Inside the limit of glenohumeral motion is a *second dashed line*, which for lesser elevations without humeral rotation represents glenohumeral positions that do not result in capsular tension. *(Modified from Harryman DT II, Lazarus MD, Sidles JA, and Matsen FA III: Pathophysiology of shoulder instability. In McGinty JB, Caspari RB, Jackson RW, and Poehling GG [eds]: Operative Arthroscopy, 2nd ed. Philadelphia: Lippincott-Raven, 1996, p 680.)*

Points A, B, C, D, E, and F represent glenohumeral positions for routine daily activities. Three of these positions—lifting a gallon overhead (C), washing the opposite shoulder (F), and hand behind the head (maximal rotation in mid-elevation) (B)—are performed at the end range of glenohumeral motion; otherwise, most activities are recorded in the functional midrange.

Point A, scratching the back; point B, tucking in a shirt; point C, hand behind the head; point D, lifting a gallon to the top of the head; point E, placing a coin on the shelf at shoulder height; point F, hand to mouth; point G, washing the back of the opposite shoulder.

and (3) adhesions within the extra-articular HSMI or STMI.[195] Restrictions of these soft tissues may occur independently or in combination.

Glenohumeral Joint, Capsule, and Ligaments

The glenohumeral articular capsule remains lax while performing motions in the midrange. In cadaveric tests, Harryman and associates measured torsional resistance of the glenohumeral joint with an intact capsule and a cuff tendon preparation.[132] In the midrange of glenohumeral motion, the capsular tissue remained essentially free of tension until the terminal degrees of range were approached (Fig. 20-4). The end range, therefore, was defined by increased tension in the static restraints of the capsule and its ligaments. The majority of motions performed during work and activities of daily living are carried out in humeroscapular positions away from the extremes of range (see Fig. 20-3).[136,246]

Glenohumeral motion is limited by the length of the capsuloligamentous checkreins. In a biomechanical study of eight intact cadaveric shoulders, Moskal and colleagues measured the range of glenohumeral positions in which the capsular structures were "tension free."[206] Tension free was defined in the cadaver as the range of glenohumeral rotation exerting less than 0.5 N-m of humeral torque with an intact capsule (see Fig. 20-4). Complete capsular division circumferentially about the glenoid increased the limits of tension-free elevation and internal and external rotation. Forward elevation increased by an average of 15% in all planes tested. External rotation increased 22% in posterior planes but only 9% in anterior planes. Nonarticular abutment did not result from increased over-rotation. Only a moderate increase in motion occurred after capsular division, presumably because the excursion of the rotator cuff tendons restrained glenohumeral rotation (Fig. 20-5). Conversely, the capsule and its ligaments would appear to protect the rotator cuff tendons from excessive tensile loads at the extremes of rotation because they limit motion to a smaller arc.

A contracted capsule reduces glenohumeral rotational motion.[132] In a cadaveric study, eight shoulders underwent posterior capsular plication. The ranges of forward elevation, internal rotation, and horizontal adduction became limited. The motions of external rotation with and without elevation, abduction, and adduction remained unaffected. Furthermore, tightening of the capsule increased the torque necessary to achieve an elevated position (see Fig. 20-4).[132] Release of the tight capsule would be predicted to relieve this condition. The concept of releasing localized or generalized capsular contractures to increase range is not new and has been used clinically at open surgery for decades.[166,195,199,212,224]

A released capsule increases joint laxity, but increased laxity does not lead to instability. In the cadaver shoulder, Moskal and colleagues found anterior, posterior, and inferior translational laxity of the humeral head to be increased an average of 15 mm in each direction after complete capsular release.[195,206] Clinical and experimental data have shown that releasing or surgically tightening the rotator interval capsule increases or decreases posterior and inferior translational laxity, respectively (Fig. 20-6).[133,319] Lippitt and associates and Lazarus and colleagues have shown that the humeral head, which is stabilized within the glenoid concavity by compressive loads and resistance to a displacing force, is augmented by increased depth and the presence of the glenoid labrum and thickened peripheral glenoid cartilage.[175,184] Releasing the capsule and its ligaments in vivo should therefore increase laxity but not lead to instability.

Specific regions of the glenohumeral joint capsule and their identified ligaments are responsible for limiting end range rotations (Table 20-2). Early investigators found that the anterior capsular ligaments tighten at maximal external rotation. The anterosuperior capsule in the rotator interval contains the coracohumeral ligament and superior glenohumeral ligament and assumes tension with humeral external rotation in the unelevated extremity.[100,133,319] The middle glenohumeral ligament and the anterosuperior band of the inferior glenohumeral ligament become taut with maximal external rotation in midrange and full abduction, respectively.[305,311] The inferior capsular sling becomes taut in full humeral elevation, with tension shifting in orientation along the cruciate lines (anterior and posterior) with external and internal rotation, respectively.[226,319] The posterosuperior capsule

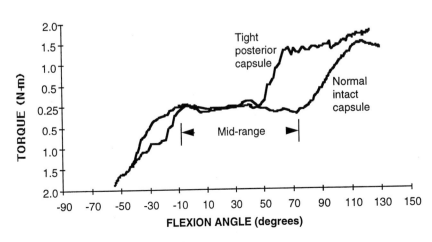

■ **Figure 20-4**

In the midrange of glenohumeral motion, the capsule and ligaments are not under tension. As the humerus is elevated (e.g., extreme flexion or extension), the cuff and capsule become tight near the end range of motion, where capsular torsion increases for each incremental degree of elevation. Torsional loads become increased only in the midrange of motion when a portion of the capsule is tight. *(Modified from Harryman DT II, Lazarus MD, Sidles JA, and Matsen FA III: Pathophysiology of shoulder instability. In McGinty JB, Caspari RB, Jackson RW, and Poehling GG [eds]: Operative Arthroscopy, 2nd ed. Philadelphia: Lippincott-Raven, 1996, p 679.)*

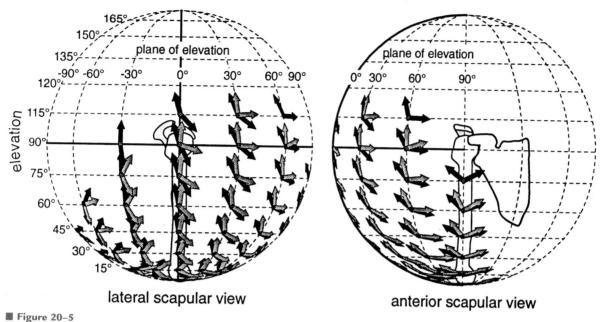

■ Figure 20–5

Global diagrams graphically summarizing the mean rotational data measured from eight cadaveric shoulders before and after capsular release. An increase in the motions of rotation and elevation before *(gray arrows)* and after *(black arrows)* total capsular release are depicted. Even after capsular release, only an average of approximately 20 degrees of gain in motion occurs, thus indicating that other soft tissue such as the intact rotator cuff secondarily restrains glenohumeral motion. *(From Harryman DT II, Sidles JA, and Matsen FA III: Arthroscopic management of refractory shoulder stiffness. Arthroscopy 13:133-147, 1997.)*

TABLE 20–2. Capsule and Ligaments Limiting Glenohumeral Motions

Capsule and Ligaments	Glenohumeral Motions
Rotator interval capsule (RIC) Coracohumeral ligament (CHL) Superior glenohumeral ligament (SGHL)	Flexion, extension, adduction at low elevation, external rotation at low elevation
Middle glenohumeral ligament (MGHL)	External rotation at mid elevation
Inferior glenohumeral ligament (IGHL)	External rotation at high elevation
Inferior capsular sling (ICS)	Abduction and high elevation
Posteroinferior glenohumeral ligament (PIGHL)	Internal rotation at high elevation
Posterosuperior capsule (PSC)	Internal rotation at low elevation

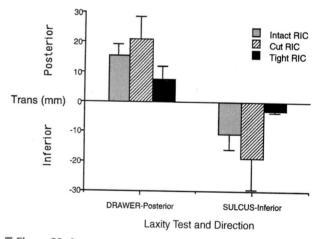

■ Figure 20–6

A tight rotator interval capsule (RIC) restricts normal joint laxity. Release of the RIC will increase translation and range in tight shoulders (see text). *(From Harryman DT II, Lazarus MD, Sidles JA, and Matsen FA III: Pathophysiology of shoulder instability. In McGinty JB, Caspari RB, Jackson RW, and Poehling GG [eds]: Operative Arthroscopy, 2nd ed. Philadelphia: Lippincott-Raven, 1996, p 687.)*

becomes taut with internal rotation at the side, and tension is shifted inferiorly to the posteroinferior capsule with increasing angles of elevation.[132,195]

A contracture of any given portion of the capsule will restrict range as though the end range constraint were invoked prematurely (see Fig. 20–4). Pathologic contractures of isolated regions of the capsule have been identified[129,135,212,228,239,307] or intentionally created, as with some instability procedures. Asymmetric tightness of the capsule may cause obligate pathologic translation of the humeral head.[133,195] Anatomically, a normal glenohumeral joint displays true ball-and-socket mechanics, with the humeral head remaining centered within the glenoid fossa throughout its midrange.[134,255] In the cadaver, however, when the posterior capsule was surgically tight-ened, forward flexion caused consistent anterosuperior translation of the humeral head.[132] A posterior capsular contracture, therefore, may cause significant "impingement" with compression of the rotator cuff against the coracoacromial arch (Fig. 20–7). Clinically, a similar pathomechanical phenomenon (also called "capsular constraint") can occur in shoulders after excessively tight anterior instability repairs (Fig. 20–8). Chronic asymmetric tightness can result in greater joint reaction forces directed to the opposite side of the glenoid and can cause excessive wear, posterior erosion, and osteoarthrosis.[139]

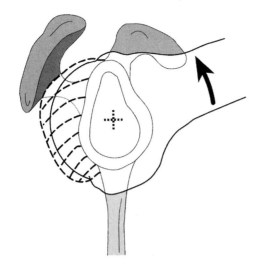

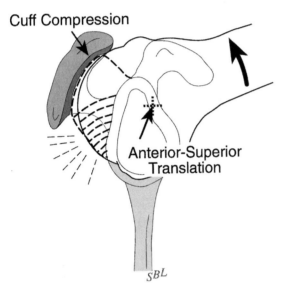

Cuff Compression

Anterior-Superior Translation

SBL

■ **Figure 20–7**

Tightness of the posterior capsular region causes anterosuperior translation of the humeral head. The rotator cuff becomes entrapped between the humeral head and the coracoacromial arch. A posterior capsular contracture may therefore initiate or potentiate subacromial compression and abrasion of the rotator cuff. *(Modified from Matsen FA III, Lippitt SB, Sidles JA, and Harryman DT II: Practical Evaluation and Management of the Shoulder. Philadelphia: WB Saunders, 1994, pp 19-109.)*

Matsen and colleagues have called this pathologic process *capsulorrhaphy arthropathy*.[195] To eliminate clinical pathologic restrictions, authors have advocated specific open or arthroscopic surgical release of the contracted capsule and ligaments.*

Humeroscapular Motion Interface

In 1934, Codman stated that "The subacromial bursa itself is the largest in the body and the most complicated in structure and in its component parts. It is in fact, a secondary scapulohumeral joint, although no part of its

*See references 135, 166, 195, 212, 228, 239, 254, 286, 307, 318.

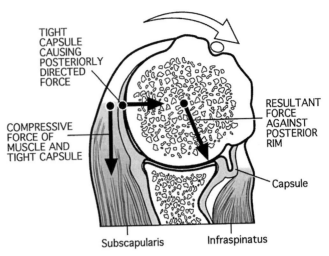

■ **Figure 20–8**

Rotation of the humeral head is associated with capsular tightening at the end range of motion. The asymmetrically tight capsule opposes a load or displacement directed toward itself and attempts to translate the humeral head toward the opposite side of the glenoid. This stabilizing force is referred to as the "capsular constraint mechanism." The tense capsule also applies a load to compress the humeral head into the glenoid fossa. The resultant force vector is directed against the opposite side of the glenoid. *(From Harryman DT II, Lazarus MD, Sidles JA, and Matsen FA III: Pathophysiology of shoulder instability. In McGinty JB, Caspari RB, Jackson RW, and Poehling GG [eds]: Operative Arthroscopy, 2nd ed. Philadelphia: Lippincott-Raven, 1996, p 686.)*

surface is cartilage."[65] He also believed that the roughly hemispheric shape of the coracoacromial arch was "almost a counterpart in size and curvature of the articular surface of the true joint." Matsen and Romeo have extended Codman's auxiliary joint concept and defined the HSMI as a sliding surface between the deep side of the deltoid, the acromion, and the coracoid process and its tendons and the superficial side of the humerus, rotator cuff, and long head of the biceps tendon and its sheath (Fig. 20–9).[195,278] If pathologic conditions such as adhesions secondary to trauma or surgery spot-weld across or obliterate the HSMI, shoulder motion will be limited.

Romeo and associates measured humeroscapular motion in vivo in five normal shoulders.[278] The relative motion between the proximal end of the humerus and the deltoid, coracoid, and its tendons was determined from serial axial magnetic resonance imaging (MRI) views in sequential increments over the full range of external to internal rotation. The maximal average interfascial sliding motion approached 3 cm (29.1 mm) and occurred at the level of the widest axial section of the humeral head. Interfascial motion varied with the site measured until no relative motion was present distally at the level of the deltoid tuberosity.

In clinical practice, humeroscapular stiffness after trauma, immobilization, or surgery is partly related to adhesions within the HSMI.[195] At repeat surgery, dense adhesions have been identified between the acromion and the bursal surface after rotator cuff repair and under the coracoid, conjoined tendon, and deltoid after anterior instability repair. Attempts to restore normal interfacial sliding motion after a surgical repair of the rotator cuff is difficult when shoulder stiffness is secondary to adhesions in the HSMI.[112]

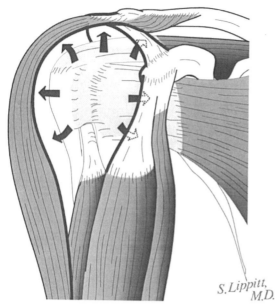

■ **Figure 20–9**

The humeroscapular motion interface is an important continuum of interfacial sliding surfaces, including the deep sides of the deltoid, the acromion, and the coracoid process and its tendons and the superficial side of the humerus, rotator cuff, long head of the biceps tendon, and its sheath. *(Modified from Matsen FA III, Lippitt SB, Sidles JA, and Harryman DT II: Practical Evaluation and Management of the Shoulder. Philadelphia: WB Saunders, 1994, pp 19-109.)*

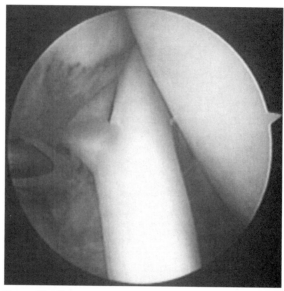

■ **Figure 20–10**

Arthroscopic glenohumeral joint view showing an intra-articular adhesion binding the biceps tendon to the contracted rotator interval. *(From Harryman DT II: Shoulders: Frozen and stiff. Instr Course Lect 42:247-257, 1993.)*

The long head of the biceps tendon is unique in position about the shoulder. The root of the biceps is a structural extension of the glenohumeral articular surface and forms part of the glenohumeral articular motion surface. Like a monorail system, the humeral head and its bicipital tendon groove move along the tendon, and normal biceps glide is necessary for full glenohumeral range. All glenohumeral motion is accompanied by gliding or rotation of the bicipital groove on the surface of the biceps tendon. If synovitis is present within the glenohumeral joint or tendon sheath, adhesions can spot-weld the long head of the biceps tendon to the cuff, capsule, or groove (Fig. 20–10).[129,135,228] Pasteur in 1932, followed by Lippman, Neviaser, Hitchcock and Bechtol, and DePalma, reported peritendinous adhesions that caused a variable degree of impairment in motion of the tendon within its groove in patients with frozen shoulder.[81,145,185,213,243] They recommended either lysis of adhesions or excision of the biceps to restore motion.

Unrestricted humeral motion along the biceps tendon is essential to maintain the full range of glenohumeral motion. If this monorail assemblage is blocked, the range of glenohumeral motion will be limited.[195] Basta and colleagues used a mathematical model and a cadaveric shoulder instrumented with a 6-degree-of-freedom spatial sensor to experimentally verify the effect of limited biceps tendon excursion on glenohumeral motion.[15] They found that the bicipital groove translated 50 mm along the biceps tendon with maximal intra-articular tendon length in external rotation and minimal intra-articular tendon length in maximal elevation.

Adhesion or tenodesis of the biceps tendon in situ within the bicipital groove after injury, inflammation, or surgical incorporation could potentially limit maximal recovery of significant useful glenohumeral motion. Basta and coworkers performed tenodesis of the biceps tendon in situ at three different angles of humeral rotation. Positions of tenodesis with increasing internal rotation demonstrated greater restriction in motion (Fig. 20–11).

Scapulothoracic Motion

Studying the contribution of scapulothoracic motion to total humerothoracic motion has proved difficult. Much of this difficulty lies in accurately tracking the scapula. Past investigators determined that scapulothoracic motion is responsible for approximately a third of humerothoracic elevation (see Fig. 20–3).[103,153] Poppen and Walker defined scapular motion according to the radiographic position of the glenoid, but such a definition of motion has limited usefulness for clinical examination.[255] Pearl and colleagues designed a hand-held scapula locator to help determine the scapular plane, position, and motion of the shoulder.[247] Harryman and associates pinned electromagnetic sensors to the scapula and humerus in eight volunteers and recorded humerothoracic, scapulothoracic, and glenohumeral motion.[134] Scapular spine motion was described relative to the thoracic anatomic axes in terms of the plane of elevation, angle of elevation, and angle of rotation. The limits of scapulothoracic motion were determined: maximal scapulothoracic elevation was 56 ± 8 degrees, the plane of maximal scapular elevation was 59 ± 10 degrees forward of the coronal plane (about 30 degrees forward of the nominal "plane of the scapula" determined radiographically), and the plane of scapular motion varied widely, with a range from +83 degrees (flexion) to −95 degrees (extension) for low angles. They also found that scapular

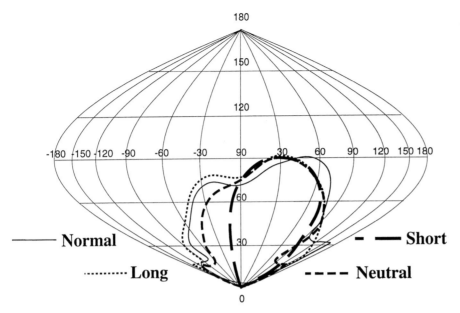

■ **Figure 20–11**
Tethering the intact long head of the biceps restricts glenohumeral motion. This global diagram shows the maximal limit of normal scapulohumeral motion in elevation and plane (humerus in maximal internal humeral rotation). The relative limits in plane and elevation for each in situ tenodesis preparation (short, neutral, long intra-articular biceps length) are exposed for comparative examination against a normal, nontenodesis preparation.

motion was constantly realigned on the thorax in response to load transfer from the torso to the extremity and vice versa (Fig. 20-12).

Recent evidence points to the complexity of scapulothoracic motion. In an in vivo study, McClure and colleagues measured active and passive scapulothoracic arcs in normal volunteers.[197] They used a direct measurement technique to illustrate the three-dimensional motion of the scapula during dynamic arm motions. During active scapular plane elevation of the arm, the scapula is upwardly rotated (50 ± 4.8 degrees), tilted posteriorly around a medial lateral axis (30 ± 15.0 degrees), and externally rotated around a vertical axis (24 ± 12.8 degrees). Reversal of these motions in a slightly different pattern occurs during lowering of the arm.

Because loss of glenohumeral range (e.g., after shoulder fusion) can result in an accommodative increase in scapulothoracic range,[136] we would also predict that a contracture in the scapulothoracic musculature or a loss of scapulothoracic motion (e.g., after scapulothoracic fusion) may demand greater range from the glenohumeral joint. Although it is a challenge to clinically measure scapulothoracic motion accurately, Nicholson recorded excessive scapular upward rotation (elevation) during active attempts at humeral elevation in patients with frozen shoulder.[223]

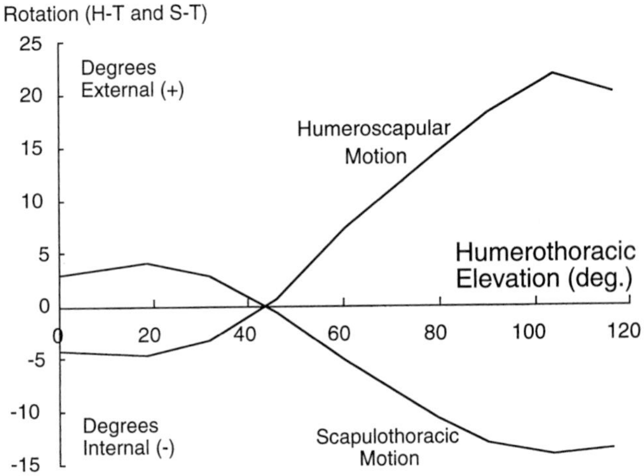

DIAGNOSTIC CRITERIA

A frozen shoulder, or primary stiffness, implies a glenohumeral contracture that occurs after minimal or no trauma and arises as a fibrotic process intrinsic to the glenohumeral joint capsule. A post-traumatic stiff shoulder, or secondary stiffness, is an extrinsic process that requires initiation from a traumatic precursor or other condition. Each of these diagnoses appear to have a different underlying pathology, history, and treatment. In addition, they may not be mutually exclusive. Although a post-traumatic stiff shoulder may originate as an

Rotation (H-T and S-T)

■ **Figure 20–12**
Graphic data from a subject with the transmitter fixed to the thorax and the magnetic field oriented to the anatomic axes. Spatial motion sensors were pinned to the scapula and humerus for tracking motion in three dimensions. The data show that glenohumeral and scapulothoracic motion is in constant balance, presumably to maintain maximal efficiency in transfer of load from the extremity to the torso and vice versa.

extracapsular process, subsequent capsular contracture may soon develop. Alternatively, on rare occasion, inflammation and adhesions have been identified in the subacromial bursa in association with idiopathic frozen shoulder.[129]

Idiopathic Frozen Shoulder

The lack of consensus regarding nomenclature and classification has in part originated from the confusion surrounding the necessary and sufficient diagnostic criteria for frozen shoulder. Many authors have suggested criteria that often refer to guidelines of measured range. These motion arcs have been defined in terms of

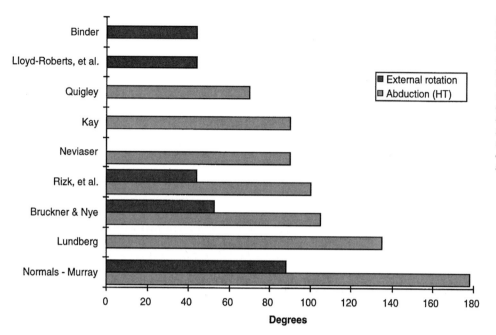

■ **Figure 20–13**
Investigators have recommended specific thresholds of limited motion to diagnose frozen shoulder. The most frequent motion criteria have been set according to abduction in the coronal plane or the degree of external rotation (all motions adjusted to humerothoracic [HT] range relative to normal controls defined by Murray and associates[209]).

humerothoracic planes of elevation (coronal abduction or sagittal flexion) and humeroscapular arcs of rotation (internal and external rotation). Traditional measurements assess humerothoracic motion between the arm and the thorax along anatomic axes, and some have attempted to isolate glenohumeral motion while stabilizing the scapulothoracic articulation to exclude motion.

On review of the literature, we might easily conclude that a restricted motion of approximately 50% is a reasonable mean among investigators who cite humerothoracic or scapulohumeral motion criteria for diagnosis.* Various authors have included a given set of diagnostic criteria for frozen shoulder (Fig. 20–13). These criteria lead to some confusion because the percent loss in range is clearly a measure of severity. Some authors define restrictive motion in a single motion arc and others in multiple planes. For example, Neviaser, Kay, Binder and associates, and Lloyd-Roberts and French included criteria that described, on average, a 50% limitation relative to normal in abduction or external rotation.[25,161,186,216,217] In contrast, Rizk and Pinals set four motion criteria, including combined abduction, forward elevation, and external and internal rotation, with relative percentages of normal ranging from 55% to 80%.[275]

Because motion restrictions are typically isolated to the scapulohumeral articulation, precise quantification of glenohumeral range should be attempted. Pearl and coauthors[248] suggested elevating the humerus in the scapular plane 45 degrees to assume the midpoint of joint motion and capsular laxity and from there performing maximal external and internal rotation to assess the degree of restricted motion isolated to the glenohumeral joint (Fig. 20–14). An arc of rotation restricted to less than 50% correlated significantly with a frozen shoulder. The present authors have not attempted to define a specific threshold for measured ranges but instead rely on histor-

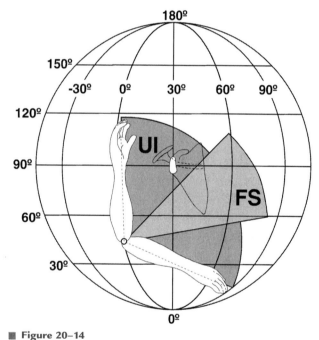

■ **Figure 20–14**
Global diagram showing humeral elevation of 45 degrees in the plane of the scapula (30-degree humerothoracic plane). The *shaded* rotational range measures the uninvolved (UI) side against the affected side limited by a frozen shoulder (FS). *(Courtesy of M. Pearl, M.D.[248])*

ical information, examination of patterns of motion restriction relative to the normal shoulder, and radiographic criteria. Similar to others,[45,178] we have combined multiple measured ranges of standard motion mathematically into a composite ratio to allow meaningful comparisons between groups of patients (see "Examination").

Other descriptive criteria have been deemed essential to diagnose a frozen shoulder. Kessel's criteria were unique in that no threshold of limited range was specified; instead, they required symptoms of spontaneous onset

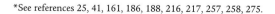

*See references 25, 41, 161, 186, 188, 216, 217, 257, 258, 275.

with progressive loss of glenohumeral motion, no identifiable associated illness, and normal radiographs.[164] Bruckner and Nye as well as Lloyd-Roberts and French included symptomatic night pain for a duration of 1 and 3 months, respectively.[41,186] Neviaser's criteria demand an ancillary arthrogram in addition to historic and clinical findings.

Our necessary and sufficient diagnostic criteria[195] for an idiopathic frozen shoulder embody some features similar to those described by Kessel[164] and include

1. A history of restricted shoulder motion without previous major injury or reconstructive surgery
2. An examination demonstrating global stiffness (i.e., restricted motion in all directions not accompanied by loss of strength, stability, or joint smoothness)
3. Plain radiographs with normal cartilaginous joint space and no focal periarticular abnormalities (osteopenia may be seen)

If uniform criteria such as these are applied to define an idiopathic frozen shoulder, other investigators can correctly differentiate clinical entities grouped under the general guise of "scapulohumeral periarthritis," "frozen shoulder," or "adhesive capsulitis."

Post-traumatic Stiff Shoulder

The earliest description of shoulder stiffness occurring after trauma was recorded by Malgaigne, who wrote in regard to minor nondisplaced extracapsular fractures about the shoulder.[88] In 1859 he said,

> . . . there remains long afterwards a stiffness, and a difficulty in moving the shoulder; and however great care may be taken, the motion of elevation of the arm will always remain limited; at least I have in no case seen it perfectly restored, even after the lapse of from eleven to fifteen months.

Reeves coined the term the *post-traumatic stiff shoulder* and referred to the clinical features described by Robert Jones and Lovett in 1923.[159,261]

Less controversy and confusion surround the nomenclature of this clinical entity; however, some investigators, such as Neviaser and Neviaser, have introduced an alternative classification.[219] They included stiffness that originated from trauma but was not associated with capsular contracture under the heading "the stiff and painful shoulder." Other classification alternatives, such as Kay's "early capsulitis" and Withers's "irritative capsulitis," border on being related to a post-traumatic stiff shoulder by virtue of less severe restrictions in motion, but they clearly were not defined for association with trauma.[161,330] Finally, the division of secondary frozen shoulders described by Lundberg includes all manifestations of post-traumatic stiff shoulders.[188]

Some shoulder stiffness is typical after intrinsic injuries to the soft tissues or articulations surrounding the shoulder. Restriction in shoulder motion has been reported after simple contusions, glenohumeral subluxations, dislocations, fracture-dislocations, acromioclavicular joint injury, clavicular and scapular fractures, and especially subcapital fractures of the humerus in the elderly.[71,116] Partial restrictions in motion may also occur in association with soft tissue injury.

Reports of partial motion loss in specific patterns are more frequent in the recent literature. These patterns are most often seen post-traumatically, usually after low-level, repetitive trauma. Neer recognized an asymmetric manifestation associated with repetitive injury that he called "impingement syndrome" and encouraged therapeutic stretching in forward elevation, internal rotation, and cross-body adduction.[210] Thomas and associates reported three cases with atraumatically induced stiffness in forward flexion and internal rotation, yet the inferior recess and joint capacity on arthrography was normal, and no specific lesion was identified at arthroscopy.[306] Ticker and coauthors reported the findings of nine patients who had painful stiffness and a discrete loss of forward elevation and internal rotation in abduction. At arthroscopy, these patients were found to have a thickened posterior capsule.[307] In a recent review of the senior author's first 30 patients from an ongoing prospective study of refractory shoulder stiffness, 11 experienced partial restriction in motion that was attributed to a posterior capsular contracture.[135] In each of these patients, an associated pathologic process was identified, with seven having a partial-thickness rotator cuff tear. In a review of 90 patients who eventually underwent surgical capsular release, the initial degree of stiffness after an injury (60 shoulders), as opposed to those with an idiopathic onset (30 shoulders), was significantly less for the motions of flexion, external rotation at the side, and external and internal rotation in 90 degrees of abduction (Table 20–3).[130]

Surgical procedures are widely recognized as a cause of shoulder stiffness. Anterior or posterior capsulorrhaphy, inferior capsular shift, and rotator cuff repairs are typical examples of iatrogenic tightening of the glenohumeral capsule that produce predictable limitations in motion. Occasionally, this restricted motion can lead to pathologic changes in the glenohumeral joint.[139] Repair of a defect in the supraspinatus or infraspinatus tendon often limits motions such as internal rotation and cross-body adduction.[195,344] Major trauma requiring surgery to repair soft tissue tears or reconstruction of the proximal end of the humerus often results in combined intra-articular and extra-articular adhesions.[110] Bush and Hansen advocated incorporating the intact biceps tendon into rotator cuff

TABLE 20–3. Comparative Motion Ranges of Frozen and Post-traumatic Stiff Shoulders (*N* = 117)

Motions	Noninjured (49)	Injured (68)	ANOVA Dunn
FE	104 ± 20	118 ± 30	P = .007
ERS	13 ± 20	32 ± 25	P < .0001
ERA	37 ± 24	56 ± 29	P = .0004
IRA	12 ± 18	32 ± 19	P < .0001
IRB	6 ± 3	6 ± 3	NSD
XBA	25 ± 7	24 ± 8	NSD

FE, forward elevation; ERS, external rotation at side; ERA, external rotation in abduction; IRA, internal rotation in abduction; IRB, internal rotation up the back; XBA, cross-body adduction; NSD, no significant difference.

reconstructions, which would have the potential to cause motion restriction.[53,127] The degree of stiffness and the direction of limited range may reflect the presence of adhesions in the extra-articular HSMI, contractures in musculotendinous units, and fibrosis of the articular capsule.

Our necessary and sufficient diagnostic criteria[195] for a post-traumatic stiff shoulder (or postsurgical) include

1. A history of injury, repetitive low-level trauma, or surgery with an onset of stiffness that functionally restricts use of the extremity
2. An examination with limited shoulder motion in a specific direction, multiple directions, or globally
3. Radiographs with a normal cartilaginous joint space

In shoulders that become symptomatic after an injury, pronounced restrictions in shoulder motion may occur asymmetrically or globally. Although the history, examination, and management of a post-traumatic stiff shoulder may be different from that of an idiopathic frozen shoulder, the long-term symptoms of post-traumatic stiffness and their progression may not be appreciably different. Motion loss in isolated directions may progress to global limitation in motion, depending on the severity of the injury or the length of disability. We are unaware whether stiffness of this type recovers without intervention or whether a loss in range becomes accepted by adaptation.

Although a post-traumatic stiff shoulder may have less homogeneity than an idiopathic frozen shoulder with regard to a historical mechanism or severity, the recommended diagnostic criteria are easily applied to both categories at all levels of expertise and do not require special ancillary tests. Additional specific diagnostic criteria for study of certain post-traumatic subgroups, such as a posterior capsular contracture or postsurgical stiff shoulder, are easily formulated. It is worthwhile recognizing that almost all cases of shoulder stiffness fit the basic criteria described and that wide application would allow meaningful comparison for prospective evaluation and treatment.

EPIDEMIOLOGY

To determine the exact incidence of a specific type of shoulder stiffness in the general population, investigators must prospectively define the entity with specific diagnostic criteria and establish age- and sex-matched controls.[45] Small but significant differences in measured shoulder range have been established for adults in early and later age groups.[63,209] Clarke and associates found slightly greater shoulder range for women than for men,[63] but data from Murray and coworkers neither confirmed this finding nor noted differences in side or dominance.[209]

Studies with stringent diagnostic criteria for frozen shoulder have defined the incidence of frozen shoulder in the general population as slightly greater than 2%. Reliable data were collected by Lundberg, who sampled a local hospital patient population, and by Bridgman, who reviewed 600 outpatients.[37,188] Pal and associates found a 5% incidence and Sattar and Luqman detected a 3% incidence of clinical signs and symptoms of frozen shoulder in 75 and 100 nonpatient controls, respectively.[240,285] In a study that included 100 geriatric inpatients, Chard and Hazleman found a 3% prevalence of painful stiff shoulder.[59] An accurate incidence of idiopathic frozen and post-traumatic stiff shoulder in a cross-section of a specified general population has yet to be determined.

FACTORS THAT PREDISPOSE THE SHOULDER TO STIFFNESS

Age Prevalence

The bulk of adults who seek care for a stiff shoulder, whether idiopathic or post-traumatic in origin, are generally between 40 and 60 years of age (Fig. 20–15).[41,128,195,208,263] It is unusual for an idiopathic frozen shoulder to develop in patients younger than 40 years unless insulin-dependent diabetes has been present since childhood. In a large study, Lundberg noted a slightly

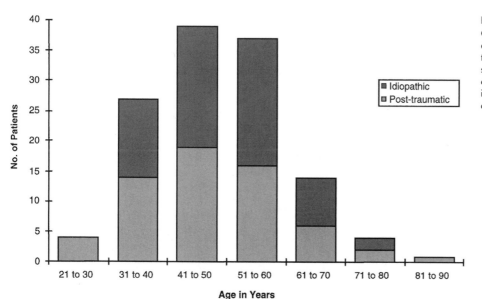

■ **Figure 20–15**

Graph depicting the age at initial evaluation for 126 patients with a frozen[64] or post-traumatic stiff shoulder[62] as defined by our diagnostic criteria.[195] No differences were found in the mean age between these two diagnoses.

higher mean age for men (55) than women (52).[188] A difference in age according to sex or type of stiffness, however, has not been evident in the senior author's series of 126 patients with refractory shoulder stiffness.[130] Our mean age was 50 years for both diabetic and nondiabetic patients and 50 years for either sex. The mean age of patients with the post-traumatic and idiopathic subclassifications was 49 and 50 years, respectively.

Injuries

Many patients in whom "idiopathic" shoulder stiffness develops can associate a minor traumatic incident contemporary with the onset of symptoms.[65,84,198] Of course, the distinct trauma of a fracture, rotator cuff tear, or surgical procedure, for example, is easily documented and classified within the post-traumatic category.

In a significant number of patients who have painful stiffness after a rotator cuff strain or a repetitive overuse injury, "impingement syndrome" is often diagnosed. On closer inspection, the history and physical examination of these patients typically fit within the post-traumatic classification, and these patients are suffering from a contracture of the posterior capsule.[129,132,135,195,307]

Non-shoulder Surgery

Although stiffness after shoulder surgery is expected and typically addressed after surgical procedures performed in the vicinity of the shoulder girdle, postoperative therapy to recover motion may be neglected or resisted by a patient who undergoes other types of surgery. Common examples include axillary node and cervical neck dissection, both of which are known causes of impaired shoulder motion postoperatively, especially when combined with radiation therapy.[244,294] Cardiac catheterization in the axilla, coronary artery bypass grafting with sternotomy, and thoracotomy may also restrict shoulder range because of severe pain after the procedure.[252] In addition, frozen shoulder may be triggered by interventional cardiology, such as cardiac catheterization through the brachial artery[230] or placement of an ipsilateral, subpectoral cardiac defibrillator.[52] The incidence of frozen shoulder developing in a male patient population undergoing cardiothoracic surgery has been estimated at 3.3%.[312]

Immobility

After a minor strain, injury, surgery, or other painful source, it may seem logical to rest and immobilize the part, especially when inflammation may be involved. However, in adults, when the shoulder is immobilized, it is at risk of becoming stiff.[122,157,217,295] Bruckner and Nye performed a prospective study to evaluate factors that placed neurologic patients (mostly after subarachnoid hemorrhage) at greater risk for adhesive capsulitis.[41] Over a 6-month period of observation, frozen shoulder developed in 25% of these patients. They identified five risk factors that could be linked primarily to a significant period of immobility of the affected upper extremity.

The majority of patient referrals for shoulder stiffness to an orthopaedic specialist occur subsequent to a recommended rest period imposed by the referring physician. In a review of patients referred to Binder and colleagues, 75% were initially told to rest the shoulder instead of gentle exercises being prescribed to maintain mobility.[25] Only half of these patients received advice in regard to care of their painful shoulder after an initial assessment from their primary care physician.

Diabetes Mellitus

Patients with diabetes mellitus are at much greater risk for the development of limited joint motion, not only in the shoulder but in other joints as well.[279] The incidence of frozen shoulder in diabetics averages approximately 10% to 20% but may be as high as 35%.* Diabetics who have been insulin dependent for many years have a much greater frequency of frozen shoulder and, in up to 42%, have bilateral shoulder involvement.[37,101,205] Patients with diabetes of childhood onset may have symptoms of stiffness in the fifth decade of life, but if adult-onset diabetics are included (type 1 plus type 2 diabetes mellitus), the age at onset is similar to that of the general population (Fig. 20–16). Diabetics with frozen shoulder are more likely to have organ involvement.[11]

Insulin-dependent diabetics with joint stiffness in the hands and other major articulations are categorized as having limited joint motion syndrome.[279] High circulating blood glucose levels may actually accelerate "aging" of certain proteins in the body by triggering a series of chemical reactions that form and accumulate irreversible cross-links between adjacent protein molecules.[42,146,191] This pathway, which leads to diffuse arthrofibrosis, is termed nonenzymatic glycosylation. Diabetics who have cheiroarthropathy (a waxy thickening and induration of the skin associated with flexion contractures of the fingers) and a frozen shoulder have a higher incidence of retinopathy and bilateral shoulder involvement (77%),[101] and joint stiffening is found more commonly in those with skin changes.[292] Rarely, shoulder stiffness has been reported to antedate diabetic symptoms.[287] Finally, the longer that a patient has been taking insulin, the greater the risk of shoulder stiffness developing[205] and the greater the resistance to all treatment modalities.[101,285]

Lequesne and coworkers found 17 patients with glucose intolerance out of 60 new patients with idiopathic frozen shoulder.[182] Therefore, an attentive clinician should inquire into the family history of all patients in whom frozen shoulder has been newly diagnosed, and consideration should be given to performing an oral glucose tolerance test or other diabetic workup in those affected. Anecdotally, patients with a frozen shoulder often have a family history of diabetes, even if they themselves do not have the disease. Because of the refractory nature of shoulder stiffness in long-term insulin-dependent diabetics, early intervention has been considered appropriate to prevent progressive disability.[101,228,285]

---

*See references 11, 37, 101, 182, 188, 205, 240, 241, 285, 334.

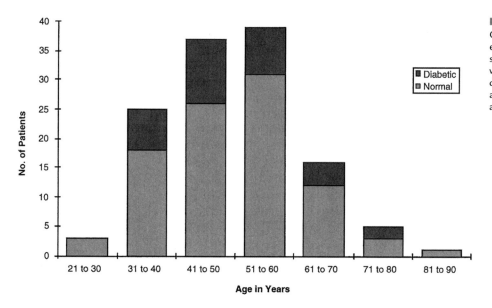

■ **Figure 20–16**
Graph depicting the age at initial evaluation for 126 patients with shoulder stiffness divided by those with or without diabetes.[195] No differences were found in the mean age between patients with diabetes[32] and those without diabetes.[92]

Cervical Disease

Degeneration of the cervical intervertebral disks between C5-C6 and C6-C7 has been noted to be more frequent in patients with shoulder stiffness than in a similarly age-matched control group.[335] The peak age incidence of frozen shoulder and cervical disk degeneration is similar.[160] In other studies, frozen shoulder was noted to develop more frequently in patients with degenerative disk disease of the cervical spine.[116,188,199] Finally, patients with symptomatic cervical radiculitis and a painful shoulder, with or without a fixed joint contracture, experienced less pain and regained pain-free range when cervical traction was added to exercises.[62]

Thyroid Disorders

The rare manifestation of bilateral frozen shoulders has been reported in both hyperthyroidism and hypothyroidism.[33,201,300,334] Because of potential activation within the sympathetic nervous system, Wohlgethan has postulated that hyperthyroidism, frozen shoulder, and shoulder-hand syndrome are linked disorders.[331] Resolution of shoulder stiffness has occurred after thyroidectomy and stabilization of the thyroid hormone level.[235,331]

Cardiac Disease

For many years, clinicians have been keen to associate ischemic heart disease and shoulder stiffness.[9,34,95,198,334] Furthermore, frozen shoulder has been reported to persist years after coronary artery occlusion.[9] On review of 133 consecutive cases of myocardial infarction, Ernstene and Kinell found 17 whose original complaint was unrelenting pain in the shoulder region.[95] Because of this relationship, a good cardiac examination is justified to rule out an unrecognized coronary thrombosis. Similarly, shoulder-hand syndrome, an autonomic dystrophy, can be a sequel to myocardial infarction in 10% to 30% of cases.[203]

Pulmonary Disorders

Saha reported that frozen shoulder was more frequent in those afflicted with emphysema and chronic bronchitis, but he was unable to correlate the severity or the duration of illness with the finding of frozen shoulder.[283] In 1959, Johnston reported that the incidence of frozen shoulder was 3.2% in pooled populations of sanatorium patients with tuberculosis.[157] In patients undergoing treatment of tuberculosis, Good and coworkers associated cases of frozen shoulder and the use of isoniazid therapy.[111]

Neoplastic Disorders

Bronchogenic carcinoma and Pancoast's tumors of the lung parenchyma have been known to cause deep shoulder aching and a neuritic type of pain.[94,143] Other occult neoplastic tumors, masked by symptoms attributed to a frozen shoulder, include chest wall tumors and primary or metastatic carcinoma of the humerus.[80,198,214]

Neurologic Conditions

Riley and colleagues documented a 13% incidence of frozen shoulder in patients with Parkinson's disease versus a 1.7% rate in age-matched controls.[271] They also highlighted that in 8% of patients surveyed, the first symptom of Parkinson's disease was shoulder stiffness, which could occur up to 2 years before the onset of generalized symptoms. Brachial neuritis, a painful neuritic condition also known as Parsonage-Turner syndrome, has also been associated with frozen shoulder.[24] Patients with cerebral hemorrhage and cerebral tumors have likewise been shown to be at increased risk for frozen shoulder.[41,335] Even compressive neuropathies such as thoracic outlet syndrome and palsy of the accessory nerve or suprascapular nerve have been associated with the onset of frozen shoulder.[39,169,244]

In patients who have had a cerebrovascular event or traumatic brain injury, a wide variety of shoulder conditions that in part include some degree of stiffness have been loosely grouped under the heading of "stroke shoulder." At least 30% of patients with hemiplegia secondary to stroke or other causes experience shoulder pain and may be prone to shoulder stiffness.[29,118] The causes of hemiplegic shoulder pain are multifactorial; however, the association with frozen shoulder has been found to be as high as 77%.[273] It was postulated by Griffin that "careless handling of the paralyzed upper limb at any time after the onset of hemiplegia can precipitate shoulder injury and pain."[118] Wanklyn and associates also found that patients who required transfer assistance were more likely to suffer from hemiparetic shoulder pain.[316] Bruckner and Nye reported a 25% incidence of frozen shoulder in neurosurgical patients who had suffered subarachnoid hemorrhage.[41] They found that the subsequent development of adhesive capsulitis was associated with impaired consciousness, hemiparesis, intravenous infusion, older age, and depression. In a hemiparetic patient, the clinician may find it difficult to distinguish between shoulder stiffness caused by capsular constraint versus muscular spasticity or a combination of the two.[316] A form of sympathetically maintained pain, shoulder-hand syndrome, occurs in as many as 30% to 40% of stroke patients and can be terribly disabling.

Personality Disorders

In 1934, Codman described four patients with frozen shoulder who "were a little run-down without anything particular the matter."[65] This "run-down" condition may predispose an individual to chronic shoulder stiffness.[227,257] Coventry dubbed some individuals with the "periarthritic personality," which was a character disposition susceptible to frozen shoulder and in whom treatment was more difficult.[72] A person with this personality was characterized as hyperemotional and unable to tolerate pain. He went on to say that "they expect someone else to get them well and refuse to take the initiative in the recovery, a manifestation of their passivity." Many years later, however, Wright and Haq found no evidence of a characteristic personality disorder when using the Maudsley Personality Inventory to test 186 patients who had a frozen shoulder and controls.[334] Fleming and associates also profiled the personality type of 56 patients with a frozen shoulder by using the Middlesex Hospital Questionnaire and found that women had significantly greater anxiety levels than controls did.[102]

Tyber used lithium and amitriptyline to treat 55 patients with painful shoulder syndromes and found a significantly greater prevalence of depression that responded along with the shoulder pain to these medications.[313] He entertained the theory that "a painful shoulder syndrome may be a clinical entity of psychogenic origin." In response to Tyber, Sullivan recommended that the physician "should not be detracted from giving proper and early treatment to the painful shoulder."[299]

Although it may be reasonable to say that patients with chronically painful shoulder stiffness may over time lose their tolerance to cope with chronic pain, especially when treatment measures are unsuccessful, the mental health

of patients with shoulder stiffness appears to be normal. Matsen and Harryman reviewed their combined data collected at the University of Washington Shoulder Clinic for results of the mental health score on the Short Form 36 (SF-36) health status questionnaire for 295 patients with a frozen shoulder[175] or post-traumatic stiff shoulder.[120,130] They found that patients with frozen shoulder scored within 95% and post-traumatic patients with stiff shoulder scored within 88% of the mean for normal age-matched controls. Although these patients in pain may appear depressed, anxious, or passive or aggressive, they are probably no different from the general population.

Reaction to Medication

Recent reports suggest that treatment with certain medications can be complicated by the development of frozen shoulder. Good and colleagues associated cases of frozen shoulder with the use of isoniazid therapy for pulmonary tuberculosis.[111] Grasland and coworkers described eight cases of frozen shoulder developing secondary to treatment of human immunodeficiency virus (HIV) infection with protease inhibitors.[115] Specifically, all patients received the drug indinavir as part of their regimen and did not have any other risk factors for frozen shoulder. Peyriere and colleagues also reported frozen shoulder developing after treatment of HIV with indinavir.[251] Similar findings have been reported by other investigators,[181,339] as well as after treatment with barbiturates,[196] flouroquinones,[104] and nelfinavir.[82] Treatment of gastric carcinoma with the MMP inhibitor marimastat has been linked to the development of frozen shoulder.[152]

DIAGNOSTIC EVALUATION

One would think that the diagnosis of frozen shoulder should be easy. Indeed, as will be discussed, the history is usually clear, few diagnostic examination maneuvers are required, and even fewer diagnostic modalities are necessary. Nonetheless, in a recent informal pole of 24 residents each completing a 2-month rotation on the Thomas Jefferson University Shoulder and Elbow Service, frozen shoulder was chosen as the most frequently misdiagnosed problem in patients referred for a second opinion. This quick, but informative study suggests that a high index of suspicion is necessary for this condition.

History

Clinical Features of Idiopathic Frozen Shoulder

Frozen shoulder is classically characterized by three stages, although their nomenclature and description vary among authors.[130,141,208] A patient with an idiopathic frozen shoulder may have complaints and physical findings typical for this diagnosis, but the practitioner's clinical acumen is challenged to discriminate the exact stage or appropriate duration of symptoms or findings. An initial bilateral manifestation of shoulder stiffness may be a clue to systemic disease, yet even with unilateral

TABLE 20-4.   Differential Diagnoses of Shoulder Stiffness (Including Associated Diseases)

Extrinsic Causes		Intrinsic Causes

Neurologic
Parkinson's disease
Autonomic dystrophy (RSD)
Intradural lesions
Neural compression
  Cervical disk disease
  Neurofibroma
Foraminal stenosis
Neuralgic amyotrophy
Hemiplegia
Head trauma
 	
Muscular
Poliomyositis
 	
Cardiovascular
Myocardial infarction
Thoracic outlet syndrome
Cerebral hemorrhage
 	
Infectious
Chronic bronchitis
Pulmonary tuberculosis
 	
Metabolic
Diabetes mellitus
Thyroid disease
Progressive systemic sclerosis (scleroderma)
Paget's disease
 	
Neoplastic
Pancoast's tumor
Lung carcinoma
Metastatic disease
 	
Inflammatory
Rheumatologic disorders (see Table 19–1)
Polymyalgia rheumatica
	Trauma
	Surgery
	  Axillary node dissection, sternotomy,
	    thoracotomy
	Fractures
	  Cervical spine, ribs, elbow, hand, etc.
	
	Medications
	Isoniazid, phenobarbital
	
	Congenital
	Klippel-Feil syndrome
	Sprengel's deformity
	Glenoid dysplasia
	Atresia
	Contractures
	  Pectoralis major
	  Axillary fold
	
	Behovioral
	Depression
	Hysterical paralysis
	
	Referred Pain
	Diaphragmatic irritation
	Gastrointestinal disorders
	  Esophagitis
	  Ulcers
	  Cholecystitis
		Bursitis
		Subacromial
		Calcific tendinitis
		Snapping scapula
		
		Biceps Tendon
		Tenosynovitis
		Partial or complete tears
		SLAP lesions
		
		Rotator Cuff
		Impingement syndrome
		Partial rotator cuff tears
		Complete rotator cuff tears
		
		Instability—Glenohumeral
		Recurrent dislocation, anterior and posterior
		Chronic dislocation
		
		Arthritides
		Glenohumeral and acromioclavicular
		  Osteoarthritis
		  Rheumatoid
		  Psoriatic
		  Infectious
		  Neuropathic
		
		Trauma
		Fractures
		  Glenoid
		  Proximal humerus
		Surgery
		  Postoperative shoulder, breast, head, neck,
		    chest
		
		Miscellaneous
		Avascular necrosis
		Hemarthrosis
		Osteochondromatosis
		Suprascapular nerve palsy

RSD, reflex sympathetic dystrophy; SLAP, superior labral, anterior-posterior.

involvement, a prudent physician should consider the possibility of frequently associated diseases in the differential diagnosis (Table 20-4). Reports of bilateral involvement range from 10% in the general population to as high as 40% in those with insulin-dependent diabetes.[25,263]

A frozen shoulder rarely recurs in the same shoulder unless an injury or disease process predisposes the joint to repeat episodes of stiffness.[84,122,130,165,188,201] In patients without diabetes, frozen shoulder on the opposite side may develop in up to 20% of patients.[189,272]

Painful Phase: "Freezing"

As mentioned previously, the clinical expression of frozen shoulder is segmented into three phases. The painful phase begins when a patient initially notices the onset of aching pain, which often begins at night and persists during the day.[130,141,208] Sudden jolts or attempts at rapid motion exponentially punctuate the chronic discomfort. Typically, no precipitating incident is elicited, but occasionally the patient recalls a specific event such as a trivial injury, a flu shot, or a head cold that settled into the neck. As symptoms progress, fewer extremity positions remain comfortable, and those that are tolerable typically leave the arm dependent at the side in a medially rotated, resting position. The ache is unrelated to activity and may

be worse at rest, especially at night. Lying on the affected shoulder prevents sleep or soon awakens the afflicted person. Reeves wrote that this phase lasts between 2 and 9 months.[263]

Pathologically, this phase corresponds to the acute synovitis and capsulitis discussed previously. Patients will often hold their shoulder in a position of adduction and humerothoracic internal rotation because this is the neutral isometric position of relaxed tension for the inflamed glenohumeral capsule. In addition, because of nonspecific pain, patients are often treated with a period of immobilization, thus further placing the arm in an adducted and internally rotated position and worsening the stiffening process.

Progressive Stiffness Phase: "Frozen"

The phase of progressive stiffness is said to last between 3 and 12 months and ultimately gives rise to what was classically described by Codman[65] as a frozen shoulder.[141,263] Stiffness progresses to the extent that shoulder motion becomes limited in all planes. Pain is usually less than in the initial inflammatory phase, is often much more focused, and may be noted only while reaching. Many patients will continue to give a history of night pain.

Activities of daily living are severely restricted (Fig. 20–17). Common complaints, therefore, are an inability to tuck in a shirt, fasten a bra, scratch the back, wash the top of the opposite shoulder, reach away from the body, or reach overhead. An inability to sleep comfortably on the side is a universal complaint, possibly related to decreased glenohumeral laxity.

During this stage, the diagnosis of frozen shoulder is made more easily. The history must therefore be directed toward ruling out associated conditions (see Table 20–4). The patient should be questioned specifically about glucose tolerance and a family history of diabetes mellitus. A history of neck stiffness or paresthesias in the upper extremity may be a clue to the presence of underlying cervical disk disease. The presence of pulmonary or cardiac symptoms should be sought.

As time passes, the pain diminishes and a narrow comfort zone exists, albeit within severely restricted motion limits. Specifically, patients often feel little or no pain while using the shoulder within its permitted range. Any attempts to reach outside the restricted range or sudden movements that demand shock absorption (e.g., hammering) are associated with pain. Once the degree of stiffness has reached a plateau, a steady state exists during which the patient gets no worse and no better. Although this phase is said to last anywhere between 3 and 12 months, it can become refractory and last much longer.[129,135,228,318]

Resolution Phase: "Thawing"

The final stage of idiopathic frozen shoulder is the resolution or thawing phase, characterized by a slow gain in motion and comfort.[141] Although this phase has been described as lasting for as short a time as 4 weeks, for most patients months to years may be required to achieve functional motion and comfort. Typically, motion slowly improves over a period of 12 to 42 months. Several authors, however, have reported a significant number of patients with persistent symptoms lasting for as long as 6 years to as many as 10 years from the onset of disease (Fig. 20–18 and see the section on natural history).[63,290]

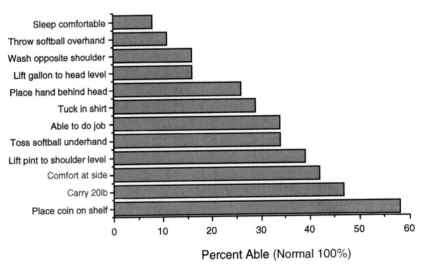

■ Figure 20–17
Shoulder function as depicted on the Simple Shoulder Test self-assessment examination for the first 30 patients of a prospective study who had recalcitrant shoulder stiffness.[135]

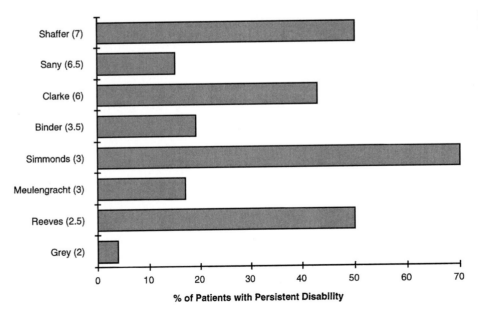

■ Figure 20–18
Graph showing the percentage of patients with persistent symptoms in studies that have more than 2 years of follow-up (years in parentheses after the first author). Symptoms typically extend well beyond the normal period expected for complete recovery.

The treatment challenge is recovery of full range and normal function. The patient's symptoms may resolve with or without aggressive treatment, but motion restrictions often persist.[25,141]

Clinical Features of Post-traumatic Stiff Shoulder

By definition, a patient with a post-traumatic stiff shoulder will have a history of a significant antecedent trauma. Common etiologic factors are a proximal humeral fracture, severe soft tissue contusion, rotator cuff injury, or previous surgery. Most often, patients have been subjected to prolonged immobilization after the traumatic event, including a lengthy postoperative immobilization. Previous operative reports are helpful in understanding limitations, and the symptoms before and after surgery should be noted.

Patients in whom shoulder stiffness develops after a rotator cuff strain typically display a pattern of restricted asymmetric range on forward elevation, internal rotation, and cross-body adduction.[129,195,307] The clinical findings are often confused with "impingement syndrome," but many of these patients do not exhibit subacromial roughness and crepitation on examination. Motion restrictions are related to contracture of the posterior capsule.[132] On repetitive elevation, the rotator cuff or biceps tendons may become abraded, thereby leading to subacromial roughness.[195] A shoulder that has sustained a severe eccentric load to the rotator cuff may have incurred partial disruption of tendon fibers. Partial rotator cuff tears, which are typically found on the deep surface of the supraspinatus or infraspinatus, are notoriously painful and often associated with posterior capsular contractures.[135]

Postsurgical stiffness is either intentional or an inadvertent consequence of postoperative healing. Some surgical procedures are designed to limit glenohumeral or scapulothoracic range. For example, the Putti-Platt procedure for recurrent anteroinferior shoulder instability shortens the capsule and imbricates the subscapularis tendon, intentionally limiting external rotation to prevent the shoulder joint from attaining a potentially unstable position.[237] Hawkins and Angelo have shown, however, the deleterious long-term effect of causing excessive asymmetric tightness, which can ultimately result in destructive capsulorrhaphy arthropathy.[139] Other procedures such as anterior or posterior capsular shifts for instability, rotator cuff repair, and prosthetic arthroplasty may also cause intrinsic tightening of the articular capsule and rotator cuff.

Open shoulder surgery almost always violates the motion plane external to the joint. On healing, adhesions between the external surface of the rotator cuff and proximal end of the humerus and the deep surface of the deltoid, coracoacromial arch, and conjoined tendon (the so-called HSMI) are often identified.

If limited motion results after a surgical procedure, examination will reveal either a specific pattern of exaggerated stiffness or global restriction. Anterior surgical approaches that imbricate the anterior capsule and subscapularis effectively limit external rotation, whereas stiffness after rotator cuff surgery is typically global, but with an accentuated posterior capsular stiffness pattern.

Examination

Examination of a patient with a painful stiff shoulder begins with both shoulders exposed. The positions of the head, neck, torso, and shoulder girdles are checked for proper alignment and symmetry. Note especially the height of each shoulder to look for a spasmodically elevated or weak droopy shoulder, and inspect the muscular contour for localized atrophy.

The cervical spine is palpated for local tenderness and muscle spasm, starting at the occiput and continuing down the spinous processes and along the paracervical muscles. It is important to palpate the musculature around the supraclavicular region and scapulas, especially near the posterosuperior angle of the scapular spine. Palpation should also be performed while the neck and shoulder are ranged. A complete cervical examination includes inspection for signs of radiculopathy and a thorough neurologic and vascular examination of both upper extremities.

The shoulder examination begins with observation and palpation. Patients with chronic painful stiffness typically experience tenderness diffusely about the subacromial region and biceps tendon and toward the deltoid insertion. Most report persistent discomfort around the deltoid tuberosity, even without the application of local pressure.

In patients with shoulder stiffness, it is preferable to test the strength of the rotator cuff and deltoid with the arm at the side. A steady gentle force is applied to resist a patient's attempt to isometrically rotate internally and externally, abduct, forward-elevate, extend, and adduct. If range will accommodate testing, the supraspinatus and the deltoid may also be tested against resistance in elevation. Isolated weakness in specific rotations may be indicative of a rotator cuff tear, and ultrasound or MRI may be indicated. It is also important to test the strength of the distal musculature in the upper part of the arm, forearm, and hand after examining these areas for swelling, texture, and color changes. Most patients with an insidious onset of global stiffness do not exhibit signs of weakness but do experience moderate discomfort on forceful contraction. Although a rotator cuff tear and a true frozen shoulder never coexist (by definition), stiffness is commonly seen with partial cuff tears and, much less frequently, may be associated with full-thickness tears.

Active range of motion is observed from the anterior and posterior vantages, and six standard motion arcs as assigned by the ASES[13] are recorded. Passive range is also checked at the end point of each range to assess the glenohumeral and scapulothoracic contributions to total humerothoracic range. The six ranges of the ASES that are typically measured include (Fig. 20–19A to E) (1) forward elevation in the sagittal plane (FE, degrees), (2) external rotation at the side (ERS, degrees), (3) external rotation at 90 degrees of coronal plane abduction (use maximal abduction if unable to assume 90 degrees) (ERA, degrees), (4) internal rotation in coronal plane abduction (use maximal abduction if unable to assume 90 degrees) (IRA, degrees), (5) cross-body adduction (measure the span between the antecubital fossa and the opposite shoulder) (XBA, centimeters), and (6) internal rotation up the back

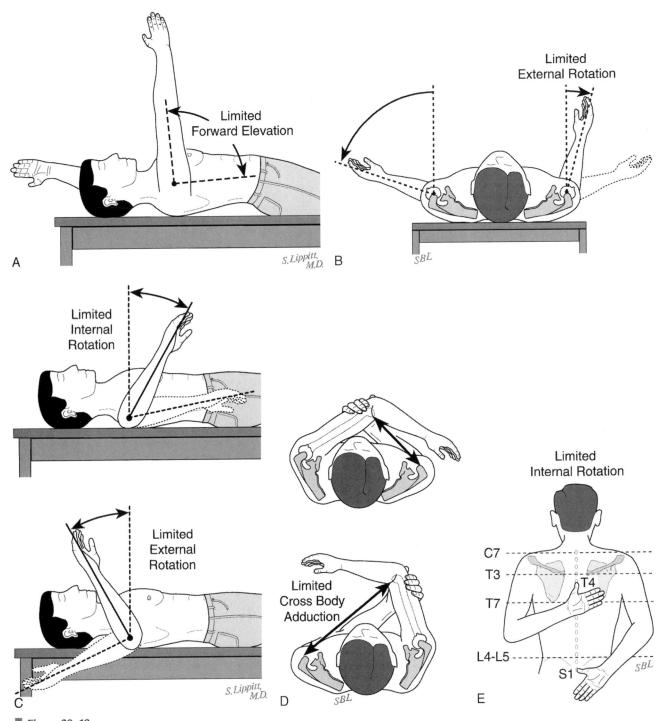

■ **Figure 20–19**

A, Active humerothoracic elevation is performed supine in the sagittal plane with comfortable rotation. A goniometer is placed in line with the humerus and long axis of the thorax for measurement. **B,** Active external rotation at the side is easily performed supine with the elbow one handbreadth from the thorax. A goniometer is placed in line with the forearm and perpendicular to the surface of the table. **C,** Active external and internal rotation in the coronal plane abduction is performed supine. A goniometer is placed in line with the forearm and perpendicular to the surface of the table. **D,** Active assisted cross-body adduction is performed supine with the opposite unaffected extremity pulling the elbow toward the opposite shoulder. The distance between the antecubital fossa and the opposite shoulder is recorded in centimeters. **E,** Active internal rotation up the back is performed in the upright position. The highest spinous process reached with the thumb tip is recorded.

(record the tip of the thumb at the highest spinous process) (IRB). Some investigators also include abduction in the coronal or scapular plane, but because this measurement also requires external rotation to achieve the maximal arc and thus combines two motions, it has not been included in the ASES standard examination. Ranges are always recorded for both extremities. The six motions measured provide a global representation of the capsule inasmuch as each represents a different capsular region. These regions are listed in Table 20-2. Comparison with the unaffected side can facilitate the diagnosis of specific or global contractures. Knowledge of the locations of capsular involvement has important implications for directing treatment.

Clinical analysts have proposed alternative methods to simplify the measurement of shoulder motion and to characterize the quantity of motion in a single factor. One author suggested a simple modification of the conventional shoulder wheel to provide the therapist, patient, and physician with an objective assessment of shoulder range.[12] Other investigators have calculated a single number based on two to six measured ranges.[45,129,135,178] These measures often prove useful in monitoring a patient's progress or response to treatment and afford simple comparison. Combined measures, however, do not allow independent characterization of an isolated or specific group of motions. In clinical practice, knowledge of ranges that are most affected or least responsive to

treatment assists in directing care. Single-number factors are therefore of limited clinical use.

To accommodate all future combinations of independently measured motion arcs, we recommend recording six active motions at each visit and comparing these measurements with those of the opposite extremity (Fig. 20–20A and B). Each motion measured for the symptomatic shoulder is divided by the range of the asymptomatic shoulder to yield a ratio in which unity indicates functional symmetry with the opposite side. Graphics for a particular range (see Fig. 20–20A and B) or a stiffness ratio (Fig. 20–21) can be generated to show patients their progress or final assessment relative to others. The mean ratios of total capsular stiffness (TCS), posterior capsular stiffness (PCS), or anterior capsular stiffness (ACS) for a specific shoulder can be calculated by combining the ratios for specific ranges and dividing by the total number as shown:

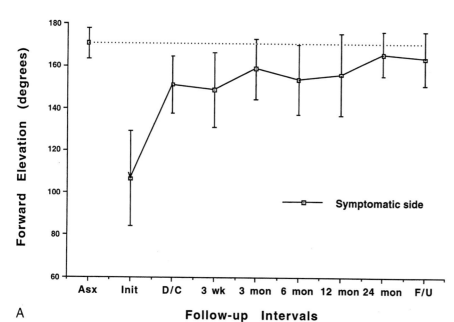

A

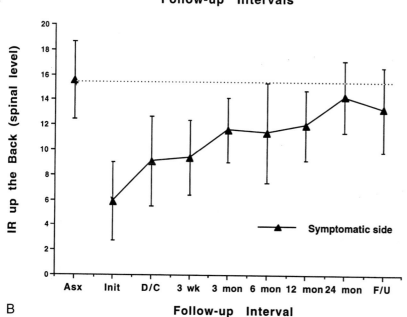

B

■ **Figure 20–20**

A, Marked improvement in range of forward elevation occurred after arthroscopic capsular release. Range recovered rapidly for the motion of forward elevation when compared with five other measured ranges (contrast with internal rotation up the back, see **B**). The results of 30 patients with a 2-year follow-up (mean ± 1 SD) are presented. Asx, asymptomatic side; D/C, range at hospital discharge; F/U, range at longest follow-up; Init, range before release.
B, Compare the rate of improvement after arthroscopic capsular release for internal rotation up the back against forward elevation (**A**). Internal rotation was improved least after release but slowly increased by the 2-year follow-up (mean ± 1 SD). *(From Harryman DT II, Sidles JA, and Matsen FA III: Arthroscopic management of refractory shoulder stiffness. Arthroscopy 13:133-147, 1997.)*

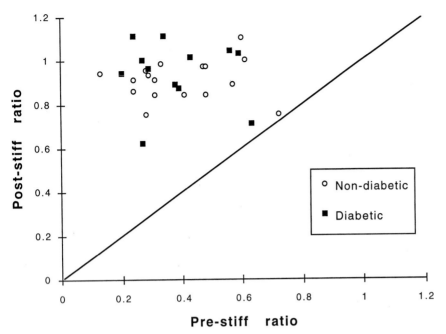

■ **Figure 20–21**
Graph of preoperative and postoperative stiffness ratios for each patient at the longest follow-up interval. No patient's motion worsened after arthroscopic capsular release (ASCR). The mean improvement in motion for all patients was greater than 90% of the asymptomatic shoulder. The distance from the diagonal for each point above the line is indicative of the relative improvement after ASCR for each patient. *(From Harryman DT II, Sidles JA, and Matsen FA III: Arthroscopic management of refractory shoulder stiffness. Arthroscopy 13:133-147, 1997.)*

The stiffness ratio (SR) is the symptomatic range divided by the asymptomatic range.

TCS:

$$TCS_{SR} = (FE_{SR} + ERS_{SR} + ERA_{SR} + IRA_{SR} + IRB_{SR} + XBA_{SR})/6$$

PCS:

$$PCS_{SR} = (FE_{SR} + IRB_{SR} + XBA_{SR})/3$$

ACS:

$$ACS_{SR} = (ERS_{SR} + ERA_{SR})/2$$

Note that no range is ever recorded as 0 degrees; instead, 1 degree is recorded to avoid numerators that yield a meaningless number. When the stiffness ratio is unity, range is symmetric. These ratios could also be used for studies of bilateral stiffness but require the use of normal age-adjusted means[63,209] for comparison; otherwise, improvement after release will appear excessive relative to the opposite side.

Individual ranges and combined ratios were used to test whether differences in the severity of stiffness or the pattern of stiffness could be characterized in groups with different pathologies. Patients with an idiopathic frozen shoulder typically have global restrictions in range. With two notable exceptions, a post-traumatic stiff shoulder often exhibits decreases in motion in all ranges. These exceptions are (1) a postsurgical stiff shoulder after anterior reconstructions for instability and (2) a post-traumatic posterior capsular contracture after a rotator cuff strain or partial rotator cuff tear.

One-hundred seventeen patients with refractory shoulder stiffness have been enrolled prospectively into a specific management protocol (Fig. 20–22). A complete evaluation that included the six ranges listed earlier was performed on each patient at the initial visit. Patients were

separated according to established diagnostic criteria[195] into those with a frozen shoulder (49) and those with a post-traumatic stiff shoulder (68). Patients whose stiffness developed after an injury had significantly less overall stiffness ($P < .02$; TCS = 0.48) than did those whose stiffness developed insidiously (TCS = 0.38). Patients whose stiffness developed after an injury had significantly less restriction in flexion, external rotation at the side, external rotation in abduction, and internal rotation in abduction (see Table 20–3). No significant differences were noted for the range of internal rotation up the back and cross-body adduction, although these groups were distinctly different. This lack of statistically significant differences for posterior capsular motions may be attributed to the scapulothoracic contribution associated with measurement.

Clarke and associates measured the shoulder motion of normal individuals and those with painful stiff shoulders.[63] They compared the motion of stiff shoulders with that of age- and sex-matched normal control shoulders and expressed the reduction in range of movement for the stiff shoulders as a percentage of the control population. Their method provides an opportunity to relate the severity of restricted range in patients who suffer from bilateral shoulder stiffness.

Supplementary Clinical Assessment

Blood Tests

After a thorough history and physical examination, the clinician must decide whether hematologic tests are necessary. A routine patient with shoulder stiffness does not need laboratory studies for diagnosis or management.[28,272] A blood count, differential smear, and an erythrocyte sedimentation rate (ESR), however, should be requested when a recent change in the patient's health status has

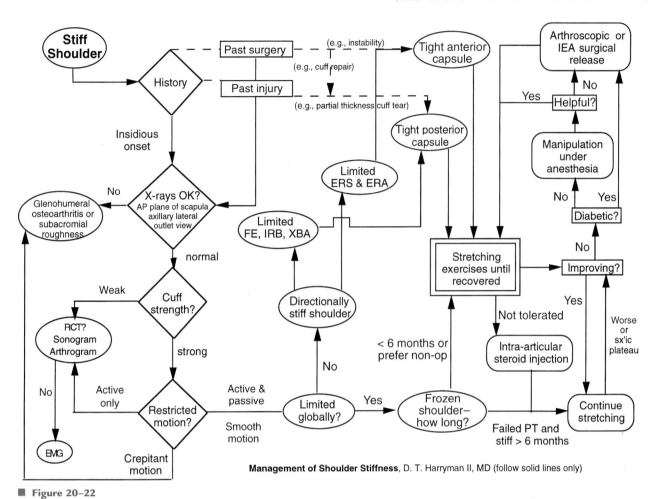

■ Figure 20–22
Evaluation and treatment algorithm for a stiff shoulder. AP, anteroposterior; EMG, electromyelogram; ERA, external rotation in abduction; ERS, external rotation at the side; PT, physical therapy; RCT, rotator cuff tear; XBA, cross-body adduction.

occurred. Lequesne and colleagues found an abnormal glucose tolerance test result in 28% of new patients with a frozen shoulder; therefore, this test should be considered, especially in those with a positive family history of diabetes.[182] In a prospective study of 50 patients with a diagnosis of primary frozen shoulder, Bunker and Esler measured the serum lipid levels and compared them with those of age- and sex-matched controls.[50] They found significantly elevated fasting serum triglyceride and cholesterol levels in the frozen shoulder group.

Investigators have searched for specific blood indices or markers that would be useful to predict the severity of disease and to monitor the progression or outcome of treatment. As with other chronic inflammatory processes, we might expect an elevated ESR. A few reports have indicated that the ESR was elevated in up to 20% of patients with a frozen shoulder and demonstrated some response to treatment.[25,201,260,281] In clinical practice and in more recent studies, however, the ESR has not proved to be reliable or useful when either evaluating the patient or monitoring the response to anti-inflammatory drugs or steroid agents.[164,338] Other serum factors have also been investigated. Bulgen and associates reported on the immune status of 40 patients in whom frozen shoulder was diagnosed.[44] They found that pretreatment increased immune complex levels and decreased cell-mediated indicators

when compared with a control group. Eight months after diagnosis, each patient was retested, and values tended to approach control levels. Others have studied the presence of the HLA-B27 histocompatibility antigen in patients with a frozen shoulder, but on extended review, the marker was identified no more frequently than in the control group.[276,288,295,338]

Noninvasive Imaging

Routine Radiographs

Radiographs are essential to diagnose a frozen or post-traumatic stiff shoulder.[195] Plain radiographs are needed to rule out abnormalities in the bone (e.g., tumor, malunion), in the joint (e.g., arthritic collapse, chronic dislocation), or in the local soft tissues (e.g., calcific deposit or heterotopic ossification) (Fig. 20–23A to C). For a postsurgical stiff shoulder, radiographs may reveal orthopaedic hardware, malpositioning of which may be a factor in the patient's stiffness. Narrowing of the clear space between the subchondral surface of the humeral head and the glenoid may indicate early degenerative arthritis.

It is important to obtain at least two orthogonal views of the joint to rule out occult fractures, loose bodies,

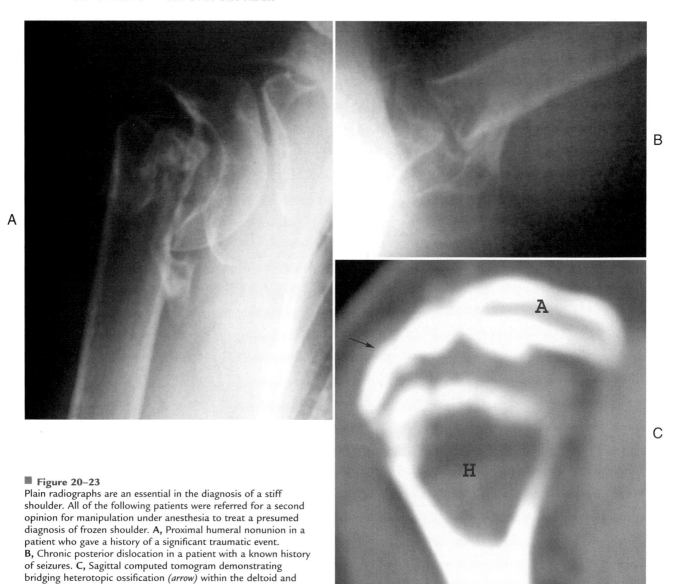

■ Figure 20–23
Plain radiographs are an essential in the diagnosis of a stiff
shoulder. All of the following patients were referred for a second
opinion for manipulation under anesthesia to treat a presumed
diagnosis of frozen shoulder. **A,** Proximal humeral nonunion in a
patient who gave a history of a significant traumatic event.
B, Chronic posterior dislocation in a patient with a known history
of seizures. **C,** Sagittal computed tomogram demonstrating
bridging heterotopic ossification *(arrow)* within the deltoid and
subacromial space in a patient with stiffness after a rotator cuff
repair. A, acromion; H, humeral head.

humeral head displacement, and blocking osteophytes.
The shoulder screening series should include

1. An anteroposterior radiograph perpendicular to the
plane of the scapula with the humerus positioned in 35
degrees of external rotation (relative to the plane of the
scapula)
2. The same view with internal rotation to the body
3. A true axillary lateral view

If the patient has a history of previous rotator cuff
surgery, a supraspinatus outlet view is included to assess
any postoperative acromial changes.

Routine shoulder radiographs in patients with shoulder stiffness are typically normal.[25] Decreased bone
density of the humeral head, however, is a fairly frequent
finding on radiographs of patients with frozen shoulder
syndrome and may be related to prolonged disuse.[25,189,267]
Lundberg and Nilsson found approximately 50% loss of
bone in a short period in 74 cases of frozen shoulder.[189]
They attributed this loss in bone mass to an inflammatory

process because the degree of loss could not be explained
by disuse and immobilization alone. Radiographic
changes in bone structure may often be seen postoperatively, such as after an acromioplasty. Narrowing of the
subacromial space has been observed in patients who have
stiffness associated with rotator cuff disease.[25]

When sentinel clues on the history and physical examination indicate a potential risk in regions extrinsic to the
shoulder, it is important to obtain routine cervical spine
films (e.g., radicular symptoms/signs), a chest radiograph
(e.g., cough or chest pain), or radiographs of the entire
humerus (e.g., bone pain or tenderness below the deltoid
tuberosity). If symptoms are unrelenting, atypical, or
unresponsive, a high index of suspicion for systemic
disease is necessary.

Bone Scans

A bone scan is rarely indicated in the evaluation of a
frozen shoulder because it has not proved to be useful in

diagnosis, management, or prognosis. Bone scan has been reported to be positive in as many as 96% of frozen shoulder patients.[315] Binder and colleagues used diphosphonate scans and found that 90% of their patients with a frozen shoulder had increased uptake on the symptomatic side and almost a third demonstrated a 50% increase over baseline activity on the unaffected side.[26] They did not, however, find an association between bone scan activity and the severity of disease, duration of symptoms, arthrographic findings, or ultimate outcome.

Most investigators using radionuclide scanning have reported use of technetium 99m (^{99m}Tc) pertechnetate or methylene diphosphonate in the frozen shoulder. Shoulder pain and increased ^{99m}Tc-pertechnetate uptake have been related, but not shoulder pain and ^{99m}Tc-methylene diphosphonate uptake.[298] Capsular uptake on a technetium bone scan is usually in the posterior plane in patients with a frozen shoulder, as opposed to anterior uptake in patients with subacromial pathology, although less than 80% of the patients had positive scans at all.[64] Even though a bone scan may not show differences in uptake between a frozen shoulder and autonomic reflex dystrophy, it has proved to be useful in distinguishing these conditions because the hand, the wrist, and the entire limb may show increased uptake in the latter.[171] Finally, Wright and associates found that 4 of 10 patients with adhesive capsulitis in whom the symptoms resolved rapidly in response to corticosteroid injections also had positive bone scans, but this association has not been duplicated.[333] The only clinical indication for ordering a bone scan is the rare circumstance in which the history suggests a possible underlying osseous neoplastic process.

Magnetic Resonance Imaging

In recent years, MRI has been used in the clinical assessment of stiff shoulder. Emig and colleagues reported on the characteristics of MRI in 10 patients with a frozen shoulder versus normal shoulders.[92] In those in whom a frozen shoulder was diagnosed, they found a combined thickness of the joint capsule and synovium of greater than 4 mm. They did not note significant differences in the volume of intra-articular fluid seen on the MRI scan or in the thickness of the rotator cuff and rotator interval capsule. In another study that used MRI, Bernageau and associates did find an increased thickness of the rotator cuff, as well as synovitis and bursitis, in patients undergoing hemodialysis who had chronic shoulder stiffness for more than 6 months.[22]

The use of intravenous gadolinium may improve the diagnostic capability of MRI in patients with a frozen shoulder. Connell and colleagues noted soft tissue density showing variable enhancement in the rotator interval and partially encasing the biceps anchor after gadolinium administration on MRI.[66] The same study demonstrated thickening and gadolinium enhancement of the axillary pouch. Carrillon and coworkers used intravenous gadolinium before MRI and demonstrated enhancement of the synovial lining in frozen shoulder patients.[56] Tamai and Yamato found enhancement of the joint capsule after intravenous gadolinium injection, and this finding was not seen in patients with subacromial impingement.[304] A

study comparing findings on MR arthrography in patients with and without frozen shoulder did not detect any specific diagnostic findings of frozen shoulder with this diagnostic tool.[192]

Although several studies clearly demonstrate some characteristic findings in frozen shoulder patients on MRI, this technique has not proved essential in the diagnosis or management of patients with stiff shoulder. Indications for MRI in this setting are infrequent and include concern about underlying rotator cuff integrity or the possibility of a soft tissue or osseous pathologic process.

Ultrasound

A few investigators have reported on the use of dynamic sonography in the evaluation of adhesive capsulitis.[99,282] Ryu and colleagues noted that the main sonographic feature of frozen shoulder was a constant limitation of the sliding movement of the supraspinatus tendon against the scapula.[282] They reported 91% sensitivity, 100% specificity, and an accuracy of 92% when compared with arthrography as the gold standard for diagnosis. Because of the noninvasive method and accuracy in detecting adhesive capsulitis, they claimed that "dynamic sonography is a reliable technique for the diagnosis for this condition." As with MRI, ultrasound is not a required diagnostic study and is usually indicated only for evaluation of the rotator cuff in those few patients in whom physical examination indicates the possibility of coexisting stiffness and a rotator cuff tear.

Arthrography

Intra-articular Pressure Measurement

In 1957, after Neviaser revealed the contracted nature of the articular capsule in patients with frozen shoulder, Kernwein and associates performed arthrographic studies in 12 patients with this diagnosis.[163] On open biopsy they found that the capsule and coracohumeral ligament were very contracted, thickened, and inelastic. They also noted the presence of subacute inflammation. Later, Neviaser described the arthrographic findings of adhesive capsulitis, which included decreased joint capacity, obliteration of the reflected axillary fold, and variable filling of the bicipital tendon sheath.[214] Other studies using arthrography added more findings, such as frequent obliteration of the subscapularis bursa, poor visualization of the biceps sheath, a joint capacity of less than 10 to 12 mL, dye filling short of the humeral neck, and a moth-eaten appearance of the capsular insertion on the humerus.* Arthrography has also been used to demonstrate the presence and location of joint capsule disruption during pressure injection and manipulation under anesthesia (MUA).[4,96,164,188,261,295] In an attempt to enhance arthrography, injection of air and contrast was touted to be superior to contrast alone for reasons of improved visualization along the margins of the joint and capsule and improved patient tolerance.[109,308]

---

*See references 4, 142, 164, 187, 188, 215, 218, 261, 266, 325.

Lundberg and others showed a positive correlation between arthrographic contraction of the axillary pouch and range of motion.[142,164,188,216,221,261] A legitimate correlation can only be accomplished, however, by controlling for a defined volume of contrast medium or measurement of intra-articular pressure during injection. Lundberg claimed that a normal range of motion could be detected in a shoulder joint that on arthrography showed a greatly decreased capacity and complete obliteration of the axillary pouch and subscapularis bursa.[188] Although contracture of the axillary pouch has been well documented,[214,284] the extent of posterior capsule distention has not been assessed in the post-traumatic stiff shoulder even though contracture of the posterior pouch has been seen clinically in relative isolation.[129,135,307] Itoi and Tabata found only mild correlation between external and internal rotation and anterior capsular and axillary pouch filling of the dye, respectively.[154]

Intra-articular volume and pressure have also been correlated with restriction of shoulder range.[164,188,216,261] Resnik and associates observed a gradual increase in pressure after arthrographic fluid injection in normal individuals but a rapid increase in pressure in patients with adhesive capsulitis.[268] They found that in normal shoulders, the intra-articular pressure in a resting position was less than 0 mm Hg. With dynamic contraction and elevation, pressure typically rose to above 90 mm Hg with the arm overhead, whereas patients with a contracted shoulder or a defect in the rotator cuff peaked in the range of 60 mm Hg. The early rise in pressure with elevation of the extremity[137] and the marked increase in pressure on continuous intra-articular fluid injection point to a decrease in compliance of the capsule.[164,225,261,268]

Proponents of arthrography claim its usefulness in standardizing classification and in selecting patients for clinical research.[187,199,213,221] Reeves and Neviaser and Neviaser explain the use of arthrographic findings to differentiate between a true frozen shoulder and a post-traumatic or painful stiff shoulder.[219,261] We have found that our diagnostic criteria are sufficient to differentiate these conditions.[195] No correlation between arthrographic findings and treatment outcome has been found.[26,187] As seen with intra-articular injection studies, the presence of a contracted joint volume does not mitigate against the clinical findings of a frozen shoulder.[188,214] In summary, arthrography has little contemporary use in the diagnostic workup of a stiff shoulder.

Arthroscopy

Many reports illustrate how arthroscopy has been used in cases of shoulder stiffness to (1) evaluate pathologic changes in the glenohumeral joint and subacromial space, (2) recognize problems associated with shoulder stiffness (e.g., a tendon or labral tear), and (3) determine the local effects of closed manipulation.* We should, however, keep in mind what Neviaser has written: "Arthroscopy is not a means of establishing a diagnosis."[220]

Arthroscopic detection of a frozen shoulder begins with introduction of the trocar through the posterior part of the capsule. Shoulders with a contracted and fibrotic capsule typically require additional insertional force.[135,220,228] On entry, the contracted space restricts not only visibility but also the ability to maneuver about the joint. In the early phases, a mild to moderate red inflammatory synovitic carpet of variable thickness is evident, especially under the rotator interval capsule along the biceps tendon root, superior labrum, and posterior capsule (Fig. 20-24).[121,129,135,221,327]

Neviaser described four arthroscopic stages of adhesive capsulitis and proposed that these stages could be used to guide treatment planning.[220] His stages are (1) a mild erythematous synovitis, (2) acute synovitis with adhesions in the dependent folds of the synovial lining, (3) maturation of adhesions with less reactive synovitis, and (4) chronic adhesions without synovitis. Other arthroscopists have found the articular surface free of capsular adhesions and have rarely identified adhesions in the recesses or dependent fold.[121,135,228,327] These clinical observations detract from the "adhesive" nature of the capsular process and lend credence to proliferative fibrosis leading to capsuloligamentous contractures.

Arthroscopic findings immediately after a successful manipulative release have been noted to include hemarthroses; avulsion of the inferior capsule, usually adjacent or peripheral to the labrum (Fig. 20-25); tears in the rotator interval capsule with occasional labral avulsions; and capsular tears anterosuperiorly or anteroinferiorly.[89,135,220,228,231,254,314]

Arthroscopists are also quick to point out its usefulness in identifying associated intra-articular pathology that had not been identified by history or clinical exami-

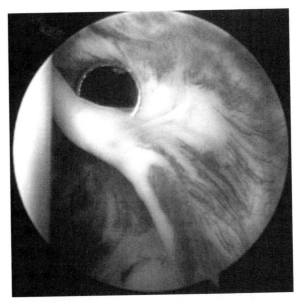

■ **Figure 20–24**
Arthroscopic view of inflamed hypervascular synovial proliferation along the biceps tendon root, rotator interval capsule, and posterosuperior capsule. Note that the proximal biceps tendon and root are adherent to the undersurface of the synovium and deep capsular layer under the rotator cuff (note that the synovium fails to wrap around the biceps as in a mesosynovium).

---

*See references 35, 121, 220, 228, 229, 231, 254, 318, 327, 328.

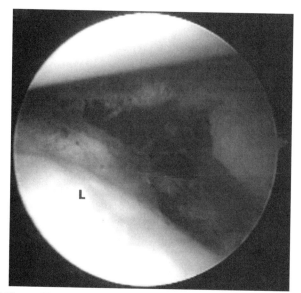

■ **Figure 20–25**

The contracted inferior capsule was avulsed away from the inferior peripheral articular labrum (L) during manipulation. Inferior capsular tears are often found to extend anteriorly and posteriorly through the recesses.

nation.[135,228,254] Arthroscopy affords the opportunity to recognize these pathologies and direct proper rehabilitation once the stiffness has resolved, if necessary.

Examination under Anesthesia

Sometimes the clinical history and examination fail to fit the diagnostic criteria, yet particular elements seem appropriate to a frozen or post-traumatic stiff shoulder. For example, an apprehensive or sensitive patient might have a fixed restraint and no restriction in shoulder range, but muscle spasm or an inability to actively relax prevents an adequate passive motion examination. These patients are typically younger than 40 years, and some have had previous surgery. For these patients we consider examination after the administration of a regional or general anesthetic to eliminate inhibitory painful or anxious reflexes. In our experience, we have found some without any motion restrictions or, rarely, a partial limitation and severe grinding secondary to articular damage with associated anterior or posterior instability. Appropriate rehabilitation exercises or further surgical treatment is then arranged.

NATURAL HISTORY OF SYMPTOMS AND OUTCOME

For any diagnosis, treatment decisions are based on a known course of a disease. Effective treatment is begun only when it is believed that it will positively change the natural history of the disease. The natural history of idiopathic or post-traumatic frozen shoulder, however, is not entirely known and remains controversial inasmuch as the majority of long-term follow-up reports were performed in conjunction with evaluation of the patient's response to a particular treatment regimen.

For years, much of the literature has referred to idiopathic frozen shoulder as a self-limited disease.[65,263,322] Even these studies, however, describe the process as lasting 12 to 18 months before resolution.[117,122,188,329,330] Others have described residual pain or stiffness that may or may not be significantly disabling many years after a frozen shoulder.[25,117,263,290] Differentiation of these outcomes is critical when deciding on the appropriate treatment. If indeed frozen shoulder is a process that will resolve independent of treatment, only palliative treatment is necessary and patients should be encouraged to accommodate their temporary disability. If, however, frozen shoulder is a debilitating, long-standing, and sometimes permanent process, aggressive treatment should begin immediately after diagnosis.

Most patients cannot tolerate a chronically painful extremity during their productive years of life and are concerned about the possibility of permanent dysfunction developing. Patients expect the physician to not only diagnose the condition but also prognosticate how long it will take to recover. Studies with follow-up of more than 2 years and as long as 7 years have consistently demonstrated persistent symptoms in a large percentage of patients (see Fig. 20–18). Meulengracht and Schwartz monitored 65 patients for 3 years and found that 23% had persistent pain and limitation of shoulder motion.[201] Reeves monitored 41 patients for more than 4 years and identified residual stiffness in more than 60%, with 12% of this group displaying severe restriction in motion.[261]

Discrepancy may exist between a patient's perspective of functional limitation and measured motion restrictions. At a 3.5-year follow-up, Binder and coworkers found objective motion restriction in 16 of 40 patients, yet only a few recognized symptomatic functional impairment.[25] This result was quite different from the findings of Shaffer and colleagues. They monitored 68 patients with frozen shoulder for approximately 7 years. On objective motion measurement, 30% were restricted when compared with the opposite unaffected side, yet 50% complained of persistent pain or stiffness.[290]

Further discrepancy occurs when evaluating the symptomatic and functional disturbance caused by a frozen shoulder in the presence of comorbidities. Wolf and Green analyzed the influence of several comorbidities on the self-reported functional status of patients with frozen shoulder.[332] Increasing numbers of comorbidities were associated with worsening scores on the Disabilities of the Arm, Shoulder, and Hand (DASH) survey, Simple Shoulder Test (SST), and SF-36 health status survey. It is clear that the presence of comorbidities can influence patients' perception of their disability and probably alters their response to treatment.

Some prospective studies intended to demonstrate a particular benefit of one treatment over another, only to find that either all or none of the treatment regimens shorten the duration of frozen shoulder, concluded that patients would have recovered with or without intervention.[16,45,74,83] In stark contrast, other authors, who performed comparative studies to demonstrate the benefit of one treatment over another, suggested that early diagnosis plus early treatment results in early recovery.[25,140,263] Carette and colleagues demonstrated in a randomized controlled study that either of two treatment wings resulted in improvement whereas a placebo saline injection group had none.[55] Finally, Helbig and coworkers and Harryman and colleagues observed that the degree of disability and the duration of symptoms before treatment in patients without diabetes had no influence on the final outcome, but that treatment appeared to effectively abbreviate the disease course.[135,142]

Regression analyses have been performed to assess significant variables that would best prognosticate the course of disease. Dominant arm involvement has been reported as a good prognostic indicator, whereas patient occupation, ability to work, duration of stiffness, associated injuries, and the treatment program used did not achieve statistical significance when analyzed against other outcome measures.[25,63,135] The finding of an associated intrinsic pathology such as a partial-thickness rotator cuff tear[135] or insulin-dependent diabetes of more than 10 years' duration would tend to indicate a poorer prognosis.[101,155,205]

The preponderance of evidence suggests that frozen shoulder is not a self-limited process and, if untreated, can result in persistent and permanent pain and disability. Treatment is therefore indicated for all patients who can participate in the required therapeutic regimens.

TREATMENT

The choice of treatment of shoulder stiffness should always be aligned according to the duration and severity of symptoms to avoid undertreatment or overtreatment. Because shoulder stiffness often develops in response to a known variety of initiating factors, it is important to consider the potential cause or underlying disease and the appropriate timing of treatment in the context of the patient's needs, risk factors, and tolerance. Two examples follow.

Treating the Source of the Pain

If a frozen shoulder develops subsequent to painful cervical radiculitis, it is most appropriate to primarily address the herniated cervical disk to eliminate the source of pain while encouraging a gentle shoulder stretching program instead of first manipulating the shoulder to restore full range. The symptoms in the neck will probably prevent adequate shoulder rehabilitation after manipulation.

Treating the Stiffness

If a patient has a small rotator cuff tear and shoulder stiffness develops secondarily, it is important to treat the shoulder stiffness as the primary problem to fully recover range of motion before considering a rotator cuff repair. A rotator cuff tear may improve with rehabilitation alone, and a repair is often a "shoulder-tightening" procedure that may result in increased stiffness postoperatively.

These examples enumerate cases with a recognizable "cause and effect" of shoulder stiffness. After the differential diagnosis has been exhausted, however, we are frequently left with idiopathic stiffness that on its own must always be treated aggressively to prevent progression of disease. A specific plan that follows an appropriate algorithm and presents the least risk to the patient is best (see Fig. 20–22).

In the painful phase of shoulder stiffness, it is often beneficial to reduce discomfort by using methods that do not involve narcotics. Ice or heat, rest or activity, support or traction, electrical or ultrasonic stimulation, chiropractic mobilization, and many other "modalities" have been used to reduce pain, but few have shown significant benefit relative to another.

In the review of treatment that follows, there are six major groups of therapeutic approaches, each of which includes a variety of therapeutic regimens. These six treatment categories are

1. Supportive treatment, including observation and passive external modalities such as immobilization, heat, ice, diathermy, ultrasound, transcutaneous electrical nerve stimulation (TENS), and massage
2. Medications given orally, topically, and parenterally (locally and intra-articularly), such as nonsteroidal anti-inflammatory agents, analgesics, narcotics, neuroleptics, enzymatic preparations, and corticosteroids
3. Stretching exercises or traction applied by the patient, mechanically by a device, or by an assistant, typically consisting of gentle stretching, with or without muscle activity
4. Injections of fluid, arthrographic dye, or medications (e.g., long-acting anesthetic agents with or without corticosteroids) for the purpose of joint distention to release capsular contracture (brisement)
5. Manipulative therapy with or without anesthesia to release adhesions or contracted structures
6. Surgical release of adhesions or contracted structures by open or arthroscopic means

Prophylaxis

The primary method of treatment of either a frozen or post-traumatic stiff shoulder is the same—prevention! The initial challenge is to avoid the natural tendency of most treating physicians to immobilize a painful extremity until comfort returns. The period of enforced immobilization, though provisionally somewhat comforting to the patient, will prolong and worsen the capsular contracture, delay diagnosis of an underlying condition, and may begin a self-propagating spiral of unrelenting shoulder pain, immobilization, and predictable motion loss.

Analgesics

Nonsteroidal anti-inflammatory drugs or salicylates and even nonsalicylate analgesics such as acetaminophen are said to be effective in alleviating the painful distress of shoulder stiffness.[27,40,272] The degree of relief from stiff shoulder conditions has been used frequently to test and compare a wide range of nonsteroidal anti-inflammatory medications.[32,87,97,113,151]

Analgesics and suitable anti-inflammatory agents can be given systemically or applied locally.[222] Binder and colleagues found that patients experienced greater pain relief with nonsalicylate analgesics than with nonsteroidal agents.[27] Lee and associates were able to show that patients who performed exercises regularly demonstrated greater improvement when analgesics were added.[177] The use of analgesics should therefore be combined with an early gentle stretching exercise program.

Injections

Injections are often offered in an attempt to directly suppress or potentially eliminate the irritative source of the pain. Because an inflammatory phase is part of the pathophysiologic evolution of these painful conditions, the use of corticosteroids has often been advocated. However, their use is not without risk or morbidity. The literature is extremely controversial regarding the benefit of this treatment.

Periarticular Injections

Well-localized painful periscapular areas are defined as "trigger points" or "tender points." Trigger point injections are generally performed about the subscapularis tendon and the periscapular musculature to reduce symptoms of myofascial pain or fibrositis.[310] Some clinicians inject these painful sites with local anesthetics such as lidocaine or bupivacaine admixed with a steroid such as hydrocortisone. The effectiveness of these treatments is unknown to the authors.

Injections in other sites at the point of maximal tenderness about the shoulder and the periarticular region have been tried and found to be unsuccessful in providing long-term benefit or pain relief.[147,207] On the other hand, Steinbrocker and Argyros reported rather surprising results: 85% restoration of function in 95% of 42 patients after multiple injections into the supraspinatus tendon, subdeltoid bursa, bicipital tendon, and joint capsule.[297] No control group, however, was provided.

Paired Injections

A paired injection refers to a local anesthetic and steroid given intra-articularly and into the subacromial bursa in an attempt to eliminate "pain and inflammation." Using comparative treatment regimens, studies by Richardson and by Bulgen and coworkers failed to show a significant difference or improvement in pain relief and increase in shoulder movement at follow-up examination after paired injections with deposition of steroids.[45,269] Possibly, an inaccurate injection location is responsible for the poor response. Richardson monitored attempts at intra-articular injection with radiopaque dye and noted that the majority of physicians were unsuccessful in delivering the fluid into the shoulder joint.[269] Weiss and Ting recommended routine use of arthrography to deliver an intra-articular dose of steroids.[325]

In England, Dacre and associates compared the use of local steroids and physiotherapy in a prospective, randomized, observer-blind trial to assess the cost and efficacy of conventional nonoperative therapy for a painful stiff shoulder. Their results show that local steroid injections were as effective as physiotherapy alone or in combination. They provided rapid treatment and were less expensive. In uncomplicated cases, a local steroid injection was the most cost-effective treatment.[74]

Patients referred to our clinic are often relieved when we assure them that our primary treatment will not involve repetitive steroid injections. We believe that steroid injections are overused and that patients should not be treated with an exhaustive series of injections to reduce pain. We recognize that other investigators, however, have found injections of methylprednisolone to be significantly beneficial.[281]

Intra-Articular Injections

Macnab proposed an autoimmune hypothesis for the frozen shoulder whereby the degenerative tendon of the supraspinatus releases proteinaceous fragments that invoke an inflammatory foreign body response in the glenohumeral joint.[190] Assuming this hypothesis to be true, steroids may suppress the painful inflammatory response. On the other hand, the deleterious effects of intra-articular steroids on tendon metabolism and articular hyaline cartilage are well documented.[77,162,303]

Studies that evaluate the response to intra-articular injections generally combine the injection with other treatment modalities and rarely compare the efficacy of repository steroids alone. Williams and associates compared repetitive intra-articular injections of hydrocortisone acetate with serial stellate ganglion blocks, but all patients were also instructed in an exercise program and given analgesics.[329] At follow-up, the investigators were unable to demonstrate improvement in half the patients who received steroids, and no significant differences in treatment groups were found. In a combined comparative treatment study, Lee and colleagues failed to show a benefit of combined intra-articular hydrocortisone injections and exercise versus heat and exercise; however, overall, they found that patients improved more than those who used analgesics alone.[178]

Cyriax and Trosier found no benefit of intra-articular hydrocortisone injections, and Quin reported that his experience with these injections in the treatment of frozen shoulder was not encouraging.[73,259] Quin went on to say, however, that "a local injection of hydrocortisone may give some relief of pain in cases of frozen shoulder, but it has very little effect in restoring movement."[259] A recent meta-analysis suggested little evidence of a beneficial role of corticosteroid injection for idiopathic frozen shoulder.[43]

Some investigators are advocates of intra-articular steroid injections for painful shoulder stiffness.[325] Hollingworth and colleagues were able to demonstrate that intra-articular steroid injections were more advantageous than trigger point injections.[147] They reported that a quarter of the patients with frozen shoulder received benefit from an intra-articular injection whereas none of the other patients who received the other treatment were relieved. Thomas and associates demonstrated a 50% improvement in pain scores after intra-articular injection and only a 13% increase in range of motion.[306] Some investigators have failed to demonstrate an improvement in the rate of recovery in shoulder range.[259] Conversely, Arslan and Celiker, in a controlled study, demonstrated similar improvement in motion when comparing steroid injection and physiotherapy, although the study numbers were small.[8] Carette and coworkers demonstrated a statistically significant improvement after treatment with a corticosteroid injection plus exercise versus exercise alone or placebo treatment.[55]

Though usually safe, intra-articular injections pose a small risk of infection. Over the past 8 years, we have seen six cases of chronic sepsis referred to our practice after steroid and arthrographic injection. In some of these cases, the only treatment possible was shoulder fusion. Seradge and Anderson reported a case of fatal clostridial myonecrosis that occurred after an intra-articular injection of steroids in the shoulder.[289] With these data in mind, it behooves the practitioner to prepare the skin and handle the procedure as though it were surgical.

Occasionally, a patient is unable to tolerate physical therapy exercises solely because of intractable pain. In this circumstance, an intra-articular steroid injection might provide enough relief for the patient to tolerate an exercise program. If a steroid injection appears to be indicated, remember that the use of steroids in diabetic patients often causes blood glucose fluctuations and may incur a greater risk of infection. We do not advocate the routine use of intra-articular steroid injections for the treatment of shoulder stiffness.

Physiotherapy

Physiotherapy in the form of gentle, firm stretching exercises in various planes of motion has been proved to be effective in the relief of pain and recovery of range of motion in up to 90% of patients with chronic frozen shoulder.[242] In 226 frozen shoulders treated with stretching exercises alone, Watson-Jones found that only 5% failed to regain satisfactory range within 6 months.[322] He recommended 3 minutes of active stretching each hour. Griggs and coworkers demonstrated satisfactory results in 90% of 75 patients who completed a stretching program for frozen shoulder.[119] Only seven of their patients required more aggressive intervention. The therapeutic advantage of performing passive stretching in abduction in addition to active exercises was confirmed by Nicholson.[223] Physical therapy has been shown to improve health-related quality of life.[83]

Occasionally, physiotherapy has been demonstrated to be inadequate in relieving symptomatic stiffness and has been shown to actually exacerbate the condition. Rizk and associates reported on patients who received physical therapy along with other modalities, and only 60% achieved the ability to sleep pain free after 5 months' duration.[272] Up to a third of Hazleman's patients who were treated by physiotherapy alone experienced an increase in their pain, and only half of this group significantly improved with exercises.[140]

Other therapeutic modalities such as the application of ice packs or ice massage, microwaves, short waves, and heat lamps have not proved to be particularly beneficial in any specific phase of shoulder stiffness. Often, however, heat is applied to increase the extensibility of tight capsular tissues before range-of-motion stretching therapy.[180] A double-blind trial designed to test the efficacy of ultrasound in patients with tendinitis, bursitis, and adhesive capsulitis of the shoulder found little or no benefit when combined with range-of-motion exercises or nonsteroidal anti-inflammatory medications.[86] Although ultrasound also provides an increase in temperature that should augment tissue flexibility, these treatments did not offer any specific advantage over heat and therapeutic exercises in a short-term follow-up study performed by Quin.[260]

Therapeutic exercises are often combined with stimuli in an attempt to overload and distract the mind away from painful sensations. Echternach demonstrated a significant improvement in the recovery of motion in a comparative study using "audio analgesia" as an adjunct to mobilization in patients with chronic frozen shoulder.[90] He also reported a reduction in the number of treatments necessary for recovery. Similarly, Rizk and colleagues used TENS to diminish pain as opposed to exercises alone and found a significant improvement and early recovery of shoulder range.[272]

In most patients, physiotherapy can be successfully performed as a strictly home-based program. At our institution, we refer to this program as the Jackins program after our therapist Sarah Jackins (Fig. 20–26A to D). A single instructional visit to a physical therapist is often adequate, with monthly visits to the physician and therapist to determine whether the symptoms and range of motion are improving. At each visit the patient should demonstrate the motions, and the range is recorded by the same examiner. A comparison is made with the values from the previous visit and with the opposite side. Ongoing encouragement from the family, physician, and therapist is extremely valuable, and once treatment is initiated, the physician's role often becomes that of a cheerleader.

We stress daily and frequent home therapy exercises with the Jackins exercise program.[108,129,195] The four cornerstones of this program are patient motivation, frequency, consistency, and the four quadrants of capsular stretch. We recommend 10 repetitions of each exercise, held for 10 seconds each stretch, performed five times each day. This exercise program must be performed gently against the limits of tolerance. We favor frequency over forcefulness and avoid the "no pain, no gain" regimen.

Short periods of exercise with increased frequency have proved to be therapeutic.[25,187,195,322] Leffert and others have emphasized that the patient must assume primary responsibility and tolerate the discomfort that comes along with the exercise program to recover fully.[72,179,195,199,213]

We do not recommend performing any light-resistance strengthening or a muscle-toning exercise program until the patient has recovered functional range and comfort.[195]

Distention Arthrography or Brisement

Intra-articular fluid injection has been used to (1) evaluate intra-articular pressure, (2) measure joint compliance in response to a fluid challenge, and (3) measure the

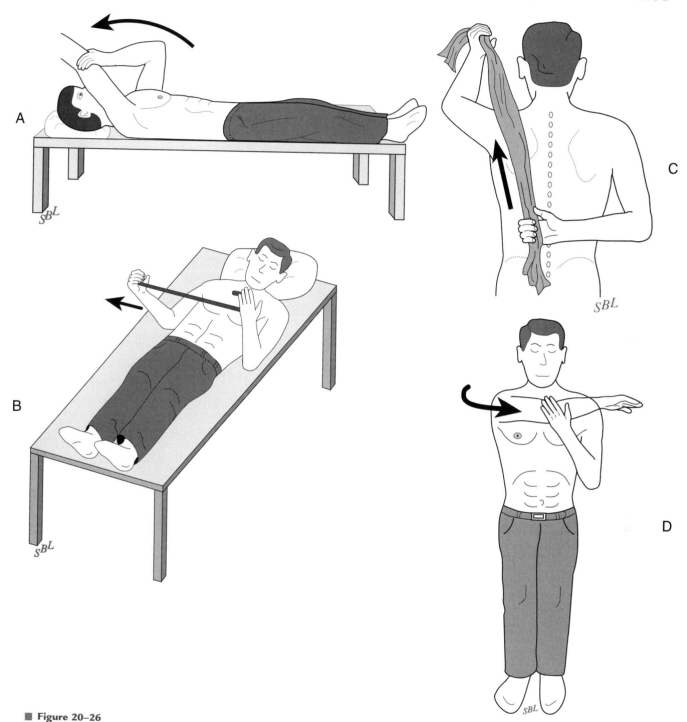

■ Figure 20–26

The Jackins stretching program. **A,** Forward elevation stretch. **B,** External rotation stretch. **C,** Internal rotation stretch. **D,** Cross-body stretch. *(From Matsen FA III, Lippitt SB, Sidles JA, and Harryman DT II: Practical Evaluation and Management of the Shoulder. Philadelphia: WB Saunders, 1994.)*

capacity and maximal limit of progressively increased intra-articular pressure until the contracted gleno-humeral capsule ruptures. This technique received wide attention as an option in the treatment of frozen and post-traumatic stiff shoulder. On a literature review of these methods, most studies profess an extremely low risk and a high benefit ratio.[4,69,96,124,173,204,234,261,291] Many of these

studies include therapeutic exercise, which is probably a confounding variable.

Lundberg reported that Payr in 1931 was the first to describe the use of "brisement," a distensible capsular stretching and rupturing technique.[188,245] Since then, brisement has become a common outpatient procedure used in surgical and radiographic suites and even office practice. In a review of the literature, only a single study did not find a significant improvement in the degree of pain or an increase in motion at a follow-up of 1 to 3 months. Corbeil and associates conducted a double-blind, prospective study of 45 patients with frozen shoulder to compare the therapeutic efficacy of nondistention and distention arthrography in combination with intra-articular steroid injection.[70] Initially, they found that 80% of the patients experienced a diminution in nocturnal pain with both treatment regimens. During the initial months, range of motion was significantly improved, but after 3 months, no significant difference in the degree of pain or range of motion could be found between the two treatment regimens. In a critical literature review, Alvado and coworkers questioned the quality of much of the capsular distention literature but still thought that the literature supported the use of this technique versus intra-articular injection alone.[2] In a small, prospective, randomized study, Gam and colleagues confirmed improved comfort and function in patients treated with distention and corticosteroid injection versus steroid alone.[105]

The procedure is performed by insufflating the glenohumeral joint with incremental injections of fluid so that intra-articular pressure is progressively increased to greater than 800 mm Hg and up to a maximum of 1500 mm Hg.[121,137,261] During the initial injection phase, an arthrogram is often obtained to confirm intra-articular instillation of fluid. Some authors instill a volume of approximately 60 to 100 mL followed by manipulation to produce hydrostatic distention of the joint capsule.[69] Reeves found that disruption occurs at the weakest point in the capsule, namely, the subcoracoid bursa or the biceps tendon sheath.[261]

Sharma and associates compared the results of brisement and MUA and found significantly better results after distention.[291] In distinct opposition, Reeves, when analyzing time until resolution of disease, found that distention arthrography compared unfavorably with MUA.[261,262] Reeves also compared the results of this procedure in patients with a frozen or post-traumatic stiff shoulder.[262] In post-traumatic stiff shoulders, Reeves found less severe joint restriction and a poorer response to serial distention, as opposed to 67% recovery by 6 months after treatment in those with a frozen shoulder. A reputable cadre of investigators have performed distention arthrography and claim that hydraulic distention is relatively noninvasive, simple to perform, and an effective mechanism in achieving symptomatic lasting relief of frozen shoulder.[96,274,291,295]

Andren and Lundberg noted that the good results associated with joint distention are seen primarily in patients without severe restriction in motion and in those in whom moderate joint distention was successful before rupture.[4] They also found that relief of pain may occur without improvement in motion and that the procedure may be repeated at a later date to achieve additional improvement in function. Older and coworkers demonstrated that although distention arthrography alone did not seem to provide relief of pain, it did serve as an adjunct to range-of-motion exercises.[234]

Like Corbeil and associates,[70] the authors have used distention arthrography and failed to find lasting benefit.

Our patients with severe motion restriction eventually returned for further treatment. Because the entire capsule in a frozen shoulder is involved in the inflammatory process and subsequent capsular fibrosis, a treatment that has been found to only rupture the anterior capsule and not specifically reduce inflammation or lengthen the contracted capsule seems an unlikely solution.

Prolonged Traction

Kottke and colleagues explained that the attachments between collagen fibers show high resistance to suddenly applied tension, but that they relax or creep when exposed to prolonged tension.[170] Applying this logic to the awake patient, Rizk and associates exerted prolonged traction with a pulley and weights to the affected upper extremity in 28 frozen shoulders and compared the results with those of 28 shoulders treated by heat and therapeutic exercises. Although both groups demonstrated improvement in range of motion, the increase was significantly greater in those who were treated with progressive abduction traction while pain was controlled with TENS.[272]

Neurologic Blockade

In 1941, Wertheim and Rovenstine were the first to report on the use of suprascapular nerve blockade for relief of shoulder pain.[326] Later, Koppell and Thompson explained that the suprascapular nerve supplied not only motor but also sensory innervation to the external rotators and the shoulder joint.[169] They hypothesized that the suprascapular nerve might be the source of pain in patients with frozen shoulder and performed a suprascapular block in 20 cases, with substantial pain relief within 24 hours in the majority. Because of the dramatic response to these blocks, they surmised that the suprascapular nerve was inflamed and the apparent source of pain in these conditions. In more recent reports from the anesthesiology literature, other authors have recommended a suprascapular block with a local anesthetic and steroid to relieve pain.[57,76,114]

Wassef studied the use of suprascapular nerve blockade to manage a frozen shoulder associated with reflex sympathetic dystrophy.[320] He found not only a significant increase in comfort with an improvement in the patient's tolerance to deep pressure on the shoulder joint but also an improved passive range of motion when blocks were repeated twice weekly for a total of two to four treatments. This treatment, however, has not been proved to offer any advantage over other treatment modalities.

Recently, Dahan and colleagues randomized patients suffering from frozen shoulder to either a suprascapular nerve block group or a placebo cohort.[75] At 1 month after injection, the treatment group patients had significantly less pain than those in the control group. Improved comfort, however, did not translate into increased range or better function. As with other studies, patients were also instructed in a home stretching program, which somewhat equilibrates the groups and can confuse the results. Jones and Chattopadhyay compared suprascapular nerve blockade with intra-articular corticosteroid injection and found quicker return of comfort and function in the nerve block group.[158]

Isolated Alternative Methods

Ultrasound

Ultrasound is widely used to treat patients with painful shoulder conditions, but its use may not be justified. In a prospective study, ice and ultrasonic application were compared in a series of patients with frozen shoulder syndrome, and no significant advantage of one treatment over the other was appreciated.[125] In a double-blind comparison, patients with painful shoulder stiffness were randomized into one of three treatment groups: ultrasound, conventional therapeutic exercises, and nonsteroidal anti-inflammatory drugs plus exercises.[86] Ultrasound offered no benefit over the other methods.

Intra-articular Protein Instillation

Leardini and colleagues performed intra-articular injections of hyaluronic acid into painful shoulders in which either osteoarthritis or adhesive capsulitis was diagnosed.[176] Though short in follow-up, the authors reported rapid and significant improvement in joint mobility and comfort. The results, however, were not compared with those of a control group. Rovetta and Monteforte randomized patients into sodium hyaluronate plus steroid versus steroid alone for the treatment of frozen shoulder.[280] Both groups also received physical therapy. Although the authors believed that hyaluronate may offer some benefit, both treatment groups substantially improved. Enzymes such as α-chymotrypsin and hylase have also been injected into the shoulder, but the beneficial results are obscured by the combination with physiotherapy.[10,21]

Salmon Calcitonin

In a prospective study that included 50 cases of frozen shoulder divided into three etiologic groups, Waldburger and associates demonstrated a statistically significant effect on pain reduction in patients treated with early mobilization associated with subcutaneous salmon calcitonin injection versus physiotherapy alone.[315] This improvement was noted only in patients with post-traumatic frozen shoulders and not in those that were idiopathic or neurologic in origin. Other investigators have noted a similar benefit of pain reduction with salmon calcitonin used for frozen shoulder, as well as other presumed inflammatory conditions of the shoulder.[6]

Roentgen Therapy

In surprisingly large series,[5,30,38,138,342] radiation proved to be effective in eliminating pain from shoulder stiffness in up to 70%, but the long-term risks were not considered. Quin compared radiation therapy with ultrasound or heat and physiotherapy and did not find a treatment advantage.[260] In a prospective study of 233 patients with periarthritis, Hassenstein identified improvement in only 26%.[138] The authors agree with Coventry, who in 1953 surmised that radiotherapy did not have much effect on chronic forms of frozen shoulder.[72] Radiotherapy is no longer used in the United States for the treatment of idiopathic frozen shoulder. Radiation is used occasionally in association with shoulder stiffness secondary to heterotopic ossification to prevent a recurrence of ectopic bone after surgical resection (see later under "Open Surgical Release").

Acupuncture

In patients with frozen shoulder who had received conventional physiotherapy with limited success, six acupuncture treatment sessions were required to achieve an excellent response and complete recovery.[93] Lin and associates randomly divided 150 patients with frozen shoulder into three groups treated with electroacupuncture (EAP), regional nerve block (RNB), and a combination of both treatments.[183] They found that the combined EAP and RNB method resulted in significantly high pain control with a long duration and better range of motion than either EAP or RNB alone did. Finally, Sun and associates randomized patients into either physiotherapy or therapy plus acupuncture groups.[301] These investigators demonstrated a statistically significant improvement in Constant scores after acupuncture treatment in comparison to therapy alone.

Other Modalities

Common modalities such as massage and electrophysiotherapy or more atypical modalities such as hyperbaric oxygen and magnetotherapy have been tried.[7,31,78,120] Taken together, these studies, which attempt to compare and evaluate the effect of one alternative treatment against another, lack rigid diagnostic criteria and a control population. None of these treatments would fit into a standard treatment algorithm.

Operative Treatment

When a patient with a stiff shoulder remains symptomatic and fails a minimum of 6 months of appropriate nonoperative treatment, manipulative or surgical intervention is usually considered. All patients should be aware that no treatment cures all cases and that more aggressive methods incur a greater risk of morbidity. In addition, although we discuss each of these procedures as separate treatment entities, in fact they are frequently combined to provide for maximal restoration of motion.

It is reasonable to again state that of patients who continue to have a significant loss of shoulder motion, less than 5% to 20% remain functionally disabled with persistent symptomatic impairment.[25,63,263,293] Often, many of these refractory patients are insulin-dependent diabetics. For recalcitrant frozen shoulders, aggressive surgical release by open or arthroscopic methods may be the only option.[129,135,179,198,228,254,286,318]

For all surgical procedures, we recommend the use of an interscalene brachial plexus block with or without an indwelling interscalene catheter either as the primary anesthetic or as an adjunct to general anesthesia. For an idiopathic frozen shoulder that requires surgical intervention, a single interscalene injection is our standard. This regional long-lasting anesthetic allows the patient to tolerate passive motion immediately after the procedure. As an additional benefit, for as long as 6 to 8 hours after completion of the procedure, the surgeon can return to the patient to demonstrate the full range of motion achieved. The block is generally effective for 12 hours or more when long-acting bupivacaine is combined with epinephrine, and with this regimen, all surgical interventions for idiopathic frozen shoulder are performed on an outpatient basis.

As will be discussed, surgical interventions for a post-traumatic and, in particular, a postsurgical stiff shoulder are less successful than for an idiopathic frozen shoulder. In these cases, we routinely use an indwelling interscalene catheter with continuous interscalene anesthesia and an overnight hospital stay. This approach permits an aggressive mobilization program. Pollock and associates have found a significant advantage in recovered motion with the use of indwelling catheters in a large series of patients.[254]

Manipulation under Anesthesia

For well over a century, MUA has been the primary mode of treatment recommended for a persistent frozen shoulder.[88,256] Although the effectiveness of this treatment has been documented by several studies,[122,123,142,330] others have denounced its use.[60,81,179,200] Most of those who shun manipulation cite complications that deterred their favor of the method.

Manipulation is primarily indicated for patients who are worsening after at least 3 months of an appropriate nonoperative exercise regimen or after failure to respond to a 6-month exercise program.[129,135,165,188] Kessel and associates suggested that patients who were symptomatic for more than 6 months before manipulative treatment achieved a greater degree of improvement than did those who had a shorter duration of symptoms.[165] Manipulation is generally contraindicated in patients with severe osteopenia of the humerus and long-term diabetes mellitus (longer than 20 years).[129,135,155]

Complications of manipulation do occur, although the cumulative reported risk of an inadvertent event is less than 1%. Reported complications of the procedure include subscapularis and rotator cuff rupture,[81] surgical neck and humeral shaft fracture,[123] and dislocation.[60,258] We have also treated a patient who was referred with a complete brachial plexus palsy after manipulation that resulted in an anterior/inferior dislocation. Given that many patients with frozen shoulders will suffer from osteopenia of the proximal part of the humerus,[232] the risk of fracture after manipulation is not unexpected. The reported rate of recurrent stiffness is between 5% and 20%; however, most of the studies monitored patients for approximately 6 months.[306,330] Janda and Hawkins

reported an unacceptably high rate of recontracture after manipulation in patients with long-term insulin-dependent diabetes.[155]

The immediate effects of manipulation on structures about the shoulder have been observed at open and arthroscopic surgery. At open surgery, Neviaser and DePalma separately recorded tears in the subscapularis muscle and tendon along with disruption of the anterior and inferior capsule. Tears have also been observed in the supraspinatus tendon and the long head of the biceps tendon.[199,262]

The technique of shoulder manipulation is typically performed under an interscalene brachial plexus block or a general anesthetic, but it has been performed as an outpatient treatment and with a local injection combined with hydrostatic distention.[69] The standard technique is performed by applying a constant controlled force to the proximal end of the humerus while holding the scapula stable. Sudden force causes greater risk to normal structures.[142] Most authors recommend an initial abduction force[123,257]; however, Charnley recommended against this maneuver before achieving external rotation to avoid a shoulder dislocation.[60] A crepitant disruptive release of the articular capsule is considered to be a good prognostic sign because immediate full motion is usually recovered.[128,165,258] Increased force should not be applied if a crepitant release does not ensue under constantly applied force.[129,188] Placzek and colleagues recommended a translational force instead of a rotational force, which they believed lessened the chance of fracture and gave results similar to those of traditional manipulation.[253] If the recovered motion is not symmetrical to the opposite side or recurs in a short time postoperatively, repeat manipulation may be necessary and indicated.[122,128,142]

After manipulation is completed, many authors have recommended injecting the shoulder with a corticosteroid to limit early healing of the capsular disruption and to diminish the local inflammation and pain associated with the procedure,[123,128,129,135,142] although its use has not been definitively proved to enhance the outcome.[167] Quigley demonstrated in more than 100 cases that no medication other than codeine was required in the immediate postmanipulation period to control pain.[258] Thomas and associates randomly allocated 30 patients with frozen shoulders to two groups, one with manipulation and steroid use and the other with intra-articular steroids alone.[306] They found that the group treated by manipulation and steroid injection retained significantly greater movement (40% versus 13%) and had less pain at follow-up (80% versus 47%) than did those treated by steroid injection alone. Weiser performed manipulation under a local anesthetic with three to five treatment sessions and noted full recovery in 60%.[324]

The reported results of shoulder manipulation alone or in combination with steroid injection are extremely variable, with a range of 25% to over 90% of patients significantly improved by 3 months after manipulation and an average of 70% improved by 6 months.* Recently,

---

*See references 23, 67, 122, 123, 128, 142, 144, 161, 186, 188, 238, 258, 259, 262, 265, 306, 323, 324.

Dodenhoff and colleagues found that 94% of 37 patients who underwent MUA were satisfied with their result, but that 12.8% of patients retained significant persistent disability.[85] Othman and Taylor, in a review of 74 patients who underwent MUA, found that significant improvement in range and comfort occurred as early as 3 weeks postoperatively.[238] Reichmister and Friedman demonstrated a success rate of 97% after MUA, although 8% of patients required a second manipulation.[265] However, Lundberg noted no change in the time course of disease after manipulation.[188]

Manipulation may also be performed under local anesthesia after infiltrating the glenohumeral joint with a substantial volume of local anesthetic.[107,187,324] Some of these authors also recommend subacromial injection and arthrographic visualization before and after manipulation. These reports claim successful relief of pain and recovered motion in approximately two thirds of patients; however, a greater percentage were relieved of discomfort alone.

A variety of postmanipulation management regimens have been recommended. After successful manipulation, systemic steroids have been given but are not recommended because of the potential side effects and lack of lasting benefit.[18,186,201] Some authors put the extremity into immediate passive motion. As an alternative to passive motion, Neviaser described attaching the arm to the bed in a position of abduction and external rotation, similar to that originally described by Codman.[65,217] Although the use of prolonged traction may stretch out residual contractures and promote range, it may require significant narcotic analgesia.[65,221] Moreover, this maneuver selectively stretches only one region of the contracted capsule, specifically, the anteroinferior portion, with the remaining sections of capsule left in a position of potential recontracture. While still under a regional interscalene block, our patients are instructed in a four-quadrant capsular stretching program (refer to Jackins' stretching program).[129,135] Neviaser has recommended a 3- to 5-day inpatient visit.[217] He also suggested that after discharge, the patient should maintain the abducted and externally rotated position at night for 3 weeks to eliminate stiffness.

Manipulation and Arthroscopy

Although MUA clearly has its place, it also has several disadvantages. One of these disadvantages is the lack of a synovectomy. If, as we have discussed previously, synovitis is one of the precipitating factors that leads to capsular fibrosis, persistent synovitis after MUA may be one of the factors leading to recurrence of contracture. Several investigators have therefore investigated arthroscopy with joint lavage and synovectomy after MUA as a technique to decrease the chance of failure.[3,54,61,149,172,202,254,327]

Andersen and colleagues reviewed 25 patients who underwent combined MUA and arthroscopy for frozen shoulder.[3] Seventy-five percent regained full motion and 79% were pain free. Pollock and coworkers demonstrated an 83% success rate with this algorithm, although recalcitrant patients did undergo release of the coracohumeral ligament.[254]

Open Surgical Release

Codman originally described open release of adhesions in the subacromial and subdeltoid bursa.[65] Neviaser found it necessary to perform an arthrotomy through an anterior axillary approach in patients whose stiffness recurred after MUA.[217] He, like his father, recommended release of periarticular adhesions and the tightly contracted articular capsule from the humeral head, especially in the location of the axillary fold.[213]

Lippman asserted that open lysis of adhesions about the long head of the biceps tendon would liberate the shoulder from restricted motion.[185] Continuing in this mode, Simmonds performed complete excision of the biceps long head tendon in cases of intractable frozen shoulder, but with no improvement in range of motion.[293] He also noted that there were no intra-articular adhesions between the articular capsule and the surface of the joint.

In patients who failed to improve after gentle manipulation, Harmon performed soft tissue release of contracted tissues about the joint in eight patients and found the results to be similar to those of closed manipulation in all except two patients with intractable stiffness.[128] Alternatively, Harmon treated 30 cases of shoulder stiffness with excision of the acromion and the acromioclavicular joint. In all cases, restoration of active abduction to 160 degrees or more was achieved by 3 months after surgery.

McLaughlin described release of the biceps tendon and subscapularis as treatment of shoulder contracture.[199] Leffert recommended surgical release of the structures responsible for restricted motion when a patient failed to improve after 6 months of a nonoperative therapeutic regimen.[179] Matsen and Kirby found that surgical release of the capsule was safer than closed manipulation in patients with recalcitrant stiffness and osteoporosis that did not respond to 6 months of home exercise therapy.[194] Kieras and Matsen reported on open release in the management of refractory frozen shoulder in 12 patients, 4 of whom were insulin-dependent diabetics.[166] The duration of preoperative symptoms and treatment averaged 16 months. The average flexion improved from 73 degrees (range, 20 to 95) to 132 degrees (range, 90 to 150). The average external rotation improved from 3 degrees (range, 5 to 25) to 45 degrees (range, 15 to 60). Pain was decreased or eliminated in all patients at 2-year follow-up. No complications occurred, and all patients returned to work.

In 1957, Kernwein and colleagues performed open release of the capsule and coracohumeral ligament in 4 of 12 patients with frozen shoulder and found that these tissues were markedly thickened and inelastic.[163] In 1987 and in 1990, Nobuhara and coauthors reported on dysfunctional range in shoulders with a tight rotator interval capsule, which was remarkably relieved in 21 shoulders by local release of this contracture.[224] Ozaki and associates treated 17 of 365 patients who had recalcitrant chronic shoulder stiffness, and at surgery, the major tether restricting glenohumeral movement was identified as a contracture of the coracohumeral ligament within the rotator interval capsule.[239] Release of this contracted structure relieved pain and restored motion in all patients.

They also noted that the long head of the biceps was inflamed and stenosed beneath the contracted coracohumeral ligament and rotator interval capsule.

In patients in whom severe stiffness and a marked internal rotation contracture developed after a stroke, Braun and associates performed excision of the subscapularis tendon and incision of the pectoralis major insertion while preserving the anterior capsule.[36] Of 13 patients who were treated in this manner, 3 were not improved but 10 regained 90 degrees of abduction, 20 degrees of external rotation, and complete pain relief within 2 months postoperatively.

Omari and Bunker recently published their results of open release in 25 patients.[236] These patients came from an initial group of 75, and they had failed both therapy and manipulation, so they were the most affected patients. Surgical findings included a contracted, fibrotic coracohumeral ligament, which was excised as part of the procedure. Good or excellent results were seen in 20 of 25 patients, with diabetic patients having worse results.

Our current indication for open surgical release includes cases that cannot be managed by arthroscopic capsular release and subacromial lysis of adhesions. Often, the indication is a post-traumatic surgical stiff shoulder. For example, a patient with stiffness after a Putti-Platt repair may have severe intra- and extra-articular postsurgical contractures and is best managed by open release of the HSMI, lengthening of the subscapularis tendon, and release of the contracted articular capsule. Advantages of open surgical release include (1) access to the entire HSMI, (2) lengthening of musculotendinous subscapularis contractures, and (3) excision of heterotopic ossification or bone spurs (Fig. 20–27).[129,166]

Open surgical release also has significant disadvantages and risks. It can be technically difficult to achieve a complete posterior capsule release by open means. Postoperative pain and the need to protect a repaired or lengthened subscapularis tendon inhibit the patient from performing the unrestricted full-range stretching program necessary to maintain all the motion achieved under anesthesia. Finally, extended hospitalization may be necessary for pain control.

As an alternative to open release of contracted tissues, Baumann offers a method of denervating the ventral aspect of the shoulder capsule to cause an immediate and progressive decrease or total elimination of shoulder pain.[17] He reported on 20 shoulders treated in this fashion, with 85% having painless mobilization and total rehabilitation of joint function. This experience, however, has not been duplicated.

Arthroscopic Surgical Release

The earliest report of actually using arthroscopic equipment to perform a partial arthroscopic surgical release of a contracted articular capsule was by Conti in France in 1979.[68] He divided the rotator interval capsule with a trocar and forceps, instilled a corticosteroid, and performed gentle manipulation of the shoulder. Sixteen of 18 patients fully recovered within 3 weeks and 2 other

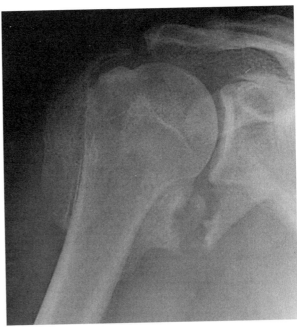

■ **Figure 20–27**
Radiograph of a patient with severe shoulder stiffness secondary to heterotopic ossification associated with a head injury. This condition is best treated by complete capsular release, excision of heterotopic ossification, lysis of adhesions in the humeroscapular motion interface, and subscapularis tendon lengthening.

patients recovered by 3 to 6 months. Using a similar technique, Ogilvie-Harris and Wiley reported arthroscopic "freeing up" with a blunt instrument and in some cases cutting of the anterior capsule in a controlled manner to improve recalcitrant stiffness in patients with a frozen shoulder.[231] Eleven of the 81 patients were diabetic, and in those, the results were less satisfactory.

Early reports that used arthroscopic methods in the treatment of stiff shoulder generally combined examination of the glenohumeral joint with joint distention to stretch the tight capsular constraints and manipulation. In 1980, Wiley and Older were the first to report this procedure in 10 patients, all of whom were relieved of their symptom.[328] In 1991, Hsu and Chan performed a prospective study of 75 patients and demonstrated that arthroscopic distention or manipulation combined with physiotherapy was significantly better than physiotherapy alone.[149] They recommended arthroscopic distention over manipulation because it was controllable and provided valuable insight into the intra-articular pathology.

Ogilvie-Harris and associates compared manipulation with arthroscopic release in patients with resistant frozen shoulder.[228] Arthroscopic division of tight structures was performed in four steps that included (1) resection of the inflammatory synovium in the rotator interval, (2) division of the anterior/superior glenohumeral ligament and anterior capsule, (3) division of the subscapularis tendon, and (4) division of the inferior capsule. At 2- to 5-year follow-up, patients treated by arthroscopic division had significantly better pain relief and restoration of function than did those who underwent arthroscopy and manipulation. Patients with diabetes initially did worse, but the final outcome was similar to that of patients without diabetes. These authors suggest that patients with diabetes may benefit from early intervention. In a later study reviewing the results of arthroscopic release in 17 diabetic patients, Ogilvie-Harris and Myerthall found that 13 of 17 had no pain and symmetrical motion, thus demonstrating the efficacy of this treatment option in the diabetic population.[230]

Pollock and associates found that arthroscopy served as a useful adjunct to MUA in the treatment of resistant frozen shoulder.[254] They performed manipulation under interscalene brachial plexus block anesthesia followed by an arthroscopic examination, sectioning of the coracohumeral ligament, and débriding of the glenohumeral joint as well as the subacromial space. Twenty-five of 30 shoulders treated in this manner had satisfactory results (83%); however, satisfactory results were obtained in only 64% of a subgroup of patients with diabetes mellitus. Yamaguchi and coworkers reported similar results with implantation of an intra-articular pain pump containing 0.5% bupivacaine after arthroscopic release[337]; 95% of patients achieved complete, painless range of motion.

Segmuller and associates reported a short-term (13.5 months) follow-up study of arthroscopic inferior capsulotomies performed with cutting diathermy.[286] More than 50% of their patients were found to have persistent stiffness in internal rotation, yet 88% were satisfied with their outcome and 87% had good to excellent results by Constant score. Other investigators have reported success with partial release for idiopathic frozen shoulder.[20]

A more aggressive and complete release of chronic refractory capsular contractures of the shoulder has been reported in several studies.[135,156,168,250,318,321] Morbidity was minimal when compared with the open surgical procedure, and early pain relief was achieved with few recurrent cases of refractory stiffness. Complications have been reported, including anterior dislocation[318] immediately postoperatively with subsequent recovered stability and excellent motion, complete axillary nerve palsy,[135] which also fully recovered at follow-up examination, and in most studies, reports of recurrence of contracture, which can occur in as many as 11% of patients.[321]

Pearsall and coworkers discussed release of the intra-articular portion of the subscapularis tendon during arthroscopic capsular release.[249,250] In an anatomic study, the authors determined the feasibility of this technique, and in 35 patients who underwent the procedure, only 1 may have demonstrated symptoms of subscapularis insufficiency postoperatively. Whether this aspect of capsular release is truly necessary is unknown because most studies yield excellent results without subscapularis release.

Harryman and associates demonstrated a remarkable improvement in six of nine health status scores on the SF-36 general health survey and excellent recovery of function on all questions of the SST after arthroscopic capsular release.[135] Warner and associates showed similar results with the Constant score.[318] Harryman and colleagues reported no difference between diabetic and nondiabetic patients in all outcome measures; however,

three patients in whom recurrent refractory stiffness developed were insulin-dependent diabetics.[135] In summary, arthroscopic capsular release is safe and effective in the management of refractory idiopathic global capsular fibrosis.[307,318]

The arthroscope can also be a useful tool in the posttraumatic stiff shoulder, including the postsurgical stiff shoulder, though to a less degree than for idiopathic frozen shoulder. Gerber and colleagues reviewed their results of arthroscopic capsular release in 45 shoulders, 21 of which were postsurgical and 15 post-traumatic.[106] They demonstrated significant improvement in pain scores, range of motion, and Constant scores for the group as a whole. When stratifying results by etiology, however, patients with idiopathic frozen shoulder did better than those with a post-traumatic or postsurgical etiology of their stiffness. Regardless of the etiology, ultimate outcome was most related to the degree of preoperative motion loss. In a similar report, Holloway and coworkers reported excellent results after arthroscopic capsular release in 50 patients, although less improvement in pain, range of motion, subjective function, and satisfaction was noted in patients with stiffness secondary to a postsurgical etiology.[148]

Combined Modes of Treatment

A consensus exists among authors who have written about current management of stiff shoulder in that the initial treatment should consist of gentle range-of-motion exercises in a patient-managed program of stretching exercises in conjunction with analgesics.[27,130,141,150,179,343] If this initial program is unsuccessful in improving comfort or range of motion, several treatment options may be considered next. There is no agreement, however, on the next best step along a treatment algorithm. A nonsurgical option such as injection of steroids or arthrography with distention is often preferred before more aggressive manipulative or surgical options.[98,295] For patients in whom this treatment has been unsuccessful or for investigators who have not found brisement to be advantageous, manipulative treatment has been the next step. Many recommend that shoulder manipulation be reserved for shoulders that have not responded to 6 months of consistent exercises and that have demonstrated persistent symptomatic stiffness.[60,129,188,194,217] Although some orthopaedists condemn this procedure because of rare complications, the overall morbidity is low.

For a patient with recalcitrant stiffness in whom manipulation may be contraindicated, an arthroscopic or open surgical alternative is considered next, depending, of course, on the patient's pathology and the surgeon's experience with the technical approach. For most clinicians, an arthroscopic or open release is preferred for a recalcitrant idiopathic frozen or post-traumatic stiff shoulder.[60,129,135,188,193,194,217,317]

No matter what method is selected for a given patient, it is important to consider the patient's medical and psychological profile, the functional impact of delayed recovery on earning potential, and the most economical and effective approach. It is imperative that investigators collect long-term follow-up data because the functional and objective restrictions of chronic shoulder stiffness persist for years after the onset of disability.[63] Finally, in patients who have recovered from shoulder stiffness or in those who are at greater risk for shoulder stiffness, it is fundamental that a preventive stretching exercise program be the primary goal.[129,130,141,208]

■ AUTHORS' PREFERRED TREATMENT

NONOPERATIVE TREATMENT

Once a thorough history and physical examination have been completed and other treatable conditions frequently associated with painful shoulder stiffness have been addressed, a simple nonoperative program should begin. Our initial management includes a trial of analgesics, anti-inflammatory medications, and therapeutic stretching exercises for 3 to 6 months. We initiate the Jackins stretching program even if patients say that they "had therapy" and especially when they are unable to recall or demonstrate their previous exercise regimen.

JACKINS' EXERCISE PROGRAM

Our preferred stretching program consists of four basic passive or active assisted stretching exercises performed by the patient.[195] Each exercise is completed 10 times during five sessions a day, with each session lasting 5 minutes. Before stretching, it is often helpful to apply heat to the stiff shoulder to increase flexibility and relax tight musculature.

Jackins recommends that three of the four exercises be performed supine, but they can also be performed standing or sitting (see Jackins' stretching program, Fig. 20-26).[195] In each direction, a push against the firm end point of range is maintained for a minimal count of 10. Severe pain should be avoided. After all the stretching exercises are finished, pain should subside to the previous baseline and gradually diminish after regular daily sessions. If pain and stiffness worsen with exercise, it is preferable to reduce the intensity of the stretch, but not the frequency.

The contralateral extremity is used to assist each motion. Humeral elevation should be performed close to the sagittal plane while allowing the limb to rotate as necessary to achieve maximal range. Alternatively, this motion may be duplicated with the use of a pulley, especially when it is impossible to assist elevation with the opposite extremity. External rotation is performed supine by placing a cane between the hands while the elbow is held close to the body and then applying pressure to rotate the affected extremity away from the body. Alternatively, while standing, external rotation is assisted by placing the arm against a door jam and twisting the body away from the arm. To perform the cross-body stretch in either the supine, sitting, or standing position, the affected extremity is grasped behind the elbow and pulled across the chest toward the opposite shoulder. It is best to begin with the elbow low and then stretch to a higher level in a cross-body (horizontal) adduction motion. Internal rotation is performed by putting the hand behind the buttock and pulling the wrist up the back with the opposite extremity or by using a towel to connect the hands similar to drying the back. Alternatively, a door handle may be grasped behind the buttock, and with a deep knee bend, an internal rotation stretch is performed.

If the pain becomes unbearable and exercises are not tolerated in any direction or if painful stiffness increases even with regular exercises, it is often useful to inject the glenohumeral joint with 7 mL of a local, long-acting anesthetic (bupivacaine 0.5%) and 1 mL of a repository steroid (40 mg of methylprednisolone). Our experience with intra-articular steroids agrees with previous studies that quote effective pain reduction but no long-term advantage.[128] We use it solely to enable the patient to perform the stretching regimen with greater comfort.

We do not advance to isometric strengthening exercises until the majority of motion and comfort has been restored. Use of the symptomatic extremity in all daily activities speeds rehabilitation along.[128] All patients must assume responsibility for their own 7-day-a-week exercise program.[179] Generally, it is unnecessary for a patient to see a therapist more than once a week to monitor progress, receive encouragement, and ensure that stiffness and pain are not increasing. Usually, the program is performed exclusively at home and, as a home exercise program, has been demonstrated to improve patient self-assessed comfort and function.[233]

EXAMINATION UNDER ANESTHESIA AND MANIPULATIVE RELEASE

Our indications for examination under anesthesia with gentle MUA are the following:

1. Inability to perform any stretching exercises because of severe pain, usually after a failed attempt with local intra-articular anesthetic and steroid instillation (diagnostically useful to determine whether stiffness actually exists)
2. Increasing painful global stiffness after 12 weeks of regular Jackins' exercises (usually after intra-articular steroid injection)
3. Absolutely no improvement in comfort, with global stiffness present after 18 to 24 weeks of regular Jackins' exercises

The purpose of the examination under anesthesia portion of this procedure is to confirm that the apparent restrictions in range are true physical boundaries and are not established solely by pain, fear of instability, muscular spasm, or even hysterical psychosis. All these examples have been manifested as "stiffness" in our clinic and have initially deceived us. For example, a patient with frank instability may voluntarily or involuntarily hold the extremity tight at the side, never relaxing enough for an adequate examination. Often, we are suspicious because the patient's age, history, or body language fails to fit typical patterns (see Table 20-4). Under anxiolytic relaxation or even an anesthetic paralyzing agent, the fixed physical restriction disappears.

MUA is contraindicated and surgical release is considered in the following cases:

1. A gentle manipulative force is inadequate to recover full range.
2. No improvement or worsening in range or comfort occurs after a previous manipulation.
3. The patient has significant osteopenia, a rotator cuff tear, or long-term insulin-dependent diabetes mellitus (e.g., more than 20 years).

Should manipulation be performed in a post-traumatic stiff shoulder? Consider the "not too unusual" example of stiffness occurring after a rotator cuff repair. How is a surgeon to know which tissue has the greater resistance to rupture—the combined strength of the contracted capsule and HSMI adhesions or the healing rotator cuff insertion? Similarly, consider stiffness that occurs after nonoperative treatment of a proximal humeral fracture. The dense adhesions within the HSMI are extremely resistant to manipulative force while the healing fracture may still be vulnerable. Stiffness that occurs secondary to trauma, especially when the trauma is previous surgery, is therefore a relative contraindication to MUA.

EXAMINATION AND MANIPULATION TECHNIQUE

The purpose of the MUA portion of this procedure is to perform a traumatic capsular rupture. We prefer to manipulate the shoulder under an interscalene anesthetic block for the reasons previously discussed. With the patient supine, we compare the passive range of motion of the stiff extremity and the opposite side in the five arcs previously described in the physical examination section. If the patient is awake, we can also add internal rotation up the back with the patient sitting. These ranges are our passive reference motions used for later comparison.

Gentle manipulative force is applied to the stiff extremity in the following order. We begin by elevating the extremity with a "two-finger" force applied in the sagittal plane while allowing free rotation. Brute force should be avoided or serious injury can occur. Force is applied to the humerus close to the shoulder to diminish the lever arm. With constant pressure, this stretch usually results in a palpable and audible release of contractures associated with disruption of the inferior capsule.[82,128,213] If a crepitant give does not occur, manipulation is discontinued and the surgeon may proceed with an arthroscopic or open capsular release.

If full forward elevation is successfully achieved, we proceed with MUA. With the arm elevated at shoulder level, the humerus is then adducted under the chin and across the body by pushing with a "two-finger" force to release the posteroinferior capsule. Next, the arm is abducted to the coronal plane with the arm elevated at shoulder level. In this position, internal rotation is applied to stretch the posterior capsule and soft tissues. The arm is then slowly lowered toward the side holding internal rotation with the elbow extended and the forearm pronated as required in the supine position. If the patient can sit up, internal rotation up the back works even better.

The arm is returned to the abducted position, and external rotation is performed to release the anteroinferior capsule. Each position should be held until the range is comparable to that of the normal opposite side. The surgeon should have absolute control over scapular position to ensure that motion gains are truly glenohumeral. Once symmetrical external rotation is obtained in abduction, the elbows are slowly lowered together to the side matching full external rotation to release the anterior capsule. If symmetrical range to the opposite side is obtained, an intra-articular steroid (40 mg of methylprednisolone) is injected to end the procedure (unless contraindicated). If persistent asymmetry exists, the surgeon should then proceed to an arthroscopic or open capsular release.

AFTERCARE

The patient meets with a therapist immediately postoperatively to review the home stretching program. Before the patient is discharged but while the interscalene block is still intact, a member of the surgical team will range the patient's shoulder to demonstrate the full passive arc achieved. This visible cue motivates the patient to begin stretching immediately.

The home exercise program is continued until the patient regains complete motion, usually in 6 to 12 weeks. If a patient begins to lose motion, supervised therapy is begun. Otherwise, all of the postoperative program is done by the patient as a home exercise program.

SURGICAL TREATMENT

Only patients who have failed a satisfactory nonoperative treatment course and an attempt at manipulation (unless contraindicated) should be considered for surgical release. Noncompliance with an exercise program is not an indication for surgical treatment. Patients who are intolerant of exercises or insufficiently motivated to perform them will rarely improve with nonoperative or operative treatment.

Some patients should not be treated surgically. Contraindications include significant depression, autonomic dystrophy, poor health, and those who defy improvement for secondary gain. Although the indications for open and arthroscopic surgical release are similar, each has unique aspects; in addition, in special cases we have even found it useful to combine these methods. Patients who are sensitive to fluid challenges (e.g., a diabetic with cardiac or renal insufficiency) may not be able to tolerate the fluid extravasation that occurs during arthroscopic release. Patients with a contracted articular capsule and extensive extra-articular adhesions, such as those with a posttraumatic or postsurgical stiff shoulder (e.g., after percutaneous pin treatment of humeral fractures), may require an arthroscopic capsular release and an open extra-articular release to lyse adhesions in the HSMI.

OPEN RELEASE

The major advantage of an open surgical release is the opportunity to safely palpate and visualize adhesions outside the joint. When rotating the extremity and palpating between tissue planes, it becomes easier to identify tight bands that restrict motion. For example, in a postsurgical stiff shoulder secondary to arthroplasty or anterior instability surgery, it is not unusual to find adhesions between the subscapularis, the coracoid, and the conjoined tendon. The other primary advantage of this technique is the ability to surgically lengthen a contracted subscapularis.

Although accurate release of the contracted articular and rotator interval capsule, the glenohumeral and coracohumeral ligaments, the biceps, and the subscapularis tendons can be accomplished under direct vision, this approach has significant disadvantages. In tight shoulders, it may be difficult to release the contracted posterior capsule via the open approach. Another major disadvantage of the open surgical procedure is the postoperative pain that may inhibit early passive and active assisted motion and prevent timely hospital discharge. Finally, with an open release via an anterior approach, external rotation stretching could result in rupture of the subscapularis.

Our primary indication for an open release is significant loss of motion that occurs after a surgical procedure performed through an anterior approach. Such procedures include anterior instability repair, open reduction of fractures, and glenohumeral arthroplasty. In all of these conditions, the potential exists for significant subscapularis contracture. This procedure is performed under regional anesthesia, and an indwelling interscalene catheter is placed for continuous postoperative interscalene anesthesia.

Technique

The procedure begins with careful examination under anesthesia directed at accurately defining directions of motion restriction. We recommend the same measurements as during the initial physical examination (see "Examination"). In addition, similar measurements are recorded for the normal shoulder. For a post-traumatic stiff shoulder, we do not begin with gentle MUA. The dense adhesions that form within the HSMI are resistant to manipulation.

A standard deltopectoral approach is performed. The preferred approach is to use the previous incision because the bulk of the surgical adhesions are likely to be there. If the incision was placed in such a way to make complete mobilization of the deltopectoral interval difficult, the old incision is ignored and an incision is made directly over the deltopectoral interval. The clavipectoral fascia is divided just lateral to the conjoined tendon and muscle. This split is continued proximally up to but not through the coracoacromial ligament.

The procedure begins with mobilization of the HSMI. This technique can often be quite challenging inasmuch as the dense scar prevents accurate identification of the interface. Because this plane is defined as a "motion interface," it can be identified by visualizing motion of the rotator cuff tendons. Specifically, we use a test that we refer to as the "roll–no roll test."[129,195] Simply by rotating the humerus, the plane between the underlying rotator

cuff and the overlying deltoid and conjoined tendon is identified. As motion improves, identification of this interval is facilitated. Often, the thick scar requires sharp dissection and excision. As an alternative, the interface can be identified by entering the subacromial space, thus defining the subdeltoid plane. Interface scar includes the thickened subacromial bursa, which should be excised. Excision of scar tissue between the conjoined tendon and the underlying subscapularis is more challenging because of the close proximity of the axillary nerve and major neurovascular structures. Resection of adhesions is best accomplished by externally rotating the humerus and presenting the adhesions to the lateral aspect of the conjoined tendon. With excision, further external rotation is permitted to present more adhesions. Dissection medial to the conjoined tendon should be avoided. The goal of release should be excision of all scar, with the HSMI left both free and completely smooth. Interface release is complete when the surgeon can pass a finger over all surfaces of the rotator cuff and palpate the axillary nerve both anteriorly on the superficial surface of the subscapularis and posteriorly as it exits the quadrangular space. The entire bursal surface of the rotator cuff should then be visualized and palpated to ensure that the cuff is intact.

Attention is next given to division of the subscapularis tendon and entrance to the glenohumeral joint. If the shoulder can externally rotate more than 40 degrees after mobilization of the HSMI, a simple subscapularis tenotomy can be accomplished. More often, subscapularis lengthening is required. Three options are available for lengthening the subscapularis. It is critical to choose the technique of subscapularis lengthening at this juncture because once division of the tendon is begun, the choices are limited. The choice depends on the degree of contracture and the thickness of the subscapularis tendon.

The simplest choice for subscapularis lengthening, and the authors' preferred option, is division of the subscapularis tendon from its insertion on the lesser tuberosity with subsequent repair of the tendon to the humeral articular margin (subscapularis recession or slide). The technique begins by passing a small elevator through the rotator interval and into the joint. The elevator is then passed behind the combined subscapularis and anterior capsule while protecting the long head of biceps tendon. The thick upper rolled border of the subscapularis is then identified. Using sharp dissection, the upper rolled border is excised from the lesser tuberosity, and care is taken to not leave any subscapularis tendon attached. Subscapular release is then carried distally while always ensuring that the complete tendon is included in the release. As the subscapularis is divided, the anterior capsular insertion is exposed. By sharp dissection the anterior capsule is released from its attachment at the humeral articular margin. The capsule remains united with the deep surface of the subscapularis. Approximately at the level of the anterior humeral circumflex vessels, the subscapularis attachment becomes muscular. By passing a small Darrach retractor superior to the vessels and subscapularis muscle, the inferior capsule can be exposed while protecting the axillary nerve. The inferior capsule is then released from its humeral insertion. On closure, the subscapularis is repaired to drill holes placed at the humeral articular margin. This technique will gain approximately 1 cm in subscapularis length, which will correlate with a gain in rotation of approximately 20 degrees.[131,195]

By placing a Fukuda humeral head retractor into the joint, the anterior glenoid rim is exposed. With sharp dissection, the anterior capsule is incised just lateral to its labral insertion. The incision is carried through the superior, middle, and anterior bands of the inferior glenohumeral ligaments. While protecting the axillary nerve, the inferior capsule is incised. Because the subscapularis tendon with the associated lateral aspect of the anterior glenohumeral capsule will be repaired on closure, we believe that an incision into the capsule itself constitutes the actual release. Care must be taken to ensure that the incision remains lateral to the glenoid labrum to preserve the labral attachment and its contribution to glenohumeral stability.

The advantage of subscapularis recession or slide is that the tendon keeps its full thickness and therefore has less risk of postoperative rupture. The main disadvantage is that the amount of length gain is limited to 1 cm.

The second option for subscapularis lengthening and open release is a coronal Z-plasty of the combined subscapularis and anterior capsule, as described by Neer (Fig. 20–28).[211] A small elevator is passed through the rotator interval and deep to both the subscapularis tendon and the anterior capsule. This maneuver will help gauge the combined thickness of the anterior structures. With sharp dissection, the superficial surface of the subscapularis tendon is longitudinally divided just medial to its insertion at the lesser tuberosity. When half of the combined thickness of the tendon/capsule is incised, the superficial flap is elevated medially to the level of the anterior glenoid labrum, at which point the anterior capsule is longitudinally incised. While protecting the axillary nerve with a small Darrach retractor, the incision is carried through the inferior capsule, always preserving the glenoid labral attachment. On closure, the medial edge of the capsule is repaired to the lateral edge of the coronal split with heavy nonabsorbable suture. Two centimeters of length and hence 40 degrees of rotation can be gained by this technique.

The final option for lengthening the anterior capsule and subscapularis is an inside-out lengthening. Although this technique is the least desirable of the three choices, it is the only one that can be chosen in retrospect, after a subscapular and capsular incision has already been made. The anterior capsule is incised just lateral to the glenoid labrum as earlier. If at that point it becomes clear that subscapularis lengthening is necessary, the anterior capsule is divided from the deep surface of the subscapularis in a medial-to-lateral direction to 1 cm from the subscapularis and capsular arthrotomy incision, with the natural union between these structures left intact. By repairing the medial capsular edge to the humeral articular margin through bone tunnels, a lengthening of 2 cm (40 degrees) can be achieved.

Unfortunately, tendon-lengthening methods can be a disadvantage because of weakened subscapularis integrity

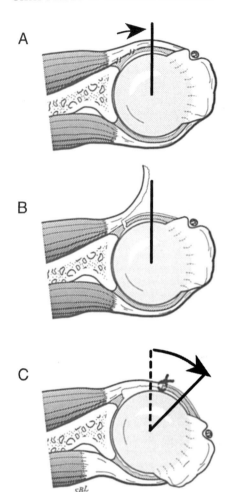

■ **Figure 20–28**

A, A contracted subscapularis and anterior capsule limit external rotation. **B,** The subscapularis tendon is incised from the lesser tuberosity laterally. The capsule is incised from the labrum medially. **C,** At the conclusion of the procedure, the lateral end of the subscapularis tendon is sutured to the medial end of the capsule, thereby resulting in substantial lengthening of these structures. As a rule of thumb, each centimeter of length gained by this procedure increases external rotation by approximately 20 degrees. *(From Matsen FA III, Lippitt SB, Sidles JA, and Harryman DT II: Practical Evaluation and Management of the Shoulder. Philadelphia: WB Saunders, 1994.)*

and a repair that must be protected from forceful stretch for 6 to 8 weeks. In a review of 35 patients with postoperative subscapularis insufficiency, 3 had undergone previous subscapularis lengthening for severe refractory global shoulder stiffness.[341] In two cases, the integrity of the subscapularis tendon could not be restored.

Once the subscapularis and anterior capsule have been divided, posterior capsular release is begun. With the lip of the Fukuda retractor placed behind the posterior glenoid rim, the hole in the retractor provides access to the posterior capsule. A long-handled scalpel is inserted through the retractor, and the posterior capsule is incised just lateral to the posterior labrum. By moving the Fukuda retractor superior and inferior or rotating the handle, the entire posterior capsule is released.

Before subscapularis repair, regardless of the lengthening technique, the subscapularis requires mobilization on all surfaces (a 360-degree release). Release of the coraco-humeral ligament is an important component of this mobilization. By applying traction to the subscapularis, the coracohumeral ligament becomes taut at its coracoid origin. With either sharp dissection or heavy scissors, the coracohumeral ligament is released from the coracoid. Adhesions in the subcoracoid recess and subscapular attachments to the anterior glenoid must be completely incised. The superficial surface was cleared of adhesions during the initial humeroscapular interface release. Finally, the more dangerous inferior release is accomplished with a finger used to palpate and protect the axillary nerve during incision of the scar. After release, the lengthened subscapularis is repaired with heavy, nonabsorbable suture. Intraoperative external rotation is noted and set as the limit during postoperative rehabilitation.

Aftercare

The patient is admitted for a 1- to 2-day hospital stay, depending on the degree of preoperative motion loss. Continuous interscalene anesthesia is used throughout the stay. The shoulder is gently put through range of motion at the bedside daily, and a global capsular stretching program is begun immediately. On the morning of discharge, the interscalene catheter is bloused with 20 mL of 0.5% bupivacaine. The patient continues to stretch the shoulder at home as often as possible. For a severe post-surgical stiff shoulder, the exercise program is recommended every hour while awake. Patients are encouraged to use the arm for all activities of daily living, and their overhead reaching is limited. If subscapularis lengthening was performed, internal rotation against resistance, as in closing a door, is restricted for the first 6 weeks postoperatively. Only if the patient begins to lose motion is formal therapy initiated.

The most important aspect of the postoperative regimen is ensuring concentration on motion only. Too often, patients are referred to supervised physical therapy with orders to "evaluate and treat." This vague recommendation will probably lead to a generalized program, including treatment modalities, weight training, and resistance exercises. These exercises not only take time away from the real beneficial stretching program but may also be detrimental. If supervised therapy is ordered, therapists should be encouraged to concentrate only on motion exercises. Use of a pulley, in addition to the program as outlined, can be of some benefit. Therapists and patients should also be encouraged to use general aerobic conditioning as part of the postoperative program. Strengthening exercises are begun only when motion is symmetrical in all directions.

ARTHROSCOPIC RELEASE

Conventional management strategies often fail to yield consistent or prompt return of comfort and function. We have used an approach to the evaluation and management of glenohumeral stiffness that involves arthroscopic release of capsular contractures for the most refractory shoulder stiffness.

The main advantages of this approach include the following:

1. Accurate and complete release of the contracted capsular structures
2. Ability to perform a synovectomy
3. Improved mobility of musculotendinous units without compromising their integrity
4. Minimal postoperative pain by avoiding an open incision
5. An opportunity to identify other intrinsic pathology that may have initiated or contributed to the pain leading to shoulder stiffness
6. Aggressive active and passive motion can be encouraged immediately
7. Some ability to excise adhesions in the HSMI

The objective of an arthroscopic capsular release is a direct intra-articular capsular release, including the anterior glenohumeral ligaments, the rotator interval capsule, the coracohumeral ligament, and the posterior and inferior capsule. Subacromial release of bursal adhesions can also be accomplished.

In certain cases, an arthroscopic capsular release is absolutely contraindicated. Contraindications include

1. Patients unable to understand or cooperate with a stretching motion program
2. Patients who cannot tolerate the surgical stress of a fluid challenge (e.g., renal or cardiac failure)

A relative contraindication includes patients with reflex sympathetic dystrophy or cervical radiculopathy because pain may significantly restrict rehabilitation exercises.

Finally and most importantly, a relative contraindication is lack of experience of the surgeon. To perform a complete, circumferential capsular release is technically difficult. The contracted joint volume makes visualization poor. Hypertrophic synovium often bleeds and obscures visualization. Once the capsular incision begins, fluid extravasation causes collapse of the viewing space. Finally, the axillary nerve is dangerously close. These factors make the procedure technically among the most challenging in all of shoulder arthroscopy, and it should not be undertaken by a novice arthroscopist.

Technique of Arthroscopic Capsular Release

Before starting arthroscopy, 1 mL of 1:1000 injectable epinephrine is added to each 3-L bag of saline. The tools required for the procedure include one or two smooth diaphragm cannulas (5.5-mm outer diameter), a capsular elevator, a straight and 20-degree-angled capsular release forceps, a bipolar electrocautery and ablation instrument, and a motorized synovial resector blade.

We perform the procedure in the half-sitting beach chair position on a specifically designed arthroscopy positioner. The osseous anatomy is marked on the skin along with all potential portals because later soft tissue swelling will make portal localization difficult. The posterior portal is created just superior to the standard posterior portal to allow space for a second inferior posterior portal.

A blunt, tapered-tip trocar is advanced to penetrate the stiff posterior capsule. On removal of the trocar, the synovial "string" sign confirms intra-articular placement of the scope. If manipulation was attempted before arthroscopy, blood may be present and lavage will be required to visualize the biceps tendon and rotator interval. With the "outside-in technique," an 18-gauge spinal needle is used to choose a location for an anteroinferior portal. This portal should be just superior to the upper rolled border of the subscapularis and have a slight lateral-to-medial angulation. The degree of synovitis and the pathologic findings seen about the biceps, labrum, capsule, and ligaments are recorded. Synovitis of the superior recess is resected. An ablator is used liberally to keep bleeding to a minimum. The biceps is palpated to ensure normal glide out of the groove. If it is scarred to the overlying supraspinatus, it is released from the superior glenoid rim. The arthroscope is then switched to the anterior portal. Capsular release proceeds according to the following steps (Fig. 20–29).

1. POSTERIOR CAPSULAR RESECTION

The posterior capsule should always be released first because fluid extravasation is limited posteriorly by the intact rotator cuff musculature, which is not the case after releasing the anterior rotator interval capsule. The posterosuperior capsule is viewed by looking through the anterior portal. A complete synovectomy is performed posteriorly. Care is taken to not penetrate the capsule during synovectomy because keeping the capsular plane "clean" will assist in release (Fig. 20–30A).

Capsular forceps are placed inside the joint through a posterior diaphragmed cannula. The cannula is partially withdrawn outside the joint, and the forceps are opened to capture the capsule at the edge of the portal in the jaw of the biter. The capsule is lifted toward the joint away from the rotator cuff muscle fibers and sectioned approximately 1 cm peripheral to the labrum. Closed capsular forceps are advanced outside the capsule to separate the muscular fibers from the capsule. Capsular resection is continued into the superior recess while avoiding the biceps root, labrum, and supraspinatus muscle.

Next, the scope is angled to view the capsule inferior to the posterior portal. The technique described earlier is used to transect the posterior capsule. Often, it is useful to switch to a 70-degree scope to view more of the posteroinferior recess. It is wise to discontinue this portion of the release when it becomes too difficult to see the tip of the forceps. Cutting posteroinferiorly without seeing the tip risks bleeding or injury to the axillary nerve.

Once the posterior capsular release is completed, the capsular ends are resected for approximately 0.5 cm both medially and laterally. Care is taken to avoid shaving the now-exposed supraspinatus and infraspinatus muscles because bleeding will occur. In addition, the labrum and labral attachment should be preserved to prevent instability (Fig. 20–30B).

Although an ablator can be used to cut the capsule, it is not our recommended technique. The ablation instrument tends to "melt" the cut capsular ends to the overlying rotator cuff musculature, thus making later resection of the capsular ends difficult. If one chooses to use an ablation-type instrument, as capsular division proceeds more inferiorly, the ablator should be abandoned to avoid thermal injury to the axillary nerve.

2. INFERIOR CAPSULAR RESECTION

While viewing through the anterosuperior portal, a posteroinferior portal is created. The location of this portal is approximately 2 cm inferior and 1 cm lateral to the original posterior (now posterosuperior) portal. The location is chosen with a spinal needle such that the angle of attack of a straight-biting capsular release forceps will be parallel to the capsule. The 30-degree scope is switched to the posterosuperior portal and angulated inferiorly. A second smooth-diaphragmed cannula is placed in the posteroinferior portal. The cannula is advanced into the joint at the inferior extent of the previous posteroinferior capsular resection. After insertion of the forceps, the cannula is retracted outside the capsule. The straight forceps is advanced outside the capsule to free it from muscle or the axillary nerve. The jaws of the forceps are opened and retracted until the cutting jaw is inside the capsule (Fig. 20–30C).

Inferior resection continues anteriorly along the inferior recess adjacent to the labrum. The axillary nerve is visualized in the majority of cases (Fig. 20–30D). To avoid injury to the nerve, release is best conducted within 1 cm of the glenoid rim.[340] The capsule may be attached to the underlying triceps and division of the superior triceps fibers to ensure that complete capsular division is appropriate.[91] As capsular division proceeds anteriorly, the

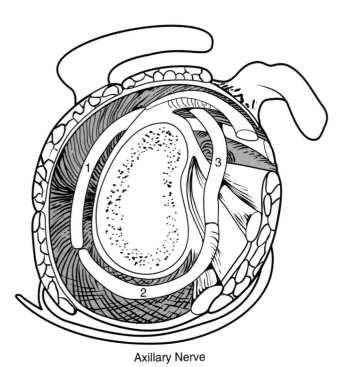

■ Figure 20–29
Diagram depicting the typical sequence of performing capsular release about the glenohumeral joint: (1) posterior, (2) axillary recess, and (3) rotator interval and subscapularis.

Axillary Nerve

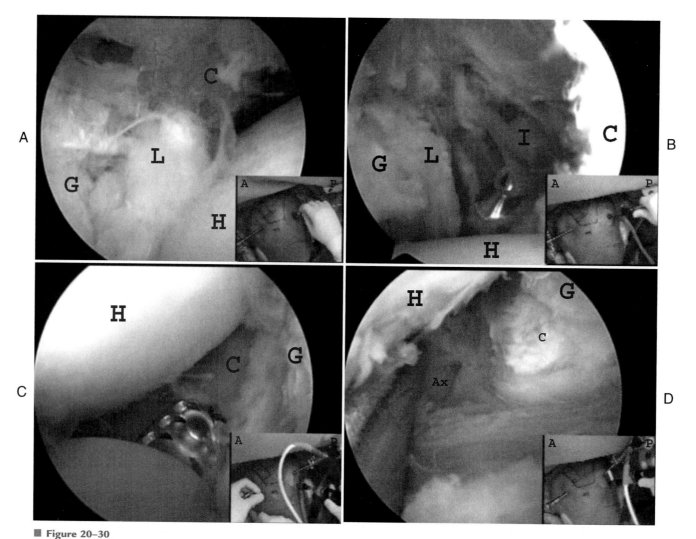

■ **Figure 20–30**

Technique for arthroscopic capsular release. A, anterior; Ax, axillary nerve; B, biceps tendon; C, capsule; G, glenoid; H, humeral head; I, infraspinatus muscle; L, glenoid labrum; P, posterior; R, rotator interval capsule; S, subscapularis. **A,** Posterior capsule as viewed from the anterior portal. Release of the capsule progresses in a superior direction in a line approximately 1 cm lateral to the glenoid labrum. **B,** The posterior capsule is released from the superior recess to the posteroinferior recess, and the capsular edges are resected to expose the underlying cuff musculature. **C,** A posteroinferior portal is established. The arthroscope is placed in the posterosuperior portal and the instruments in the posteroinferior portal to allow access to a contracted axillary recess. **D,** The inferior capsule is released as far anterior as can be visualized, usually completely through the anterosuperior band of the inferior glenohumeral ligament. Care is taken to protect the axillary nerve, which is commonly seen.

Continued

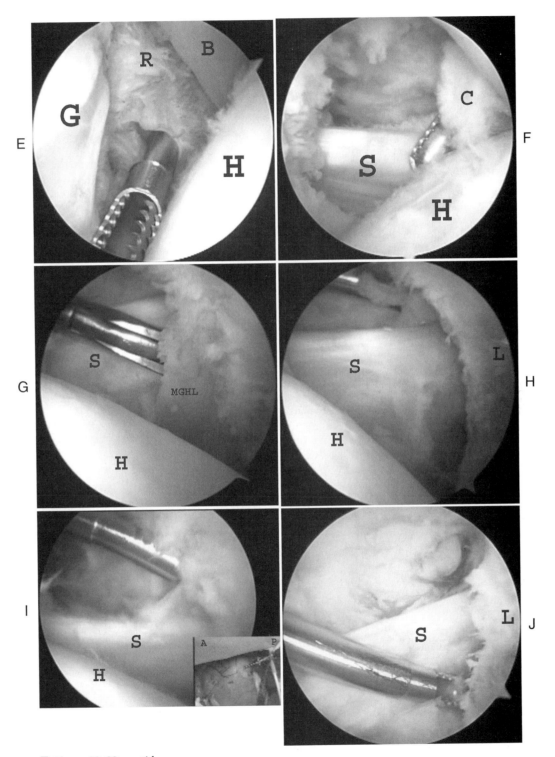

■ **Figure 20–30, cont'd.**
E, The rotator interval capsule is released in an inferior-to-superior direction, just lateral to the glenoid labrum. This direction of release is used to connect with the previous posterosuperior release. **F,** Release of the superior rotator interval is complete when both the coracoacromial ligament and the conjoined tendon are visualized. **G,** The middle glenohumeral ligament (MGHL) is released as it crosses the subscapularis tendon. **H,** Once the MGHL is resected, rotator interval release is complete. **I,** The subscapularis is commonly encased in adhesions, well medial into the subcoracoid recess. **J,** Adhesions about the subscapularis are resected with either a motorized shaver or an ablator. A 70-degree arthroscope is helpful in viewing medially into the recess.

arthroscope can be advanced anteriorly as well, and visualization of the anteroinferior capsule is improved. The remaining fibers of the anterosuperior band of the inferior glenohumeral ligament can now be divided with up-biting forceps. The edges of the cut capsule are resected with a motorized shaver, with care taken to keep the aggressive side of the instrument facing superiorly, away from the axillary nerve, and using suction sparingly.

3. ROTATOR INTERVAL RESECTION

The capsular forceps are placed into the joint through the cannula in the rotator interval (Fig. 20–30E). The cannula is withdrawn, and the superior glenohumeral ligament is transected. The anterosuperior release continues in a posterior direction to connect with the previous posterosuperior release. The labrum and root of the biceps tendon must remain intact (Fig. 20–30F). Next, the middle glenohumeral ligament is resected at the point where it crosses the subscapularis tendon (Fig. 20–30G and H). If the anterosuperior band of the inferior glenohumeral ligament was not completely released during inferior capsular division, it can be visualized and released by switching to a 70-degree arthroscope to continue anteroinferior capsular transection. Rotator interval release is complete when the coracoacromial ligament and conjoined tendon are visualized. The subcoracoid recess is often contracted or obliterated by synovitis. All attachments along the upper rolled border of the subscapularis tendon should be resected with a combination of a motorized shaver and ablator (Fig. 20–30I and J). If necessary, a 70-degree arthroscope is used to visualize the subscapularis down into the subcoracoid recess.

4. GLENOHUMERAL CLEAN-UP AND DIAGNOSTIC EXAMINATION

A motorized shaver is inserted inside the joint to thoroughly remove residual synovitis and resected debris. At this point, the shoulder should have excellent motion and a formal diagnostic examination can be done. Often, this is the first opportunity to fully visualize the rotator cuff insertion.

5. SUBACROMIAL SPACE

The arthroscope is inserted into the subacromial space to visualize the bursal side of the cuff. Generally, no surgical release or débridement is necessary for idiopathic frozen shoulders. In stiffness of post-traumatic or post-surgical origin, adhesions are released with capsular forceps or an ablator and resected with a motorized shaver. If the cause of stiffness was previous rotator cuff repair, this aspect of the procedure can be surprisingly challenging. The arthroscope and shaver should alternate between posterior, lateral, and anterior portals to provide a complete view of the subacromial bursa and ensure complete resection of adhesions.[19] If loose suture material is encountered, it is removed. The coracoacromial arch is left untouched unless otherwise indicated by significant roughness or by the presence of an inferiorly directed bony protrusion.

After Release

Arthroscopic release is followed by an intra-articular injection of methylprednisolone (40 mg). It is unnecessary to put steroids in the subacromial space because they are contiguous after release of the rotator interval. After arthroscopy, the portals are closed and bulky dressings are applied.

Although extravasated fluid prevents immediate full range, postoperative motion is measured and gentle manipulation is performed. In this way, symmetrical motion to the opposite side can be more reasonably ensured and a "fully aware" patient can participate. The patient is immediately started on a self-managed passive stretching program. Later during the same day, a repeat manipulation is performed at the patient's bedside while the interscalene block is still effective to free up residual adhesions and allow the patient to assist with and observe the recovered motion.

Before being discharged from the hospital, the patient is reminded how to perform the Jackins exercise program. Discharge from the hospital occurs the day of surgery for an idiopathic frozen shoulder and the following day for a stiff shoulder of post-traumatic origin. As with open release, continuous interscalene anesthesia is used overnight for a post-traumatic stiff shoulder, with an anesthetic bolus given before discharge.

COMBINED OPEN AND ARTHROSCOPIC RELEASE

Because patients with a post-traumatic stiff shoulder may have secondary capsular contracture and because both open release and arthroscopic release have benefits and drawbacks, we have performed combined open and arthroscopic release in select patient groups. The advantages of combining the procedures are as follows:

1. Ability to adequately release the HSMI through an incision
2. Complete capsular access through the arthroscope, including access to the posterior capsule
3. Ability to perform a complete release without having to incise the subscapularis or rotator cuff
4. Ability to resect ectopic bone or remove prominent or loose hardware
5. Decreased postoperative pain and faster rehabilitation

The primary indication for a combined arthroscopic and open release is a postsurgical stiff shoulder, primarily after anterior acromioplasty or rotator cuff repair. These patients usually have a previous deltoid-splitting incision and have severe scar formation on the HSMI. In addition, these individuals often have associated posterior capsular contracture, particularly after rotator cuff repair. Neither open nor arthroscopic release will adequately mobilize these shoulders. Combined release is also indicated for long-standing post-traumatic stiff shoulders, in which secondary capsular contracture can be expected. Finally, the combined technique is indicated for shoulder stiffness after proximal humeral fractures, where associated capsular contracture is usually evident.

Technique

A thorough examination under anesthesia is performed to define specific motion restrictions and assign probable locations of pathology. Glenohumeral arthroscopy is accomplished next, and a selective arthroscopic capsular release is performed, with attention directed to the regions identified by the history and examination as having capsular contracture.

Open HSMI release is performed next. If a superior, deltoid-splitting approach was previously used, the deltoid is again divided in the same plane. The deltoid split should extend proximal to the acromion process and distally to just proximal to the palpable subdeltoid reflection of the subacromial bursa because the axillary nerve is distal to this reflection.[19] Splitting the deltoid without incision from the acromion usually provides sufficient exposure. A self-retaining retractor placed deep to the deep deltoid fascia usually reveals a hypertrophic and thickly adherent subacromial bursa. A complete subacromial bursectomy is performed, and scar tissue between the bursal surface of the rotator cuff and the coracoacromial arch is excised. By rotating the arm, adhesions deep to the deltoid are excised, again taking care to not stray distal to the subdeltoid bursal reflection. A periosteal elevator or flat retractor is passed into the supraspinatus and infraspinatus fossae to break adhesions between the superficial surface of these muscles and the overlying deltoid. When the HSMI is free enough to pass a finger deep to the conjoined tendon anteriorly and to the quadrangular space posteriorly, the procedure is completed. On completion, the bursal surface of the rotator cuff should be inspected for tears.

Aftercare

The same care is required as after arthroscopic capsular release.

SUMMARY

The initiating etiology of capsular fibrosis still remains a mystery, but active investigations in cellular and molecular physiology may yield many clues in the near future. When treating a stiff shoulder, the physician must understand the major types of shoulder stiffness, their manifestations, the pathologic mechanism, and the location affecting function. We recommend use of the following simple definitions:

Frozen shoulder: An idiopathic global limitation of humeroscapular motion resulting from contracture and loss of compliance of the glenohumeral joint capsule.

Post-traumatic stiff shoulder: A limitation in humeroscapular motion occurring after an injury or low-level repetitive trauma or as part of an accompanying condition that results in a contracture of structures participating in the glenohumeral or humeroscapular motion interfaces.

Differentiation of stiffness into defined groups helps customize an individual's treatment within a logical framework. Investigators are also able to establish homogeneous treatment groups for analysis.[130] Classification is useful in planning treatment because shoulders that become stiff are best treated by corrective measures that address any intra- or extra-articular pathologic process contributing to the stiffness.

Tissue biopsies have helped distinguish fibrosis as the common lesion causing mechanical stiffness and the clinical manifestations of shoulder stiffness. The authors suggest attaching a specific descriptor to the term fibrosis that is associated with the pattern of clinical findings or the anatomic site of pathology. Terminology such as global capsular fibrosis, posterior capsular fibrosis, or interfascial fibrosis would accurately describe distinct clinically diagnosable entities and reflect recognizable pathophysiology.

Recovery from a stiff shoulder depends on motivating a patient to actively participate in nonoperative management. The Jackins exercise program leads to early resumption of functional activities. In patients with chronic or progressive global stiffness, manipulation may be indicated. Only patients with stiff shoulders refractory to nonsurgical treatment should be considered for surgical release by open or arthroscopic means. If necessary, operative management combined with an aggressive rehabilitation program can provide significant relief of pain and restoration of shoulder motion.

REFERENCES

1. Aitman TJ and Todd JA: Molecular genetics of diabetes mellitus. Baillieres Clin Endocrinol Metab 9:631-656, 1995.
2. Alvado A, Pelissier J, Benaim C, et al: [Physical therapy of frozen shoulder: Literature review.] Ann Readapt Med Phys 44:59-71, 2001.
3. Andersen NH, Sojbjerg JO, Johannsen HV, et al: Frozen shoulder: Arthroscopy and manipulation under general anesthesia and early passive motion. J Shoulder Elbow Surg 7:218-222, 1998.
4. Andren L and Lundberg BJ: Treatment of rigid shoulders by joint distention during arthrography. Acta Orthop Scand 36:45-53, 1965.
5. Angiolini G, Pasquinelli V, and Putti C: La roentgenterapia nella cura della periartrite della spalla. Minerva Med 56:504-508, 1965.
6. Appelboom T: Calcitonin in reflex sympathetic dystrophy syndrome and other painful conditions. Bone 30(suppl):84S-86S, 2002.
7. Arenberg AA: [Oxygen therapy of brachio-scapular periarthritis.] Vestn Khir Im I I Grek 107:126-127, 1971.
8. Arslan S and Celiker R: Comparison of the efficacy of local corticosteroid injection and physical therapy for the treatment of adhesive capsulitis. Rheumatol Int 21:20-23, 2001.
9. Askey JM: The syndrome of painful disability of the shoulder and hand complicating coronary occlusion. Am Heart J 22:1-12, 1941.
10. Awad T, Losada M, and Losada A: [Treatment of scapulo-humeral periarthritis with alpha-chymotrypsin and rehabilitation.] Rev Med Chil 5:372-376, 1967.
11. Balci N, Balci MK, and Tuzuner S: Shoulder adhesive capsulitis and shoulder range of motion in type II diabetes mellitus: Association with diabetic complications. J Diabetes Complications 13:135-140, 1999.
12. Bansil CK: Modification to the conventional wheel for measuring the range of movements of the shoulder joint. Med J Zambia 9:111-113, 1975.
13. Barrett WP, Franklin JL, Jackins SE, et al: Total shoulder arthroplasty. J Bone Joint Surg Am 69:865-872, 1987.
14. Baslund B, Thomsen BS, and Jensen EM: Frozen shoulder: Current concepts. Scand J Rheumatol 19:321-325, 1990.
15. Basta J, Harryman DT II, and Sidles JA: Is biceps glide essential to glenohumeral motion? Paper presented at the 64th Annual Meeting of the American Academy of Orthopaedic Surgeons, 1997, San Francisco.
16. Baum J: Joint pain. It isn't always arthritis. Postgrad Med 85:311-321, 1989.
17. Baumann F: Ventral capsular denervation: An operative treatment of periarthropathia humero-scapularis. Arch Orthop Trauma Surg 98:13-17, 1981.
18. Bayley JIL and Kessel L: Treatment of the frozen shoulder by manipulation: A pilot study. In Shoulder Surgery. Berlin: Springer-Verlag, 1982, pp 118-123.
19. Beals TC, Harryman DT 2nd, and Lazarus MD: Useful boundaries of the subacromial bursa. Arthroscopy 14:465-470, 1998.

20. Beaufils P, Prevot N, Boyer T, et al: Arthroscopic release of the glenohumeral joint in shoulder stiffness: A review of 26 cases. French Society for Arthroscopy. Arthroscopy 15:49-55, 1999.
21. Bellmann H, Zacharias J, Hasert V, et al: [Use of hylase "Dessau" in periarthritis humero-scapularis (Duplay syndrome).] Zentralbl Chir 94:1288-1304, 1969.
22. Bernageau J, Bardin T, Goutallier D, et al: Magnetic resonance imaging findings in shoulders of hemodialyzed patients. Clin Orthop 304:91-96, 1994.
23. Bierner SM: Manipulation in the treatment of frozen shoulder. Orthopedics 12:356, 380-381, 1989.
24. Billey T, Dromer C, Vedrenne C, et al: [Parsonage-Turner syndrome complicated by sympathetic dystrophy syndrome with adhesive capsulitis of the shoulder. Apropos of 2 cases.] Rev Rhum Mal Osteoartic 59:765-767, 1992.
25. Binder AI, Bulgen DY, Hazleman BL, et al: Frozen shoulder: A long-term prospective study. Ann Rheum Dis 43:361-364, 1984.
26. Binder AI, Bulgen DY, Hazleman BL, et al: Frozen shoulder: An arthrographic and radionuclear scan assessment. Ann Rheum Dis 43:365-369, 1984.
27. Binder A, Hazleman BL, Parr G, et al: A controlled study of oral prednisolone in frozen shoulder. Br J Rheumatol 25:288-292, 1986.
28. Bland JH, Merrit JA, and Boushey DR: The painful shoulder. Semin Arthritis Rheum 7:21-47, 1977.
29. Bohannon RW, Larkin PA, Smith MB, et al: Shoulder pain in hemiplegia: Statistical relationship with five variables. Arch Phys Med Rehabil 67:514-516, 1986.
30. Bollini V: [Roentgen therapy of painful shoulder. Indications and results.] Minerva Orthop 22:367-370, 1971.
31. Bosch Olives V, Llurba Llurba J, and Peinado Vistuer A: [Electrophysiotherapy in the treatment of a frozen shoulder.] Rev Esp Reum Enferm Osteoartic 12:149-156, 1967.
32. Boussina I, Gunther W, and Mart'i MR: Double-blind multicenter study comparing meclofenamate sodium with indomethacin and placebo in the treatment of extra-articular rheumatic disease. Arzneimittelforschung 33:649-652, 1983.
33. Bowman CA, Jeffcoate WJ, Pattrick M, et al: Bilateral adhesive capsulitis, oligoarthritis and proximal myopathy as presentation of hypothyroidism. Br J Rheumatol 27:62-64, 1988.
34. Boyle-Walker KL, Gabard DL, Bietsch E, et al: A profile of patients with adhesive capsulitis. J Hand Ther 10:222-228, 1997.
35. Bradley JP: Arthroscopic treatment for frozen capsulitis. Oper Tech Orthop 1:248-252, 1991.
36. Braun RM, West F, Mooney V, et al: Surgical treatment of the painful shoulder contracture in the stroke patient. J Bone Joint Surg Am 53:1307-1312, 1971.
37. Bridgman JF: Periarthritis of the shoulder and diabetes mellitus. Ann Rheum Dis 31:69-71, 1972.
38. Bronzini C: [Roentgenotherapeutic methods in Duplay's disease.] Minerva Radiol 13:630-632, 1968.
39. Brown C: Compressive, invasive referred pain to the shoulder. Clin Orthop 173:55-62, 1983.
40. Bruckner FE: Frozen shoulder (adhesive capsulitis). J R Soc Med 75:688-689, 1982.
41. Bruckner FE and Nye CJ: A prospective study of adhesive capsulitis of the shoulder ("frozen shoulder") in a high risk population. Q J Med 50:191-204, 1981.
42. Bucala R, Makita Z, Koschinsky T, et al: Lipid advanced glycosylation: Pathway for lipid oxidation in vivo. Proc Natl Acad Sci U S A 90:6434-6438, 1993.
43. Buchbinder R, Green S, and Youd JM: Corticosteroid injections for shoulder pain. Cochrane Database Syst Rev CD004016, 2003.
44. Bulgen DY, Binder A, Hazleman BL, et al: Immunological studies in frozen shoulder. J Rheumatol 9:893-898, 1982.
45. Bulgen DY, Binder AI, Hazleman BL, et al: Frozen shoulder: Prospective clinical study with an evaluation of three treatment regimens. Ann Rheum Dis 43:353-360, 1984.
46. Bulgen DY and Hazleman BL: Immunoglobulin-A, HLA-B27, and frozen shoulder. Lancet 2:760, 1981.
47. Bulgen DY, Hazleman BL, and Voak D: HLA-B27 and frozen shoulder. Lancet 1:1042-1044, 1976.
48. Bulgen D, Hazleman B, Ward M, et al: Immunological studies in frozen shoulder. Ann Rheum Dis 37:135-138, 1978.
49. Bunker TD and Anthony PP: The pathology of frozen shoulder. A Dupuytren-like disease. J Bone Joint Surg Br 77:677-683, 1995.
50. Bunker TD and Esler CN: Frozen shoulder and lipids. J Bone Joint Surg Br 77:684-686, 1995.
51. Bunker TD, Reilly J, Baird KS, et al: Expression of growth factors, cytokines and matrix metalloproteinases in frozen shoulder. J Bone Joint Surg Br 82:768-773, 2000.
52. Burke MC, Drinan K, Kopp DE, et al: Frozen shoulder syndrome associated with subpectoral defibrillator implantation. J Interv Card Electrophysiol 3:253-256, 1999.
53. Bush LF: The torn shoulder capsule. J Bone Joint Surg Am 57:256-259, 1975.
54. Bynum CK and Tasto J: Arthroscopic treatment of synovial disorders in the shoulder, elbow, and ankle. Am J Knee Surg 15:57-59, 2002.
55. Carette S, Moffet H, Tardif J, et al: Intraarticular corticosteroids, supervised physiotherapy, or a combination of the two in the treatment of adhesive capsulitis of the shoulder: A placebo-controlled trial. Arthritis Rheum 48:829-838, 2003.
56. Carrillon Y, Noel E, Fantino O, et al: Magnetic resonance imaging findings in idiopathic adhesive capsulitis of the shoulder. Rev Rhum Engl Ed 66:201-206, 1999.
57. Carron H: Relieving pain with nerve blocks. Geriatrics 33:49-57, 1978.
58. Champion GD, Saxon JA, and Kossard S: The syndrome of palmar fibromatosis (fasciitis) and polyarthritis. J Rheumatol 14:1196-1198, 1987.
59. Chard MD and Hazleman BL: Shoulder disorders in the elderly (a hospital study). Ann Rheum Dis 46:684-687, 1987.
60. Charnley J: Periarthritis of the shoulder. Postgrad Med 35:384-388, 1959.
61. Chen SK, Chien SH, Fu YC, et al: Idiopathic frozen shoulder treated by arthroscopic brisement. Kao Hsiung J Med Sci 18:289-294, 2002.
62. Cinquegrana OD: Chronic cervical radiculitis and its relationship to "chronic bursitis." Am J Phys Med Rehabil 47:23-30, 1968.
63. Clarke GR, Willis LA, Fish WW, et al: Preliminary studies in measuring range of motion in normal and painful stiff shoulders. Rheumatol Rehabil 14:39-46, 1975.
64. Clunie G, Bomanji J, and Ell PJ: Technetium-99m-MDP patterns in patients with painful shoulder lesions. J Nucl Med 38:1491-1495, 1997.
65. Codman EA: The Shoulder. Boston: Todd, 1934, pp 216-224.
66. Connell D, Padmanabhan R, and Buchbinder R: Adhesive capsulitis: Role of MR imaging in differential diagnosis. Eur Radiol 12:2100-2106, 2002.
67. Connolly J, Regen E, and Evans OB: Management of the painful, stiff shoulder. Clin Orthop 84:97-103, 1972.
68. Conti V: Arthroscopy in rehabilitation. Orthop Clin North Am 10:709-711, 1979.
69. Coombes WN: Distension-manipulation for the treatment of adhesive capsulitis (frozen shoulder syndrome). Clin Orthop 188:309-310, 1984.
70. Corbeil V, Dussault RG, Leduc BE, et al: [Adhesive capsulitis of the shoulder: A comparative study of arthrography with intra-articular corticotherapy and with or without capsular distension.] Can Assoc Radiol J 43:127-130, 1992.
71. Cotta H and Correll J: [The post-traumatic frozen shoulder.] Unfallchirurgie 8:294-306, 1982.
72. Coventry MB: Problem of the painful shoulder. JAMA 151:177-185, 1953.
73. Cyriax J and Trosier O: Hydrocortisone and soft tissue lesions. BMJ 2:966-968, 1953.
74. Dacre JE, Beeney N, and Scott DL: Injections and physiotherapy for the painful stiff shoulder. Ann Rheum Dis 48:322-325, 1989.
75. Dahan TH, Fortin L, Pelletier M, et al: Double blind randomized clinical trial examining the efficacy of bupivacaine suprascapular nerve blocks in frozen shoulder. J Rheumatol 27:1464-1469, 2000.
76. Dangoisse MJ, Wilson DJ, and Glynn CJ: MRI and clinical study of an easy and safe technique of suprascapular nerve blockade. Acta Anaesthesiol Belg 45:49-54, 1994.
77. Darlington LG and Coomes EN: The effects of local steroid injection for supraspinatus tears. Rheumatol Rehabil 16:172-179, 1977.
78. Degen IL: [Magnetotherapy of brachio-scapular periarthritis.] Ortop Travmatol Protez 34:66-68, 1974.
79. Demaziere A and Wiley AM: Primary chest wall tumor appearing as frozen shoulder. Review and case presentations. J Rheumatol 18:911-914, 1991.
80. Denham RHJ and Dingley AFJ: Conservative management of periarthritis of the shoulder. J Indiana State Med Assoc 62, 1969.
81. DePalma AF: Loss of scapulohumeral motion (frozen shoulder). Ann Surg 135:193-204, 1952.
82. de Witte S, Bonnet F, Bonarek M, et al: Adhesive capsulitis of the shoulder in an HIV patient treated with nelfinavir. AIDS 16:1307-1378, 2002.
83. Dickson JA and Crosby EH: Periarthritis of the shoulder: An analysis of two hundred cases. JAMA 99:2252-2257, 1932.
84. Di Fabio RP and Boissonnault W: Physical therapy and health-related outcomes for patients with common orthopaedic diagnoses. J Orthop Sports Phys Ther 27:219-230, 1998.
85. Dodenhoff RM, Levy O, Wilson A, et al: Manipulation under anesthesia for primary frozen shoulder: Effect on early recovery and return to activity. J Shoulder Elbow Surg 9:23-26, 2000.
86. Downing DS and Weinstein A: Ultrasound therapy of subacromial bursitis. A double blind trial. Phys Ther 66:194-199, 1986.
87. Duke O, Zecler E, and Grahame R: Anti-inflammatory drugs in periarthritis of the shoulder: A double-blind, between-patient study of naproxen versus indomethacin. Rheumatol Rehabil 20:54-59, 1981.
88. Duplay ES: De la periarthrite scapulo-humerale. Rev Frat Trav Med 53:226, 1896.
89. Duralde XA, Jelsma RD, Pollock RG, et al: Arthroscopic treatment of resistant frozen shoulder. Arthroscopy 9:345, 1993.
90. Echternach JL: Audioanalgesia as an adjunct to mobilization of the chronic frozen shoulder. Phys Ther 46:839-846, 1966.
91. Eiserloh H, Drez D Jr, and Guanche CA: The long head of the triceps: A detailed analysis of its capsular origin. J Shoulder Elbow Surg 9:332-335, 2000.
92. Emig EW, Schweitzer ME, Karasick D, et al: Adhesive capsulitis of the shoulder: MR diagnosis. AJR Am J Roentgenol 164:1457-1459, 1995.
93. Ene EE and Odia GI: Effect of acupuncture on disorders of musculoskeletal system in Nigerians. Am J Chin Med 11:106-111, 1983.
94. Engleman RM: Shoulder pain as a presenting complaint in upper lobe bronchogenic carcinoma. Report of 21 cases. Conn Med 30:273-276, 1966.

95. Ernstene AC and Kinell J: Pain in the shoulder as a sequel to myocardial infarction. Arch Intern Med 66:800-806, 1940.

96. Esposito S, Ragozzino A, Russo R, et al: [Arthrography in the diagnosis and treatment of idiopathic adhesive capsulitis.] Radiol Med (Torino) 85:583-587, 1993.

97. Famaey JP and Ginsberg F: Treatment of periarthritis of the shoulder: A comparison of ibuprofen and diclofenac. J Intern Med Res 12:238-243, 1984.

98. Fareed DO and Gallivan WR Jr: Office management of frozen shoulder syndrome. Treatment with hydraulic distension under local anesthesia. Clin Orthop 242:177-183, 1989.

99. Fernandes MS and Pinto AC: Ombros dolorosos. Acta Med Port 3:229-234, 1990.

100. Ferrari DA: Capsular ligaments of the shoulder. Anatomical and functional study of the anterosuperior capsule. Am J Sports Med 18:20-24, 1990.

101. Fisher L, Kurtz A, and Shipley M: Association between cheiroarthropathy and frozen shoulder in patients with insulin-dependent diabetes mellitus. Br J Rheumatol 25:141-146, 1986.

102. Fleming A, Dodman S, Beer TC, et al: Personality in frozen shoulder. Ann Rheum Dis 35:456-457, 1975.

103. Freedman L and Munro RR: Abduction of the arm in the scapular plane: Scapular and glenohumeral movements. A roentgenographic study. J Bone Joint Surg Am 48:1503-1510, 1966.

104. Freiss S, Lecocq J, Isner ME, and Vautravers P: Frozen shoulder and fluoroquinones. Two case reports. Bone Joint Spine 67:245-259, 2000.

105. Gam AN, Schydlowsky P, Rossel I, et al: Treatment of "frozen shoulder" with distension and glucocorticoid compared with glucocorticoid alone. A randomised controlled trial. Scand J Rheumatol 27:425-430, 1998.

106. Gerber C, Espinosa N, and Perren TG: Arthroscopic treatment of shoulder stiffness. Clin Orthop 390:119-128, 2001.

107. Gilula LA, Schoenecker PL, and Murphy WA: Shoulder arthrography as a treatment modality. AJR Am J Roentgenol 131:1047-1048, 1978.

108. Goldberg BA, Scarlat MM, Harryman DT 2nd: Management of the stiff shoulder. J Orthop Sci 4:462-471, 1999.

109. Goldman AB and Ghelman B: The double contrast shoulder arthrogram: A review of 158 studies. Radiology 127:655-663, 1978.

110. Goldman RT, Koval KJ, Cuomo F, et al: Functional outcome after humeral head replacement for acute three- and four-part proximal humeral fractures. J Shoulder Elbow Surg 4:81-86, 1995.

111. Good AE, Green RA, and Zarafonetis CJD: Rheumatic symptoms during tuberculosis therapy: Manifestation of isoniazid toxicity? Ann Intern Med 63:800-897, 1965.

112. Gore DR, Murray MP, Sepic SB, et al: Shoulder-muscle strength and range of motion following surgical repair of full-thickness rotator cuff tears. J Bone Joint Surg Am 68:266-272, 1986.

113. Gotter G: Comparative evaluation of tenoxicam and piroxicam in the treatment of humeroscapular periarthritis. Eur J Rheumatol Inflamm 9:95-97, 1987.

114. Grabovoi AF, Grishko AI, Rodichkin VA, et al: [Blockade of the suprascapular nerve in the complex treatment of humero-scapular periarthritis.] Vestn Khir 136:65-66, 1986.

115. Grasland A, Ziza JM, Raguin G, et al: Adhesive capsulitis of shoulder and treatment with protease inhibitors in patients with human immunodeficiency virus infection: Report of 8 cases. J Rheumatol 27:2642-2646, 2000.

116. Greinemann H: [The painful frozen shoulder (author's transl).] Unfallchirurgie 6:239-244, 1980.

117. Grey RG: The natural history of "idiopathic" frozen shoulder. J Bone Joint Surg Am 60:564, 1978.

118. Griffin JW: Hemiplegic shoulder pain. Phys Ther 66:1884-1893, 1986.

119. Griggs SM, Ahn A, and Green A: Idiopathic adhesive capsulitis. A prospective functional outcome study of nonoperative treatment. J Bone Joint Surg Am 82:1398-1407, 2000.

120. Gusarova SA: [Massage in humeroscapular periarthrosis.] Med Sestra 48:36-38, 1989.

121. Ha'eri GB and Maitland A: Arthroscopic findings in the frozen shoulder. J Rheumatol 8:149-152, 1981.

122. Haggart GE, Digman RJ, and Sullivan TS: Management of the "frozen" shoulder. JAMA 161:1219-1222, 1956.

123. Haines JF and Hargadon EJ: Manipulation as the primary treatment of the frozen shoulder. J R Coll Surg Edinb 27:271-275, 1982.

124. Halverson L and Maas R: Shoulder joint capsule distension (hydroplasty): A case series of patients with "frozen shoulders" treated in a primary care office. J Fam Pract 51:61-63, 2002.

125. Hamer J and Kirk JA: Physiotherapy and the frozen shoulder: A comparative trial of ice and ultrasonic therapy. N Z Med J 83:191-192, 1976.

126. Hannafin JA, DiCarlo ED, Wickiewicz TL, et al: Adhesive capsulitis: Capsular fibroplasia of the glenohumeral joint. J Shoulder Elbow Surg 3:5, 1994.

127. Hansen PE: Biceps transfer intra-position grafting in massive rotator cuff tears. In Burkhead WZ (ed): Rotator Cuff Disorders. Baltimore: Williams & Wilkins, 1996, pp 349-355.

128. Harmon PH: Methods and results in the treatment of 2580 painful shoulders. Am J Surg 95:527-544, 1958.

129. Harryman DT II: Shoulders: Frozen and stiff. Instr Course Lect 42:247-257, 1993.

130. Harryman DT II, Lazarus MD, and Rozencwaig R: The stiff shoulder. In

Rockwood CA Jr and Matsen FA 3rd (eds): The Shoulder. Philadelphia: WB Saunders, 1998, pp 1064-1112.

131. Harryman DT II, Sidles JA, et al: Pathophysiology of shoulder instability. In McGinty JB (ed): Operative Arthroscopy. Philadelphia: JB Lippincott, 1996, pp 677-693.

132. Harryman DT II, Sidles JA, Clark JM, et al: Translation of the humeral head on the glenoid with passive glenohumeral motion. J Bone Joint Surg Am 72:1334-1343, 1990.

133. Harryman DT II, Sidles JA, Harris SL, et al: The role of the rotator interval capsule in passive motion and stability of the shoulder. J Bone Joint Surg Am 74:53-66, 1992.

134. Harryman DT II, Sidles JA, and Matsen FA III: Laxity of the normal glenohumeral joint: A quantitative in vivo assessment. J Shoulder Elbow Surg 1:66-76, 1992.

135. Harryman DT II, Sidles JA, and Matsen FA III: Arthroscopic management of refractory shoulder stiffness. Arthroscopy 13:133-147, 1997.

136. Harryman DT II, Walker ED, and Harris SL: Residual motion and function after glenohumeral or scapulothoracic arthrodesis. J Shoulder Elbow Surg 2:275-285, 1993.

137. Hashimoto T, Suzuki K, and Nobuhara K: Dynamic analysis of intraarticular pressure in the glenohumeral joint. J Shoulder Elbow Surg 4:209-218, 1995.

138. Hassenstein E, Nusslin F, Hartweg H, et al: [Radiation therapy of humeroscapular periarthritis.] Strahlentherapie 155:87-93, 1979.

139. Hawkins RJ and Angelo RL: Glenohumeral osteoarthrosis: A late complication of the Putti-Platt repair. J Bone Joint Surg Am 72:1193-1197, 1990.

140. Hazleman BL: The painful stiff shoulder. Rheum Phys Med 11:413-421, 1972.

141. Hazleman BL: Frozen shoulder. In MS (ed): Watson Surgical Disorders of the Shoulder. New York, Churchill-Livingstone, 1991, pp 167-179.

142. Helbig B, Wagner P, and Dohler R: Mobilization of frozen shoulder under general anaesthesia. Acta Orthop Belg 49:267-274, 1983.

143. Herbut PA and Watson JS: Tumor of the thoracic inlet producing the Pancoast syndrome. A report of seventeen cases and a review of the literature. Arch Pathol 42:88-103, 1946.

144. Hill JJ Jr and Bogumill H: Manipulation in the treatment of frozen shoulder. Orthopedics 11:1255-1260, 1988.

145. Hitchcock HH and Bechtol CO: Painful shoulder. J Bone Joint Surg Am 30:263-273, 1948.

146. Hogan M, Cerami A, and Bucala R: Advanced glycosylation end products block the antiproliferation effect of nitric oxide. Role in the vascular and renal complications of diabetes mellitus. J Clin Invest 90:1110-1112, 1992.

147. Hollingworth GR, Ellis RM, and Hattersley TS: Comparison of injection techniques for shoulder pain: Results of a double blind, randomised study. BMJ 287:1339-1341, 1983.

148. Holloway GB, Schenk T, Williams GR, et al: Arthroscopic capsular release for the treatment of refractory postoperative or post-fracture shoulder stiffness. J Bone Joint Surg Am 83:1682-1687, 2001.

149. Hsu SY and Chan KM: Arthroscopic distension in the management of frozen shoulder. Int Orthop 15:79-83, 1991.

150. Hulstyn MJ and Weiss AP: Adhesive capsulitis of the shoulder. Orthop Rev 22:425-433, 1993.

151. Huskisson EC and Bryans R: Diclofenac sodium in the treatment of painful stiff shoulder. Curr Med Res Opin 8:350-353, 1983.

152. Hutchinson JW, Tierney GM, Parsons SL, et al: Dupuytren's disease and frozen shoulder induced by treatment with a matrix metalloproteinase inhibitor. J Bone Joint Surg Br 80:907-908, 1998.

153. Inman VT, Saunders JB, and Abbot LC: Observations on the function of the shoulder joint. J Bone Joint Surg Am 26:1-30, 1944.

154. Itoi E and Tabata S: Range of motion and arthrography in the frozen shoulder. J Shoulder Elbow Surg 1:106-112, 1992.

155. Janda DH and Hawkins RJ: Shoulder manipulation in patients with adhesive capsulitis and diabetes mellitus: A clinical note. J Shoulder Elbow Surg 2:36-38, 1993.

156. Jerosch J: 360 degrees arthroscopic capsular release in patients with adhesive capsulitis of the glenohumeral joint—indication, surgical technique, results. Knee Surg Sports Traumatol Arthrosc 9:178-186, 2001.

157. Johnston JTH: Frozen shoulder syndrome in patients with pulmonary tuberculosis. J Bone Joint Surg Am 41:877-882, 1959.

158. Jones DS and Chattopadhyay C: Suprascapular nerve block for the treatment of frozen shoulder in primary care: A randomized trial. Br J Gen Pract 49:39-41, 1999.

159. Jones R and Lovett RW: Orthopedic Surgery. New York: Williams & Wood, 1923, p 59.

160. Kamieth H: Radiology of the cervical spine in shoulder periarthritis. Z Orthop Ihre Grenzgeb 100:162-167, 1965.

161. Kay NR: The clinical diagnosis and management of frozen shoulders. Practitioner 225:164-167, 1981.

162. Kennedy JC and Willis RB: The effects of local steroid injections on tendons: A biomechanical and microscopic correlative study. Am J Sports Med 4:11-21, 1976.

163. Kernwein GA, Rosenberg B, and Sneed WA: Arthrographic studies of the shoulder. J Bone Joint Surg Am 39:1267-1279, 1957.

164. Kessel L: Disorders of the Shoulder. New York: Churchill-Livingstone, 1982, p 82.

165. Kessel L, Bayley I, and Young A: The upper limb: The frozen shoulder. Br J Hosp Med 25:334, 336-337, 339, 1981.
166. Kieras DM and Matsen FA III: Open release in the management of refractory frozen shoulder. Orthop Trans 15:801-802, 1991.
167. Kivimaki J and Pohjolainen T: Manipulation under anesthesia for frozen shoulder with and without steroid injection. Arch Phys Med Rehabil 82:1188-1190, 2001.
168. Klinger HM, Otte S, Baums MH, et al: Early arthroscopic release in refractory shoulder stiffness. Arch Orthop Trauma Surg 122:200-203, 2002.
169. Koppell HP and Thompson WAL: Pain and the frozen shoulder. Surg Gynecol Obstet 109:92-96, 1959.
170. Kottke FJ, Pauley DL, and Ptak RA: The rationale for prolonged stretching for correction of shortening of connective tissue. Arch Phys Med Rehabil 47:345-352, 1966.
171. Kozin F: Two unique shoulder disorders. Adhesive capsulitis and reflex sympathetic dystrophy syndrome. Postgrad Med 73:207-210, 214-216, 1983.
172. Kuptniratsaikul S, Kuptniratsaikul V, Tejapongvorachai T, et al: A capsular dilatation facilitated shoulder manipulation for treating patients with frozen shoulder. J Med Assoc Thai 85(suppl 1):S163-S169, 2002.
173. Laroche M, Ighilahriz O, Moulinier L, et al: Adhesive capsulitis of the shoulder: An open study of 40 cases treated by joint distention during arthrography followed by an intraarticular corticosteroid injection and immediate physical therapy. Rev Rhum Engl Ed 65:313-319, 1998.
174. Laumann U: The so-called "periarthritis humeroscapularis"—possibilities of an operative treatment. Arch Orthop Trauma Surg 97:27-37, 1980.
175. Lazarus MD, Yung SW, Harryman DT II, et al: The effect of a chondral-labral defect on glenoid concavity and glenohumeral stability. A cadaveric model. J Bone Joint Surg Am 78:94-102, 1996.
176. Leardini C, Perbellini A, Franceschini M, et al: Intra-articular injections of hyaluronic acid in the treatment of painful shoulder. Clin Ther 10:521-526, 1988.
177. Lee M, Haq AM, Wright V, et al: Periarthritis of the shoulder: A controlled trial of physiotherapy. Physiotherapy 59:312-315, 1973.
178. Lee PN, Lee M, Haq AM, et al: Periarthritis of the shoulder: Trial of treatments investigated by multivariate analysis. Ann Rheum Dis 33:116-119, 1974.
179. Leffert RD: The frozen shoulder. Instr Course Lect 34:199-203, 1985.
180. Lehman JF, Warren CG, and Scham SM: Therapeutic heat and cold. Clin Orthop 99:207-245, 1974.
181. Leone J, Beguinot I, Dehlinger V, et al: Adhesive capsulitis of the shoulder induced by protease inhibitor therapy. Three new cases. Rev Rhum Engl Ed 65:800-801, 1998.
182. Lequesne M, Dang N, Bensasson M, et al: Increased association of diabetes mellitus with capsulitis of the shoulder and shoulder-hand syndrome. Scand J Rheumatol 6:53-56, 1977.
183. Lin ML, Huang CT, Lin JG, et al: [A comparison between the pain relief effect of electroacupuncture, regional nerve block and electroacupuncture plus regional nerve block in frozen shoulder.] Acta Anaesthesiol Sin 32:237-242, 1994.
184. Lippitt SB, Vanderhooft JE, Harris SL, et al: Glenohumeral stability from concavity-compression: A quantitative analysis. J Shoulder Elbow Surg 2:27-35, 1993.
185. Lippman RK: Frozen shoulder; periarthritis; bicipital tenosynovitis. Arch Surg 47:283-296, 1943.
186. Lloyd-Roberts GC and French PR: Periarthritis of the shoulder. BMJ 1:1569-1571, 1959.
187. Loyd JA and Loyd HM: Adhesive capsulitis of the shoulder: Arthrographic diagnosis and treatment. South Med J 76:879-883, 1983.
188. Lundberg BJ: The frozen shoulder. Clinical and radiographical observations. The effect of manipulation under general anesthesia. Structure and glycosaminoglycan content of the joint capsule. Local bone metabolism. Acta Orthop Scand Suppl 119:1-59, 1969.
189. Lundberg BJ and Nilsson BE: Osteopenia in the frozen shoulder. Clin Orthop 60:187-191, 1968.
190. Macnab I: Rotator cuff tendinitis. Ann R Coll Surg Engl 53:271-287, 1973.
191. Makita Z, Radoff S, Rayfield EJ, et al: Advanced glycosylation end products in patients with diabetic nephropathy [see comments]. N Engl J Med 325:836-842, 1991.
192. Manton GL, Schweitzer ME, Weishaupt D, et al: Utility of MR arthrography in the diagnosis of adhesive capsulitis. Skeletal Radiol 30:326-330, 2001.
193. Massoud SN, Pearse EO, Levy O, et al: Operative management of the frozen shoulder in patients with diabetes. J Shoulder Elbow Surg 11:609-613, 2002.
194. Matsen FA III and Kirby RM: Office evaluation and management of shoulder pain. Orthop Clin North Am 13:453-475, 1982.
195. Matsen FA III, Lippitt SB, Sidles JA, et al: The stiff shoulder. In Practical Evaluation and Management of the Shoulder. Philadelphia: WB Saunders, 1994, pp 19-109.
196. Mattson RH, Cramer JA, and McCutchen CB: Barbiturate-related connective tissue disorders. Arch Intern Med 149:911-914, 1989.
197. McClure PW, Michener LA, Sennett BJ, et al: Direct 3-dimensional measurement of scapular kinematics during dynamic movements in vivo. J Shoulder Elbow Surg 10:269-277, 2001.
198. McLaughlin HL: On the "frozen" shoulder. Bull Hosp Jt Dis 12:383-393, 1951.
199. McLaughlin HL: The "frozen shoulder." Clin Orthop 20:126-131, 1961.
200. Melzer C, Wallny T, Wirth CJ, et al: Frozen shoulder—treatment and results. Arch Orthop Trauma Surg 114:87-91, 1995.
201. Meulengracht E and Schwartz M: The course and prognosis of periarthritis humeroscapularis with special regard to cases with general symptoms. Acta Med Scand 143:350-360, 1952.
202. Midorikawa K, Hara M, Emoto G, et al: Arthroscopic débridement for dialysis shoulders. Arthroscopy 17:685-693, 2001.
203. Minter WT: The shoulder-hand syndrome in coronary disease. JAMA 56:45-49, 1967.
204. Morency G, Dussault RG, Robillard P, et al: [Distention arthrography in the treatment of adhesive capsulitis of the shoulder.] Can Assoc Radiol J 40:84-86, 1989.
205. Moren-Hybbinette I, Moritz U, and Shersten B: The clinical picture of the painful diabetic shoulder—natural history, social consequences and analysis of concomitant hand syndrome. Acta Med Scand 221:73-82, 1987.
206. Moskal MJ, Harryman DT II, Romeo AA, et al: Glenohumeral motion after complete capsular release. Arthroscopy 15:408-416, 1999.
207. Murnaghan GF and McIntosh D: Hydrocortisone in painful shoulder—a controlled trial. Lancet 2:798-801, 1955.
208. Murnaghan JP: Adhesive capsulitis of the shoulder: Current concepts and treatment. Orthopedics 11:153-158, 1988.
209. Murray MP, Gore DR, Gardener GM, et al: Shoulder motion and muscle strength of normal men and women in two age groups. Clin Orthop 192:268-273, 1985.
210. Neer CS II: Anterior acromioplasty for the chronic impingement syndrome in the shoulder. J Bone Joint Surg Am 54:41-50, 1972.
211. Neer CS II: Shoulder Reconstruction. Philadelphia: WB Saunders, 1990, pp 328, 421-427.
212. Neer CS II, Satterlee CC, Dalsey RM, et al: The anatomy and potential effects of contracture of the coracohumeral ligament. Clin Orthop 280:182-185, 1992.
213. Neviaser JS: Adhesive capsulitis of the shoulder. J Bone Joint Surg Am 27:211-222, 1945.
214. Neviaser JS: Arthrography of the shoulder joint. J Bone Joint Surg Am 44:1321-1330, 1962.
215. Neviaser JS: Adhesive capsulitis and the stiff and painful shoulder. Orthop Clin North Am 11:327-331, 1980.
216. Neviaser RJ: Arthrography of the Shoulder. Springfield, IL: Charles C Thomas, 1975, pp 60-66.
217. Neviaser RJ: Painful conditions affecting the shoulder. Clin Orthop 173:63-69, 1983.
218. Neviaser RJ: Radiologic assessment of the shoulder. Plain and arthrographic. Orthop Clin North Am 18:343-349, 1987.
219. Neviaser RJ and Neviaser TJ: The frozen shoulder. Diagnosis and management. Clin Orthop 223:59-64, 1987.
220. Neviaser TJ: Arthroscopy of the shoulder. Orthop Clin North Am 18:361-372, 1987.
221. Neviaser TJ: Adhesive capsulitis. Orthop Clin North Am 18:439-443, 1987.
222. Newton DR: The management of non-articular rheumatism. Practitioner 208:64-73, 1972.
223. Nicholson GG: The effects of passive joint mobilization on pain and hypomobility associated with adhesive capsulitis of the shoulder. Orthop Sports Phys Ther 6:238-246, 1985.
224. Nobuhara K, Sugiyama D, Ikeda H, and Makiura M: Contracture of the shoulder. Clin Orthop 254:105-110, 1990.
225. Nobuhara K, Supapo AR, and Hino T: Effects of joint distention in shoulder diseases. Clin Orthop 304:25-29, 1994.
226. O'Brien SJ, Neves MC, Arnoczky SP, et al: The anatomy and histology of the inferior glenohumeral ligament complex of the shoulder. Am J Sports Med 18:449-456, 1990.
227. Oesterreicher W and van Dam G: Social psychological researches into brachialgia and periarthritis. Arthritis Rheum 7:670-683, 1964.
228. Ogilvie-Harris DJ, Biggs DJ, Fitsialos DP, and MacKay M: The resistant frozen shoulder. Manipulation versus arthroscopic release. Clin Orthop 319:238-248, 1995.
229. Ogilvie-Harris DJ and D'Angelo G: Arthroscopic surgery of the shoulder. Sports Med 9:120-128, 1990.
230. Ogilvie-Harris DJ and Myerthall S: The diabetic frozen shoulder: Arthroscopic release. Arthroscopy 13:1-8, 1997.
231. Ogilvie-Harris DJ and Wiley AM: Arthroscopic surgery of the shoulder. A general appraisal. J Bone Joint Surg Br 68:201-207, 1986.
232. Okamura K and Ozaki J: Bone mineral density of the shoulder joint in frozen shoulder. Arch Orthop Trauma Surg 119:363-367, 1999.
233. O'Kane JW, Jackins S, Sidles JA, et al: Simple home program for frozen shoulder to improve patients' assessment of shoulder function and health status. J Am Board Fam Pract 12:270-277, 1999.
234. Older MWJ, McIntyre JL, and Lloyd GJ: Distention arthrography of the shoulder joint. Can J Surg 19:203-207, 1976.
235. Oldham BE: Periarthritis of the shoulder associated with thyrotoxicosis. N Z Med J 29:766-770, 1959.
236. Omari A and Bunker TD: Open surgical release for frozen shoulder: Surgical findings and results of the release. J Shoulder Elbow Surg 10:353-357, 2001.
237. Osmond-Clarke H: Habitual dislocation of the shoulder: The Putti-Platt operation. J Bone Joint Surg Br 30:19-25, 1948.

238. Othman A and Taylor G: Manipulation under anaesthesia for frozen shoulder. Int Orthop 26:268-270, 2002.

239. Ozaki J, Nakagawa Y, Sakurai G, et al: Recalcitrant chronic adhesive capsulitis of the shoulder. Role of contracture of the coracohumeral ligament and rotator interval in pathogenesis and treatment. J Bone Joint Surg Am 71:1511-1515, 1989.

240. Pal B, Anderson J, Dick WC, et al: Limitation of joint mobility and shoulder capsulitis in insulin and non–insulin dependent diabetes mellitus. Br J Rheumatol 25:147-151, 1986.

241. Pal B, Griffiths ID, Anderson J, et al: Association of limited joint mobility with Dupuytren's contracture in diabetes mellitus. J Rheumatol 14:582-585, 1987.

242. Parsons JL, Shepard WL, and Fosdick WM: DMSO: An adjutant to physical therapy in the chronic frozen shoulder. Ann N Y Acad Sci 141:569-571, 1967.

243. Pasteur F: Les algies de l'epaule et la physiotherapie. J Radiol Electrol 16:419-426, 1932.

244. Patten C and Hillel AD: The 11th nerve syndrome. Accessory nerve palsy or adhesive capsulitis? Arch Otolaryngol Head Neck Surg 119:215-220, 1993.

245. Payr E: Gelenk-"sperren" und "ankylosen"; über die "Schultersteifen" verschiedener Urasche und die sogenannte "Periarthritis humero-scapularis." Ihre Behandlung Zentralbl Chir 58:2993, 1931.

246. Pearl ML, Harris SL, Lippitt SB, et al: A system for describing positions of the humerus relative to the thorax and its use in the presentation of several functionally important arm positions. J Shoulder Elbow Surg 1:113-118, 1992.

247. Pearl ML, Jackins S, Lippitt SB, et al: Humeroscapular positions in a shoulder range-of-motion examination. J Shoulder Elbow Surg 1:296-305, 1992.

248. Pearl ML, Wong K, and Frank C: Restrictions of glenohumeral motion in patients with frozen shoulders. Presented at the Sixth International Congress on Surgery of the Shoulder, Helsinkia, Finland, 1995.

249. Pearsall AW, Holovacs TF, and Speer KP: The intra-articular component of the subscapularis tendon: Anatomic and histological correlation in reference to surgical release in patients with frozen-shoulder syndrome. Arthroscopy 16:236-242, 2000.

250. Pearsall AW, Osbahr DC, and Speer KP: An arthroscopic technique for treating patients with frozen shoulder. Arthroscopy 15:2-11, 1999.

251. Peyriere H, Mauboussin JM, Rouanet I, et al: Frozen shoulder in HIV patients treated with indinavir: Report of three cases. AIDS 13:2305-2306, 1999.

252. Pineda C, Arana B, Martinez-Lavin M, et al: Frozen shoulder triggered by cardiac catheterization via the brachial artery. Am J Med 96:90-91, 1994.

253. Placzek JD, Roubal PJ, Freeman DC, et al: Long-term effectiveness of translational manipulation for adhesive capsulitis. Clin Orthop 356:181-191, 1998.

254. Pollock RG, Duralde XA, Flatow EL, and Bigliani LU: The use of arthroscopy in the treatment of resistant frozen shoulder. Clin Orthop 304:30-36, 1994.

255. Poppen NK and Walker PS: Normal and abnormal motion of the shoulder. J Bone Joint Surg Am 58:195-201, 1976.

256. Putnam JJ: The treatment of a form of painful periarthritis of the shoulder. Boston Med Surg 107:536-539, 1882.

257. Quigley TB: Checkrein shoulder. A type of "frozen shoulder." N Engl J Med 250:188-192, 1954.

258. Quigley TB: Indications for manipulation and corticosteroids in the treatment of stiff shoulders. Surg Clin North Am 43:1715-1720, 1969.

259. Quin CE: Frozen shoulder: Evaluation of treatment with hydrocortisone injections and exercises. Ann Phys Med 8:22-29, 1965.

260. Quin CE: Humeroscapular periarthritis. Observations on the effects of x-ray therapy and ultrasonic therapy in cases of "frozen shoulder." Ann Phys Med 10:64-69, 1969.

261. Reeves B: Arthrography of the shoulder. J Bone Joint Surg Br 48:424-435, 1966.

262. Reeves B: Arthrographic changes in frozen and post-traumatic stiff shoulders. Proc R Soc Med 59:827-830, 1966.

263. Reeves B: The natural history of the frozen shoulder syndrome. Scand J Rheumatol 4:193-196, 1975.

264. Refior HG: [Clarification of the concept humeroscapular periarthritis.] Orthopade 24:509-511, 1995.

265. Reichmister JP and Friedman SL: Long-term functional results after manipulation of the frozen shoulder. Md Med J 48:7-11, 1999.

266. Resnick D: Shoulder arthrography. Radiol Clin North Am 19:243-253, 1981.

267. Resnick D: Shoulder pain. Orthop Clin North Am 14:81-97, 1983.

268. Resnik CS, Fronek J, Frey C, et al: Intra-articular pressure determination during glenohumeral joint arthrography. Preliminary investigation. Invest Radiol 19:45-50, 1984.

269. Richardson AT: The painful shoulder. Proc R Soc Med 68:731-736, 1975.

270. Riedel R: Versteifung des Shultergelenkes durch Hangenlassen des Armes. Munch Med Wochenschr 63:1397, 1916.

271. Riley D, Lang AE, Blair RD, et al: Frozen shoulder and other shoulder disturbances in Parkinson's disease. J Neurol Neurosurg Psychiatry 52:63-66, 1989.

272. Rizk TE, Christopher RP, Pinals RS, et al: Adhesive capsulitis (frozen shoulder): A new approach to its management. Arch Phys Med Rehabil 64:29-33, 1983.

273. Rizk TE, Christopher RP, Pinals RS, et al: Arthrographic studies in painful hemiplegic shoulders. Arch Phys Med Rehabil 65:254-256, 1984.

274. Rizk TE, Gavant ML, and Pinals RS: Treatment of adhesive capsulitis (frozen shoulder) with arthrographic capsular distension and rupture. Arch Phys Med Rehabil 75:803-807, 1994.

275. Rizk TE and Pinals RS: Frozen shoulder. Semin Arthritis Rheum 11:440-452, 1982.

276. Rizk TE and Pinals RS: Histocompatibility type and racial incidence in frozen shoulder. Arch Phys Med Rehabil 65:33-34, 1984.

277. Rodeo SA, Hannafin JA, Tom J, et al: Immunolocalization of cytokines and their receptors in adhesive capsulitis of the shoulder. J Orthop Res 15:427-436, 1997.

278. Romeo AA, Loutzenheiser T, Rhee YG, et al: The humeroscapular motion interface. Clin Orthop 350:120-127, 1998.

279. Rosenbloom AL: Limitation of finger joint mobility in diabetes mellitus. J Diabetes Complications 3:77-87, 1989.

280. Rovetta G and Monteforte P: Intraarticular injection of sodium hyaluronate plus steroid versus steroid in adhesive capsulitis of the shoulder. Int J Tissue React 20:125-130, 1998.

281. Roy S and Oldham R: Management of painful shoulder. Lancet 1:1322-1324, 1976.

282. Ryu KN, Lee SW, Rhee YG, et al: Adhesive capsulitis of the shoulder joint: Usefulness of dynamic sonography. J Ultrasound Med 12:445-449, 1993.

283. Saha NC: Painful shoulder in patients with chronic bronchitis and emphysema. Am Rev Respir Dis 94:455-456, 1966.

284. Samilson RL, Raphael RL, Post L, et al: Arthrography of the shoulder joint. Clin Orthop 20:21-32, 1961.

285. Sattar MA and Luqman WA: Another duration-related complication of diabetes mellitus. Diabetes Care 8:507-510, 1985.

286. Segmuller HE, Taylor DE, Hogan CS, et al: Arthroscopic treatment of adhesive capsulitis. J Shoulder Elbow Surg 4:403-408, 1995.

287. Seibold JR: Digital sclerosis in children with insulin-dependent diabetes mellitus. Arthritis Rheum 25:1357-1361, 1982.

288. Seignalet J, Sany J, Caillens JP, et al: [Lack of correlation between frozen shoulder and HLA-B27 (author's transl).] Sem Hop Paris 57:1738-1739, 1981.

289. Seradge H and Anderson MG: Clostridial myonecrosis following intra-articular steroid injection. Clin Orthop 147:207-209, 1980.

290. Shaffer B, Tibone JE, and Kerlan RK: Frozen shoulder. A long-term follow-up. J Bone Joint Surg Am 74:738-846, 1992.

291. Sharma RK, Bajekal RA, and Bhan S: Frozen shoulder syndrome. A comparison of hydraulic distension and manipulation. Int Orthop 17:275-278, 1993.

292. Sherry DD, Rothstein RRL, and Petty RE: Joint contractures preceding insulin-dependent diabetes mellitus. Arthritis Rheum 25:1362-1364, 1982.

293. Simmonds FA: Shoulder pain with particular reference to the frozen shoulder. J Bone Joint Surg Am 31:834-838, 1949.

294. Simon L, Pujol H, Blotman F, et al: [Aspects of the pathology of the arm after irradiation of breast cancer.] Rev Rheum Mal Osteoartic 43:133-140, 1976.

295. Simon WH: Soft tissue disorders of the shoulder. Frozen shoulder, calcific tendinitis, and bicipital tendinitis. Orthop Clin North Am 6:521-539, 1975.

296. Smith SP, Devaraj VS, and Bunker TD: The association between frozen shoulder and Dupuytren's disease. J Shoulder Elbow Surg 10:149-151, 2001.

297. Steinbrocker O and Argyros TG: Frozen shoulder: Treatment by local injections of depot corticosteroids. Arch Phys Med Rehabil 55:209-213, 1974.

298. Stodell MA, Nicholson R, Scot J, et al: Radioisotope scanning in painful shoulder syndromes. Ann Rheum Dis 38:496, 1979.

299. Sullivan JD: Painful shoulder syndrome. Can Med Assoc J 111:505, 1974.

300. Summers GD and Gorman WP: Bilateral adhesive capsulitis and Hashimoto's thyroiditis. Br J Rheumatol 28:451, 1989.

301. Sun KO, Chan KC, Lo SL, et al: Acupuncture for frozen shoulder. Hong Kong Med J 7:381-391, 2001.

302. Suzuki K, Attia ET, Hannafin JA, Rodeo SA, et al: The effect of cytokines on the migration of fibroblasts derived from different regions of the canine shoulder capsule. J Shoulder Elbow Surg 10:62-67, 2001.

303. Sweetnam R: Corticosteroid arthropathy and tendon rupture. J Bone Joint Surg Br 51:397-398, 1969.

304. Tamai K and Yamato M: Abnormal synovium in the frozen shoulder: A preliminary report with dynamic magnetic resonance imaging. J Shoulder Elbow Surg 6:534-543, 1997.

305. Terry GC, Hammon D, France P, and Norwood LA: The stabilizing function of passive shoulder restraints. Am J Sports Med 19:26-34, 1991.

306. Thomas D, Williams RA, and Smith DS: The frozen shoulder: A review of manipulative treatment. Rheumatol Rehabil 19:173-179, 1980.

307. Ticker JB, Warner JJ, and Beim GM: Recognition and treatment of refractory capsular contracture of the shoulder. Arthroscopy 16:673-674, 2000.

308. Tielbeek AV and van Horn JR: Double-contrast arthrography of the shoulder. Diagn Imaging 52:154-162, 1983.

309. Todd JA: Genetic analysis of type 1 diabetes using whole genome approaches. Proc Natl Acad Sci U S A 92:8560-8565, 1995.

310. Travell JG and Simmons DG: Myofascial Pain and Dysfunction: Trigger Point Manual. Baltimore: Williams & Wilkins, 1983, pp 410-424.

311. Turkel SJ, Panio MW, Marshall JL, et al: Stabilizing mechanisms preventing anterior dislocation of the glenohumeral joint. J Bone Joint Surg Am 63:1208-1217, 1981.

312. Tuten HR, Young DC, Douoguih WA, et al: Adhesive capsulitis of the shoulder in male cardiac surgery patients. Orthopedics 23:693-696, 2000.

313. Tyber MA: Treatment of the painful shoulder syndrome with amitriptyline and lithium carbonate. Can Med Assoc J 111:137-140, 1974.

314. Uitvlugt G, Detrisac DA, Johnson LL, et al: Arthroscopic observations before and after manipulation of frozen shoulder. Arthroscopy 9:181-185, 1993.

315. Waldburger M, Meier JL, and Gobelet C: The frozen shoulder: Diagnosis and treatment. Prospective study of 50 cases of adhesive capsulitis. Clin Rheumatol 11:364-368, 1992.

316. Wanklyn P, Forster A, and Young J: Hemiplegic shoulder pain (HSP): Natural history and investigation of associated features. Disabil Rehabil 18:497-501, 1996.

317. Warner JJ: Frozen shoulder: Diagnosis and management. J Am Acad Orthop Surg 5:130-140, 1997.

318. Warner JJ, Allen A, Marks PH, et al: Arthroscopic release for chronic, refractory adhesive capsulitis of the shoulder. J Bone Joint Surg Am 78:1808-1816, 1996.

319. Warner JJ, Deng XH, Warren RF, and Torzilli PA: Static capsuloligamentous restraints to superior-inferior translation of the glenohumeral joint. Am J Sports Med 20:675-685, 1992.

320. Wassef MR: Suprascapular nerve block. A new approach for the management of frozen shoulder. Anaesthesia 47:120-124, 1992.

321. Watson L, Dalziel R, and Story I: Frozen shoulder: A 12-month clinical outcome trial. J Shoulder Elbow Surg 9:16-22, 2000.

322. Watson-Jones R: Simple treatment of stiff shoulders. J Bone Joint Surg Br 45:207, 1963.

323. Weiser HI: [Mobilization under local anesthesia for painful primary frozen shoulder.] Harefuah 90:215-219, 1976.

324. Weiser HI: Painful primary frozen shoulder mobilization under local anesthesia. Arch Phys Med Rehabil 58:406-408, 1977.

325. Weiss JJ and Ting YM: Arthrography-assisted intra-articular injection of steroids in treatment of adhesive capsulitis. Arch Phys Med Rehabil 59:285-287, 1978.

326. Wertheim HM and Rovenstine EA: Suprascapular nerve block. Anesthesiolgy 2:541-545, 1941.

327. Wiley AM: Arthroscopic appearance of frozen shoulder. Arthroscopy 7:138-143, 1991.

328. Wiley AM and Older MW: Shoulder arthroscopy. Investigations with a fibrooptic instrument. Am J Sports Med 8:31-38, 1980.

329. Williams NE, Siefert MH, Cuddigan JHB, et al: Treatment of capsulitis of the shoulder. Rheumatol Rehabil 14:236, 1975.

330. Withers RJW: The painful shoulder: Review of one hundred personal cases with remarks on the pathology. J Bone Joint Surg Am 31:414-417, 1949.

331. Wohlgethan JR: Frozen shoulder in hyperthyroidism. Arthritis Rheum 30:936-939, 1987.

332. Wolf JM and Green A: Influence of comorbidity on self-assessment instrument scores of patients with idiopathic adhesive capsulitis. J Bone Joint Surg Am 84:1167-1173, 2002.

333. Wright MG, Richards AJ, and Clarke MB: ^{99m}Tc pertechnetate scanning in capsulitis. Lancet 2:1265-1266, 1975.

334. Wright V and Haq AM: Periarthritis of the shoulder. I. Aetiological considerations with particular reference to personality factors. Ann Rheum Dis 35:213-219, 1976.

335. Wright V and Haq AM: Periarthritis of the shoulder. II. Radiological features. Ann Rheum Dis 35:220-226, 1976.

336. Xie KY, Zhao GF, and Lu JM: Treatment of 103 cases of periarthritis of the shoulder by acupoint laser irradiation. J Tradit Chin Med 8:265-266, 1988.

337. Yamaguchi K, Sethi N, and Bauer GS: Postoperative pain control following arthroscopic release of adhesive capsulitis: A short-term retrospective review study of the use of an intra-articular pain catheter. Arthroscopy 18:359-365, 2002.

338. Young A: Immunological studies in the frozen shoulder. In Bayley J and Kessel L (eds): Shoulder Surgery. Berlin: Springer-Verlag, 1982, pp 110-113.

339. Zabraniecki L, Doub A, Mularczyk M, et al: Frozen shoulder: A new delayed complication of protease inhibitor therapy? Rev Rhum Engl Ed 65:72-74, 1998.

340. Zanotti RM and Kuhn JE: Arthroscopic capsular release for the stiff shoulder. Description of technique and anatomic considerations. Am J Sports Med 25:294-298, 1997.

341. Ziegler DW, Harryman DT II, and Matsen FA III: Subscapularis insufficiency in the previously operated shoulder. Paper presented at the 12th Open Meeting of the American Shoulder and Elbow Surgeons, 1996, Atlanta.

342. Zilberberg C and Leveile-Nizerolle M: La radiographie anti-inflammatoire dans 200 cas de periarthrite scapulo-humerale. Sem Hop Paris 52:909-911, 1976.

343. Zuckerman JD and Cuomo F: Frozen shoulder. In Matsen FA 3rd, Fu FH, and Hawkins RJ (eds): The Shoulder: A Balance of Mobility and Stability. Rosemont, IL: American Academy of Orthopedic Surgeons, 1993, pp 253-268.

344. Zuckerman JD, Leblanc JM, Choueka J, et al: The effect of arm position and capsular release on rotator cuff repair. J Bone Joint Surg Br 73:402-405, 1991.

CHAPTER 21

MUSCLE RUPTURES AFFECTING THE SHOULDER GIRDLE

Todd W. Ulmer, M.D., and Peter T. Simonian, M.D.

• • • •

Injury to muscle structures is exceedingly common, yet many of these injuries remain poorly described and ill defined. Most injuries are not identified as the cause of significant long-term disability unless they involve complete disruption of the muscle or its attachments. Fortunately, this complication is much less common than when a rupture involves the tendon, such as in rotator cuff tears. Interference with function, particularly diminution of strength, has previously been the major means of confirming muscular injury, together with palpable deficiency or major atrophy of the muscle substance. The exact pathologic process, however, has seldom been defined because muscle strains and minor disruptions rarely require the surgical exposure that allows documentation of pathology. Recently, computed tomography (CT) and magnetic resonance imaging (MRI) have provided methods of visualizing muscle injuries not hitherto possible. Whereas in the past relatively few muscle injuries of the shoulder girdle have been described, such injuries will undoubtedly be recorded more often and more precisely in the future.

Brickner and Milch[8] described muscle ruptures as being caused by (1) active contraction of a muscle, (2) contraction of an antagonist, (3) increase in tearing over cohesive power, (4) asynchronous contraction, or (5) the additional muscular force of another muscle.

Basically, however, one may consider most significant muscle ruptures as occurring when an actively contracting muscle group is overloaded by the application of a resisting load or external force that exceeds tissue tolerance. When such overload occurs, the muscle fibers are torn and the muscle sheath is disrupted, thus leading to a palpable defect in the muscle. The defect can heal only by the formation of scar tissue. Effective surgical repair of muscle injury is very difficult to accomplish.

GENERAL PRINCIPLES OF RUPTURE OF THE MUSCULOTENDINOUS UNIT

The classic experiments performed by McMaster[51] demonstrated the relative strength of a muscle, tendon, and bone preparation. He suspended the gastrocnemius of the amputated limb of an adult rabbit. A wire was passed through the femur, and increasing weight was attached to the os calcis until rupture occurred. Between 10 and 21 kg of weight, the unit ruptured. In the seven preparations successfully tested, rupture occurred at the insertion with associated bony avulsion in three cases; two ruptured at the origin, again with bony avulsion; and the others ruptured through either the muscle belly or the musculotendinous junction. McMaster could produce a rupture of the tendon midsubstance only after 50% of its substance had been divided. The normal tendon appears to be the strongest component of the musculotendinous unit, a finding that was confirmed by Cronkite.[14]

The site of rupture may be influenced by the rate of loading. In 1971 Welsh and coworkers,[98] while testing a tendon-bone system in the rabbit, found that lower rates of loading were associated with rupture at the tendon-bone junction. At higher rates, the tendon broke at the site of clamping, and the strength of the tendon-bone junction was found to be more secure.

Similar studies have been undertaken in stimulated muscle.[24] The energy absorbed by the muscle before disruption was twice as great with prestimulation. Indeed, Safran and associates[81] have demonstrated experimentally that in rabbit muscle preconditioned with isometric stimulation, more tension developed and a greater change in length was required before failure occurred.

Another point to note is that muscles that cross two joints are subject to stretch at each joint and are therefore more vulnerable to injury. Likewise, muscles with a higher percentage of type II fibers are also more susceptible.[23]

Other factors that should be considered include the mechanism of injury, which may well influence the site of rupture. For example, in rupture of the pectoralis major, McEntire and associates[50] noted that direct trauma more commonly resulted in muscle belly rupture, whereas indirect trauma was more likely to produce rupture distally. Similarly, although rupture of the long head of the biceps is common and rupture at the insertion is well recognized, rupture of the biceps muscle belly is exceedingly rare. However, as many as 48 complete belly ruptures were described by Heckman and Levine[36] in parachutists, in whom the injury was caused by direct trauma from the static line.

The site of rupture is also influenced by anatomic factors peculiar to the shoulder. Rupture occurs most commonly in the tendons of the long head of the biceps

1173

and the rotator cuff. The intra-articular course of the former and impingement and impaired vascularity of the latter predispose them to rupture.

The role of anabolic steroids in predisposing to muscle rupture also bears consideration, especially in bodybuilding, weightlifting, and throwing athletes.[97,100] In 1992, Miles and coworkers[53] conducted experiments on 24 male rats in which anabolic steroids and exercise were used as variables. Biomechanical tests revealed stiffer tendons in the group of rats receiving stanozolol intramuscularly than in the rats that did not receive steroid injections. In addition, "The energy at the time when the tendon failed, the toe-limit elongation, and the elongation at the time of first failure were all affected significantly."[53] Examination via electron microscopy revealed alterations in the size of collagen fibrils in rats receiving stanozolol in comparison to the control group. In a similar study, Wood and associates[100] found that the crimp pattern of collagen was shorter and the angle between collagen fibrils longer in the tendons of rats treated with anabolic steroids. On the basis of the aforementioned results, it can be speculated that steroids play a role in altering both the structure and the pattern of collagen fibrils, in turn causing a stiffer and weaker musculotendinous junction that is more likely to rupture.

Clinically, rupture of the quadriceps tendon mechanism above the knee has been seen in power-lifting professionals who have been using anabolic steroids. Similarly, the authors have seen rupture of the pectoralis major at the musculotendinous junction in weight-training athletes indulging in a high intake of steroids.

Overall, however, rupture of the muscles of the shoulder girdle is uncommon. The literature does not abound with reports of such involvement. In this chapter, a comprehensive overview of the subject is presented with an account of lesions of the pectoralis major, deltoid, triceps, biceps, serratus anterior, coracobrachialis, subscapularis, supraspinatus, infraspinatus, and teres major muscles.

RUPTURE OF THE PECTORALIS MAJOR

Historical Review

Rupture of the pectoralis major, first described by Patissier[73] in 1822, is a relatively rare injury. In 1972, a comprehensive review of the literature by McEntire and colleagues[50] revealed only 45 cases, to which they added 11 more. However, only 22 of the 56 patients had undergone surgical exploration, and 1 case of rupture was confirmed at autopsy. Thus, actual confirmation of the lesion was lacking in 33 patients, and cases of congenital absence of the pectoralis major may have been represented in this group. Since then, 167 additional cases have been published in the literature, at least 104 of which have been confirmed surgically.

Anatomy

The pectoralis major arises in a broad sheet as two distinct heads—an upper clavicular head and a lower sternocostal head—that spread to a complex trilaminar insertion along the lateral lip of the bicipital groove. A portion of the sternocostal head spirals on itself to produce the round appearance of the anterior axillary fold, with the result that the lowermost fibers are inserted most proximally on the humerus and in a crescent into the capsule of the shoulder joint. McEntire and associates[50] attribute the infrequency of complete rupture of the pectoralis major to the layered form of the muscle and its complex insertion.

Classification

Pectoralis major ruptures may be classified according to the extent and site of the rupture. Type 1 ruptures consist of a contusion or sprain; type 2 represents partial ruptures; and type 3 includes complete rupture of the muscle origin, muscle belly, musculotendinous junction, or tendon or avulsion of the insertion.

Partial tears are more common than complete tears, with partial tears usually occurring at the musculotendinous junction and complete tears tending to occur at the tendon-bone interface.[50] Most cases are undoubtedly partial, but 90 of the 104 cases reported since 1972 that came to surgery were complete. In these reports the predominant lesion was avulsion from the humerus in 78 cases. Avulsion from the musculotendinous junction occurred in 17 cases, tendinous ruptures accounted for 3 cases, and only 2 cases involved rupture of the muscle itself.

Incidence and Mechanisms

Rupture of the pectoralis major muscle was believed to be rare, with only infrequent reports in the literature until the 1970s. McEntire and colleagues[50] reviewed the literature in 1972 and concluded that the injury probably occurs much more frequently than reports would indicate. The approximately 167 cases that have been reported during the past 30 years account for nearly 75% of the 223 cases reported in the literature. The problem has been reported exclusively in males. Although the injury has occurred in patients ranging in age from newborn to 79 years old, the majority occur between the ages of 20 and 40.

Rupture of the pectoralis major follows extreme muscle tension or direct trauma, or a combination of both. Of the 56 cases reviewed by McEntire and coworkers,[50] excessive muscle tension caused 37 injuries and direct trauma caused 9. A combination of the two mechanisms was the cause in four cases, and spontaneous rupture was reported in three instances. In the more recent literature, excess tension injury was the cause in 152 patients, and direct injury occurred in 5 cases. The most common mechanism of injury has been associated with weightlifting (46%), with approximately 30% of the injuries resulting from the bench press exercise. Injuries arising from the bench press accounted for four of nine cases reported by Zeman and associates,[101] 9 of 19 cases reported by Kretzler and Richardson,[40] 9 of 15 patients recorded by Connell,[12] and 10 of 17 cases examined by

Schepsis and coworkers.[83] (Injuries sustained during rugby play accounted for 12 of 22 cases reported by Hanna and associates.[32])

Wolfe and associates,[99] supported by cadaver and clinical studies, provide an explanation for the high rate of injury with bench pressing. Their patients describe the rupture occurring when the bar is at its lowest point with the shoulders extended to 30 degrees. At this point the fibers of the lowest portion of the sternal head become disproportionately stretched. Elliot and associates[19] have shown by electromyographic studies that the pectoralis major muscle is maximally activated at the initiation of the lift with the humerus in the extended position. Wolfe and associates[99] believe that the application of maximal load to inferior fibers stretched to an extreme mechanical disadvantage produces rupture of these fibers. Continued loading then increases the tension on the remaining fibers of the sternal head, which fail. This explanation may account for the increased incidence of rupture of the sternal head during weightlifting. Another common mechanism of injury occurs when a person attempts to break a fall and severe force is applied to a maximally contracted pectoralis major muscle.

There also appears to be a correlation between the mechanism of injury and the site of rupture. Direct trauma causes tears of the muscle belly, whereas excessive tension causes avulsion of the humeral insertion or disruption at the musculotendinous junction. Wrestlers have a propensity to disrupt the muscle at its upper sternoclavicular portion.

Clinical Findings

In the case of an acute injury, a history of excessive muscle stress, a direct blow, or a crush, injury in the shoulder region is associated with severe, sharp, and often burning pain and a tearing sensation at the site of rupture. This is a major and severe injury that is accompanied by significant swelling and ecchymosis. Immediate shoulder dysfunction is apparent.

The physical findings depend on the site of rupture. If the muscle is injured in its proximal portion, the swelling and ecchymosis are usually noted on the anterior part of the chest wall on the involved side. The muscle belly retracts toward the axillary fold and causes a prominent bulge. Rupture in the distal portion may cause swelling and ecchymosis in both the arm and the chest; the body of the muscle bulges on the chest, and such bulging causes the axillary fold to become thin (Fig. 21–1). The shoulder is tender at the site of rupture, and a visible or palpable defect is usually present. Zeman and coworkers[101] described one patient in whom the tendon felt intact through to its humeral insertion. At surgery, however, a complete tear was found at the musculotendinous junction (Fig. 21–2), with an overlying fascial layer giving the impression of an intact tendon. These authors cautioned that the lack of a palpable defect in the axilla is not a reliable sign of continuity of the pectoralis major muscle. Resisted adduction and internal rotation of the arm are weak and accompanied by accentuation of the defect and pain. Indeed, in cases initially seen late after injury, this finding is the predominant sign, with the palpable defect being confirmatory of the pathologic process involved.

X-ray and Laboratory Evaluation

Radiographs generally fail to reveal any bone abnormality, but loss of the normal pectoralis major shadow has been described as a reliable sign of rupture. Soft tissue shadowing is visible when a significant hematoma is present, whereas ultrasound may be useful when confirming the site of rupture. Recent reports suggest that

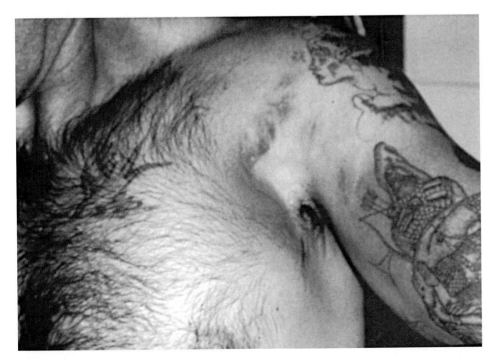

■ **Figure 21–1**
Rupture of the pectoralis major in a 30-year-old weightlifter. *(Courtesy of J. J. Brownlee, M.D.)*

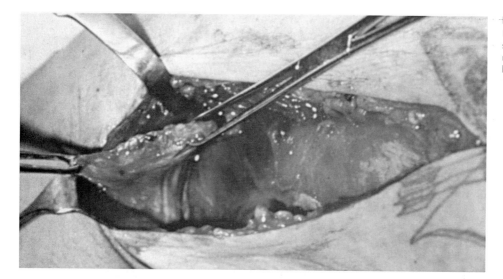

■ Figure 21–2
Findings at surgery in the case shown in Figure 21-1. The pectoralis major tendon is avulsed from its humeral insertion *(right)*.

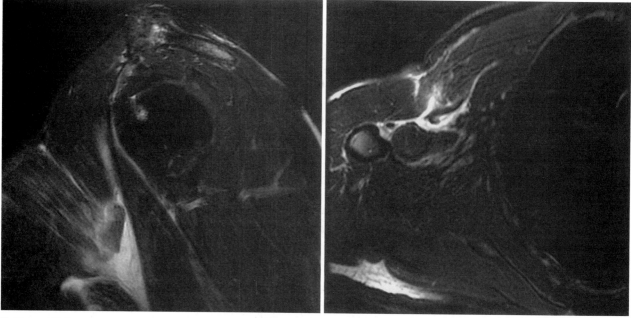

■ Figure 21–3
Magnetic resonance images of pectoralis major tendon avulsion from its humeral insertion.

MRI is superior to CT and should be the modality of choice for assessment of pectoralis major injury.[11] It has been suggested that partial tears can be distinguished from complete tears by MRI and that acute tears can be differentiated from chronic tears.[11] Acute tears demonstrate hemorrhage and edema (Fig. 21-3), whereas chronic tears demonstrate fibrosis and scarring on MRI.[11] MRI may be used to monitor interval healing when patients are treated conservatively and to evaluate muscle quality before return to competitive sports.

Complications

The most sinister documented complication of pectoralis major rupture is sepsis involving the associated hematoma. Noted in three reported cases,[61,69,73] sepsis directly caused the death of one patient and led to death of a second from pneumonia. A patient described by Pai and Simison[69] was remarkable in having a temperature of only 37.5° C and a white blood cell count of 11,500/cm³ despite 1500 mL of frank pus being drained. β-Hemolytic streptococci were cultured. Pseudocyst formation in a hematoma has been described by Ronchetti,[80] and associated neuromuscular injuries have also been reported. Kawashima and associates[39] described a patient with a crush injury, total rupture of the pectoralis major at the musculotendinous junction, and hypoesthesia of the C6-C8 and T1 dermatomes of the affected extremity. Several associated muscle injuries have also been described, including rupture of the anteromedial portion of the adjacent deltoid, pectoralis minor rupture, and rotator cuff tears. Additional injuries in one patient included a fractured humerus and compound fractures of both forearm bones. Purnell[79] has described myositis ossificans in a patient seen 4 months after rupture, and Smith[88] reported the development of rhabdomyosarcoma 10 years after rupture of the pectoralis major at the same site.

Treatment

Methods

Partial rupture of the pectoralis major or lesions of the muscle belly respond to conservative treatment with initial icing and rest to control the hematoma. The early application of heat and ultrasound and a program of shoulder-mobilizing exercises (both passive and active assisted) help restore shoulder function. Unresisted stretching exercises should be included early in the rehabilitation program, but resisted strengthening should await a 6-week recovery with restoration of good shoulder mobility and settling of all pain.

Surgical Treatment

Complete rupture of the pectoralis major demands early surgical treatment in an active athlete. The results of late repair, although they may be satisfactory, are not as good as when primary repair is undertaken.[16]

Tendinous avulsion can be repaired by anatomic reattachment with heavy sutures through drill holes in the humeral cortex. When some tendon remains attached to the humerus, Orava and coworkers[67] have described an effective method of treatment by end-to-end repair of the tendons and reinforcement of the repair with retention sutures into bone.

Tears of the musculotendinous junction can be sutured directly; however, the shredding of tissue structure associated with muscle substance tears offers poor substance for repair, and only imperfect results can be anticipated with this injury.

Results of Treatment

In 1970, Park and Espiniella[71] reviewed 31 patients reported in the literature. Surgical treatment produced an excellent result in 80% of patients, and 10% had good results. This outcome compared most favorably with the good results reported in only 58% of patients who were treated nonoperatively. These authors stated that in the nonoperative group, varying degrees of weakness of adduction and internal rotation were present. However, over time the teres major, subscapularis, deltoid, and latissimus dorsi slowly take over the function of the pectoralis major. Three cases have been reported of wrestlers returning to successful careers after nonoperative treatment. However, Gudmundsson[30] reported that normal power is rarely achieved in these instances. More recently, Zeman and colleagues[101] described nine athletes who had rupture of the pectoralis major. Surgical treatment was undertaken in four cases; all patients had excellent results. In the five patients treated nonoperatively, residual weakness was present in all cases; one professional boxer could not return to boxing, and two weightlifters had good results but were not entirely happy because of persistent weakness.

Kretzler and Richardson[40] undertook repair in 16 of 19 patients, and 13 patients reported full return of strength. This study included two patients who underwent repair as late as $5\frac{1}{2}$ years after the injury. Although full strength was not achieved in these patients, significant improvement was reported. One patient demonstrated improvement in horizontal adduction strength from 50% to 80% and the other from 60% to 84%. The authors believe that with diligent freeing of adhesions and firm fixation to the humerus, late repair is worthwhile.

Scott and associates[84] recommended conservative treatment on the basis that late repair is possible in patients in whom dynamometry indicates persistent weakness. However, they believed that all four patients tested by dynamometry, one of whom underwent repair, had complete rupture of just the sternocostal head and that these injuries would be expected to perform better than total rupture. Wolfe and colleagues[99] tested six patients who had chronic tears, including four with complete tears. In the four patients with complete tears, the peak torque in horizontal adduction was 74% of the normal side, and performance on repetitive testing showed 60% of the normal side at low speed and 76% of the normal side at high speed. Late repair yielded satisfactory results. The authors recommend acute repair for complete tears in patients who require their upper extremity for high-tension activities or sports.

Jones and Matthews[38] classified the outcomes in the literature into one of three grades, depending on range of movement, power, and pain. If the results of those who had surgery within 1 week of injury are compared with those of a combined group of patients who had delayed or no surgery, the results of early surgery are much better ($P < .001$).

Hanna and associates[32] examined 22 patients with complete tears of the pectoralis major by objective strength and subjective functional outcome measures. Injuries sustained in athletic activities were the mechanism in 19 of the 22 cases. Ten patients treated by surgical repair were compared with 12 patients treated nonoperatively. In the group treated surgically, the injured arm regained an average of 99% and 97% of the strength of the uninjured arm as assessed by dynamometer testing of peak torque and work, respectively, whereas patients treated nonsurgically regained 56% of the strength of the uninjured arm. Only one patient who did not undergo repair returned to full function.

Schepsis and associates[83] reported on 17 patients with pectoralis major injuries; 4 were treated nonoperatively and 13 were treated by surgery. They found an overall satisfaction rating of 96% in the acute surgical group, 93% in the chronic surgical group, and 51% in the nonoperative group. On isokinetic testing, adduction strength was found to be 102% of the opposite side in the acute surgical group, 94% in the chronic surgical group, and 71% in the nonoperative group. They concluded that there were no significant differences in outcome between patients treated operatively for acute or chronic injuries, but that surgically treated patients fared significantly better than patients treated nonoperatively.

In a meta-analysis of 112 cases of pectoralis major rupture, Bak and colleagues[6] calculated 88% excellent or good results for patients treated surgically versus 27% for patients treated conservatively. They also found that significantly more patients had an excellent outcome when surgery was performed within 8 weeks of the injury than when surgery was delayed. They concluded that surgical treatment, preferably within the first 8 weeks after the injury, has a significantly better outcome than conservative treatment or delayed repair does.

■ PREFERRED TREATMENT

For major avulsions of the musculotendinous junction or tendinous insertion in all but sedentary patients, we recommend early surgical treatment. We treat ruptures of the muscle belly or partial tears nonoperatively.

RUPTURE OF THE DELTOID

Historical Review

The deltoid muscle is probably the single most important muscular structure in the shoulder girdle. Satisfactory function of the shoulder cannot be anticipated if this muscle is irrevocably injured or its nerve supply is compromised. Luckily, rupture of the deltoid muscle itself is a relatively uncommon clinical entity. First described by Clemens[11] in 1913 in a railway worker, reports in the literature have been sparse since then. In 1919, Davis[16] reported one case in which the deltoid became detached after suppuration of its bony origin as a result of osteomyelitis of the clavicle. Gilcreest and Albi[29] described two further cases in 1939. In 1972, McEntire and co-workers[50] reported a case associated with rupture of the pectoralis major. In 1975, Samuel and associates[82] described a single case, and in 1976, Pointud and colleagues[76] described a further case, both reported in the French literature. Both patients had received multiple injections of steroids—in the first case, 18 injections for a frozen shoulder, and in the second case, approximately 12 per year for several years in association with a rotator cuff tear. In the latter case the patient also received radiotherapy, and this treatment, combined with injections of steroids in direct contact with the deltoid, resulted in disruption of the middle third of the deltoid. Management was conservative.

Panting and Hunter[70] reported two deltoid ruptures in elderly patients in 1983, and Morisawa and associates[58] reported two instances of deltoid muscle rupture associated with rotator cuff tears. One patient was 71 years old and the other was 80 years old; neither had an associated traumatic injury, although one did have repeated hydrocortisone injections. One patient was treated surgically with resection of the thinned portion and a side-to-side repair and achieved excellent motion at 3 months. In their review, the authors noted that most of the patients had sclerotic changes and an osteophyte at the greater tuberosity and postulated that upward migration of the humeral head in the presence of a massive rotator cuff tear

combined with an osteophyte on the greater tuberosity may cause repeated friction and degeneration of the deltoid.

In 2002, Allen and Drakos[3] described a 31-year-old professional cricket player (fast bowler) who suffered partial detachment of the deltoid muscle without concomitant rotator cuff injury. This patient appears to be the first report of deltoid muscle detachment without an associated rotator cuff tear. The authors suggested that the windmill action of the bowling motion places significant force on the deltoid muscle and can lead to partial detachment of the deltoid muscle. The patient did well with conservative management.

The literature does not abound with reports of deltoid rupture. Indeed, the rarity of this type of injury was exemplified in the Mayo Clinic series of 1014 cases of musculotendinous rupture described by Anzel and colleagues[5] in which no cases were unveiled.

Anatomy

The deltoid is a multipennate muscle arising from the outer aspect of the anatomic "horseshoe" formed by the spine of the scapula, the acromion, and the outer end of the clavicle. It enfolds the shoulder and encloses the rotator cuff, with insertion on the outer aspect of the humerus. The motor supply from the axillary or circumflex nerve reaches the muscle posteriorly on its undersurface.

Mechanism

Minor strains of the deltoid are common in athletic activity, particularly in throwing sports. The anterior deltoid may be injured in the acceleration phase of throwing when forward body movement and forcible contraction are simultaneously applied to an already stretched musculotendinous unit. In the follow-through phase at the end of forward motion of the arm, the posterior deltoid must restrain the shoulder and is vulnerable to injury.

Complete traumatic disruption of the deltoid, as the literature reviewed indicates, is rare. Indeed, the trauma to the deltoid most commonly seen in clinical practice is associated with misguided shoulder surgery, particularly if the deltoid is detached from the acromion and becomes dehiscent. The posterior approach to the shoulder, in which the deltoid is released from the spine of the scapula, is a major culprit in this regard.

In instances in which traumatic rupture of the deltoid has occurred, the rupture inevitably involves the application of a major external force to an already maximally contracted deltoid muscle.

Clinical Findings

Examination findings vary with the site of rupture. If the muscle is avulsed from its origin, the normal deltoid contour is lost, and the patient has weakness in abduction, flexion, or extension, depending on the involved part. If the rotator cuff is also deficient, contraction of the remaining deltoid will cause the humeral head to protrude in the direction of the deltoid deficiency.

If the lesion is located near the deltoid insertion, a defect may be palpable along with an associated mass that becomes firmer on contraction of the deltoid muscle.

Methods of Treatment

Minor strains and partial lesions of the deltoid muscle can be handled nonoperatively. Local icing in the acute phase followed by heat, mobilization of the shoulder, stretching, and gentle strengthening over a 6-week period will usually restore the shoulder to full activity.

In the management of complete disruptions, no published experience is available to guide us. If such an injury is observed, consideration should be given to prompt surgical exploration in an effort to restore the structure anatomically. However, unless the injury is an avulsion from bone, the repair is likely to be weak. Midsubstance muscle injuries are difficult to suture effectively.

Delay in repair with associated retraction and scarring makes the situation even more difficult. In 1919, Davis[16] first reported the management of a chronic defect of the anterior deltoid with a broad graft of fascia from the thigh. He recommended retaining a thick layer of subcutaneous fat to prevent the formation of adhesions between the rotator cuff and the fascial implant. Clearly, late salvage of this injury is not satisfactory; if deltoid ruptures are to be dealt with satisfactorily, early identification and prompt surgical repair are mandatory.

Postoperative care after such surgery is vital. Abduction or flexion splinting to relieve the tension on the repair is maintained for 6 weeks or so before mobilization is commenced, and a strengthening program is not introduced for 6 to 8 weeks after intervention.

■ PREFERRED TREATMENT

We carry out early surgical treatment in cases involving complete disruption of a third or more of the deltoid substance. Tears and strains of lesser degree are treated nonoperatively. The problem of compromise of the deltoid origin by previous surgery is a difficult one. When an acromionectomy has been performed, reconstruction is not possible because the important anterolateral deltoid has lost its origin. With symptomatic failure of deltoid reattachment after acromioplasty, we consider re-exploration, mobilization of the superficial and deep aspects of the muscle, and repair back to the acromion. Postoperative protection is necessary to avoid active flexion and passive extension.

RUPTURE OF THE TRICEPS

Historical Review

In 1868, Partridge[72] reported the first case of rupture of the triceps in a patient who fell partly on the roadway and partly on the sidewalk and struck the left arm just above

and behind the elbow joint. He observed a $^3/_4$-inch-long depression and a slight wound above and behind the elbow, in addition to tenderness over the triceps tendon. The arm was held extended and quiet for 1 week, after which passive motion commenced. Only eight more cases were reported in the next 100 years before Tarsney[92] added seven cases; this author clarified the mechanism of injury and emphasized the importance of the presence of avulsed bony fragments on the lateral radiograph when confirming the diagnosis. Although Tarsney described one patient with the combination of triceps rupture and fracture of the radial head, it was Levy and colleagues[43] who drew attention to this combination in 1978. In 1982 Levy and associates[44] reported on 16 patients with triceps rupture, 15 of whom had associated radial head fractures and 1 had a fracture of the capitellum.

Anatomy

The triceps muscle consists of two aponeurotic laminae. The long head arising from the inferior glenoid neck and the lateral head from the humerus converge to form the superficial lamina, which commences at about the middle of the muscle and covers its lower half. The tendon inserts into the posterior portion of the upper surface of the olecranon.

The medial head lies deep and arises from a broad origin on the humerus; it inserts both directly into the olecranon and indirectly via the superficial lamina formed from the other two heads. A few fibers are inserted into the posterior capsule of the elbow joint to retract it during extension.

Incidence and Mechanisms

Rupture of the triceps muscle is a rare injury, and only 50 cases have been reported in the literature. Patients with renal osteodystrophy are at greater risk of sustaining triceps rupture with bony avulsion.[21,77] The condition may result from either indirect injury or a direct blow. Of the 40 cases in which the mechanism of injury is known, 29 (75%) resulted from an indirect injury (the application of excessive tension to the muscle fibers), 7 (17%) from a direct blow, and 3 (8%) from a combination of both. The usual cause of injury is a fall onto the outstretched hand. This mechanism was evident in 8 of 15 cases collected by Tarsney[92] and in 13 of 16 cases presented by Levy and coworkers[44] in which the mechanism was known.

Most direct injuries are a result of the elbow striking a fixed object, but crush injury has also been described.[56] There appears to be no correlation between the mechanism of injury and the site of disruption of the triceps.

Clinical Findings

The patient gives a history of a direct blow or indirect injury, as described earlier. Particularly with an indirect injury, the patient may report a tearing sensation about the elbow. Pain, swelling, and weakness of elbow extension are commonly noted.

On examination a palpable defect is present, usually in the triceps tendon, along with associated swelling and often bruising. The patient exhibits an inability to actively extend the elbow when the rupture is complete. If a fracture of the radial head has also occurred, tenderness and swelling are present over the fracture site and may dominate the clinical picture.[44]

X-ray Evaluation

Radiographs may be helpful in confirming triceps avulsion. In six of seven patients described by Tarsney and in 12 of 16 patients in Levy's series, avulsion fragments from the olecranon were present. Radiographs are also important in excluding associated injuries. Radial head fracture is a common associated finding,[44] and fracture of the distal end of the radius and ulna has also been reported.[41]

Complications

Levy and colleagues[44] emphasized the association of radial head fracture with triceps rupture, which was present in 15 of 16 of their patients. Hence they recommended that all patients with a radial head fracture be carefully assessed to exclude injury to the triceps tendon.

A most unusual complication described in 1987 by Brumbuck[9] involved avulsion of the origin of the lateral head of the triceps with an associated compartment syndrome. Partial ulnar nerve palsy following a direct blow that resulted in rupture of the triceps tendon has also been described.[2] A year later, tenderness was still present over the ulnar nerve together with hypoesthesia of the ulnar distribution; at surgery, the nerve was found to be enclosed in a bed of adhesions. Transposition of the ulnar nerve was carried out.

Methods of Treatment

In complete rupture of the triceps tendon, experience with nonoperative treatment is limited. In 1962, Preston and Adicoff[77] described a patient with hyperparathyroidism who had suffered avulsion of the quadriceps tendons bilaterally and rupture of the triceps tendon with an avulsed bone fragment. The elbow was not immobilized, and in the 14 months after injury the patient was described as having little disability with ordinary activity. In a case described by Anderson and Le Cocq[4] in which a 27-year-old woman had struck her triceps region against the gearshift of a car, the result was poor. After 1 year she still lacked 10 degrees of extension and had tenderness over the rupture site. Her triceps strength was reduced by approximately half. Exploration revealed a completely ruptured tendon that had healed by scarring in an elongated position. After excision of the scar and shortening of the tendon, she achieved an excellent result with almost normal power. Sherman and coworkers[87] described a 24-year-old patient (a bodybuilder) who was examined 3 months after injury. Resisted extension of the arm was markedly weak in comparison to the opposite side. Cybex testing revealed a 42% extensor deficit at 60 degrees per

second. After surgical repair at 6 months, normal function was eventually achieved. A patient described by Tarsney[92] was originally treated with a plaster cast with the elbow flexed to 90 degrees. Although the patient regained some active extension initially, at 4 months she had increased weakness. Examination confirmed a palpable defect and loss of extension of the elbow. Delayed repair resulted in return of full motion and power. In 1992, O'Driscoll[65] reported a patient with complete intramuscular rupture of the long head of the triceps that was treated nonoperatively. The patient's isometric strength was normal, but endurance testing was reduced by 5% to 10%. Nonoperative treatment was recommended for all except those who require significant endurance strength in elbow extension.

Sheps and colleagues[86] in 1997 reported a 13-year-old boy with an intramuscular rupture of the long head of the triceps muscle. Despite Cybex testing indicating a large extension and pronation deficit, the patient had no significant functional weakness and remained active without any significant disability following conservative management.

■ PREFERRED TREATMENT

We prefer surgical treatment of both early and late injuries. Although our method of repair has varied somewhat, fixation with heavy suture material via drill holes in the olecranon is effective. In one patient treated by the authors, the avulsed fragment was large enough to fix with Kirschner wires and a tension band wire, with supplementary sutures in the damaged tendon and muscle yielding sound fixation. The arm is immobilized in a cast at 30 degrees for a period of 4 weeks before mobilization.

RUPTURE OF THE BICEPS

Lesions of the biceps tendon are discussed in detail in Chapter 19. This section focuses on rupture of the biceps muscle.

Historical Review

In documenting the history of biceps muscle rupture, we have had difficulty in confirming the site of the lesion. While reviewing the predominantly European literature, Gilcreest noted that of 81 cases of biceps rupture, only 15 had come to surgery. Difficulty in locating the site of rupture clinically is highlighted by the comments made in 1935 by Haldeman and Soto-Hall,[31] who noted this problem in recent tears of the biceps.

The hematoma produced by a tear in the upper part of the tendon gravitates downward through the sheath to the region of the belly, where it becomes clinically evident. The ecchymosis and tenderness suggest that the tear took place at the musculotendinous junction.

Many of the early cases of "muscle rupture" are likely to have been tears of the long head. In 1900, Loos[45] believed that 19.5% of ruptures of the biceps were actually ruptures of the long head and 43.6% occurred at the musculotendinous junction of the long head; 15.1% were total muscle ruptures, whereas 21.8% were partial muscle ruptures. In 1922 Gilcreest[27] stated, "According to most writers, about 66% are believed to occur in the muscle substance." Clearly, these figures for muscle rupture are much too high; certainly, however, the earlier literature contains well-documented cases of muscle rupture. In 1928, Conwell[13] described a 38-year-old man who sustained a traction injury to the limb while holding a drill handle. Surgery revealed complete rupture of both bellies of the biceps in the middle third, with the margins of the rupture being quite smooth, as though cut by a knife.

In 106 biceps ruptures in 100 patients, Gilcreest[27] diagnosed complete rupture of the entire muscle in 6, partial rupture in 1, complete rupture of the muscle of the long head in 3, and partial rupture in 5. In addition, one complete rupture of the muscle of the short head and one partial rupture were diagnosed.

In 1941, Tobin and associates[93] described rupture of the biceps muscle in parachutists. In 1978, Heckman and Levine[36] reported on 48 parachutists with rupture of the biceps muscle, thus making this series the largest by far in the literature.

A ruptured biceps muscle was noted by Bricknell[7] in a British parachutist who achieved complete functional recovery and no loss of muscle power with conservative treatment. Both DiChristina and Lustig[10] and Moorman and coworkers[57] reported cases of biceps rupture suffered in water-skiing accidents, the latter resulting in neurovascular disruption of the musculotendinous unit as it was displaced into the forearm.

Incidence and Mechanisms

Rupture of the biceps muscle was thought to be a rare injury. The lesion was overdiagnosed in the early literature for reasons stated earlier, and the figures are therefore misleading. In the older literature, indirect injury from traction applied to a contracting biceps muscle is described. More recently, reports in the literature involve examples of direct injury in military parachutists.[36,93] In the period from 1973 to 1975, Heckman and Levine[36] encountered more than 50 patients with closed transection of the biceps in a population of 40,000 paratroopers undertaking a total of over 10,000 parachute jumps each year.

The mechanism of injury is essentially the same for all parachutists. A 2-cm-wide woven nylon strap (the static line) is attached to the paratrooper's pack and the aircraft. The paratrooper jumps, and when a force of 6.33 kg/cm (80 lb/in²) is applied to the casing of the parachute, it comes free and allows the parachute to open. If the static line is positioned incorrectly in front of the arm, a severe force may be applied over the biceps, especially if the arm is simultaneously abducted after pushoff.

Clinical Findings

The patient gives a history of direct or indirect injury, as described earlier. A tearing or popping sensation in the

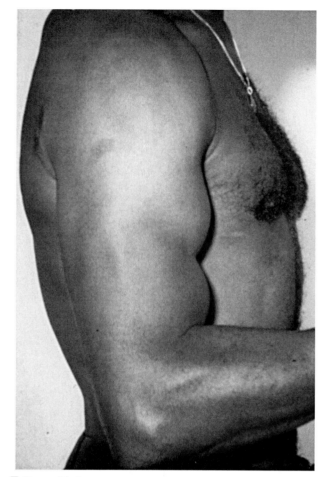

■ Figure 21–4
Biceps muscle rupture in a weightlifter.

arm often accompanies an indirect injury, followed by severe pain, swelling, and loss of strength. Gilcreest[28] states that the pain is more intense with muscle rupture than with tendon rupture. A visible and palpable defect in the muscle may also be present (Fig. 21–4), particularly if the patient is seen early, before significant hematoma and swelling occur. Gilcreest also states that the humerus may be felt beneath the skin in the defect, presumably with the brachialis interposed. Extensive ecchymosis and pronounced bruising are often noted. Weakness is present, and its severity depends on the extent of rupture. In the paratroopers described by Heckman and Levine, the skin always showed some degree of contusion or abrasion but had no laceration. These authors stated that although immediate, marked local hemorrhage and swelling occur, the defect may be difficult to appreciate immediately and the degree of the injury may not be recognized. After the acute hematoma and swelling subside, however, the severity of the injury can more readily be appreciated.

X-ray Evaluation

In Heckman and Levine's series,[36] radiographs at the time of injury were negative, except in one patient with an associated scapular neck fracture. The recent literature has offered numerous reports that support the authors' predictions regarding the usefulness of both ultrasound and MRI in confirming biceps ruptures.[20,46,48,78,94,96] The superior soft tissue contrast resolution of these diagnostic tools in comparison to radiography not only allows for confirmation of a diagnosis but can also portray the extent of the muscle injury.

Complications

Musculocutaneous nerve injury was common in Heckman and Levine's series.[36] Although none of their patients showed alterations in sensation with respect to the distribution of the lateral cutaneous nerve of the forearm, electromyographic studies were positive in 9 of 11 patients studied. On follow-up, 1 year later, two patients had normal electromyograms, six had signs of re-establishment of the nerve supply to the muscle, and one had persistent denervation. Two patients showed denervation of only one head of the biceps at 3 and 4 months after injury and were expected to recover. The authors concluded that contusion of the musculocutaneous nerve is frequent but permanent paralysis of the muscle rarely occurs.

The results of inadequately treated rupture of the biceps muscle were well documented by Heckman and Levine.[36] They evaluated 28 male paratroopers an average of 19 months after injury. Twenty-five patients displayed weakness of the arm and fatigue, especially with activity requiring rapid, repeated elbow flexion. Seventeen patients complained of an unsightly cosmetic defect, and 12 experienced pain, generally when using the muscle. The maximal force generated by elbow flexion at 90 degrees as measured with an ergometer was 53% of that of controls.

Methods of Treatment

Heckman and Levine[36] treated 20 patients whom they allocated to one of two treatment regimens. Ten patients underwent acute surgical repair within 72 hours of injury. The muscle was explored through an anteromedial approach. The typical lesion found in all cases was transection of the belly with an intact fascial envelope, with the space within the fascia being filled with blood. The hematoma was evacuated and the muscle belly was reapproximated with double right-angled sutures of heavy catgut reinforced with a U-shaped flap of biceps fascia. The elbow was then immobilized in acute flexion for 4 weeks and at 90 degrees for an additional 2 weeks. The second group of 10 patients was treated by aspiration and splinting. It appeared to the authors that the intrafascial hematoma was the primary obstruction to closure of the muscle gap. Because it was seen at surgery that the hematoma could be aspirated with a 16-gauge needle and the muscle gap closed with acute elbow flexion, this treatment method was used. After aspiration, the elbow was immobilized in a cast in acute flexion for 6 weeks; range-of-motion exercises were then begun.

At follow-up 8.8 months after surgery or 7.1 months after aspiration, muscle power was virtually identical—76.5% and 77% of normal, respectively. Both were superior to the 53% of normal found in the original, untreated group. In one patient in the surgical group a deep wound infection developed and required débridement, intravenous antibiotics, and secondary wound closure. In view of the equal strength of the two groups and the lack of complications with aspiration and splinting, this latter treatment was favored.

Delayed treatment gives only fair results. Heckman and Levine[36] undertook repair in six patients at 4 to 18 months. The musculocutaneous nerve was intact in the base of the wound in all cases. Scar tissue was noted to be denser in those operated on later. At 6 months, three of five patients showed improved power (an average of 42% of normal power improving to 57%), and the appearance was somewhat improved.

Interestingly, Leighton and associates,[42] expanding on previous work by Agins and colleagues,[1] revealed differences between complete repair of dominant and nondominant extremities after operative treatment of distal biceps tendon ruptures. Testing of dominant extremities showed full return of forearm supination strength as well as elbow flexion strength. In nondominant repaired extremities, a 14% supination strength deficit in expected values and a 14% flexion strength deficit (both corrected for dominance) were noted. Interestingly, after excision of the disrupted biceps brachii from the arm of a 15-year-old boy, Moorman[57] noted no loss of strength on supination of the forearm or glenohumeral flexion 1 year after the injury, although a deficit of strength on flexion of the elbow was noted. Endurance differences were not significant. Leighton and associates[42] suggested that although dominant extremities are more likely to achieve normal function after repair, nondominant extremities may require intense rehabilitation to achieve maximal strength.

■ PREFERRED TREATMENT

For patients seen with biceps rupture in the acute phase, we prefer aspiration of the hematoma and immobilization of the elbow in acute flexion for 6 weeks. For subacute ruptures, we favor open repair and immobilization in acute flexion for 4 weeks and flexion at 90 degrees for 2 weeks. When a significant delay before initial examination has occurred, we base the decision to repair the muscle on the patient's occupation, functional deficit, and concern regarding cosmesis. The prognosis in such cases is guarded.

RUPTURE OF THE SERRATUS ANTERIOR

Although traumatic winging of the scapula as a result of injury to the long thoracic nerve is not uncommon, with several hundred cases reported in the English literature, rupture of the serratus anterior muscle is extremely uncommon. Fitchet[22] was the first to report on injury to the serratus anterior muscle; in 1930 he described five cases, although the diagnosis was not confirmed surgically in any, nor was electrodiagnostic equipment available to exclude injury to the long thoracic nerve. In 1940, Overpeck and Ghormley[68] reported five additional cases of suspected rupture of the serratus anterior muscle. They believed that the severity of the pain was helpful in differentiating muscle rupture from long thoracic nerve palsy in that trauma to the muscle produced more severe pain than that seen with involvement of the nerve alone. Again, the cases were not confirmed surgically or electro-diagnostically.

In 1981, Hayes and Zehr[35] provided the first report of a surgically proven traumatic avulsion of the serratus anterior muscle. Their patient, a 25-year-old man who was driving an all-terrain vehicle that rolled over, sustained a mild cerebral contusion, a fractured jaw, and an injury to the right shoulder that resulted in a displaced fracture of the inferior angle of the scapula. The exact mechanism of injury was uncertain. He was treated in a sling, and at 2 weeks winging of the scapula was noted. The winging persisted; after returning to work as a carpenter several months later, he noted that the arm tired easily and was weak, particularly when working with the arm in front or overhead. He was also troubled by a grating sensation under the scapula. These symptoms persisted, and after 9 months he underwent exploration. The findings included rupture of both the rhomboideus major and serratus anterior muscles. The tendinous attachment of the serratus anterior to the separated inferior pole fragment remained intact. The inferior pole was excised, and both muscles were reattached to the freshened border of the scapula with No. 1 silk sutures. A Velpeau sling was used postoperatively, and the shoulder was protected for 6 weeks. Full strength was regained, with no further winging of the scapula, and the patient returned to his former occupation. Hayes[34] has subsequently treated a second patient who rolled a car over and sustained a similar avulsion of the inferior pole of the scapula. He experienced pain and weakness in his work as a welder and greatly improved after repair.

In 1986, a third case of rupture of the serratus anterior was described by Meythaler and colleagues[52] in a 64-year-old man with severe rheumatoid arthritis. His injury occurred with two episodes of rolling over in bed while the shoulder was flexed and abducted. Winging of the scapula was evident clinically, along with marked infrascapular swelling and ecchymoses that extended along the lateral chest wall. Nerve conduction studies were normal in the long thoracic nerve, as was electromyography. Treatment was conservative, with rest followed by an intensive physiotherapy program. After 16 weeks the patient was independent in activities of daily living, but the winging persisted. In this case, several predisposing factors existed. Gross restriction of glenohumeral joint movement resulted in increased stress on the serratus anterior, which was already weakened by chronic prednisone therapy and type 2 muscle atrophy associated with rheumatoid arthritis. Salicylate-induced coagulopathy may have contributed to the hematoma.

From the limited experience with disruption of the serratus anterior muscle reported in the literature, the authors advocate surgical repair in all except elderly and debilitated patients.

RUPTURE OF THE CORACOBRACHIALIS

In 1939, Gilcreest and Albi[29] stated that they were unable to find any recorded case of rupture of the coraco-brachialis in the literature. However, they reported a single case that was due to direct violence, and at surgery they discovered a rupture of the belly of the muscle. The patient had experienced considerable impairment of function in the arm; he was reported to make a complete recovery postoperatively. In 1941, a second case was described by Tobin and colleagues[93] in which a parachutist sustained a direct injury caused by his static line. No cases were included in the series of 1412 muscle ruptures reported by Anzel and coworkers[5] from the Mayo Clinic. This lesion appears to be rare. Acute repair is recommended in young, active patients.

RUPTURE OF THE SUBSCAPULARIS

In 1835, Smith[89] first reported an isolated tear of the subscapularis tendon in a cadaver. Speed[90] reported two patients in whom rupture of the subscapularis tendon had been diagnosed clinically but was not treated surgically. Gilcreest and Albi[29] reported one rupture found at surgery, but no details of the site of rupture were available.

Partial rupture of the subscapularis in association with anterior dislocation of the glenohumeral joint is well documented.[17,33,59,91] The part of the muscle that appears particularly vulnerable is the lower quarter, where the insertion may be directly from muscle into bone.[17,91] Of 45 patients operated on for recurrent anterior dislocation, Symeonides[91] reported six ruptures of the lower quarter of the subscapularis; 24 patients had partial rupture of the muscle at various other points. Partial rupture of the subscapularis muscle has also been produced in cadavers by anterior dislocation of the shoulder.[17,91] The presence of the muscle injury has been used as a rationale for immobilization in internal rotation after acute anterior dislocation of the shoulder.

McAuliffe and Dowd[49] reported a case of complete avulsion of the subscapularis insertion in a 54-year-old woman after she fell directly onto her shoulder. It was not possible to dislocate the shoulder under general anesthesia. After reattachment at the fragment with nylon sutures, the patient regained full movement and returned to her normal activities in 3 months.

In the recent literature four larger studies have been published on isolated rupture of the subscapularis tendon. In 1991, Gerber and Krushell[26] reported on 16 men, 3 of whom had previously undergone surgery. The average age of the patients was 51 years. The injury was caused by violent external rotation of the adducted arm in seven cases and by violent hyperextension in six cases. Two injuries occurred in motor vehicle accidents, and only one was associated with an anterior dislocation. All patients complained of pain anteriorly that was troublesome at night, and all had pain and weakness when the arm was used above and below the shoulder level. The authors describe the "liftoff" test, which was abnormal in 12 of 13 patients tested. One patient had limitation of internal rotation such that performance of the test was not possible. Weakness of internal rotation was noted in 13 of 14 patients tested, and passive external rotation was increased in 10 of 16 patients. The long head of the biceps was dislocated medially in nine patients and ruptured in two patients. Ultrasound, CT arthrography, and MRI scanning all correctly predicted the surgical diagnosis. The authors recommend ultrasound examination first and the addition of MRI in questionable cases. All 16 patients underwent surgery, mainly by the recommended deltopectoral approach, with care taken to protect the axillary and musculocutaneous nerves because the tendon stump was mobilized. The early results of repair were very encouraging.

In 1994, Nove Josserand and associates[64] published a report of 21 cases of isolated subscapularis rupture, all of which were confirmed surgically. Also in the French literature, Nerot and colleagues[62] reported 25 rotator cuff tears that predominantly involved the subscapularis. When coracohumeral impingement is evident, the authors advise a high index of suspicion for subscapularis rupture.

Gerber and colleagues[25] in 1996 reported the results of operative repair of isolated rupture of the subscapularis tendon in 16 patients. Patients who had an avulsion of the lesser tuberosity or postoperative avulsion were excluded. Operative treatment consisted of transosseous reinsertion of the tendon to a trough created at the lesser tuberosity. Thirteen patients subjectively rated the result as excellent or good. The average functional score of the shoulder, as assessed according to the system of Constant, was 82% of the average age- and gender-matched normal value. The capacity of the patients to work in their original occupations had increased from an average of 59% of full capacity preoperatively to an average of 95% postoperatively. The most consistent preoperative findings were increased passive excessive external rotation and an inability to maintain passive maximal internal rotation actively. The results suggested that a long delay (greater than 36 months) between injury and repair adversely affected the ultimate outcome. In summary, a significant number of isolated subscapularis ruptures have been reported in the recent literature, and it is apparent that the lesion is more common than previously thought.

Rupture of the subscapularis after first-time dislocation of the shoulder predisposes to recurrent instability. Neviaser and associates[63] evaluated 37 patients older than 40 years who sustained rotator cuff tears with primary anterior dislocation of the shoulder. Anterior instability developed in 11 patients from this group as a result of rupture of the subscapularis tendon and anterior capsule. Stability was restored with repair of the capsule and subscapularis. In 1993, Moeckel and colleagues[55] addressed the problem of instability in a review of 236 total shoulder replacements from the Hospital for Special Surgery. Instability developed in 10 patients, anteriorly in 7 of them. This instability was due to rupture of the subscapularis tendon. Despite repair, three patients continued to have instability.

In 1994, Patten[74] reported the MRI findings in nine patients with surgically confirmed rotator cuff tears that predominantly or exclusively involved the subscapularis tendon. The contours of the subscapularis tendon were poorly defined, and the tendon itself was of abnormally high signal intensity on T2-weighted images. Discontinuity and frank retraction of the tendon were evident in seven patients (78%). Thickening of the distal portion of the tendon was present in three cases and calcification in one. Five patients had medial dislocation of the tendon.

In 1999, Pfirrmann and associates[75] retrospectively reviewed MR arthrograms of the shoulder in 50 patients. Two radiologists analyzed the images and found a sensitivity of 91% and a specificity of 86%/79% (reader 1/reader 2) for the diagnosis of tears of the subscapularis tendon. Several signs were specific (90% to 100%) but insensitive (29% to 62%): leakage of contrast material onto the lesser tuberosity, fatty degeneration of the subscapularis muscle, and abnormality in the course of the long biceps tendon.

Tung and colleagues[95] in 2001 reported on signs of subscapularis tendon tears on MRI. They performed a retrospective review of 16 patients with isolated tears of the subscapularis tendon confirmed at surgery or arthroscopy. Primary signs of subscapularis tendon tear were present on MRI in 94% of surgically confirmed tears, although a preoperative diagnosis was made in only 31% of cases. The most common appearance on MRI (63%) was a full-thickness tear involving the superior third of the tendon with a relatively normal appearance of the inferior two thirds. Associated findings on MRI include medial displacement or abnormal signal of the biceps tendon and superior glenoid labral tears.

RUPTURE OF THE SUPRASPINATUS

Rupture of the supraspinatus muscle at the musculotendinous junction was reported by Hertel and Lambert[37] in 1998. The injury occurred in a 34-year-old man after falling from a bicycle and was associated with osseous avulsion of the infraspinatus. The patient was initially examined 6 years after the injury, and an end-to-end repair was performed. Full active elevation was regained by 12 weeks postoperatively, but a rerupture occurred 5 months after surgery when the patient fell from a ladder.

RUPTURE OF THE INFRASPINATUS

In 1990, Motta and Carletti[60] reported spontaneous rupture of the infraspinatus muscle from its scapular insertion. The injury occurred in a young women after a fall from a chair, with the mechanism being forced internal rotation and adduction of the shoulder. The patient was treated conservatively and had no limitation of shoulder movement 1 year later.

RUPTURE OF THE TERES MAJOR

Maldjian and associates[47] reported an isolated tear of the teres major muscle that occurred as a result of a waterskiing injury produced by a sudden forward force caused by the tow rope jerking the patient's arm forward. MRI demonstrated disruption of the teres major muscle fibers near its insertion site on the humerus, but the rotator cuff was intact. The authors describe why the teres major muscle might be particularly vulnerable to damage from this mechanism of injury. A discussion of treatment and outcome is not presented.

CONCLUSION

Muscle ruptures are not common, yet they can produce substantial disability after a direct or indirect injury to the shoulder or arm. Surgical repair is difficult because of the problem of suturing muscle tissue directly; however, repair in the acute phase is recommended whenever possible. Such repair can be further assisted by immobilization in a position that approximates the edges of the torn muscle. Careful protected exercise programs can then be initiated to further ensure optimal rehabilitation.

REFERENCES

1. Agins HJ, Chess J, Hoekstra D, and Teitge R: Rupture of the distal insertion of the biceps brachii tendon. Clin Orthop 233:34-38, 1988.
2. Albo A: Ruptured pectoralis major tendon: A case report on delayed repair with muscle advancement. Acta Orthop Scand 65:652-653, 1994.
3. Allen AA and Drakos MC: Partial detachment of the deltoid muscle. Am J Sports Med 30:133-134, 2002.
4. Anderson KJ and Le Cocq JF: Rupture of the triceps tendon. J Bone Joint Surg Am 39:444-446, 1957.
5. Anzel H, Covey KW, Weiner AD, et al: Disruption of muscles and tendons: An analysis of 1,014 cases. Surgery 45:406-414, 1959.
6. Bak K, Cameron EA, and Henderson J: Rupture of the pectoralis major: A meta-analysis of 112 cases. Knee Surg Sports Traumatol Arthrosc 8:113-119, 2000.
7. Bricknell MCM: Traumatic rupture of biceps brachii—a hazard of military parachuting. J R Army Med Corps 137:144-145, 1991.
8. Brickner WM and Milch H: Ruptures of muscles and tendons. International Clinics, vol II, Series 38-7, 1997.
9. Brumbuck RJ: Compartment syndrome complicating avulsion of the origin of the triceps muscle: A case report. J Bone Joint Surg Am 69:1445-1447, 1987.
10. DiChristina DG and Lustig KA: Rupture through the short head of the biceps muscle belly. Clin Orthop 277:139, 1992.
11. Clemens H: Traumatische Hemie des M. deltoideus. Dtsch Med Wochenschr 39:2197, 1913.
12. Connell DA, Potter HG, Sherman MF, and Wickiewicz TL: Injuries of pectoralis major muscle: Evaluation with MRI imaging. Radiology 210:785-791, 1999.
13. Conwell HL: Subcutaneous rupture of the biceps flexor cubiti; report of one case. J Bone Joint Surg 10:788-790, 1928.
14. Cronkite AE: The tensile strength of human tendons. Anat Rec 64:173-186, 1936.
15. Danielsson L: Ruptur av. m. pectoralis major en brottningsskada. Nord Med 72:1089, 1964.
16. Davis CB: Plastic repair of the deltoid muscle. Surg Clin 3:287-289, 1919.
17. Delport HP and Piper MS: Pectoralis major rupture in athletes. Arch Orthop Trauma Surg 100:135-137, 1982.
18. DePalma AF, Cooke AJ, and Prabhaker M: The role of the subscapularis in recurrent anterior dislocations of the shoulder. Clin Orthop 54:35, 1967.
19. Elliot BC, Wilson GJ, and Kerr GK: A biomechanical analysis of the sticking region in the bench press. Med Sci Sports Exerc 21:450-462, 1989.
20. Falchook FS, Zlatkin MB, Erbacher GE, et al: Rupture of the distal biceps tendon: Evaluation with MR imaging. Acta Orthop Belg 59:426-469, 1993.
21. Farrar EL and Lippert FG: Avulsion of the triceps tendon. Clin Orthop 161:242, 1981.
22. Fitchet SM: Injury of the serratus magnus (anterior) muscle. N Engl J Med 303:818-823, 1930.
23. Garrett WE Jr, Califf JC, and Bassett FH III: Histochemical correlates of hamstring injuries. Am J Sports Med 12:98-103, 1984.
24. Garrett WE Jr, Safran MR, Scaber AV, et al: Biomechanical comparison of stimulated and nonstimulated skeletal muscle pulled to failure. Am J Sports Med 15:448-454, 1987.
25. Gerber C, Hersche O, and Farron A: Isolated rupture of the subscapularis tendon. Results of operative repair. J Bone Joint Surg Am 78:1015-1023, 1996.
26. Gerber C and Krushell RJ: Isolated rupture of the tendon of the subscapularis muscle. Clinical features in 16 cases. J Bone Joint Surg Br 73:389-394, 1991.
27. Gilcreest EL: Rupture of muscles and tendons, particularly subcutaneous rupture of biceps flexor cubiti. JAMA 84:1819-1822, 1922.
28. Gilcreest EL: The common syndrome of rupture, dislocation and elongation of the long head of the biceps brachii; analysis of 200 cases. Surg Gynecol Obstet 58:322-324, 1934.
29. Gilcreest EL and Albi P: Unusual lesions of muscles and tendons of the shoulder girdle and upper arm. Surg Gynecol Obstet 68:903-917, 1939.
30. Gudmundsson B: A case of agenesis and a case of rupture of the pectoralis major muscle. Acta Orthop Scand 44:213-218, 1973.
31. Haldeman K and Soto-Hall R: Injuries to muscles and tendons. JAMA 104:2319-2324, 1935.
32. Hanna CM, Glenny AB, Stanley SN, and Caughey MA: Pectoralis major tears: Comparison of surgical and conservative treatment. Br J Sports Med 35:202-206, 2001.
33. Hauser FDW: Avulsion of the tendon of subscapularis muscle. J Bone Joint Surg Am 36:139-141, 1954.
34. Hayes JM: Personal communication, 1988.
35. Hayes JM and Zehr DJ: Traumatic muscle avulsion causing winging of the scapula. J Bone Joint Surg Am 63:495-497, 1981.
36. Heckman JD and Levine MI: Traumatic closed transection of the biceps brachii in the military parachutist. J Bone Joint Surg Am 60:369-372, 1978.
37. Hertel R and Lambert SM: Supraspinatus rupture at the musculotendinous junction. J Shoulder Elbow Surg 7:432-435, 1998.
38. Jones MW and Matthews JP: Rupture of pectoralis major in weight lifters: A case report and review of the literature. Injury 19:219, 1988.
39. Kawashima M, Sato M, Torisu T, et al: Rupture of the pectoral major: Report of 2 cases. Clin Orthop 109:115-119, 1975.
40. Kretzler HH Jr and Richardson AB: Rupture of the pectoralis major muscle. Am J Sports Med 17:453-458, 1989.
41. Lee MLH: Rupture of triceps tendon. BMJ 2:197, 1960.
42. Leighton MM, Bush-Joseph CA, and Bach BR Jr: Distal biceps brachii repair: Results in dominant and nondominant extremities. Clin Orthop 317:114-121, 1995.
43. Levy M, Fishel RE, and Stern GM: Triceps tendon avulsion with or without fracture of the radial head—a rare injury. J Trauma 18:677-679, 1978.
44. Levy M, Golderg I, and Meir I: Fracture of the head of the radius with a tear or avulsion of the triceps tendon. J Bone Joint Surg Br 64:70-72, 1982.
45. Loos: Beitr Z Klin Chir 29:410, 1900.
46. Lozano V and Alonso P: Sonographic detection of the distal biceps tendon rupture. J Ultrasound Med 14:389-391, 1995.
47. Maldjian C, Adam R, Oxberry B, et al: Isolated tear of the teres major: A waterskiing injury. J Comput Assist Tomogr 24:594-595, 2000.
48. Mayer DP, Schmidt RG, and Ruiz S: MRI diagnosis of biceps tendon rupture. Comput Med Imaging Graph 16:345-347, 1992.
49. McAuliffe TB and Dowd GS: Avulsion of the subscapularis tendon: A case report. J Bone Joint Surg Am 69:1454, 1987.
50. McEntire JE, Hess WE, and Coleman S: Rupture of the pectoralis major muscle. J Bone Joint Surg Am 54:1040-1046, 1972.
51. McMaster PF: Tendon and muscle ruptures. Clinical and experimental studies and locations of subcutaneous ruptures. J Bone Joint Surg 15:705-722, 1933.
52. Meythaler JM, Reddy NM, and Mitz M: Serratus anterior disruption: A complication of rheumatoid arthritis. Arch Phys Med Rehabil 67:770-772, 1986.
53. Miles J, Grana W, Egle D, et al: The effect of anabolic steroids on the biomechanical and histological properties of rat tendon. J Bone Joint Surg Am 74:411-422, 1992.
54. Miller MD, Johnson DL, Fu FS, et al: Rupture of the pectoralis major muscle in a collegiate football player. Am J Sports Med 21:475-477, 1993.
55. Moeckel BH, Altchek DW, Warren RF, et al: Instability of the shoulder after arthroplasty. J Bone Joint Surg Am 75:492-497, 1993.
56. Montgomery AH: Two cases of muscle injury. Surg Clin 4:871, 1920.
57. Moorman CT, Silver SG, Potter HG, and Warren RF: Proximal rupture of the biceps brachii with slingshot displacement into the forearm. J Bone Joint Surg Am 78:1749, 1996.
58. Morisawa K, Yamashita K, Asami A, et al: Spontaneous rupture of the deltoid muscle associated with massive tearing of the rotator cuff. J Shoulder Elbow Surg 6:556-558, 1997.
59. Moseley HF and Overgaard B: The anterior capsular mechanism in recurrent anterior dislocation of the shoulder. J Bone Joint Surg Br 44:913, 1962.
60. Motta F and Carletti T: Spontaneous rupture of the infraspinatus muscle. Int Orthop 14:351-353, 1990.
61. Moulonguet G: Rupture spontanée du grand pectoral chez un vieillard. Enorme hematome. Mort Bull Mem Soc Anat Paris 94:24-28, 1924.
62. Nerot C, Jully JL, and Gerard Y: Rotator cuff ruptures with predominant involvement of the subscapular tendon. Chirurgie 291:103-106, 1993-1994.
63. Neviaser RJ, Neviaser TJ, and Neviaser JS: Anterior dislocation of the shoulder and rotator cuff rupture. Clin Orthop 291:103-106, 1993.
64. Nove Josserand L, Levigne C, Noel E, and Walch G: Isolated lesions of the subscapularis muscle. A propos of 21 cases. Rev Chir Orthop Reparatrice Appar Mot 80:595-601, 1994.
65. O'Driscoll SW: Intramuscular triceps rupture. Can J Surg 35:203-207, 1992.
66. Ohashi K, El-Khoury GY, Albright JP, and Tearse DS: MRI of complete rupture of the pectoralis major muscle. Skeletal Radiol 25:625-628, 1996.
67. Orava S, Sorasto A, Aalto K, and Kvist H: Total rupture of the pectoralis major muscle in athletes. Int J Sports Med 5:272-274, 1984.
68. Overpeck DO and Ghormley RK: Paralysis of the serratus magnus muscle. JAMA 114:1994-1996, 1940.

69. Pai VS and Simison AJ: A rare complication of pectoralis major rupture. Aust N Z J Surg 65:694-695, 1995.

70. Panting AL, Hunter MH: Spontaneous rupture of the deltoid [abstract]. J Bone Joint Surg Br 65:518, 1983.

71. Park JY and Espiniella JL: Rupture of pectoralis major muscle: A case report and review of literature. J Bone Joint Surg Am 52:577-581, 1970.

72. Partridge: A case of rupture of the triceps cubiti. Med Times Gaz 1:175-176, 1868.

73. Patissier P: Traite des Maladies des Artisans. Paris: 1822, pp 162-164.

74. Patten RM: Tears of the anterior portion of the rotator cuff (the subscapularis tendon): MR imaging findings. AJR Am J Roentgenol 162:351-354, 1994.

75. Pfirrmann CWA, Zanetti M, Weishaupt D, et al: Subscapularis tendon tears: Detection and grading at MR arthrography. Radiology 213:709-714, 1999.

76. Pointud P, Clerc D, Manigand G, and Deparis M: Rupture spontanée du deltoide. Nouv Presse Med 6:2315-2316, 1976.

77. Preston FS and Adicoff A: Hyperparathyroidism with avulsion of three major tendons. N Engl J Med 266:968-971, 1962.

78. Ptasznik R and Hennessy O: Abnormalities of the biceps tendon of the shoulder: Sonographic findings. AJR Am J Roentgenol 164:409-414, 1995.

79. Purnell R: Rupture of the pectoralis major muscle: A complication. Injury 19:284, 1988.

80. Ronchetti G: Rottura sottocutanea parziale del muscolo grand pettorale con formazione di pseudocistie ematica. Minerva Chir 14:22-28, 1959.

81. Safran MR, Garrett WE Jr, Scaber AV, et al: The role of warm-up in muscular injury prevention. Am J Sports Med 16:123-129, 1988.

82. Samuel J, Levernieux J, and de Seze S: A propos d'un cas de rupture du deltoide. Rev Rhum Mal Osteoartic 42:769-771, 1975.

83. Schepsis AA, Grafe MW, Jones HP, and Lemos MJ: Rupture of the pectoralis major muscle: Outcome after repair of acute and chronic injuries. Am J Sports Med 28:9-15, 2000.

84. Scott BW, Wallace WA, and Barton MA: Diagnosis and assessment of pectoralis major rupture by dynamometry. J Bone Joint Surg Br 74:111-113, 1992.

85. Shellock FG, Mink J, and Deutsch AL: MR Imaging of muscle injuries. Appl Radiol 1:11-16, 1994.

86. Sheps D, Black GB, Reed M, and Davidson JM: Rupture of the long head of the triceps muscle in a child. J Trauma 42:318-320, 1997.

87. Sherman OH, Snyder SJ, and Fox JM: Triceps avulsion in a professional body builder: A case report. Am J Sports Med 12:329, 1984.

88. Smith FC: Rupture of the pectoralis major muscle: A caveat. Injury 19:282-283, 1988.

89. Smith HG: Pathological appearances of seven cases of injury of the shoulder joint with remarks. Am J Med Sci 16:219-224, 1835.

90. Speed K: Personal communication to Gilcreest, 1939.

91. Symeonides PP: The significance of the subscapularis muscle in the pathogenesis of recurrent anterior dislocation of the shoulder. J Bone Joint Surg Br 54:476-483, 1972.

92. Tarsney FF: Rupture and avulsion of the triceps. Clin Orthop 83:177-183, 1972.

93. Tobin WJ, Cohen LJ, and Vandover JT: Parachute injuries. JAMA 117:1318-1321, 1941.

94. Tomczak R, Friedrich JM, Haussler MD, and Wallner B: [Sonographic diagnosis of diseases of the bicep muscle of arm.] Rontgenpraxis 45:145-149, 1992.

95. Tung GA, Yoo DC, and Levine SM: Subscapularis tendon tear: Primary and associated signs on MRI. J Comput Assist Tomogr 25:417-424, 2001.

96. Van Leersum M and Schweitzer ME: Magnetic resonance imaging of the biceps complex. Magn Reson Imaging Clin N Am 2:77-86, 1993.

97. Visuri T and Lindholm H: Bilateral distal biceps tendon avulsions with use of anabolic steroids. Med Sci Sports Exerc 26:941-944, 1994.

98. Welsh RP, Macnab I, and Riley V: Biomechanical studies of rabbit tendon. Clin Orthop 81:171-177, 1971.

99. Wolfe SW, Wickiewicz TL, and Cavanaugh JT: Ruptures of the pectoralis major muscle. An anatomic and clinical analysis. Am J Sports Med 20:587-593, 1992.

100. Wood TO, Cooke PH, and Goodship AE: The effect of exercise and anabolic steroids on the mechanical properties and crimp morphology of the rat tendon. Am J Sports Med 16:153-158, 1988.

101. Zeman SC, Rosenfeld RT, and Lipscomb PR: Tears of the pectoralis major muscle. Am J Sports Med 7:343-347, 1979.

BIBLIOGRAPHY

Albo A: Ruptured pectoralis major tendon: A case report on delayed repair with muscle advancement. Acta Orthop Scand 65:642-643, 1994.

Bach BR Jr, Warren RF, and Wickiewicz TL: Triceps rupture: A case report and literature review. Am J Sports Med 15:285-289, 1987.

Bach NR, Warren RF, and Fronck K: Disruption of the lateral capsule of the shoulder: A cause of recurrent dislocation. J Bone Joint Surg Br 70:74, 1988.

Bakalim G: Rupture of the pectoralis major muscle: A case report. Acta Orthop Scand 36:274-279, 1965.

Bayley I, Fisher K, Tsitsui H, and Matthews J: Functional biofeedback in the management of habitual shoulder instability. Paper presented at the 3rd International Conference on Surgery of the Shoulder, Oct 28-30, 1986, Fukuoka, Japan.

Bennett BS: Triceps tendon ruptures. J Bone Joint Surg Am 44:741-774, 1962.

Berson BL: Surgical repair of pectoralis major rupture in an athlete. Am J Sports Med 7:348-351, 1979.

Blondi J and Bear TF: Isolated rupture of the subscapularis tendon in an arm wrestler. Orthopaedics 11:647-649, 1988.

Borchers E and Iontscheff P: Die subkutane Ruptur des grossen Brustmuskels ein wenig bekanntes aber typisches Krankheitsbild. Zentralbl Chir 59:770-774, 1932.

Bowerman JW and McDonnell EJ: Radiology of athletic injuries; baseball. Radiology 116:611, 1975.

Brownlee JJ: Rupture of the pectoralis major: A case report. Paper presented at a meeting of the New Zealand Orthopaedic Association, Oct 1987.

Buck JE: Rupture of the sternal head of the pectoralis major: A personal description. J Bone Joint Surg Br 45:224, 1963.

Butters AC: Traumatic rupture of the pectoralis major. BJM 2:652-653, 1941.

Cougard P, Petitjean D, Hamoniere G, and Ferry C: Rupture traumatique complète du muscle grand pectoral. Rev Chir Orthop 71:337-338, 1985.

Coughlin EJ and Baker DM: Management of shoulder injuries in sport. Conn Med 29:723-727, 1965.

de Rouguin B: Rupture of the pectoralis major muscle: Diagnosis and treatment: A propos of 3 cases. Rev Chir Orthop Reparatrice Appar Mot 78:248-250, 1992.

Dragoni S, Giombini A, Candela V, and Rossi F: Isolated partial tear of subscapularis muscle in a competitive water skier: A case report. J Sports Med Phys Fitness 34:407-410, 1994.

Dunkelman NR, Collier F, Rook JL, et al: Pectoralis major muscle rupture in windsurfing. Arch Phys Med Rehabil 75:819-821, 1994.

Egan TM and Hall H: Avulsion of the pectoralis major tendon in a weight lifter: Repair using a barbed staple. Can J Surg 30:434, 1987.

Guerterbock P: Zerreissung der Sehn des M. triceps brachii. Arch Klin Chir 265:256-260, 1981.

Hayes WM: Rupture of the pectoralis major muscle: Review of the literature and report of two cases. J Int Coll Surg 14:82-88, 1950.

Heimann W: Uber einige subkutane Muskel- und Sehnenverletzungen van den oberen Gliedmassen. Monatschr Unfallh 15:266-279, 1908.

Holleb PD and Bach BR Jr: Triceps brachii injuries. Sports Med 10:273-276, 1990.

Jens J: The role of subscapularis muscle in recurring dislocation of the shoulder. J Bone Joint Surg Br 46:780, 1964.

Kehl T, Holzach P, and Matter P: Rupture of the pectoralis major muscle. Unfallchirurg 90:363-366, 1987.

Kingsley DM: Rupture of pectoralis major: Report of a case. J Bone Joint Surg 28:644-645, 1946.

Knaack WHL: Die subkutanen Verletzungen der Muskeln Veroffentl. Geb Mil Sanitatswesens 16:1-123, 1900.

Kuniichi A and Takehiko T: Muscle belly tear of the triceps. Am J Sports Med 12:484, 1984.

Lage J de A: Ruptura do musculo grande pectoral. Rev Hosp Clin 6:37-40, 1951.

Law WB: Closed incomplete rupture of pectoralis major. BJM 2:499, 1954.

Letenneur M: Rupture sous-cutanée du muscle grand pectoral: Guérison complète en quinze jours. Gaz de Hop 35:54, 1862.

Lindenbaum BL: Delayed repair of a ruptured pectoralis major muscle. Clin Orthop 109:120-121, 1975.

Liu J, Wu JJ, Chang CY, Chou YE, and Lo WE: Avulsion of the pectoralis major tendon. Am J Sports Med 20:366-368, 1922.

MacKenzie DB: Avulsion of the insertion of the pectoralis major muscle. S Afr Med J 60:147-148, 1981.

Malinovski I: Rare case of rupture of the pectoralis major at its attachment with process of the humerus. Voyenno Med J 153:136-138, 1885.

Mandl F: Ruptur des Musculus pect. maor. Wien Med Wochenschr 75:2192, 1925.

Manjarris J, Gershuni DH, and Moitoza J: Rupture of the pectoralis major tendon. J Trauma 25:810-811, 1985.

Marmor L, Bechtol CO, and Hall CB: Pectoralis major muscle function of sternal portion and mechanism of rupture of normal muscle: Case reports. J Bone Joint Surg Am 43:81-87, 1961.

Maydl K: Veber subcutane Muskel- und Sehrserrisungen, sowie Rissferacturer mit Berucksichtigung de Analogen, dirche directe Gewalt enstandenen und offerien Verletzungen. Dtsch Z Chir 17:306-361, 1882; 18:35-139, 1883.

McKelvey D: Subcutaneous rupture of the pectoralis major muscle. BJM 2:611, 1928.

Mendoza Lopez M, Cardoner Parpal JC, Sanso Bardes F, and Coba Sotes J: Lesions of the subscapular tendon regarding two cases in arthroscopic surgery (published erratum appears in Arthroscopy 1994). Arthroscopy 9:671-674, 1993.

Newmark H III, Olken SM, and Halls J: Ruptured triceps tendon diagnosed radiographically. Australas Radiol 29:60-63, 1985.

Nikitin GD, Linnik SA, and Filippov KV: Allotendoplasty in rupture of the pectoralis major muscle. Ortop Travnatol Protez 9:47-48, 1987.

O'Donoghue DH: Injuries to muscle tendon unit. Am Surg 29:190-200, 1963.

Pantazopoulos T, Exarchov B, Stavrov Z, et al: Avulsion of the triceps tendon. J Trauma 15:827-829, 1975.

Parkes M: Rupture of the pectoralis major muscle. Ind Med 12:226, 1943.

Penhallow D: Report of a case of ruptured triceps due to direct violence. N Y Med J 91:76-77, 1910.

Pirker H: Die Verletzungen durch Muskelzug. Ergebn Chir Orthop 25:553-634, 1934.

Pulaski EJ and Chandlee BH: Ruptures of the pectoralis major muscle. Surgery 10:309-312, 1941.

Pulaski EJ and Martin GW: Rupture of the left pectoralis major muscle. Surgery *25*:110-111, 1949.

Recht J, Docquier J, Soete P, and Forthomme JP: Avulsion-fracture of the subscapular muscle. Acta Orthop Belg *57*:312-316, 1991.

Redard P, cited by Deveny P: Contribution à l'étude des ruptures musculaires [thesis No. 423:12]. Paris, 1878.

Regeard A: Étude sur les ruptures musculaires [thesis No. 182:51]. Paris, 1880.

Rijnberg WJ and Van Ling B: Rupture of the pectoralis major muscle in bodybuilders. Arch Orthop Trauma Surg *112*:104-105, 1993.

Rio GS, Respizzi S, and Dworzak F: Partial rupture of the pectoralis major muscle in athletes. Int J Sports Med *11*:85-87, 1990.

Schechter LR and Gristina AG: Surgical repair of rupture of the pectoralis major muscle. JAMA *188*:1009, 1964.

Searfoss R, Tripi J, and Bowers W: Triceps brachii rupture: Case report. J Trauma *16*:244-245, 1976.

Smart A: Rupture of pectoralis major. Guys Hosp Gaz *2*:61, 1873.

Solokoff L and Hough AJ Jr: Pathology of rheumatoid arthritis and allied disorders. *In* McCarthy DJ (ed): Arthritis and Allied Conditions: A Textbook of Rheumatology, 10th ed. Philadelphia: Lea & Febiger, 1985, pp 571-592.

Stimson H: Traumatic rupture of the biceps brachii. Am J Surg *29*:472-476, 1935.

Thielemann FW, Kley U, and Holz U: Isolated injury of the subscapular muscle tendon. Sportverlets Sportschaden *6*:26-28, 1992.

Tietjen R: Closed injuries of the pectoralis major muscle. J Trauma *20*:2623-2624, 1980.

Urs ND and Jani DM: Surgical repair of rupture of the pectoralis major muscle: A case report. J Trauma *16*:749-750, 1976.

Von Eiselberg A: Cited by Mandl.

Weinlechner J: Uber subcutane Muskel, Sehnen und Knochenrisse. Wien Med Blatter *4*:1561-1565, 1881.

CHAPTER 22

TUMORS AND RELATED CONDITIONS

Ernest U. Conrad III, M.D.

• • • •

Management of musculoskeletal tumors, which represent approximately 10% of all orthopaedic diagnoses, is a broad and complex topic.[149] This chapter emphasizes the initial assessment and evaluation because of the typical delay and difficulty in reaching an accurate diagnosis. The classification, staging, and imaging of these lesions represent, in a broad sense, many of the improvements achieved in the last 10 to 15 years. A review of the salient radiographic and clinical features of the more common lesions is included without an in-depth discussion of any particular lesion. The principles of biopsy and surgical resection, the definition and significance of surgical margins, and the classification of resections and reconstructions are all discussed. Most of the surgical reconstructive techniques (e.g., allografts, arthrodesis, and arthroplasty) presented have only short follow-up to date and should be considered accordingly. Many molecularly based biologic findings relevant to musculoskeletal tumors have occurred in the last 4 to 5 years and are discussed briefly. Tumors involving the shoulder girdle are distinguished clinically by concern over a potential increased risk of tumor recurrence and loss of function in this particular anatomic location and a definite increased difficulty in achieving good functional recovery after proximal humeral resection.

HISTORICAL REVIEW

The term "sarcoma" was used by Abernethy in the 19th century to describe tumors that have a "firm and fleshy feel." Sarcoma refers to malignancies of mesenchymal, or connective tissue, origin. In that early period, sarcomas were lesions of the extremities and were confused with osteomyelitis and other conditions. Even the most accomplished professors of surgery demonstrated little interest in the recognition of sarcomas as malignancies distinct from carcinomas, and consequently, little previous work involving classification or treatment was conducted.

An exception to that rule was Samuel W. Gross (1837 to 1884), a well-known surgeon, pathologist, and anatomist at the Jefferson Medical College in Philadelphia, who authored one of the first works that attempted to deal with the classification of various sarcomas, their salient features, indications for treatment, and prognosis. Gross was one of the first persons in the world to identify sarcomas as a distinctly different group of tumors from carcinomas.[83] With the discovery and development of radiographs (1893), various lesions of bone were beginning to attract attention. Gross was one of the first to appropriately identify sarcomas as locally invasive, extremity tumors, with frequent metastases to the lungs and infrequently demonstrating lymphatic or hepatic metastases. These unusual lesions were associated with a history of trauma in half the cases and, according to Gross, required radical amputation or resection. In retrospect, his description of these first cases is remarkable for its clinical accuracy.

The scientific and technical developments in radiology, surgery, and medicine in the early 20th century resulted in significant advances in orthopaedics, which were reflected in improvements in the care of fractures, infections, and tumors. At that time, pathologists and surgeons such as John Ewing (New York), Ernest A. Codman (Boston), and James Bloodgood (Baltimore) became interested in various tumors of bone.[110] Treatment of sarcomas varied greatly during those early years, but management of these unusual and difficult tumors gradually became more uniform as lesions were recognized histologically and radiographically as distinct entities. The same process of classifying sarcomas into histologic subtypes based on molecular subtype continues today. Surgical treatment also improved with developments in pathology and radiology. Aggressive ablative surgery for sarcomas was first recommended by Gross in his classic article on sarcomas[1] and was followed by various reports in the early 20th century of various innovative surgical techniques.[85,108] Linberg's classic article in 1928 regarding interscapulothoracic resections[112] for malignancies of the shoulder joint reported on aggressive surgery for skeletal tumors. Since these early reports, dramatic advances in imaging, chemotherapy, pathology, and surgical technique have resulted in improved survival and allowed more limb-sparing surgery.

In the 20th century, Dallas B. Phemister (1882 to 1951) of the University of Chicago was one of the first surgeons in North America to demonstrate a special interest in limb-sparing or "limb salvage" surgery as we know it today.[156] Phemister reviewed the American College of

Surgeons' records for osteosarcoma in 1938 and found that only 4 of 86 extremity cases (4.6%) were treated with a limb-sparing resection.[156] Other reports of limb-sparing surgery at that time described variable results in terms of morbidity and mortality.[143,156] The popularity of "limb salvage" surgery reached its zenith in the 1970s and 1980s with an emphasis on the need for appropriate tumor resection and good functional results.

The specialty of musculoskeletal oncology has crystallized from improvements in radiographic "staging" studies, chemotherapy, pathology, and surgery. One of the most significant developments has involved the evolution of a histologic grading system for sarcomas of bone and soft tissue that allows assessment of a patient's prognosis according to the stage of the tumor and the proposed treatment.[61,84,162] It is one of the only systems that appropriately reflect a patient's prognosis based on the most significant determinants of that prognosis: its mitotic index, histologic subtype, and histologic pleomorphism. It is a system that has demonstrated more predictability than previous grading systems have. New cDNA genotyping of tumors has allowed improved histologic subtyping and the ability to identify molecular defects.[146]

Limb-sparing procedures, when properly executed, involve innovative reconstructive techniques to achieve an arthroplasty or arthrodesis associated with reasonable functional results. The indications for and assessment of these procedures in terms of functional results and tumor recurrence are discussed briefly. Although the true worth of some of these procedures, in many cases, remains to be determined, the value of an accurate classification system for sarcomas and coordinated multidisciplinary treatment of musculoskeletal neoplasms is obvious. Sarcomas are unusual tumors that require complex treatment. Their rarity and complexity have been major reasons for their haphazard treatment in the past. Recent advancements in description of the molecular phenotypes of these tumors and in assessment of their corresponding grade and molecular imaging[88] allow more accuracy in both tumor subtyping and decisions regarding the treatment of high-grade tumors.

ANATOMY

Many anatomic considerations are involved in the treatment of musculoskeletal tumors. In the shoulder girdle, these considerations are amplified by the proximity of the brachial plexus and major vessels of the upper extremity to the humerus, scapula, and chest wall. The implications of these anatomic points involve many aspects of the treatment and prognosis of shoulder neoplasms.

Although an evaluation of musculoskeletal tumors frequently refers to the various anatomic compartments of the region involved, the exact anatomy of the compartments about the shoulder remains poorly defined. The compartments of the shoulder (Fig. 22–1) include the deltoid compartment, the posterior scapular compartment (supraspinatus, infraspinatus, teres minor, and teres major), the subscapular compartment (subscapularis), the anterior pectoral compartment (pectoralis minor and major), the anterior humeral compartment (biceps and

coracobrachialis), the lateral humeral compartment (brachialis), the posterior humeral compartment (medial, lateral, and long head of the triceps), and the intra-articular compartment of the glenohumeral joint. Little work has been done on the true containment or integrity of these compartments, and their boundaries are theoretical. Although they are anatomically based, their actual potential for containment remains untested.

Many anatomic clues are helpful in making the initial diagnosis in patients with an unknown musculoskeletal lesion. For instance, Ewing's sarcoma typically develops in the shaft or diaphysis of the humerus; it rarely occurs in the metaphysis of a long bone. On the other hand, the epicenter of an osteogenic sarcoma is rarely located in the shaft and is usually found in the metaphysis. Similarly, whether a lesion is intra-articular or extra-articular is important for several reasons. Intra-articular tumors are very unusual because most lesions have their epicenter in bone or in the soft tissues outside a joint. An intra-articular lesion is more likely to represent a degenerative, traumatic, or other nontumorous diagnosis. The fact that a tumor might involve a joint primarily or secondarily is significant from the point of view of treatment because it requires more complex, extra-articular resection. Secondary involvement of a joint by an intraosseous malignancy is usually a late phenomenon associated with a longer diagnostic delay or a more aggressive lesion and a worse prognosis (see the section "Staging and Classification of Tumors").[61,199]

Difficult locations for neoplasms in the shoulder girdle include those of the brachial plexus or lesions involving the axillary brachial vessels. Both the plexus and the axillary vessels are contained within their own sheaths, which can eventually be penetrated or infiltrated by an aggressive lesion. Primary tumors of the brachial plexus (neurosarcomas) are usually manifested as a brachial plexus nerve deficit on clinical examination. Any patient with distinct peripheral nerve symptoms associated with a shoulder mass should be assumed to have nerve involvement until demonstrated otherwise. Biopsy of that type of lesion is therefore very likely to involve that nerve and result in further nerve loss. Lesions involving the axillary or brachial vessels require magnetic resonance imaging (MRI) and arteriography to define the precise extent of involvement.

The shoulder girdle is unique in that it has one of the largest and most well-defined muscle compartments in the body, that is, deltoid muscle. To function normally, the shoulder is dependent on a well-innervated deltoid and rotator cuff, in addition to adequate glenohumeral stability. The deltoid, like most muscle compartments, has anatomic subdivisions (acromial, clavicular, scapular), but grossly it is a well-defined muscle that is easily resectable, though extremely difficult to reconstruct functionally. Perhaps the most important anatomic consideration involved in the treatment of shoulder tumors is the anatomy of the axillary nerve and its relationship to the deltoid and the placement of shoulder incisions, biopsies, and so forth. Injuries to the axillary nerve during tumor resection or biopsy may result in almost total loss of deltoid function. Thus, the location of the axillary nerve at the time of biopsy and during resection has great

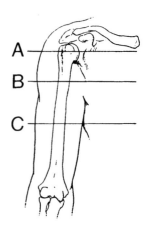

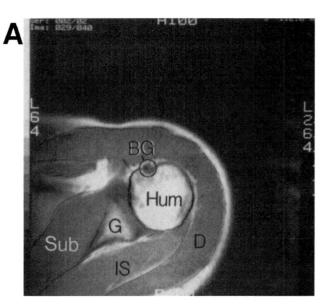

Transverse (axial) MRI image at the level of glenoid.

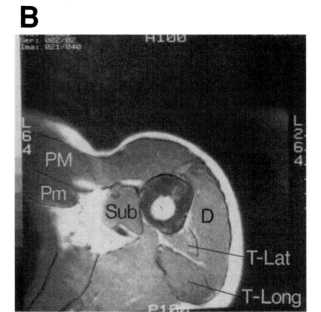

Transverse (axial) MRI image at the level of the proximal humerus.

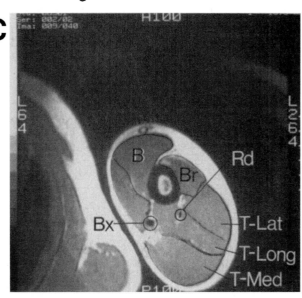

Transverse (axial) MRI image at the level of the mid-humerus.

D - Deltoid
Ax - Axillary vessels
TM - Teres Major
PM - Pectoralis Major
CB - Coracobrachialis
Md - Median Nerve
Hum - Humeral Head

Pm - Pectoralis Minor
BG - Bicipital groove
G - Glenoid
Sub - Subscapularis
B - Biceps brachii
Bx - Brachial vessels
IS - Infraspinatus

T-Lat - Triceps
          (lateral head)
T-Med - Triceps
          (mid-head)
T-Long - Triceps
          (long head)
Br - Brachialis
Rd - Radial Nerve

■ Figure 22–1
Shoulder anatomy on axial magnetic resonance imaging.

significance. In general, the functional prognosis for tumors of the shoulder girdle is much better if the axillary nerve, deltoid, and rotator cuff are preserved. Whereas glenohumeral joint mechanics can be replaced by shoulder arthroplasty, reconstruction of the deltoid or rotator cuff is much more difficult.

STAGING AND CLASSIFICATION OF TUMORS

Staging

The early classification system for musculoskeletal tumors was popularized by Lichtenstein, who classified tumors according to basic histologic categories.[111] It was useful in identifying general trends in diagnosis and prognosis, but this descriptive histologic system had limited significance for determining adjuvant treatment (e.g., chemotherapy, radiation therapy) and prognosis.

One of the greatest contributions to the improved treatment of sarcomas today has been the development of a staging system that assists in the selection of treatment, assessment of prognosis, and evaluation of results. Such a classification system was introduced by Enneking in 1980,[61] adopted by the Musculoskeletal Tumor Society, and subsequently accepted, with modifications, by the National Institutes of Health Sarcoma Consensus Study Group as the staging system for all sarcomas.[162] It represents a combined assessment of the histologic, or "surgical," grade (G), the anatomic site of primary disease (T), and the presence or absence of metastases (M). Surgical grading is based on histologic assessment, with a lesion identified as benign (G0), low grade malignant (G1), or high grade malignant (G2) (Tables 22-1 and 22-2).

The original concept of the staging system as devised by Enneking represented a departure from the staging system of the American Joint Committee for Cancer Staging and End-Results,[3] originally designed for the evaluation of various carcinomas. Enneking thought that that system correlated poorly with the natural history of sarcomas. He described the salient features of sarcomas with reference to their distinction from carcinomas and the significance of those features regarding staging.[3,61,162]

Most sarcomas, in contrast to carcinomas, were described as having a similar natural history, one of progressive local invasion and eventual hematogenous pulmonary metastasis. The surgical treatment of sarcomas of the extremities is significantly different from that of lesions of the head and neck, retroperitoneum, trunk, and abdomen. Appropriate surgery with or without radiation therapy remains the definitive treatment of the primary disease for most sarcomas. However, surgery must be combined with systemic chemotherapy to be curative. Chemotherapy or radiation therapy without surgery is rarely, if ever curative for the primary lesion. It remains, however, an important adjuvant and palliative method of treatment.

The extent of disease in the Enneking system is defined by the "anatomic setting." Compartmentalization, or compartmental escape, is an important characteristic of sarcomas, in contrast to previous classification systems

TABLE 22-1.   Surgical Staging System: Bone Tumors

Stage Grouping					
IA	T1	N0	M0	G1,2	Low grade
IB	T2	N0	M0	G1,2	Low grade
IIA	T1	N0	M0	G3,4	High grade
IIB	T2	N0	M0	G3,4	High grade
III	T3	N0	M0	Any G	
IVA	Any T	N0	M1a	Any G	
IVB	Any T	N1	Any M	Any G	
	Any T	Any N	M1b	Any G	

Used with the permission of the American Joint Committee on Cancer (AJCC), Chicago. From Greene FL, Page DL, Fleming ID, et al: AJCC Cancer Staging Manual, 6th ed, Stage Groupings for Bone. New York: Springer-Verlag, 2002 (www.springer-ny.com).

TABLE 22-2.   Surgical Staging System: Soft Tissue Tumors

Stage Grouping					
I	T1a	N0	M0	G1-2	G1	Low
I	T1b	N0	M0	G1-2	G1	Low
I	T2a	N0	M0	G1-2	G1	Low
I	T2b	N0	M0	G1-2	G1	Low
II	T1A	N0	M0	G3-4	G2-3	High
II	T1b	N0	M0	G3-4	G2-3	High
II	T2a	N0	M0	G3-4	G2-3	High
III	T2b	N0	M0	G3-4	G2-3	High
IV	Any T	N1	M0	Any G	Any G	High or Low
IV	Any T	N0	M1	Any G	Any G	High or Low

Used with the permission of the American Joint Committee on Cancer (AJCC), Chicago. From Greene FL, Page DL, Fleming ID, et al: AJCC Cancer Staging Manual, 6th ed, Stage Groupings for Soft Tissue Sarcoma. New York: Springer-Verlag, 2002 (www.springer-ny.com).

and other tumors (carcinomas). It was postulated that the anatomic site (T) was the greatest factor in prognosis because it represented a composite of the following characteristics: anatomic site, rate of growth, and delay in diagnosis. The primary extent of disease is limited by the natural boundaries of the anatomic compartment in which the lesion is located. A lesion located in the anterior of the thigh is contained by the fascial envelope of the quadriceps compartment until progressive growth causes it to extend beyond the natural boundary. When extension occurs, the patient has a worse prognosis and a higher risk of metastatic disease because of the presence of a more aggressive tumor. Lesions that develop in poorly compartmentalized anatomic sites (e.g., groin, popliteal fossa, perivascular space) are, by the nature of that site, poorly compartmentalized and usually associated with a worse prognosis.

The histologic grading system proposed for sarcomas by the Enneking system was simplified to a two-grade system, that of high-grade versus low-grade histology. No allowance for intermediate-grade histology was made because there was no intermediate surgical treatment. This system required the pathologist to classify all sarcomas as either high-grade or low-grade lesions, which contradicts most classic sarcoma grading systems, in which high-, low-, and intermediate-grade histology is typically described. Grading remains a topic of controversy today, especially for soft tissue sarcomas, because they do occur as intermediate-grade lesions in certain cases. The system has subsequently been modified to include intermediate-grade soft tissue tumors. The basic concept, however, remains a valid one, and intermediate-grade soft tissue tumors remain a treatment paradox regarding indications for chemotherapy. Tumor grading should not be based on the histologic type alone. The theory that some histologic diagnoses always represent high-grade lesions and a worse prognosis, regardless of their histologic grade, is not generally accepted.

In the original Enneking staging system, the prognosis for a patient with regional lymph node involvement was believed to be as poor as that for a patient with pulmonary metastasis. Therefore, either lymph node metastasis or pulmonary metastasis was represented by stage III disease.

The strength of the Enneking staging system is its simplicity. By emphasizing high-grade versus low-grade histology and by limiting the number of tumor stages (IA, IB, IIA, IIB, III), this system is simple enough to be used by a wide group of specialists and allows for a variety of treatments. The Enneking system uses a subtly, but significantly different numbering system for benign and malignant disease. Benign disease is denoted as grade 1, 2, or 3, depending on whether it is a latent, active, or aggressive tumor (see Table 22–1). A latent benign lesion does not show active growth. An active lesion shows active growth but is confined within the compartment defined by the surrounding natural boundaries. An aggressive lesion has the potential to penetrate or violate natural boundaries, such as cortical bone, periosteum, or fascial compartments, and to remain locally aggressive without metastasizing. Theoretically, only malignant tumors (by definition) have the ability to metastasize; a contradiction in terms is presented by the ability of histologically "benign" giant cell tumors to "metastasize" to the lung in a few cases. Other aggressive benign tumors (chondroblastoma) have also demonstrated lung metastases in a small number of cases.

Malignant tumors are denoted as stage I, II, III, or IV (see Table 22–1),[81] depending on the histologic grade (G), primary tumor extent (T), regional nodes (N), or the presence of metastases (M). Thus, a IA lesion is malignant, low grade, and intracompartmental. A IIA lesion is high grade and intracompartmental, and IIB is high grade and extracompartmental (see Table 22–1). Grade IV lesions are metastatic regardless of the grade or anatomic site of the lesion. Benign tumors are graded as 1 (inactive), 2 (active), or 3 (aggressive). The system is somewhat different for soft tissue (see Table 22–2).[82]

The anatomic or surgical site classification (T) defines the primary lesion in relation to its position in the anatomic compartment of origin. Tumors are described as encapsulated (T0), intracompartmental (T1), or extracompartmental (T2). This designation is based on the Enneking compartmental theory, in which an anatomic compartment is described as a space or potential space defined by natural boundaries.[61] Tumors contained within an anatomic compartment may violate the boundaries of the compartment with growth—usually a sign of an aggressive benign or malignant tumor. Active benign tumors are typically well encapsulated (T0) and intracompartmental, whereas aggressive benign lesions may be poorly encapsulated but remain intracompartmental (T1). Low-grade malignant lesions are typically intra-

compartmental (T1), whereas extracompartmental lesions (T2) usually represent high-grade malignancies. Extracompartmental tumors may extend from one compartment into another or from one compartment into a surrounding extrafascial plane, or they may arise within a poorly compartmentalized, extracompartmental space. Poorly compartmentalized anatomic spaces include perivascular areas such as the subsartorial space of the common femoral artery, the popliteal fossa, the antecubital fossa, or the midhand, midfoot, axilla, or groin.

The stage of the lesion and the surgical margin achieved by a procedure are associated with a certain local recurrence rate as described in the work of Enneking (see the section "Surgical Margin" and Table 22–5). These recurrence rates are based on an extensive retrospective review of the literature and reflect the risk of local recurrence after surgical resection without the use of adjuvant treatment. A benign aggressive (stage 3) lesion treated with a wide margin has a recurrence rate of 10% or less. This recurrence rate reflects surgical treatment alone and does not take into account the lower recurrence rate associated with surgery and adjuvant treatment, as performed for most malignant conditions. High-grade malignant tumors (IIB), such as a typical osteosarcoma, require at least a wide surgical margin that includes a surrounding cuff of normal tissue to avoid a local recurrence.

After careful anatomic staging of the tumor, the appropriate surgical procedure can be predicted by considering the grade of the lesion and the extent of involvement at the primary site (stage). The difficulty of that resection will also become apparent from this evaluation. A patient's prognosis and risk for local recurrence can similarly be assessed by considering the grade of the tumor and the surgical margin achieved at the time of the surgical procedure. This "articulation" or correlation of the tumor "stage" and the "surgical margin" allows an assessment of the risk of local recurrence as a result of the procedure and margin achieved.

Thorough initial evaluation and staging, before treatment, remain the crucial ingredients for a successful outcome. Without these initial studies and an adequate and accurate biopsy, a successful treatment plan is unlikely. A universally accepted staging classification system is important to direct patient care and adequately assess clinical results regarding disease-free status. This initial staging philosophy remains one of the major contributions of the Enneking staging system to patient care.

The staging evaluation involves an assessment by various radiographic studies to determine the precise anatomic extent of the primary disease, in addition to whether regional or distant metastases have occurred. Typical staging studies include plain radiographs, technetium bone scan, computed tomographic (CT) scans, MRI, and other studies that better define a lesion's location. A total body bone scan is the best study to assess the extent of the primary bone lesion and the possibility of metastatic disease.[90,195,199] CT scans are excellent for visualizing cortical geography and bone involvement at the primary site on a two-dimensional plane.[61] CT scanning of the lung is routinely carried out in most institutions to assess possible pulmonary metastasis, and it is a more sensitive method than plain radiographs.

MRI is indicated for evaluating soft tissue disease, intramedullary bony disease, and spinal or pelvic lesions.[207] The soft tissue or neurovascular margins are best assessed by MRI because it is much more sensitive than CT scanning for evaluating soft tissue margins. MRI does image the peripheral inflammatory "reactive zone" with a bright signal that may or may not contain a tumor. Similarly, the radiologist may over-read soft tissue margins when interpreting malignancies such as osteosarcoma and Ewing's sarcoma[207] because of the inability to distinguish inflammation from tumor on MRI.

Tumor imaging has always been an essential ingredient for success in limb salvage surgery, particularly for malignant tumors in which the malignancy involves bone or soft tissue. This importance of imaging is especially true for tumors in the shoulder area because of the increased complexity of proximal humeral and shoulder girdle tumors. Although MRI is clearly the optimal imaging modality for demonstrating anatomic detail and extent of tumor involvement in both bone and soft tissue malignancies, the current "state of the art" for assessing a tumor's degree of malignancy and response to chemotherapy is quantitative positron emission tomography (PET) using fluorodeoxyglucose (see Fig. 22–2A to C). PET scans have the benefit of being quantifiable; that is, the technique can be validated to yield a specific numerical value, typically referred to as the standard uptake value (SUV). The SUV gives an indication of the tumor's degree of malignancy and activity. This assessment is valuable in terms of grading tumors up front, evaluating response to treatment, assessing heterogeneity, and assessing local recurrences. Although PET scans are relatively early in their development for sarcoma applications, there is no doubt that these scans are valuable studies for assessing tumor grade, response to treatment, and the possibility of recurrence, and they are used routinely in most major centers today.

Classification of Tumors

Although the histologic classification of tumors has limitations in predicting the prognosis and directing treatment,[88] it does serve a purpose in identifying tumor or sarcoma subtypes and their general tendencies. Knowledge of a tumor's histologic type and the age of the patient

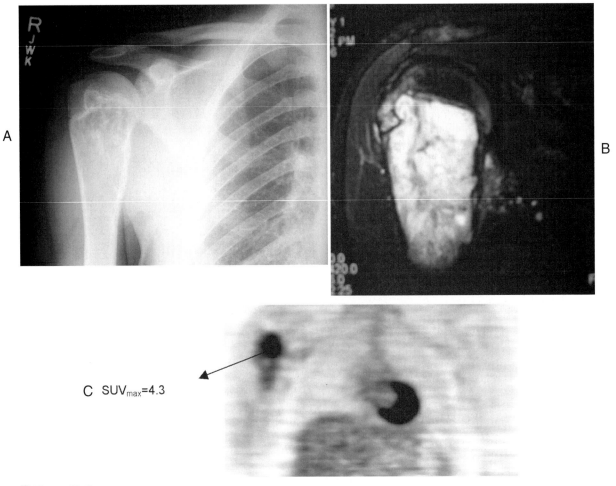

C SUV$_{max}$=4.3

■ Figure 22–2
Pretreatment, preresection imaging of a 16-year-old boy with an osteogenic sarcoma of the proximal aspect of the right humerus. Imaging includes a plain radiograph (A), magnetic resonance imaging (B), and a positron emission tomographic scan (C) showing a standard uptake value maximum (SUV$_{max}$) of 4.3.

are quite helpful in making a reliable tentative diagnosis in many patients, especially when the x-ray appearance is added to that information. The most common lesions of bone, cartilage, and soft tissue are described here in order to discuss their general histologic, radiographic, and clinical characteristics. The clinical scenario of patient age, type of radiographic abnormality, and type of tissue involvement can, in many cases, lead to a significant and limited differential diagnosis.

Benign Osseous Lesions

Osteoid Osteoma

Benign osseous lesions of the shoulder are uncommon. Osteoid osteoma and osteoblastoma occur in the proximal part of the humerus or scapula in 10% to 15% of cases and, when they do occur, favor the proximal end of the humerus or glenoid.[53,94] Osteoid osteoma typically displays the classic symptom of night pain, which is relieved by salicylates. Radiographically, it is characterized by a large area of reactive bone surrounding a small radiolucent "nidus." On technetium bone scan, osteoid osteoma has impressive increased activity, and the central nidus can be visualized as a distinct cortical hole on CT scanning or tomography. Plain x-ray tomography may also be an effective diagnostic tool for localizing many osteoid osteomas. Histologically, this lucent nidus is a well-demarcated, small area of immature, very active osteoblastic tissue. Preoperative localization is an extremely important strategy to avoid intraoperative difficulty in locating these lesions and thus in minimizing local recurrences.

Osteoblastoma

Some clinicians regard osteoblastoma as a larger version of osteoid osteoma ("giant osteoid osteoma"), and it is typified by a large lucent area of osteoblastic tissue surrounded by a thin, sclerotic, reactive rim of bone.[53] Radiographically, osteoblastoma is generally seen as a lucent lesion that has expanded the overlying cortex into a thin rim. As with osteoid osteoma, osteoblastoma may be difficult to localize radiographically and requires careful preoperative imaging to avoid recurrence. Osteoblastoma, unlike osteoid osteoma, also occurs in an aggressive (stage 3) form that is less well defined radiographically, has a high recurrence rate, and may have a histologic appearance that is difficult to distinguish from low-grade osteosarcoma. Technetium bone scanning and CT scans are good imaging techniques for both these lesions.

Myositis Ossificans

Myositis ossificans is a benign, reactive, bone-forming process that develops intramuscularly or in the "areolar tissues" (tendon, ligament, capsule, fascia) adjacent to bone. It may occur with or without a history of trauma and, in the latter instance, may be referred to as pseudomalignant myositis ossificans of the soft parts.[147] The pseudomalignant form is typically seen as a symptomatic enlarging soft tissue mass that develops in the second decade of life, and it occurs in the shoulder in 15% of cases.

The typical radiographic appearance is an osseous density in soft tissue that demonstrates peripheral radiographic maturity or margination of the mass, separated from adjacent cortical bone by a narrow zone of uninvolved soft tissue. This characteristic histologic margination or zonation phenomenon (peripheral maturity) reflects the fact that the more active (immature) osteoblastic tissue is located centrally in the lesion, in contrast to other neoplasms, which have their most active histologic area peripherally. Isotope scans of myositis ossificans demonstrate high uptake peripherally that may continue for 8 to 12 weeks or until spontaneous maturation occurs. Excision before that time is associated with a high recurrence rate.

In some patients, myositis ossificans may be confused with osteosarcoma or a soft tissue sarcoma, but these tumors do not demonstrate the same zonation or peripheral margination phenomenon, nor do they have the same radiographic characteristics. When the proper diagnosis is uncertain, optimal management includes a complete radiographic evaluation and careful clinical observation rather than a hasty or premature excision or biopsy (which may be difficult to interpret).[33] The radiographic differential diagnosis for myositis ossificans includes extraosseous or parosteal osteosarcoma, synovial sarcoma, vascular lesions, and calcification of soft tissue secondary to necrosis or inflammation.

Malignant Osseous Lesions

Osteosarcoma

Osteosarcoma is the most common primary sarcoma of bone (excluding multiple myeloma). It is the most frequent primary sarcoma occurring in the shoulder, followed by Ewing's sarcoma and chondrosarcoma. In the past, it has typically developed in the adolescent age group, although a significant percentage of patients are young adults in their third decade of life.

Classic osteosarcoma is a high-grade, aggressive tumor that develops in metaphyseal bone, typically as a stage IIB lesion and usually with an extraosseous soft tissue component present at initial evaluation.[53,95,111] The typical patient has intrinsic bone pain at night that is frequently unrelated to activity. The average duration of symptoms at initial assessment is 3 to 6 months, which reflects the subtle nature of the preliminary symptoms and the need for early recognition of intraosseous pain and night pain as warning symptoms.[49]

Approximately 10% to 15% of all osteosarcomas occur in the proximal part of the humerus, whereas 1% to 2% develop in the scapula or clavicle.[32,63,95,111] The typical radiograph for osteosarcoma has a sunburst or osteoblastic pattern, with penetration of the adjacent cortex (Fig. 22–3A). Osteosarcomas usually have increased activity on bone scan (Figure 22–3B), and a soft tissue mass is seen on CT scan (Fig. 22–3C) and MRI (Fig. 22–3D). Arteriography is no longer the technique of choice for evaluating soft tissue involvement but may be performed to evaluate for major vessel involvement or for response to intra-arterial chemotherapy (Fig. 22–3E). Variants of

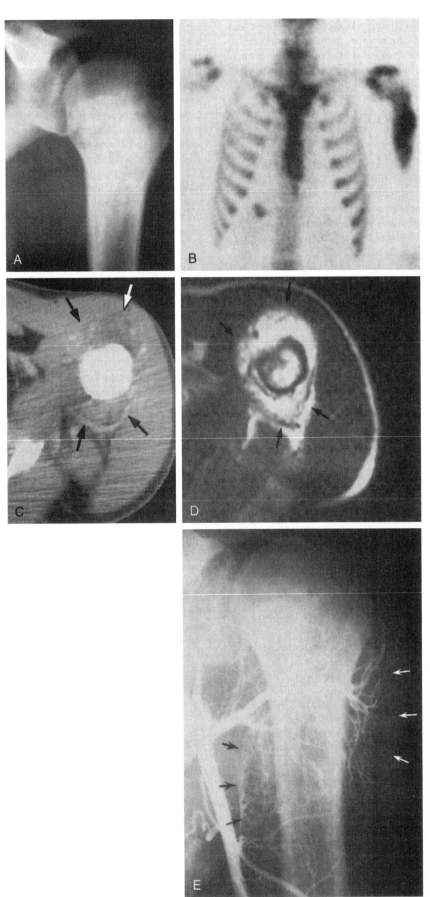

■ **Figure 22–3**

A, Plain radiograph of an osteosarcoma of the proximal end of the humerus suggesting minimal soft tissue involvement by tumor. **B,** Bone scan of the same lesion demonstrating significant extension proximally and distally in the humerus. **C,** Computed tomographic (CT) scan of the same patient that does not demonstrate the extent of soft tissue extension *(arrows)*. **D,** Magnetic resonance imaging (MRI) through the same area of the humerus demonstrating circumferential soft tissue involvement *(arrows)* with much better visualization than achieved by the CT scan. **E,** Arteriogram obtained for intra-arterial chemotherapy demonstrating some soft tissue disease *(arrows)* but with less sensitivity than MRI has.

osteosarcoma other than the classic type include telangiectatic (vascular) osteosarcoma,[133] secondary osteosarcoma (Paget's disease or radiation induced), and various low-grade lesions such as periosteal and parosteal osteosarcoma.[63,212,213] The basic histologic criterion for the diagnosis of classic osteosarcoma includes a malignant stroma-producing (spindle cells) tumor or immature, neoplastic osteoid.[32,95,111] The overall survival rate for patients with osteosarcoma at 5 years of follow-up is approximately 70% with appropriate chemotherapy and surgery.[145] Prognostic factors for survival remain debatable; however, histologic necrosis at resection and the size of the tumor are probably the most significant variables.[36]

Benign Cartilaginous Lesions

Osteochondroma

The incidence of cartilaginous tumors in the shoulder is second only to those occurring about the pelvis.[49] Solitary osteochondroma, or exostosis, is the most common benign tumor of the shoulder; approximately a fourth of all exostoses occur in the proximal part of the humerus. Osteochondromas actually represent a developmental abnormality arising from the peripheral growth plate and are typically active, benign (stage 2) lesions during skeletal growth. The plain radiograph is usually diagnostic in demonstrating a smooth excrescence of metaphyseal cancellous bone that is confluent and continuous with normal metaphyseal bone (Fig. 22–4). Exostoses may appear as pedunculated, stalk-like lesions or as flat, sessile lesions. Concern regarding a possible secondary chondrosarcoma may arise in adult patients with pain, an enlarging soft tissue mass, or intraosseous bony erosions.

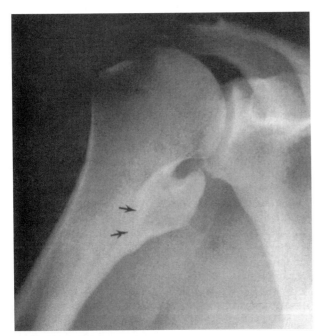

■ **Figure 22–4**
Osteochondroma of the proximal end of the humerus demonstrating "confluence" of normal metaphyseal bone into the lesion *(arrows)*.

Evidence of a thickened cartilaginous cap (>1 cm) on CT scan, in association with a soft tissue mass, pain, or radiographic evidence of possible malignant degeneration, suggests a secondary chondrosarcoma. The risk of a secondary chondrosarcoma arising out of an exostosis is approximately 1% per lesion, although rates as high as 10% to 30% have been referred to in the literature regarding secondary malignancy in patients with multiple hereditary exostoses.[188]

Exostoses are typically diagnosed in the skeletally immature. An enlarging or symptomatic exostosis should be considered with caution in the skeletally mature because parosteal osteosarcoma is an alternative diagnosis in that situation. Treatment of a solitary exostosis involves excision through the base of the lesion. In the sessile form, care should be taken to excise the cartilaginous cap to avoid a recurrence. The most common complication of an exostosis is iatrogenic or surgical injury to the adjacent growth plate or neurovascular structures at the time of excision. Adequate surgical exposure should be emphasized, especially for proximal humeral and proximal femoral lesions, which are usually large and adjacent to the major neurovascular bundle of that extremity.

The diagnosis of secondary chondrosarcoma arising out of an exostosis is unusual and best made on a preoperative CT scan demonstrating a thickened "cap" or enlarging soft tissue mass and not by biopsy. Cartilage histology is very difficult to interpret, and thus the diagnosis of a secondary malignancy is best made clinically and radiographically. The transition from benign to malignant is usually a protracted one involving relatively subtle histologic changes. The finding of a cartilage cap thicker than 1 cm should serve as a warning of at least a low-grade chondrosarcoma.

Chondroblastoma

Chondroblastoma, or Codman's tumor, is an unusual benign, cartilaginous tumor that occurs in the proximal humeral epiphysis (25% of cases) as a round or oval lesion containing fine calcifications surrounded by a reactive bony margin.[35,93,105] It occurs in the skeletally immature, and histologically it consists of aneurysmal tissue, "chicken wire" calcifications, and immature "paving stone" chondroblasts. Chondroblastoma occurs as an active, benign stage 2 lesion, although it also has a more aggressive stage 3 form. Treatment usually involves extensive intralesional curettage, which results in a large subchondral defect of the humeral head that requires an autogenous bone graft to prevent subchondral and cartilaginous collapse. The radiographic appearance of this epiphyseal lesion is usually typical, and it develops in adolescents or young adults. The differential diagnosis includes a simple cyst, eosinophilic granuloma, osteomyelitis, or an aneurysmal bone cyst.

Periosteal Chondroma

Periosteal chondroma is another benign cartilaginous lesion of the proximal end of the humerus that is usually located just proximal to the deltoid insertion of the lateral humeral shaft. It is typically manifested as a minimally symptomatic or asymptomatic mass that is radiographically evident as a sessile lesion with a distinct, well-defined margin of reactive cortex underlying the radiolucent cartilaginous mass.[35] Marginal excision results in a cortical defect of the humerus that may or may not require bone grafting. The differential diagnosis includes periosteal osteosarcoma, which does not have the well-defined underlying sclerotic cortex. Periosteal osteosarcoma is a more aggressive intracortical lesion that may extend into the medullary canal in a small percentage of cases.

Enchondroma

Solitary enchondroma is a benign, central cartilaginous lesion that is most commonly found in the small tubular bones of the hand but also occurs in the proximal end of the humerus in 10% to 15% of cases.[9,50,96] As a benign lesion, enchondromas are asymptomatic and require no treatment. When they occur adjacent to a joint that is symptomatic for degenerative reasons, clinical assessment of bone pain related to the enchondroma may be difficult. This scenario is not uncommon, and it makes the initial evaluation of intraosseous cartilage tumors difficult because intrinsic bone pain is an important symptom suggestive of a low-grade malignancy. Thus, the ability to distinguish intraosseous from intra-articular symptoms is a difficult but necessary challenge. The typical radiographic appearance of a benign enchondroma is that of a central lucent lesion with a well-defined bony margin and intrinsic calcifications. Figure 22–5 presents such a lesion in a 35-year-old woman with rotator cuff symptoms and a heavily calcified benign cartilage lesion.

Malignant Cartilaginous Lesions

Chondrosarcoma

Chondrosarcoma may develop de novo as a primary chondrosarcoma, or it may arise out of a preexisting benign cartilage lesion and is then referred to as secondary chondrosarcoma. Secondary chondrosarcoma occurs in young adults, accounts for approximately 25% of all chondrosarcomas, and may be found in patients with a preexisting enchondroma, osteochondroma, multiple enchondromatosis (Ollier's disease),[104,105,191] or multiple hereditary exostosis.[71] The radiographic evidence of a secondary, or low-grade, chondrosarcoma arising out of such a lesion includes enlarging radiolucent areas within the lesion or endosteal cortical erosions along the cortical margins (Fig. 22–6). Technetium bone scans are typically moderately "hot" for both enchondroma and low-grade chondrosarcoma and are not helpful in distinguishing one from the other. Microscopic evaluation of cartilage lesions is not diagnostic in a large percentage of cases. Histologic characteristics suggestive of malignancy include cellularity, pleomorphism, and evidence of mitotic activity, such as double-nucleated lacunae. These findings are subtle, and the histologic evidence for low-grade chondrosarcoma versus enchondroma is frequently incomplete and inconclusive.[50,104] This confusion has led to use of the term "grade one-half chondrosarcoma" to describe cartilage tumors that are histologically borderline between low-grade chondrosarcoma and benign enchondroma. In

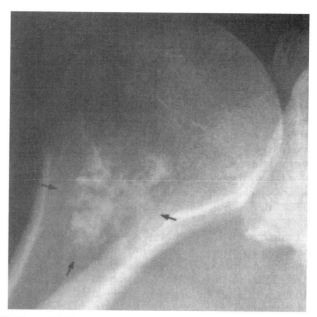

■ **Figure 22–5**

Plain radiograph of a 35-year-old woman with rotator cuff symptoms and an incidental benign enchondroma. There is no involvement or erosion of the endosteal cortical surface *(arrows)*.

most patients, the diagnosis of low-grade chondrosarcoma is best made radiographically by assessing whether there is evidence of endosteal erosions created by active cartilaginous tumor growth. Low-grade, or secondary, chondrosarcomas are unique among intraosseous tumors in the difficulty in interpreting their light microscopic picture.

Primary chondrosarcoma is more commonly seen in the middle decades of life, and its incidence in the shoulder is second to that in the pelvis or hip joint.[13,52,73,119,161] These tumors are typically manifested as intraosseous lesions with a poorly defined margin and faint intrinsic calcifications. Less commonly, a primary chondrosarcoma may arise from the surface of a bone or joint. Its clinical and radiographic appearance is very subtle, and a diagnostic delay of 6 to 12 months is not uncommon. Approximately two thirds of primary chondrosarcomas are also low grade and may have the appearance of benign, encapsulated cartilage lesions. High-grade lesions are more invasive, have a higher metastatic rate, and usually occur in long-standing lesions as a "dedifferentiated" chondrosarcoma.[27,33,70,127] As a general rule, low-grade chondrosarcomas may be treated surgically with curettage and grafting, whereas high-grade tumors deserve surgical resection and subsequent reconstruction.

Synovial Dysplasias

Cartilaginous loose bodies typically arise out of a proliferative synovium in a reactive metaplastic process known as synovial chondromatosis (or osteochondromatosis).[137] It most commonly affects large joints (knee, elbow, shoulder, hip) in young adults and results in multiple small, cartilaginous, intra-articular loose bodies as the process matures. In the few cases in which the nodules form a

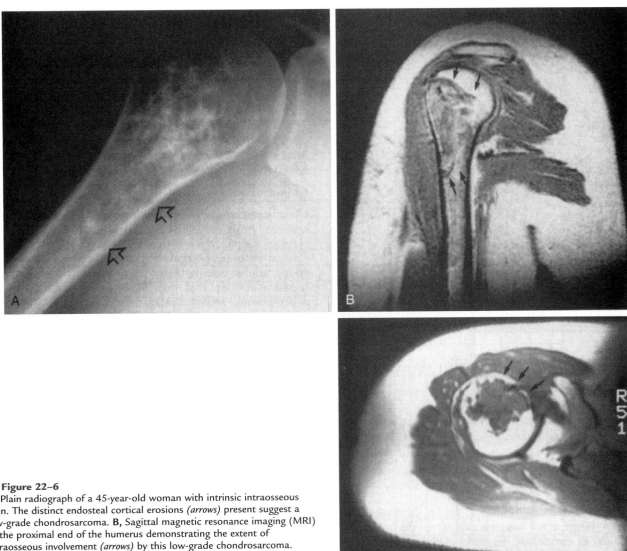

■ **Figure 22–6**

A, Plain radiograph of a 45-year-old woman with intrinsic intraosseous pain. The distinct endosteal cortical erosions *(arrows)* present suggest a low-grade chondrosarcoma. **B,** Sagittal magnetic resonance imaging (MRI) of the proximal end of the humerus demonstrating the extent of intraosseous involvement *(arrows)* by this low-grade chondrosarcoma. **C,** Axial (transverse) MRI scan through the humeral head demonstrating distinct bone erosions *(arrows)*.

compact mass of cartilage, it may be confused with a low-grade, periarticular or juxta-articular chondrosarcoma. An intra-articular location favors the benign diagnosis of synovial chondromatosis; consequently, determining whether it is intra-articular or extra-articular is sometimes one of the preoperative goals. In such cases, MRI or CT scanning with or without arthrography might pinpoint the exact site of involvement. Synovial chondromatosis is typically a slowly progressive, degenerative disease that ultimately leads to joint destruction. It requires aggressive total synovectomy to prevent persistence or recurrence, and in older patients with degenerative disease, it is well treated with joint excision and replacement. A few reports in the literature associate malignant transformation with long-standing synovial chondromatosis.[140]

Another disease associated with proliferating synovium is pigmented villonodular synovitis.[163] It is generally associated with a boggy, inflammatory synovitis, with or without bony erosions, in adolescents or young adults.

Histologically, it is an aggressive synovial-histiocytic process that defies description as inflammatory or neoplastic. Treatment requires aggressive complete synovectomy for the diffuse form of the disease. Various forms of radiation therapy have been used in some centers with acceptable early clinical results.[201] As a general rule, the long-term prognosis for synovial sarcoma is poor, with a high local recurrence rate and incidence of lung metastasis.

Miscellaneous Intraosseous Tumors

Simple Bone Cyst

Simple bone cysts, or unicameral bone cysts, occur most commonly in children between the ages of 4 and 12. Figure 22–7 presents a simple cyst in the humerus of an 8-year-old. Although the lesion appeared somewhat expansile and thus suggested an aneurysmal bone cyst,

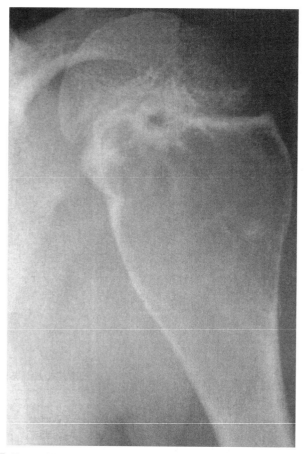

the cortices remained intact, clear fluid was aspirated, and the cyst healed after the intraosseous injection of steroids. Simple bone cysts are well-defined, central, radiolucent lesions arising in the metaphysis adjacent to the physis (active) and, with maturation, migrate distally into the diaphysis (latent). They typically involve the proximal part of the humerus (50%), contain straw-colored fluid, and may be confused with an aneurysmal bone cyst.[57,82,117,143,148,184]

The treatment of choice consists of pressure measurement of the cyst, aspiration, and intraosseous steroid injection. The result is complete healing of the cystic area in approximately 50% of cases and partial healing in 45%[174] Approximately three fourths of patients require multiple injections.[184] Complete repair after injection is most common in more inactive cysts with lower pressure. Varying results in more recent reports have cast some doubt on the efficacy of steroid injections for simple bone cysts, especially when associated with a venogram at the time of injection of dye into the lesion.[82] Recurrence or persistence of the cyst after surgical curettage and bone grafting occurs in approximately 30% of cases. This relatively high local recurrence rate may be lowered by the addition of liquid nitrogen freezing to the curettage.[189] Some diagnostic overlap occurs between aneurysmal and simple cysts in children because some simple cysts can

have hemorrhagic fluid and yet do not contain aneurysmal tissue.

Aneurysmal Bone Cyst

Aneurysmal bone cyst, nonossifying fibroma, and fibrous dysplasia are all benign lesions that may also occur in the shoulder. Aneurysmal bone cysts are not uncommon in the proximal end of the humerus, but because of their widespread occurrence as a "secondary" lesion engrafted on other tumors (simple cyst, giant cell tumor, chondroblastoma), the true incidence is unknown. The radiographic hallmark is that of a lucent, expansile metaphyseal lesion. Treatment includes curettage plus bone grafting,[10,58] which is associated with a recurrence rate of 20% to 30%. Aneurysmal bone cysts can have an aggressive appearance and should have a careful biopsy performed before curettage to exclude the possibility of telangiectatic osteosarcoma.

Fibrous Dysplasia

Fibrous dysplasia is a congenital dysplasia of bone that frequently surfaces as a painful lesion secondary to pathologic fracture, microfracture, or the subtle, intrinsic, diaphyseal weakness resulting from pathologic bone. The typical plain radiograph demonstrates a ground-glass density with cortical thickening. Figure 22–8A and B are the plain radiograph and CT scan, respectively, of the humerus of a 20-year-old woman with severe polyostotic fibrous dysplasia. She had a history of chronic pseudarthroses (see Fig. 22–8A) that had persisted despite bracing. When associated with symptoms or pathologic fracture, diaphyseal involvement usually requires intramedullary fixation rather than bone grafting because cancellous bone graft is consistently "consumed" by the dysplastic process and is ineffective in resolving the weakened dysplastic process. Histologically, fibrous dysplasia demonstrates a furnace of dysplastic bone activity with similar, impressive increased activity on bone scan.[87,89,98,109,205]

Nonossifying Fibroma

Nonossifying fibroma is a benign fibrous lesion that appears radiographically as an eccentric, well-defined, lucent lesion that has a scalloped border abutting the adjacent cortex (Fig. 22–9). It is more commonly found in the lower than the upper extremity. When the lesion is smaller than 2 cm, it may be referred to as a fibrous cortical defect. When larger than 3 cm or occupying more than half the transverse diameter of the bone, these lesions are at risk for pathologic fracture. The majority of nonossifying fibromas probably heal spontaneously and require no treatment. Treatment is reserved for lesions with atypical radiographs (requiring biopsy) or for symptomatic or larger lesions (>3 cm) that require treatment to prevent a pathologic fracture.[4]

Giant Cell Tumor

Giant cell tumor of bone is a common lesion in young adults that develops primarily in the distal end of the femur or proximal part of the tibia (60% to 70%), but it

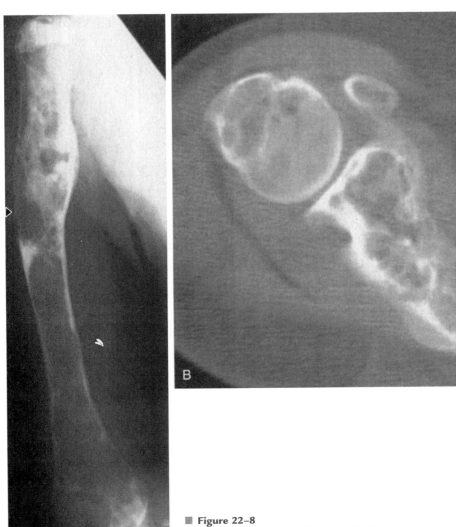

■ **Figure 22–8**
A, A 20-year-old woman with fibrous dysplasia of the humerus and a chronic pseudarthrosis *(arrow)* resistant to bracing. **B,** Computed tomographic scan of the proximal part of the humerus and scapula in the same patient demonstrating part of her extensive polyostotic disease involving the humerus and scapula while sparing the glenohumeral joint.

may also occur in the proximal end of the humerus in 5% to 10% of cases. It is a radiolucent, epiphyseal or metaphyseal tumor that most commonly has a distinct bony margin and is frequently associated with extensive subchondral bone erosion. It is typically a stage 2 active lesion (60% of cases) but also shows up as a more aggressive, benign stage 3 tumor in 20% of cases. Treatment alternatives for giant cell tumor include curettage with or without local adjuvant treatment versus marginal resection. The local recurrence rate after curettage alone is 20% to 30% for active lesions versus 5% after marginal resection.[24,30,34,76,135] Local adjuvant therapy used in conjunction with curettage includes the application of phenol, bone cement (cementation), or liquid nitrogen (cryotherapy). Histologically, "benign" giant cell tumor has demonstrated a potential for pulmonary metastasis in a very small percentage of cases.[30,77,116,124,126,128,154,155] The radiographic differential diagnosis in an adult includes aneurysmal bone cyst, metastatic adenocarcinoma, lymphoma, chondrosarcoma, and osteomyelitis.

Reticuloendothelial Tumors

Tumors of reticuloendothelial origin include a category of intraosseous lesions that arise from marrow stem cells and lesions of similar histology. They are also referred to as round cell or small, blue cell tumors. This category of tumors or abnormalities includes diagnoses such as leukemia, lymphoma,[208] neuroblastoma, histiocytosis, rhabdomyosarcoma, Ewing's sarcoma, infection, and in adults, multiple myeloma and metastatic adenocarcinoma.

Multiple Myeloma

Multiple myeloma is the most common primary malignancy of bone and typically occurs in the middle decades of life, with the shoulder girdle involved in 5% to 10% of cases.[39,77] The most common site of involvement is the axial skeleton, but multiple distinct lesions develop in the extremities in a significant number of patients and may require surgical stabilization to prevent impending frac-

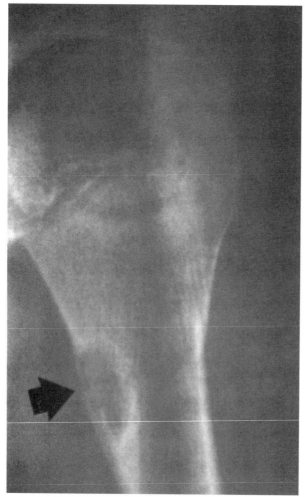

■ **Figure 22–9**
A small eccentric, juxtacortical, nonossifying fibroma manifested as a pathologic fracture *(arrow)*.

ture if medical treatment has failed. In patients who have a solitary intraosseous myeloma or plasmacytoma of the shoulder at initial evaluation, biopsy is indicated for diagnostic reasons. Elevated serum calcium levels, anemia, serum protein electrophoresis, or a distinctly cold bone scan may suggest the diagnosis of myeloma before biopsy in a patient with a solitary lesion or unknown diagnosis. The overall prognosis is poor; however, newer treatments involving aggressive chemotherapy and plasma cell antibodies offer hope for the future. Figure 22–10A is the plain radiograph of a 42-year-old man in apparent good health but experiencing shoulder pain. Coronal (Fig. 22–10B) and transverse (Fig. 22–10C) MRI views demonstrate a suprascapular soft tissue lesion that extends anteriorly and posteriorly to the scapula. The preoperative diagnosis was a probable soft tissue sarcoma. Open biopsy was diagnostic for multiple myeloma with extensive bone disease. The patient died suddenly 1 week after the biopsy, with an undocumented serum calcium level. All patients with the diagnosis of myeloma need to have careful evaluation of their serum electrolytes for the possibility of hypercalcemia.

Ewing's Sarcoma

The second most common intraosseous malignancy in adolescence is Ewing's sarcoma, an aggressive marrow cell tumor that appears as a permeative diaphyseal tumor that is poorly marginated and typically associated with a large, soft tissue mass.[6,56] Figure 22–11A demonstrates such a "permeative" lesion in the humeral diaphysis of a 16-year-old with a typically hot bone scan (Fig. 22–11B) and an associated soft tissue mass (Fig. 22–11C). Ewing's sarcoma today is primarily treated with aggressive chemotherapy and surgical resection or radiation therapy, depending on the size and location of the primary lesion.

Miscellaneous Dysplasias

Gaucher's Disease

Gaucher's disease is an uncommon metabolic disorder of the reticuloendothelial system and glucocerebroside-glycolipid metabolism that affects the liver, spleen, and bone marrow.[75] The disease has an increased incidence in the Jewish population and occurs most commonly in the first 3 decades of life and without sexual preference. Patients typically experience pain secondary to bone involvement and marrow infiltration, which occurs most commonly in the femoral head, with a high degree of bilaterality. The disease in many ways represents a form of avascular necrosis of the femoral head. The humeral head is the second most common site of involvement, and radiographic changes include osteopenia, diaphyseal or medullary expansion, and cortical erosions. The differential diagnosis includes osteomyelitis in the acute setting and round cell tumors in the nonacute setting. Surgical treatment involves internal fixation for fracture prophylaxis, joint replacement in adults when indicated, and appropriate management of femoral head necrosis in children.

Paget's Disease

Paget's disease (osteoporosis circumscripta, osteitis deformans) occurs after the fourth decade and has a slight preponderance in men.[101] Geographically, it appears to have a higher incidence in Great Britain, Europe, Australia, and the United States, whereas it is relatively rare in India and most parts of Asia. Paget's disease develops most commonly in the pelvis, skull, lumbosacral spine, femur, and humerus. It can occur in a polyostotic or a monostotic form and is usually evident at the time of initial evaluation. The typical radiographic picture shows cortical thickening and rarefaction, followed by pathologic microfracture and diaphyseal bowing (Fig. 22–12A). The differential diagnosis in an adult includes metastatic adenocarcinoma, osteosarcoma, and osteomyelitis. Patients should be assessed by evaluation of serum alkaline phosphatase and urinary hydroxyproline levels, a total body bone scan, and a CT scan or MRI.

Patients with Paget's disease undergoing orthopaedic surgery should, in general, be pretreated. Paget's disease itself is best managed medically with diphosphonates or calcitonin. Sarcoma arising out of Paget's disease is

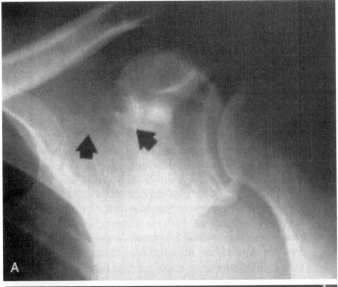

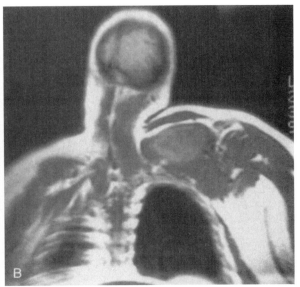

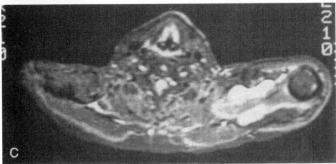

■ **Figure 22–10**

A, A 42-year-old man with left shoulder pain and a lytic scapular lesion *(arrows)*. **B,** Coronal magnetic resonance imaging (MRI) in the same patient demonstrates a suprascapular soft tissue mass. **C,** An axial MRI view of the same patient shows a lesion wrapped anteriorly and posteriorly over the scapula.

characterized by a history of progressive pain and a bony lytic lesion (see Fig. 22–12B) associated with a soft tissue mass. "Pagetoid sarcoma" is a rare variant of osteosarcoma with a 5-year mortality of 80% to 90%.[160] Paget's sarcoma is best managed by ensuring a radical surgical margin because of the diffuse nature of the process of Paget's disease and the difficulty of assessing the extent of sarcomatous changes.

Figure 22–12A and B present early and late radiographs of Paget's disease in the proximal end of the humerus. The lytic lesion, combined with a history of increasing arm pain, served notice of an early secondary osteosarcoma that showed up 3 months later with a more impressive lytic lesion in the proximal part of the humerus (see Fig. 22–12C). Paget's disease affected the full humerus, and the bone scan (Fig. 22–12D) was of little help in demarcating bony margins or osseous involvement by this secondary, or pagetoid, osteosarcoma.[111] MRI and CT scans again demonstrate the soft tissue and bony extent of disease in the proximal part of the humerus (Fig. 22–12E and F).

Benign Soft Tissue Tumors

Lipoma

Lipomas may occur intramuscularly or within normal fat planes of the axilla or the subscapular or other perivascular spaces. They frequently appear in the anterior deltoid as a large, soft, nontender, intramuscular mass.[55] A few lipomas may be tender or firm or have an equivocal history of a change in size. On MRI or CT scan, a benign lipoma usually has a uniform, fatty consistency. Clinically, a liposarcoma has a firmer, denser consistency than a lipoma does. If a lipoma feels very dense or firm clinically, MRI should be performed for further evaluation. If MRI demonstrates areas of distinctly different density, a biopsy should precede marginal excision to exclude the possibility of a liposarcoma.

Hemangioma

Hemangiomas typically appear as "enlarging" intramuscular lesions in a child or young adult and are best visualized by MRI. If they are intimately involved with a major vessel, they should also be evaluated with an arteriogram. These lesions do not usually pose diagnostic or surgical problems, with the exception of large hemangiomas or hemangiomatosis of skeletal muscle. These are aggressive, congenital lesions that are frequently unresectable because of extensive neurovascular and soft tissue involvement.[2,54] Many of these extensive lesions result in amputations because of painful, dysvascular, or infected extremities. Most of these lesions are best diagnosed by open biopsy after MRI, CT scan with contrast, or arteriography. Well-localized lesions are more easily resected

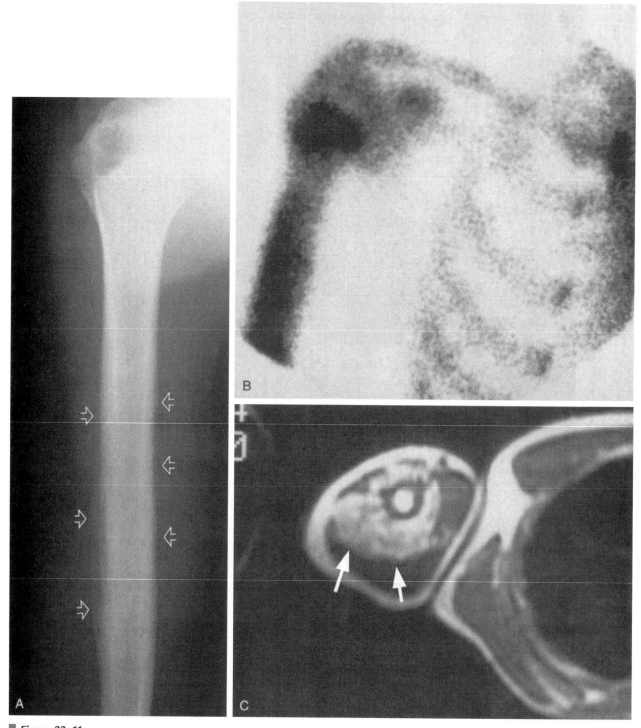

■ **Figure 22–11**

A, Permeative diaphyseal lesion demonstrating a periosteal reaction in a 16-year-old boy *(arrowheads)*. The open biopsy was consistent with Ewing's sarcoma. **B,** A bone scan of the same lesion demonstrates significant activity in the humerus. **C,** Axial magnetic resonance imaging demonstrates a circumferential soft tissue mass *(arrows)* typical of Ewing's sarcoma.

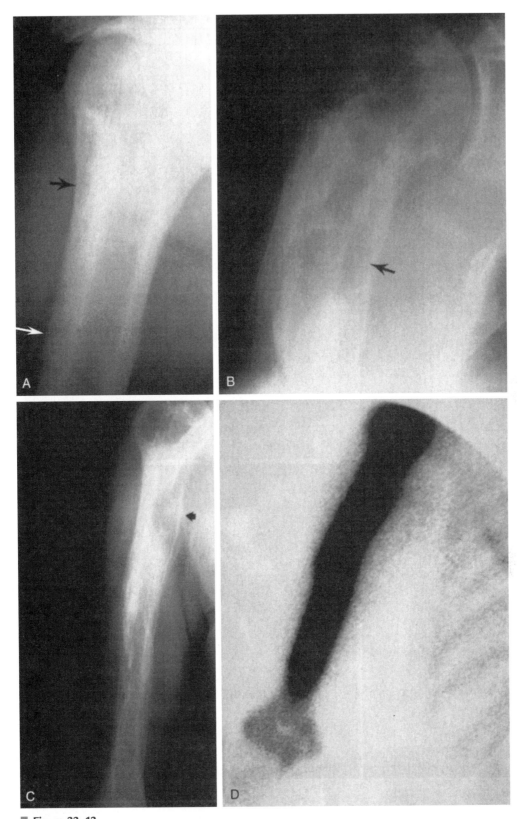

■ Figure 22–12
A, Early Paget's disease of the proximal part of the humerus demonstrating cortical thickening and
rarefaction *(arrows)*. **B,** The same patient was evaluated years later for shoulder pain and a lytic lesion of
the humerus *(arrow)* consistent with a secondary osteosarcoma. **C,** Several months later, this lytic process
had become larger *(arrow)* and was associated with a large soft tissue mass (sarcoma). **D,** Bone scanning
demonstrates intense humeral activity without distinguishing involvement by Paget's disease from
sarcomatous changes.

Continued

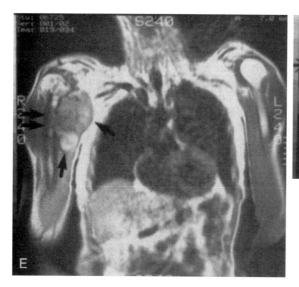
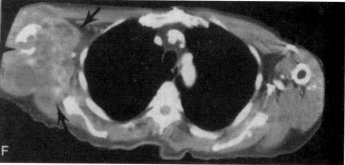

■ **Figure 22–12, cont'd**
E, Coronal magnetic resonance imaging shows a large soft tissue mass arising out of the proximal end of the humerus *(double arrows)* and extending into the axilla. **F,** Computed tomography also demonstrates this secondary osteosarcoma with gross destruction of the proximal end of the humerus *(arrows).*

than the more extensive congenital lesions. Embolization has had mixed results in halting the progression of disease.

Fibromatosis

Fibromatosis (desmoid) is a locally aggressive (stage 2 or 3) lesion found in young children, teenagers, and young adults. These lesions have a firm consistency on clinical examination and may be associated with osseous erosions or invasion of a neurovascular bundle. Many of these lesions recur locally because of inadequate preoperative staging, underestimation of their potential for local recurrence, and an inadequate surgical margin. The literature reveals considerable confusion and contradiction regarding the natural history of fibromatosis. Spontaneous regression as described in some publications is unusual except in some congenital forms, and the natural history of lesions in adolescents is progressive growth and recurrence after marginal resection. These lesions rarely demonstrate pulmonary metastasis, and chemotherapy is not usually efficacious, although indications for chemotherapy do exist.[48,64,65,166] The congenital form of the disease is referred to as congenital fibrosarcoma primarily because of its very impressive histologic cellularity. The adolescent version is best referred to as aggressive fibromatosis and behaves as an active aggressive lesion. Preoperative and postoperative MRI studies are mandatory in these patients to fully assess the soft tissue involvement. Bone scans should also be carried out if there is any doubt about secondary bone involvement. The essence of treatment of fibrous dysplasia remains adequate resection and radiation therapy.

Soft Tissue Sarcomas

Soft tissue sarcomas occur in the upper extremity in approximately a third of all cases. They are frequently misdiagnosed initially as benign lesions and suffer a contaminated marginal resection before a definitive biopsy. Soft tissue sarcomas are characterized by four fairly typical

TABLE 22–3.   Sarcoma: Signs and Symptoms

Bone	Soft Tissue
Bone pain	Firm mass
Night pain	Nontender mass
Pain (unrelated to joint motion)	Large (5 cm) or enlarging
Tender, soft tissue mass	Deep or subfascial

From Enneking WF, Spanier SS, and Goodman MA: A system for the surgical staging of musculoskeletal sarcoma. *Clin Orthop 153:*105-120, 1980.

clinical characteristics. They generally have a firm consistency, are deep to the superficial muscular fascia, are larger than 5 cm, and are nontender (Table 22–3). Adequate staging before biopsy is important for soft tissue sarcomas, just as it is for bone sarcomas (Fig. 22–13). Open biopsy is preferred in such lesions rather than needle biopsy to diagnose both the histologic type and the histologic grade of the lesion.

The most common soft tissue sarcoma in adults is malignant fibrous histiocytoma, which occurs most often in older adults (50 to 70 years).[26,65,216] Liposarcoma[66,164,193] typically occurs in the lower extremities in young adults as a large lesion with a histology ranging from low grade to high grade or pleomorphic. Synovial sarcoma[220] is a less common lesion associated with faint soft tissue calcifications, a juxta-articular location, and a high metastatic rate. Fibrosarcoma, rhabdomyosarcoma,[134] leiomyosarcoma, clear cell sarcoma, and epithelioid lesions are other, less common soft tissue malignancies.[67] Regardless of the tissue type, the grade of the lesion and the anatomic location of the primary tumor are the most significant factors determining prognosis and treatment. Soft tissue sarcomas of intermediate-grade histology are problematic to treat because of a variable prognosis and response to chemotherapy. There has been some early experience with flow cytometry in identifying more active (aneuploid) tumors, and this knowledge may prove helpful in the future in subclassifying or grading intermediate-grade tumors. Synovial sarcoma, epithelioid sarcoma, and rhabdomyosarcoma are characterized as soft tissue sarcomas

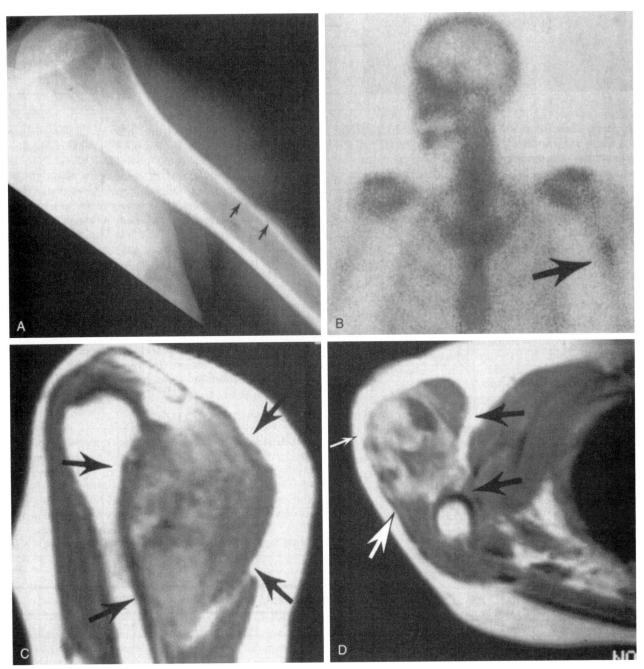

■ **Figure 22–13**

A, Plain radiograph of a 55-year-old woman with a large soft tissue sarcoma at the deltoid. The cortical irregularity at the deltoid insertion *(arrows)* is suggestive of bone invasion. **B,** A bone scan demonstrates distinct bone involvement at the deltoid tubercle with increased uptake *(arrow)*. **C,** Sagittal magnetic resonance imaging (MRI) shows a large mass *(arrows)* abutting against the proximal part of the humerus. **D,** Axial MRI also suggests posterior humeral cortical invasion by a large deltoid malignant fibrous histiocytoma *(arrows)*.

with a high incidence (10% to 20%) of regional lymph node metastasis and a poor prognosis,[41,62,113,172,173,200,206] but survival is generally recognized as being closely related to an individual tumor's histologic grade.[180]

INCIDENCE OF NEOPLASMS

Malignant tumors arising within the musculoskeletal system are rare and account for 0.5% to 0.7% of all malig-

nancies.[25] They are relatively more common in children, in whom they represent 6.5% of all cancers. Although the incidence of soft tissue sarcomas has little apparent sexual or racial predilection, osteosarcoma and Ewing's sarcoma have demonstrated a slight male preference (1.3 to 1.0).[31,92] Approximately 4500 new cases of soft tissue sarcoma occur in the United States each year, with an incidence of 1.8 per 100,000, or approximately 18 cases per million. The number of new bone and cartilage or skeletal malignancies is similar. Various sources estimate that 1000 to

2000 new cases of osteosarcoma occur annually in the United States.[25,32,177] The true incidence of most of these tumors remains somewhat speculative.

The most common tumor of the adult musculoskeletal system is metastatic adenocarcinoma, most frequently from the kidney, lung, breast, or prostate.[46] The most common primary malignancy of bone is multiple myeloma, a plasma cell malignancy usually diagnosed by the medical oncologist rather than the orthopaedic surgeon.[77] Multiple myeloma has an incidence that is approximately twice that of osteosarcoma. Exclusive of multiple myeloma, the most common primary malignant tumor of bone is osteosarcoma. If both benign and malignant primary lesions of the musculoskeletal system are included, cartilaginous tumors are the most common primary lesion (benign and malignant) of the skeletal system.[31]

Age is a very important characteristic in the occurrence and distribution of tumors. The overall distribution of tumors by age in decades (Figs. 22–14 and 22–15) demonstrates a preponderance of benign tumors in the skeleton of growing children; 58% of all benign lesions occur in the second and third decades. Malignant tumors of the skeleton have a peak incidence in adolescents and middle-aged adults.[32,46,177] Osteosarcoma and Ewing's sarcoma are the most frequent malignant bone tumors in adolescents. In adults, osteosarcoma and chondrosarcoma occur with an incidence second to multiple myeloma and metastatic adenocarcinoma. Osteosarcoma represents approximately 40% of all primary malignancies of bone, chondrosarcoma accounts for 20%, and Ewing's sarcoma accounts for 12.5%.[32,46,177]

The incidence of tumors by anatomic location is best estimated by review of the works of Enneking[57] and Dahlin.[32] The overall incidence of primary sarcomas in the shoulder is approximately 15%.[35,57] Lesions of the shoulder are the third most common overall site for sarcomas, behind the hip-pelvis (1) and the knee (distal femoral and proximal tibial areas) (2). In general, one third of all sarcomas affect the upper extremity.[170] Most shoulder tumors develop in the proximal part of the humerus (68.6% to 71.5%) (Fig. 22-16). Tumors of the shoulder girdle occur in the clavicle (6% to 10% of all cases) and in the scapula (18% to 24%) to a much less common degree.[32,46]

CLINICAL FEATURES

Despite refinements and developments in the field of musculoskeletal oncology, patients with musculoskeletal malignancies in general experience a 3- to 6-month history of symptoms before an accurate diagnosis is made. The challenge for the general practitioner is to predict the diagnosis based on the initial history, physical examination, and plain radiographs. Most of these lesions have a subtle onset, and their initial diagnosis requires attention to certain details and an understanding of a few hallmark signs. The patient's initial assessment remains the first and a crucial step to a successful evaluation and treatment plan. In fact, in 70% to 80% of cases, it is possible to correctly diagnose and recognize most malignancies based on the initial history, physical examination, and plain radiographs.[46]

Patients with an intraosseous malignancy almost always have pain. The challenge to the physician is to distinguish between the pain of malignancy and the other more common types of musculoskeletal pain secondary to degenerative joint disease, overuse, inflammatory joint disease, trauma, sepsis, and so forth. The hallmark symptom of an intraosseous malignancy is that of pain at

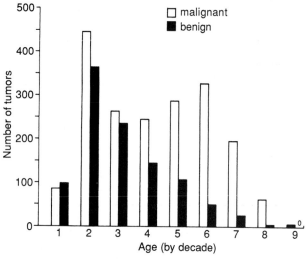

■ **Figure 22–14**
Distribution of musculoskeletal tumors by age.

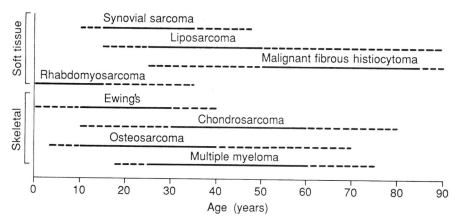

■ **Figure 22–15**
Sarcomas versus age.
(Adapted from Enzinger FM and Weiss SW: Soft Tissue Tumors. St Louis: CV Mosby, 1983.)

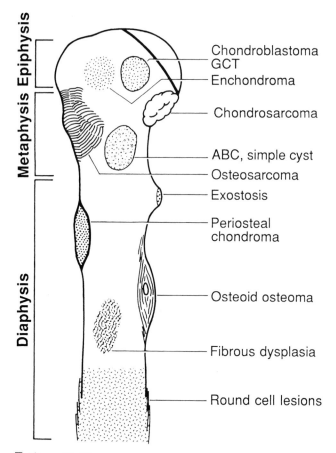

■ Figure 22–16
Common tumors of the proximal end of the humerus. ABC, aneurysmal bone cyst; GCT, giant cell tumor.

Labels in figure:
Epiphysis / Metaphysis / Diaphysis

Chondroblastoma
GCT
Enchondroma

Chondrosarcoma

ABC, simple cyst
Osteosarcoma

Exostosis

Periosteal chondroma

Osteoid osteoma

Fibrous dysplasia

Round cell lesions

night or pain at rest (see Table 22–3). Any patient who experiences a symptom of significant pain at night should be very carefully assessed radiographically at the time of the first evaluation. A patient with night pain or pain at rest, coupled with plain radiographic studies that demonstrate an osseous "abnormality" of any kind, should be further imaged with a technetium bone scan as a matter of routine. Some patients with inflammatory or degenerative joint disease will complain of pain at night, but in general, pain at night as a prominent symptom, paired with abnormal plain films, is very suggestive of a possible tumor.

Other pertinent findings in the history that may be helpful include a strong family history of malignancy (adenocarcinoma or sarcoma) or a history of a previous malignancy in the patient that may now be metastatic to the skeleton. Weight loss and general malaise may be significant symptoms for metastatic disease, and the physician should initiate a workup to further evaluate the patient's general health. It is unusual, however, for a patient to have generalized symptoms or metastatic disease as the initial symptom of a sarcoma.

Musculoskeletal neoplasms present a clinical challenge to the orthopaedist in determining whether a patient has intraosseous pain or intra-articular pain. This distinction is not readily apparent in the early diagnosis of most intraosseous tumors. A careful physical examination can sometimes elicit findings consistent with joint tenderness, impingement, or weakness, thus suggesting some sort of intra-articular process. It is unusual for sarcomas to extend into a joint, and the presence of joint findings or symptoms is more consistent with trauma, degenerative disease, or some other non-neoplastic process. In general, intra-articular processes are exacerbated by physical activities and joint motion (see the section on physical examination). Similarly, some patients have referred pain that may lead to an erroneous diagnosis of shoulder pain that has really originated from the cervical spine or have hip pain that originates in the lumbar spine. The challenge of determining whether a particular patient's problem is intraosseous or intra-articular requires a careful musculoskeletal evaluation, which is usually best accomplished by an orthopaedist.

A careful orthopaedic examination is important when evaluating all patients but is vital when evaluating a patient with difficult symptoms. Every adult patient who is evaluated specifically for a possible neoplasm should have a careful general examination of the head and neck, cardiopulmonary status, abdomen, spine, breasts (women), and prostate (men), as well as an examination for lymphadenopathy. This sort of general examination is most appropriate for adults older than 35 to 40 years, who are more likely to have metastatic adenocarcinoma. In addition to a specific examination to evaluate patients for a possible neoplasm, all patients should have a complete general musculoskeletal examination to evaluate for joint range of motion, strength, stability, and so forth. Regional adenopathy should be routinely checked on examination and will be found to be present with many tumors. It is usually an inflammatory phenomenon, reactive to the tumor. However, lymph node adenopathy larger than 1 cm should be evaluated further by MRI, and biopsy should be performed before definitive resection of the primary tumor is attempted.

Patients with an aggressive intraosseous malignancy usually have bone tenderness and a mass. The primary site may be deep and well covered by muscle and may be difficult to palpate. Usually, careful palpation will demonstrate the presence or absence of any soft tissue mass. However, low-grade intraosseous lesions may not involve the soft tissues. The ability to elicit joint findings is more suggestive of an intra-articular, traumatic, inflammatory, or degenerative process. Thus, joint tenderness or stiffness can be a very helpful finding. Extension of an intraosseous malignancy medially toward the major neurovascular bundle, which is close to the humerus, may preclude limb-sparing surgery and is associated with a worse prognosis. The extent of involvement of the soft tissues on physical examination is an important finding to follow in addition to radiographic imaging. Clinical involvement of the soft tissues can yield important information for directing the MRI scan and other studies. In general, the soft tissue mass produced by an intraosseous malignancy is relatively subtle as an early clinical finding and requires some attention on examination. If an osseous sarcoma is manifested as a large soft tissue mass, more care should be taken when evaluating the extent of soft tissue involvement if limb-sparing surgery is planned.

Soft tissue sarcomas most commonly have a history of a mass. Most soft tissue sarcomas, in contradistinction to intraosseous malignancies, are not painful. All soft tissue lesions should be carefully evaluated for the four characteristics of a soft tissue sarcoma: nontender mass, firm consistency, deep or subfascial location, and larger than 5 cm in size (see Table 22–3). Exceptions occur, but as a general rule, these guidelines are very reliable in the initial evaluation of various soft tissue lesions. The most reliable clinical sign for a soft tissue sarcoma is the consistency or density of the lesion. For instance, the most common soft tissue tumor in an adult is a lipoma, which may be large, deep in location, and nontender; however, its consistency will usually indicate whether it is malignant. Lipomas are typically very soft with the consistency of normal fat, whereas liposarcomas are usually firm. The ability to distinguish the consistency of a soft tissue mass can be a somewhat subtle, but important finding. Anything with a consistency more dense than normal fat should be evaluated carefully. Lipomas that feel firmer than normal fat or larger than 10 cm should be evaluated by MRI; intramuscular lesions that are firmer than normal muscle should also be evaluated by MRI. If a soft tissue mass is thought to be cystic, it is reasonable and advisable to attempt careful aspiration in the clinic to document whether that lesion contains fluid. Repeated or multiple aspirations are not advised and will lead only to contamination of a possible soft tissue sarcoma.

In summary, all patients with a possible musculoskeletal neoplasm (or an unknown diagnosis) should have a complete general and musculoskeletal examination with an emphasis on the joints and soft tissues. Always put your hand on the patient and consider the possibility of a mass when examining a patient with a difficult problem. Always consider the challenges of referred pain. The size of any soft tissue mass should be carefully measured and recorded in the chart to give an objective finding for further follow-up. It is also helpful to take a photograph in the clinic for future reference. The most common omission in the general physical examination of patients without a known tumor diagnosis is failure to detect an obvious primary site of involvement for an adenocarcinoma (e.g., abdominal mass, prostatic mass). The most common mistake on the initial orthopaedic examination is failure to detect the true location of the abnormality (referred pain) or failure to detect a soft tissue mass.

Routine clinical follow-up for a patient with a malignancy is important to detect progressive disease at an early stage. After the immediate postoperative evaluation, patients with high-grade sarcomas are generally monitored every 3 months for 2 years, every 6 months for another 2 years, and every year thereafter. Frequent clinical follow-up is important to detect metastatic or recurrent disease at an early stage, thus enhancing further treatment. Frequent follow-up is also advisable in patients with undiagnosed skeletal pain. Such follow-up is most appropriate in an adult who has significant joint symptoms and normal-appearing plain radiographs. If the plain radiographs are not consistent with the patient's symptoms, a total body technetium bone scan is well indicated to rule out a possible neoplasm. On the other hand, most patients who have a small (<5 cm) soft tissue mass can be monitored without biopsy or MRI without significant danger of missing a possible malignancy. Similarly, intraosseous lesions that appear benign on plain radiographs or lesions that are picked up incidentally in the evaluation of a patient with intra-articular shoulder pathology can easily be monitored if the plain radiographs are well demarcated and the lesions are obviously benign. If the initial plain radiographs are equivocal, a bone scan and CT scan or MRI are indicated to determine whether the lesion is active and a biopsy needs to be performed or whether it can be monitored clinically. For instance, most low-grade, calcified, or cartilaginous intraosseous lesions can be safely monitored at 6-month intervals.

X-RAY AND LABORATORY EVALUATION

The orthopaedist's interpretation of the initial plain radiographs is an important step in the early diagnosis of most musculoskeletal tumors. When dealing with intraosseous or skeletal lesions, the orthopaedist should have a system for evaluating the initial plain radiographs and formulating the initial diagnosis. Every bone lesion has a characteristic location, margin, and density that typify it radiographically. These three radiographic characteristics are important in describing a lesion's growth rate and intrinsic density.[57] These concepts originated in a different format from that of Jaffee,[99] who first posed the questions "What is the lesion's density?"; "What is it doing to bone?"; "What is the bone doing to it?"; and "What is its location?" when evaluating radiographs. This approach helps focus attention on a lesion's growth rate, its degree of activity, and thus its malignant potential. With these three characteristics in mind, the initial plain radiographs can be interpreted with the correct diagnosis in most cases.

Location

Where is the lesion located? Is it in the epiphysis, metaphysis, or diaphysis? Are there multiple metastatic sites or one primary site of involvement? For example, an aggressive metaphyseal tumor in an adolescent is very likely to be an osteosarcoma, whereas a diaphyseal lesion is much more likely to be Ewing's sarcoma. Whether the lesion is central or eccentric with the bone is also important information. Nonossifying fibroma is almost always eccentric, whereas cartilaginous lesions (enchondroma) are usually centrally located.

Margin

The margin of the lesion on plain radiographs is the best reflection of that lesion's growth rate at the time of the initial evaluation. It refers to the margin or interface between the lesion and surrounding normal bone. If a tumor is slow growing, it will have a distinct or sclerotic margin that demonstrates the ability of the surrounding normal bone to react to it, thus marginating, or walling off, that lesion. A sclerotic or distinct peripheral bony margin indicates a slow-growing or benign lesion and is not generally seen with malignant or aggressive benign tumors. This type of margin reflects the ability of bone to respond to a slowly growing tumor. At the other end of the spectrum is a lesion that is not well marginated and does not have a sclerotic rim of reactive bone around it. This pattern reflects a more rapidly growing tumor that enlarges at a rate that is faster than normal bone can react to it. The best example of an aggressive lesion that infiltrates or percolates through bone is the permeative lesion of Ewing's sarcoma or any intramedullary round cell tumor or small blue cell tumor of bone. Round cell tumors occur more commonly in children, and the differential diagnosis includes lymphoma, leukemia, Ewing's sarcoma, rhabdomyosarcoma, neuroblastoma, histiocytosis, Wilms' tumor, and acute osteomyelitis. In contrast, the differential diagnosis for round cell tumors in adults includes metastatic carcinoma, Ewing's sarcoma, multiple myeloma, lymphoma, and osteomyelitis.

Density

The intrinsic density of a lesion within bone or soft tissue is another piece of information that contributes to the initial diagnosis. Is the lesion making bone, cartilage (calcifications), fibrous dysplasia (ground-glass density), or soft tissue (clear)? A truly cystic (or fluid-filled) lesion is most likely to be a benign or infectious lesion in bone or soft tissue, and this cystic nature may be determined clinically or demonstrated by staging studies.

Thus, complete assessment of a patient with a musculoskeletal lesion involves a careful evaluation of both the clinical and radiographic findings. The complex anatomy and frequency of referred pain make many diagnoses in the shoulder a challenge. Knowledge and awareness of the typical symptoms, physical findings, and radiographic clues for sarcomas are essential for successful treatment.

Appropriate initial radiographs for evaluating most patients include a well-exposed, properly positioned film. Accepting poor-quality radiographs can lead to disaster. It is essential that a well-exposed radiograph of the shoulder be obtained in all patients, especially those with persistent symptoms who may be failing conservative treatment for what is believed to be an intra-articular glenohumeral problem. Without a doubt the best initial staging diagnostic study for evaluating a possible intraosseous malignancy is a technetium bone scan. The best staging study for a soft tissue lesion is MRI. CT scans are routinely used for ruling out lung metastasis in addition to initial plain chest radiographs for all patients who have probable soft tissue or bone malignancies.

The staging studies involved in assessing a high-grade intraosseous lesion, such as an osteosarcoma, include bone scan, MRI of the extremity, CT scan of the extremity, and CT of the lung. MRI is indicated to assess the degree of soft tissue involvement and the neurovascular bundle margin before and after biopsy and induction chemotherapy. CT scan of the extremity remains a good study to assess the degree of bony cortical involvement. A total body bone scan should be carried out in all patients with musculoskeletal malignancies to assess the presence of distant bone metastases and the extent of primary disease. Diagnostic strategies for evaluation of possible skeletal metastases have been reviewed.[175]

Possible tumor involvement of the neurovascular bundle and brachial plexus is best assessed by MRI, whereas arteriography is now reserved specifically for lesions located adjacent to a major vessel. Arteriography has also been used in the past to assess the extent of soft tissue involvement by sarcomas, but it has been more or less replaced at present by MRI. Other modalities for assessing the extent of soft tissue sarcomas have included gallium scans, which have generally been considered to have inferior resolution quality when compared with MRI.

Evaluation of possible chest wall involvement by shoulder lesions remains a difficult task. Such involvement is best assessed by CT scanning, MRI, and bone scans. If rib uptake is noted on the bone scan, bony chest wall involvement is obvious. It is somewhat unusual for proximal humeral malignancies to have chest wall involvement. However, chest wall involvement may well occur with soft tissue lesions that have extended from the brachial plexus, axilla, or scapula.

Metabolic imaging using radioisotopes such as fluorodeoxyglucose and others has received greater attention over the last several years. Such studies are potentially useful in grading tumors (high versus low grade), assessing the response to chemotherapy, and evaluating patients for residual minimal disease.

Laboratory

In general, laboratory studies for sarcomas are not of great assistance in making the initial diagnosis. The most common exception is serum alkaline phosphatase, which is frequently elevated in osteosarcoma or Paget's disease.[106] Measurement of serum acid phosphatase or prostate-specific antigen levels and urinalysis (microscopic hematuria) are helpful in the evaluation of possible malignancies of the prostate or kidney.[153] A hematocrit, white blood cell count, and erythrocyte sedimentation rate (ESR) are well indicated in evaluating for possible sepsis, although both the white blood cell count and the ESR may be nonspecifically elevated with various tumors and the hematocrit may be nonspecifically low. Any patient who has plasmacytoma or multiple myeloma in the differential diagnosis should have serum calcium and serum electrolytes checked preoperatively to detect hypercalcemia. In addition, these patients should undergo a serum and urine protein electrophoresis study to evaluate their immunoglobulin profile.[99]

Routine laboratory studies (e.g., liver enzymes) are checked in the standard follow-up of patients with a musculoskeletal malignancy; however, it is unusual for a sarcoma to metastasize to the liver, and thus liver enzymes are rarely elevated secondary to tumor. Elevated liver enzymes can occur for other reasons (hepatitis) and are included in routine follow-up blood work for that reason. It is useful to evaluate liver enzymes and complete blood counts in all sarcoma patients to assess a patient's general medical health.

COMPLICATIONS OF TUMORS

Pathologic Fractures

One of the most significant complications of a musculoskeletal tumor is that of pathologic fracture, the majority of which are secondary to metastatic adenocarcinoma. Approximately a third of all diagnosed cases of breast, pulmonary, thyroid, renal, and prostatic carcinoma include skeletal metastases.[11,68,86,215] Although the most common site for metastasis is the axial skeleton, approximately 25% of all metastases are located in the shoulder girdle.

Surgery may be indicated to obtain a primary diagnosis by open biopsy or to achieve internal fixation for fracture prophylaxis. Patients with an established tumor diagnosis and lytic lesions representing bone metastases should, in general, be treated with chemotherapy and radiation therapy first, if the evidence indicates that that particular lesion is likely to respond to that treatment. Metastatic lesions that are generally considered to be resistant to radiation therapy or chemotherapy or lesions that have failed similar previous treatment should be treated surgically (e.g., renal cell carcinoma). Surgical stabilization or internal fixation is indicated in any patient with an impending or completed pathologic fracture who can tolerate a general anesthetic and has a life expectancy of at least 1 month. Coaptation splinting, as an alternative to surgery, does a relatively poor job of relieving fracture symptoms in the humerus because of persistent rotational instability. Figure 22–17 shows a pathologic fracture of the proximal part of the humerus in a 65-year-old patient with extensive metastatic disease. His pain was unrelieved with coaptation bracing, and he was treated surgically with methylmethacrylate and short Ender rods placed through the fracture site. His poor medical status and limited life expectancy (several months) dictated this more conservative surgical procedure rather than the usual treatment of hemiarthroplasty. Even patients with widespread metastatic disease can benefit greatly from a careful, but aggressive approach to the management of pathologic fractures versus impending fractures.

Intraosseous sarcomas that result in a pathologic fracture represent less than 10% of all sarcomas, and although they present a challenge, they are no longer considered to be an absolute indication for immediate amputation. Another problem seen is that of fractures occurring after a poorly designed biopsy, thus emphasizing the need for careful biopsy procedures. An additional problem arises in patients with Ewing's sarcoma, in whom a late fracture can develop in a diaphyseal lesion that has previously been irradiated. Such lesions should be stabilized prophylactically with an intramedullary rod to prevent possible fracture if there is any evidence of an impending fracture. Fractures through irradiated bone are unlikely to heal and should be internally fixed or resected as soon as possible. Fibrous dysplasia is another example of pathologic bone that may require intramedullary fixation to prevent repeated fractures and progressive deformity. Intramedullary fixation is the method of choice because of its biomechanical superiority. Plating with screws is vastly inferior to intramedullary fixation of impending or completed pathologic diaphyseal lesions.

DIFFERENTIAL DIAGNOSIS

The shoulder girdle is an area that presents a challenge to the diagnosis of many different conditions. Its close relationship with the cervical spine and brachial plexus can present a formidable challenge in differentiating cervical spine problems from shoulder problems. The complexity of the soft tissue anatomy of the glenohumeral joint and the difficulty of distinguishing intra- from extra-articular diagnoses are significant, even for the most skilled orthopaedist. The confusion that may arise can delay the diagnosis of various musculoskeletal tumors for a significant period of time.

The differential diagnosis for various musculoskeletal lesions includes the lesions identified in Table 22–4. Although the categories of trauma, tumor, infection, and inflammatory or degenerative disease include the diagnosis in most cases, various dysplastic, hematologic, and metabolic problems are important and require a more extensive evaluation. Certainly, the process of separating out difficult problems starts with an accurate and thorough history and physical examination.

Trauma as the cause of lesions of the musculoskeletal system obviously often includes a history of an injury, but "incidental" trauma is also frequently associated with sarcomas, although no causal relationship has been demonstrated. Chronic injuries or stress fractures are often a more subtle and challenging diagnosis but are less common in the shoulder than in the lower extremity. Figure 22–18 demonstrates a degenerative condition of the sternoclavicular joint in an area that does not easily lend itself to imaging techniques; this degenerative lesion with an apparent soft tissue mass could be misinterpreted as a possible neoplasm of the proximal part of the clavicle. An understanding of the pathology of the sternoclavicular joint is of great assistance in interpreting diagnostic studies of this area.

Infections are a common problem in healthy young children who suffer from acute hematogenous osteomyelitis or septic arthritis. In fact, the differential diagnosis for any lesion in a child should always include infection as a possible cause. Acute hematogenous osteomyelitis is an unusual problem in adults because osteomyelitis usually develops in adults as a result of

TABLE 22–4. Differential Diagnosis of Musculoskeletal Lesions

1. Trauma (subtle, bony, acute, or chronic)
2. Tumor (benign or malignant, primary or metastatic)
3. Infection (bacterial, viral, fungal, or venereal)
4. Inflammatory disease (rheumatoid arthritis, gouty arthropathy, collagen vascular disease, pigmented villonodular synovitis)
5. Degenerative disease (osteoarthritis)
6. Dysplasias (fibrous dysplasia, Paget's disease, multiple hereditary exostoses, neurofibromatosis)
7. Hematologic disorders (hemophilia, histiocytosis, myeloproliferative disorder)
8. Metabolic disorders (osteomalacia, rickets, hyperparathyroidism, renal osteodystrophy)

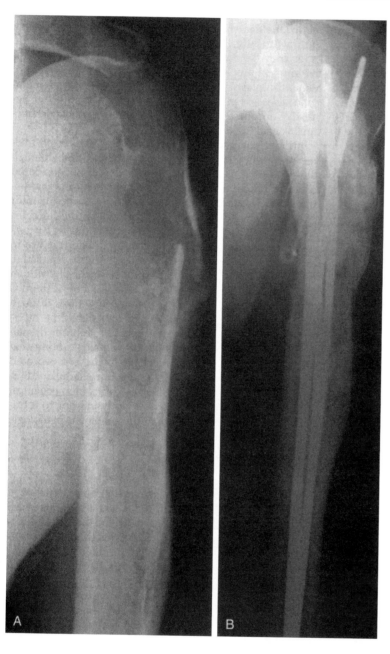

■ **Figure 22–17**
A, Metastatic adenocarcinoma of the lung in a 65-year-old man with extensive metastatic disease and a pathologic fracture. **B,** Conservative surgical stabilization in this patient involved cementation and placement of a rod through the fracture site.

traumatic wounds, surgical complications, or chronic decubitus ulcers. Tuberculous or fungal infections are an even greater diagnostic and treatment challenge, and a culture should be performed in all patients with suspected infections. In general, tuberculous infections have an unimpressive amount of reactive bone on radiographs and a chronic history. Whenever an infectious problem is being considered, a biopsy specimen should be sent in addition to abundant, appropriate material for culture. Some necrotic soft tissue tumors contain pus and strongly resemble a soft tissue abscess. The old adage "always biopsy an infection and culture a tumor" remains good advice as a general rule in the evaluation of any lesion.

Inflammatory and degenerative disease is usually associated with typical findings on plain radiographs such as a joint space narrowing, subchondral sclerosis, and cyst formation. Clinically, it can be very difficult to distinguish inflammatory or degenerative disease from a subtle neoplasm. The differential diagnosis can also be difficult in children, in whom pauciarticular juvenile rheumatoid arthritis in its initial manifestation can be very difficult to distinguish from septic arthritis or other soft tissue tumors.

The most common dysplasias of bone masquerading as neoplasms include fibrous dysplasia in children and Paget's disease in adults. These are usually polyostotic "tumors" that actually represent dysplasias of bone. Fibrous dysplasia and Paget's disease can frequently be diagnosed by evaluating plain radiographs and bone scans, as can many of the polyostotic syndromes. Both fibrous dysplasia and Paget's disease may require

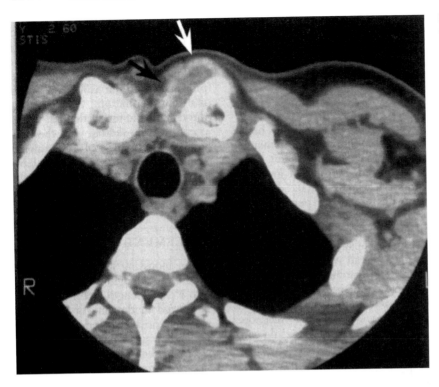

■ **Figure 22–18**
Computed tomographic scan of the sternoclavicular joint in a patient with degenerative joint disease, an effusion, and a soft tissue mass consisting of redundant synovium *(arrows)*. This area is difficult to image and could be misinterpreted as a neoplasm.

intramedullary fixation to treat chronic, pathologic, painful, and weak long bones. Secondary malignancies are unusual and associated with increasing pain and obvious x-ray changes. Other dysplasias include multiple hereditary exostoses and enchondromatoses.

Hematologic disorders (excluding myeloma) that may masquerade as tumors occur most commonly in children or young adults with the various histiocytoses, hemophilia, and other blood dyscrasias. The least aggressive form of histiocytosis is eosinophilic granuloma, which is truly the "great imitator" in children because it can masquerade as a tumor. Eosinophilic granuloma occurs in the diaphysis and is usually seen as a solitary lesion in a healthy child. However, it may occur as multiple lesions, and when diagnosed in a young child (2 years or younger), there is always the concern that the initial lesion may signal the presence of other lesions in the more severe form of the syndrome, such as Hand-Schüller-Christian disease (older children) or Letterer-Siwe disease (infants). Similarly, classic hemophilia or factor VIII deficiency, though uncommon, may show up initially as a solitary knee effusion (septic knee). Therefore, it is important to obtain an accurate history, and questions should be asked specifically about previous bleeding problems in other family members in order to make the diagnosis.

Metabolic disorders in adults can also be difficult diagnoses to make. Adult patients with osteomalacia may have a stress fracture, a hot bone scan, equivocal staging studies, and a risk factor in their history (e.g., renal disease, gastrointestinal malabsorption). The syndromes of renal osteodystrophy, osteomalacia, and osteoporosis are unlikely to show up as a problem of the upper extremity, but they remain an important part of any complete differential diagnosis. Patients with osteomalacia frequently have diffuse manifestations of their disease (e.g.,

vertebral fractures, osteopenia) and may require a full metabolic workup: serum calcium, PO_4, serum and urinary hydroxyproline, vitamin D, parathyroid hormone levels, bone scan, densitometry, and a tetracycline-labeled iliac crest biopsy.

BIOPSY, RESECTIONS, RECONSTRUCTIONS, AND MANAGEMENT OF SPECIFIC LESIONS

Biopsy

The management and treatment of any malignancy begins with a sound histologic diagnosis. Biopsy is recommended for all suspicious abnormalities of bone and soft tissue, although as previously discussed, biopsy of low-grade cartilage and fatty tumors is not usually indicated. Although every institution has its own experiences and prejudices regarding biopsy for sarcomas, open, or incisional, biopsy is nevertheless regarded by most as the standard method.[196] Incisional biopsy is an operative technique that involves incising a small wedge-shaped piece of tissue from the tumor for histologic evaluation. Its primary advantage over a closed, or needle, biopsy is the acquisition of a larger, more adequate specimen, which is especially important in the face of the challenging diagnosis of sarcoma. However, open or incisional biopsies do carry a risk of tumor contamination from postoperative hemorrhage. It is important that the surgical principles of incisional biopsy be strictly observed in the shoulder, just as in any other anatomic site. A dissecting hematoma after any biopsy can easily contaminate otherwise normal tissue and expand the necessary margin for resection, or it can contaminate nearby major neurovascular structures such as the brachial plexus or brachial vessels and thus preclude the possibility of a limb salvage type of resection. Needle biopsies have become a preferred technique in most medical centers with an established sarcoma program. This technique is now preferred for both soft tissue and osseous lesions.

Mankin and colleagues, under the auspices of the Musculoskeletal Tumor Society,[123] carried out a retrospective comparison of 329 cases of sarcoma on which biopsies were performed in a referring (primary or secondary) hospital versus those done in a setting with experience in the biopsy of sarcomas. The study concluded that biopsy-related problems were three to five times more frequent in the outside referring hospital than in the treatment center. The referring hospitals without sarcoma experience had a higher incidence of major diagnostic errors, nonrepresentative biopsies, wound complications, treatment alterations, changes in results, and changes in final results. Finally, the incidence of unnecessary amputations was 4.5% of all the cases. This sort of study may be prejudiced in favor of the tertiary institutions by the fact that most patients were difficult cases that had been referred for treatment, but the study does emphasize a high complication rate for biopsies and the need for careful planning and execution. Higher complication rates and more diagnostic errors do occur in less experienced centers because of the complexity of the diagnosis and treatment of sarcomas. The best management for all patients with sarcomas is to have the biopsy carried out in an experienced center where the definitive treatment will be rendered.[44] A follow-up review of biopsy complications in sarcoma patients suggests that biopsy complications have increased. The best surgical approach for a biopsy of the proximal part of the humerus has traditionally been through the anterior substance of the deltoid (Fig. 22–19). The deltopectoral groove should be avoided because any hematoma after the biopsy might enter the groove, spread proximally into the axilla, and lead to considerable proximal contamination. Approaching malignant lesions through the anterior deltoid requires resection of that portion of the deltoid with the definitive procedure but minimizes the risk of contamination; thus, this is the traditional site for an incisional biopsy of the proximal end of the humerus. Tumor contamination after the biopsy is a significant problem even in experienced hands, and the following principles of technique should be observed.[196]

Placement of the Incision

When biopsying lesions in the extremities, the surgeon should use a longitudinal (not transverse) incision, usually 4 to 5 cm in length (see Fig. 22–19). The incision should be placed in the line of the proposed future definitive resection so that it does not contaminate the lines of a possible future amputation. Around the scapula or clavicle, as in the pelvic girdle, an oblique or transverse incision is appropriate; however, as a general rule, all extremity tumors should be biopsied through a longitudinal incision.

Contamination by Tumor Hematoma

If possible, always perform a biopsy of a tumor at its most superficial and accessible site. An incisional biopsy technique should involve as little soft tissue dissection as possible. A marginal, or excisional, biopsy should be reserved only for obviously benign lesions (e.g., lipoma) or for small (2 to 3 cm) lesions. Similarly, always biopsy the lesion away from a major neurovascular bundle or joint to avoid contaminating these structures and thus precluding a need for limb-sparing surgery. This precaution is especially important in the proximal part of the humerus and shoulder because of the proximity of the brachial vessels and brachial plexus.

Before wound closure, strict hemostasis should be carefully accomplished. The use of a tourniquet is not possible in the shoulder, and even in areas where one is used, it should be released before wound closure to achieve hemostasis. Very vascular malignant lesions (e.g., angiosarcoma, myeloma, hypernephroma, or Ewing's sarcoma) in the shoulder may prove to be a challenge regarding hemostasis. In these situations, packing the wound with various coagulant materials in addition to a pressure dressing may prove helpful in enhancing hemostasis. The use of surgical drains or the practice of leaving the wound open after an open biopsy is associated with a higher incidence of wound contamination or infection and is not an accepted method of management. After achieving hemostasis, the surgeon should meticulously close the biopsy wound and carefully close the deep and superficial layers to prevent late wound dehiscence. The skin is best closed with a subcuticular closure to minimize skin contamination and enable a smaller ellipse of skin to be excised with the main tumor specimen at the time of definitive resection.

Adequacy of the Specimen

Before awakening the patient, it is important to wait for the pathologist to confirm the adequacy of the specimen

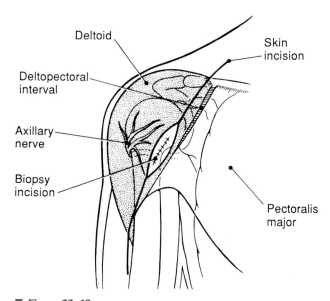

■ **Figure 22–19**
Biopsy of the proximal end of the humerus.

by frozen section under the microscope. Although it may not be possible to make a definitive diagnosis by frozen section in every case, it is possible to determine whether the specimen has diagnostic or lesional tissue and thus whether it is an adequate specimen. Bacterial and fungal cultures should be obtained routinely, in addition to sending tissue for special stains, electron microscopy, flow cytometry,[120] or immunohistochemistry. As a general rule, it is advisable to biopsy infections and culture tumors. If there is some doubt about the location of a biopsy site in the extremity, pelvis, or spine, an intraoperative radiograph with an appropriate marker should be taken before the biopsy. In many cases of osteogenic sarcoma, it is not necessary to biopsy the bone to obtain adequate tissue. A biopsy of a bone lesion can frequently be obtained from its soft tissue extension, thus avoiding fenestration of that bone and the complications of postoperative fracture and further contamination from osseous bleeding.

Open versus Closed Biopsy

The alternatives to an incisional, or open, biopsy include a marginal, or excisional, biopsy or closed needle biopsy. Excisional biopsy is not an accepted method for any lesion that may be malignant. It is an acceptable biopsy technique only when used to excise a small lesion (<3 cm) or to excise a lesion that is obviously benign (e.g., lipoma). Marginal excisional biopsy of a small lesion produces little more contamination than an incisional biopsy and is thus an adequate technique for that size of lesion. Marginal excision of a tumor, however, is best indicated for benign lesions. Small (<5 cm) soft tissue sarcomas do develop in the upper extremity, and if there is concern or confusion about a lesion, consultation with a specialist before the biopsy is the appropriate approach.[47]

Needle biopsy is the recommended method for use on most tumors.[16,139,185] The disadvantage is the small size of the specimen and the difficulty of assessing whether a lesion is high grade or low grade.[8,16] The attraction of needle biopsy is that it avoids the operative setting and is achievable in the clinic, thus giving a quick diagnosis that may be useful in initiating preoperative chemotherapy if a lesion is obviously high grade. The disadvantage remains that of sampling error, which has been reported in approximately 25% to 30% of cases.[196] Needle biopsy is the preferred method for biopsy of osteosarcoma when the radiographs are typical and only a tissue diagnosis (malignant stroma or osteoid) is required. It has the advantage of a small bony fenestration, thus minimizing both the potential for postbiopsy hemorrhage and the risk of pathologic fracture. The best indications for needle biopsy include the following:

1. **To achieve a "tissue and grade" diagnosis** (i.e., metastasis, recurrence, or confirming an otherwise classic manifestation). In experienced medical centers, needle biopsy is now a relatively reliable method for grading soft tissue sarcomas.
2. **For cystic lesions or abscesses**. Cystic lesions are not usually malignancies, and in children, needle biopsy is a good way to quickly rule out possible infections. It is

the preferred method of diagnosing and treating many cystic lesions. If purulent drainage is not obvious, beware of soft tissue sarcomas with central necrosis; a definitive open biopsy should accompany any surgical drainage procedure.
3. **For vertebral or pelvic tumors**. Needle biopsy is an appropriate technique for vertebral and pelvic lesions to avoid the more extensive open biopsy. Most of these lesions are biopsied under CT guidance in the radiology department.

The instruments required for needle biopsy are not complex. Needle biopsy of soft tissue sarcomas typically involves the use of a trocar cutting needle that delivers a small strip of tissue. Larger trephine or bone marrow needles (3 to 5 mm in diameter) are used for bone lesions. The skinny-needle technique for soft tissue tumors uses a 22-gauge needle for a cytologic smear; this smear requires interpretation by an experienced cytopathologist.

Immediately proceeding with definitive resection after an open biopsy is a treatment alternative that offers the advantage of minimizing the risk of postbiopsy hematoma and contamination. It requires appropriate intraoperative precautions, such as a change in gowns, gloves, instruments, and operative drapes, between the biopsy and the definitive resection. The issue of whether it is prudent to proceed with a definitive surgical resection immediately after the frozen section histologic diagnosis depends on the lesion involved and the confidence level of the pathologist giving the diagnosis. This course of action requires careful planning and a confident, well-informed pathologist at the time of the frozen section biopsy. It is not a reasonable alternative for patients who are candidates for preoperative adjuvant therapy or when the differential diagnosis includes radiosensitive tumors such as lymphomas, which are not treated by resection. When there is doubt regarding whether a lesion is malignant or benign, high grade or low grade, treatment should be delayed until a definitive diagnosis is reached.

Biopsies are a challenging aspect of sarcoma management because of both the rarity and the complexity of diagnosing and treating these lesions. Although biopsy appears to be a technically small operative procedure, it represents a significant hurdle to achieving an appropriate and successful treatment plan. The complexity of the diagnosis of most sarcomas requires that this significant, initial step in the treatment be carried out in a center experienced in the management of sarcomas.[44] Biopsy is recommended for all tumors, except when dealing with low-grade chondrosarcoma (versus enchondroma) and lipomatous soft tissue tumors.

Surgical Resections about the Shoulder Girdle

Surgical Margin

Appropriate surgery remains the definitive treatment of most sarcomas at their primary site. Surgical treatment is

TABLE 22–5. Surgical Margins

Surgical Margin	Surgical Procedure	Result
Intralesional	Piecemeal debulking or curettage	Leaves macroscopic tumor
Marginal	Excision of tumor and pseudocapsule through reactive zone	Leaves microscopic tumor
Wide	Excision of tumor, pseudocapsule, reactive zone, and a cuff of normal tissue	Risk of leaving microscopic tumor
Radical	Extracompartmental procedure removes tumor, pseudocapsule, reactive zone, and entire compartment	Minimal risk of residual microscopic tumor

From Enneking WF, Spanier SS, and Goodman MA: A system for the surgical staging of musculoskeletal sarcoma. Clin Orthop 153:105-120, 1980.

best described by separately defining the tumor resection part of the procedure and the reconstructive part of the procedure. These two aspects of any surgical procedure for a tumor are potentially conflicting in their objectives, and great care should be taken to ensure that the resection is not minimized or compromised to facilitate the reconstructive part of the procedure and thus enhance function. Resection must take precedence over reconstruction to achieve a cure. It is imperative that these two procedures remain separate in principle. In some institutions, different surgeons carry out these two parts of the procedure to achieve that goal.

When discussing the probable success of a procedure in terms of local tumor control, the resection procedure is best defined by the surgical margin achieved. The surgical margin describes the efficacy of the procedure in terms of possible future tumor recurrence.[102] Assessing and describing the surgical margin require a cooperative effort by both the surgeon and the pathologist, who must immediately review the surgical specimen. The four fundamental types of margins are intracapsular, marginal, wide, and radical (Table 22–5 and Fig. 22–20).

An intracapsular, or intralesional, surgical margin describes an inadequate margin resulting from a resection that violates the tumor's pseudocapsule and runs through the tumor, with gross residual tumor left behind. It involves a partial and incomplete excision of tumor. In general, such debulking procedures are grossly inadequate and not indicated for any tumor.

A marginal surgical margin (see Fig. 22–20) involves a plane of dissection through the reactive zone located between the tumor and normal tissue. The reactive zone refers to areolar tissue surrounding the tumor that is compressed and inflamed by tumor invasion and enlargement. Although it is located outside a tumor's pseudocapsule, it potentially contains foci of microscopic tumor, and thus dissection through this plane is associated with a high recurrence rate, especially when dealing with high-grade malignant tumors. This reactive or inflammatory zone usually demonstrates a significant decrease in activity with appropriate chemotherapy.

A wide margin (see Fig. 22–20) involves a surgical procedure that excises the tumor, its pseudocapsule, the surrounding reactive zone, and a cuff of normal tissue. The dissection remains outside the zone of reactive tissue, and thus the tumor specimen contains a cuff of normal tissue around its entire circumference. No specifications or requirements have been determined for the thickness of this cuff of normal tissue. According to this system, however, it is generally believed that a wide margin extends at least 1 to 2 cm.

TABLE 22–6. Recurrence Rate by Surgical Margin versus Stage

Surgical Margin	Benign			Malignant			
	1	2	3	IA	IB	IIA	IIB
Intracapsular	0%	30%	50%	90%	90%	100%	100%
Marginal	0%	0%	50%	70%	70%	90%	90%
Wide	0%	0%	10%	10%	30%	50%	70%
Radical	0%	0%	0%	0%	0%	10%	20%

Adapted from Enneking WF: Musculoskeletal Tumor Surgery. New York: Churchill-Livingstone, 1983, p 99.

A radical margin (see Fig. 22–20) involves an en bloc excision of tumor, its pseudocapsule, the reactive zone, and the entire compartment within which it is contained.

A malignant intraosseous tumor of the proximal end of the humerus treated with a radical surgical margin requires excision of the entire humerus. A similar lesion of the deltoid treated with a radical surgical margin would involve a procedure that includes total excision of the deltoid compartment from origin to insertion. The surgical margin is defined by its worst or closest margin. If a specimen has primarily a wide margin but is marginal in one aspect, it is described as marginal and not as a wide margin. Each particular surgical margin may be achieved by local resection or by amputation (see Fig. 22–20). Determination of the surgical margin is the critical step that allows the surgeon to integrate the surgical treatment with the staging system and thus outline treatment and assess clinical results. By assessing the surgical margin and the stage of the lesion, a prediction of local recurrence can be based on past experience (Table 22–6).

Limb Salvage Surgery

The surgical treatment of high-grade sarcomas of bone may involve amputation or limb salvage. In the skeletally immature with significant growth potential remaining, amputation is preferable to resection, although expandable prostheses are also available. These metallic arthroplasties have an extendible screw mechanism that can be lengthened at intervals to allow for skeletal growth. Limb salvage surgery is a reasonable alternative to amputation when a wide surgical margin is achievable and enough soft tissue is preserved to allow a reasonably good functional result. In most cases, the functional criteria for limb-sparing surgery are stricter than the criteria for tumor control. Sufficient functional muscle mass is required to

LIMB SALVAGE RESECTION

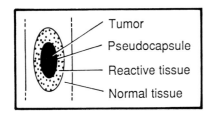

- Tumor
- Pseudocapsule
- Reactive tissue
- Normal tissue

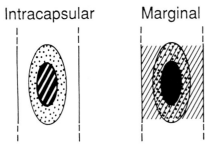

Intracapsular   Marginal

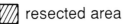 resected area

Wide   Radical

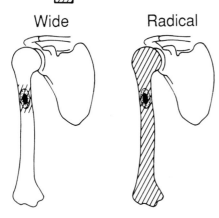

AMPUTATION

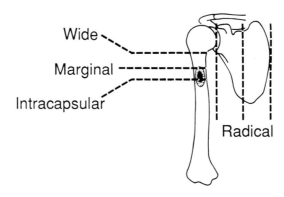

Wide

Marginal

Intracapsular

Radical

■ **Figure 22–20**
Surgical margins.

obtain a reasonable functional result and to avoid wound complications.[198]

Limb salvage, or limb-sparing, resections of the shoulder girdle are generally indicated for neoplasms that have no major neurovascular involvement and have enough remaining bone stock proximally and distally to allow a reasonable reconstruction. In addition, adequate soft tissue coverage and deltoid function are required to avoid wound complications and achieve sufficient functional results.[1,42,45,59,115,142,156] The most common restrictions for effective limb salvage involve the adequacy of nerve involvement or soft tissue coverage.

Patients with soft tissue sarcomas or bony sarcomas of the proximal part of the humerus with considerable soft tissue extension are challenging limb salvage candidates. The brachial neurovascular structures and glenohumeral joint are not infrequently involved by tumor, and careful preoperative staging is essential before deciding on a surgical plan or attempting limb salvage procedures. High-grade malignant tumors of the proximal end of the humerus are typically extracompartmental lesions (IIB) that require a wide surgical resection to achieve a cure. Patients who undergo marginal resections for high-grade malignancies are at risk for local recurrence in most cases, no matter how efficacious their adjuvant chemotherapy. Thus, a typical IIB osteosarcoma of the proximal end of the humerus requires a wide surgical resection for an adequate margin. In fact, many, if not most resections for osteosarcoma involve a marginal margin at some part of the resected specimen. That marginal margin remains an adequate margin if the patient has had an adequate response to preoperative chemotherapy. Determining appropriate surgical candidates and the feasibility of a wide surgical resection preoperatively is accomplished by the preoperative staging studies. Most osteosarcomas show up as IIB lesions with soft tissue involvement by the tumor. The amount of soft tissue involvement and the proximity of the medial neurovascular bundle present a preoperative challenge to determining candidates for limb salvage. Another preoperative challenge for high-grade sarcomas involves assessment of the extent of bone disease and whether disease extends into the glenohumeral joint. If the joint is involved, an extracapsular or extra-articular resection is indicated, with resection of the glenoid en bloc with the capsule of the glenohumeral joint and the remainder of the proximal end of the humerus. Preoperative tasks include assessing for distant, metastatic disease and determining the extent of bone and soft tissue margins with the planned resection.[142]

The primary site of a tumor to some extent predicts certain resection and reconstruction tendencies. High-grade sarcomas of the proximal part of the humerus are likely to have a close relationship to the medial neurovascular bundle (brachial plexus or brachial artery or vein), axillary nerve, deltoid, or glenohumeral joint. Chest wall involvement with these tumors is less common and usually occurs as a late finding after involvement of the medial neurovascular structures. Obviously, the best limb salvage candidates are those with primary bone tumors that have minimal extraosseous extension. Soft tissue sarcomas of the shoulder region are easily resected when located in the deltoid, but deltoid resection precludes

arthroplasty as a reasonable alternative because of the subsequent loss of active abduction. The following classification system is useful for describing these different resections and the various reconstructive principles (Fig. 22–21).

Type 1—Short Proximal Humeral Resection

Type 1 resections, or short proximal humeral resections, are proximal to the deltoid insertion of the humerus (see Fig. 22–21). These resections are intra-articular; that is, the bone resection includes the humeral head, and the proximal plane of resection goes through the glenohumeral joint. These resections may or may not involve an en bloc resection of the abductor mechanism. The abductor mechanism refers to the rotator cuff, deltoid muscle, and its (axillary) innervation. Sacrifice of any part of this composite results in significantly weakened abduction and a significant change in the expectation of postoperative function (see various reconstructive procedures). Axillary nerve injury or resection is a common consideration because of its strategic location at the inferior and posterior aspect of the humeral neck.

The deltoid muscle inserts into the humerus at approximately 10 to 14 cm from the articular surface of the proximal humeral head. Removal of the deltoid insertion from the humerus involves a reconstructive procedure with greater complications and a longer rehabilitation period than does a procedure without detachment of the deltoid insertion. Such deltoid resections for shoulder tumors are in fact rarely indicated in today's sarcoma environment. Thus, bone resections distal to the deltoid insertion are associated with more complications or more limited functional results. If the deltoid and rotator cuff are preserved along with their respective innervations, good active abduction can be achieved postoperatively and a better functional result can be expected after the reconstruction. Sacrifice of the rotator cuff, the deltoid, its innervation, or its vascular supply leads to a significant reduction in potential shoulder abduction. There is a great difference between resections of the proximal end of the humerus that include the deltoid muscle, axillary nerve, or rotator cuff and those that do not. Proximal humeral resections including a part of the abductor mechanism are referred to in this classification system as type 1B humeral resections (see Fig. 22–21). Resections of the humerus that do not sacrifice a part of the abductor mechanism are referred to as type 1A resections. This subclassification of A (preservation of an active abductor mechanism) and B (resection or sacrifice of a part of the abductor mechanism) is also used to classify the other resection types as described.

Type 2—Long Proximal Humeral Resections

Type 2 resections (see Fig. 22–21) refer to proximal humeral resections in which the distal osteotomy is made distal to the deltoid insertion. This type usually includes proximal humeral resections longer than 12 cm. They are referred to as type 2A or 2B, depending on whether they spare or include (respectively) the abductor mechanism with the resection. Type 1 or type 2 resections of the

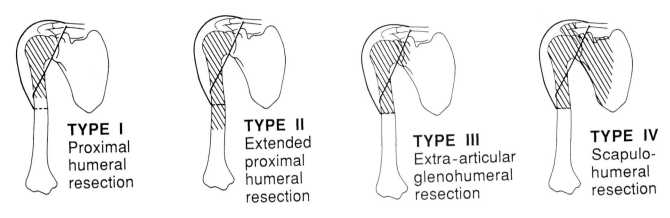

Scapular Resections

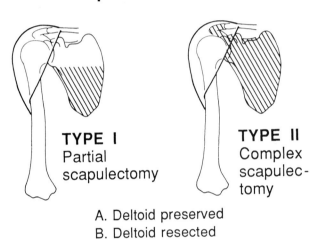

A. Deltoid preserved
B. Deltoid resected

■ **Figure 22–21**
Classification of shoulder resections.

proximal part of the humerus may be reconstructed with an arthroplasty or an arthrodesis, depending on whether the potential for active abduction remains after the resection. Type 2, or long humeral, resections have a longer rehabilitative period and a greater overall incidence of complications or more limited functional results because of the long bone reconstruction and the need for reattachment of the deltoid.

Type 3—Glenohumeral Resections

Type 3 resections of the proximal end of the humerus extend to the glenoid side of the glenohumeral joint in an extra-articular or extracapsular fashion (see Fig. 22–21). The proximal bone resection is through the base of the glenoid or scapular neck. If enough bone stock remains in the glenoid area, an arthroplasty or arthrodesis may be achieved, depending on the competency of the abductor mechanism. Without a good abductor mechanism, an arthrodesis is preferable, but adequate bone stock must exist in the lateral portion of the scapula, either at the acromion or at the remaining scapular neck or glenoid area. Type 3 resections are typically carried out for a high-

grade malignancy of the proximal part of the humerus or humeral head with intra-articular invasion, as can occur with osteosarcoma or chondrosarcoma. Indications for type 3 glenohumeral resections occur relatively rarely.

Type 4—Scapulohumeral Resections

Type 4 resections refer to scapulohumeral resections of the proximal end of the humerus and scapula (see Fig. 22–21), including the classic Tikhoff-Linberg procedure, which involves a full scapular resection with resection of the humeral head.[12,69,112,125] An extended Tikhoff-Linberg resection refers to a complete scapular resection with a lengthy proximal humeral resection. The resection may or may not include a portion of the deltoid or abductor mechanism (A or B). Modifications of the original Tikhoff-Linberg procedure involve a subtotal scapular resection en bloc along with extra-articular resection of the proximal end of the humerus. These large resections are typically carried out for high-grade lesions of the proximal part of the humerus with glenohumeral joint involvement. One criterion for a Tikhoff-Linberg procedure, as with any limb-sparing surgery, is lack of involvement of the neurovascular structures (brachial artery, vein, and brachial plexus). The procedure entails a large scapular resection that is usually left without reconstruction.

Scapulohumeral resections are an example of a limb-sparing procedure that results in very limited postoperative function. They are accepted well by the patient when the functional limitations are fully discussed before surgery. Postoperatively, patients typically have varying degrees of proximal humeral stability and a well-innervated, functional hand and elbow. Elbow motion depends on the degree of postoperative humeral stability. In this setting, where the surgical alternative is an amputation, many patients are satisfied with this limited degree of function. Patients frequently prefer to retain the extremity even with limited functional expectations. When the patient is well informed preoperatively and a functional hand persists postoperatively, the patient's subjective evaluations are quite good despite limited functional results.[12,69,112,125]

Types 1 and 2—Scapular Resections

Scapular resections may be classified as partial type 1 or complex type 2 resections, depending on whether they include the glenoid (complex) or not (partial) (see Fig. 22-21). Partial resections of the scapula are associated with relatively high functional results postoperatively, as opposed to the more restricted functional performance after complex or complete resections of the scapula.[22,130,211] This classification system does not include other, less common resections about the shoulder such as various partial or intercalary resections of the humerus that may or may not involve reconstruction. These resections are associated with excellent function postoperatively when the surrounding neurovascular structures and the abductor mechanism are preserved. Partial resection of the humerus may be undertaken for less aggressive benign lesions, such as periosteal chondroma or chondroblastoma. Generally, these partial resections lead to superior functional results. Partial resection of the scapula and clavicle is also unusual and may be undertaken for malignant or benign lesions.[184,185] Partial and complete scapular resections are associated with surprisingly good functional results, even in the absence of reconstruction.

Reconstructive Procedures of the Shoulder

Three basic choices are available for reconstruction after limb-sparing resection of the shoulder: arthroplasty, arthrodesis, or a flail shoulder (Fig. 22-22). A flail shoulder is defined as one that lacks functional motor power and stability. It is functionally inferior to arthroplasty or arthrodesis but superior to a painful arthroplasty or arthrodesis. A flail shoulder, such as the shoulder that results after a Tikhoff-Linberg procedure, is an acceptable result for a patient who has undergone a large scapulohumeral resection for an aggressive tumor and is satisfied with limited shoulder and elbow function. Elbow motion is limited by instability of the proximal end of the humerus, and thus stabilization of the proximal end of

the humerus significantly enhances function of both the elbow and the hand. Multiple techniques have been attempted in the past to stabilize the remaining humerus to the chest wall. The original technique of using an intramedullary rod sutured to a proximal rib was discontinued because of migration of the rod into the wound flaps.[22] In addition, suspension of the midhumerus to the remaining clavicle to achieve some degree of stability has also been carried out. The best method of stabilization involves reattachment of any remaining proximal musculature to the proximal end of the humerus. Although a flail shoulder is not functionally attractive, it does allow generous tumor resection and is usually associated with predictable relief of pain. It remains a viable alternative after large resections and for the complications of a painful, infected, or failed arthroplasty or arthrodesis. However, a flail joint is unstable, in the true sense of the word, and an attempt should be made to limit instability by soft tissue reconstruction whenever possible.[12,69,112,125,150]

The choice of arthroplasty versus arthrodesis after shoulder resection should be considered carefully with the patient before surgery. A patient's personality, vocation, lifestyle, and handedness all affect the decision, and these factors should be taken into account. In general, an arthroplasty requires active abduction and glenohumeral stability, both of which call for a competent, functional abductor mechanism. What constitutes a functionally competent abductor mechanism is a source of some debate. The abductor mechanism has three basic anatomic components: the deltoid muscle, the rotator cuff muscles (supraspinatus, infraspinatus, and teres minor), and their respective blood supply (circumflex and suprascapular vessels) and innervation (axillary and suprascapular nerves). Resection or injury of the axillary nerve after resection or biopsy of the humerus is not uncommon, and the loss of deltoid function has significant functional consequences. A well-innervated deltoid is the minimal requirement for a functional, stable arthroplasty. Loss of rotator cuff function has, in the past, required a constrained or semiconstrained arthroplasty, which is associated with greater complications, and may have served as an indication for arthrodesis.[158] Newer reconstructive procedures have achieved functional arthroplasties with various unconstrained prostheses using oversized humeral components instead of constrained glenohumeral designs.[132] These techniques and others have improved results significantly over the previous high failure rates in earlier series (50%), but they lack long-term follow-up.[7,79,144,157]

Currently, techniques of arthroplasty involve the use of metallic, ceramic, or osteochondral allograft implants.* The increasing use of allograft transplantation[121,122,152] has had two major effects on the reconstruction of humeral resections. First, it has increased the length of the proximal part of the humerus that can be reconstructed, thus expanding the indications for limb salvage procedures. Previously, resections were limited to those that could be reconstructed with an autogenous fibular graft or a cus-

---

*See references 21, 32, 97, 103, 157, 167, 181, 182, 194, 218.

Arthroplasty

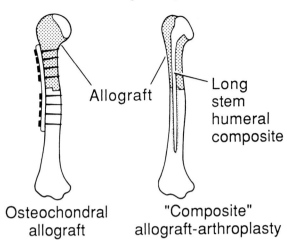

Allograft

Long
stem
humeral
composite

Osteochondral
allograft

"Composite"
allograft-arthroplasty

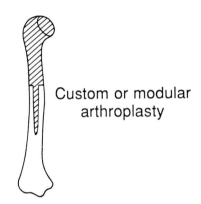

Custom or modular
arthroplasty

Arthrodesis

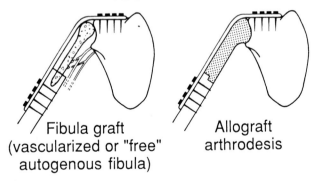

Fibula graft
(vascularized or "free"
autogenous fibula)

Allograft
arthrodesis

■ **Figure 22–22**
Reconstruction alternatives.

tomized long-stemmed humeral component. It is now possible to replace resections within 8 cm of the distal end of the humerus. Second, allograft reconstructions may be a more reasonable reconstructive alternative in a younger patient because of their potential as a biologic structure. An allograft reconstruction offers the advantages of enhanced soft tissue attachment to the graft, bone union to the remaining humerus, and the potential for transplantation of viable cartilage. The relative complications of an allograft versus a prosthetic reconstruc-

tion have not yet been demonstrated to be significantly different.

Arthroplasty reconstructions after tumor resection involve the choice of an allograft,[157] a metallic[15] or ceramic[15,181,190,194] prosthesis, or a combination of an allograft and a prosthesis, referred to as a "composite" reconstruction (Fig. 22–23).[165] This "composite" reconstruction involves an allograft that is fixed with a long-stemmed humeral component through the graft and cemented into the remaining humeral bone stock. Composite proximal

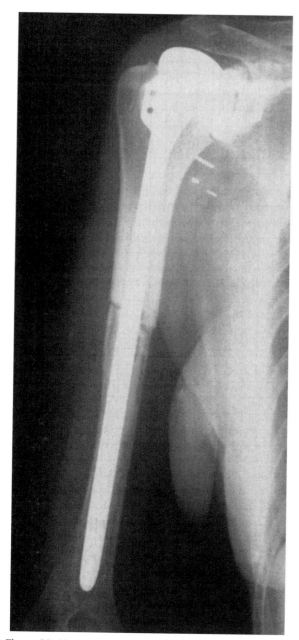

■ Figure 22–23

"Composite" reconstruction of the proximal part of the humerus.

humeral allografts are the preferred type of allograft reconstruction because of the relatively high (50%) failure rate with osteochondral grafts. It can be cemented or press-fitted into the allograft or the remaining humerus. With this type of reconstruction, reattachment of the deltoid or rotator cuff to the allograft is a distinct advantage over reattachment to metallic prostheses. Thus, these reconstructions have the potential for enhanced stability, strength, motion, and function. However, the preliminary results of transplanted allograft rotator cuff and other allograft ligaments show a high failure rate.[79]

The greatest challenge after a proximal humeral hemi-arthroplasty reconstruction with an allograft is reconstruction of the surrounding soft tissues. Great care has

to be taken in reconstructing the glenohumeral joint capsule, the rotator cuff, and the deltoid insertion at the time of transplantation. The processes of bone ingrowth and remodeling, soft tissue attachment, graft fixation, revascularization, and cartilage survival remain areas of active research and clinical investigation. Graft fracture, infection, rejection, and instability are still serious potential complications that occur in 20% to 30% of all patients.[121,122,152]

The reconstructive alternative to allograft transplantation is a custom prosthetic implant of acceptable metal or ceramic.* Prosthetic implants offer the advantage of strength and custom fit and are an excellent alternative, especially in older patients. To date, the functional results of arthroplasties in the proximal end of the humerus have been excellent for both composite reconstructions and metallic implants.[15,165,190,192] As yet, no studies have described comparative differences in function, infection, and revision surgery for these procedures. Newer modular prosthetic designs provide the attractive alternative of a readily available implant that can be customized to the resection defect intraoperatively without delay. These prostheses are newer designs with as yet little clinical follow-up, but they appear to have considerable application in reconstructing the humerus after tumor resection.[165]

When the deltoid muscle is sacrificed by resection, the best reconstructive choice is an arthrodesis. As a technique, arthrodesis has changed significantly. An arthrodesis after tumor resection may be achieved with various bone graft materials, including free or vascularized autogenous fibular grafts or allograft transplantation.[28,29,71,176,214] Resections of 5 to 6 cm or less may be reconstructed with autogenous cancellous grafts from the iliac crest, with or without some shortening of the humerus itself.[18,19,202,214] The remaining humerus should be buttressed against the acromion and may or may not be offset from the glenoid with autogenous grafts. Resections of the humerus up to 20 cm in length may be reconstructed with a vascularized autogenous fibular graft. Free (nonvascularized) autogenous fibular grafts may be used for defects less than 12 cm.[187] Nonvascularized fibular grafts longer than 12 cm are associated with a high incidence of graft fracture.[18]

Frozen allograft is a reasonable alternative graft material for shoulder arthrodesis. However, its use has been reported in several series with short follow-up, and it may be associated with potential problems such as an increased risk of nonunion or loss of fixation after nonunion.[218] The use of postoperative radiation therapy or chemotherapy has deleterious effects on the bone union of any reconstruction. Patients with high-grade lesions who need an arthrodesis are immediately at even higher risk for nonunion and fracture if they receive postoperative radiation therapy. Most surgeons consider postoperative radiation therapy a contraindication to an allograft arthrodesis.

Internal fixation of an arthrodesis is best achieved with the use of a long-angled custom plate that enables

*See references 15, 21, 32, 97, 103, 157, 165, 167, 181, 182, 190, 192, 194, 218.

patients to avoid prolonged postoperative immobilization and permits enhanced fixation and positioning of the fusion. Such long-angled plates are required for long humeral resections, whereas shorter, more conventional plates may be used for shorter humeral resections.[29] Newer implants to enhance fixation of the proximal end of the humerus to the scapula are currently being evaluated clinically.

The use of a long-angled plate with adequate purchase of the scapula and remaining humerus has improved postoperative function by avoiding immobilization with a postoperative shoulder spica cast. Proper positioning of the plate on the scapular spine, acromion, and lateral border of the humerus is crucial to achieve proper positioning of the arm and adequate postoperative function. Intraoperative positioning remains a demanding part of the procedure and significantly affects the rotational position of the arm by its orientation proximally and distally. When such a plate is used, at least eight cortices are required for adequate distal humeral fixation. Likewise, scapular fixation requires four to five good scapula screws to prevent failure of fixation proximally. Careful positioning of the plate at the acromion is necessary to avoid prominence and wound complications. Spica cast immobilization is not required postoperatively if adequate fixation is achieved, as it is in most cases.[29] Postoperatively, patients may use a sling with a soft bolster under the elbow. They begin exercises to improve rhomboid and periscapular strength 6 weeks after surgery and may carefully begin abduction exercises at 8 weeks.[29]

The greatest functional disadvantage of an arthrodesis is the restriction of rotation inherent in the procedure. Most patients are happy with the functional results and obtain adequate abduction (70 to 80 degrees) postoperatively. Limited abduction after arthrodesis usually reflects prolonged immobilization, poor rehabilitation, or a persistent or painful nonunion. The abduction that does occur after arthrodesis is at the scapulothoracic interval and is powered by the rhomboids and other scapular muscles. Patients who are not candidates for an arthroplasty are frequently good candidates for an arthrodesis because their alternative reconstructive choice is usually a flail shoulder.[28,29,72,176]

Scapular resections are unusual procedures that may involve partial or complex resections.[22,37,130,151,179,183,211] Complex scapular resections in this classification system (see Fig. 22–21) involve a portion of the glenoid. Some experience has been gained in prosthetic replacement of the scapula after total scapulectomy.[40] Reconstruction with a scapular prosthesis requires the humeral head replacement to articulate with the prosthetic glenoid. According to the most recent report of this procedure, the ideal indication for such a prosthesis is a partial scapulectomy.[40] Eckhard and colleagues[40] reported a series of eight patients treated by endoprosthetic replacement of the scapula for various malignant or benign aggressive lesions. The follow-up on these patients was limited (20 months' mean follow-up), and 50% achieved acceptable (good to excellent) functional results. As yet, scapular prosthetic replacement remains a somewhat experimental procedure for which only early, short-term clinical results have been reported. Partial and complete scapulectomies

achieve remarkably good functional results without reconstructive procedures beyond soft tissue closure.

Management of Specific Lesions

Aggressive Benign Bone Tumors

The surgical treatment of active or aggressive bone tumors presents a greater challenge when the tumor occurs adjacent to significant structures such as a major nerve or vessel, a joint or joint surface, or an active growth plate. Aggressive benign lesions of bone with significant subchondral bone loss frequently present the greatest challenge in preserving a functional joint.

Aggressive and active benign tumors are typified in the adult by benign giant cell tumor of bone, which occurs in the proximal part of the humerus in 15% to 20% of cases. The choice of treatment for such a lesion includes resection versus intralesional curettage. The latter is usually associated with the use of a local adjuvant to enhance the opportunity to kill the tumor. Various local adjuvants that have been used in the recent past include the application of liquid nitrogen (cryosurgery) or phenol (phenolization), the placement of methylmethacrylate (cementation), and various forms of cauterization. Wide surgical resection offers the lowest risk of tumor recurrence but, to some extent, diminishes joint function. For that reason, the slightly less effective intralesional procedures are preferred when associated with a relatively low rate of tumor recurrence (10%). Experience with curettage and cryosurgery has demonstrated a lower recurrence rate (<10%) than with other forms of local adjuvant treatment, and it may be the preferred intralesional treatment.[30,77]

Surgical resection is more effective in controlling tumor and is the preferred method for more aggressive or recurrent lesions. Reconstructions after humeral head resection usually involve an allograft or a custom or modular arthroplasty. Thus, a larger resection that enhances tumor control requires a larger, more complicated reconstruction.

Aggressive benign soft tissue tumors are best exemplified by aggressive fibromatosis in young adults; these lesions also require a wide surgical margin to minimize the risk of recurrence. Lesions that are juxtaposed to a major neurovascular structure may be treated with a marginal surgical resection in addition to radiation therapy. Radiation therapy appears to be efficacious in minimizing the recurrence rate after marginal resection, despite controversy to the contrary.

Low-Grade Malignancies of Bone

Chondrosarcoma

Chondrosarcoma is the most common low-grade malignancy of bone. It occurs frequently in the proximal part of the humerus and presents a clinical challenge in interpreting the source of pain (intra-articular versus extra-articular) and early radiographic signs of malignancy. The definitive treatment of low-grade chondrosarcoma is usually intralesional curettage. Chemotherapy and radio-therapy have no added benefit in the treatment of an intermediate- or low-grade intraosseous lesion such as chondrosarcoma. Patients in whom local recurrence develops after surgery can also be treated surgically for the local recurrence, but if multiple recurrences appear, restaging and adjuvant therapy should be considered.

The appropriate surgical treatment of a low-grade intraosseous chondrosarcoma that is well contained within the cortices of the proximal end of the humerus is intralesional curettage with or without cryosurgery. The functional results of an intralesional procedure are grossly superior to those of resection and reconstruction. Control of tumor is better with resection than with any intralesional procedure, although it is not usually required. Most chondrosarcomas that are intraosseous in the proximal part of the humerus are low grade and may be treated with curettage alone. A significant proportion of these patients have local recurrence over a period of 5 to 10 years; thus, curettage should include some type of adjuvant treatment to optimize tumor control.

Resection of a chondrosarcoma involving the gleno-humeral joint necessitates an extra-articular resection of the shoulder. This procedure is more difficult and requires a total shoulder arthroplasty. The risk of a contaminated surgical margin is higher with this procedure; however, the alternative tumor procedure is either an inadequate, contaminated resection or a forequarter amputation.

Intermediate- or high-grade chondrosarcomas are less common and require a wide surgical margin and appropriate arthroplasty reconstruction. These higher-grade malignancies cannot reasonably be treated by intralesional procedures with or without local adjuvant therapy because of an increased risk of local recurrence and metastatic disease. The results of chemotherapy for high-grade chondrosarcoma are quite limited, but chemotherapy is nonetheless indicated.

High-Grade Malignancies of Bone

Osteosarcoma

High-grade malignant lesions of bone, such as osteosarcoma, are best treated by preoperative (induction) chemotherapy, reassessment of the response to chemotherapy (restaging), surgical resection, and postoperative chemotherapy.[36,145,168,197] Osteosarcoma of the proximal end of the humerus is usually best reconstructed with a composite allograft reconstruction. Postoperative chemotherapy is tailored or adjusted, depending on the degree of necrosis in the surgical tumor specimen. This type of treatment was first developed in the Sloan Kettering T10 methotrexate protocol and has become the standard treatment of osteosarcoma in many centers.[36,168,198] Controlled studies specifically evaluating the true significance of preoperative chemotherapy, the significance of the histologic response to that preoperative therapy, and the effect of postoperative tailoring of chemotherapy have demonstrated statistical significance with the degree of histologic necrosis.[36] We do not know how much of a histologic response to chemotherapy is required to improve survival. We do not know which tumor types respond to

which drugs. We do not know which drug combinations are more efficacious (cisplatin versus methotrexate). We do not know whether the intra-arterial administration of chemotherapy has a greater effect on tumor. There are proponents for many of these theories, but very few well-controlled studies.[36]

Adequate evidence does exist to demonstrate improved survival with the addition of chemotherapy to surgery.[14] Experience with radiation therapy as the primary treatment of osteosarcoma has been limited, and such therapy does not have a significant role in the curative treatment of osteosarcoma in most centers today. Although more aggressive chemotherapy has achieved a significant increase in survival, many of the significant studies have yet to be carried out.[23,100,141,219] In addition, the protocols for managing metastatic pulmonary disease remain to be written. Although it is apparent that pulmonary resection aids survival, its integration with chemotherapy has been poorly defined.[20,73,78,131,186]

Ewing's Sarcoma

Treatment of Ewing's sarcoma today is somewhat similar to treatment of osteosarcoma in that preoperative induction chemotherapy is delivered after a histologic diagnosis is obtained with an appropriate biopsy.[78,138,170,204,209,219] The location from which the biopsy sample is taken is very important in Ewing's sarcoma because of the high risk of pathologic fracture after radiation therapy. Although treatment of Ewing's sarcoma 10 years ago involved a combination of chemotherapy and radiation therapy, several studies documenting a high local recurrence rate, especially with large tumors (>10 cm), have led to a greater emphasis on surgical treatment of the disease.[170] Thus, lesions that are surgically resectable, especially when larger than 8 to 10 cm, are frequently treated with preoperative chemotherapy, restaging, and surgical resection. A wide surgical margin should be the goal of surgical resection, but surgical margins are more difficult to assess with Ewing's sarcoma. If the surgical resection is marginal, postoperative radiation therapy is indicated. Patients with Ewing's sarcoma typically have a large soft tissue mass that usually demonstrates impressive shrinkage with a reasonable response to chemotherapy.[170,209] Patients in whom shrinkage of the inflammatory border of the soft tissue portion of Ewing's sarcoma is not apparent probably have lesions that are not responding well to chemotherapy and should be reassessed very carefully, both preoperatively and postoperatively. The total treatment protocol for Ewing's sarcoma usually involves approximately 12 months of treatment (chemotherapy).

Amputation may be indicated for the treatment of young patients with Ewing's sarcoma and significant growth potential remaining if they have a lesion in the lower extremity.[210] The alternative is to treat that patient with chemotherapy and radiation therapy, which will usually result in physeal arrest and a discrepancy in leg length. The morbidity may be significant after radiation treatment of lower extremity lesions in young children with Ewing's sarcoma.[107,138,204,219] In addition, these patients have one of the highest risks for secondary sarcomas, such as osteosarcoma, arising from their radiation field.[118,145] In the upper extremity, Ewing's sarcoma not infrequently occurs in the proximal end of the humerus, and surgical resection of the humerus with an intercalary allograft reconstruction is usually indicated for most patients.

Soft Tissue Sarcomas

Soft tissue sarcomas may occur as high-, low-, or inter-mediate-grade neoplasms. Low- and intermediate-grade soft tissue sarcomas with adequate surgical margins are best treated by surgical resection and postoperative radi-ation therapy. Worrisome surgical margins may serve as an indication for preoperative radiation therapy. High-grade soft tissue sarcomas have been treated in the past with preoperative radiation therapy followed by surgical resection and chemotherapy.[5] Local recurrence has not been a significant problem (<10%), whereas pulmonary metastases have posed a problem (10% to 30%). The insti-tution of preoperative radiation therapy usually delays surgical resection by approximately 7 to 8 weeks. Chemotherapy in this setting is given postoperatively and is not usually possible until 2 to 3 weeks after resection or 10 to 12 weeks after the institution of treatment. Because of this delay in chemotherapy and the real problems of pulmonary metastases, chemotherapy may be given pre-operatively to assess the histologic response and treat sys-temic disease. Postoperative therapy is adjusted according to the histologic response and is given 2 to 3 weeks after surgery. Radiation therapy is indicated for marginal surgical margins and is integrated with postoperative chemotherapy.

■ AUTHOR'S PREFERRED METHODS OF TREATMENT

BIOPSY

Biopsy of musculoskeletal tumors will always be the initial and probably one of the most important steps in the evaluation and treatment of these challenging lesions. The biopsy site should always be placed in the line of a possible future resection and should not be performed before an adequate clinical evaluation and diagnostic radiographic staging studies have been completed. When the staging studies and the clinical findings of the patient are suggestive of a particular lesion, a needle biopsy is the preferred method. A fairly reliable, tentative diagnosis can be made after the staging studies have been completed. This diagnosis can then be easily confirmed with a needle biopsy. Thus, most classic osteosarcomas have fairly typical radiographic findings and can easily be diagnosed with a needle biopsy. However, when a lesion's diagnosis is still uncertain, even after initial staging studies, an open biopsy provides the best diagnosis. In that situation, the more generous the biopsy specimen, the easier the diag-nosis. Providing enough of a biopsy specimen without contaminating an extremity remains a challenge even for an experienced oncology surgeon. In general, the biopsy

should be performed by the surgeon who will carry out the definitive resection.

SURGICAL CHOICES

In terms of treatment choices, three different categories of lesions remain a challenge in today's setting: (1) aggressive benign lesions such as giant cell tumor, (2) low-grade malignant lesions such as chondrosarcoma, and (3) high-grade malignant lesions such as osteosarcoma or Ewing's sarcoma.

Giant cell tumor, in many cases, is a difficult lesion to treat because it is locally aggressive and destructive to the adjacent joint. It is a difficult tumor to grade histologi-cally and radiographically, and the specific indications for various surgical treatments are nebulous. In most cases, curettage is indicated for all benign tumors. Curettage supplemented with liquid nitrogen freezing (cryosurgery) may be a better method of treatment in terms of control-ling the tumor. Aggressive recurrent lesions will not be resolved with curettage alone and require curettage with liquid nitrogen freezing or a wide surgical resection. The experience with curettage and liquid nitrogen has been good regarding tumor control and function of the extremity.[30,77] It requires very careful intraoperative mon-itoring of the patient for both embolic precautions and protection of soft tissues and neurovascular structures. It should be carried out only by someone experienced in the technique and is best combined with a subchondral bone graft and internal fixation or cementation of the remain-ing bone defect. Patients should be advised of the risks and benefits of cryosurgery versus wide resection in the treatment of a giant cell tumor. Resection is clearly indi-cated for benign tumors that recur after multiple attempts at curettage. In many clinical settings, either pro-cedure is a reasonable alternative.

Low-grade malignancies are typified by low-grade chondrosarcomas, which are difficult lesions to define his-tologically. Microscopically, a low-grade chondrosarcoma is defined by increased cellularity, binucleated lacunae, and microscopic bone resorption, in addition to the clin-ical radiographic picture of endosteal cortical resorption and bone destruction. Most of these low-grade lesions are located at the metaphyseal-diaphyseal junction in intramedullary or cancellous bone. In general, surgical treatment is indicated for only symptomatic patients (intraosseous pain). Biopsy is unreliable as a diagnostic procedure for this problem. When the diagnosis is uncer-tain, the patient is much better off being monitored care-fully with repeat radiographs every 3 to 6 months and a repeat CT scan or MRI. A low-grade chondrosarcoma of the extremities (secondary chondrosarcoma) is a very low-grade malignancy in the typical case, with very little threat of pulmonary metastasis. It can be comfortably moni-tored clinically with little or no risk to the patient. A biopsy specimen of such a low-grade cartilaginous lesion is frequently difficult to interpret and may result in an equivocal histologic diagnosis with regard to its malig-nant grade or potential. Thus, the diagnosis of a benign versus a low-grade malignant lesion is best made in the clinical setting rather than in the pathology department. This is a rare exception to the general rule of relying on the histologic evaluation of all musculoskeletal lesions to define their true nature.

Treatment of a low-grade malignancy (chondrosarcoma) is similar to that of an aggressive benign lesion (giant cell tumor). Curettage alone is associated with a very high (70% to 80%) recurrence rate for low-grade malignancies, although recurrence may take 5 to 10 years to show up. Thus, curettage alone is really, in the strict sense of the word, an inadequate form of treatment. Lesions that have failed to respond to previous curettage procedures should be treated by resection to minimize multiple recurrences and wider contamination. For most patients, curettage with freezing (cryosurgery) is indicated before resection.

HIGH-GRADE TUMORS AND PREOPERATIVE CHEMOTHERAPY

High-grade malignancies in the shoulder have a distribution similar to those in other sites, with the most common lesions being osteosarcoma and Ewing's sarcoma. Most patients with a high-grade malignancy of bone or soft tissue are best treated with chemotherapy before surgical resection to minimize local recurrence and to attempt to evaluate tumor response. The Sloan Kettering T10 protocol of preoperative chemotherapy was the first to use methotrexate-based therapy in high dosage (combination of methotrexate, cisplatin, and doxorubicin [Adriamycin]) given before surgical resection and then tailored postoperatively according to the histologic response of the tumor specimen. It has been effective in significantly improving the 5-year survival rate for osteosarcoma in several different clinical studies. Five-year survival rates went from 25% to 30% previously to a current rate of approximately 50% to 60%. Other improvements in treatment (e.g., radiology, pathology, surgery) have also contributed to this improved survival rate. The chemotherapy protocols are complex and demand a multidisciplinary setting with real communication between the chemotherapist and the surgeon. Preoperative chemotherapy is also used for Ewing's sarcoma, that is, preoperative chemotherapy followed by surgery and then by maintenance chemotherapy. When a patient with Ewing's sarcoma appears to have a lesion that will have a close or marginal surgical margin, the alternative treatment choice for that patient is chemotherapy and radiation therapy without surgery or chemotherapy with preoperative radiation therapy and surgical resection. The pendulum has more or less swung away from radiation therapy and toward surgical resection for Ewing's sarcoma because of higher recurrence rates after radiation treatment of the primary site alone. Ewing's sarcomas smaller than 8 to 10 cm may be reasonably treated with chemotherapy and radiation therapy in some settings. However, lesions larger than 8 to 10 cm require surgical resection and chemotherapy with or without radiation therapy as the definitive treatment of their primary disease. Many experienced musculoskeletal tumor surgeons believe that radiation therapy has no role at all in the treatment of Ewing's sarcoma, especially in a young child with a juxtaepiphyseal lesion that should be treated with an amputation to maximize survival. The dilemma of when to use radiation therapy for Ewing's

sarcoma persists; however, higher local recurrence rates and greater morbidity in young patients have resulted in little enthusiasm for radiation therapy as the treatment of primary disease, especially in the skeletally immature.

Soft tissue sarcomas are also best treated with preoperative chemotherapy, surgery, and further postoperative chemotherapy. The benefit of preoperative chemotherapy for soft tissue sarcomas is the early systemic treatment of a systemic disease, minimization of local recurrences, and the opportunity to evaluate the tumor specimen for response to chemotherapy. Most patients with a soft tissue sarcoma have microscopic circulating tumor cells in their bloodstream. A delay in the institution of systemic chemotherapy may represent a deleterious delay in systemic treatment. Such delay explains a significant pulmonary metastasis rate despite adequate local control with any treatment. Protocols that call for radiation therapy before surgical resection and chemotherapy for soft tissue sarcomas usually result in a 6-week delay in the institution of chemotherapy and a higher wound complication rate.[17] At the University of Washington, we have therefore elected to administer preoperative chemotherapy for all high-grade soft tissue sarcomas, followed by restaging and surgical resection after three cycles of chemotherapy. If the surgical margin is marginal, patients also receive postoperative radiation therapy interposed with their postoperative chemotherapy. Other similar protocols elsewhere have replaced preoperative radiation therapy with preoperative chemotherapy.

Much has been written and proclaimed about limb-sparing procedures.[60,159] In fact, it is relatively easy to carry out a limb-sparing procedure in the current context of preoperative chemotherapy and to achieve adequate local control without recurrence at the primary tumor site. It is a much greater challenge, however, to carry out limb-sparing procedures and have a good or excellent functional result after that procedure. Thus, soft tissue involvement may be more important than bone and joint involvement. A good functional result requires well-innervated muscle, adequate soft tissue, and a stable joint. If the soft tissues, strength, and stability of the reconstruction are inadequate, the emotional and financial investment in limb-sparing surgery is probably not warranted. When appropriately carried out, limb-sparing procedures do not increase a patient's risk for local recurrence or diminish the patient's chance for survival.[198] These procedures should, however, be very carefully planned and coordinated in the treatment of all patients. Surgical complications need to be limited enough to enable resumption of chemotherapy within 2 to 3 weeks after surgery.

Because of the emotional effect of losing an extremity, most patients are naturally drawn to the idea of limb salvage surgery. The responsibility of outlining the true risks and benefits of such a procedure rests with the surgeon, who will transmit his own prejudices. The gold standard for comparison is an amputation, and the total rehabilitation time should be compared with the limited recovery time of an upper or lower extremity amputation (6 months). These comparisons and differences should be well thought out beforehand so that a clear picture can be presented to the patient. In the final analysis, tumor control should be emphasized, and any attempt at limb salvage should stress stabilization and mobilization to maximize the functional results. These problems are challenging and require challenging treatments, and only experience and a carefully coordinated team approach will meet that challenge.

All these treatment protocols are logistically complex and demand a close relationship between the chemotherapist, surgical oncologist, and radiation therapist. The specialized treatment of these patients also requires a clinical nurse specialist to serve as a clinical coordinator and a source of continuity for patients. It is very difficult to treat sarcoma patients only occasionally and do it well.

REFERENCES AND BIBLIOGRAPHY

1. Albee FH: The treatment of primary malignant changes of bone by radical resection and bone graft replacement. JAMA 107:1693, 1936.
2. Allen PW and Enzinger FM: Hemangioma of skeletal muscle. Cancer 29:8, 1972.
3. American Joint Committee for Cancer Staging and End-Results Reporting: Manual for Staging of Cancer. Chicago: American Joint Committee, 1977.
4. Arata MA, Peterson HA, and Dahlin DC: Pathologic fractures through non-ossifying fibromas. J Bone Joint Surg Am 63:980-988, 1981.
5. Azzarelli A, Quagliuolo V, Casali P, et al: Preoperative doxorubicin plus ifosfamide in primary soft-tissue sarcomas of the extremities. Cancer Chemother Pharmacol 31(suppl):210-212, 1993.
6. Bacci G, Picci P, Gherlinzoni F, et al: Localized Ewing's sarcoma of bone: Ten years' experience at the Istituto Ortopedico Rizzoli in 124 cases treated with multimodal therapy. Eur J Cancer Clin Oncol 21:163-173, 1985.
7. Barrett WP, Franklin JL, Jackins SE, et al: Total shoulder arthroplasty. J Bone Joint Surg Am 69:865-872, 1987.
8. Barth RJ Jr, Merino MJ, Solomon D, et al: A prospective study of the value of core needle biopsy and fine needle aspiration in the diagnosis of soft tissue masses. Surgery 112:536-543, 1992.
9. Bauer HC, Brosjo O, Kreicbergs A, et al: Low risk of recurrence of enchondroma and low-grade chondrosarcoma in extremities: 80 patients followed for 2-25 years. Acta Orthop Scand 66:283-288, 1995.
10. Beisecker JL, Marcove RC, Huvos AG, and Moke V: Aneurysmal bone cysts: A clinicopathologic study of 66 cases. Cancer 26:615, 1970.
11. Berrettoni BA and Carter JR: Mechanisms of cancer metastasis to bone. J Bone Joint Surg Am 68:308-312, 1986.
12. Bickels J, Wittig JC, Kollender Y, et al: Limb-sparing resections of the shoulder girdle. J Am Coll Surg 194:422-435, 2002.
13. Bjornsson J, Unni KK, Dahlin DC, et al: Clear cell chondrosarcoma of bone: Observations in 47 cases. Am J Surg Pathol 8:223-230, 1984.
14. Bleyer WA, Haas JE, Feigl P, et al: Improved 3-year disease-free survival in osteogenic sarcoma: Efficacy of adjunctive chemotherapy. J Bone Joint Surg Br 64:233-238, 1982.
15. Bos G, Sim FH, Pritchard DJ, et al: Prosthetic proximal humeral replacement: The Mayo Clinic experience. In Enneking WF (ed): Limb Salvage in Musculoskeletal Oncology. (Bristol-Myers/Zimmer Orthopaedic Symposium.) New York: Churchill Livingstone, 1987, p 61.
16. Broders AC: The microscopic grading of cancer. In Pack GT and Arrel IM (eds): Treatment of Cancer and Allied Diseases. New York: PB Hoeber, 1964.
17. Bujko K, Suit HD, Springfield DS, et al: Wound healing after preoperative radiation for sarcoma of soft tissues. Surg Gynecol Obstet 176:124-134, 1993.
18. Burchardt H, Busbee GA III, and Enneking WF: Repair of experimental autologous grafts or cortical bone. J Bone Joint Surg Am 57:814-819, 1975.
19. Burchardt H, Jones H, Glowczewskie F, et al: Freeze dried allogenic segmental cortical bone grafts in dogs. J Bone Joint Surg Am 60:1081-1090, 1978.
20. Burgers JMV, Breur K, van Dobbenburgh OA, et al: Role of metastatectomy without chemotherapy in the management of osteosarcoma in children. Cancer 45:1664-1668, 1980.
21. Burrows HJ, Wilson JN, and Scales JT: Excision of tumors of humerus and femur, with restoration by internal prostheses. J Bone Joint Surg Br 57:140, 1975.
22. Burwell HN: Resection of the shoulder with humeral suspension for sarcoma involving the scapula. J Bone Joint Surg Br 47:300, 1965.
23. Campanacci M, Bacci G, Bertoni F, et al: The treatment of osteosarcoma of the extremities: Twenty years' experience at the Istituto Ortepedico Rizzoli. Cancer 48:1569-1581, 1981.
24. Campanacci M, Baldini N, Boriani S, and Sudanese A: Giant-cell tumor of bone. J Bone Joint Surg Am 69:106-114, 1987.
25. Cancer Patient Survival, Report No. 5. U.S. Department of Health, Education and Welfare. Publication No. (NIH) 77-992, 1976.
26. Capanna R, Bertoni F, Bacchini P, et al: Malignant fibrous histiocytoma of bone: The experience at the Rizzoli Institute: Report of 90 cases. Cancer 54:177-187, 1984.
27. Capanna R, Bertoni F, Bettelli G, et al: Dedifferentiated chondrosarcoma. J Bone Joint Surg Am 70:60-69, 1988.
28. Cofield R: Glenohumeral arthrodesis. J Bone Joint Surg Am 61:673, 1979.
29. Conrad EU and Enneking WF: Shoulder arthrodesis following tumor resection. Paper presented at the 53rd Annual Meeting of the American Academy of Orthopaedic Surgeons, February 1986, New Orleans.
30. Conrad EU III, Enneking WF, and Springfield DS: Giant cell tumor treated with curettage and cementation. In Limb Salvage in Musculoskeletal Oncology. New York: Churchill Livingstone, 1987, p 626.
31. Dahlin DC: Bone Tumors: General Aspects and Data on 6,221 Cases, 3rd ed. Springfield, IL: Charles C Thomas, 1978, pp 3-17.
32. Dahlin DC: Bone Tumors: General Aspects and Data on 6,221 Cases, 3rd ed. Springfield, IL: Charles C Thomas, 1978, pp 156-175.
33. Dahlin DC and Beabout JW: Dedifferentiation of low-grade chondrosarcomas. Cancer 28:461-466, 1971.
34. Dahlin DC, Cupps RE, and Johnson EW Jr: Giant cell tumor: A study of 195 cases. Cancer 25:1061-1070, 1970.
35. Dahlin DC and Ivins JC: Benign chondroblastoma: A study of 125 cases. Cancer 30:401-413, 1972.
36. Davis AM, Bell RS, Goodwin PJ: Prognostic factors in osteosarcoma: A critical review. J Clin Oncol 12:423-431, 1994.
37. DeNancrede CBG: The end results after total excision of the scapula. Ann Surg 50:1, 1909.
38. DeSantos LA, Murray SA, and Ayaler AG: The value of percutaneous needle biopsy in the management of primary bone tumors. Cancer 43:735-744, 1979.
39. Durie BGM and Salmon SE: A clinical staging system for multiple myeloma. Correlation of measured myeloma cell mass with presenting clinical features, response to treatment and survival. Cancer 36:842-854, 1975.
40. Eckardt JJ, Eilber FR, Jinnah RH, and Mirra JM: Endoprosthetic replacement of the scapula, including the shoulder joint, for malignant tumors: A preliminary report. In Enneking WF (ed): Limb Salvage in Musculoskeletal Oncology. New York: Churchill Livingstone, 1987, pp 542-553.
41. Eilber FR, Eckhardt J, and Morton DL: Advances in the treatment of sarcomas of the extremity: Current status of limb salvage. Cancer 54:2695-2701, 1984.
42. Eilber FR, Morton DL, Eckardt JJ, et al: Limb salvage for skeletal and soft tissue sarcomas. Cancer 53:2579, 1984.
43. Eiselsberg A: Zur Heilung Groesserer. Defects der Tibia durch Gestielte Haut-Periost-KnochenLappen. Arch Klin Chir 55:435, 1897.
44. Enneking WF: The issue of the biopsy [editorial]. J Bone Joint Surg 644:1119-1120, 1982.
45. Enneking WF: Functional evaluation of reconstruction after tumor resection. Paper presented at the Second International Workshop on the Design and Application of Tumor Prostheses for Bone and Joint Reconstruction, 1983, Vienna.
46. Enneking WF: Musculoskeletal Tumor Surgery. New York: Churchill Livingstone, 1983, pp 1-60.
47. Enneking WF: Biopsy. In Musculoskeletal Tumor Surgery. New York: Churchill Livingstone, 1983, pp 185-201.
48. Enneking WF: Fibromatosis. In Musculoskeletal Tumor Surgery. New York: Churchill Livingstone, 1983, pp 760-773.
49. Enneking WF: Cartilaginous lesions in bone. In Musculoskeletal Tumor Surgery. New York: Churchill Livingstone, 1983, pp 875-997.
50. Enneking WF: Enchondroma. In Musculoskeletal Tumor Surgery. New York: Churchill Livingstone, 1983, pp 878-892.
51. Enneking WF: Periosteal chondroma. In Musculoskeletal Tumor Surgery. New York: Churchill Livingstone, 1983, pp 913-919.
52. Enneking WF: Primary chondrosarcoma. In Musculoskeletal Tumor Surgery. New York: Churchill Livingstone, 1983, pp 945-964.
53. Enneking WF: Osseous lesions originating in bone. In Musculoskeletal Tumor Surgery. New York: Churchill Livingstone, 1983, pp 1021-1123.
54. Enneking WF: Vascular lesions. In Musculoskeletal Tumor Surgery. New York: Churchill Livingstone, 1983, pp 1175-1190.
55. Enneking WF: Lipoma. In Musculoskeletal Tumor Surgery. New York: Churchill Livingstone, 1983, pp 1225-1240.
56. Enneking WF: Ewing's sarcoma. In Musculoskeletal Tumor Surgery. New York: Churchill Livingstone, 1983, pp 1345-1380.
57. Enneking WF: Simple cyst. In Musculoskeletal Tumor Surgery. New York: Churchill Livingstone, 1983, pp 1494-1513.
58. Enneking WF: Aneurysmal bone cysts. In Musculoskeletal Tumor Surgery. New York: Churchill Livingstone, 1983, pp 1513-1530.
59. Enneking WF: Modified system for functional evaluation of surgical management of musculoskeletal tumors for limb salvage. In Enneking WF (ed): Musculoskeletal Oncology. New York: Churchill Livingstone, 1987.
60. Enneking WF, Dunham W, Gebhardt MC, et al: A system for the functional evaluation of reconstructive procedures after surgical treatment of tumors of the musculoskeletal system. Clin Orthop 286:241-246, 1993.
61. Enneking WF, Spanier SS, and Goodman MA: A system for the surgical staging of musculoskeletal sarcoma. Clin Orthop 153:106, 1980.
62. Enneking WF, Spanier SS, and Malawer MM: The effect of the anatomic setting on the results of surgical procedures for soft parts sarcoma of the thigh. Cancer 47:1005-1022, 1981.

63. Enneking WF, Springfield DS, and Gross M: The surgical treatment of parosteal osteosarcoma in long bones. J Bone Joint Surg Am 67:125-135,1985.

64. Enzinger FM and Weiss SW: Fibromatoses. In Soft Tissue Tumors. St Louis: CV Mosby, 1983, p 45.

65. Enzinger FM and Weiss SW: Malignant fibrohistiocytic tumors. In Soft Tissue Tumors. St Louis: CV Mosby, 1983, p 166.

66. Enzinger FM and Weiss SW: Liposarcoma. In Soft Tissue Tumors. St Louis: CV Mosby, 1983, p 242.

67. Enzinger FM and Weiss SW: Rhabdomyosarcoma. In Soft Tissue Tumors. St Louis: CV Mosby, 1983, p 338.

68. Fidler IJ and Hart IR: Biological diversity in metastatic neoplasms: Origins and implications. Science 217:998-1003, 1982.

69. Francis KC and Worcester JN Jr: Radical resection for tumors of the shoulder with preservation of a functional extremity. J Bone Joint Surg Am 44:1423-1429, 1962.

70. Frassica FJ, Unni KK, Beabout JW, and Sim FH: Differentiated chondrosarcoma. A report of the clinicopathological features and treatment of 78 cases. J Bone Joint Surg Am 68:1197, 1986.

71. Garrison RC, Unni KK, McLeod RA, et al: Chondrosarcoma arising in osteochondroma. Cancer 49:1890-1897, 1982.

72. Gebhardt MC, McGuire MH, and Mankin HJ: Resection and allograft arthrodesis for malignant bone tumors of the extremity. In Enneking WF (ed): Lung Salvage in Musculoskeletal Oncology. New York: Churchill Livingstone, 1987.

73. Gitellis S, Bertoni F, Chieti PP, et al: Chondrosarcoma of bone. J Bone Joint Surg Am 63:1248-1256, 1981.

74. Glasser DB, Lane JM, Huvos AG, et al: Survival, prognosis, and therapeutic response in osteogenic sarcoma: The Memorial hospital experience. Cancer 69:698-708, 1992.

75. Goldblatt J, Sacks S, and Beighton P: The orthopaedic aspects of Gaucher disease. Clin Orthop 137:208, 1978.

76. Goldenberg RR, Campbell CJ, and Bonfiglio M: Giant-cell tumor of bone: An analysis of two hundred and eighteen cases. J Bone Joint Surg Am 52:619-663, 1970.

77. Goodman MA: Plasma cell tumors. Clin Orthop 204:87-92, 1986.

78. Goorin AM, Deloney MJ, Lack EE, et al: Prognostic significance of complete surgical resection of pulmonary metastases in patients with osteogenic sarcoma: Analysis of 32 cases. J Clin Oncol 2:425-430, 1984.

79. Gore DR, Murray MP, Sepic MS, and Gardner GM: Shoulder-muscle strength and range of motion following surgical repair of full-thickness rotator-cuff tears. J Bone Joint Surg Am 68:266, 1986.

80. Greene FL, Page DL, Fleming ID, et al: AJCC Cancer Staging Manual, 6th ed, Stage Groupings for Soft Tissue Sarcoma. New York: Springer-Verlag, 2002.

81. Greene FL, Page DL, Fleming ID, et al: AJCC Cancer Staging Manual, 6th ed, Stage Groupings for Bone. New York: Springer-Verlag, 2002.

82. Griffith M, Betz RR, Mardjetko S, et al: Review of Treatment of Unicameral Bone Cysts. Paper presented at the annual meeting of the American Association of Orthopaedic Surgeons, Feb 8, 1988, Atlanta.

83. Gross SW: Sarcoma of the long bones: Based upon a study of one hundred and sixty-five cases. Clin Orthop 18:17-57, 1975.

84. Guillou L, Coindre JM, Bonichon F, et al: Comparative study of the National Cancer Institute and French Federation of Cancer Centers Sarcoma Group grading systems in a population of 410 adult patients with soft-tissue sarcoma. J Clin Oncol 15:350-362, 1997.

85. Hardin CA: Interscapulothoracic amputations for sarcomas of the upper extremity. Surgery 49:355, 1961.

86. Harrington KD: Metastatic disease of the spine. J Bone Joint Surg Am 68:1110-1115, 1986.

87. Harris WH, Dudley HR Jr, and Barry RJ: The natural history of fibrous dysplasia: An orthopaedic, pathological and roentgenographic study. J Bone Joint Surg Am 44:207-233, 1962.

88. Hawkins DS, Rajendran JG, Conrad EU III, et al: Evaluation of chemotherapy response in pediatric bone sarcomas by F-18 fluorodeoxy-D-glucose positron emission tomography. Cancer 94:3277-3284, 2002.

89. Henry A: Monostotic fibrous dysplasia. J Bone Joint Surg Br 51:300-306, 1969.

90. Hudson TM, Schakel M, Springfield DS, et al: The comparative value of bone scintigraphy and computed tomography in determining bone involvement by soft-tissue sarcomas. J Bone Joint Surg Am 66:1400-1407, 1984.

91. Huvos AG, Rosen G, Dabska M, and Marcove RC: Mesenchymal chondrosarcoma: A clinicopathologic analysis of 35 patients with emphasis on treatment. Cancer 51:1230-1237, 1983.

92. Huvos AG: Bone Tumors: Diagnosis, Treatment and Prognosis. Philadelphia: WB Saunders, 1979.

93. Huvos AG: Chondroblastoma. In Huvos AG (ed): Bone Tumors: Diagnosis, Treatment and Prognosis. Philadelphia: WB Saunders, 1979.

94. Huvos AG: Osteoid osteoma. In Huvos AG (ed): Bone Tumors: Diagnosis, Treatment and Prognosis. Philadelphia: WB Saunders, 1979, pp 8-46.

95. Huvos AG: Osteogenic sarcoma. In Huvos AG (ed): Bone Tumors. Philadelphia: WB Saunders, 1979, pp 47-93.

96. Huvos AG: Osteochondroma and enchondromas. In Huvos AG (ed): Bone Tumors: Diagnosis, Treatment and Prognosis. Philadelphia: WB Saunders, 1979, pp 139-170.

97. Imbriglia JE, Negr CS, and Dick HM: Resection of the proximal one half of the humerus in a child for chondrosarcoma. J Bone Joint Surg Am 60:262, 1978.

98. Jaffe HL: Fibrous dysplasia. In Tumors and Tumorous Conditions of the Bones and Joint. Philadelphia: Lea & Febiger, 1958, pp 117-142.

99. Jaffe HL: Tumors and Tumorous Conditions of the Bone and Joints. Philadelphia: WB Saunders, 1979.

100. Jaffe N, Prudich J, Knapp J, et al: Treatment of primary osteosarcoma with intra-arterial and intravenous high-dose methotrexate. J Clin Oncol 1:428-431, 1983.

101. Kanis JA and Gray RE: Long term follow-up observations on treatment in Paget's disease of bone. Clin Orthop 217:99-125, 1987.

102. Klapp R: Ueber einen Fall Ausgedehnter Knochev-transplantation. Dtsch Z Chir 54:576, 1900.

103. Koelbel R, Rohlmann A, and Bergmann G: Biomechanical considerations in the design of a semi-constrained total shoulder replacement. In Bayley I and Kessel L (eds): Shoulder Surgery. Berlin: Springer-Verlag, 1982.

104. Kreicbergs A, Boquist L, Borssen B, and Larsson SE: Prognostic factors in chondrosarcoma: A comparative study of cellular DNA content and clinicopathologic features. Cancer 50:577-583, 1982.

105. Lane JM, Hurson B, Boland PJ, and Glasser DB: Osteogenic sarcoma, ten most common bone and joint tumors. Clin Orthop 204:93-110, 1986.

106. Levine AM and Rosenberg SA: Alkaline phosphatase levels in osteosarcoma tissue as related to prognosis. Cancer 44:2291-2293, 1979.

107. Lewis RJ, Marcove RC, and Rosen G: Ewing's sarcoma: Functional effects of radiation therapy. J Bone Joint Surg Am 59:325-331, 1977.

108. Lexer E: Die Gesamte Widerherstellungs Chirurgie. Leipzig: Barth, 1931.

109. Lichtenstein L: Polyostotic fibrous dysplasia. Arch Surg 36:874-898, 1938.

110. Lichtenstein L: Preface to the First Edition. General remarks, classification of primary tumors of bone. In Bone Tumors. St Louis: CV Mosby, 1959, pp 6-34.

111. Lichtenstein L: Bone Tumors, 4th ed. St Louis: CV Mosby, 1972.

112. Linberg BF: Interscapulothoracic resection for malignant tumors of the shoulder joint region. J Bone Joint Surg 10:344, 1928.

113. Lindberg RD, Martin RG, Romsdahl MM, and Barkley HT Jr: Conservative surgery and postoperative radiotherapy in 300 adults with soft-tissue sarcomas. Cancer 47:2391-2397, 1981.

114. Linder L: Reaction of bone to the acute chemical trauma of bone cement. J Bone Joint Surg Am 59:82, 1977.

115. Lugli T: The facts of an exceptional intervention and the prosthetic method. Clin Orthop 133:215-218, 1978.

116. Malawer MM, Dunham WK, Zaleski T, and Zielinski CJ: Cryosurgery in the management of benign (aggressive) and low grade malignant tumors of bone: Analysis of 40 consecutive cases. Paper presented at the 53rd Annual Meeting of the American Academy of Orthopedic Surgeons, February 1986, New Orleans.

117. Malawer MM, McKay DW, Markle B, et al: Analysis of 40 consecutive cases of unicameral bone cysts treated by high pressure Renografin injection and intracavitary methylprednisolone acetate: Prognostic factors and hemodynamic evaluation. Paper presented at the 52nd Annual Meeting of the American Academy of Orthopaedic Surgeons, 1985, Las Vegas, NV.

118. Mameghan H, Fisher RJ, O'Gorman-Hughes D, et al: Ewing's sarcoma: Long-term follow-up in 49 patients treated from 1967 to 1989. Int J Radiat Oncol Biol Phys 25:431-438, 1993.

119. Mankin HJ, Cantley KD, Lipielo L, et al: The biology of human chondrosarcoma. I. Description of the cases, grading, and biochemical analyses. J Bone Joint Surg 62:160-176, 1980.

120. Mankin HJ, Connor JF, Schiller AL, et al: Grading of bone tumors by analysis of nuclear DNA content using flow cytometry. J Bone Joint Surg Am 67:404-413, 1985.

121. Mankin HJ, Doppelt SH, Sullivan TR, and Tomford WW: Osteoarticular and intercalary allograft transplantation in the management of malignant tumors of bone cancer. Cancer 50:613-630, 1982.

122. Mankin HJ, Fogelson FS, Thrasher AA, et al: Massive resection and allograft transplantation in the treatment of malignant bone tumors. N Engl J Med 294:1247-1255, 1976.

123. Mankin HJ, Lange TA, and Spanier SS: The hazards of biopsy in patients with malignant primary bone and soft-tissue tumors. J Bone Joint Surg Am 64:1121-1127, 1982.

124. Marcove RC: A 17-year review of cryosurgery in the treatment of bone tumors. Clin Orthop 163:231-233, 1982.

125. Marcove RC, Lewis MM, and Huvos AG: En bloc upper humeral-interscapular resection: The Tikhoff-Linberg procedure. Clin Orthop 124:219-228, 1977.

126. Marcove RC, Lyden JP, Huvos AC, and Bullough PB: Giant-cell tumor treated by cryosurgery. A report of twenty-five cases. J Bone Joint Surg Am 55:1633-1644, 1973.

127. Marcove RC, Mike V, Hutter RVP, et al: Chondrosarcoma of the pelvis and upper end of femur. An analysis of factors influencing survival time in one hundred and thirteen cases. J Bone Joint Surg Am 54:561-572, 1972.

128. Marcove RC, Stovell P, Huvos AC, et al: The use of cryosurgery in the treatment of low and medium grade chondrosarcoma: A preliminary report. Clin Orthop 122:147-156, 1977.

129. Marcove RC, Weis LD, Vaghaiwall MR, et al: Cryosurgery in the treatment of giant cell tumors of bone. A report of 52 consecutive cases. Cancer 41:957-969, 1978.

130. Marhade G, Monastryrski J, and Steuner B: Scapulectomy for malignant tumors, function and shoulder strength in five patients. Acta Orthop Scand 56:332, 1985.

131. Martini N, Huvos AG, Mike V, et al: Multiple pulmonary resections in the treatment of osteogenic sarcoma. Ann Thorac Surg 12:271-280, 1971.
132. Matsen FA III: Personal communication, January 1988.
133. Matsuno T, Unni KK, McLeod RA, and Dahlin DC: Telangiectatic osteosarcoma. Cancer 38:2538-2547, 1976.
134. Maurer HM, Moon T, Donaldson M, et al: The intergroup rhabdomyosarcoma study. Cancer 40:2015, 1977.
135. McDonald DJ, Sim FH, McLeod RA, and Dahlin DC: Giant-cell tumor of bone. J Bone Joint Surg Am 68:235-242, 1986.
136. McKenzie DH: The fibromatoses: A clinicopathologic concept. BMJ 4:777, 1972.
137. Milgram JW: Synovial osteochondromatosis. J Bone Joint Surg Am 59:792-901, 1977.
138. Miser J, Kinsella T, Tsokos M, et al: High response rate of recurrent childhood tumors to etoposide (VP16), ifosfamide (IFOS0, and mesna (MES) uroprotection. Proc Soc Clin Oncol 5:209, 1986.
139. Moore TM, Meyers MH, Patzakis MJ, et al: Closed biopsy of musculoskeletal lesions. J Bone Joint Surg Am 61:375-380, 1979.
140. Mullins F, Berard CW, and Eisenberg SH: Chondrosarcoma following synovial chondromatosis. Cancer 18:1180, 1965.
141. Murray JA, Jessup K, Romsdahl M, et al: Limb salvage surgery in osteosarcoma: Early experience at M.D. Anderson Hospital. Proceedings of NIH Consensus Development Conference on Limb-Sparing Treatment of Adult Soft Tissue Sarcomas and Osteosarcoma. U.S. Department of Health and Human Services, Public Health Services, NIH Cancer Treatment Symposia, vol 3, 1985.
142. National Institutes of Health, Consensus Development Panel: Limb-sparing treatment of adult soft-tissue sarcomas and osteosarcomas. JAMA 254:1791-1794, 1985.
143. Neer CS, Francis KC, Kiernan HA, et al: Current concepts in the treatment of solitary unicameral bone cysts. Clin Orthop 97:40-51, 1973.
144. Neer CS, Watson KC, and Stanton FJ: Recent experience in total shoulder replacement. J Bone Joint Surg Am 64:319-337, 1982.
145. Nicholson HS, Mulvihill JJ, and Byrne J: Late effects of therapy in adult survivors of osteosarcoma and Ewing's sarcoma. Med Pediatr Oncol 20:6-12, 1992.
146. Nielsen TO, West RB, and van de Rijn, et al: Molecular characterization of soft tissue tumors: A gene expression study. Lancet 359:1307, 2002.
147. Ogilvie-Harris DJ, Hans CB, and Fornasier VL: Pseudomalignant myositis ossificans: Heterotopic new bone formation without a history of trauma. J Bone Joint Surg Am 62:1274-1283, 1980.
148. Oppenheimer WL and Galleno H: Operative treatment versus steroid injection in the management of unicameral bone cysts. J Pediatr Orthop 4:1-7, 1984.
149. Orthopaedic Practice in the U.S. 1986-1987. Chicago, American Academy of Orthopaedic Surgeons, Department of Professional Affairs, 1987.
150. Pack GT, McNeer G, and Coley BL: Interscapulo-thoracic amputation for malignant tumors of the upper extremity. Surg Gynecol Obstet 74:161, 1942.
151. Papaioannou AN and Francis KD: Scapulectomy for the treatment of primary malignant tumors of the scapula. Clin Orthop 41:125, 1965.
152. Parrish FF: Treatment of bone tumors by total excision and replacement with massive autologous and homologous grafts. J Bone Joint Surg Am 48:968-990, 1966.
153. Paulson DF, Perez CA, and Anderson T: Cancer of the kidney and ureter. In DeVita VT, Hellman S, and Rosenberg SA (ed): Cancer: Principles and Practice of Oncology, 2nd ed. Philadelphia: JB Lippincott, 1985, pp 895-905.
154. Persson BM, Ekelund L, Lovdahl R, and Gunterberg B: Favourable results of acrylic cementation for giant cell tumors. Acta Orthop Scand 55:209-214, 1984.
155. Persson BM and Wouters HW: Curettage and acrylic cementation in surgery of giant cell tumors of bone. Clin Orthop 120:125-133, 1976.
156. Phemister DB: Conservative bone surgery in the treatment of bone tumors. Surg Gynecol Obstet 70:355, 1940.
157. Poppen NK and Walker PS: Forces at the glenohumeral joint in abduction. Clin Orthop 135:165-170, 1978.
158. Post M, Haskell SS, and Jablon M: Total shoulder replacement with a constrained prosthesis. J Bone Joint Surg Am 62:327-335, 1980.
159. Postma A, Kingma A, De Ruiter JH, et al: Quality of life in bone tumor patients comparing limb salvage and amputation of the lower extremity. J Surg Oncol 51:47-51, 1992.
160. Price CHG and Golde W: Paget's sarcoma of bone: A study of eighty cases. J Bone Joint Surg Br 51:205-224, 1969.
161. Pritchard DJ, Lunke RJ, Taylor WF, et al: Chondrosarcoma: A clinicopathologic and statistical analysis. Cancer 45:149-157, 1980.
162. Proceedings of NIH Consensus Development Conference on Limb-Sparing Treatment of Adult Soft Tissue Sarcomas and Osteosarcoma. Bethesda, MD, U.S. Department of Health and Human Services, Public Health Services, NIH Cancer Treatment Symposia, vol 3, 1985.
163. Rao A, Srinvasa V, and Vincent J: Pigmented villonodular synovitis (giant-cell tumor of the tendon sheath and synovial membrane): A review of eighty-one cases. J Bone Joint Surg Am 66:76-94, 1984.
164. Reszel PA, Soule EH, and Coventry MB: Liposarcomas of the extremities and limb girdles: A study of 222 cases. J Bone Joint Surg Am 48:229, 1966.
165. Rock M: Intercalary allograft and custom Neer prosthesis after en bloc resection of the proximal humerus. In Enneking WF (ed): Limb Salvage in Musculoskeletal Oncology. (Bristol-Myers/Zimmer Orthopaedic Symposium.) New York: Churchill Livingstone, 1987, p 586.
166. Rock MG, Pritchard DJ, Reiman HM, et al: Extra-abdominal desmoid tumors. J Bone Joint Surg Am 66:1369-1374, 1984.
167. Rock MG, Sim FH, and Chao EYS: Limb salvage procedures for primary bone tumors of the shoulder. In Bateman JE and Welsh RP (eds): Surgery of the Shoulder. Philadelphia: BC Decker, 1984.
168. Rosen G: Neoadjuvant chemotherapy for osteogenic sarcoma. A model for treatment of malignant neoplasm. Recent Results Cancer Res 103:48-157, 1986.
169. Rosen G, Caparros B, Huvos AC, et al: Preoperative chemotherapy for osteogenic sarcoma: Selection of postoperative adjuvant chemotherapy based upon the response of the primary tumor to preoperative chemotherapy. Cancer 49:1221-1230, 1982.
170. Rosen G, Caparros B, Nirenberg A, et al: Ewing's sarcoma. Ten-year experience with adjuvant chemotherapy. Cancer 47:2204-2213, 1981.
171. Rosenberg SA, Fyle MW, Conkle D, et al: The treatment of osteosarcoma. II. Aggressive resection of pulmonary metastases. Cancer Treat Rep 63:753-762, 1979.
172. Rosenberg SA, Kent H, Cost J, et al: Prospective randomized evaluation of the role of limb sparing surgery, radiation therapy, and adjuvant chemoimmunotherapy in the treatment of adult soft tissue sarcomas. Surgery 84:62-69, 1978.
173. Rosenberg SA, Suit FD, and Baker LH: Sarcoma of soft tissue. In DeVita VT, Hellman S, and Rosenberg SA (eds): Cancer: Principles and Practice of Oncology, 2nd ed. Philadelphia: JB Lippincott, 1985, pp 1243-1293.
174. Rougraff BT and Kling TJ: Treatment of active unicameral bone cysts with percutaneous injection of demineralized bone matrix and autogenous bone marrow. J Bone Joint Surg Am 84:921-929, 2002.
175. Rougraff BT, Kneisl JS, and Simon MA: Skeletal metastases of unknown origin. A prospective study of a diagnostic strategy. J Bone Joint Surg Am 75:1276-1281, 1993.
176. Rowe CR: Re-evaluation of the position of the arm in arthrodesis of the shoulder in the adult. J Bone Joint Surg Am 56:913, 1974.
177. Rubin P: Clinical Oncology, 6th ed. American Cancer Society, 1983.
178. Rydholm A: Management of patients with soft-tissue tumors: Strategy developed at a regional oncology center. Acta Orthop Scand Suppl 203:3-76, 1983.
179. Ryerson EW: Excision of the scapula: Report of a case with excellent functional result. JAMA 113:1958, 1939.
180. Saddegh MK, Lindholm J, Lundberg A, et al: Staging of soft-tissue sarcomas. Prognostic analysis of clinical and pathological features. J Bone Joint Surg Br 74:495-500, 1992.
181. Salzer M, Knahr K, Locke H, et al: A bioceramic endoprosthesis for the replacement of the proximal humerus. Arch Orthop Trauma Surg 93:169-184, 1979.
182. Salzer M, Zweymueller K, Locke H, et al: Further experimental and clinical experience with aluminum oxide endoprosthesis. J Biomed Mater Res 10:847, 1976.
183. Samilson RL, Morris JM, and Thompson RW: Tumors of the scapula: A review of the literature and an analysis of 31 cases. Clin Orthop 58:105, 1968.
184. Scaglietti O, Marchetti PG, and Bartolozzi P: The effects of methylprednisolone acetate in the treatment of bone cysts. Results of three years follow-up. J Bone Joint Surg Br 61:200-204, 1970.
185. Schajowicz F and Derquie JC: Puncture biopsy in lesions of the locomotor system: Review and results in 4050 cases, including 941 vertebral punctures. Cancer 21:5331-5487, 1968.
186. Schaller RT Jr, Haas J, Schaller J, et al: Improved survival in children with osteosarcoma following resection of pulmonary metastases. J Pediatr Surg 17:546-550, 1982.
187. Schauffler RM: Transplant of the upper extremity of the fibula to replace the upper extremity of the humerus. J Bone Joint Surg 8:723, 1926.
188. Schmale GA, Conrad EU III, and Raskind WH: The natural history of hereditary multiple exostoses. J Bone Joint Surg Am 76:986-992, 1994.
189. Schreuder HWB, Conrad EU III, Bruckner JD, et al: The treatment of simple bone cysts in children with curettage and cryosurgery. J Pediatr Orthop 17:814-820, 1997.
190. Sekera J, Ramach W, Pongracz N, et al: Experience with ceramic and metal implants for the proximal humerus in cases of malignant bone tumor. In Enneking WF (ed): Limb Salvage in Musculoskeletal Oncology (Bristol-Myers/Zimmer Orthopaedic Symposium.) New York: Churchill Livingstone, 1987, p 211.
191. Shapiro F: Ollier's disease: An assessment of angular deformity, shortening, and pathological fracture in twenty-one patients. J Bone Joint Surg Am 64:95-103, 1982.
192. Shibata T: Reconstruction of skeletal defects after the Tikhoff-Linberg procedure using aluminum ceramic endoprosthesis and stabilization of the shoulder. In Enneking WF (ed): Limb Salvage in Musculoskeletal Oncology (Bristol-Myers/Zimmer Orthopaedic Symposium.) New York: Churchill Livingstone, 1987, p 553.
193. Shiu MH, Castro EB, Hajdu SI, and Fortner JG: Results of surgical and radiation therapy in the treatment of liposarcoma arising in an extremity. AJR Am J Roentgenol 123:577, 1975.
194. Sim FH, Chao EYS, Prichard DJ, and Salzer M: Replacement of the proximal humerus with a ceramic prosthesis: A preliminary report. Clin Orthop 146:161, 1980.

195. Simon MA and Bos GD: Epiphyseal extension of metaphyseal osteosarcoma in skeletally immature individuals. J Bone Joint Surg Am 62:195-204, 1980.
196. Simon MA: Biopsy of musculoskeletal tumors. J Bone Joint Surg Am 64:1253-1257, 1982.
197. Simon MA: Current concepts review: Causes of increased survival of patients with osteosarcoma: Current controversies. J Bone Joint Surg Am 66:306-310, 1984.
198. Simon MA, Aschliman MA, Thomas N, and Mankin HJ: Limb-salvage treatment versus amputation for osteosarcoma of the distal end of the femur. J Bone Joint Surg Am 68:1331-1337, 1986.
199. Simon MA and Hecht JD: Invasion of joints by primary bone sarcomas in adults. Cancer 50:1649-1655, 1982.
200. Simon MA, Spanier SS, and Enneking WF: The management of soft-tissue tumors of the extremities. J Bone Joint Surg Am 60:317-327, 1976.
201. Sledge CB, Atcher RW, Shoetkeoff S, et al: Intra-articular radiation synovectomy. Clin Orthop 182:37-40, 1984.
202. Smith WS and Struhl S: Replantation of an autoclaved autogenous segment of bone for treatment of chondrosarcoma. Long-term follow-up. J Bone Joint Surg Am 70:70, 1988.
203. Springfield D: Liposarcoma. Clin Orthop 289:50-57, 1993.
204. Springfield DS and Pagliarulo C: Fractures of long bones previously treated for Ewing's sarcoma. J Bone Joint Surg Am 67:477-481, 1985.
205. Stewart MJ, Gilmer WS, and Edmonson AS: Fibrous dysplasia of bone. J Bone Joint Surg Br 44:302-318, 1962.
206. Suit HD, Proppe KH, Mankin HJ, et al: Preoperative radiation therapy for sarcoma of soft tissue. Cancer 47:2267-2274, 1981.
207. Sundaram M, McGuire MH, Herbold DR, et al: Magnetic resonance imaging in planning limb-salvage surgery for primary malignant tumors of bone. J Bone Joint Surg Am 68:809-819, 1986.
208. Sweet D, Mass DP, Simon MA, and Shapiro CM: Histiocytic lymphoma of bone: Current strategy for orthopaedic surgeons. J Bone Joint Surg Am 63:79-84, 1981.
209. Thomas PRM, Perez CA, Neff JR, et al: The management of Ewing's sarcoma: Role of radiotherapy in local tumor control. Cancer Treat Rep 68:703-710, 1984.
210. Toni A, Neff JR, Sudanese A, et al: The role of surgical therapy in patients with nonmetastatic Ewing's sarcoma of the limbs. Clin Orthop 286:225-240, 1993.
211. Turnbull A, Blumencranz P, and Fortner J: Scapulectomy for soft tissue sarcoma. Can J Surg 21:37, 1981.
212. Unni KK, Dahlin DC, and Beabout JW: Periosteal osteogenic sarcoma. Cancer 37:2467-2485, 1976.
213. Unni KK, Dahlin DC, McLeod RA, et al: Interosseous well-differentiated osteosarcoma. Cancer 40:1337-1347, 1977.
214. Weiland AJ, Daniel RK, and Riley CH: Application of the free vascularized bone graft in the treatment of malignant or aggressive bone tumors. Johns Hopkins Med J 140:85, 1977.
215. Weiss L and Gilbert HA: Bone Metastases. Boston: GK Hall, 1981.
216. Weiss SW and Enzinger FM: Malignant fibrous histiocytoma: An analysis of 200 cases. Cancer 41:2250-2266, 1978.
217. Wilkins RM, Pritchard DJ, Burgert EO, and Unni KK: Ewing's sarcoma of bone—experience with 140 patients. Cancer 58:2551-2555, 1986.
218. Wilson PD and Lance EM: Surgical reconstruction of the skeleton following segmental resection for bone tumors. J Bone Joint Surg Am 47:1629, 1965.
219. Winkler K, Beron G, Kotz R, et al: Neoadjuvant chemotherapy for osteogenic sarcoma: Results of a cooperative German/Austrian study. J Clin Oncol 2:617-624, 1984.
220. Wright PH, Sim FH, Soule EH, and Taylor WF: Synovial sarcoma. J Bone Joint Surg Am 64:112-122, 1982.

CHAPTER 23

SEPSIS OF THE SHOULDER: MOLECULAR MECHANISMS AND PATHOGENESIS

Robin R. Richards, M.D., F.R.C.S.C.

• • • •

Shoulder sepsis can have a devastating impact on shoulder function, particularly if diagnosis and treatment are delayed or inadequate. The general principles in the pathogenesis of shoulder sepsis are similar to those pertaining to all intra-articular infections. Pathogens can enter a joint by three fundamental pathways: (1) spontaneous hematogenous seeding via the synovial blood supply, (2) contiguous spread from adjacent metaphyseal osteomyelitis via the intra-articular portion of the metaphysis, and (3) penetration of the joint by trauma, therapy, or surgery (Fig. 23–1). Susceptibility to infection is determined by the adequacy of host defenses. Spontaneous bacteremia, trauma, and surgery present an opportunity for inoculation of the joint, particularly if local or systemic conditions are favorable for infection. Shoulder sepsis is relatively uncommon because of normal defense mechanisms, the use of antibiotic prophylaxis, and a good local blood supply.

Certain patient groups with immune system depression or aberrations are at increased risk for infection. Patients with rheumatoid disease can manifest a spontaneous and somewhat cryptic sepsis in joints.[73,88] Diabetics, infants, children, the aged, patients with vascular disease, drug abusers, and patients with human immunodeficiency virus are at increased risk for infection with specific organisms, as are patients with hematologic dyscrasia and neoplastic disease. Joint infection requires a threshold inoculum of bacteria and can be facilitated by damaged tissue, foreign body substrata, and the acellularity of cartilage surfaces. Total joint arthroplasties are at potential risk because of the presence of metallic and polymeric biomaterials and the decreased phagocytic ability of macrophages in the presence of methylmethacrylate. Biomaterials and adjacent damaged tissues and substrata are readily colonized by bacteria in a polysaccharide biofilm that is resistant to macrophage attack and penetration of antibiotic.[57,65,68] With antibiotic prophylaxis, published infection rates of total joint arthroplasty are low—1% to 5%, depending on the device and the location.[32,71,111] However, once infected, biomaterials and damaged tissues are exceedingly resistant to treatment.

Clinical infection in normal or immunosuppressed patients involves the maturation of an inoculum of known pathogens (e.g., *Staphylococcus aureus* or *Pseudomonas aeruginosa*) or the transformation of nonpathogens (*Staphylococcus epidermidis*) to a septic focus of adhesive, virulent organisms. Such transformation can occur in the presence of and be potentiated by the surface of biomaterials,[65,67,68] damaged tissue[112] and defenseless cartilage matrix surfaces.[158]

HISTORY

The experience in shoulder infection has paralleled that in other large joints, though with less frequency. The work of outstanding scientists such as Louis Pasteur (1822-1895), Joseph Lister (1827-1912), and Robert Koch (1843-1910) in the last quarter of the 19th century ushered in the modern age of bacteriology and an early understanding of intra-articular sepsis. Koch's experiments with culture media at the Berlin Institute for Infectious Disease verified the role of the tubercle bacillus in musculoskeletal infection. In 1893, Péan attempted to reconstruct the tuberculous shoulder of a 30-year-old man by using a prosthetic replacement made of platinum and rubber.

The latter part of the 19th century also saw the development of the concept of antisepsis. Lister maintained that sepsis was the main obstacle to significant advances in surgery. He documented a dramatic drop in cases of empyema, erysipelas, hospital gangrene, and surgical infection through the use of antiseptic techniques. Although popularization of antiseptic technique in the surgical theater greatly reduced the rate of complications from infection, it was not until the 1930s that specific antimicrobial therapy was discovered. In 1935, a German bacteriologist, Gerhard Domagk, discovered that sulfonamides protected mice against fatal doses of hemolytic staphylococci. Sulfonamides were soon used for infection in patients, with excellent results.

Although the history of bacteriology, antiseptic techniques in surgery, and the development of antibiotics are well documented, very little of the early literature relates specifically to infections about the shoulder. In Codman's book *The Shoulder*, published in 1934, infection of the shoulder and, in particular, osteomyelitis of the proximal part of the humerus were considered very rare lesions.[32] Codman cited a report by King and Holmes in 1927 in which a review of 450 consecutive symptomatic shoulders evaluated at Massachusetts General Hospital revealed five cases of tuberculosis of the shoulder, one luetic infection

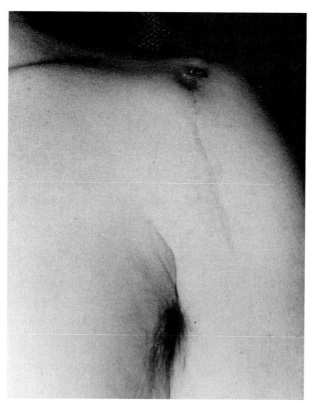

■ Figure 23–1
Sinus communicating with a prosthetic shoulder joint. A chronic low-grade infection developed in this patient after undergoing total shoulder arthroplasty.

of the shoulder, three unspecified shoulder infections, and two cases of osteomyelitis of the proximal end of the humerus. The rarity of tubercular lesions of the shoulder was documented through the results of four large series of tuberculosis involving the musculoskeletal system (Townsend, 21 of 3244 cases; Whitman, 38 of 1833 cases; Young, 7 of 5680 cases; Billroth, 14 of 1900 cases). As microbial culturing and identification techniques developed in the early 20th century, streptococcal and staphylococcal species were more frequently identified as the causative agents in shoulder infection.

SEPTIC ANATOMY OF THE SHOULDER

A review of shoulder anatomy reveals specific structural relationships that are intimately linked to the pathogenesis of joint sepsis and osteomyelitis. The circulation of the proximal end of the humerus and periarticular structures (particularly the synovium) and the intricate system of bursae about the shoulder are critical factors.

Classically, the age-dependent manifestations of hematogenous osteomyelitis and septic arthritis of the shoulder (and other large joints such as the hip and knee) have been attributed to vascular development about the growth plate and epiphysis. The most detailed studies of vascular development in this area have been performed on the proximal part of the femur but are analogous to the same development about the proximal part of the humerus. Experimental work by Trueta[154] demonstrated

that before 8 months of age, the nutrient artery system and the epiphyseal ossicle are in direct vascular communication across the growth plate. This observation was believed to account for the frequency of infection involving the epiphyseal ossicle and subsequent joint sepsis in infants. At some point between 8 and 18 months of age (an average of 1 year), the growth plate forms a complete barrier to direct vascular communication between the metaphysis and epiphysis. The last vestiges of the nutrient artery turn down acutely at the growth plate and reach sinusoidal veins. At this point blood flow "slows down," thereby creating an ideal medium for the proliferation of pathogenic bacteria.[155]

In the adult shoulder, the intra-articular extent of the metaphysis is located in the inferior aspect of the sulcus and is intracapsular for approximately 10 to 12 mm.[31] Infection of the proximal metaphysis, once established, may gain access to the shoulder joint via the haversian and Volkmann canals at the nonperiosteal zone (Fig. 23–2). With obliteration of the growth plate at skeletal maturity, anastomoses of the metaphyseal and epiphyseal circulation are again established.

In his study of the vascular development of the proximal end of the femur, Chung did not find evidence of direct communication between the metaphyseal and epiphyseal circulation across the growth plate in any age group.[30] Chung's work demonstrated a persistent extraosseous anastomosis between the metaphyseal and epiphyseal circulation on the surface of the perichondral ring. He found no evidence of vessels penetrating the growth plate in the infant population and attributed apparent changes in the arterial supply with age to enlargement of the neck and ossification center.

Branches of the suprascapular artery and the circumflex scapular branch of the subscapular artery from the scapular side of the shoulder anastomose with the anterior and posterior humeral circumflex arteries from the humeral side of the shoulder. This anastomotic system supplies the proximal portion of the humerus by forming an extra-articular and extracapsular arterial ring. Vessels from this ring traverse the capsule and form an intra-articular synovial ring. This fine anastomosis of vessels in the synovial membrane is located at the junction of the synovium and articular cartilage. This subsynovial ring of vessels was first described by William Hunter in 1743 and named the circulus articuli vasculosus.[82] At the transitional zone, synovial cells become flattened over this periarticular vascular fringe. Fine arterioles at this boundary acutely loop back toward the periphery. Again, blood flow at this level may decrease, which provides a site for the establishment of an inoculum of pathogenic organisms. Rather than hemodynamic changes, however, it is more probable that receptor-specific, microbe–to–cell surface interactions potentiate the infectious process.

Another consideration in the septic anatomy of the shoulder is communication between the joint space and capsule and the system of bursae about the shoulder. Anteriorly, there is direct communication between the capsule and the subscapular bursa located just below the coracoid process. Posteriorly, the capsule communicates with the infraspinatus bursa. A third opening in the capsule occurs at the point at which the tendon of the

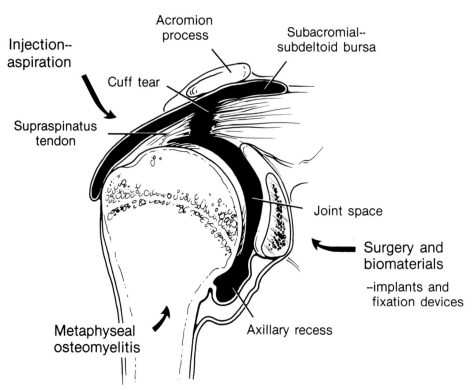

long head of the biceps enters the shoulder. From the transverse humeral ligament to its entry into the shoulder capsule, the tendon of the long head of the biceps is enveloped in folds of synovium. Intentional or inadvertent injection of the subscapular bursa, the infraspinatus bursa, or the tendon of the long head of the biceps provides the potential for intra-articular bacterial inoculation. Injection of the subacromial/subdeltoid bursa in the presence of a rotator cuff tear (degenerative or traumatic) provides another potential setting for bacterial contamination of the joint.

Ward and Eckardt reported on four subacromial/subdeltoid bursa abscesses.[162] Three of the four patients were chronically ill and debilitated, and in these patients the bursal abscesses coexisted with clinically diagnosed mild to resolving glenohumeral pyarthrosis. The symptoms and signs of these abscesses were minimal in all four patients. Ward and Eckardt found that computed tomography (CT) or magnetic resonance imaging (MRI) may be of help in detecting abscesses and planning treatment.

Microanatomy and Cell Biology

The hyaline cartilage of the articular surface is essentially acellular and consists of horizontally arranged collagen fibers in proteoglycan macromolecules. The boundaries of the joint cavity are composed of richly vascularized, cellular synovial tissue. It has been suggested that collagen fibers and the glycoprotein matrix, rather than the synovium, are the target substrata for microbial adhesion and colonization.[144,158]

Some synovial cells are phagocytic and appear to combat infection as part of the inflammatory response.

Microscopic examination of infected joints in a rabbit model indicated predominant colonization of cartilaginous rather than synovial surfaces.[158] Receptors for collagen have been identified on the cell surface of certain strains of *S. aureus*.[144] The infrequent occurrence of bacteria on synovial tissue may reflect the innate resistance of synovial cells to colonization, lack of appropriate synovial ligands, or functional host defense mechanisms at the synovial level.[18] The subintimal vascularized layer contains fibroadipose tissue, lymphatic vessels, and nerves. Ultrastructural studies of the synovial subintimal vessels reveal that gaps between endothelial cells are bridged by a fine membrane. The synovial lining does not have any epithelial tissue and, therefore, does not have a structural barrier (basement membrane) to prevent the spread of infection from synovial blood vessels to the joint. The synovial lining in the transition zone is rarely more than three or four cell layers thick, thus placing the synovial blood vessels in a superficial position. Intra-articular hemorrhage caused by trauma, combined with transient bacteremia, may be implicated as a factor in the pathogenesis of joint sepsis. Hematogenous seeding can allow bacterial penetration of synovial vessels and produce an effusion consisting primarily of neutrophils that release cartilage-destroying lysosomal enzymes.

Articular (hyaline) cartilage varies from 2 to 4 mm in thickness in the large joints of adults. This avascular, aneural tissue consists of a relatively small number of cells and chondrocytes and an abundant extracellular matrix. The extracellular matrix contains collagen and a ground substance composed of carbohydrate and noncollagenous protein and has a high water content. The chondrocytes are responsible for the synthesis and degradation of matrix components and are therefore ultimately responsible for the biomechanical and biologic properties of articular cartilage. Collagen produced by the chondrocytes accounts for more than half the dry weight of adult articular cartilage (type II). Individual collagen fibers, with a characteristic periodicity of 640 Å, vary from 300 to 800 Å in diameter, depending on their distance from the articular surface.

The principal component of the ground substance produced by chondrocytes is a protein polysaccharide complex termed *proteoglycan.* The central organizing molecule of proteoglycan is hyaluronic acid. Numerous glycosaminoglycans (mainly chondroitin sulfate and keratin sulfate) are covalently bound from this central strand. Glycosaminoglycans carry considerable negative charge. The highly ordered array of electronegativity on the proteoglycan molecule interacts with large numbers of water molecules (small electric dipole). Approximately 75% of the wet weight of articular cartilage is water, the majority of which is structured by the electrostatic forces of the proteoglycan molecule.

The structure of articular cartilage varies relative to its distance from the free surface. For purposes of description, the tissue has been subdivided into zones that run parallel to the articular surface. Electron microscopy of the free surface reveals a dense network of collagen fibers (40 to 120 Å in diameter) that is arranged tangentially to the load-bearing surface and at approximately right angles to each other. This dense, mat-like arrangement, the lamina obscurans, is acellular.

Zone 1 contains large bundles of collagen fibers that are approximately 340 Å thick and lie parallel to the joint surface and at right angles to each other (Fig. 23-3).[156] This zone, the lamina splendins, has little or no intervening ground substance and contains the highest density of collagen. Chondrocytes in zone 1 are ellipsoid in shape and oriented parallel to the articular surface. They show little electron microscopic evidence of metabolic activity.

In zone 2, the collagen consists of individual, randomly oriented fibers of varying diameter. The chondrocytes in zone 2 tend to be more spherical and larger than those of zone 1; their abundant mitochondria and extensive endoplasmic reticulum suggest greater metabolic activity. The proteoglycan-collagen ratio in zone 2 is much higher than that near the surface.

In zone 3, the collagen fibers are thicker, often in the range of 1400 Å, and tend to form a more orderly

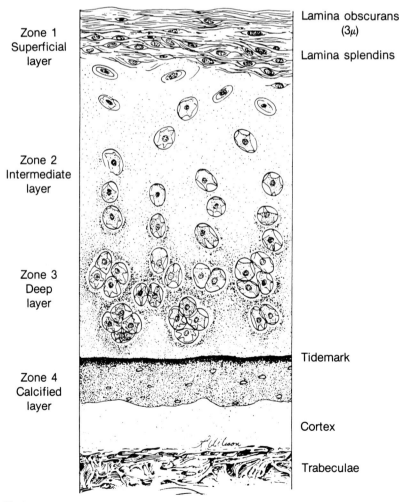

Zone 1
Superficial
layer

Zone 2
Intermediate
layer

Zone 3
Deep
layer

Zone 4
Calcified
layer

Lamina obscurans
(3μ)

Lamina splendins

Tidemark

Cortex

Trabeculae

■ **Figure 23-3**
Zones of adult articular cartilage. *(Modified from Turek SL: Orthopaedics: Principles and Their Application. Philadelphia: JB Lippincott, 1977.)*

meshwork that lies radial to the articular surface. The chondrocytes in zone 3 are larger and tend to be arranged in columns, often appearing in groups of two to eight cells. The cells are noted to have enlarged Golgi complexes, many mitochondria, and an extensively developed endoplasmic reticulum, thus indicating a high degree of metabolic activity.

Bone is a composite structure that incorporates calcium hydroxyapatite crystals in a collagen matrix grossly similar to synthetic composites or to partially crystalline polymers. Devitalized bone provides a passive substratum for bacterial colonization and ultimate incorporation of its proteinaceous and mineral constituents as bacterial metabolites.[70] S. aureus binds to bone sialoprotein, a glycoprotein found in joints, and it produces chondrocyte proteases that hydrolyze synovial tissue.[138]

CLASSIFICATION

Intra-articular sepsis may be classified in order of pathogenesis and frequency as (1) directly hematogenous, (2) secondary to contiguous spread from osteomyelitis, or (3) secondary to trauma, surgery, or intra-articular injection (Fig. 23–4 and Table 23–1). Most joint infections are caused by hematogenous spread, although direct contamination is not uncommon with trauma. Inoculation of the joint with bacteria can occur in association with

TABLE 23–1. Classification of Osteomyelitis and Intra-articular Sepsis
Hematogenous
Contiguous spread
Osteomyelitis
Soft tissue sepsis
Vascular insufficiency
Direct inoculation
Trauma with or without a foreign body or biomaterials
Surgery with or without a foreign body or biomaterials

intra-articular injection of steroids, local anesthetics, or synthetic joint fluid. Infection rates after arthroscopy are also low and range from 0.4% to 3.4%.[19] Armstrong and Bolding[7] reported that sepsis following arthroscopy can be associated with inadequate arthroscope disinfection and the use of intraoperative intra-articular corticosteroids.

Osteomyelitis of the humerus may spread intra-articularly, depending on the age of the patient, the type of infecting organism, and the severity of the infection. Osteomyelitis of the clavicle or scapula is uncommon, although it can occur after surgery and internal fixation, from retained shrapnel fragments, or in heroin addicts.[23,94,103,145,170] Brancos and colleagues reported that S. aureus and P. aeruginosa were the etiologic agents in 75% and 11% of episodes of septic arthritis in heroin addicts.[22] The sternoclavicular joint was involved more commonly than the shoulder joint. Septic arthritis of the shoulder has been reported by Chaudhuri and associates after mastectomy and radiotherapy for breast carcinoma.[29] Lymphedema was present in all cases. The infection had a subacute onset in all cases, and delay in diagnosis led to destruction of the joint in all but one patient.

Hematogenous osteomyelitis, though common in children,[109] is uncommon in adults until the sixth decade or later and is usually associated with a compromised immune system. Intravenous drug use is associated with the development of osteomyelitis in adults. Direct spread from wounds or foreign bodies, including total joint and internal fixation devices, is the most common etiology for shoulder sepsis in adults. Gowans and Granieri have noted the relationship between intra-articular injection of hydrocortisone acetate and the subsequent development of septic arthritis.[64] Kelly and associates noted that two of their six patients had a history of multiple intra-articular injections of corticosteroid.[89] Ward and Goldner[163] reported that chronic disease was present in more than half of their 30 cases of glenohumeral pyarthrosis and that 4 cases were associated with ipsilateral forearm fistulas for arteriovenous dialysis. Soft tissue infection about the shoulder can also be manifested in the form of pyomyositis, sometimes occurring as a result of hematogenous spread.[42] Aglas and coworkers reported sternoclavicular joint arthritis as a complication of subclavian venous catheterization.[1] Their two patients responded to antibiotic treatment. Glenohumeral pyarthrosis has been observed after acupuncture.[92] Lossos and colleagues[99] reported that associated medical conditions were present in the majority of their patients with septic arthritis of the shoulder.

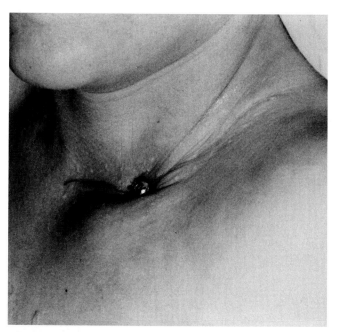

■ Figure 23–4
Internal fixation visible over the clavicle. The patient had a clavicular nonunion that was treated by internal fixation and bone grafting. An infection developed and resulted in wound breakdown and exposure of the internal fixation. The patient was treated by removal of the internal fixation and dressing changes. The wound healed, without recurrence of drainage over a 6-year period. Infection is not uncommon in the area of the clavicle and the acromioclavicular joint because of the thin soft tissue envelope that overlies the clavicle and the acromioclavicular joint.

PATHOGENIC MECHANISMS OF SEPTIC ARTHRITIS AND OSTEOMYELITIS

Surfaces as Substrata for Bacterial Colonization

The pathogenesis of bone and joint infections is related, in part, to preferential adhesive colonization of inert substrata whose surfaces are not integrated with healthy tissue composed of living cells and intact extracellular polymers, such as the articular surface of joints or damaged bone (Fig. 23–5).[20,70,76,137,165] Almost all natural biologic surfaces are lined by cellular epithelium or endothelium. The exceptions are intra-articular cartilage and the surface of teeth. Mature enamel is the only human tissue that is totally acellular; it is primarily composed of inorganic hydroxyapatite crystals (96% by weight), with a small amount of water (3%) and organic matrix (<1%).[8] Proteins in the organic matrix are distributed between the hydroxyapatite crystals and form a framework that strengthens the enamel by decreasing its tendency to fracture or separate. These proteins are unique among mineralized tissue because they are not a fibrous collagen protein like that found in bone, dentin, and cementum or in cartilage but are similar to the keratin family of proteins.[8]

Cartilage and enamel are readily colonized by bacteria because they lack the protection afforded by natural desquamation or by intact extracapsular polysaccharides that is provided by an active cellular layer. Their acellular surfaces are similar to many of those in nature for which bacteria have developed colonizing mechanisms. Certain strains of *S. aureus* adhere to specific sites on collagen fibrils, a process that is mediated by specific surface receptor proteins. Dissimilarities in surface structure are probably responsible for the specificity of colonization of bacterial species on these surfaces.

Enamel is mostly crystalline and inorganic, and cartilage is organic and noncrystalline. Enamel contains no collagen, whereas collagen is ubiquitous in cartilage and bone. Because it contains collagen receptors, *S. aureus* is the natural colonizer of cartilage, not enamel.[78,149] The specificity of colonization is also modulated in part by lectins and by host-derived synovial fluid, blood, and serum, conditioning films of protein, and polysaccharide macromolecules.

Whereas colonization of teeth by *Streptococcus mutans* and other organisms is a natural polymicrobial process and may be symbiotic or slowly destructive, bacterial colonization of articular cartilage is unnatural and rapidly destructive. The acellular cartilage matrix and inanimate biomaterial surfaces offer no resistance to colonization by *S. aureus* and *S. epidermidis*, respectively. The invasion and gradual destruction of cartilage observed over time support clinical observations of the course of untreated septic arthritis (Fig. 23–6).[78,140,141] The acellular cartilaginous surfaces of joints are particularly vulnerable to sepsis because they allow direct exposure to bacteria from open trauma, surgical procedures, or hematogenous spread. This mechanism parallels previous observations on the mechanism of osteomyelitis that suggest that adhesion of bacteria to dead bone or cartilage (surfaces not protected by living cells) via receptors and extracellular polysaccharides is a factor in pathogenesis.[70,143]

Intra-articular Sepsis

The articular cavity is a potential dead space that can provide a favorable environment for bacterial growth. In this avascular and relatively acellular space, host defense mechanisms are at a disadvantage. Synovial cells are not actively antibacterial, although they are somewhat

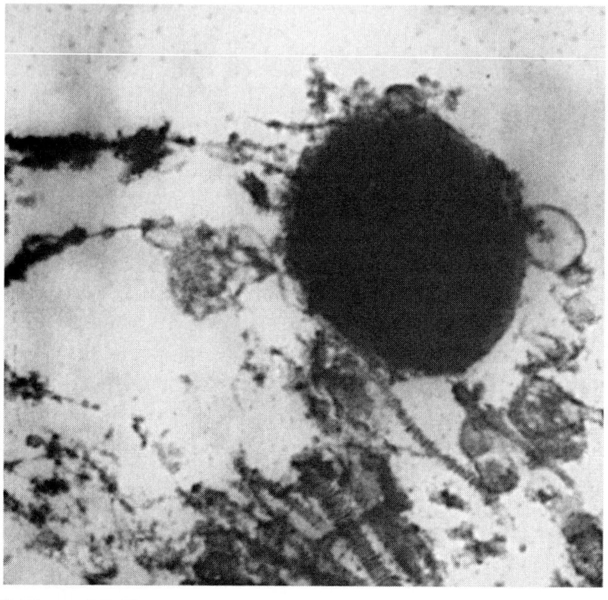

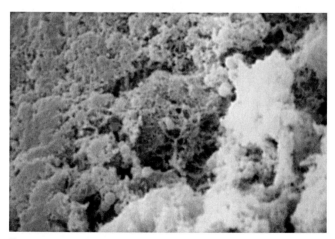

■ **Figure 23–5**
Photoelectromicrograph of rabbit articular cartilage illustrating direct contact of bacteria with collagen fiber. *(From Voytek A, Gristina AG, Barth E, et al: Staphylococcal adhesion to collagen in intra-articular sepsis. Biomaterials 9:107-110, 1988.)*

■ **Figure 23–6**
A photoelectromicrograph of articular cartilage at 7 days demonstrates destructive changes occurring beneath matrix-enclosed cocci. *(From Voytek A, Gristina AG, Barth E, et al: Staphylococcal adhesion to collagen in intra-articular sepsis. Biomaterials 9:107-110, 1988.)*

phagocytic. White blood cells must be delivered to the area and lack a surface for active locomotion. Under such conditions it is expected that phagocytic action is impaired, especially against encapsulated organisms.

Spontaneous intra-articular sepsis of the shoulder is caused by random hematogenous bacterial seeding. The synovial vasculature is abundant, and the vessels lack a limiting basement membrane. Bacteremia, especially with *Neisseria gonorrhoeae,* increases the risk of intra-articular spread. Contiguous spread from adjacent and intracapsular metaphyseal osteomyelitis also occurs. Surgery, arthroscopy, total joint replacement, aspirations, and steroid injections can also result in direct inoculation of bacteria into the intra-articular space. The presence of foreign bodies from trauma or after surgery (stainless steel, chrome cobalt alloys, ultra-high-molecular-weight polyethylene, and methylmethacrylate) increases the possibility of infection by providing a foreign body nidus for colonization and thereby allowing antibiotic-resistant colonization to occur.[68,70] The presence of a foreign body also lowers the size of the inoculant required for sepsis and perturbs host defense mechanisms.

Septic arthritis of the shoulder most frequently involves the glenohumeral joint. The acromioclavicular and sternoclavicular joints are occasionally infected in specific patient groups or after steroid injections for arthritis. Direct contamination from open wounds is also possible. Sternoclavicular sepsis is more common in drug addicts and usually involves gram-negative organisms, specifically, *P. aeruginosa.* Involvement of *S. aureus, Escherichia coli, Brucella,* and *N. gonorrhoeae* has also been reported.

Septic arthritis of the shoulder represents up to 14% of all septic arthritis cases.[105] In earlier studies, the incidence was 3.4%.[89] A more elderly population, increased trauma, and the common use of articular and periarticular steroids may be factors in this epidemiology (Fig. 23–7). The primary causal organism of shoulder sepsis is *S. aureus.* Sepsis in immunocompromised patients may be polyarticular as well as polymicrobial. Ten percent of cases of septic arthritis involve more than one joint, and such involvement is likely to occur in children.

Osteomyelitis

Hematogenous osteomyelitis accounts for 80% to 90% of cases of osteomyelitis in children. Contiguous osteomyelitis is more common in adults and occurs as a result of surgery and direct inoculation. In persons older than 50 years, contiguous osteomyelitis and disease related to vascular insufficiency are predominant.

Osteomyelitis is usually caused by one organism in children and by mixed organisms (*S. aureus* and gram-negative and anaerobic bacteria) in adults. Of the bones of the shoulder, the humerus is most frequently involved in osteomyelitis. The clavicle is occasionally involved in drug addicts as a result of hematogenous spread. The scapula is rarely involved; infection usually occurs by direct inoculation or contiguous spread (Table 23–2).

Epps and associates[43] reviewed 15 patients who had sickle cell disease and osteomyelitis affecting 30 bones. *S.*

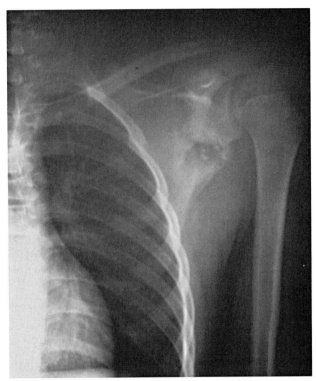

■ **Figure 23–7**
Staphylococcal osteomyelitis of the scapula secondary to closed trauma and hematologic seeding with abscess formation. The shoulder joint is not involved. *(Courtesy of the Department of Radiology, Wake Forest University Medical Center, Winston-Salem, NC.)*

TABLE 23–2.   Frequency of Joint Involvement in Infectious Arthritis (%)*

Joint	Bacterial (Suppurative)		Mycobacterial§	Viral
	Children†	Adults‡		
Knee	41	48	24	60
Hip	23	24	20	4
Ankle	14	7	12	30
Elbow	12	11	8	20
Wrist	4	7	20	55
Shoulder	4	15	4	5
Interphalangeal and metacarpal	1.4	1	12	75
Sternoclavicular	0.4	8	0	0
Sacroiliac	0.4	2	0	0

*More than one joint may be involved; therefore, the percentage exceeds 100%.
†Compiled from Nelson and Koontz[114] and Jackson and Nelson.[83]
‡Compiled from Kelly and colleagues,[91] Argen and colleagues,[5] and Gifford and associates.[58]
§Compiled from Smith and Sanford[139] and Medical Staff Conference.[106]
From Mandell L, Douglas KG Jr, and Bennett JE (eds): Principles and Practice of Infectious Diseases, 2nd ed. New York: John Wiley, 1985, p 698.

aureus was isolated on culture of specimens of bone from 8 of the 15 patients, *Salmonella* from 6, and *Proteus mirabilis* from 1. Accordingly, it appears that *Salmonella* is not always the principal causative organism of osteomyelitis in patients who have sickle cell disease.

MICROBIAL ADHESION AND INTRA-ARTICULAR SEPSIS

An understanding of microbial adhesion is required for complete clinical and therapeutic insight into joint sepsis. Studies of bacteria in marine ecosystems indicate that they tend to adhere in colonies to surfaces or substrata. The number of bacteria that can exist in a given environment is directly related to stress and nutrient supply.[169] Because surface attachment rather than a floating or suspension population is a favored survival strategy, it is the state of the major portion of bacterial biomasses in most natural environments[126] and is a common mode of microbial life in humans.

Bacterial attachment to surfaces is influenced by proteinaceous bacterial receptors and by an extracapsular exopolysaccharide substance within which bacteria aggregate and multiply.[34] Once bacteria have developed a biofilm-enclosed, adhesive mode of growth, they become more resistant to biocides,[126] antiseptics,[104] antibiotics,[63] antagonistic environmental factors,[34] and host defense systems.[10,63,165] Free-floating, nonadhesive bacteria or microbes that lack a well-developed outer layer or exopolysaccharide are more susceptible to host-clearing mechanisms[10,133] and lower concentrations of antibacterial agents.[63]

Gibbons and van Houte first described the significance of this adhesive phenomenon in the formation of dental plaque.[57] In diseases such as gonococcal urethritis,[154] cystic fibrosis,[168] and endocarditis, bacterial colonization and propagation occur along endothelial and epithelial surfaces. The association between bacterial growth on biomaterial surfaces and infection was first described in 1963.[72] Microbial adhesion and associated phenomena also explain the foreign body effect, in which susceptibility to infection is increased in the presence of a foreign body. Infections centered on foreign bodies are resistant to host defenses and treatment and tend to persist until the infecting locus is removed.[70] Foreign bodies include implanted biomaterials, fixation materials, prosthetic monitoring and delivery devices, traumatically acquired penetrating debris and bone fragments,[67] and compromised tissues.[67,68,70]

Molecular Mechanisms in Adhesion

Initial bacterial attachment or adhesion depends on the long-range physical forces characteristic of the bacterium, the fluid interface, and the substratum. Specific irreversible adhesion, which occurs after initial attachment, is based on time-dependent adhesin-receptor interactions and the synthesis of extracapsular polysaccharide.[85] Biomaterial surfaces present sites for environmental interactions that are derived from their atomic structures (Fig. 23-8).[153] Metallic alloys have a thin (100 to 200 Å) oxide

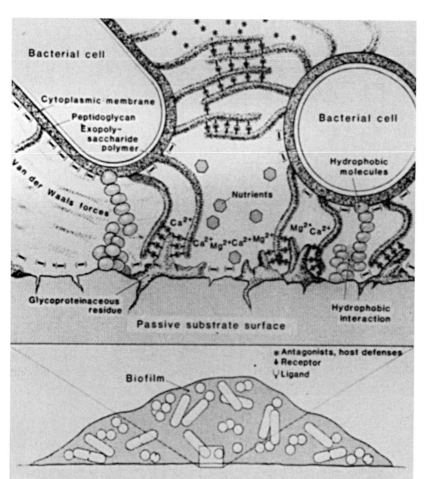

■ **Figure 23–8**
Mechanism of bacterial adherence. At specific distances, the initial repelling forces between like charges on the surfaces of bacteria and substrate are overcome by attracting van der Waals forces, and there are hydrophobic interactions between molecules. Under appropriate conditions, extensive development of exopolysaccharide polymers occurs and allows ligand-receptor interaction and proteinaceous binding of bacteria to the substrate. *(From Gristina AG, Oga M, Webb LX, and Hobgood CD: Adherent bacterial colonization in the pathogenesis of osteomyelitis. Science 228:990-993, 1985. Copyright 1985 by the American Association for the Advancement of Science.)*

layer that is the true biologic interface.[2,87] The surfaces of polymers and metals are modified by texture, manufacturing processes, trace chemicals, and debris and also by host-derived ionic, polysaccharide, and glycoproteinaceous constituents (conditioning films). The finite surface structure of conditioning film in a human is specific for each individual biomaterial, type of tissue cell, and local host environment.[2,9] Biomaterial surfaces may also act as catalytic hot spots for molecular and cellular activities.[2,87] In addition, tissue cells and matrix macromolecules provide substrata for bacterial colonization. Bacteria have developed adhesins or receptors that interact with tissue cell surface structures (Fig. 23–9).

Subsequent to or concomitant with initial attachment, fimbrial adhesins *(E. coli)* and substratum receptors may interact, as in bacteria–to–tissue cell pathogenesis or for the production of glycoproteinaceous conditioning films that immediately coat implants.[9] A pivotal factor is the production and composition of the extracellular polysaccharide polymer, which tends to act like a glue.[169] After colony maturation, cells on the periphery of the expanding biomass may separate or disaggregate and disperse, a process that is moderated by colony size, nutrient conditions, and hemodynamic or mechanical shear forces; in natural environments, disaggregation is a survival strategy. In humans, however, it is involved in the pathogenesis of septic emboli. Disaggregation (dispersion) and its parameters may explain the phenomenon of intermittent or short-term "bacterial showers" or disseminated bacterial emboli.

BACTERIAL PATHOGENS

The following organisms are involved in septic arthritis and osteomyelitis of the shoulder and are listed in order of frequency.[89]

Bacteria:
S. aureus
S. epidermidis, Streptococcus group B
E. coli, P. aeruginosa, Haemophilus influenzae type B
N. gonorrhoeae, Mycobacterium tuberculosis
Salmonella and *Pneumococcus* species
Yersinia enterocolitica[152]

Reported Associations:
Rheumatoid arthritis—*Listeria monocytogenes*[157]
Renal transplant—*Aspergillus fumigatus*[50]
Newborns and pregnant women—Group B β-hemolytic *Streptococcus agalactiae*[53]
Lymphedema—*Pasteurella multocida.*[45]
Systemic lupus erythematosus, septic arthritis—*Mycobacterium xenopi*[127]
Chronic vesicoureteral reflux—*E. coli*[41]

Fungi:
Actinomyces
Blastomyces
Coccidioides
Candida albicans
Sporothrix schenckii

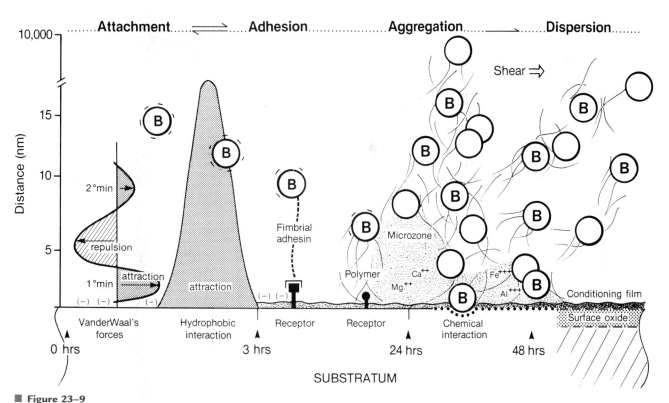

■ **Figure 23–9**

Molecular sequence in bacterial (B) attachment, adhesion, aggregation, and dispersion at the substratum surface. A number of possible interactions may occur, depending on the specificities of the bacteria or substratum system (graphics, nutrients, contaminants, macromolecules, species, and materials). *(From Gristina AG: Biomaterial-centered infection: Microbial adhesion versus tissue integration. Science 237:1558-1595, 1987. Copyright 1987 by the American Association for the Advancement of Science.)*

H. influenzae type B is most frequently isolated in children younger than 2 years and is rarely found in children older than 5 years. Group B *Streptococcus*, gram-negative bacilli, and *S. aureus* are common infecting organisms in the neonatal period. *S. aureus* is most common in adults, and *N. gonorrhoeae* is common in adults younger than 30 years.[55] Hemolytic streptococci are the most common streptococci in adults and children. Hematogenous septic arthritis in infants is primarily streptococcal, whereas hospital-acquired infections are primarily staphylococcal but may also feature *Candida* and gram-negative organisms, especially in infants.[132] Lavy and coauthors[96] reported on 19 children younger than 2 years with *Salmonella* septic arthritis of the shoulder. The authors concluded that low nutritional status was a factor in the development of bacteremia in their patients.

Gram-negative bacilli such as *E. coli* and *P. aeruginosa* are found in approximately 15% of joints, especially in association with urinary tract infection, diabetes,[11] or debilitating disease. *M. tuberculosis* involves the knee, hip, ankle, and wrist more frequently than the shoulder. *Mycobacterium marinum* is found in marine environments. The occurrence of *M. tuberculosis* is rare today.[14,145] *Blastomyces* usually spreads from osteomyelitis to the intra-articular space. *C. albicans* may spread via the hematogenous route in debilitated patients or directly from steroid injections. Pneumococcal septic arthritis seems to be predominantly a disease affecting the elderly.[16]

S. aureus is often the major pathogen in biometal, bone, joint, and soft tissue infections and is the most common pathogen isolated in osteomyelitis when damaged bone or cartilage acts as a substratum.[70] The predominance of *S. aureus* in adult intra-articular sepsis[119] may be explained by its ubiquity as a tissue pathogen seeded from remote sites, its natural invasiveness and toxicity, and its receptors for collagen, fibronectin, fibrinogen, and laminin. *S. epidermidis* is most frequently involved when the biomaterial surface is a polymer or when a polymer is a component of a complex device (extended-wear contact lenses,[137] vascular prostheses,[165] an artificial heart,[65] and total joint prostheses).

Studies of chronic adult osteomyelitis have revealed polymicrobial infection in more than two thirds of cases.[25,70] The most common pathogens isolated have included *S. aureus*, *S. epidermidis*, and *Pseudomonas*, *Enterococcus*, *Streptococcus*, *Bacillus*, and *Proteus* species. Polymicrobial infections therefore appear to be an important feature of substratum-induced infections, are probably present more often than realized, and can also be a feature of chronic intra-articular sepsis and sinus formation.

In summary, *S. aureus* is the most common organism in septic infections and is usually spread via hematogenous seeding. *S. epidermidis* is the principal organism in biomaterial-related infections, especially those centered on polymers. Mixed (polymicrobial), gram-negative, and anaerobic infections are probably more common than past studies have indicated and are frequently associated with open wounds and sinus tracts.

CLINICAL FINDINGS

Symptoms and Signs

Pain, loss of motion, and effusion are early signs of infection. Shoulder effusion is difficult to detect and often missed. Motion is painful, and the arm is adducted and internally rotated. Radiographs may show a widened glenohumeral joint space and later signs of osteomyelitis (Fig. 23–10). Systemic signs include fever, leukocytosis, and changes in the sedimentation rate. The symptoms of immunosuppressed and rheumatoid patients may be muted.

The sternoclavicular joint may be involved, and such involvement should be suspected in patients younger than 50 years who have unilateral enlargement without trauma. Gonococcal and staphylococcal infections have been reported. Intravenous drug addicts are susceptible to infection by gram-negative organisms, especially *P. aeruginosa* and *Serratia marcescens*. The acromioclavicular joint is rarely involved in sepsis but may be contaminated by steroid injections. Wound infection is not uncommon after surgical resection of the distal part of the clavicle for osteoarthritis, probably because of the proximity of the joint to the overlying skin and lack of an intervening muscle layer.

Gabriel and colleagues reported a 5-week-old male infant who had a brachial plexus neuropathy and paralysis of the upper extremity secondary to septic arthritis of the glenohumeral joint and osteomyelitis of the proximal part of the humerus.[51] They pointed out that pseudoparalysis of a limb associated with sepsis is a well-documented phenomenon. Similarly, muscular spasm associated with pain caused by infection can lead to apparent weakness. True nerve paralysis associated with osteomyelitis is uncommon, and documentation by electrodiagnostic studies is rare. Permanent weakness

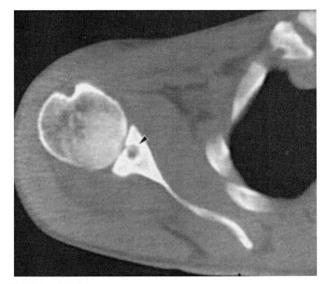

■ **Figure 23–10**

Staphylococcal osteomyelitis of the scapula. The *arrow* indicates an abscess secondary to infection caused by intra-articular steroid injection. *(Courtesy of Mark Warburton, M.D., High Point, NC.)*

persisted in their patient even though the glenohumeral joint and proximal part of the humerus were surgically drained. Possible causes of plexus neuropathy associated with infection include ischemic neuropathy from thrombophlebitis of the vasa nervorum, arterial embolism, hyperergic or hypersensitivity reactions, and local compression from abscess formation. Rankin and Rycken reported bilateral dislocations of the proximal end of the humerus as a result of septic arthritis.[123] Miron and colleagues have also reported transient brachial plexus palsy associated with suppurative arthritis of the shoulder.[108]

Total Shoulder Replacement

Sepsis after total joint replacement of the shoulder is relatively uncommon because of prophylactic antibiotic use and the excellent blood supply of the surrounding soft tissues. Symptoms of infection include pain, loss of motion, and subluxation. Pain relief is so universal after total shoulder replacement that infection should be suspected if pain or radiolucency around the cement mantle, or both, are present.

Rheumatoid Arthritis

Patients with chronic rheumatoid arthritis are susceptible to spontaneous septic arthritis.[73,88] Because the active destructive process of the rheumatoid arthritis masks the septic condition, detection of infection is often delayed. The onset of septic arthritis should be suspected when the clinical course of a rheumatoid patient worsens acutely, especially if the disease is long term. When infection is present, the patient experiences a sudden aggravation of pain and swelling and increased temperature in the joint. Sudden chills may also occur. The physician should emphasize to patients with chronic rheumatoid arthritis (and to other caregivers) that a sudden exacerbation of symptoms warrants investigation.

Differential Diagnosis

Roentgenograms are not very useful for early diagnosis because septic arthritis does not significantly alter the bone destruction attributable to rheumatoid arthritis and because bone and joint radiographic changes are delayed. Other acute arthritic disorders, including gout, pseudogout, rheumatic fever, juvenile rheumatoid arthritis, neuropathic arthropathy,[100] and the oligoarthritic syndromes, may imitate or mask sepsis. Trauma and tumors may cause adjacent joint effusions and must be considered.

LABORATORY EVALUATION

Culture plus analysis of synovial fluid is critical for diagnosis. Aspiration of the joint should always be performed when sepsis is suspected. X-ray control of aspiration is indicated if the approach is difficult because of total joint replacements. Injection of saline or a simultaneous arthrogram of the glenohumeral joint may be helpful in certain cases. When the results of culture are negative and the diagnosis is difficult to make, an arthroscopic biopsy can be useful. A synovial biopsy and culture for acid-fast organisms and fungi should be performed in patients with chronic monarticular arthritis, especially those with tenosynovitis.

Viral infection must be considered when bacteria cannot be identified. Smith and Piercy report that viral arthritis is associated with rubella, parvovirus, mumps, hepatitis B, and lymphocytic choriomeningitis.[138] In a person with multiple joint involvement and systemic manifestations consistent with viral infection, serologic confirmation of the infection should be obtained because it is not usually possible to isolate the virus from joint fluid.

Synovial Fluid Analysis

If septic arthritis is suspected, synovial fluid should be examined. Septic arthritis is probable if the leukocyte count is usually more than 50,000 cells/mm³, the glucose level is low, and more than 75% of the cells are polymorphonuclear. These findings are beyond the range compatible with uncomplicated rheumatoid arthritis.[161] In bacterial infections, aspiration may yield 10 mL or more of fluid. Synovial joint fluid is usually opaque or brownish, turbid, and thick, but it may be serosanguineous in 15% of cases with poor mucin clot. Protein levels are elevated, primarily because of an elevated white blood cell count (usually greater than 50,000 and often as great as 100,000 and primarily composed of neutrophils).[161] Half of adults and a lower percentage of children will have a joint fluid glucose level that is 40 mg less than the level of glucose in serum drawn at the same time.[83,136,160] These findings are more common later in infection. Polymorphonuclear leukocytes are dominant (90%). Counts over 100,000/mm³ are typical of staphylococcal and acute bacterial infection. Monocytes are more predominant in mycobacterial infections. Rheumatoid, rheumatic, and crystalline joint diseases also elevate leukocytes, but the presence of these diseases does not exclude concomitant sepsis. Crystal examination is needed to rule out gout or pseudogout.

The results of Gram stain are positive approximately 50% of the time, but false-positive findings do occur.[159] Positive joint cultures occur in 90% of established bacterial septic arthritis cases and in 75% of patients with tubercular arthritis.[159] Blood cultures should also be obtained, and the results are positive in approximately 50% of patients with acute infection. Some prosthesis-centered infections are difficult to detect unless tissue biopsy samples are obtained and prepared for culture (Table 23–3).

Specimens should be taken for culture of gram-positive, gram-negative, aerobic, and anaerobic bacteria; mycobacteria; and fungi. The laboratory technique and choice of media should be based on the type of antibiotic given and the special nutrient requirements of suspected bacteria. The use of blood agar is routine; chocolate agar is the best medium for culturing *Neisseria* and *Haemophilus* species. Thayer-Martin media may be used to isolate gonococcal organisms, but because it contains vancomycin and colistin methanesulfonate, *Haemophilus* species or other

TABLE 23–3. Synovial Fluid Findings in Acute Pyogenic Arthritis

Joint Fluid Examination	Noninflammatory Fluids	Inflammatory Fluids	
		Noninfectious	Infectious
Color	Colorless, pale yellow	Yellow to white	Yellow
Turbidity	Clear, slightly turbid	Turbid	Turbid, purulent
Viscosity	Not reduced	Reduced	Reduced
Mucin clot	Tight clot	Friable	Friable
Cell count (per mm³)	200–1000	3000–10,000	10,000–100,000
Predominant cell type	Mononuclear	PMN	PMN
Synovial fluid–blood glucose ratio	0.8–1.0	0.5–0.8	<0.5
Lactic acid	Same as plasma	Higher than plasma	Often very high
Gram stain for organism	None	None	Positive*
Culture	Negative	Negative	Positive*

*In some cases, especially in gonococcal infection, no organisms may be demonstrated.
PMN, polymorphonuclear leukocyte.
From Schmid FR: Principles of diagnosis and treatment of bone and joint infections. *In* McCarty DJ (ed): Arthritis and Allied Conditions: A Textbook of Rheumatology. Philadelphia: Lea & Febiger, 1985, p 1638.

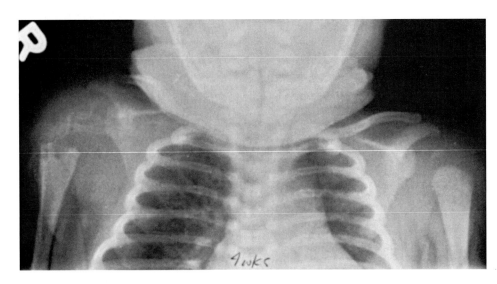

■ **Figure 23–11**
Septic arthritis of the right shoulder with destruction and widening of the proximal end of the humerus. Also note healing of a right clavicular fracture. Organism: β-hemolytic streptococci. (*Courtesy of the Department of Radiology, Wake Forest University Medical Center, Winston-Salem, NC.*)

mixed flora will not grow on it.[131] Sabouraud medium is specific for fungi. An egg-glycerol-potato and synthetic agar combination is used to culture mycobacteria.[131] Centrifugation is recommended for detection of mycobacteria (which are less frequently present) if sufficient fluid can be obtained. The magnitude of anaerobic septic arthritis has been underestimated in the past.[46]

Radiographic, Ultrasound, Computed Tomographic, Magnetic Resonance Imaging, and Isotope Techniques

Radiographs and CT scans of a septic shoulder may indicate changes ranging from widening to subluxation and from bone destruction to new bone formation (Figs. 23–11 to 23–13). Ultrasound is useful in assisting aspiration and in assessing the infected shoulder joints.[60] Positive technetium bone scanning has been reported in 75% to 100% of septic arthritis cases, but technetium, gallium, and indium scans are not always consistent.[56,107,171] Schmidt and colleagues found that the results of technetium bone scans performed in children with septic arthritis were frequently negative.[132] Indium scans may be more accurate indicators of sepsis, but conclusive data are lacking. Indium scintigraphy for osteomyelitis should be preceded by a positive result on a technetium scan. If the result of an indium scan is negative, infection is unlikely. A positive result on an indium scan increases the specificity of the diagnosis. Indium uptake should be evaluated against the normal reticuloendothelial background.[171] False-negative results can occur in neonates and during the acute phase of osteomyelitis.[54]

Gupta and Prezio found that the specificity of nuclear scintigraphy using ^{99m}Tc-phosphonates, ^{67}Ga-citrate or ^{111}In-labeled leukocytes for diagnosing musculoskeletal infection could be improved if two nucleotide studies were used in conjunction.[75] The main limitation of scintigraphic investigations is their limited spatial resolution, which makes the results inexact. Furthermore, such studies may take hours to days to complete.

CT is useful in identifying small early lytic lesions caused by osteomyelitis that might be obscured on ordinary radiographs. The diagnosis of sternoclavicular joint sepsis and clavicular osteomyelitis may be improved with CT because it overcomes the tissue overlap problem that

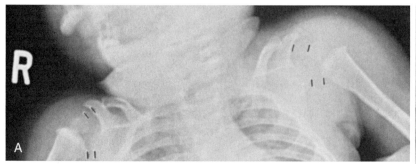

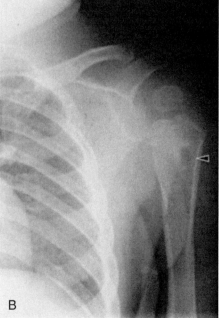

■ **Figure 23–12**
A, Early intra-articular sepsis of the left shoulder. Note the widening of the joint space (markers) in comparison to the opposite side. **B,** Late intra-articular sepsis. Note the radiolucent lesion and osteomyelitis of the proximal end of the humerus *(arrow)*. Organisms: *Staphylococcus epidermidis,* β-hemolytic streptococci, and *Bacillus subtilis.*

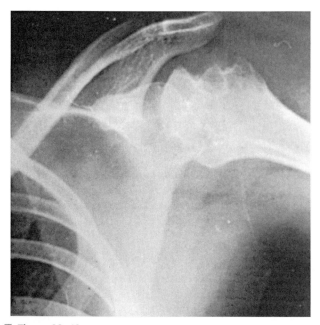

■ **Figure 23–13**
Cystic lesions in the humeral head consistent with tuberculosis sicca in a 19-year-old woman. *(From DePalma AF [ed]: Surgery of the Shoulder, 3rd ed. Philadelphia: JB Lippincott, 1983.)*

occurs with ordinary radiographs; however, CT does not offer much advantage in imaging the humerus. MRI may facilitate differentiation of acute from chronic osteomyelitis and may help detect evidence of active infection in the presence of chronic inflammation or post-traumatic lesions.[15,151] Early changes of osteomyelitis cause an accumulation of fluid, inflammatory cells, and exudate in the marrow and produce a focus of low signal intensity within bright, fatty marrow. In chronic osteomyelitis, large areas of abnormal or low signal on MRI may indicate an area of possible sequestration and

hyperemia, especially along sinus tracts.[35] Capsular distention of articular cartilage and fluid-filled spaces are clearly visible on MRI, as are damaged surfaces, loose bodies, and avascular regions. MRI can be sensitive in early detection and specific for the localization and identification of sequestra.[47,77,130] De Boeck and coworkers reported on the utility of MRI in detecting pyomyositis.[36] MRI was useful in excluding other pathologic processes such as infectious arthritis, osteomyelitis, hematoma, thrombophlebitis, and malignant tumor. MRI is helpful in pregnant patients because it provides a highly sensitive method of detecting skeletal infection without exposing the fetus to ionizing radiation. Ultrasound can also be used to advantage in defining abscess formation.[146] Widman and associates[166] report that ultrasound can be used to differentiate septic arthritis of the acromioclavicular joint from septic arthritis of the shoulder joint.

Hopkins and colleagues assessed the role of gadolinium-enhanced MRI in providing diagnostic information beyond that given by nonenhanced MRI in the evaluation of musculoskeletal infectious processes.[79] They found that gadolinium-enhanced MRI was a highly sensitive technique that was especially useful for distinguishing abscesses from surrounding cellulitis or myositis. Lack of contrast enhancement ruled out infection with a high degree of certainty. However, these authors point out that contrast enhancement cannot be used to reliably distinguish infectious from noninfectious inflammatory conditions. In their study, gadolinium-enhanced MRI was found to have very high sensitivity (89% to 100%) and accuracy (79% to 88%) in the diagnosis of various infectious lesions in the musculoskeletal system. However, its specificity (46% to 88%) was not as high. Tehranzadeh and coauthors reported on the use of MRI in diagnosing osteomyelitis.[151] In several comparative studies, MRI has been more advantageous in detecting the presence and determining the extent of osteomyelitis than have scintigraphy, CT, and conventional radiography.

COMPLICATIONS

Inadequately treated intra-articular sepsis or osteo-myelitis may result in recurrent infection, contiguous spread, bacteremia, distant septic emboli, anemia, septic shock, and death. Delayed diagnosis with adequate treatment may result in joint surface destruction, contractures, subluxation, arthritis, and growth aberrations (Fig. 23-14).[118] Inflammation, bacterial products, and lysosomal enzymes break down cartilage.[93] Within weeks, bacterial antigens stimulate destructive inflammation that may persist after the infection is treated. Bacterial endotoxins are chemotactic, and bacterial proteolytic enzymes further destroy surfaces. Increased intra-articular pressure also causes ischemia. In addition, thrombotic events are stimulated by burgeoning infection, with further destruction of the joint and adjacent bone. Long-term complications of chronic osteomyelitis can include amyloidosis, nephrotic syndrome, and epidermal carcinoma.

TREATMENT

Most clinicians agree that systemic antibiotic therapy should begin immediately after the diagnosis of septic arthritis, but there is less agreement on subsequent therapy. Repeated needle aspiration has been recommended as primary treatment[91,160]; however, the author believes that drainage by urgent arthroscopy or arthrotomy is the treatment of choice, especially for the shoulder.[86,124] Forward and Hunter[49] reported the use of a small arthroscope in the treatment of septic arthritis of the shoulder in infants. Stutz and colleagues[148] reported that septic arthritis in 78 joints (including 10 shoulders) could be treated with arthroscopic irrigation and systemic antibiotic therapy in 91% of affected joints. Jerosch and associates reported the successful treatment of septic arthritis by arthroscopy in 12 patients ranging in age from 4 to 57 years.[84]

In general, the literature suggests that treatment of septic arthritis by repeated needle aspiration and appropriate intravenous antibiotics may be adequate except for the hip. However, conclusive studies of initial surgical drainage versus needle aspiration are lacking. A retrospective study comparing 55 infected joints treated by needle aspiration with 18 joints treated surgically concluded that 60% of surgically treated patients had sequelae whereas 80% of medically treated patients recovered completely.[59] However, it must be noted that the only randomized prospective study comparing aspiration with arthrotomy[142] found no difference in outcome. These authors studied 61 children in Malawi with septic arthritis of the shoulder. Both groups received antibiotics for 6 weeks, and most of the infections were due to *Salmonella*.

Most orthopaedic surgeons believe that the anatomy of the shoulder and the nature of shoulder sepsis demand surgical treatment. Septic arthritis that does not rapidly and progressively respond to medical management should be surgically drained. Sternoclavicular infections in drug abusers usually involve bone and joint. For these patients, needle aspiration has not been useful in establishing the diagnosis. However, surgical drainage has been helpful in providing the pathogen. It also allows débridement of necrotic bone and permits drainage of abscesses, which are often present.[12,125]

Gelberman and associates reported a satisfactory outcome in 8 of 10 patients with septic arthritis of the shoulder when treatment was begun 4 weeks or less after the symptoms appeared.[55] Six of the eight satisfactory

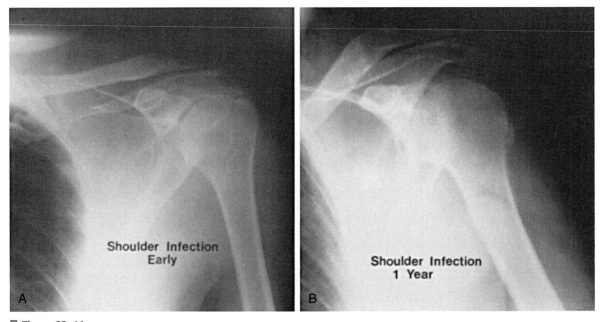

■ **Figure 23–14**
Hematogenous osteomyelitis secondary to intra-articular sepsis. **A,** Minimal radiolucency of the proximal part of the humerus 2 weeks after the probable onset of infection. **B,** After arthrotomy, antibiotic treatment, and resolution of infection, the radiograph reveals periosteal new bone formation and joint contracture. Organism: *Staphylococcus aureus*.

results from Gelberman's series were in patients who had infection with either *Streptococcus* or coagulase-negative *Staphylococcus*. Gelberman and coworkers attributed the poor results in eight patients to delay in diagnosis, although six of the poor results were in patients infected with *S. aureus*. Pfeiffenberger and Meiss[120] reported that in their series of 28 patients with bacterial infection of the shoulder, favorable results could be obtained only if the diagnosis was made early. Bettin and coworkers[17] found early diagnosis to be the most important factor determining the final outcome of septic arthritis in their 35 elderly patients.

Leslie and colleagues reviewed 18 cases of septic arthritis of the shoulder in adults.[98] The patients ranged in age from 42 to 89 years. All except one patient had at least one serious associated disease. Eight patients had an injection or aspiration of the shoulder before the development of their infection. The diagnosis was delayed in 17 of the 18 patients. At the time of admission to the hospital, the erythrocyte sedimentation rate was always elevated but body temperature and the white blood cell count were not. After treatment, the functional result was usually poor. Only five patients regained forward flexion to 90 degrees or more. Eight patients had no active motion of the glenohumeral joint, and two patients died. Arthrotomy appeared to have resulted in a better outcome than repeated aspiration did.

Smith and Piercy reported that the characteristics of patients with bacterial arthritis for whom a poor outcome is expected include age older than 60 years, preexisting rheumatoid arthritis, infection in the shoulder, duration of symptoms before treatment of longer than 1 week, involvement of more than four joints, and persistently positive cultures after a 7-day course of appropriate antibiotic therapy.[138]

Intra-articular sepsis should be treated in a timely manner.[141] Variables that influence the selection of treatment methods include the duration of infection, host immune status, types of infecting organisms, and the presence of foreign bodies or adjacent osteomyelitis. The most critical factors in treatment are the infecting organism and the presence of a foreign body.

Osteomyelitis of the proximal metaphysis may either precede or be secondary to septic arthritis of the glenohumeral joint (Fig. 23–15). Therefore, drilling of the metaphysis has been recommended for pediatric septic glenohumeral arthritis to rule out osteomyelitis and allow adequate decompression of the bone.

Leslie and coworkers noted that five of six patients with septic arthritis who had rotator cuff tears had a marked discrepancy between active and passive shoulder motion.[98] They thought that the poor functional results recorded in these six patients may have been more a reflection of the rotator cuff tear than damage to the articular cartilage as a result of infection. Septic arthritis following rotator cuff surgery may rarely result in exposure of the humeral head and sinus formation. In such cases, interposition of a muscle flap may be required, as has been described for the closure of infected sternotomy wounds.[44]

Immobilization is usually recommended for septic arthritis. However, Salter and colleagues' study of septic arthritis in a rabbit model indicated that the use of continuous passive motion was superior to immobilization or intermittent active motion.[129] Possible explanations for these results include prevention of bacterial adhesion, enhanced diffusion of nutrients, improved clearance of lysosomal enzymes and debris from the infected joints, and stimulation of chondrocytes to synthesize the various components of the matrix.

The majority of children do well after treatment of septic shoulder arthritis. In a study of nine children with glenohumeral arthritis, Schmidt and associates suggested surgical treatment with exploration of the biceps tendon sheath.[132] Growth center damage is possible. Lejman and colleagues[97] reported that almost all patients had reduced motion as a sequela of septic arthritis occurring during the first 18 months of life. Although only 7% of the humeral heads were normal in their series of 42 patients, range of motion could not be predicted from the shape of the humeral head.

The prognosis for adults with septic arthritis of the shoulder is poor, but shoulders treated soon after the onset of symptoms may do well. Poor results are associated with delayed diagnosis, virulent (gram-negative) infecting organisms, persistent pain, drainage, osteomyelitis, and destruction of the joint. Bos and coworkers concluded that in their series of eight children who had neonatal septic arthritis of the shoulder, early diagnosis and treatment were associated with a more favorable outcome.[21]

Gonococcal septic arthritis may be polyarticular. Fever is low grade, with temperatures usually below 102° F. Articular and periarticular structures become swollen, stiff, and painful, followed by desquamation of skin over the joints. During septicemia, a macular rash or occasionally a vesicular rash occurs in one third of patients, but such rash can also be caused by *Neisseria meningitidis*, *Haemophilus*, and *Streptobacillus*.[26,135] Organisms are not common in joint fluid and, therefore, are not isolated in most cases. The general picture of gonococcal septic arthritis is less acute than that of staphylococcal infection. Gonococcal arthritis responds well to systemic antibiotic therapy and needle aspiration; however, in refractory cases, arthrocentesis may be required.

The antimicrobial agents used to treat joint infections generally achieve intra-articular levels equal to or greater than serum levels, except for erythromycin and gentamicin (Table 23–4). Accordingly, intra-articular antibiotics are not generally advocated. In osteomyelitis, antibiotic penetration into bone is unreliable.[116] Clindamycin achieves higher bone levels than cephalothin or methicillin does. When healthy (nonsequestrated) bone in children is being treated, delivery of antibiotics to the infected site is likely. The opposite situation exists in adults, the aged, vascularly compromised patients, and patients with chronic osteomyelitis, sequestration, and sinus formation. Animal studies have suggested that antibiotic combinations (e.g., oxacillin and aminoglycosides) may be more effective in osteomyelitis.[116] The quinolone group of antibiotics may be useful because of its broad spectrum of activity against staphylococci, *Pseudomonas* species, and gram-negative bacteria.[38] These agents achieve excellent local levels in living and dead bone. The emergence of mutant strains may occur but can

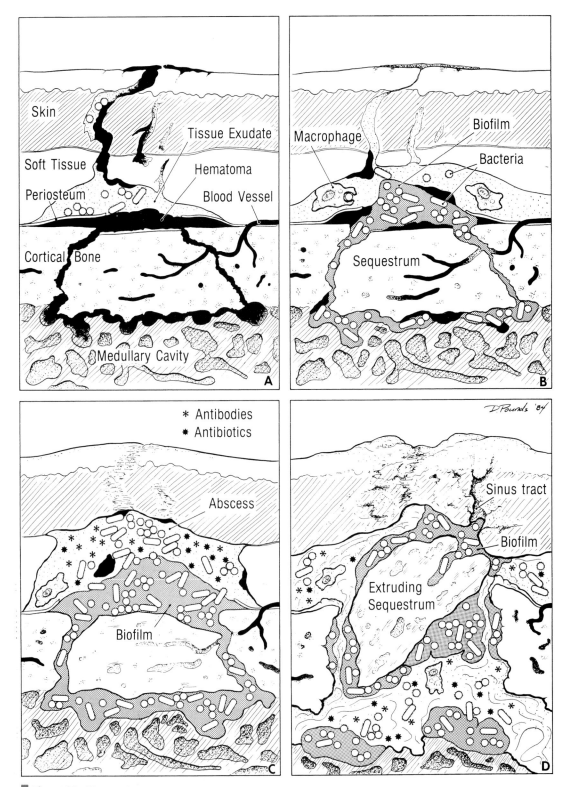

■ **Figure 23–15**

The sequence of pathogenesis in osteomyelitis. **A,** The initial trauma produces soft tissue destruction and bone fragmentation, as well as wound contamination by bacteria. In closed wounds, contamination may occur by hematogenous seeding. **B,** As the infection progresses, bacterial colonization occurs within a protective exopolysaccharide biofilm. The biofilm is particularly abundant on the devitalized bone fragment, which acts as a passive substratum for colonization. **C,** Host defenses are mobilized against the infection but are unable to penetrate or be effective in the presence of the biofilm. **D,** Progressive inflammation and abscess formation eventually result in the development of a sinus tract and, in some cases, ultimate extrusion of the sequestrum that is the focus of the resistant infection. *(From Gristina AG, Barth E, and Webb LX: Microbial adhesion and the pathogenesis of biomaterial-centered infections. In Gustilo RB, Gruninger RP, and Tsukayama DT [eds]: Orthopaedic Infection. Diagnosis and Treatment. Philadelphia: WB Saunders, 1989, pp 3-25.)*

TABLE 23-4.   Empirical Antibiotic Therapy for Septic Arthritis

Age	Preferred	Alternative
<2 Months: no organism on stain	Oxacillin and aminoglycoside	Cefazolin and aminoglycoside
2 Months to 5 years: no organism	Nafcillin and chloramphenicol	Cefuroxime
5–15 Years: no organism	Nafcillin or oxacillin	Cefazolin or vancomycin
>40 Years: no organism	Nafcillin ± aminoglycoside	Cefazolin ± aminoglycoside
<2 Months: gram-positive cocci	Oxacillin or nafcillin	Cephalothin or cephapirin
<2 Months to 40 years: gram-negative bacilli	Aminoglycoside	Cefotaxime
>2 Months: gram-positive cocci	Nafcillin or oxacillin	Cefazolin, cephalothin, vancomycin, clindamycin
2 Months to 5 years: gram-negative coccobacilli	Cefotaxime or ampicillin and chloramphenicol	Chloramphenicol alone; trimethoprim-sulfamethoxazole
15–40 Years: gram-negative cocci	Treat for *Neisseria gonorrhoeae*	
>40 Years: gram-negative bacilli	Ticarcillin plus aminoglycoside	Cefotaxime ± aminoglycoside

From American Medical Association, Division of Drugs and Toxicology: Anti-microbial therapy for common infectious diseases. *In* Drug Evaluations Annual 1995. Chicago: American Medical Association, 1995, pp 1277–1282.

be reduced by intelligent use of quinolones in combination with other antibiotics.

Mader and coauthors reported that antibiotic selection should be based on in vitro sensitivity testing and that the drug exhibiting the highest bactericidal activity with the least toxicity and lowest cost should be chosen.[101] Surgical treatment must convert an infection with dead bone to a situation with well-vascularized tissues that are readily penetrated by blood-borne antibiotics. The length of antibiotic therapy is empirical and depends on the clinical response of the patient. Several (4 to 6) weeks of treatment has become a standard length for empirical reasons. Dirschl and Almekinders reported that combined intravenous and oral antibiotic therapy has become accepted as a standard treatment of osteomyelitis in children.[39] The duration of intravenous antibiotic therapy has ranged from 3 to 14 days in various series. Adequate serum concentrations of the oral antibiotic must be documented before the patient is discharged from the hospital. Close outpatient follow-up is imperative, and treatment should be continued for 4 to 6 weeks. Treatment should be prolonged if the erythrocyte sedimentation rate does not fall below 20 mm/hr after 6 weeks.

Oral therapy for osteomyelitis in adults has lagged behind that of children, although some studies have demonstrated that the results are generally good. Oral antibiotic therapy has obvious economic advantages over intravenous therapy and as such is very desirable. The route of antibiotic delivery is probably not important as long as the infecting organism is susceptible to the antibiotic and the antibiotic is delivered to the tissues in adequate concentration to eradicate infection. The serum bactericidal titer is used as a method of determining the adequacy of therapy. This titer is defined as the maximal dilution of the patient's serum that will kill more than 99.9% of the infecting organisms in vitro. The serum bactericidal titer is useful for ensuring adequate antimicrobial activity, absorption, and compliance.

Intravenous therapy is generally continued for more than 3 weeks for septic arthritis and for more than 4 to 6 weeks for osteomyelitis and is monitored by systemic signs, white blood cell counts, and sedimentation rates.[117] Surgical débridement is the mainstay of therapy for septic arthritis and osteomyelitis of the shoulder. The logic is as follows: (1) toxic products, damaged tissue, and foreign bodies must be removed to prevent damage and to treat infection effectively, and (2) laboratory studies have shown that the minimal inhibitory and bactericidal concentrations needed to treat surface-adherent bacterial populations are 10 to 100 times higher than those for suspension populations.[69,95,118] These findings suggest that it is possible to clear bacteremia or bacteria suspended in synovial fluid but very difficult to sterilize an infected cartilaginous joint surface or sequestrum covered with debris without administering toxic levels of antibiotics.

Antibiotic-impregnated beads (gentamicin or tobramycin) may be indicated in certain cases of osteomyelitis and articular sepsis.[24,48,61] Removal at 6 to 12 weeks is suggested. In special cases, closed suction and irrigation may be used for short periods (<3 days) in septic joints if necessary, provided that the system does not allow retrograde contamination. However, the literature does not indicate a definite advantage with this treatment, and it is seldom required in de novo joint sepsis because adequate antibiotic levels can be achieved systemically.

Open wounds involving joints are by definition contaminated, even though bacteria are not always detected. Type 3 open fractures, especially those involving joints, have a very high rate of infection. There are indications that these infections should be treated with either cefazolin or a combination of cefazolin and gentamicin.[116] Intravenous amphotericin B remains the preferred drug in patients with deep systemic fungal infections.[39]

Infection after Shoulder Arthroplasty

Infection occurs in less than 1% of cases after total joint arthroplasty of the shoulder (Figs. 23–16 and 23–17).[71,111] When subacute or chronic infection occurs, radiographic change in the form of radiolucency around the cement mantle, prosthesis, or both may be observed. The periarticular soft tissues may be tender, and cellulitis and sinus formation may or may not occur. The sedimentation rate is usually high. Bone and gallium scanning can be helpful in differentiating infection from loosening. Aspiration of a prosthetic shoulder joint under image intensifier control is a useful method of obtaining specimens for culture. In some cases the diagnosis can be confirmed only at surgery by culture of tissue specimens. When subacute

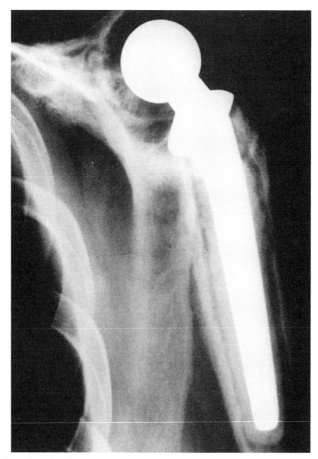

■ **Figure 23–16**
Infected total shoulder arthroplasty (radiograph of the patient shown in Fig. 23-1). The glenoid and humeral cement mantles are surrounded by large radiolucent lines. Reactive periostitis is present in the medial part of the humerus.

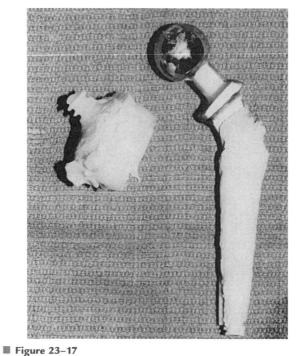

■ **Figure 23–17**
An infected total shoulder arthroplasty (same patient shown in Figs. 23-1 and 23-16). Both the humeral and glenoid components were removed. It was not difficult to remove the infected arthroplasty components because they were surrounded by purulent debris and a prolific membrane.

or chronic infection is suspected, a trial of antibiotics can be instituted. In a small percentage of patients with chronic infection, a symbiotic relationship can develop, with the long-term use of oral antibiotics depending on the severity of the infection and the patient's biologic resistance. In most cases, however, such symbiosis does not occur and removal of the component is required. Rarely, early infection may be treated with irrigation and débridement if it is due mainly to an infected hematoma. Removal of components is generally required in most cases if the infection is deep.

A Rush rod may be used as a "skeleton" on which an antibiotic-impregnated cement spacer can be constructed. The author uses 1 g of gentamycin for every 40 g of cement in constructing such spacers. The spacer is used in staged reconstruction of the shoulder after removal of the components, cement, and surrounding membrane. The timing of reimplantation of the prosthesis is dependent on the clinical course of the patient, the virulence of the organism that infected the original arthroplasty, the response of the sedimentation rate to antibiotic treatment, and closure of any sinus tracts that may have developed. In most cases, reimplantation can occur 3 to 6 months after implantation of the spacer.

All damaged tissue and methylmethacrylate should be removed if possible. The prognosis for revision total joint arthroplasty after infection is poor.[110] Fusion may be required (Fig. 23-18). Some patients may have surprisingly good function 1 year after removal of the components without fusion. Resection rather than fusion is preferred by some authors as the standard salvage method for failed, infected shoulders and elbows. The author prefers arthrodesis as a method of reconstruction after removal of prosthetic components. Delayed bone grafting may be required because of the extent of bone loss after removal of the prosthetic components.

Seitz and Damacen reported eight patients with shoulder sepsis after arthroplasty who were treated by staged exchange arthroplasty with antibiotic-impregnated methylmethacrylate spacers shaped and fitted to the patients' anatomy.[134] Intravenous antibiotic therapy was used for a minimum of 3 months. After 6 months, the patients underwent exchange prosthetic reconstruction with standard implants fixed with antibiotic-impregnated methylmethacrylate cement (Fig. 23-19). Three patients had revision of the total shoulder arthroplasty and five underwent hemiarthroplasty of the humerus with a local capsular flap to resurface the glenoid. All patients experienced substantial pain relief and improvement in function despite limited total overhead motion.

The author has minimal experience with reimplantation of a prosthesis after a prosthetic infection. It is possible that removal of the prosthesis and insertion of cement-impregnated beads or immediate reimplantation of a prosthesis with antibiotic-impregnated cement may salvage some arthroplasties after infection develops. This type of treatment is best attempted for infections caused by organisms of low virulence, such as *S. epidermidis*. The author does not recommend reimplantation of a prosthesis after infection with gram-negative bacilli or any other organism with high virulence.

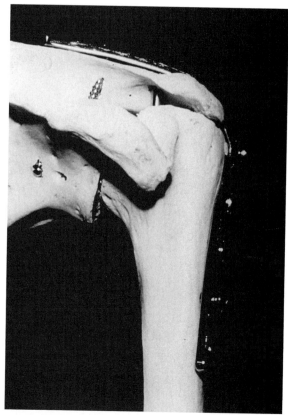

■ Figure 23-18

Shoulder arthrodesis achieved with plate fixation. Shoulder arthrodesis can be used to treat chronic glenohumeral sepsis and destruction of articular cartilage. If bone loss occurs after removal of a shoulder arthroplasty because of a tumor, curettage and bone grafting may have to be combined with internal fixation. Depending on the adequacy of the débridement and the health of the surrounding soft tissues, it may be necessary to stage débridement and bone grafting to obtain a solid arthrodesis. (*From Richards RR, Waddell JP, and Hudson AR: Shoulder arthrodesis for the treatment of brachial plexus palsy. Clin Orthop 198:250-258, 1985.*)

Prophylaxis

Antibiotic prophylaxis is effective because bacteria are cleared before they establish surface-adherent, rapidly growing populations at sites deep within bone or on biomaterials. The author suggests using antibiotic prophylaxis, such as cefazolin, 1 g intravenously at anesthesia and repeated at 4 hours.[115] The use of prophylactic antibiotics is suggested for all implant surgery, including both prosthetic and internal fixation of fractures. The antibiotic used varies according to the special conditions of each case and patient.[116] Treatment for 24 hours in clean cases is believed to be sufficient.

■ AUTHOR'S PREFERRED METHOD OF TREATMENT

Either an arthroscopic or an open approach can be used to drain the shoulder joint. If arthroscopy is to be used, the surgeon should be able to use multiple portals to facilitate drainage and insert instruments for débridement.

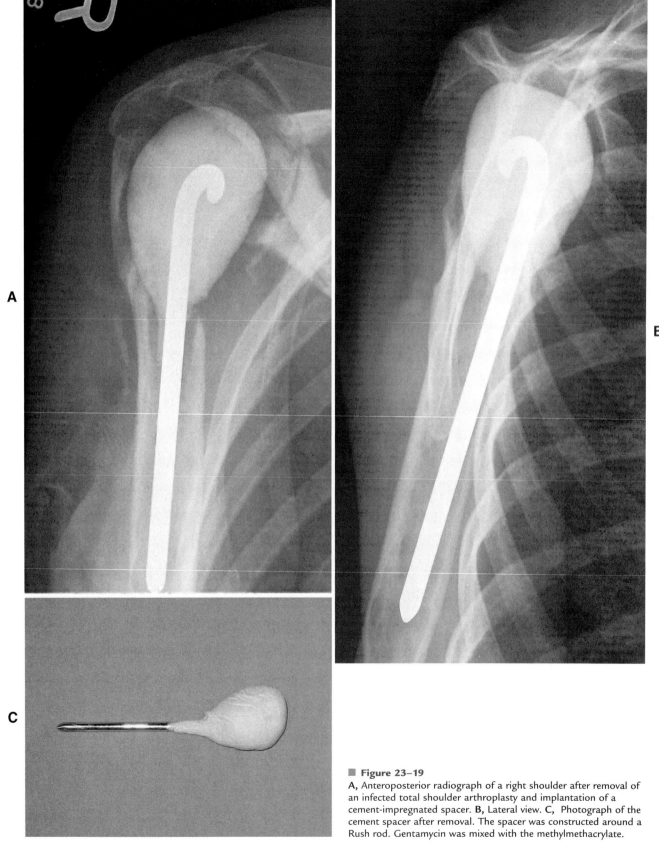

■ **Figure 23–19**

A, Anteroposterior radiograph of a right shoulder after removal of an infected total shoulder arthroplasty and implantation of a cement-impregnated spacer. **B,** Lateral view. **C,** Photograph of the cement spacer after removal. The spacer was constructed around a Rush rod. Gentamycin was mixed with the methylmethacrylate.

When performing open drainage, the author uses an anterior deltopectoral approach. The deltoid and coracoid are not detached. Infected surfaces are débrided of adherent clot and other debris. Lavage of the joint with saline or saline mixed with bacitracin is an appropriate technique. In most cases, the wound may be loosely closed and a large Hemovac inserted for 24 hours to remove postsurgical accumulations. In cases of chronic sepsis or infection with gram-negative organisms, the wound is left open. Adequate intra-articular concentrations of antibiotics can be achieved by intravenous administration.[113] The duration of antibiotic treatment varies, depending on the host and organism; 3 weeks of intravenous therapy followed by 3 weeks of oral treatment is a reasonable base. The patient's response is the key to the duration of treatment.

In summary, intra-articular shoulder sepsis presents many challenges in diagnosis and treatment. Sepsis following shoulder arthroplasty is being seen with increased frequency because of the number of arthroplasties inserted. The shoulder anatomy is unique in that bursae communicating with the joint can provide a pathway for bacteria for which cartilage is the target substratum. Successful treatment depends on the immune system response, the type of infecting organism, and early surgical débridement.

REFERENCES

1. Aglas F, Gretler J, Rainer F, and Krejs GJ: Sternoclavicular septic arthritis: A rare but serious complication of subclavian venous catheterization. Clin Rheumatol 13:507-512, 1994.
2. Albrektsson T: The response of bone to titanium implants. Crit Rev Biocompat 1:53-84, 1985.
3. American Medical Association, Division of Drugs and Toxicology: Antimicrobial therapy for common infectious diseases. In Drug Evaluations Annual 1995. Chicago: American Medical Association, 1995, pp 1277-1282.
4. Antibiotics for osteomyelitis. Lancet 1:153-154, 1975.
5. Argen RJ, Wilson DH Jr, and Wood P: Suppurative arthritis. Arch Intern Med 117:661-666, 1966.
6. Armbuster G, Slivka J, Resnick D, et al: Extraarticular manifestations of septic arthritis of the glenohumeral joint. AJR Am J Roentgenol 129:667-672, 1977.
7. Armstrong RW and Bolding F: Septic arthritis after arthroscopy: The contributing roles of intraarticular steroids and environmental factors. Am J Infect Control 22:16-18, 1994.
8. Avery JK (ed): Oral Development and Histology. Baltimore: Williams & Wilkins, 1987.
9. Baier RE, Meyer AE, Natiella JR, et al: Surface properties determine bioadhesive outcomes: Methods and results. J Biomed Mater Res 18:337-355, 1984.
10. Baltimore RS and Mitchell M: Immunologic investigations of mucoid strains of Pseudomonas aeruginosa: Comparison of susceptibility to opsonic antibody in mucoid and nonmucoid strains. J Infect Dis 141:238-247, 1980.
11. Barzaga RA, Nowak PA, and Cunha BA: Escherichia coli septic arthritis of a shoulder in a diabetic patient. Heart Lung 20:692-693, 1991.
12. Bayer AS, Chow AW, Louie JS, et al: Gram-negative bacillary septic arthritis: Clinical, radiologic, therapeutic, and prognostic features. Semin Arthritis Rheum 7:123-132, 1977.
13. Bendall RP, Jacobson SK, and Adebajo A: Septic arthropathy complicating apatite associated destructive arthritis. Ann Rheum Dis 50:1005-1007, 1990.
14. Berney S, Goldstein M, and Bishko F: Clinical and diagnostic features of tuberculous arthritis. Am J Med 53:36-42, 1972.
15. Berquist TH, Brown M, Fitzgerald R, et al: Magnetic resonance imaging: Application in musculoskeletal infection. Magn Reson Imaging 3:219, 1985.
16. Bertone C, Rivera F, Avallone F, et al: Pneumococcal septic arthritis of the shoulder. Case report and literature review. Panminerva Med 44:151-154, 2002.
17. Bettin D, Schul B, and Schwering L: Diagnosis and treatment of joint infections in elderly patients. Acta Orthop Belg 64:131-135, 1998.
18. Bhawan J, Das Tandon H, and Roy S: Ultrastructure of synovial membrane in pyogenic arthritis. Arch Pathol 96:155-160, 1973.
19. Bigliani LU, Flatow EL, and Deliz ED: Complications of shoulder arthroscopy. Orthop Rev 20:743-751, 1991.
20. Birinyi LK, Douville C, Lewis SA, et al: Increased resistance to bacteremic graft infection after endothelial cell seeding. J Vasc Surg 5:193-197, 1987.
21. Bos CF, Mol LJ, Obermann WR, and Tjin a Ton ER: Late sequelae of neonatal septic arthritis of the shoulder. J Bone Joint Surg Br 80:645-650, 1998.
22. Brancos MA, Peris P, Miro JM, et al: Septic arthritis in heroin addicts. Semin Arthritis Rheum 21:81-87, 1991.
23. Broadwater JR and Stair JM: Sternoclavicular osteomyelitis: Coverage with a pectoralis major muscle flap. Surg Rounds Orthop 2:47-50, 1988.
24. Buccholz HW and Gartmann HD: Infektionsprophylaxe und operative Behandlung der schleichenden tiefen Infektion bei der totalen Endoprothese. Chirurg 43:446-452, 1972.
25. Burch KK, Fine G, Quinn EL, and Eisses JF: Cryptococcus neoformans as a cause of lytic bone lesions. JAMA 231:1057-1059, 1975.
26. Cabot RC (ed): Case records of the Massachusetts General Hospital: An obscure general infection. Boston Med Surg J 197:1140-1142, 1927.
27. Caksen H, Ozturk MK, Uzum K, et al: Septic arthritis in childhood. Pediatr Int 42:534-540, 2000.
28. Capov I, Wechsler J, Sumbera J, et al: Pericardial abscess—a rare complication of sepsis. Acta Chir Hung 38:19-21, 1999.
29. Chaudhuri K, Lonergan D, Portek I, and McGuigan L: Septic arthritis of the shoulder after mastectomy and radiotherapy for breast carcinoma. J Bone Joint Surg Br 75:318-321, 1993.
30. Chung SMK: The arterial supply of the developing proximal end of the human femur. J Bone Joint Surg Am 58:961-970, 1976.
31. Clemente C (ed): Gray's Anatomy of the Human Body, 5th ed. Philadelphia: Lea & Febiger, 1985.
32. Codman EA: The Shoulder. Rupture of the Supraspinatus Tendon and Other Lesions in or about the Subacromial Bursa, 2nd ed. Malabar, FL: Robert E. Kreiger, 1984.
33. Cofield RH: Total shoulder arthroplasty with the Neer prosthesis. J Bone Joint Surg Am 66:899-906, 1984.
34. Costerton JW, Geesey GG, and Cheng K-J: How bacteria stick. Sci Am 238:86-95, 1978.
35. David R, Barron BJ, and Madewell JE: Osteomyelitis, acute and chronic. Radiol Clin North Am 25:1171-1201, 1987.
36. De Boeck H, Noppen L, and Desprechins B: Pyomyositis of the adductor muscles mimicking an infection of the hip. Diagnosis by magnetic resonance imaging: A case report. J Bone Joint Surg Am 76:747-750, 1994.
37. DePalma AF (ed): Surgery of the Shoulder, 3rd ed. Philadelphia: JB Lippincott, 1983.
38. Desplaces N and Acar JF: New quinolones in the treatment of joint and bone infections. Rev Infect Dis 10(suppl 1):S179-S183, 1988.
39. Dirschl DR and Almekinders LC: Osteomyelitis: Common causes and treatment recommendations. Drugs 45:29-43, 1993.
40. Dubost JJ, Soubrier M, and Sauvezie B: Pyogenic arthritis in adults. Joint Bone Spine 67:11-21, 2000.
41. Egan SC, LaSalle MD, Stock JA, and Hanna MK: Septic arthritis secondary to vesicoureteral reflux into single ectopic ureter. Pediatr Nephrol 13:932-933, 1999.
42. Ejlertsen T and Dossing K: Pneumococcal pyomyositis secondary to pneumonia. Scand J Infect Dis 29:520-521, 1997.
43. Epps CH Jr, Bryant DD 3rd, Coles MJ, and Castro O: Osteomyelitis in patients who have sickle-cell disease. Diagnosis and management. J Bone Joint Surg Am 73:1281-1294, 1991.
44. Fansa H, Handstein S, and Schneider W: Treatment of infected median sternotomy wounds with a myocutaneous latissimus dorsi muscle flap. Scand Cardiovasc J 32:33-39, 1998.
45. Fellows L, Boivin M, and Kapusta M: Pasteurella multocida arthritis of the shoulder associated with postsurgical lymphedema. J Rheumatol 23:1824-1825, 1996.
46. Fitzgerald RH, Rosenblatt JE, Tenney JH, and Bourgault A-M: Anaerobic septic arthritis. Clin Orthop 164:141-148, 1982.
47. Fletcher BD, Scoles PV, and Nelson AD: Osteomyelitis in children: Detection by magnetic resonance. Radiology 150:57-60, 1984.
48. Flick AB, Herbert JC, Goodell J, and Kristiansen T: Noncommercial fabrication of antibiotic-impregnated polymethylmethacrylate beads. Technical note. Clin Orthop 223:282-286, 1987.
49. Forward DP and Hunter JB: Arthroscopic washout of the shoulder for septic arthritis in infants. A new technique. J Bone Joint Surg Br 84:1173-1175, 2002.
50. Franco M, Van Elslande L, Robino C, et al: Aspergillus arthritis of the shoulder in a renal transplant recipient. Failure of itraconazole therapy. Rev Rhum Engl Ed 62:215-218, 1995.
51. Gabriel SR, Thometz JG, and Jaradeh S: Septic arthritis associated with brachial plexus neuropathy. J Bone Joint Surg Am 78:103-105, 1996.
52. Gamlin F, Caldicott LD, and Shah MV: Mediastinitis and sepsis syndrome following intubation. Anaesthesia 49:883-885, 1994.
53. Garcia S, Combalia A, and Segur JM: Septic arthritis of the shoulder due to Streptococcus agalactiae. Acta Orthop Belg 62:66-68, 1996.
54. Garnett ES, Cockshott WP, and Jacob J: Classical acute osteomyelitis with a negative bone scan. Br J Radiol 50:757, 1977.
55. Gelberman RH, Menon J, Austerlitz S, and Weisman MH: Pyogenic arthritis of the shoulder in adults. J Bone Joint Surg Am 62:550-553, 1980.
56. Gentry LO: Osteomyelitis: Options for diagnosis and management. J Antimicrob Chemother 21(suppl):115-128, 1988.
57. Gibbons RJ and Van Houte J: Dental caries. Annu Rev Med 26:121-136, 1975.

58. Gifford DB, Patzakis M, Ivler D, and Swezey RL: Septic arthritis due to *Pseudomonas* in heroin addicts. J Bone Joint Surg Am 57:631-635, 1975.

59. Goldenberg DL and Reed JI: Bacterial arthritis. N Engl J Med 312:764-771, 1985.

60. Gompels BM and Darlington LG: Septic arthritis in rheumatoid disease causing bilateral shoulder dislocation: Diagnosis and treatment assisted by grey scale ultrasonography. Ann Rheum Dis 40:609-611, 1981.

61. Goodell JA, Flick AB, Hebert JC, and Howe JG: Preparation and release characteristics of tobramycin-impregnated polymethylmethacrylate beads. Am J Hosp Pharm 43:1454-1460, 1986.

62. Govan JRW: Mucoid strains of *Pseudomonas aeruginosa:* The influence of culture medium on the stability of mucus production. J Med Microbiol 8:513-522, 1975.

63. Govan JRW and Fyfe JAM: Mucoid *Pseudomonas aeruginosa* and cystic fibrosis: Resistance of the mucoid form to carbenicillin, flucloxacillin and tobramycin and the isolation of mucoid variants in vitro. J Antimicrob Chemother 4:233-240, 1978.

64. Gowans JDC and Granieri PA: Septic arthritis, its relation to intra-articular injections of hydrocortisone acetate. N Engl J Med 261:502-504, 1959.

65. Gristina AG: Biomaterial-centered infection: Microbial adhesion versus tissue integration. Science 237:1558-1595, 1987.

66. Gristina AG, Barth E, and Myrvik Q: Materials, microbes, and man. The problem of infection associated with implantable devices. In Williams DF (ed): Current Perspectives on Implantable Devices. London: JAI Press, 1989.

67. Gristina AG and Costerton JW: Bacteria-laden biofilms: A hazard to orthopedic prostheses. Infect Surg 3:655-662, 1984.

68. Gristina AG and Costerton JW: Bacterial adherence to biomaterials and tissue. The significance of its role in clinical sepsis. J Bone Joint Surg Am 67:264-273, 1985.

69. Gristina AG, Hobgood CD, Webb LX, and Myrvik QN: Adhesive colonization of biomaterials and antibiotic resistance. Biomaterials 8:423-426, 1987.

70. Gristina AG, Oga M, Webb LX, and Hobgood CD: Adherent bacterial colonization in the pathogenesis of osteomyelitis. Science 228:990-993, 1985.

71. Gristina AG, Romano RL, Kammire GC, and Webb LX: Total shoulder replacement. Orthop Clin North Am 18:445-453, 1987.

72. Gristina AG and Rovere GD: An in vitro study of the effects of metals used in internal fixation on bacterial growth and dissemination. J Bone Joint Surg Am 45:1104, 1963.

73. Gristina AG, Rovere GD, and Shoji H: Spontaneous septic arthritis complicating rheumatoid arthritis. J Bone Joint Surg Am 56:1180-1184, 1974.

74. Guest SS, Kirsch CM, Baxter R, et al: Infection of a subclavian venous stent in a hemodialysis patient. Am J Kidney Dis 26:377-380, 1995.

75. Gupta NC and Prezio JA: Radionuclide imaging in osteomyelitis. Semin Nucl Med 18:287, 1988.

76. Hamill RJ, Vann JM, and Proctor RA: Phagocytosis of *Staphylococcus aureus* by cultured bovine aortic endothelial cells: Model for postadherence events in endovascular infections. Infect Immun 54:833-836, 1986.

77. Hendrix RW and Fisher MR: Imaging of septic arthritis. Clin Rheum Dis 12:459-487, 1986.

78. Holderbaum D, Spech T, Ehrhart L, et al: Collagen binding in clinical isolates of *Staphylococcus aureus.* J Clin Microbiol 25:2258-2261, 1987.

79. Hopkins KL, Li KC, and Bergman G: Gadolinium-DTPA–enhanced magnetic resonance imaging of musculoskeletal infectious processes. Skeletal Radiol 24:325-330, 1995.

80. Hoppe HG: Attachment of bacteria. Advantage or disadvantage for survival in the aquatic environment. In Marshall KC (ed): Microbial Adhesion and Aggregation. New York: Springer-Verlag, 1984, pp 283-301.

81. Hughes GM, Biundo JJ Jr, Scheib JS, and Kumar P: Pseudogout and pseudosepsis of the shoulder. Orthopedics 13:1169-1172, 1990.

82. Hunter W: Of the structures and diseases of articulating cartilage. Philos Trans R Soc Lond 42:514-521, 1743.

83. Jackson MA and Nelson JD: Etiology and medical management of acute suppurative bone and joint infections in pediatric patients. J Pediatr Orthop 2:313, 1982.

84. Jerosch J, Hoffstetter I, Schroder M, and Castro WH: Septic arthritis: Arthroscopic management with local antibiotic treatment. Acta Orthop Belg 61:126-134, 1995.

85. Jones GW and Isaacson RE: Proteinaceous bacterial adhesins and their receptors. Crit Rev Microbiol 10:229-260, 1984.

86. Karten I: Septic arthritis complicating rheumatoid arthritis. Ann Intern Med 70:1147-1151, 1969.

87. Kasemo B and Lausmaa J: Surface science aspects on inorganic biomaterials. Crit Rev Biocompat 2:335-380, 1986.

88. Kellgren JH, Ball J, Fairbrother RW, and Barnes KL: Suppurative arthritis complicating rheumatoid arthritis. BMJ 1:1193-1200, 1958.

89. Kelly PJ, Conventry MB, and Martin WJ: Bacterial arthritis of the shoulder. Mayo Clin Proc 40:695-699, 1965.

90. Kelly PJ and Fitzgerald RH Jr: Bacterial arthritis. In Braude AI, Davis CE, and Fierer J (eds): Infectious Diseases and Medical Microbiology, 2nd ed. Philadelphia: WB Saunders, 1986, pp 1468-1472.

91. Kelly PJ, Martin WJ, and Coventry MD: Bacterial (suppurative) arthritis in the adult. J Bone Joint Surg Am 52:1595-1602, 1970.

92. Kirschenbaum AE and Rizzo C: Glenohumeral pyarthrosis following acupuncture treatment. Orthopedics 20:1184-1186, 1997.

93. Klein RS: Joint infection, with consideration of underlying disease and sources of bacteremia in hematogenous infection. Clin Geriatr Med 4:375-394, 1988.

94. Krespi YP, Monsell EM, and Sisson GA: Osteomyelitis of the clavicle. Ann Otol Rhinol Laryngol 92:525-527, 1983.

95. Ladd TI, Schmiel D, Nickel JC, and Costerton JW: Rapid method for detection of adherent bacteria on Foley urinary catheters. J Clin Microbiol 21:1004-1006, 1985.

96. Lavy CB, Lavy VR, and Anderson I: *Salmonella* septic arthritis of the shoulder in Zambian children. J R Coll Surg Edinb 41:197-199, 1996.

97. Lejman T, Strong M, Michno P, and Hayman M: Septic arthritis of the shoulder during the first 18 months of life. J Pediatr Orthop 15:172-175, 1995.

98. Leslie BM, Harris JM, and Driscoll D: Septic arthritis of the shoulder in adults. J Bone Joint Surg Am 71:1516-1522, 1989.

99. Lossos IS, Yossepowitch O, Kandel L, et al: Septic arthritis of the glenohumeral joint. A report of 11 cases and review of the literature. Medicine (Baltimore) 77:177-187, 1998.

100. Louthrenoo W, Ostrov BE, Park YS, et al: Pseudoseptic arthritis: An unusual presentation of neuropathic arthropathy. Ann Rheum Dis 50:717-721, 1991.

101. Mader JT, Landon GC, and Calhoun J: Antimicrobial treatment of osteomyelitis. Clin Orthop 295:87-95, 1993.

102. Mandell GL, Douglas RG Jr, and Bennett JE (eds): Principles and Practice of Infectious Diseases, 2nd ed. New York: John Wiley, 1985.

103. Manny J, Haruzi I, and Yosipovitch Z: Osteomyelitis of the clavicle following subclavian vein catheterization. Arch Surg 106:342-343, 1973.

104. Marrie TJ and Costerton JW: Prolonged survival of *Serratia marcescens* in chlorhexidine. Appl Environ Microbiol 42:1093-1102, 1981.

105. Master R, Weisman MH, Armbuster TG, et al: Septic arthritis of the glenohumeral joint. Unique clinical and radiographic features and a favorable outcome. Arthritis Rheum 10:1500-1506, 1977.

106. Medical Staff Conference: Arthritis caused by viruses. Calif Med 119:38-44, 1973.

107. Merkel KD, Brown ML, DeWanjee MK, and Fitzgerald RH: Comparison of indium-labeled leukocyte imaging with sequential technetium-gallium scanning in the diagnosis of low-grade musculoskeletal sepsis. J Bone Joint Surg Am 67:465-476, 1985.

108. Miron D, Bor N, Cutai M, and Horowitz J: Transient brachial palsy associated with suppurative arthritis of the shoulder. Pediatr Infect Dis J 16:326-327, 1997.

109. Morrey BF and Bianco AJ: Hematogenous osteomyelitis of the clavicle in children. Clin Orthop 125:24-28, 1977.

110. Neer CS and Kirby RM: Revision of humeral head and total shoulder arthroplasties. Clin Orthop 170:189-195, 1982.

111. Neer CS, Watson KC, and Stanton FJ: Recent experience in total shoulder replacement. J Bone Joint Surg Am 64:319-337, 1982.

112. Neihart RE, Fried JS, and Hodges GR: Coagulase-negative staphylococci. South Med J 81:491-500, 1988.

113. Nelson JD: Antibiotic concentrations in septic joint effusions. N Engl J Med 284:349-353, 1971.

114. Nelson JD and Koontz WC: Septic arthritis in infants and children: A review of 117 cases. Pediatrics 38:966-971, 1966.

115. Neu HC: Cephalosporin antibiotics as applied in surgery of bones and joints. Clin Orthop 190:50-64, 1984.

116. Norden C: Experimental osteomyelitis. IV. Therapeutic trials with rifampin alone and in combination with gentamicin, sisomicin, and cephalothin. J Infect Dis 132:493-499, 1975.

117. Norden CW: A critical review of antibiotic prophylaxis in orthopedic surgery. Rev Infect Dis 5:928-932, 1983.

118. O'Meara PM and Bartal E: Septic arthritis: Process, etiology, treatment outcome: A literature review. Orthopedics 11:623-628, 1988.

119. Patzakis MJ, Wilkins M, and Moore TM: Use of antibiotics in open tibial fractures. Clin Orthop 178:31-35, 1983.

120. Pfeiffenberger J and Meiss L: Septic conditions of the shoulder—an up-dating of treatment strategies. Arch Orthop Trauma Surg 115:325-331, 1996.

121. Popa A, Fenster J, Jacob H, and Gleich S: Shoulder girdle abscess due to *Streptococcus agalactiae* complicating esophageal dilatation. Am J Gastroenterol 94:1410-1411, 1999.

122. Post M: The Shoulder: Surgical and Nonsurgical Management. Philadelphia: Lea & Febiger, 1988.

123. Rankin KC and Rycken JM: Bilateral dislocation of the proximal humeral epiphyses in septic arthritis: A case report. J Bone Joint Surg Br 75:329, 1993.

124. Rimoin DL and Wennberg JE: Acute septic arthritis complicating chronic rheumatoid arthritis. JAMA 196:617-621, 1966.

125. Roca RP and Yoshikawa TT: Primary skeletal infections in heroin users: A clinical characterization, diagnosis and therapy. Clin Orthop 144:238-248, 1979.

126. Ruseska I, Robbins J, and Costerton JW: Biocide testing against corrosion-causing oil-field bacteria helps control plugging. Oil Gas J 10:253-264, 1982.

127. Rutten MJ, van den Berg JC, van den Hoogen FH, and Lemmens JA: Nontuberculous mycobacterial bursitis and arthritis of the shoulder. Skeletal Radiol 27:33-35, 1998.

128. Sadat-Ali M: Septic arthritis of the shoulder in adults. J Bone Joint Surg Am 73:154, 1991.

129. Salter RB, Bell RS, and Keeley FW: The protective effect of continuous passive motion in living articular cartilage in acute septic arthritis: An experimental investigation in the rabbit. Clin Orthop 159:223-247, 1981.

130. Sartoris DJ and Resnick D: Magnetic resonance imaging for musculoskeletal disorders. West J Med 148:102-109, 1988.

131. Schmid FR: Principles of diagnosis and treatment of bone and joint infections. In McCarty DJ (ed): Arthritis and Allied Conditions. A Textbook of Rheumatology. Philadelphia: Lea & Febiger, 1985, pp 1627-1650.

132. Schmidt D, Mubarak S, and Gelberman R: Septic shoulders in children. J Pediatr Orthop 1:67-72, 1981.

133. Schwarzmann S and Boring JR III: Antiphagocytic effect of slime from a mucoid strain of Pseudomonas aeruginosa. Infect Immun 3:762-767, 1971.

134. Seitz WH Jr and Damacen H: Staged exchange arthroplasty for shoulder sepsis. J Arthroplasty 17(4 suppl 1):36-40, 2002.

135. Sharp JT: Gonococcal arthritis. In McCarty DJ (ed): Arthritis and Allied Conditions. A Textbook of Rheumatology, 9th ed. Philadelphia: Lea & Febiger, 1979, pp 1353-1362.

136. Sharp JT, Lidsky MD, Duffey J, and Duncan MW: Infectious arthritis. Arch Intern Med 139:1125-1130, 1979.

137. Slusher MM, Myrvik QN, Lewis JC, and Gristina AG: Extended-wear lenses, biofilm, and bacterial adhesion. Arch Ophthalmol 105:110-115, 1987.

138. Smith JW and Piercy EA: Infectious arthritis. Clin Infect Dis 20:225-231, 1995.

139. Smith JW and Sanford JP: Viral arthritis. Ann Intern Med 67:651-659, 1967.

140. Smith RL and Schurman DJ: Comparison of cartilage destruction between infectious and adjuvant arthritis. J Orthop Res 1:136-143, 1983.

141. Smith RL, Schurman DJ, Kajiyama G, et al: The effect of antibiotics on the destruction of cartilage in experimental infectious arthritis. J Bone Joint Surg Am 69:1063-1068, 1987.

142. Smith SP, Thyoka M, Lavy CB, and Pitani A: Septic arthritis of the shoulder in children in Malawi. A randomised, prospective study of aspiration versus arthrotomy and washout. J Bone Joint Surg Br 84:1167-1172, 2002.

143. Speers DJ and Nade SML: Ultrastructural studies of adherence of Staphylococcus aureus in experimental acute haematogenous osteomyelitis. Infect Immun 49:443-446, 1985.

144. Speziale P, Raucci G, Visai L, et al: Binding of collagen to Staphylococcus aureus Cowan 1. J Bacteriol 167:77-81, 1986.

145. Srivastava KK, Garg LD, and Kochhar VL: Tuberculous osteomyelitis of the clavicle. Acta Orthop Scand 45:668-672, 1974.

146. Steiner GM and Sprigg A: The value of ultrasound in the assessment of bone. Br J Radiol 65:589-593, 1992.

147. Stern GA and Lubniewski A: The interaction between Pseudomonas aeruginosa and the corneal epithelium. Arch Ophthalmol 103:1221-1225, 1985.

148. Stutz G, Kuster MS, Kleinstuck F, and Gachter A: Arthroscopic management of septic arthritis: Stages of infection and results. Knee Surg Sports Traumatol Arthrosc 8:270-274, 2000.

149. Switalski LM, Ryden C, Rubin K, et al: Binding of fibronectin to Staphylococcus strains. Infect Immun 42:628-633, 1983.

150. Tabor OB Jr, Bosse MJ, Hudson MC, et al: Does bacteremia occur during high pressure lavage of contaminated wounds? Clin Orthop 347:117-121, 1998.

151. Tehranzadeh J, Wang F, and Mesgarzadeh M: Magnetic resonance imaging of osteomyelitis. Crit Rev Diagn Imaging 33:495-534, 1992.

152. Tiddia F, Cherchi GB, Pacifico L, and Chiesa C: Yersinia enterocolitica causing suppurative arthritis of the shoulder. J Clin Pathol 47:760-761, 1994.

153. Tromp RM, Hamers RJ, and Demuth JE: Quantum states and atomic structure of silicon surfaces. Science 234:304-309, 1986.

154. Trueta J: The normal vascular anatomy of the human femoral head during growth. J Bone Joint Surg Br 39:358-394, 1957.

155. Trueta J: The three types of acute hematogenous osteomyelitis: A clinical and vascular study. J Bone Joint Surg Br 41:671-680, 1959.

156. Turek SL: Orthopaedics. Principles and Their Application. Philadelphia: JB Lippincott, 1977.

157. Ukkonen HJ, Vuori KP, Lehtonen OP, and Kotilainen PM: Listeria monocytogenes arthritis of several joints. Scand J Rheumatol 24:392-394, 1995.

158. Voytek A, Gristina G, Barth E, et al: Staphylococcal adhesion to collagen in intra-articular sepsis. Biomaterials 9:107-110, 1988.

159. Wallace R and Cohen AS: Tuberculous arthritis. A report of two cases with review of biopsy and synovial fluid findings. Am J Med 61:277-282, 1976.

160. Ward JR and Atcheson SG: Infectious arthritis. Med Clin North Am 61:313-329, 1977.

161. Ward J, Cohen AS, and Bauer W: The diagnosis and therapy of acute suppurative arthritis. Arthritis Rheum 3:522-535, 1960.

162. Ward WG and Eckardt JJ: Subacromial/subdeltoid bursa abscesses: An overlooked diagnosis. Clin Orthop 288:189-194, 1993.

163. Ward WG and Goldner RD: Shoulder pyarthrosis: A concomitant process. Orthopedics 17:591-595, 1994.

164. Watt PJ and Ward ME: Adherence of Neisseria gonorrhoeae and other Neisseria species to mammalian cells. In Beachey EH (ed): Bacterial Adherence. Receptors and Recognition, series B, vol 6. London: Chapman & Hall, 1980, pp 251-288.

165. Webb LX, Myers RT, Cordell AR, et al: Inhibition of bacterial adhesion by antibacterial surface pretreatment of vascular prostheses. J Vasc Surg 4:16-21, 1986.

166. Widman DS, Craig JG, and van Holsbeeck MT: Sonographic detection, evaluation and aspiration of infected acromioclavicular joints. Skeletal Radiol 30:388-392, 2001.

167. Wolf RF, Konings JG, Prins TR, and Weits J: Fusobacterium pyomyositis of the shoulder after tonsillitis. Report of a case of Lemierre's syndrome. Acta Orthop Scand 62:595-596, 1991.

168. Woods DE, Bass JA, Johanson WG Jr, and Straus DC: Role of adherence in the pathogenesis of Pseudomonas aeruginosa lung infection in cystic fibrosis patients. Infect Immun 30:694-699, 1980.

169. Wrangstadh M, Conway PL, and Kjelleberg S: The production and release of an extracellular polysaccharide during starvation of a marine Pseudomonas sp. and the effect thereof on adhesion. Arch Microbiol 145:220-227, 1986.

170. Wray TM, Bryant RE, and Killen DA: Sternal osteomyelitis and costochondritis after median sternotomy. J Thorac Cardiovasc Surg 65:227-233, 1973.

171. Wukich DK, Abreu SH, Callaghan JJ, et al: Diagnosis of infection by preoperative scintigraphy with indium-labeled white blood cells. J Bone Joint Surg Am 69:1353-1360, 1987.

172. Zaks N, Sukenik S, Alkan M, et al: Musculoskeletal manifestations of brucellosis: A study of 90 cases in Israel. Semin Arthritis Rheum 25:97-102, 1995.

CHAPTER 24

AMPUTATIONS AND PROSTHETIC REPLACEMENT

Douglas G. Smith, M.D.,   Robert L. Romano, M.D.,   and Ernest M. Burgess, M.D.[†]

• • • •

Amputations about the shoulder joint are infrequent. Although exact figures are not available, it is estimated that less than 5% of all major amputations occur at this level. The cross-sectional anatomy at the shoulder is complex. The standard techniques presented in this chapter are generally accepted as being based on well-established anatomic, surgical, and prosthetic considerations. Because many of these amputations are performed for complicated neoplasms and severe trauma, considerable surgical ingenuity is often required. The nature of the pathologic process requiring the amputation will direct the surgeon to emphasize plastic and reconstructive surgical principles to best use the available tissues and permit uncomplicated healing.

TYPES OF AMPUTATIONS

Amputations at the shoulder can be separated into two categories:

1. Those that ablate the extremity—through the proximal end of the humerus or by disarticulation of the glenohumeral joint, scapulothoracic amputation, or revision of congenital amputations
2. Those that preserve the distal extremity—scapulectomy, claviculectomy, and intercalary shoulder resection (Tikhoff-Linberg procedure)

Amputations through the proximal part of the humerus above the level of the axillary fold are treated as shoulder disarticulations. Function and prosthetic rehabilitation are comparable. The real advantage of retaining the head of the humerus is cosmetic; shoulder disarticulation leaves an unsightly concavity at the glenoid fossa with a sharp prominence of the acromion process, whereas the retained head of the humerus presents a more natural appearance with a rounded shoulder contour. Leaving the head of the humerus when technically possible enhances wearing of clothes and the cosmetic appearance of the shoulder.

Disarticulation of the shoulder joint, when carried out through relatively normal anatomy or when an adequate amount of remaining soft tissue is available, becomes essentially a plastic reconstructive exercise. Pliable scars, mobile soft tissues, and appropriate muscle and tendon management will be described (see sections on technique under "Specific Procedures").

Scapulothoracic amputation (forequarter amputation) is the surgical removal of the upper extremity in the interval between the scapula and the thoracic wall. Often, a short medial portion of the clavicle is retained. This amputation is a deforming procedure because the lateral neck structures slope directly onto the chest wall. It is possible, however, to recontour body form by modern cosmetic surface restoration to achieve a reasonable degree of appearance with the use of light, state-of-the-art materials so that under clothing, the unsightly trunk appearance is considerably improved.

Amputations that preserve the distal end of the extremity are rarely performed, except in certain cases of tumor, but they may occasionally be indicated for the residual effects of chronic infection or radiation damage and, in particular, for a patient who refuses ablation of the limb. Preservation of the neurovascular supply to the distal part of the extremity is, of course, a necessity. The patient will have a degree of hand and elbow function, depending on the nature of the partial shoulder resection, but will be severely limited in overall function of the limb because of an inability to appropriately position the arm and the hand. The hand can function only at the side as the extremity dangles without stability. An orthotic support may assist in hand placement. The intercalary shoulder resection was suggested by Tikhoff, a Russian surgeon; however, the procedure was first performed by Linberg. This unusual block resection of the shoulder area was developed for patients who refused a more radical procedure for certain tumors or for instances in which the tumor did not involve the neurovascular bundle and the distal end of the extremity could be preserved. It involves resection of the scapula; most of the clavicle; and the head, neck, and a portion of the proximal shaft of the humerus, as well as involved soft tissues. The distal portion of the limb, the vascular supply, and the brachial plexus are preserved.

A scapulectomy alone may be performed for primary bone tumors. Syme first described the technique in 1864.[64] Its indications are rare because the malignancy is not usually confined to the scapula itself. Adequate function without prosthetic assistance is expected, although the limb will be left weakened.

[†]Deceased.

0

A claviculectomy is also rarely used for neoplastic disease localized to the clavicle. This procedure yields a good functional result with satisfactory cosmesis, range of motion, and reasonable (though diminished) strength in shoulder abduction, flexion, and adduction.

PRECIPITATING FACTORS

The necessity for shoulder amputation results primarily from trauma and neoplasm. Such has been the case in past centuries and remains mostly true today. The great increase in amputations of the lower limb for peripheral vascular disease is not reflected at the shoulder level; rarely does ischemia result in such amputations. Aggressive fulminating infections, which until recently were seen primarily in developing countries, are being encountered with increasing frequency in the United States and Great Britain. These aggressive infections can be manifested as necrotizing fasciitis or myositis and may require shoulder-level amputation as a lifesaving, staged procedure. A high percentage of reported cases of necrotizing fasciitis occur in intravenous drug abusers, particularly in the upper limb. Mortality ranges from 15% to 30%. Early surgical excision or amputation of all involved tissues is required as a lifesaving measure.

In congenital amputation of the upper limb, revision surgery is rarely required. An occasional congenital limb defect such as phocomelia may require revision amputation. This circumstance seldom occurs, however, because even the presence of small residual fingers, including a partial hand or limb at shoulder level, may be useful in prosthetic rehabilitation. Function, not cosmesis, is the overriding consideration in such circumstances. A concentrated experience in congenital anomalies was acquired from the thalidomide disaster in England and northern Europe. Quite commonly, afflicted children were born with flipper-like, rudimentary upper limbs extending out from shoulder level; the condition was often bilateral. Management of this severe functional loss stimulated remarkable improvements in prosthetic design and terminal device control for shoulder-level ablation.

Trauma, which by far is the major cause of amputations through the shoulder area, often follows well-defined patterns. Physicians staffing major trauma centers are accustomed to occasionally seeing a worker whose arm has been caught in moving machinery and avulsed at the shoulder joint. A portion of the soft tissues of the chest wall is often torn away, with a large, ragged wound remaining. The injury can be life-threatening. Road accidents, often involving motorcycles, result in the person being thrown from the vehicle and dragged along with the arm often engaged and then torn from the body. Similarly, individuals unrestrained by seat belts are thrown from cars or trucks; their limbs are caught in the door, the steering wheel, or another part of the vehicle's machinery and severed from the body. Because these accidents are severe, multiple associated injuries are often sustained, thus complicating treatment of the shoulder avulsion. When burns accompany these injuries, reconstruction of the amputation site is particularly challenging.

SPECIFIC PROCEDURES

Amputation through the Surgical Neck and Shaft of the Humerus

Exposure is obtained through the lateral aspect of the shoulder area. The patient is placed supine on the operating table with support beneath the shoulder to allow access to the entire shoulder area. The arm is draped free. The incision begins anteriorly at the level of the coracoid process. It is carried distally, follows the anterior border of the deltoid muscle, and crosses the lateral aspect of the proximal end of the humerus just below the level of the deltoid insertion. It continues along the posterior border of the deltoid muscle to the level of the axillary fold, then transversely across the axilla to connect with the anterior of the arm (Fig. 24–1). Care should be taken to leave an adequate amount of skin, particularly in the axilla. Skin closure can be compromised when the flap is short and tight medially.

The next step is to identify, ligate, and divide the cephalic vein in the deltopectoral groove. The interval between the deltoid and the pectoralis major muscles is developed, and the deltoid muscle is retracted laterally and upward. The pectoralis major muscle is now divided at its humeral insertion and reflected medially. The pectoralis minor and coracobrachialis muscles can then be identified, with the neurovascular bundle exposed in the interval between them. The axillary artery and vein and adjacent tributaries are identified, isolated, doubly ligated, and divided.

The median, ulnar, radial, and musculocutaneous nerves are then isolated individually, drawn down into the wound gently, ligated circumferentially, and sectioned with a knife distal to the ligatures. They will then retract comfortably under the pectoralis minor muscle.

The deltoid muscle is sectioned at its insertion and further retracted proximally with the lateral skin flap. The insertions of the teres major and latissimus dorsi muscles are then identified at the bicipital groove, and the muscles are sectioned near their insertions. The long and short heads of the biceps, the triceps, and the coracobrachialis are next divided approximately ¾ inch distal to the planned level of bone section.

With the proximal end of the humerus thus isolated, it is divided at the desired level with a small-toothed, reciprocating power saw. Sharp, bony margins are rounded smooth, and the wound is thoroughly irrigated. In very short transhumeral amputations, the resulting muscle imbalance can pull the residual arm into 90 degrees of abduction. Recently, Baumgartner from Germany has recommended that surgeons consider arthrodesis in a functional position to prevent this complication in very short amputations.[5]

The limb is then removed. Closure is accomplished by drawing the long head of the triceps, together with both heads of the biceps and the coracobrachialis, over the cut end of the humerus, swinging the pectoralis major muscle laterally, and suturing it to the end of the bone without tension.

The deltoid muscle and skin flaps are tailored to an accurate closure with interrupted sutures or skin

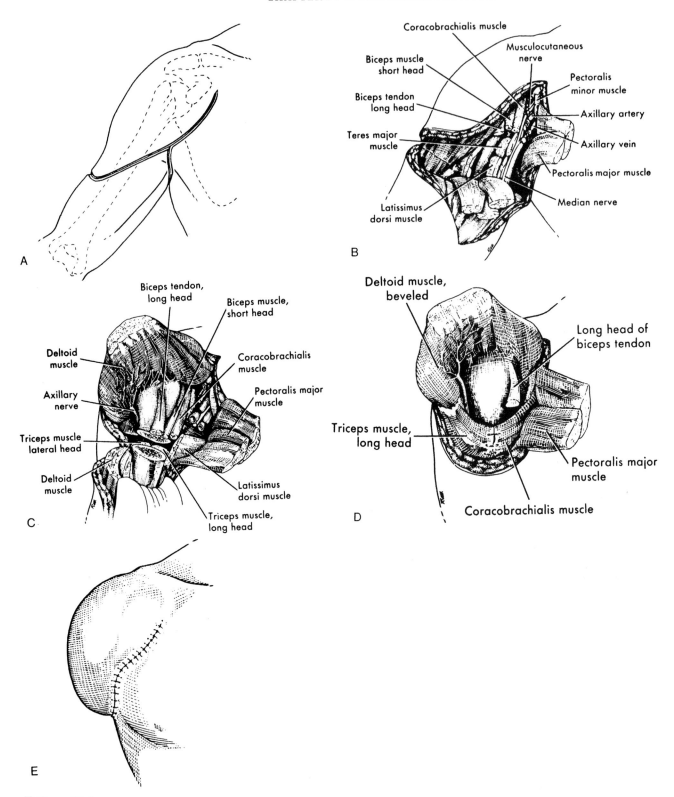

■ **Figure 24–1**
Amputation through the surgical neck of the humerus. **A,** Skin incision. **B,** Section of anterior muscles. **C,** Bone level and completed muscle section. **D,** Closure of the muscle flap. **E,** Completed amputation. *(From Tooms RE: Amputations of upper extremity. In Crenshaw AH [ed]: Campbell's Operative Orthopaedics, 7th ed. St Louis: CV Mosby, 1987. Redrawn from Slocum DB: An Atlas of Amputations. St Louis: CV Mosby, 1949.)*

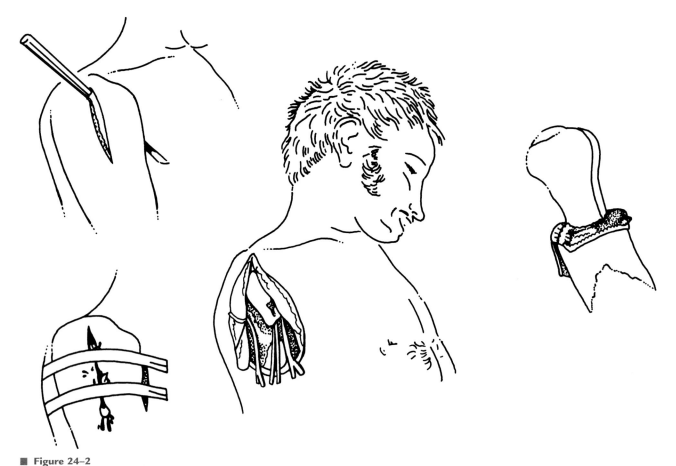

■ Figure 24–2
Modified illustration of shoulder disarticulation performed by Baron Larrey and described in 1797. *(Redrawn from Larrey DJ: Memoire sur les Amputations des Membres à La Suite des Coups de Feu Etaye de Plusieurs Observations. Paris: Du Pont, 1797.)*

clips. The wound is drained either by through-and-through drainage or by suction drainage, or by both. Supportive compression dressings are applied to assist in eliminating postsurgical dead space. Dressings are changed in 48 hours, and the drains are removed. Compressive soft dressings are continued until the wound is stable.

Disarticulation of the Shoulder

Shoulder disarticulation has been referred to in many military medical writings over the centuries. Baron Dominique Jean Larrey, military surgeon to Napoleon for 16 years, described and illustrated his technique, which established the standard of the day.[33] Baron Larrey was a skilled anatomist and an expert surgical technician; it has been said that he amputated more limbs than any surgeon before or since. He described performing 200 thigh amputations in one 24-hour period while accompanying Napoleon during the battle of Borodino. (A modified illustration of his shoulder disarticulation technique is shown in Figure 24–2.)

The patient is positioned supine with support under the affected shoulder to allow complete access to the shoulder and shoulder girdle area. The incision begins anteriorly at the coracoid process, continues along the anterior border of the deltoid muscle, and is then carried transversely across the lateral aspect of the proximal end of the humerus at the level of the deltoid muscle insertion (Fig. 24–3A). It is then continued superiorly along the posterior border of the muscle to end at the posterior axillary fold, where the two ends of the incision are joined with a second incision passing across the axilla. The cephalic vein is identified in the deltopectoral groove and ligated. The deltoid and pectoralis major muscles are separated anteriorly. The deltoid is then retracted laterally; the pectoralis major is divided at its humeral insertion and reflected medially.

The interval between the coracobrachialis and the short head of the biceps is opened to expose the neurovascular bundle (see Fig. 24–3B). The axillary artery and vein are doubly ligated independently of each other and then sectioned. The thoracoacromial artery, just proximal to the pectoralis minor muscle, is identified, ligated, and divided. The vessels then retract superiorly under the pectoralis minor muscle. The median, ulnar, musculocutaneous, and radial nerves can then be identified, drawn distally into the wound gently, ligated with a circumferential suture, and sectioned under mild tension. They then retract beneath the pectoralis minor muscle.

The coracobrachialis and short head of the biceps are next sectioned near their insertions on the coracoid process (see Fig. 24–3C). The deltoid muscle is freed from its insertion on the humerus and reflected superiorly to expose the capsule of the shoulder joint. The teres major

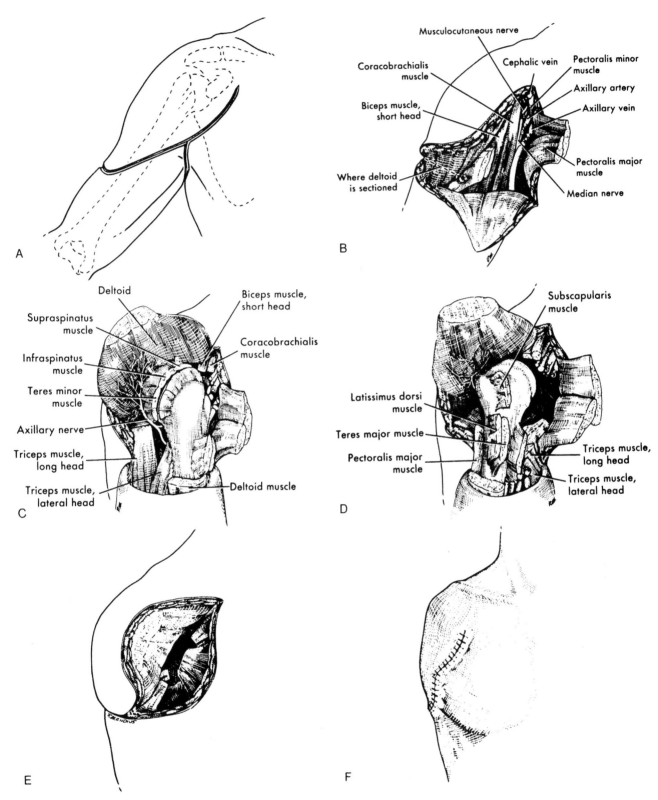

■ **Figure 24–3**

Disarticulation of the shoulder. **A,** Incision. **B,** Exposure and section of the neurovascular bundle. **C,** Reflection of the deltoid; the arm is placed in internal rotation; section of the supraspinatus, infraspinatus, and teres minor tendons and the posterior capsule; section of the coracobrachialis and biceps at the coracoid. **D,** The arm is placed in external rotation; subscapularis and anterior capsule section. **E,** Suture of muscles in the glenoid cavity. **F,** Completed amputation. *(From Tooms RE: Amputations of upper extremity. In Crenshaw AH [ed]: Campbell's Operative Orthopaedics, 7th ed. St Louis: CV Mosby, 1987. Redrawn from Slocum DB: An Atlas of Amputations, St Louis: CV Mosby, 1949.)*

and latissimus dorsi muscles are divided at their insertions, and the arm is placed in internal rotation to expose the short external rotator muscles, the posterior aspect of the shoulder joint, and the adjacent fascia. All these structures are divided.

The arm is then rotated into full external rotation, and the anterior aspect of the joint capsule, the remaining shoulder capsule, and the subscapularis muscle are sectioned (see Fig. 24–3D). The triceps muscle is divided near its insertion, and the limb is severed from the trunk by dividing the inferior capsule of the shoulder joint. The cut ends of all muscles are reflected into the glenoid cavity and sutured there to help fill the hollow left by removal of the humeral head (see Fig. 24–3E).

The deltoid muscle flap is then brought down inferiorly to permit suturing just below the glenoid (see Fig. 24–3F). Closure is accomplished without tension by using optimal wound closure technique. Drains, either suction or through-and-through, or both, are inserted and closure is carried out in layers. Compression dressings are applied to assist in eliminating any residual dead space. Scar adhesions about the site of surgery can be painful and can complicate both cosmesis and functional prosthetic fit. Drains are usually removed in 48 hours, and effective compression dressings are reapplied.

Scapulothoracic Amputation (Forequarter Amputation)

This radical procedure involves surgical removal of the entire upper limb in the interval between the scapula and the thoracic wall. Its primary indication is the presence of malignant tumors about the shoulder girdle. Because such tumors often invade the regional lymph nodes and chest wall, the operation is considered essentially a lifesaving salvage procedure. The surgery may control intractable pain for a time, although in present neoplastic management pain is best handled by a variety of medical techniques. Open ulceration and infection can further require careful planning to obtain skin and soft tissue coverage.

Most scapulothoracic amputations performed today in Western countries are carried out by surgical services specializing in neoplastic diseases. Management of connective tissue malignant tumors of the limbs has been changing dramatically over the past decade and continues to change. In those few cases in which forequarter amputation seems to be indicated, the management team should consist of oncologists, plastic and reconstructive surgeons, and orthopaedic or general surgeons. The surgery itself—except in unusual circumstances of trauma or tumor—is not complicated when carried out with the standard accepted techniques that have been used successfully for most of this century. Occasionally, staged procedures and skin or composite grafts are required to achieve wound closure.

Anterior Approach

The incision begins 4 cm lateral to the sternoclavicular articulation at a point corresponding to the lateral border of the sternocleidomastoid muscle insertion (Fig. 24–4A). It follows the entire anterior aspect of the clavicle and passes over the top of the shoulder to the spine of the scapula. At this point, the arm is flexed over the chest to rotate the scapula forward and outward so that its bony contour is outlined in greater relief. The posterior aspect of the upper incision then proceeds down over the spine to its vertical border, which it follows distally to the angle of the scapula. The lower portion of the ellipse starts in the middle third of the clavicle and passes downward in the groove between the deltoid and the pectoral muscles to the anterior axillary fold. The arm is abducted, and the incision is continued across the axilla at the level of the junction of the skin of the arm and the axillary skin. As the incision passes the posterior axillary fold, it continues medially across the back to join the upper incision at the angle of the scapula. The head is bent toward the normal side so that the sternocleidomastoid muscle may be better outlined, and the pectoralis major muscle is severed from its clavicular insertion. The dissection starts at the lateral border of the insertion and proceeds close to bone to the lateral border of the sternocleidomastoid muscle. The pectoralis major muscle is then reflected downward and medially. If further exposure is needed, the humeral insertion of the pectoralis major may be divided. The upper border of the clavicle is exposed by sectioning the superficial layer of the deep fascia along the upper border of the clavicle as far medially as the sternocleidomastoid muscle. Further dissection beneath the clavicle is carried out with a finger or a blunt curved dissector. The external jugular vein, which emerges just above the clavicle at the lateral border of the sternocleidomastoid, may be sectioned and ligated if it is in the way.

The clavicle is now divided with a Gigli or reciprocating power saw at the lateral border of the sternocleidomastoid muscle. It is not desirable to section the clavicle more medially because of the danger of injuring the veins that hug its medial inch. The clavicle is sectioned at or near the acromioclavicular joint, and the freed portion is removed (see Fig. 24–4B). If the humeral insertion of the pectoralis major muscle has not already been sectioned, this is done. This whole muscle may then be reflected downward, and the entire shoulder girdle may be retracted outward and downward so that the axillary and subclavian region is in full view. The axillary fascia is sectioned, the pectoralis minor is severed from its coracoid insertion, and the costocoracoid membrane that lies between the pectoralis minor and the subclavius is divided (see Fig. 24–4D). The second layer of deep fascia up to the level of the omohyoid muscle, the periosteum at the back of the clavicle, and the subclavius are divided to complete exposure of the neurovascular bundle. The subclavian artery is isolated, sectioned, and doubly ligated. The blood in the extremity is emptied into the general circulation by elevation; the subclavian vein is then clamped, cut, and doubly ligated. The brachial plexus is identified, and each trunk is carefully ligated circumferentially. The nerves are sectioned one by one at the cranial end of the incision and allowed to retract. The latissimus dorsi muscle and all remaining soft tissues binding the shoulder girdle to the anterior chest wall are sectioned, and the limb falls freely backward.

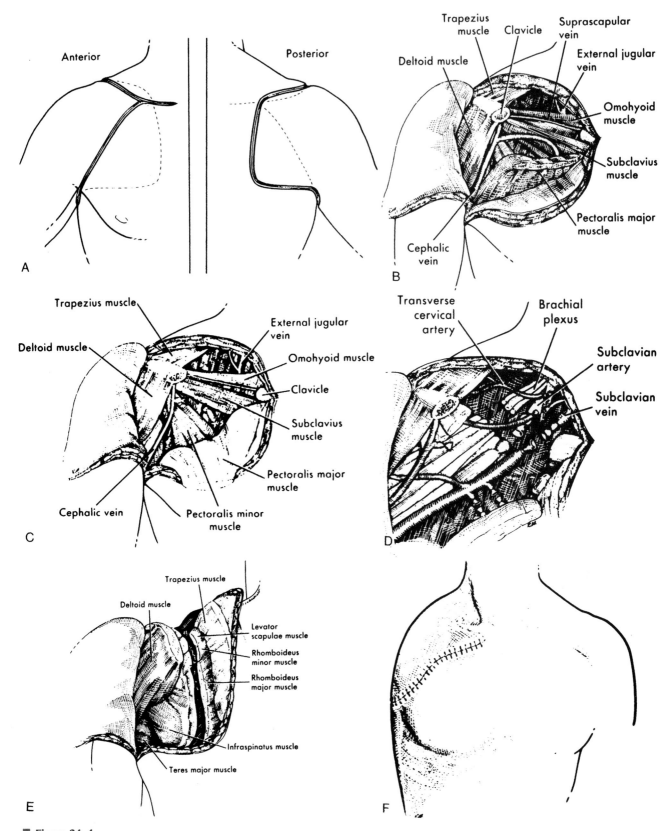

■ **Figure 24–4**
Forequarter amputation through the anterior approach. **A,** Incision. **B,** Resection of the clavicle. **C,** Lifting of the pectoral lid. **D,** Section of the vessels and nerves after incision through the axillary fascia and insertion of the pectoralis minor, the costocoracoid membrane, and the subclavius. **E,** Section of supporting muscles of the scapula. **F,** Completed amputation. *(From Tooms RE: Amputations of upper extremity. In Crenshaw AH [ed]: Campbell's Operative Orthopaedics, 7th ed. St Louis: CV Mosby, 1987. Redrawn from Slocum DB: An Atlas of Amputations. St Louis: CV Mosby, 1949.)*

Section of the Posterior Muscles

The arm is placed across the chest and held with gentle downward traction. The posterior incision is deepened through the fascia, and the skin is retracted medially. The remaining muscles fixing the shoulder girdle to the scapula are divided as they are encountered from above downward. The muscles holding the scapula to the thorax are divided (see Fig. 24-4E). The incision starts at the insertion of the trapezius to the clavicle and acromion and is carried downward along the upper border of the spine of the scapula. After sectioning, each muscle is retracted medially. The muscles along the superior angle of the vertebral border of the scapula—the omohyoid, levator scapulae, rhomboideus major and minor, and serratus anterior—are sectioned by placing double clamps near their insertions and cutting between the clamps from above downward. The extremity is removed, and hemostasis is controlled with meticulous care.

Closure

Careful inspection is made to ensure that all malignant tissue has been removed. If the pectoralis major has not, of necessity, been removed, it should be sutured to the trapezius muscle. Closure is accomplished in layers, with all remaining muscular structures grouped over the lateral chest wall to provide as much padding as possible. The skin flaps are brought together and tailored to form an accurate approximation. The wound is closed with interrupted sutures (see Fig. 24-4F), and adequate drainage is established. Dry dressings are applied, and a snug pressure dressing is placed over the lateral chest wall. The drains are removed in 48 to 72 hours, and the sutures are removed between the 10th and 14th days.

Posterior Approach

Littlewood, in 1922, described a technique of scapulothoracic amputation that requires two incisions and approaches the shoulder area from the posterior aspect (Fig. 24-5).[36] This posterior approach is considered technically easier. We have used the conventional (Berger) anterior approach for patients under our care over the years but recognize the advantages of the two-incision technique, especially in atypical cases.

The patient is positioned on the uninvolved side near the edge of the operating table (see Fig. 24-5). Two incisions are required—one posterior (cervicoscapular) and one anterior (pectoroaxillary). The posterior incision is made first. Beginning at the medial end of the clavicle, the incision extends laterally for the entire length of the bone, carries over the acromion process to the posterior axillary fold, continues along the axillary border of the scapula to a point inferior to the scapular angle, and finally curves medially to end 2 inches from the midline of the back. From the scapular muscles an entire full-thickness flap of skin and subcutaneous tissue is elevated medially to a point just medial to the vertebral border of the scapula.

Next, the trapezius and latissimus dorsi muscles are identified and divided parallel with the scapula. The same is done to the levator scapulae, the rhomboideus major and minor, and the scapular attachments of the serratus anterior and the omohyoid. As the dissection progresses, vessels are ligated when necessary, especially the branches of the transverse cervical and transverse scapular arteries. The soft tissues are then freed from the clavicle, and the bone is divided at its medial end. The subclavius muscle is also divided.

The extremity is then allowed to fall anteriorly, thus placing the subclavian vessels and the brachial plexus under tension and making identification of them easier. The cords of the plexus are clamped close to the spine, and the subclavian artery and vein are clamped, doubly ligated, and divided.

The anterior incision is then begun at the middle of the clavicle. It curves inferiorly just lateral to but parallel with the deltopectoral groove, extends across the anterior axillary fold, and finally carries inferiorly and posteriorly to join the posterior axillary incision at the lower third of the axillary border of the scapula. As the final step in the operation, the pectoralis major and minor muscles are divided and the limb is removed. The skin flaps are trimmed to allow a snug closure, and their edges are sutured with interrupted sutures of nonabsorbable material. Effective through-and-through and suction drains are inserted to eliminate any accumulation of fluid. Firm chest wall pressure dressings are required. Drains can be removed after 48 hours.

Depending on the nature and extent of the pathologic process, surgical variations may be indicated, such as the need for regional lymph node resection and soft tissue removal at the chest wall when the tumor has extended into these structures. Skin grafts, including composite tissues, may be necessary to obtain primary or secondary closure. Several recent articles highlight the use of free tissue transfer, occasionally from the distal aspect of the amputated limb, as means to obtain closure after radical tumor resection.[13]

Intercalary Shoulder Resection

Intercalary shoulder resection (the Tikhoff-Linberg technique) involves massive removal of the musculoskeletal elements of the shoulder girdle, including the scapula, the lateral three fourths of the clavicle, and a portion of the proximal end of the humerus, with extensive removal of all adjacent muscles. The neurovascular structures that supply the arm and the hand are preserved. Excessive skin is often left after this radical resection. The remaining connecting soft tissues across the former shoulder joint consist of only the axillary vessels and the brachial plexus, together with the axillary skin. Closure of the soft tissues, including the skin, is individualized according to the nature of the malignancy for which the surgery is being performed. It is necessary to stabilize the proximal part of the humerus to the remaining medial stump of the clavicle or the chest wall to prevent excessive drooping and telescoping of the arm.

This operation is rarely used in surgical practice today. A patient's refusal to allow formal amputation can, however, justify its use. A review of 19 patients from Germany with an average follow-up of over 6 years

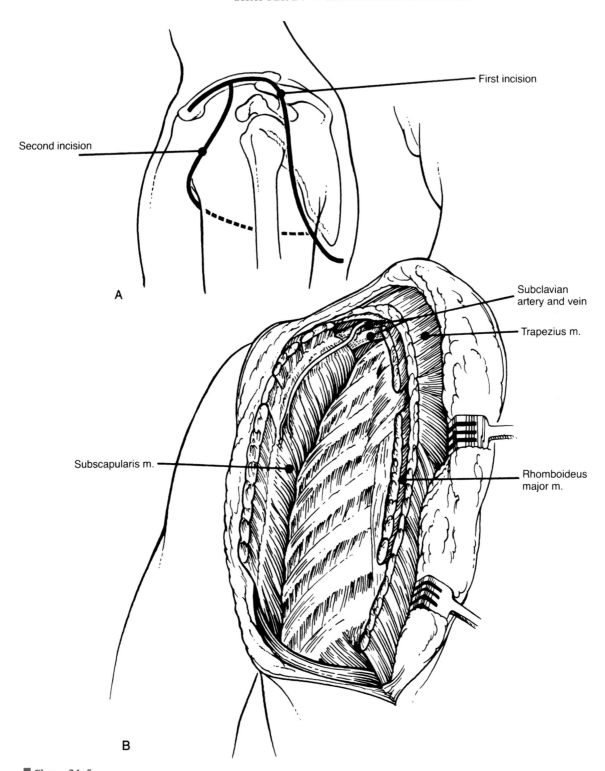

■ Figure 24–5
Forequarter amputation through the posterior approach (the Littlewood technique). *(Redrawn from Littlewood H: Amputations at the shoulder and at the hip. BMJ 1:381, 1922.)*

concluded that in spite of a 74% complication rate, the Tikhoff-Linberg procedure proved to be a valuable technique with an outcome superior to that achieved by scapulothoracic amputation.[69]

The operation is carried out with the patient in the full lateral position and lying on the uninvolved side. The

entire upper extremity, chest, and neck are prepared and draped so that the arm, shoulder, and shoulder girdle are free for manipulation and positioning. The incision resembles a tennis racquet—the "handle" extends from the medial third of the clavicle laterally, whereas the anterior limb extends downward along the deltopectoral groove to

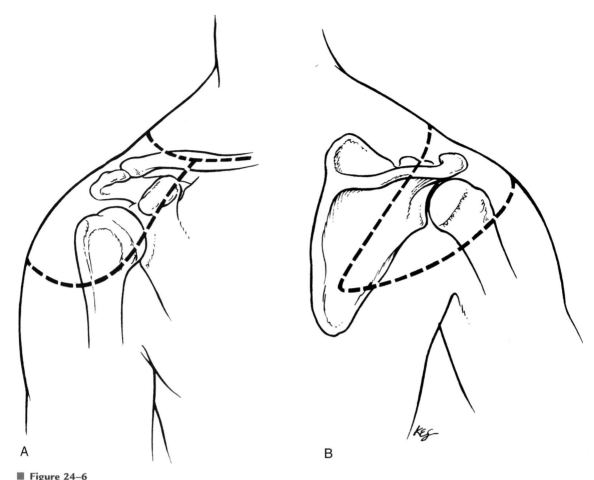

A   B

■ **Figure 24–6**
Skin incision for interscapulothoracic resection (the Tikhoff-Linberg technique). *(Redrawn from Tikhof PT: Tumor Studies. Russia, 1900.)*

the midpoint of the medial edge of the biceps, proceeds distally for 7 to 8 cm, and then curves upward to cross the lateral surface of the arm at or just below the mid-deltoid level (Fig. 24–6). From this point, the posterior limb of the "racquet" curves from the mid-deltoid area downward and medially toward the inferior angle of the scapula, where it again curves upward to join the original clavicular incision near the acromioclavicular joint.

Deeper dissection can be carried out from either an anterior or a posterior approach. We have used a combination of both approaches. In effect, this dissection combines the classic anterior technique of forequarter amputation with the posterior approach (Littlewood) technique of this surgery. The brachial plexus is preserved, as are major vessels. It is necessary to ligate the transverse cervical, suprascapular, circumflex scapular, circumflex humeral, and thoracoacromial arteries. With the scapulothoracic muscles detached and the deltoid, biceps, and triceps sectioned, the humerus can be transected at or below the surgical neck at the level selected. The biceps, triceps, and deltoid muscles are attached to the thoracic wall, and the trapezius suspends the arm as firmly as possible without compromising neurovascular integrity. The wound is drained by both suction and through-and-through drains, which are removed in 48 hours. Soft compression dressings and a Velpeau-like sling support are used postoperatively.

The skin and soft tissue resection is modified to accommodate removal of the neoplasm. The arm should be supported until sufficient scarring has occurred at the operative site to provide some stability. No attempt is made to regain a semblance of shoulder function. Rehabilitation concentrates on the neck and trunk muscles and on the arm distal to the site of amputation of the humerus. An adequate degree of hand, wrist, forearm, and elbow function can be achieved. Cosmesis is also surprisingly good in view of the massive tissue resection. The defect in the shoulder girdle and shoulder contour can be concealed with a light, modern prosthetic cosmetic restoration consisting of currently available materials—particularly the urethanes—to provide a more normal appearance of the shoulder area under clothing.

Scapulectomy

In 1864, Syme described excision of the scapula for primary bone tumors.[64] The operation is used for isolated neoplasms of the scapula, a condition that is rarely seen. Neglected, slow-growing osteocartilaginous tumors arising in the scapula may cause functional compromise sufficient to warrant excision of the scapula, which is usually accompanied by adjuvant chemotherapy and radiation. A general description of the operative technique is presented here in the realization that there is literally no standard operative approach. When the tumor has extended beyond the confines of the bone, surgery may require excision of lymph nodes in the complicated chains surrounding the shoulder girdle. Scapulectomy following a biopsy should include wide resection of the biopsy site, including skin and deep tissues.

The operation is carried out with the patient in the prone position, supported under the affected shoulder. The arm is draped free to allow movement of the humerus and scapula as the dissection proceeds. Regardless of the nature and type of incision, adequate access to the entire superior border of the scapula is mandatory.

The classic incision begins laterally at the tip of the acromion, extends posteriorly directly below the acromion spine to its midportion, and then gently curves distally across the body of the scapula to its inferior angle (Fig. 24-7). The nature of the pathologic process will determine the management of muscles and, specifically, the particular muscles that should be resected. Detaching the latissimus dorsi from the inferior angle allows the scapula to be tilted upward and outward, thus affording free access to the subscapular space.

The vertebral border of the scapula is then freed, and the remaining insertions of the inferior and middle

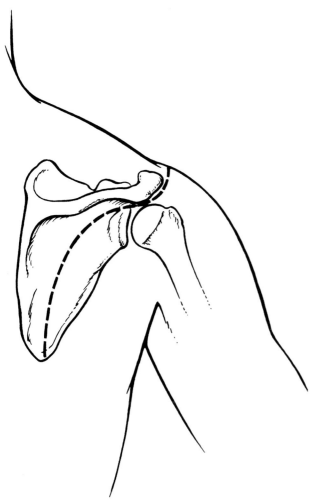

■ **Figure 24–7**
Skin incision in scapulectomy.

trapezius are detached from the spine of the scapula to expose the rhomboids for division. The superior trapezius is divided from the scapular spine, the acromion, and the distal end of the clavicle. The levator scapulae is sectioned. The superficial cervical and descending scapular vessels are identified and ligated. The suprascapular vessels and nerves are exposed, and as the scapula is lifted further laterally from the thorax, the brachial plexus and axillary vessels come into view. It is important to remove the supraspinatus, infraspinatus, and serratus anterior along with the scapula itself. The nature and extent of the pathologic process will dictate whether it is possible to preserve the acromion and the continuity of the superior trapezius-deltoid suspensory system.

The axillary border of the scapula is then approached by transection of the deltoid from the spine of the scapula and from the acromion. The teres major and the long head of the triceps muscles are transected, the subscapular artery is identified and ligated, and the underlying axillary and radial nerves are carefully preserved. Disarticulation of the acromioclavicular joint and detachment of the coracoclavicular ligaments or division of the clavicle just medial to the coracoclavicular ligaments allows the scapula to be further freed from the chest. The pectoralis minor, coracobrachialis, and short head of the biceps muscles can then be detached from the coracoid process, and the rotator cuff can be transected by external and internal rotation of the humerus. It may be appropriate to modify the level of section of the rotator cuff so that after removal of the scapula, the distal cuff can be sutured about the distal end of the clavicle to suspend and stabilize the humerus and preserve a more cosmetic shoulder outline. The wound is closed in layers over adequate drainage systems. Compression dressings are applied, and the arm is supported in a Velpeau-type dressing.

Variations of the scapulectomy technique are the rule rather than the exception. Two recent publications reviewed the results of case series of 12 and 10 patients.[47,55] These series highlight that although impairment of shoulder function will occur, hand, wrist, and elbow function is preserved, with better overall function and appearance than is the case with scapulothoracic amputation.

Claviculectomy

En bloc resection of the clavicle, though rarely indicated, has occasionally been recommended for a localized malignancy or for chronic osteomyelitis. To a large degree, the specific surgical technique depends on the type and location of the neoplasm or infection. The surgical approach is over the anterior aspect of the entire length of the clavicle and extends from the sternoclavicular joint to the acromioclavicular joint (Fig. 24–8). Biopsy sites, if present, are widely excised. Dissection is carried down to the deltoid insertion, which is divided from the clavicle, and a proximal muscular cuff is left intact. The conoid and trapezoid ligaments are divided near their clavicular attachment, and the sternocleidomastoid muscle is carefully sectioned while avoiding injury to the external jugular vein. The omohyoid muscle is retracted, and the

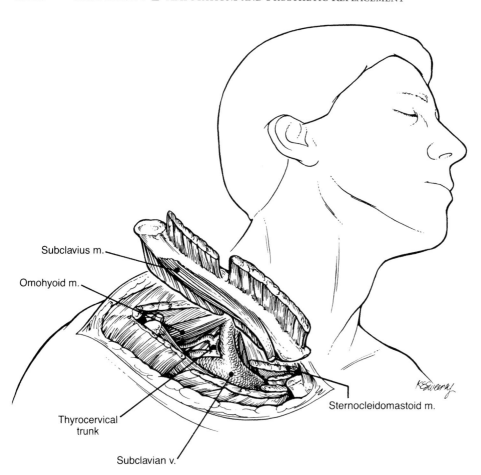

■ **Figure 24–8**
Claviculectomy. (*Redrawn from Lewis MM, Ballet FL, Kroll PG, and Bloom N: En bloc clavicular resection, operative procedure and postoperative testing of function. Clin Orthop 193:214, 1985.*)

Subclavius m.

Omohyoid m.

Thyrocervical
trunk

Subclavian v.

Sternocleidomastoid m.

pectoralis major is incised. The clavicle is then elevated with the subclavicular muscle left attached to the clavicle. The sternoclavicular capsule, sternohyoid muscle insertion, and costoclavicular ligament are all excised. Immediately adjacent vascular structures are carefully protected, and the branches of the transverse cervical artery are ligated. The clavicle is then removed.

Closure in layers, with elimination of dead spaces, is carried out over drainage. Compression dressings and a sling are applied, and drains are removed within 24 to 48 hours. The shoulder and the arm are mobilized as early as is consistent with wound healing.

Technical variations based on the site and nature of the tumor individualize the surgery to such a degree that each case must be planned surgically as a specific technical challenge. Reported series usually include only three or four cases. We have not had occasion to perform this resection-amputation.

PROSTHETIC REHABILITATION

Shoulder area amputations present the most difficult challenge for functional restoration by external prosthetic replacement. Many unilateral amputees reject a functional prosthesis because of the weight, limitations in dexterity, difficulty positioning the terminal device where it is needed, slowness of the prosthesis, and an inability to use these prosthetic devices without undue mental involvement. The requirements of providing a functional terminal device and the control to rapidly position that terminal device in space are rarely met with current prosthetic devices. Although the functional gain is less than ideal, the cosmetic deformity of shoulder-level amputations should not be underestimated. Shirts and jackets drape awkwardly on the side of the shoulder disarticulation or forequarter amputation and thus exaggerate the cosmetic deformity. Often, a lightweight cosmetic substitute or merely a prosthetic shoulder cap to re-create the normal shoulder contour can meet a patient's goals better than a heavier, functional prosthesis can. The remaining limb, whether initially dominant or not, rapidly accommodates to permit most basic activities associated with daily life.

Bilateral shoulder amputations create just the opposite functional demand. The handicap is so severe that prostheses, even though uncomfortable, heavy, and functionally crude in comparison to normal limbs, provide sufficient critically needed function to justify the training, discomfort, and inconvenience associated with their use. Children born with amelia of both upper limbs rapidly learn to use their legs and feet to substitute. Remarkable skill can be achieved. Lower limb joints, particularly the hips, ankles, and feet, develop abnormally large ranges of movement to facilitate a wide range of foot placement. The intrinsic muscles of the feet, as well as the tarsal joints, respond by adaptation to perform many grasp, hook, and pinch functions that are usually not present in feet. This adaptive substitution continues through the amputee's adult life. Though fitted with cosmetic or functional upper limb prostheses, the individual usually discards the artificial limbs in the home and work setting and uses them only for social purposes.

Adults who sustain bilateral shoulder-level amputations, in particular the elderly, often cannot develop the lower limb functional response seen in children. Some substitution can occur, although under most circumstances such a severely disabled individual requires constant attendant help.

Types of Prostheses

Prostheses for shoulder-level amputees are of four types: (1) lightweight passive, (2) body powered, (3) externally powered, and (4) hybrid combinations of body powered and externally powered. The amputee is often best served by a hybrid combination of body powering and external powering with interchangeable terminal devices, including a cosmetic hand.

The simplest artificial substitute is a lightweight passive prosthetic arm (Fig. 24–9). Though previously termed a strictly cosmetic device, we now realize the functional value of this device and avoid the term "cosmetic prosthesis." Modern designs are light, usually fabricated of urethanes or similar synthetics, with light internal or external frame rigidity (when necessary) supplied by graphite, light metals, or semirigid thermoplastics. The shoulder cap of the prosthesis is contoured to correspond to the opposite shoulder shape. Light shoulder strap suspension stabilizes the limb and prevents it from slipping off. The elbow is simple and nonfunctional and permits

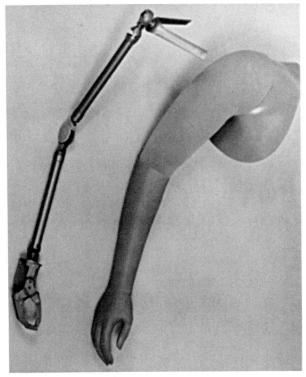

■ **Figure 24–9**
Cosmetic endoskeletal prosthetic system for shoulder disarticulation. *(Courtesy of Otto Bock Orthopedic Industry, Minneapolis, MN.)*

stable positioning at various angles by the opposite limb. The hand can be individually constructed to match the remaining hand. The psychological advantage of a light-weight passive prosthesis often plays a very important and integral part in physical rehabilitation.

These simple prosthetic limbs vary tremendously in cost. Although merely re-creating the shape and contour can be relatively cost-effective, the most elegant and detailed cosmesis can be quite expensive. They are obtained through regular prosthetic sources with the services of an aesthetic restoration artist who is responsible for the shape, texture, and surface detail, including color. Most major population centers in the United States, Canada, and Europe can provide these services. Contact with these skilled professionals is made in cooperation with conventional professional prosthetists.

This passive replacement is not entirely without function. The hand can assist in stabilizing objects on a table or workbench. In general, an active unilateral amputee will use a cosmetic prosthesis only for special social occasions and not in the course of daily work and living activities. In these instances, one should not overlook the possibility that a simple shoulder cap can improve the thoracic contours, help clothing fit better, and help the patient feel less conspicuous (Fig. 24–10A to C).

Body-Powered Functional Prostheses

A substitute limb that can perform useful functions poses a difficult engineering challenge. It requires articulation at the elbow and should permit a degree of positioning of the terminal device (wrist/hand) (Fig. 24–11). Some degree of shoulder abduction and elbow rotation is also required if positioning of the hand or hook is to operate within a significant range of usefulness. Suspending the limb and attaching it sufficiently to the body to provide stability dictates the use of a large shoulder cap, usually made of semiflexible materials, and additional straps around the trunk and across the opposite shoulder. Activation of the hand or hook is accomplished by opposite shoulder movement via a shoulder loop attached to cabling, either light, housed metal or nylon. The prosthesis can be either prepositioned and then locked or, in the case of the elbow, cable controlled (Fig. 24–12).

For years, prosthetic engineers have tried to simplify this prosthesis. Attempting to duplicate, even to a small degree, the unbelievably complex motor and sensory function of the upper limb frustrates such engineering attempts. As a result, even with present technology, body-powered limbs are rather crude, uncomfortable, and severely limited in function. More often, such limbs are designed for a special purpose, such as working at a bench or desk. When the zone of functional activity of the terminal device is confined to a relatively small area, it is more feasible to accommodate a design, thus making the prosthesis more acceptable (Figs. 24–13 to 24–16).

Externally Powered Prostheses

For the reasons just outlined, prosthetic engineers have turned to external power sources. After the thalidomide experience, which produced a considerable number of

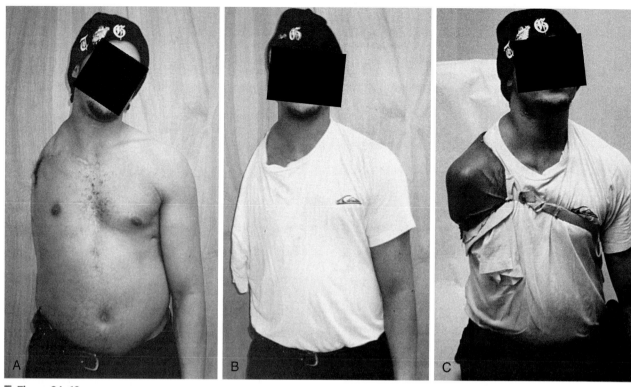

■ Figure 24–10
A, Dramatic loss of shoulder contour after forequarter amputation. **B,** Clothing drapes awkwardly and exaggerates the cosmetic deformity.
C, A simple shoulder cap prosthesis re-creates a more normal shoulder contour and improves the fit of clothing worn over the shoulder cap.
(*A-C, Courtesy of Prosthetics Research Study, Seattle.*)

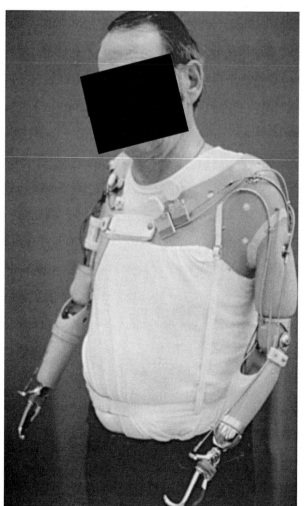

■ Figure 24–11
A cable-operated left arm with a positive-locking cable-operated elbow, positive-locking wrist rotation unit, positive-locking wrist flexion unit, and cable-operated split hook. The elbow lock is controlled by a tether to a waist belt. The locks of the two wrist components are controlled by the two nudge controls on the anterior panel of the socket. (*Courtesy of Dudley S. Childress, Ph.D., Prosthetics Research Laboratory, Northwestern University and the Orthotics and Prosthetics Clinical Services Department, Rehabilitation Institute of Chicago.*)

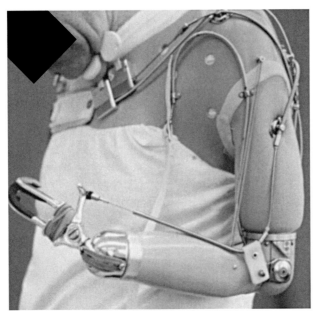

■ **Figure 24–12**
The patient is releasing the lock of the wrist flexion unit. *(Courtesy of Dudley S. Childress, Ph.D., Prosthetics Research Laboratory, Northwestern University and the Orthotics and Prosthetics Clinical Services Department, Rehabilitation Institute of Chicago.)*

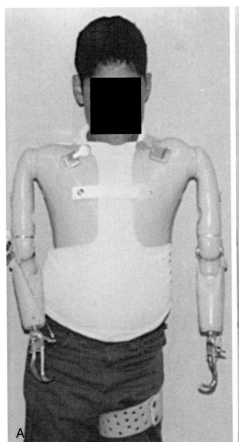

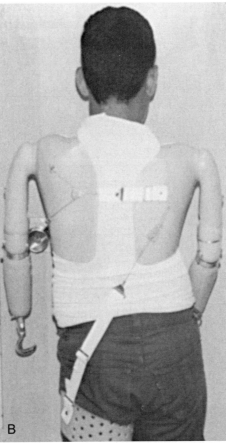

■ **Figure 24–13**
Body-powered prosthesis for bilateral phocomelia. *(Courtesy of AlphaOrthopedic Appliance Co., Los Angeles.)*

A

B

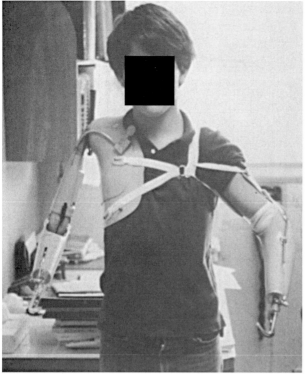

■ **Figure 24–14**
Prosthetic management for bilateral upper limb amputation: right shoulder disarticulation and left below-elbow prostheses. *(Courtesy of Eric Baron, C.P.O., University of California, Child Amputee Prosthetics Project, Los Angeles.)*

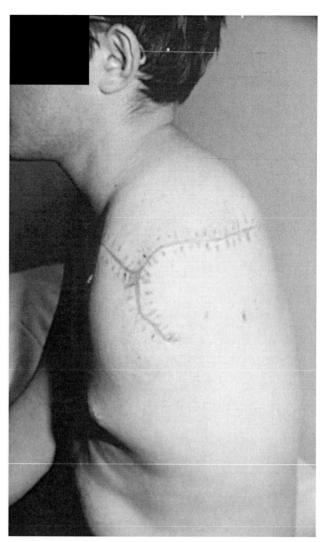

■ **Figure 24–15**
A forequarter amputee ready for prosthetic fitting.

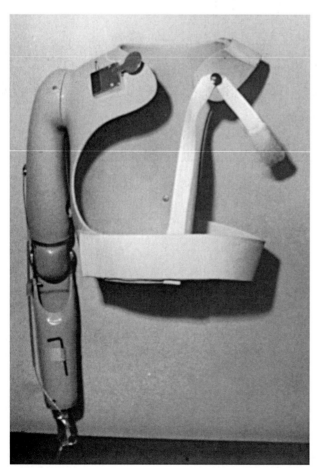

■ **Figure 24–16**
Body-powered forequarter amputation prosthesis. *(Courtesy of Alpha Orthopedic Appliance Co., Los Angeles.)*

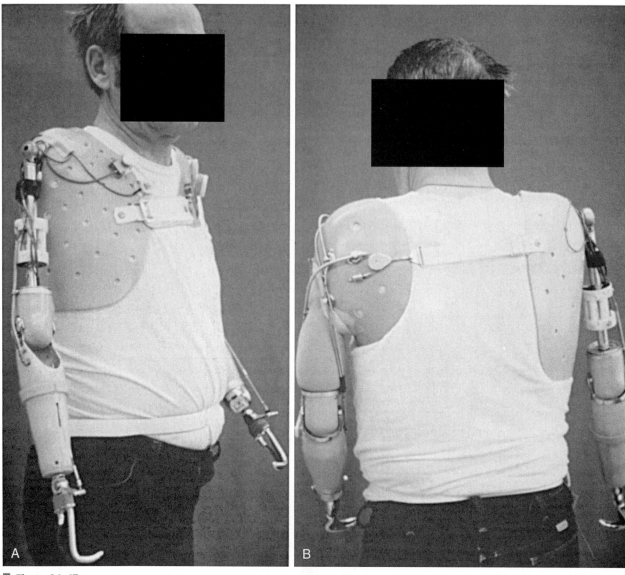

■ **Figure 24–17**

A patient with a right shoulder disarticulation, electrically powered prosthesis. The powered components are the Hosmer electric elbow and the NY/Hosmer Prehension Actuator. Both components are controlled by chin-actuated push switches near the anterosuperior border of the socket. The shoulder, turntable, and forearm rotation joints are all manually positioned friction joints. The crepe band around the forearm provides surface friction for rotation against objects. *(Courtesy of Dudley S. Childress, Ph.D., Prosthetics Research Laboratory, Northwestern University and the Orthotics and Prosthetics Clinical Services Department, Rehabilitation Institute of Chicago.)*

bilateral shoulder disarticulations, prosthetic engineers sought to activate prosthetic substitutes by using compressed gas or electricity. Though useful in the past, compressed gas systems have been discarded for lighter, more responsive electrically powered systems. In the last decade, battery technology and improved microsystems have led to smaller, lighter, and more durable devices. The current state of electronic technology has allowed considerable ingenuity in myoelectric control in which currents generated by body muscles or switches activated by small body motions control the electric motors, which in turn move the prosthesis. A number of such prosthetic systems have been developed and are commercially available worldwide.

With amputations about the shoulder, it is often most practical to seek active elbow and terminal device control only. Shoulder joint and forearm rotation are usually both positioned manually with the opposite limb. The elbow can be positioned actively by the amputee through electrical means and then stabilized in the locked position (Fig. 24–17). The terminal device is then usually operated actively through electric signals (Fig. 24–18). These highly technologic prostheses have continued to evolve from those originally developed at the University of Utah (the Utah Arm) and represent the current state of the art for this approach (Fig. 24–19). The elbow of this device can be controlled electrically, and the terminal device can be operated electrically or by body power. Hybrid limbs are also commonly worn (i.e., partially body powered and partially powered by electricity). This combination has been particularly successful in young, vigorous amputees. Even with the lightest materials, weight is still the usual limiting factor.

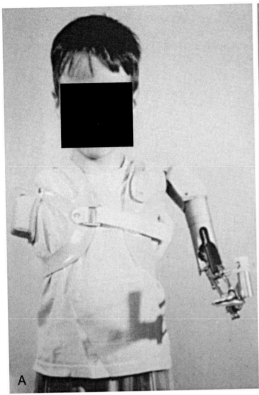

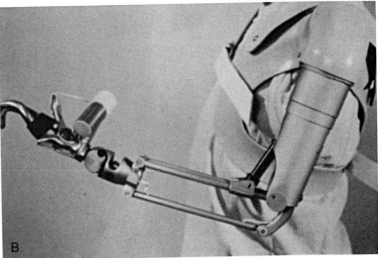

■ **Figure 24–18**
A, Child provided with a noncommercial prosthesis—the NU/Michigan Feeder Arm—with parallelogram linkage in the forearm (kinematic coupling of the elbow and wrist). **B,** The prehensor is the electrically powered Michigan Hook. *(Courtesy of Dudley S. Childress, Ph.D., Prosthetics Research Laboratory, Northwestern University and the Orthotics and Prosthetics Clinical Services Department, Rehabilitation Institute of Chicago.)*

■ **Figure 24–19**
Myoelectrical prostheses for proximal humerus/shoulder disarticulation amputations (Utah Arm). *(Courtesy of Eric Baron, C.P.O., University of California, Child Amputee Prosthetics Project, Los Angeles.)*

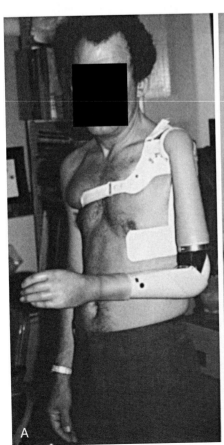

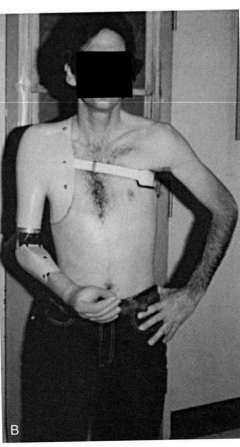

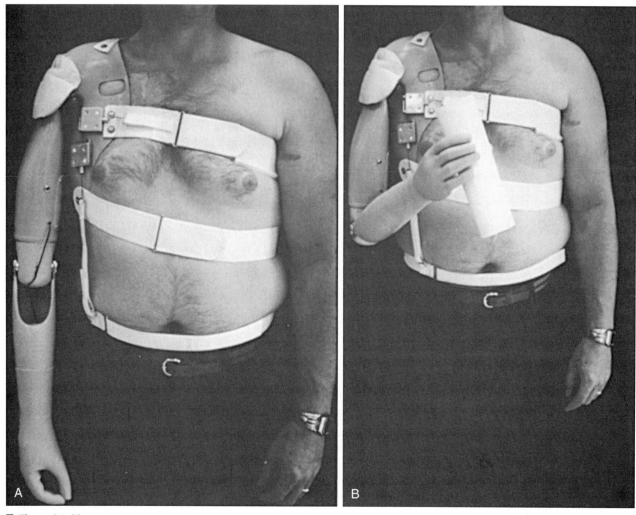

■ **Figure 24–20**
A switch-activated unilateral shoulder disarticulation prosthesis. Two four-state (off-function 1–off-function 2) switches control an electric elbow and an electric hand. Both switches are attached to the exterior of the anterior panel of the socket. The switch for the elbow is connected to a waist belt so that elevation of the shoulder moves the switch through its four states. The switch for the hand is connected to the chest strap and is operated by chest expansion. *(Courtesy of Dudley S. Childress, Ph.D., Prosthetics Research Laboratory, Northwestern University and the Orthotics and Prosthetics Clinical Services Department, Rehabilitation Institute of Chicago.)*

Recent advances have incorporated "proportional control" into externally powered prosthetic systems. Originally, the response from prosthetic limbs was "on" and "off," similar to a light switch. The elbow moved up or down or the terminal device opened or closed at one set speed. Proportional control acts like a dimmer light switch in that it grades the output response according to the intensity of the input. This advance has given the amputee the ability to move the prosthetic limb more naturally. Another development has been in augmenting traditional body-powered systems. Patients with shoulder-level amputations often lack the shoulder excursion to effectively use cable control systems and lack muscles in the residual limb to signal myoelectric sensors. Other electrical switching systems now take advantage of small body motions from the chin, chest expansion, or a change in shoulder/pelvic distance to provide the human input. Although these body motions do not usually have the excursion to power a traditional cable system, they can

signal proportional electric switches to control an externally powered prosthesis (Fig. 24-20).

Despite these technical advances, to be successful, functional prostheses require a high degree of motivation on the part of the amputee. With one remaining functional upper limb, most acts of daily living can be accomplished by the normal arm with increasing skill as training proceeds. Even after being fitted with a state-of-the-art prosthesis, users tend to gradually discard the prosthetic limb as their opposite normal limb becomes more functional. A lightweight, passive prosthesis can become the limb of choice.

Special Considerations

Postural Abnormalities

Normally, the weight of the arm and the muscle activity associated with shoulder/arm function keep the shoulders appropriately level. Unilateral hypertrophy of an upper limb, including the shoulder girdle, occurs in certain occupations and is also seen in some sports. Some people are born with a degree of shoulder-level asymmetry that involves relatively minor postural abnormalities and does not require special clothing.

When the arm is removed and the clavicle and scapula remain, the shoulder girdle elevators are unopposed by the weight of the arm and by the muscles passing across the shoulder that tend to depress the shoulder and arm. The consequence of this imbalance is an upward elevation described as "hiking" of the shoulder girdle. This "high shoulder" tends to accentuate the cosmetic loss, even when the individual is wearing a cosmetic shoulder filler or a cosmetic limb. Abnormal shoulder elevation can be countered by corrective exercises that begin as soon as they are tolerated after the amputation. Wearing of a prosthesis with its dependent weight also diminishes shoulder "hike." In most circumstances, shoulder girdle elevation is inevitable; however, its degree can be minimized by appropriate physical measures.

Removal of the entire upper limb in a growing skeleton routinely results in sharp scoliosis of the dorsal spine at the mid and upper dorsal levels. Muscular imbalance is considered to be the cause of the deformity. It may be seen to a slighter degree in an adult but is confined primarily to the growing skeleton. The combined postural deformity of upper dorsal spine scoliosis and elevation of the shoulder girdle produces asymmetry of the head and neck on the trunk, with the head appearing to be placed asymmetrically as the person stands.

In general, no corrective splinting or orthotic device successfully counteracts the postural changes associated with shoulder-level amputation. Neck and shoulder girdle exercises offer the most effective prophylaxis and treatment. The postural deficits are particularly evident with forequarter amputation. A soft, light polyurethane cosmetic restoration, either as part of a cosmetic prosthesis or used separately with the empty sleeve, will to some degree counter the unsightly upper body contour.

Amputation for Severe Brachial Plexus Injury

Management of severe brachial plexus injuries is complex, emotional, and individual. The decision to amputate all or part of the dysfunctional limb should be carefully thought out and discussed. In the authors' opinion, it is not appropriate to perform or encourage amputation at an early stage. Education, support, and visitor programs with other patients who have brachial plexus injuries tend to be most helpful. Patients need time to adapt to the injury, learn the advantages and disadvantages of retaining a nonfunctional arm, and come to terms with the hope of neurologic recovery and the practical reality of the injury.

The reason for performing an amputation, the specific level of amputation, and the expected goals can vary considerably in an incomplete plexus injury. Setting specific goals for function, cosmesis, and prosthetic use before the surgery can be very helpful for both the patient and the surgeon. Occasionally, above-elbow amputation is elected

to manage a totally dysfunctional arm after a complete brachial plexus avulsion. The advantages involve unloading the weight from the shoulder and scapulothoracic joints and removing a paralyzed arm that hinders function because it gets in the way. The necessity for shoulder arthrodesis is controversial and should be individualized. One clinical series found a slightly better rate of return to work in the group of patients with above-elbow amputation without shoulder arthrodesis. In the authors' opinion, shoulder arthrodesis makes sense only if the patient has motor control of the scapulothoracic joint and not of the glenohumeral joint. If both are flail, fusion is probably not beneficial, and if both joints have motor control, arthrodesis is not needed.

Prosthetic expectations in these patients should be very limited because prosthetic fitting adds weight to a dysfunctional shoulder girdle, often defeating one of the original goals of the amputation. A very lightweight, cosmetic prosthesis is often desired and indicated to help restore body image.

Pain

All amputees with acquired amputations have a sense that all or part of the missing limb is still present. This phantom sensation is not always described in terms of pain and is not always bothersome to the amputee. True phantom pain, a sensation that occurs in the missing limb and is described in terms of pain, does occur after some amputations. Unfortunately, phantom pain seems to be encountered in a higher percentage of persons with shoulder-level amputations than in those with lower limb amputations. This finding is particularly true with limb loss caused by trauma. Avulsion of the arm can cause severe traction trauma to nerve trunks and nerve roots up to their spinal origin. Likewise, painful neoplasms that require shoulder area amputation tend to "carry over" established pain patterns after ablation.

No direct surgical relief of these painful phenomena can be achieved, either at the time of amputation or subsequently. Careful, meticulous isolation and ligation of nerve trunks followed by sharp knife sectioning below the level of ligature has proved to be the most effective method of handling nerves at the time of surgery. The sectioned nerves should retract well under the remaining muscles and are thus protected by soft tissues. Nerve cautery and injection of the nerve ends with a long-acting local anesthetic or with tissue-destroying chemicals (e.g., phenol or absolute alcohol) have been ineffective. The transected nerve will always form a neuroma, but these neuromas tend to not be symptomatic if they retract into the deeper tissue, away from areas of pressure, scarring, and pulsating vessels. Consequently, the authors believe that the nerves should not be ligated together with the vessels.

The incidence of phantom pain in lower extremity amputations seems to be reduced by the use of perioperative epidural anesthesia. The use of axillary or intrascalene blocks to provide perioperative analgesia can lessen the perioperative opioid requirements. Early evidence has shown that blocking the sensory pathways in the perioperative period may decrease the incidence of long-term phantom pain, although this effect has not yet been proved conclusively.

When pain remains a serious problem, the best management is nonsurgical. Central neural surgery, in particular, should be avoided. High nerve division or tractotomy is almost routinely unsuccessful and, in fact, may aggravate the pain patterns. Local physical measures, including massage, cold, exercise, neuromuscular stimulation by external electrical currents, acupuncture, and regional sympathectomy, may under certain circumstances have a place in therapy when the pain is intractable. A technique that has gained some acceptance and success is the use of transcutaneous electrical nerve stimulation (TENS), either incorporated into a prosthesis or as an isolated unit. The TENS system can be worn by the amputee at night and even during the day with the battery pack attached to the belt or inside a pocket. We have used this TENS system with moderate short-term success, but patients rarely continue to use the TENS system for more than 1 year. Pharmacologic treatment has been reasonably successful with several oral agents, including gabapentin (Neurontin), amitriptyline, carbamazepine (Tegretol), phenytoin (Dilantin), and mexiletine. The appropriate use of an intravenous lidocaine challenge has been predictive of a favorable response to oral mexiletine. Unfortunately, we have not found good indicators to predict who will respond to treatment with gabapentin, amitriptyline, carbamazepine, or phenytoin. Psychological support can be beneficial, particularly when personality problems seem to accentuate the occurrence of pain. The individual needs patience and reassurance that the discomfort will decrease over time, especially when a supportive social environment is present.

REFERENCES AND BIBLIOGRAPHY

1. Abbott LC and Lucas DB: The function of the clavicle; its surgical significance. Ann Surg 140:583-599, 1954.
2. Anderson-Ranberg F and Ebskov B: Major upper extremity amputation in Denmark. Acta Orthop Scand 59:321-322, 1988.
3. Bach S, Noreng MF, and Tjellden NU: Phantom limb pain in amputees during the first 12 months following limb amputation, after preoperative lumbar epidural blockade. Pain 33:297-301, 1988.
4. Bauman PK: Resection of the upper extremity in the region of the shoulder joint. Khirurg Arkh Velyaminova 30:145-149, 1914.
5. Baumgartner R: Upper extremity amputations. Surg Tech Orthop Traumatol 55-270-C-10, 2001.
6. Berger P: Amputation du membre supéarieur dans la contiguitéa du tronc (des articulation de l'omoplate). Bull Mem Soc Nat Chir 9:656, 1883.
7. Blumenfeld I, Schortz RH, Levy M, and Lepley JB: Fabricating a shoulder somatoprosthesis. J Prosthet Dent 45:542-544, 1981.
8. Bogacki W and Spyt T: Interscapular-thoracic amputation of the arm. Nowotwory 30:261-264, 1980.
9. Burgess EM: Sites of amputation election according to modern practice. Clin Orthop 37:17-22, 1964.
10. Burton DS and Nagel DA: Surgical treatment of malignant soft-tissue tumors of the extremities in the adult. Clin Orthop 84:144-148, 1972.
11. Chappell PH: Arm amputation statistics for England 1958-88: An exploratory statistical analysis. Int J Rehabil Res 15:57-62, 1992.
12. Copland SM: Total resection of the clavicle. Am J Surg 72:280, 1946.
13. Cordeiro PG, Cohen S, Burt M, and Brennan MF: The total volar forearm musculocutaneous free flap for reconstruction of extended forequarter amputations. Ann Plast Surg 40:388-396, 1998.
14. DeNancrede CBG: End-results of total excision of the scapula for sarcoma. Ann Surg 50:1-22, 1909.
15. DePalma AF: Scapulectomy and a method of preserving normal configuration of the shoulder. Clin Orthop 4:217-224, 1954.
16. Elizaga AM, Smith DG, Sharar SR, et al: Continuous regional analgesia by intraneural block: Effect on postoperative opioid requirements and phantom limb pain following amputation. J Rehabil Res Dev 31:179-187, 1994.
17. Fanous N, Didolkar MS, Holyoke ED, and Elias EG: Evaluation of forequarter amputation in malignant diseases. Surg Gynecol Obstet 142:381-384, 1976.
18. Fisher A and Meller Y: Continuous postoperative regional analgesia by nerve sheath block for amputation surgery—a pilot study. Anesth Analg 72:300-303, 1991.
19. Flor H, Elbert T, Knecht S, et al: Phantom-limb pain as a perceptual correlate of cortical reorganization following arm amputation. Nature 375:482-484, 1995.
20. Grimes OF and Bell HG: Shoulder girdle amputation. Surg Gynecol Obstet 91:201, 1950.
21. Guerra A, Capanna R, Biagini R, et al: Extra-articular resection of the shoulder (Tikhoff-Linberg). Ital J Orthop Traumatol 11:151-157, 1985.
22. Haggart GE: The technique of interscapulothoracic amputation. Lahey Clin Bull 2:16, 1940.
23. Hall CB and Bechtol CO: Modern amputation technique in the upper extremity. J Bone Joint Surg Am 45:1717, 1963.
24. Ham SJ, Hoekstra HJ, Schraffordt KH, et al: The interscapulothoracic amputation in the treatment of malignant diseases of the upper extremity with a review of the literature. Eur J Surg Oncol 19:543-548, 1993.
25. Hardin CA: Interscapulothoracic amputations for sarcomas of the upper extremity. Surgery 49:355, 1961.
26. Harty M and Joyce JJ: Surgical approaches to the shoulder. Orthop Clin North Am 6:553-564, 1975.
27. Hau T: The surgical practice of Dominique Jean Larrey. Surg Gynecol Obstet 154:89, 1982.
28. Herberts P: Myoelectric signals in control of prostheses: Studies on arm amputees and normal individuals. Acta Orthop Scand 124(suppl):1-83, 1969.
29. Janecki CJ and Nelson CL: En bloc resection of the shoulder girdle: Technique and indications. J Bone Joint Surg Am 54:1754-1758, 1972.
30. Knaggs RL: Mr. Littlewood's method of performing the interscapulothoracic amputation [letter]. Lancet 1:1298, 1910.
31. Kneisl JS: Function after amputation, arthrodesis, or arthroplasty for tumors about the shoulder. J South Orthop Assoc 4:228-236, 1995.
32. Kochhar CL and Strivastava LK: Anatomical and functional considerations in total claviculectomy. Clin Orthop 118:199, 1976.
33. Larrey DJ: Memoire sur les Amputations des Membres à La Suite des Coups de Feu Etaye de Plusieurs Observations. Paris: Du Pont, 1797.
34. Levinthal DH and Grossman A: Interscapulothoracic amputations for malignant tumors of the shoulder region. Surg Gynecol Obstet 69:234, 1939.
35. Lewis MM, Ballet FL, Kroll PG, and Bloom N: En bloc clavicular resection, operative procedure and postoperative testing of function. Clin Orthop 193:214, 1985.
36. Littlewood H: Amputations at the shoulder and at the hip. BMJ 1:381, 1922.
37. Luiberg BE: Interscapulothoracic resection for malignant tumors of the shoulder joint region. J Bone Joint Surg 10:344-349, 1928.
38. Malawer MM, Buch R, Khurana JS, et al: Postoperative infusional continuous regional analgesia—a technique for relief of postoperative pain following major extremity surgery. Clin Orthop 266:227-237, 1991.
39. Mansour KA and Powell RW: Modified technique for radical transmediastinal forequarter amputation and chest wall resection. J Thorac Cardiovasc Surg 76:358-363, 1978.
40. Marcove RC: Neoplasms of the shoulder girdle. Orthop Clin North Am 6:541-552, 1975.
41. McLaughlin J: Solitary myeloma of the clavicle with long survival after total excision: Report of a case. J Bone Joint Surg Br 55:357, 1973.
42. McLaurin CA, Sauter WF, Dolan DM, and Harmann GR: Fabrication procedures for the open-shoulder above-elbow socket. Artif Limbs 13:46-54, 1969.
43. Melzack R: Phantom limbs. Sci Am 266:120-126, 1992.
44. Moseley HF: The Forequarter Amputation. Edinburgh: E. and S. Livingstone, 1957, p 49.
45. Nadler SH and Phelan JT: A technique of interscapulo-thoracic amputation. Surg Gynecol Obstet 122:359, 1966.
46. Neff G: Prosthetic principles in bilateral shoulder disarticulation or bilateral amelia. Prosthet Orthot Int 2:143-147, 1978.
47. Nakamura S, Kusuzaki K, Murata H, et al: Clinical outcome of total scapulectomy in 10 patients with primary malignant bone and soft-tissue tumors. J Surg Oncol 72:130-135, 1999.
48. Oible JH: Napoleon's Surgeon. London: William Heinemann, 1970.
49. Ojemann JG and Silbergeld DL: Cortical stimulation mapping of phantom limb rolandic cortex: Case report. J Neurosurg 82:641-644, 1995.
50. Pack GT: Major exarticulations for malignant neoplasms of the extremities: Interscapulothoracic amputation, hip joint disarticulations and interilioabdominal amputation: A report of end results in 228 cases. J Bone Joint Surg Am 38:249, 1956.
51. Pack GT and Baldwin JC: The Tikhoff-Linberg resection of shoulder girdle. Surgery 38:753-757, 1955.
52. Pack GT and Crampton RS: The Tikhoff-Linberg resection of the shoulder girdle: Indications for its substitution for interscapulothoracic amputation, recent data on end-results of the forequarter amputation. Clin Orthop 19:148, 1961.
53. Pack GT, Ehrlich HE, and Gentil F: Radical amputations of the extremities in the treatment of cancer. Surg Gynecol Obstet 84:1105-1116, 1947.
54. Pack GT, McNeer G, and Coley BL: Interscapulo-thoracic amputations for malignant tumors of the upper extremity: A report of thirty-one consecutive cases. Surg Gynecol Obstet 74:161, 1942.

55. Rodriguez JA, Craven JE, Heinrich S, et al: Current role of scapulectomy. Am Surg 65:1167-1170, 1999.
56. Rorabeck CH: The management of the flail upper extremity in brachial plexus injuries. J Trauma 20:491-493, 1980.
57. Roth JA, Sugarbaker PH, and Baker AR: Radical forequarter amputation with chest wall resection. Ann Thorac Surg 37:432-437, 1984.
58. Salzer M and Knahr K: Resection of malignant bone tumors. Recent Results Cancer Res 54:239-256, 1976.
59. Sauter WF: Prostheses for the child amputee. Orthop Clin North Am 3:483-494, 1972.
60. Slocum DB: Atlas of Amputations. St Louis: CV Mosby, 1949.
61. Spar I: Total claviculectomy for pathological fractures. Clin Orthop 129:236, 1977.
62. Sperling P and Rloding H: Interthoracoscapular amputation (forequarter amputation). Zentralbl Chir 106:340-343, 1981.
63. Sturup J, Thyregod HC, Jensen JS, et al: Traumatic amputation of the upper limb: The use of body-powered prostheses and employment consequences. Prosthet Orthot Int 12:50-52, 1988.
64. Syme J: Excision of the Scapula. Edinburgh: Edmonton & Douglas, 1864.
65. Tikhoff PT: Tumor Studies [monograph]. Russia, 1900.
66. Tooms RE: Amputation surgery in the upper extremity. Orthop Clin North Am 3:383-395, 1972.
67. Trishkin VA, Saakian AM, Stoliarov VI, and Kochnev VA: Interscapulothoracic amputation in treating malignant tumors of the upper extremity and shoulder girdle. Vestn Khir Im I Grek 124:75-78, 1980.
68. Turnbull A, Blumencranz P, and Fortner J: Scapulectomy for soft tissue sarcoma. Can J Surg 24:37-38, 1981.
69. Voggenreiter G, Assenmacher S, and Schmit-Neurburg KP: Tikhoff-Linberg procedure for bone and soft tissue tumors of the shoulder girdle. Arch Surg 134:252-257, 1999.
70. Ye Q, Zhao H, and Shen J: Modified en bloc resection procedure for malignant tumor of the shoulder girdle. Chung Kuo I Hsueh Ko Hsueh Yuan Hsueh Pao Acta Academiae Medicinae Sinicae 16:378-382, 1994.
71. Zachary LS, Gottlieb LJ, Simon M, et al: Forequarter amputation wound coverage with an ipsilateral, lymphedematous, circumferential forearm fasciocutaneous free flap in patients undergoing palliative shoulder-girdle tumor resection. J Reconstr Microsurg 9:103-107, 1993.
72. Zancolli E, Mitre HJ, Bick M, et al: Interscapulo-cleidothoracic disarticulation. Indications and technique. Prensa Med Argent 52:1122-1126, 1965.

CHAPTER 25

THE SHOULDER IN SPORTS

Frank W. Jobe, M.D.,   James E. Tibone, M.D.,   Marilyn M. Pink, Ph.D., P.T.,

and Christopher M. Jobe, M.D.

• • • •

Mobility of the shoulder in overhead sports is a bit like the story of Goldilocks and the Three Bears. An athlete can have too much or too little, and it is sometimes hard to get it just right. The mobility is a requisite for athletic performance, but it also leaves the shoulder vulnerable to injury. The individual needs to perform optimally while minimizing the chance of injury. The purpose of this chapter is to provide information about the shoulder to allow for optimal performance while minimizing or treating injuries. This goal is accomplished by first discussing the biomechanics of sport and injury, then the classification of instability and impingement, followed by principles of prevention and rehabilitation and common surgical procedures for shoulder problems.

BIOMECHANICS

To minimize or effectively treat injury, one must understand the tissues at risk for a given sport. In the past, athletic activities involving the arm tended to be grouped as "overhead" or "overhand" sports. This terminology evolved because much of the initial research and publication was done on baseball pitchers who threw overhand (as opposed to an underhand or sidearm pitch). Unfortunately, the work on pitchers was frequently extrapolated to other "overhead" sports. We now realize that pitchers are a paradigm unto themselves. In addition, research in swimming has proved that swimmers have tissues at risk and mechanics of injury that are specific to each of the four competitive strokes: the freestyle, butterfly, backstroke, and breaststroke. Golfers (though technically not an "overhead" sport because the shoulder rarely exceeds elevation above 90 degrees) also have specific mechanics that a clinician must understand to be of help to the athlete. Thus, the specific mechanics of each sport need to be understood by the clinician. To communicate this concept, the mechanics of the shoulder in baseball pitchers and freestyle swimmers are discussed.

Baseball Pitching

The phases of the baseball pitch that leave the shoulder most at risk for injury are late cocking, acceleration, and deceleration (Fig. 25–1).

Late Cocking

During the late cocking phase, the humerus is moving toward maximal external rotation. As it moves into external rotation, the rotator cuff tendons are rotated posteriorly (Fig. 25–2). In a pitcher with a normal shoulder, the humerus rotates externally while elevated above 90 degrees in the scapular plane. The scapular plane allows for maximal congruency of the humeral head and glenoid, as well as for the least twisting of the anterior capsule.[38]

During the late cocking phase, the infraspinatus and teres minor are quite active as they externally rotate the humerus and provide a posterior restraint to anterior subluxation.[17] The upper portion of the subscapularis also demonstrates high activity as it helps control the degree of external rotation and forms part of the "anterior wall" to help prevent anterior subluxation of the humeral head (see Fig. 25–2). Once the humerus is maximally externally rotated, the subscapularis is rotated more superiorly and can offer some superior compression of the humeral head to prevent it from migrating superiorly.[68] At this point, the supraspinatus is rotated more posteriorly and cannot offer the superior compression.

The serratus anterior is firing during late cocking as it upwardly rotates and anchors the scapula for the humerus. The levator scapulae is functioning at the opposite corner to allow for synchronous scapular motion.

Acceleration

During acceleration, the humerus internally rotates approximately 100 degrees in 0.05 second to contribute to the momentum of the ball on release.[19] Very high angular velocities and torques have been suggested to occur during this phase.[19,25,54] All of the scapular muscles are quite active as they form a stable base for humeral rotation. Of the internal rotators, the subscapularis displays the most electrical activity, followed by the latissimus dorsi.[17] Because the subscapularis inserts close to the axis of rotation, it helps keep the humeral head centered on the glenoid while it assists with internal rotation. If the subscapularis were not functioning, the humeral head could be levered anteriorly as the latissimus dorsi rotates the humerus from a more distal attachment. Thus, to prevent injury, the clinician would want to ensure that the

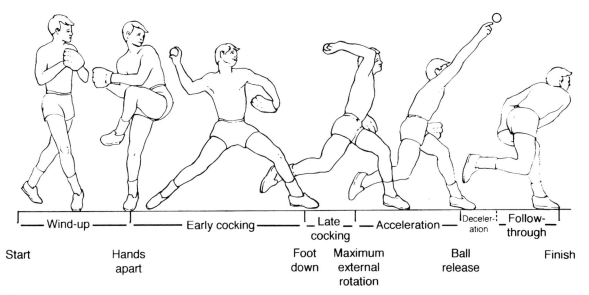

Figure 25-1
Phases of the baseball pitch. *(From Pink MM and Perry J: Biomechanics. In Jobe FW, Pink MM, Glousman RE, et al [eds]: Operative Techniques in Upper Extremity Sports Injuries. St Louis: Mosby–Year Book, 1996.)*

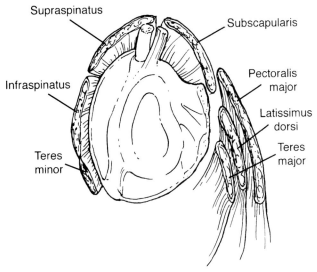

■ **Figure 25-2**
Position of the tendons and ligaments around the glenohumeral joint while in 90 degrees of abduction and 90 degrees of external rotation. With maximal external rotation, the muscles are rotated even more. *(From Pink MM and Perry J: Biomechanics. In Jobe FW, Pink MM, Glousman RE, et al [eds]: Operative Techniques in Upper Extremity Sports Injuries. St Louis: Mosby–Year Book, 1996.)*

pitcher has a stable scapular base (i.e., strong scapular muscles with endurance) and excellent strength/endurance of the subscapularis.

If a pitcher has faulty mechanics during the late cocking or acceleration phase, the humerus may move into the coronal plane (Fig. 25–3) and thereby increase the chance for anterior subluxation of the humeral head. When this position (coronal elevation above 90 degrees with maximal external rotation) is simulated in cadavers, abutment of the posterior cuff on the posterior or superior glenoid rim occurs (Fig. 25–4).[34,72] More importantly,

arthroscopic evaluation has confirmed the abutment in this position.[27,53]

Deceleration

During the deceleration phase, the excess kinetic energy that was not transferred to the ball is dissipated by controlled deceleration of the upper extremity. Once again, high forces and torques have been suggested.[25,54]

The teres minor not only demonstrates the highest level of activity of all the glenohumeral muscles during this phase, but it also functions eccentrically. The intensity of firing of the teres minor is clinically relevant in that many ball players note posterior cuff pain that can be isolated to the teres minor and reproduced in a deceleration motion. Thus, it appears that the teres minor may be vulnerable during the deceleration phase, so the clinician may want to strengthen this muscle in an arc of motion that is similar to the deceleration phase of the pitch (Fig. 25–5).

Freestyle Swimming

Approximately half of competitive swimmers will experience shoulder pain that is severe enough to prevent them from swimming for 3 weeks or more at some point in their swimming career.[62] Factors that have commonly been thought to influence this high rate of shoulder dysfunction include the extremely high number of shoulder revolutions, the extremes of shoulder range of motion necessary for each revolution, and the generalized state of joint laxity in swimmers.

A recent study investigated some of these characteristics, as well as clinical signs of shoulder pathology, in 350 competitive swimmers and age-, race-, and gender-matched controls (Pink, unpublished data). The swimmers demonstrated significantly more generalized (and

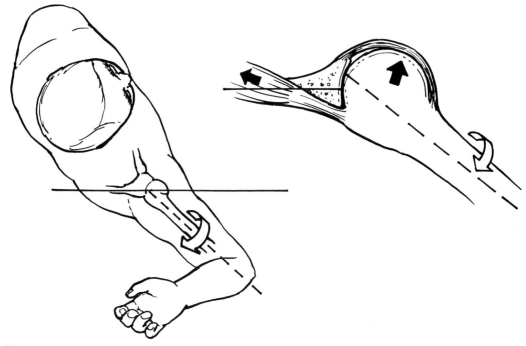

■ **Figure 25–3**
Anterior subluxation and resultant anatomic damage with the arm in the coronal plane.

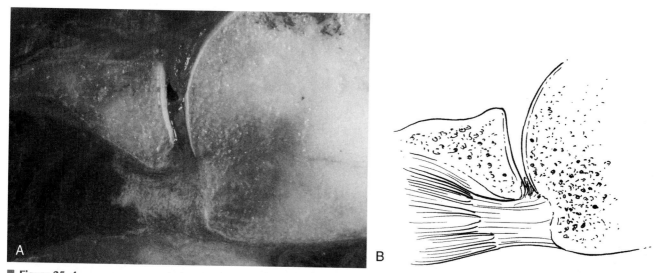

■ **Figure 25–4**
Impingement of the rotator cuff on the posterosuperior glenoid labrum during humeral abduction and maximal external rotation. **A,** Cross section from a cadaver. **B,** Schematic of **A.** *(From Jobe CM, Pink MM, Jobe FW, and Shaffer B: Anterior shoulder instability, impingement, and rotator cuff tear: Theories & concepts. In Jobe FW, Pink MM, Glousman RE, et al [eds]: Operative Techniques in Upper Extremity Sports Injuries. St Louis: Mosby-Year Book, 1996.)*

nonpathologic) laxity than the nonswimmers did. An increased prevalence of classic impingement as measured by the Hawkins and Neer tests was found in the swimmers, even though both groups reported no pain during their functional activities. It is interesting to note that the Hawkins test yielded significantly more positive results than the Neer test did, yet the swimmers did not exhibit any more shoulder instability when measured by the relocation test than the controls did. Thus, the problem involving the swimmers' shoulders appeared to not be

related to the anterior subluxation that can be found in pitchers.

One of the common positions of pain in a swimmer is the position at entry of the hand into water. This position is somewhere between the Neer and Hawkins test for impingement (Fig. 25-6). Cadaver cross sections have revealed that during the Neer test, the impingement appears to be on the undersurface of the cuff on the anterosuperior glenoid rim, whereas during the Hawkins test, the cuff appears to be compressed between the

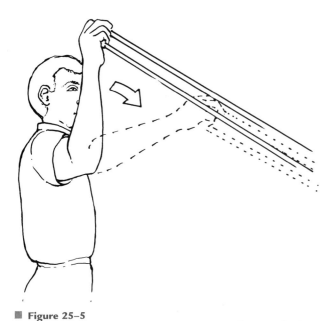

■ **Figure 25–5**
Deceleration exercise for the teres minor. *(From Pink MM, et al: Injury prevention and rehabilitation in the upper extremity. In Jobe FW, Pink MM, Glousman RE, et al [eds]: Operative Techniques in Upper Extremity Sports Injuries. St Louis: Mosby–Year Book, 1996.)*

acromion and the glenoid rim (Figs. 25–7 and 25–8).[70] Thus, the impingement in a swimmer's shoulder may be the result of a "double-squeeze'" phenomenon: compression from above and impingement from below.

One of the muscles in the swimmer's shoulder that appears to be quite vulnerable to fatigue is the serratus anterior. In an underwater electromyographic study of the freestyle stroke, the serratus anterior in swimmers with pain-free shoulders was constantly firing above 20% of the maximal manual muscle test (MMT).[55] At this intensity, the muscle is vulnerable to fatigue if no rest is provided.[48] Indeed, in swimmers with painful shoulders, muscle activity in the serratus anterior is significantly depressed (Fig. 25–9).[60] If the serratus anterior is not adequately functioning, the swimmer would be susceptible to the non-outlet type of impingement that was described by Neer.[50] Thus, a clinician would want to be certain that the serratus anterior not only demonstrates normal strength but also has good endurance.

The subscapularis is the other shoulder muscle that may be vulnerable to fatigue during the freestyle stroke in that it also constantly fires above 20% of the MMT in swimmers with normal shoulders (Fig. 25–10).[55] The constant firing of the subscapularis is easily understood when one realizes that the humerus is always in internal rotation during the stroke. (This fact alone differentiates a freestyle swimmer from a baseball pitcher, whose vulnerable position is that of maximal external rotation.) In a swimmer, the arm is positioned in neutral rotation during the midrecovery phase; however, that is as far into "external rotation" as it moves. Therefore, the clinician would want to check the strength and endurance of the subscapularis along with the serratus anterior.

With this biomechanical information as background, one can begin to see the value of understanding the normal mechanics of individual sports. The relationship of mechanics to instability and impingement will be elaborated on so that the clinician can appreciate the logic behind the surgical programs and rehabilitative principles described subsequently.

INSTABILITY AND IMPINGEMENT

Classification of Instability and Impingement

The classification and definition of impingement and instability are currently quite diverse. One of the changes since the time of the second edition of this text involves a refining of terms and classification.

This evolution was needed because impingement and instability were often used interchangeably. Within this section, the dichotomy will be discussed, followed by the current consensus and known facts. Finally, the authors' philosophy will be presented.

Terminology Dichotomy

Laxity versus Instability

Laxity is asymptomatic and instability is symptomatic. Both these characteristics are qualitatively measured, and each encompasses a spectrum rather than having one definable point. Part of the dichotomy is due to the fact that in some cases, asymptomatic laxity is greater in magnitude than is symptomatic instability.

Traumatic versus Atraumatic Instability

Traumatic instability is considered when the insult happened at one point in time. Some definable event (a fall, a hit) occurred and symptoms ensued. Atraumatic instability is considered when the cause of the symptoms takes place over a period of time (overuse, microtrauma). Nonetheless, some atraumatic shoulders have labral detachment (which had traditionally been thought of as a traumatic insult), and 25% of traumatic dislocations will also dislocate in the opposite direction.

Anterior versus Posterior Instability

The instability may be anterior or posterior. (It may also be multidirectional, but for the purpose of this discussion, the more simplistic and classic types of anterior and posterior instability will be considered.) To translate in one direction, the capsule and ligaments must be stretched on the opposite side. This relationship is the "circle" concept—that is, it is not really just one side that is affected, but rather all the connective tissue surrounding the joint. Thus, technically speaking, all instability is multidirectional.

Complexity of Structures Involved

Many times an injury is discussed as though it involves a single structure. In reality, however, associated injury is almost impossible to avoid. If the trauma (microtrauma

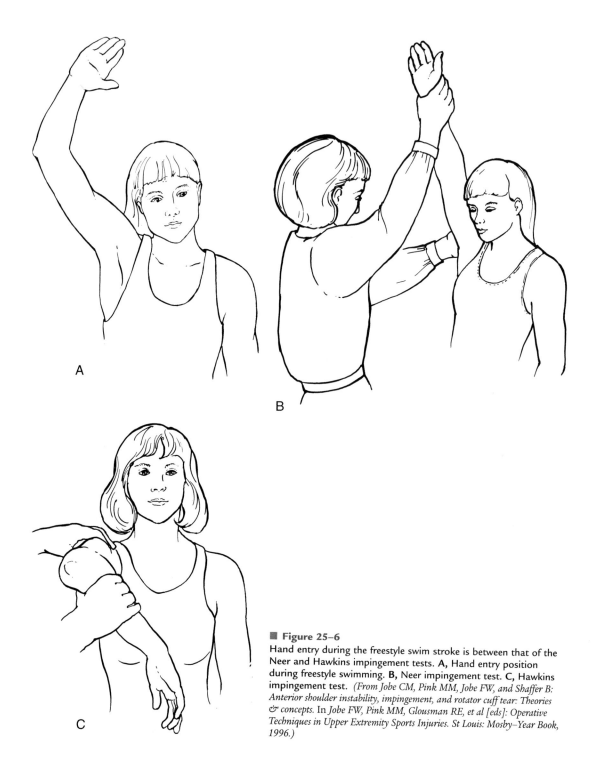

■ Figure 25–6

Hand entry during the freestyle swim stroke is between that of the Neer and Hawkins impingement tests. **A,** Hand entry position during freestyle swimming. **B,** Neer impingement test. **C,** Hawkins impingement test. *(From Jobe CM, Pink MM, Jobe FW, and Shaffer B: Anterior shoulder instability, impingement, and rotator cuff tear: Theories & concepts. In Jobe FW, Pink MM, Glousman RE, et al [eds]: Operative Techniques in Upper Extremity Sports Injuries. St Louis: Mosby–Year Book, 1996.)*

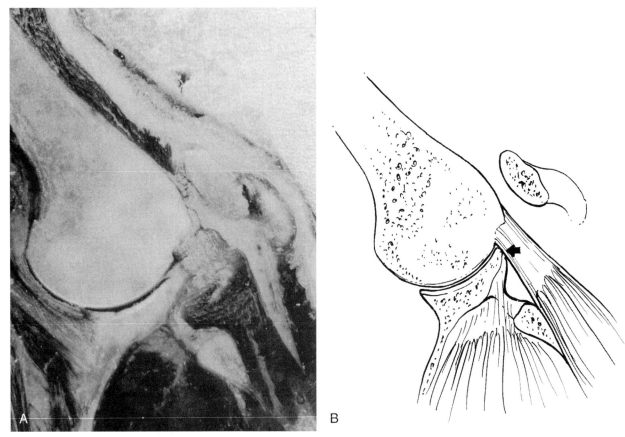

■ **Figure 25–7**
Impingement of the rotator cuff on the anterosuperior glenoid labrum during maximal humeral flexion and forceful internal rotation. **A,** Cross section of a cadaver. **B,** Schematic of A. *(From Jobe CM, Pink MM, Jobe FW, and Shaffer B: Anterior shoulder instability, impingement, and rotator cuff tear: Theories & concepts. In Jobe FW, Pink MM, Glousman RE, et al [eds]: Operative Techniques in Upper Extremity Sports Injuries. St Louis: Mosby–Year Book, 1996.)*

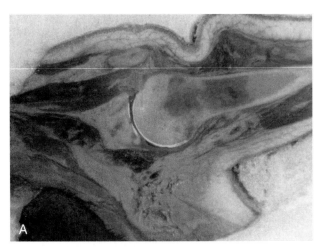

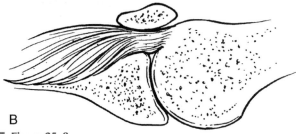

■ **Figure 25–8**
Impingement of the rotator cuff between the acromion and glenoid rim during the Hawkins test. **A,** Cross section of a cadaver. **B,** Schematic of A.

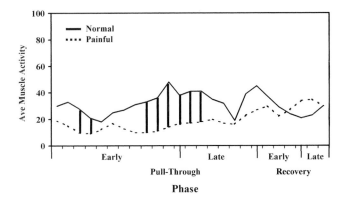

■ **Figure 25–9**
Muscle activity of the serratus anterior in swimmers with normal and painful shoulders. The *vertical lines* show periods of significant differences. *(From Pink MM and Perry J: Biomechanics. In Jobe FW, Pink MM, Glousman RE, et al [eds]: Operative Techniques in Upper Extremity Sports Injuries. St Louis: Mosby–Year Book, 1996.)*

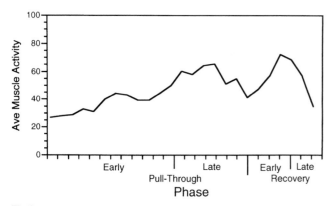

■ Figure 25–10
Muscle activity of the subscapularis in swimmers with normal shoulders.

or acute) were of such a degree that it caused injury to one structure, it would indeed have been sufficient to cause injury to other structures. Both the proximity and the interrelated functionality of the structures dictate the complexity of involvement. Therefore, rather than being manifested as a SLAP injury (detachment of the *s*uperior aspect of the *l*abrum from *a*nterior to *p*osterior) or a tendon or glenoid injury, most likely the injury involves multiple structures.

Current Consensus and Facts

Charles Neer defined outlet and non-outlet impingement in 1972.[50] Outlet impingement, the more common of the two, was defined as encroachment of the cuff by the constricting structures of the coracoacromial arch or acromioclavicular joint. Non-outlet impingement would include abnormal scapular motion (such as with serratus anterior palsy), loss of the humeral head depressors (rotator cuff tear or weakness), and a number of other etiologies.[31,32,49,51] Outlet and non-outlet types of impingement have also been referred to as primary and secondary impingement, respectively.

The impingement found in a younger athletic patient is different from that described by Neer. In his original work, Neer noted that his conclusions were drawn on observations made in older, nonathletic individuals. Hence, transferability of the information to the younger athletic population was pointedly (and accurately) avoided in the seminal 1972 work.

The impingement found in a younger athletic patient can involve the undersurface of the rotator cuff tendon impinging on the glenoid labrum. Because of the proximity of structures of the shoulder joint, contact of the tendon with the labrum is present even in a nonpathologic state. Pathology appears to be related to the degree and frequency of contact.

The majority of the model of cuff contact/impingement is based on the mechanics of the baseball pitcher, which was discussed earlier. The contact is between the undersurface of the cuff tendon and the posterosuperior labrum. The contrast between the contact/impingement areas in freestyle swimmers and baseball pitchers has also been previously discussed. Freestyle swimmers appear to be vulnerable to both the classic Neer impingement and

cuff undersurface impingement on the anterosuperior glenoid rim.[35]

Authors' Philosophy of Instability and Impingement in Baseball Pitchers

Fatigue or weakness of the anterior wall muscles (the subscapularis, pectoralis major, latissimus dorsi, and teres major) in a baseball pitcher contributes to the potential for instability, as does stretching of anterior structures such as the capsule and the glenohumeral ligaments. In addition, if the arm moves into the coronal plane (instead of the scapular plane) when abducted and externally rotated, the humeral head is levered anteriorly (see Fig. 25–3). This position is called *hyperangulation*. Each of these four factors (stretching, microtrauma, fatigue/weakness, and hyperangulation; henceforth called the Potentially Inevitable and Evil 4) has an accumulative effect on the development of instability. The overriding factors that keeps the Potentially Inevitable but Evil 4 in check are preventive exercises, scheduled periods of rest from throwing, and an emphasis on appropriate throwing mechanics. If a pitcher adheres to these principles, the potential pathologic effect of the four factors is minimized (Fig. 25–11).

If the degree of hyperangulation is not controlled by the three overriding factors (preventive exercise, scheduled rest from throwing, and good mechanics), pathology is almost certain. Any one or any combination of at least five pathologies can occur. The anterior capsule can be stretched to the point of instability. This instability can lead to SLAP lesions or internal impingement of the rotator cuff tendon. A tear of the rotator cuff tendon can ensue. Fractures of the greater tuberosity or the bony glenoid can also occur, but they are much less frequent.

The pathology resulting from the instability, or the SLAP lesion or partial cuff tear, can be minimized if identified early and if the pitcher ceases throwing while undergoing an intense and appropriate rehabilitation program. A helpful clinical test for early detection in our hands is the relocation test (Fig. 25–12).

Prevention of Injury

When discussing preventive exercise programs, once again the mechanics of the sport and the mechanisms of pathology are important to understand. In a thrower, it is essential to have as much static stability as possible, a stable scapular base, strong posterior checkreins for the humeral head, and a strong anterior wall. At present, the importance of upper extremity preventive exercises is so engrained in professional baseball that almost every pitcher is on such a program.

Static Stabilizers

The static stabilizers include the labrum, capsule, and the glenohumeral ligaments. The ligament of most concern when the arm is elevated to 90 degrees and beyond is the inferior glenohumeral ligament. It is very easy to overstretch the capsule and ligaments, and indeed, the mere repetitive act of throwing can overstretch them. Furthermore, because these structures have no contractile

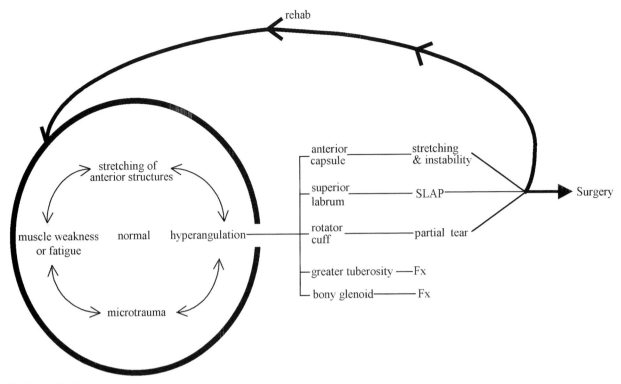

■ Figure 25–11
Instability continuum. Fx, fracture; SLAP, superior labrum, posterior and anterior lesions.

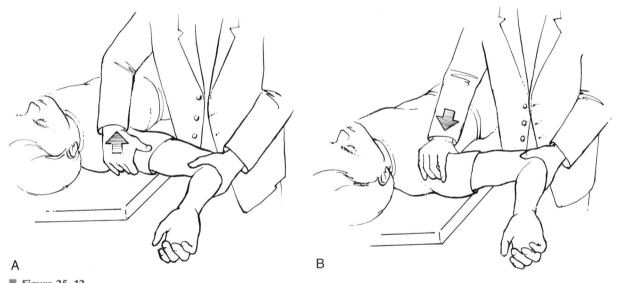

A   B

■ Figure 25–12
Relocation test. The patient is supine with the arm off the table at 90 degrees of abduction and maximal external rotation. **A,** The examiner grasps the humeral head posteriorly and pushes anteriorly. The examiner sometimes feels sliding (subluxation) of the humeral head, and this sliding typically elicits pain at the posterior joint line. **B,** The examiner grasps the humeral head anteriorly and pushes posteriorly to relocate the head and lift the rotator cuff off the posterior labrum. If the patient feels pain in the first half of the test, **A,** the pain is usually relieved in the second half of the test. *(From Jobe CM, Pink MM, Jobe FW, and Shaffer B: Anterior shoulder instability, impingement, and rotator cuff tear: Theories & concepts. In Jobe FW, Pink MM, Glousman RE, et al [eds]: Operative Techniques in Upper Extremity Sports Injuries. St Louis: Mosby–Year Book, 1996.)*

elements, once they are overstretched, there is no good noninvasive treatment that can be used to correct the problem. The clinician therefore needs to be very selective and careful about stretching the arm and would want to prescribe such stretching only for demonstrable stiffness in a particular plane of motion.

The one area that may be tight in a thrower is the posterior capsule; if too tight, it can result in obligate ante-

rior translation of the humeral head and therefore contribute to instability. Posterior capsular stretching in the scapular plane should be prescribed for any thrower with a tight posterior capsule (Fig. 25–13).

Because of the tendency for generalized ligamentous laxity in throwers, anterior and inferior capsular stretching is not recommended as a general rule. A common stretch that is performed, and the authors can think of no

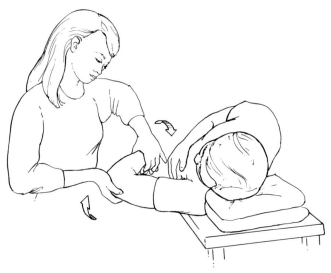

■ Figure 25–13
Posterior capsule stretch. *(From Pink MM, et al: Injury prevention and rehabilitation in the upper extremity. In Jobe FW, Pink MM, Glousman RE, et al [eds]: Operative Techniques in Upper Extremity Sports Injuries. St Louis: Mosby–Year Book, 1996.)*

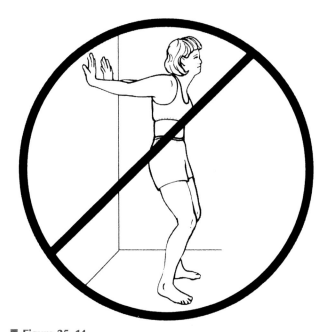

■ Figure 25–14
"Thou shalt not do this stretch." Historically, many swimmers did this stretch; however, there is a great risk for this stretch to increase anterior shoulder instability. *(From Pink MM and Tibone JE: The painful shoulder in the swimming athlete. Orthop Clin North Am 31:247-255, 2000.)*

reason to ever include it in an exercise program for an overhead athlete, is seen in Figure 25–14.

Dynamic Stabilizers

The dynamic stabilizers include the scapular muscles and the rotator cuff. If scapular asymmetry is noted during bilateral arm motion, quite likely the serratus anterior is contributing to the asymmetry. If the serratus anterior is deficient, one will notice shoulder hiking, which is the result of a normally functioning trapezius unopposed by a properly contracting serratus muscle. In this setting, the

serratus anterior is not able to provide the antagonistic anchoring activity.[6] Some people would observe the shoulder hiking and call it "excessive" scapular motion, but "excessive" would be an imprecise categorization of the motion. Other people might call it "scapular lag," which is equally imprecise. It is simply scapular asymmetry, with the serratus anterior being deficient and the upper trapezius functioning in a normal manner. However, no muscle can effectively substitute and allow controlled motion at the inferior border of the scapula. For this reason, winging and asynchronous motion will occur.

The serratus anterior has several functions. It can both protract and upwardly rotate the scapula. The upper fibers tend to be protractors, whereas the lower fibers tend to be the upward rotators.[32] The breadth of this large, flat muscle encompasses muscle fibers going in multiple directions, and hence the muscle has multiple functions. This multiplicity of function and anatomy lends itself to multiple exercises. Elevation above 120 degrees in all three planes (frontal, coronal, and scapular) is an optimal position to exercise the serratus anterior.[49] Modified pushup exercises are an excellent means to strengthen this muscle (Fig. 25–15).

The teres minor and the infraspinatus are the dynamic stabilizers of the posterior aspect of the shoulder that help hold the humeral head from translating in an anterior direction. We now know that these two muscles possess different mechanical advantages at two different elevations. The infraspinatus is primarily responsible for external rotation, humeral head depression, and approximation at lower elevations. Therefore, external rotation with the arm near the side of the body is optimal for strengthening the infraspinatus (Fig. 25–16), and external rotation with the arm at approximately 70 degrees of elevation is a more appropriate exercise for strengthening the teres minor (Fig. 25–17).

The supraspinatus is the most easily fatigued of the rotator cuff muscles.[7,29] One excellent exercise for the supraspinatus is scapular plane elevation ("scaption").[49] If this exercise is used for a preventive program, it can be done with external rotation and the arm can be elevated above the head. However, if it is being used for a rehabilitative program, the elevation should be kept well below 90 degrees to avoid impingement (Fig. 25–18). In a normal shoulder, the humeral head depressors are functioning in synchrony and keep the humeral head clear of the

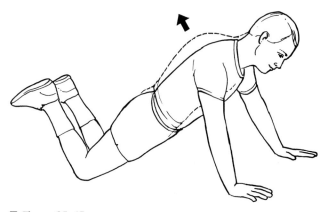

■ Figure 25–15
A pushup with a plus.

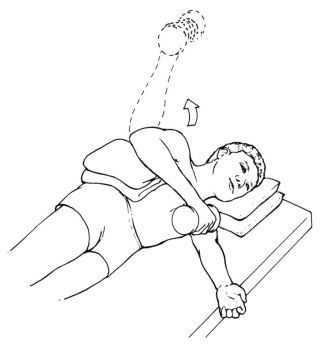

■ **Figure 25–16**
External rotation for strengthening the infraspinatus. *(From Pink MM, et al: Injury prevention and rehabilitation in the upper extremity. In Jobe FW, Pink MM, Glousman RE, et al [eds]: Operative Techniques in Upper Extremity Sports Injuries. St Louis: Mosby–Year Book, 1996.)*

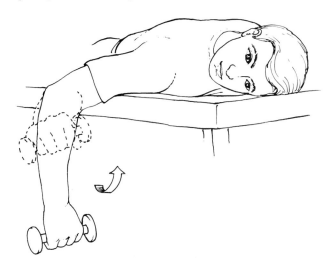

■ **Figure 25–17**
External rotation for strengthening the teres minor. *(From Pink MM, et al: Injury prevention and rehabilitation in the upper extremity. In Jobe FW, Pink MM, Glousman RE, et al [eds]: Operative Techniques in Upper Extremity Sports Injuries. St Louis: Mosby–Year Book, 1996.)*

coracoacromial arch while the arm is elevated above the head.

The subscapularis can be a difficult muscle to exercise because the latissimus dorsi and pectoralis major are also internal rotators of the glenohumeral joint. The clinician has to be certain that the subscapularis is functioning during an exercise along with these two large muscles. All three of these muscles have been considered anterior wall muscles; however, because the subscapularis inserts closest to the axis of rotation, it functions best in protecting the glenohumeral joint from anterior subluxation.

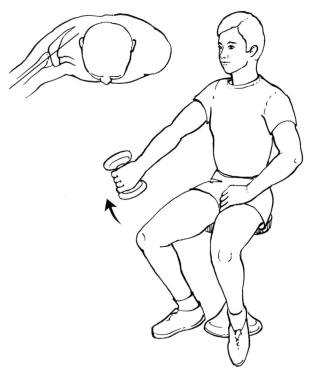

■ **Figure 25–18**
Scaption (scapular plane elevation) with internal rotation of the humerus (see also *inset*).

Experience has shown that internal rotation on an isokinetic device at high speed for a prolonged period is a good way to activate the subscapularis (Fig. 25-19). If such a device is not available, elevation in all three planes as well as the military press will activate the subscapularis.[66]

Surgical Procedures

Bristow Procedure

For many years, the Bristow procedure (developed by Helfet and modified by May) has been popular as a treatment of anteriorly dislocating shoulders. The purpose of this procedure is to reinforce the middle and inferior capsule and the glenohumeral ligament system. By transferring the tip of the coracoid process with the attached conjoined tendon, the inferior portion of the subscapularis muscle is effectively tethered during abduction and external rotation of the arm. Superior excursion of this portion of the subscapularis muscle-tendon unit is prevented, thus providing stability.

A detailed description is included here because it is still the procedure of choice in certain conditions. Within the last 10 years, other procedures have been developed, and indications for the Bristow procedure have been narrowed considerably. The primary indication for the Bristow procedure is a shoulder with a large amount of bone loss from the anterior glenoid rim.

The Bristow procedure has not been successful in patients with subluxing shoulders or those with generalized ligamentous laxity. Better procedures have been developed for many patients who would have been candidates for this operation in the past. The evolution of these newer techniques allows us to be more exacting in our selection of patients.

The Bristow procedure results in loss of humeral external rotation, which renders it unsatisfactory for treatment of the dominant arm of a thrower. Even a minimal decrease in motion usually prevents the patient from returning to high-level participation as a thrower.

The Bristow procedure has also been criticized because of hardware-related complications such as screw loosening, migration, neurovascular injuries, nonunion of the transferred coracoid, breakage, and others. Our opinion is that a technically competent surgeon can perform the procedure without significant complications. However, if the surgeon lacks the skill or the equipment to perform this procedure, it is an inappropriate surgical choice.

The choice between the Bristow and other soft tissue procedures should be based on glenoid bone deficiency. In the capsulolabral procedure, no muscles are transferred or imbricated. An athlete treated with the capsulolabral procedure will be much less likely to experience loss of external rotation, which would preclude return to high-level participation as a thrower.

The Magnuson-Stack and Putti-Platt procedures are not recommended for an athlete's dominant throwing arm under any circumstances. These procedures can tighten the shoulder to such an extent that the athlete is left with limited mobility.

Technique

The following is a detailed description of the Bristow procedure. The procedure is easily performed with the patient supine and the use of an arm board. A folded towel is placed under the scapula. In a modified axillary approach (Fig. 25–20), the deltopectoral interval is identified and developed with the cephalic vein retracted laterally. The clavipectoral fascia is likewise incised. The conjoined

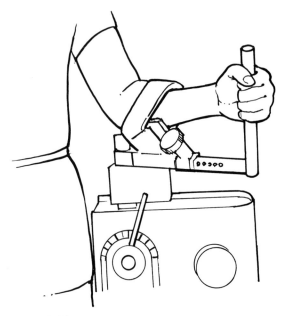

■ **Figure 25–19**
Humeral rotation on an isokinetic device.

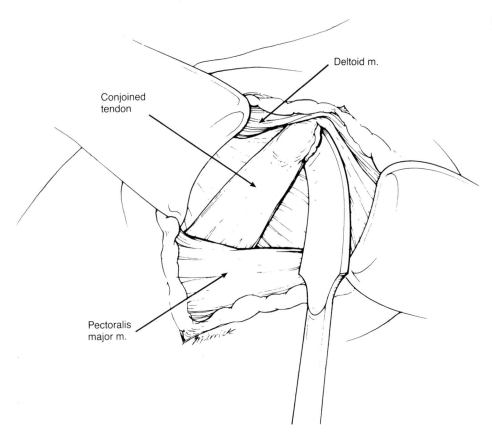

■ **Figure 25–20**
The deltopectoral interval is identified.

Conjoined tendon

Deltoid m.

Pectoralis major m.

tendon with ¼ inch of bone is removed with a curved osteotome (Fig. 25-21) and allowed to retract distally. Care must be taken to identify and protect the musculocutaneous nerve. The remaining bleeding bone edge may be rubbed with bone wax, if necessary, to secure hemostasis. The subscapularis is divided in line with its fibers with an electrocautery between its upper two thirds and lower third, beginning just medial to the bicipital groove (Fig. 25-22). Anatomic dissections performed in our laboratory have shown that the interval between the upper two thirds and the lower third lies in the internervous plane between the upper and lower subscapular nerves. This interval is therefore safe for dissection because the

branches of the upper subscapular nerve innervate the upper two thirds of the subscapularis muscle and the lower subscapular nerve innervates the lower third of the muscle.[39]

The capsule is separated from the subscapularis and incised in line with the subscapular interval. A blunt-tipped, three-pronged retractor is placed anteriorly on the scapular neck so that the following steps can be performed without damage to cartilage (Fig. 25-23). The anterior glenoid rim is débrided down to bleeding bone. With a 3.2-mm drill bit, a hole is created across the glenoid, parallel to the joint at about the 3:30 position (on the right shoulder) (Fig. 25-24). The depth is then

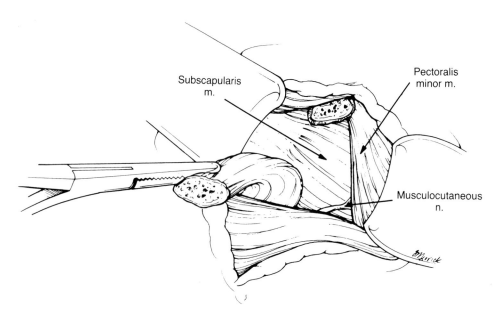

■ **Figure 25–21**
The conjoined tendon with ¼ inch of bone is removed with a curved osteotome.

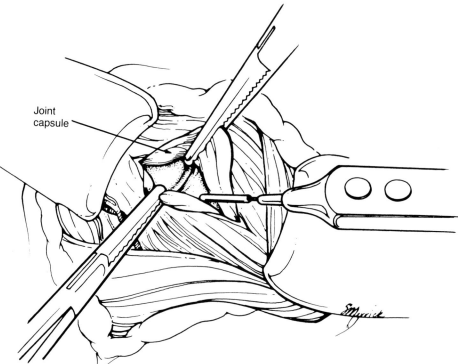

■ **Figure 25–22**
The subscapularis muscle is divided between its upper two thirds and lower third with an electrocautery.

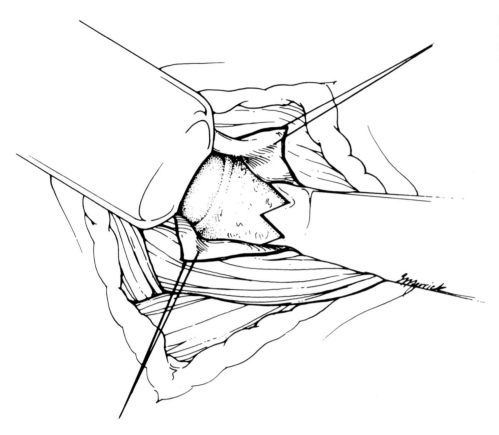

■ Figure 25–23
A blunt-tipped, three-pronged retractor is placed anteriorly on the scapular neck.

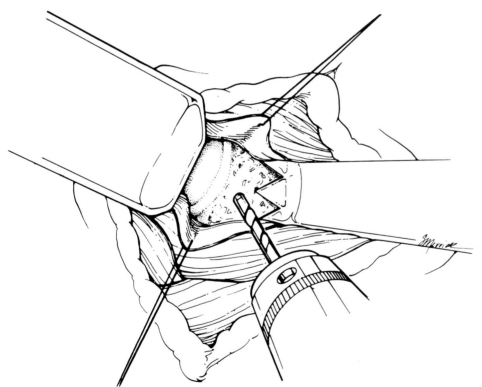

■ Figure 25–24
A 3.2-mm drill bit is used to create a hole across the glenoid, parallel to the joint.

measured with a depth gauge. The height of the bony block is added to the depth, and 5 mm is subtracted. The block is then shaped to fit snugly against the prepared surface and is secured in position with the appropriately sized malleolar screw (Fig. 25–25).

The inferior capsular flap is now pulled up and sutured to the superior capsular flap just lateral to the bony block (Fig. 25–26). Incising the inferior capsule at the glenoid rim may facilitate a tighter capsular closure if marked anteroinferior capsular redundancy is present. The shoulder is put through its range of motion. If it appears too tight, the conjoined tendon can be partially released in a controlled fashion to allow additional motion. Bleeding is controlled, and the muscles are allowed to return to their anatomic position. The wound is closed in the usual manner.

Postoperative Treatment

Postoperatively, the arm is placed in a sling, and Codman's exercises begin the next day. Motion is encouraged out of the sling within the midrange of the shoulder.

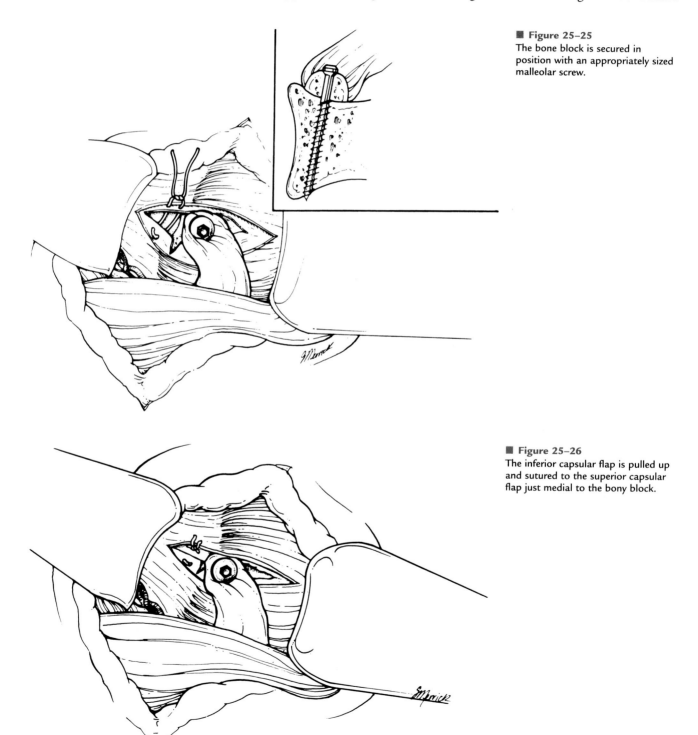

■ **Figure 25–25**
The bone block is secured in position with an appropriately sized malleolar screw.

■ **Figure 25–26**
The inferior capsular flap is pulled up and sutured to the superior capsular flap just medial to the bony block.

Care is taken to avoid forced abduction and external rotation until healing progresses. Light weights are used in the midrange only to regain strength. Strong abduction and external rotation should be avoided lest the screw be dislodged; also, use of the biceps against resistance is avoided. The bony block heals by 3 months, and more vigorous stretching and strengthening can be initiated.

Capsulolabral Reconstruction

The anterior capsulolabral reconstruction was devised for overhead throwing athletes with involvement of the dominant arm who have documented anterior instability and in whom conservative treatment has failed. Although much of the reconstruction can be explained in a logistic step-by-step process, a few decision points along the way can make the surgery more of an "art" rather than just a technique. These decision points are italicized within the text and highlighted in the following box.

"Artful" Decision Points for Anterior Cruciate Ligament Reconstruction

1. To close, or not to close, the rotator interval
2. To use, or not to use, bone anchors
3. The degree of capsule overlap (both the inferior leaf and superior leaf)

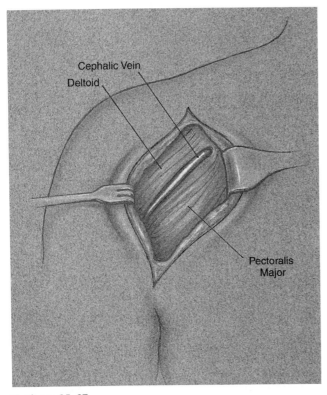

■ Figure 25–27
The incision in the right shoulder is in the skin lines of the shoulder and extends into the axilla for about ½ inch. The proximal end of the incision begins over the coracoid. The margins of the skin are mobilized so that the deltoid and pectoralis major can be identified and, if present, the cephalic vein can be seen.

Technique

The patient is placed supine on the operating table with the arm positioned on a Parker table or on two arm boards. To create stability and prominence of the humeral head, two or three folded surgical towels are placed along the vertebral border and under the scapula to elevate it and provide room to sublux the humeral head posteriorly for access to the anterior glenoid. Below the level of the coracoid, a 6- to 8-cm skin incision is made in line with a midaxillary skinfold in the relaxed skin tension lines. The skin is undermined in all directions to expose the deltopectoral fascia and interval. Meticulous hemostasis is required for proper visualization. The anterior deltoid, cephalic vein, pectoralis major, and deltopectoral groove are identified (Fig. 25–27). The deltopectoral fascia is split in line with the cephalic vein and freed along its pectoral border. The deltopectoral groove is opened with Goulet retractors while retracting the cephalic vein laterally with the deltoid, and the pectoralis major is retracted medially. The lateral border of the conjoined tendon is identified and freed from surrounding tissues (Fig. 25–28). The conjoined tendon is retracted medially with a long, narrow Richardson retractor. The superior border of the subscapularis is identified by the recess; the inferior border is identified by the anterior humeral circumflex vessels. Internal and external rotation of the humeral head helps delineate the superior and inferior margins. *At this point, the rotator interval is examined and a determination made regarding whether it needs to be closed as part of the procedure.*

With the arm in external rotation (to protect the long head of the biceps) and with the use of coagulating electrocautery, the subscapularis tendon is split in line with its fibers at its lower third (Fig. 25–29). Kocher clamps are then placed on the superior and inferior margins of the subscapularis to provide tension while the dissection

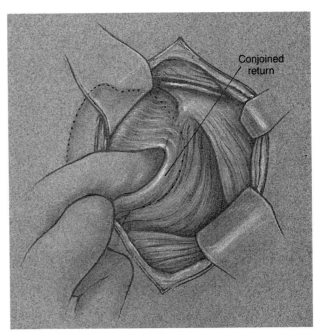

■ Figure 25–28
The conjoined tendon is identified and freed on its lateral aspect up to the coracoid so that it can be retracted medially.

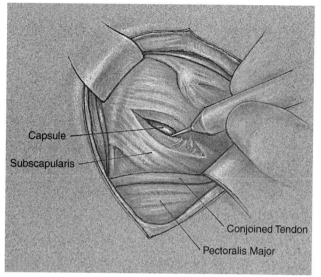

■ Figure 25–29
The subscapularis tendon is exposed. The superior and inferior borders are noted, and the upper two thirds and the lower third are identified so that the muscle can be split longitudinally in the direction of its fibers. A coagulation Bovie is used for this purpose.

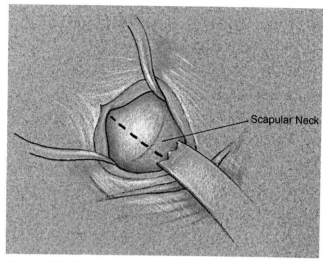

■ Figure 25–31
The capsule is split longitudinally in the same direction as the subscapularis.

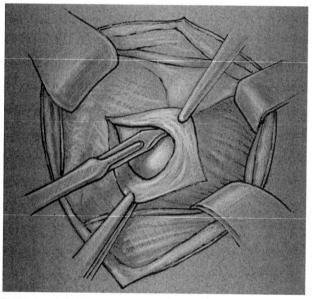

■ Figure 25–30
The split is carried down to the capsule. A knife is then used to separate the capsule from the subscapularis. The sharp section is used laterally, and the blunt section is used medially under the muscle.

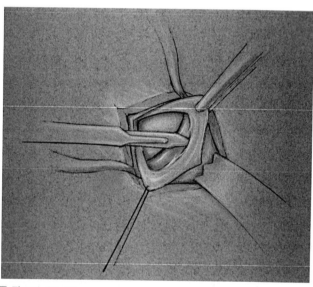

■ Figure 25–32
The incision is carried down onto the neck of the glenoid and elevated subperiosteally at that point. The labrum can be examined and removed if necessary or left in place.

progresses. With a No. 15 surgical blade, the interval between the capsule and the subscapularis is sharply defined (Fig. 25-30). Separation of the capsule and subscapularis is most easily accomplished at the myotendinous junction, where the tendon and capsule are less adherent. Meticulous dissection to define this interval is paramount. By lifting the superior and inferior edges, the interval may be more readily identified near the muscle border. Further separation superiorly, inferiorly, and medially is achieved with a soft tissue elevator and a No. 15 blade. Improved exposure to the capsule is obtained by placing a blunt-tipped, three-pronged pitchfork retractor

onto the glenoid neck, and then a modified self-retaining, long-tonged Gelpi retractor is placed beneath the superior and inferior margins of the cut subscapularis muscle and tendon laterally. Better exposure to the joint capsule and the underlying glenohumeral joint can now be appreciated.

Near the center of the humeral head, a transverse capsulotomy is made parallel to the split in the subscapularis at approximately the midjoint level (Fig. 25-31) and extended medially toward the bony glenoid rim to create a superior and inferior flap. The capsulotomy is extended onto the neck of the glenoid and the flaps are elevated subperiosteally (Fig. 25-32). Examination at this time will determine whether the labrum is severely damaged or whether a Bankart lesion is present. The capsule can also be evaluated for the amount of redundancy that needs to be corrected. It has been our experience that if the redundancy is mainly capsular and the labrum is in excellent condition, the majority of the procedure can be directed toward a capsular shift with the labrum left in place. *Whether bone anchors are used is a decision made at that time.* Generally, however, the labrum is damaged and sometimes pulled away from the bone. We have found that it is not of prime importance to save a damaged labrum. It can be trimmed or removed without compromising the end result.

As the glenohumeral joint is approached, care is taken to ensure that all the structures are carefully cleaned and separated so that at the time of closure, there is no confusion regarding which structures are approximated. To aid in identification, a stay suture is placed in both the superior flap and the inferior flap at the margin of the joint. These sutures give a reference point so that as a capsular shift is carried out, no medialization of the capsule is inadvertently produced that might compromise the end result by making the capsule too tight and thus prevent full range of motion after the repair.

With the stay sutures in hand, a two-pronged humeral head retractor can be positioned in the joint. The points of the retractor should be situated on the posterior rim, with care taken to not injure the articulating cartilage of the glenoid fossa. In the proper position, the retractor can be used as a lever to push the head posteriorly and laterally. By changing the pressure on this retractor, as well as the pressure on the pitchfork retractor, appropriate changes in position of the capsule can be made for good exposure.

After the capsule has been sufficiently cleaned and elevated from the glenoid, a half-size single-point retractor is placed on the inferior neck of the glenoid. The use of such a retractor enhances visualization immensely. The neck of the glenoid is then cleaned so that good material is present (usually some bleeding bone is desirable), and then holes are drilled for the bone anchors. The drill holes are usually placed at about the 3:00 to 3:30 position, the 4:00 to 4:30 position, and the 5:00 to 5:30 position on the right shoulder. The holes are drilled parallel to the articulating cartilage about 2 or 3 mm away from the glenoid surface (Figs. 25–33 and 25–34). Many bone anchor systems are available at the present time. We have had the most experience with the Mitek devices (Mitek Surgical Products, Norwood, MA), and we commonly use the two-pronged device with No. 2 suture. These devices are placed in position, and care is taken to aim the inferior one slightly cephalad to avoid any risk of the tip going through the posterior cortex.

The inferior flap of the capsule is then pulled superiorly. A great deal of care is taken to avoid medialization, and sutures are placed through the flap so that it can advance a predetermined amount (Fig. 25–35). The amount, of course, is determined by the degree of hyperlaxity and how much stretching was noted preoperatively. If the patient is an overhand athlete, it is very important that the capsule not be pulled too tight because if it is too tight, the athlete will never regain full range of motion.

When the capsule is properly positioned, one knot is placed in each of the three sutures and the superior flap is pulled down on top. The same sutures are used to secure

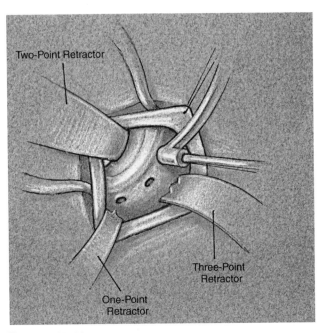

■ **Figure 25–33**
The anterior inferior rim of the glenoid is prepared, and three holes are placed next to the margin of the glenoid for placement of the bone anchors. Note the three retractors in place.

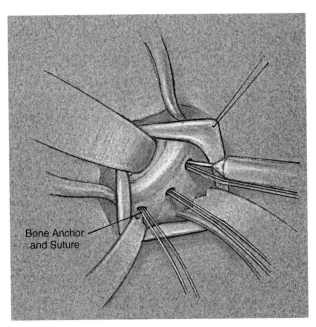

■ **Figure 25–34**
The bone anchors with No. 2 sutures are in position.

it into position. Occasionally, this flap will not reach all the way to the third anchor, but it usually extends to the second anchor. With these sutures in place, the knots cannot be tied until the two-pronged humeral head retractor is removed, after which the sutures are tied (Fig. 25–36). *At this point a judgment needs to be made about how tight the overlap should be.* It has been our custom to place the shoulder in the throwing position and see how much tightness is necessary with the arm at 90 degrees of elevation and full external rotation. Sometimes, only a very

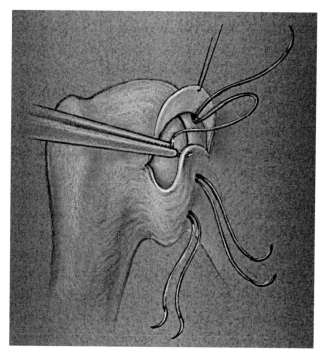

■ **Figure 25–35**
The inferior flap is pulled superiorly, and care is taken to avoid medialization so that overtightening of the capsule does not occur.

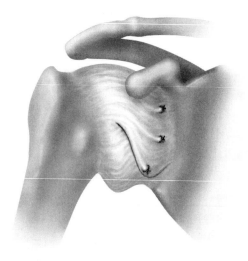

■ **Figure 25–36**
The superior flap is pulled over the top, and an adjustment is made according to the predetermined need.

small amount of flap overlap is necessary, and a single suture is usually placed just to keep the overlap in position. It is important to leave some portion of the split unsutured near the humeral head to allow range of motion so that the repair can be therapeutically adjusted postoperatively without pulling any stitches.

When this step has been accomplished, the retractors are removed and the subscapularis is closed with absorbable sutures (Fig. 25-37). The wound is usually washed with an antibiotic solution, and closure is carried out with absorbable suture for the subcutaneous tissue and 4-0 clear subcuticular nylon for the skin.

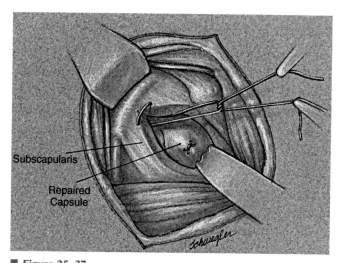

■ **Figure 25–37**
The subscapularis tendon is closed with absorbable sutures over the repair.

Postoperative Rehabilitation Program

Several years ago, patients would have been placed in an abduction brace for about 2 weeks. However, by leaving a portion of the capsular split unsutured near the humeral head, full range of motion can be regained rather quickly and achieved without the 2-week period of immobilization in the abducted position. How tight to make the repair is a matter of judgment, and such flexibility is a bonus in re-establishing range of motion (abduction and external rotation) in a thrower.

Active range of motion is begun immediately after surgery. On the first day, active elbow flexion and extension are begun along with wrist motion and ball squeezing/use of a plastic exerciser. In addition, the patient lifts the arm into flexion and places the hand on top of the head. Over the next 2 weeks, humeral flexion with the hand on the head is progressed as the elbow is gently and slowly pushed outward to move the humerus into abduction and external rotation. At 2 weeks, wand exercises are added for elevation, as are multiple-angle isometric exercises for internal rotation, external rotation, abduction, flexion, and extension. The goal is to gain optimal range of motion for the throwing athlete within 3 weeks.

If excessive connective tissue laxity in the patient is a concern, a sling may be worn and less effort applied to the flexion/abduction/external rotation exercises. By the end of 2 weeks, the sling is discarded.

Isotonic resisted exercises begin by the third week. The first group of exercises includes active resisted internal and external rotation with the use of elastic resistance bands or tubing and the arm at the side. Active shoulder extension may be performed either prone or standing while bending forward at the waist. The patient extends the arm, with the elbow straight, to the plane of the trunk. The patient should not go beyond this plane. When horizontal adduction is added 1 or 2 weeks later, the patient begins in the supine position with the humerus supported so that the exercise is performed in the scapular plane.

The second phase of the rehabilitation program emphasizes progressive strengthening, beginning with the shoulder rotators. The patient moves from elastic band resistance of increasing difficulty to side-lying external rotation with free weights. The therapist must take care to position the arm during internal rotation with a bolster under the lateral aspect of the chest wall. The patient also performs the supraspinatus exercise in a pain-free range only (see Fig. 25-18). The clinician continues strengthening the anterior deltoid. Elevation above 110 degrees can be included once the patient is able to do so with no pain.

Active horizontal abduction (with the same position options as for extension—that is, prone or leaning forward from the waist) is limited to the plane of the trunk. Scapular adduction and trunk rotation can mimic some degree of horizontal abduction and make it appear that more horizontal abduction is being accomplished than is really the case.

By the third postoperative month, eccentric rotator cuff exercises, vigorous elbow and wrist strengthening, and the military press exercise with the arms in front of the chest are all part of the program. To strengthen the serratus anterior, the patient can begin with modified hands-and-knees pushups with a plus (see Fig. 25-15). An upper extremity ergometer can also be used to strengthen the serratus anterior if the seat is set back far enough to allow exaggerated scapular protraction. The ergometer is set at low resistance.

Isokinetic training is begun when the patient is able to lift 5 to 10 lb in external rotation and 15 to 20 lb in internal rotation without pain or swelling. At about 4 months after surgery (and if isokinetic testing has verified that the involved shoulder has at least 70% of the strength of the uninvolved shoulder), the third phase—sport-specific rehabilitation—begins. For a detailed explanation of various sport-specific rehabilitation programs, see Chapter 7F in *Operative Techniques in Upper Extremity Sports Injuries.*[37] The speed of the throw will progress to about three fourths of maximal speed at about 7 months after surgery; full speed is not a reasonable goal until almost 1 year after surgery. It is important to not advance the patient too quickly in the throwing program. Time is necessary to allow adequate healing of the reconstructed tissues and adaptation to the stress placed on them during throwing.

Arthroscopy

Any discussion of sports medicine raises the question of the proper place of arthroscopy in the management of shoulder problems. When properly used, the arthroscope is an invaluable tool that provides capabilities, especially in diagnosis, not afforded by other means.

As with arthroscopy of other joints, shoulder arthroscopy can be divided into three main groups of procedures: (1) diagnostic, (2) removal or excision, and (3) reconstruction.

The arthroscopic examination can be extremely valuable and often confirms the exact nature of the disease. For example, is a subluxing shoulder secondary to labral detachment or a stretched capsule? Does the patient have any rotator cuff disease? Arthroscopy is superior to magnetic resonance imaging and other radiographic techniques in its degree of resolution in viewing intra-articular structures. In cases of instability, arthroscopy allows positioning of the shoulder to observe subluxation. These positions cannot be achieved in the magnetic resonance imaging gantry.

The question arises whether diagnostic arthroscopy can be performed under the same anesthesia as the open procedure without increasing the risk of infection. We believe that increased risk arises from fluid extravasation into the surrounding soft tissues and therefore limit diagnostic arthroscopy to the posterior portal only. We also limit the length of the arthroscopic procedure to a maximum of 5 minutes. If more portals are necessary, if more time is needed, or if excessive edema is noted, the open procedure is delayed.

Not only is diagnostic arthroscopy helpful in the treatment of an injured shoulder in an athlete, but arthroscopic removal of loose bodies or débridement of degenerative labral tears can also often be the definitive procedure. If the material removed was formerly part of a stabilizing structure (e.g., the labrum), the patient must be cautioned that although one symptomatic problem has been addressed (torn labral fragment), a second problem (instability) may be unmasked.

Arthroscopic management of SLAP lesions has become the treatment method of choice. Labral tears that are amenable to surgical repair can be anchored securely to the glenoid rim. In addition to addressing the labral pathology and stabilizing the biceps anchor, it may also eliminate the glenohumeral joint instability that can be associated with such lesions.

With regard to arthroscopic reconstructions for anterior glenohumeral instability, we consider such procedures to be techniques in development. The apparent advantage of reduced early postoperative morbidity following arthroscopy is less striking when one considers that these open procedures are among the least painful in shoulder surgery. Moreover, the duration of postoperative immobilization is much less when open stabilization procedures are performed. Therefore, arthroscopic procedures do not shorten the recovery time for these individuals.

The ideal procedure for all athletes will repair and reinforce the anterior capsule and build the anterior rim up while simultaneously adjusting the laxity of the capsule. We believe that a capsulolabral reconstruction offers the most satisfactory answer to the problem of a pathologic high-performance shoulder.[36] Because of the degree of challenge to the tissues while pitching, the open procedure affords the best results. However, for athletes in sports such as football or hockey, where the challenge is less extreme, satisfactory arthroscopic techniques are being developed by a cadre of skilled arthroscopic surgeons.

Electrothermally Assisted Capsulorrhaphy

Electrothermally assisted capsulorrhaphy (ETAC) has recently been performed for shoulder instability. The relative technical ease of the procedure had initially helped gain supporters. Moreover, the feedback of literally watching the capsule shrink in front of the surgeon's eyes has been instrumental in making converts. In addition, ETAC allowed early return to activity, and the initial short-term results were positive.[3,18,47,69,75] However, as time goes on, the results are not as positive.[16,40,45,65] The incidence of failure in the long term is much higher than usually acceptable.

The rationale for such failure appears to be at the cellular level and is related to the degree of shrinkage. If a procedure entails a large degree of shrinkage, the mechanical properties of the connective tissue are decreased.[73] Furthermore, recurrent laxity may occur as a result of deformation of capsular tissue under constant and low physiologic load (creep).[74] A high-demand patient, such as a baseball pitcher, provides a unique challenge to these tissues postsurgery. If shrinkage is applied with the intensity required to do the job by itself, it will probably fail in this type of athlete because the integrity of the tissue (decreased mechanical properties) has been compromised. If a small degree of shrinkage (less than 15%) is applied along with a suture technique, the results appear to be better than those of thermal shrinkage alone.[73] Arnoczky and Aksan pointed out that ETAC may best be used as a low-level stimulant for inducing a biologic repair response rather than as an aggressive mechanism for primary tissue shrinkage.[5] Thus, a smaller degree of shrinkage combined with a suture technique may be the most viable option for ETAC.

An additional thought to keep in mind if considering thermal shrinkage is the poor quality of tissue left behind. If it is necessary to redo a procedure, the brittle tissue left after ETAC makes any anchoring and suturing very difficult. It is the opinion of the authors that as more long-term outcome studies are published, ETAC will fall from favor for high-demand athletes. If an overhead athlete has internal impingement with anterior instability, the procedure of choice in our hands at this time is a capsular overlap performed either arthroscopically or by open means.

POSTERIOR SHOULDER PROBLEMS

Instability

Athletes very rarely suffer a posterior shoulder dislocation. If they do, they typically have repeated episodes of posterior shoulder dislocation. This injury occurs in one of two ways: (1) from overuse, which stretches out the posterior capsule, or (2) from a single traumatic episode that results in subluxation with stretching of the posterior capsule, which then recurs with repeated use of the shoulder. For example, a pitcher will stress his posterior capsule repeatedly in the follow-through phase of throwing. If he overthrows, does not warm up properly, or limits his follow-through by poor lower body mechanics, he can injure the posterior capsule, which will lead to repeated subluxation. Another example is a football offensive lineman who engages his opponent with his arms in front of his body. This mechanism can cause traumatic posterior subluxation with a pulling sensation in the posterior aspect of his shoulder. He may or may not feel the shoulder come out of joint. When he recovers from this acute injury, he notices posterior pain and difficulty with bench pressing and blocking.

On examination of an athlete with posterior instability, tenderness may be noted over the posterior shoulder joint, but tenderness may also be present over the biceps and rotator cuff tendons, as in the typical impingement syndrome. It may take a number of examinations on different occasions to ascertain that the problem is instability rather than impingement. Usually, the position of pain is in both forward flexion to 90 degrees and internal rotation. It may be possible to sublux the shoulder in this position, but if not possible, the patient should be positioned supine with the affected shoulder over the edge of the examination table. An attempt is then made, while grasping the humeral head, to sublux the humeral head posteriorly. Many athletes who are asymptomatic have posterior shoulder laxity that allows posterior subluxation on physical examination.[44] The incidence of such laxity has been documented in some series to be over 50%. Therefore, posterior subluxation present on physical examination may represent normal laxity and may not indicate pathologic instability. The examination must be correlated with the patient's symptoms and history. Occasionally, athletes in this group may be able to voluntarily sublux their shoulder posteriorly and can demonstrate the instability on clinical examination. As this maneuver is performed, a "clunk" is usually audible, which can be confusing because the audible "clunk" occurs with the reduction maneuver and not with the subluxation. The examiner must not make the mistake of thinking that the clunk is an anterior subluxation episode. These athletes, unlike voluntary subluxers, are not usually psychologically disturbed and do not use their shoulder instability for secondary gain. They can be treated exactly the same as athletes who cannot voluntarily dislocate their shoulder.

Occasionally, in a well-muscled athlete, the instability cannot be defined during the clinical examination. Examination under anesthesia, as well as arthroscopy, will usually be necessary to determine the correct diagnosis. Examination under anesthesia typically reveals anterior/posterior translation that is increased in comparison to the normal shoulder. The arthroscopic findings are commonly not striking because the only findings include capsular stretching or minor posterior labral separation or fraying. The major value of arthroscopy is assessment of the anterior glenohumeral ligaments and the labrum to determine the major direction of instability.

Pathologic findings with posterior shoulder instability are different from those with anterior instability. A true reverse Bankart lesion is usually seen in less than 5% of cases, most often in athletes involved in contact sports with a traumatic injury.[42] The labrum may be shallow and poorly developed, but it is almost always intact and not torn away from the posterior glenoid. The capsule is generally redundant. Initial management of these athletes is conservative and consists of an extensive physical therapy program. The physical therapist is instructed to strengthen the external rotators, namely, the infraspinatus and teres minor, as well as the posterior deltoid. The scapular rotators, especially the trapezius and serratus anterior, are emphasized because many athletes with posterior instability have scapular dysfunction. It is not uncommon to find mild scapular winging in these patients. This scapular winging is usually corrected with the physical therapy program. Biofeedback may have a place in this form of instability, as described by Beall and associates.[8] The exercise program usually lasts for at least 6 months. In a throwing athlete, coaches work on follow-through technique to allow the leg and trunk muscles to accept some of the stress that the athlete has been placing on the posterior of the shoulder.

With a conservative program, approximately two thirds of athletes note subjective improvement. The instability is often not eliminated, but the functional disability is improved so that the athlete can perform without any problems.[30] Management of athletes with recurrent posterior shoulder subluxation who do not respond to conservative care is controversial. The results of surgical reconstruction for posterior instability have been disappointing in the past.[28,58,64] Recent articles, however, have shown more promising results.[11,23,26,46]

Posterior Capsulorrhaphy

Our recommended procedure for athletes with posterior shoulder subluxation is posterior capsulorrhaphy. The patient is placed on the operating table in the lateral decubitus position with the involved shoulder superior and draped free. The patient is held in position with a Vacupack, supporting posts, and kidney rests. The operating table is placed in a slight reverse Trendelenburg position. The peroneal nerve should be protected at the point at which it crosses the neck of the fibula in the upper part of the leg. Diagnostic arthroscopy is usually performed to confirm the pathology and direction of instability. The patient is left in this position while the surgeon performs the posterior capsulorrhaphy. A saber incision is made on the superior aspect of the shoulder, beginning just posterior to the acromioclavicular joint and continuing posteriorly toward the posterior axillary fold (Fig. 25–38). This incision is approximately 10 cm in length. The subcutaneous tissues are undermined to expose the deltoid. The deltoid is split (Fig. 25–39) from an area on the spine 2 to 3 cm medial to the posterolateral corner of the acromion, distally approximately 5 cm. The deltoid should not be split below the level of the teres minor because the axillary nerve, which enters the deltoid at the inferior border of the teres minor, might be damaged. It is not usually necessary to reflect the deltoid from the spine or acromion, except occasionally in a well-muscled individual. The teres minor and infraspinatus are encountered below the fascia, deep to the deltoid. The interval between these muscles is not always apparent (Fig. 25–40). An important landmark, the fat stripe, marks the raphe between the two heads of the infraspinatus, which is a bipennate muscle. This raphe is more easily identified than the interval between the teres minor and infraspinatus, which is usually below the equator of the humeral head. The interval between the two heads of the infraspinatus is developed by blunt dissection. Retractors are placed to expose the posterior shoulder capsule. Care must be taken to not split the infraspinatus more than 1.5 cm medial to the glenoid to

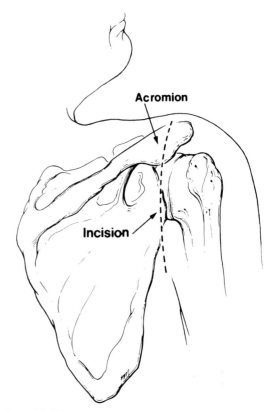

Figure 25–38
The incision is made superiorly, beginning posterior to the acromioclavicular joint and directed toward the posterior axillary fold.

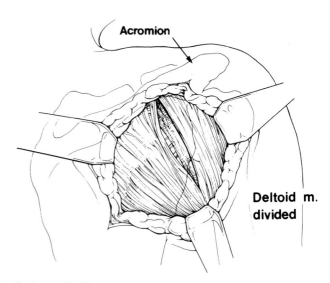

Figure 25–39
The deltoid is split 2 to 3 cm medial to the posterolateral corner of the acromion.

avoid damage to the branch of the suprascapular nerve leading to the infraspinatus (Fig. 25–41).[61]

The capsule needs to be freed from the muscles, which must be done by sharp dissection laterally because the capsule is adherent to the tendons of the teres minor and infraspinatus; medially, it can be done with a periosteal elevator. Once the capsule is sufficiently freed from the overlying muscles, a transverse arthrotomy is made in the posterior capsule in a lateral-to-medial direction down to, but not into the labrum. The joint is inspected. Two capsular flaps are developed by "T-ing" the capsule parallel to the glenoid and just adjacent to the labrum. These flaps are tagged with suture to aid in control of them. The inferior capsular flap must be developed with care because of the close proximity of the axillary nerve. If the labrum is intact, as is usually the case, the sutures can be placed directly into the labrum. (If the labrum is torn, it needs to be reflected so that suture anchors can be inserted and sutures passed through the ligamentous labrum complex, as is done for a capsulolabral reconstruction anteriorly.) The inferior capsule is then advanced superiorly and medially and attached to the glenoid labrum with No. 1 Ethibond sutures (Fig. 25–42). These sutures usually eliminate the posterior as well as any inferior instability. The superior capsular flap is then sutured over the inferior flap by advancing it inferiorly and medially (Fig. 25–43). A transverse gap may still be present in the capsule laterally; this gap is closed with interrupted mattress sutures. The two heads of the infraspinatus fall together and do not usually need any sutures. The deltoid fascia, which has been split, is then repaired (Fig. 25–44).

Postoperatively, the patient's arm and shoulder are immobilized in a position of 30 degrees of abduction, slight extension, and neutral rotation for 3 weeks.

Recently, some authors have recommended an arthroscopic posterior capsulorrhaphy. This technique is performed by repairing the posterior labrum back to the glenoid rim with suture anchors if it is torn and tensioning the posterior capsule by suturing the capsule to the labrum to decrease the posterior volume (Figs. 25–45 and 25–46). The rotator interval capsule, which is a secondary restraint to posterior instability, can also easily be addressed arthroscopically. The posterior arthroscopic repair has been performed on a limited population with short-term follow-up. Whether it will be better or worse than the conventional open technique cannot be determined at this time.

Postoperative Rehabilitation Program

Isometric exercises for the deltoid and the rotator cuff muscles are begun in the immediate postoperative period.

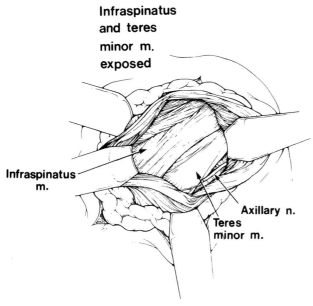

■ Figure 25–40
The teres minor and infraspinatus muscles are exposed; the axillary nerve enters the deltoid below the teres minor.

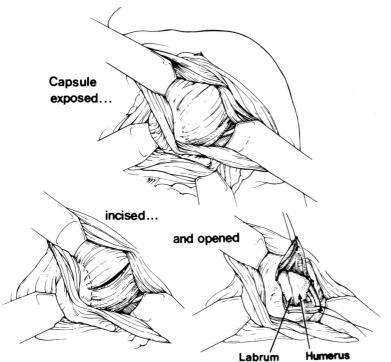

■ Figure 25–41
The capsule is exposed, and a transverse arthrotomy is made in the posterior capsule in a lateral-to-medial direction. Two capsule flaps are developed by "T-ing" the capsule parallel to the glenoid and adjacent to the labrum.

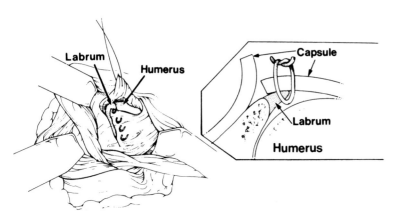

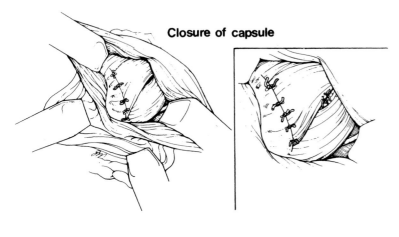

Closure of capsule

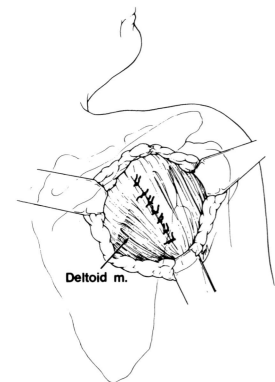

Deltoid m.

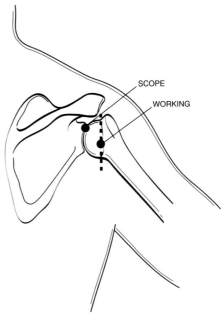

■ **Figure 25–42**
The inferior capsular flap is advanced superiorly and medially and attached to the labrum.

■ **Figure 25–43**
The superior flap is sutured over the inferior flap by advancing it inferiorly and medially. The lateral split in the capsule is closed with interrupted mattress sutures.

■ **Figure 25–45**
Posterior shoulder scope portal and "working" portal for arthroscopic posterior capsulorrhaphy.

■ **Figure 25–44**
The deltoid fascia, which has been split, is repaired.

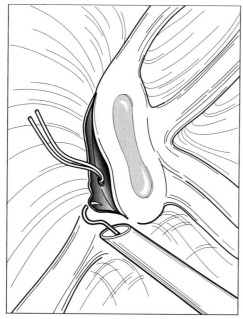

■ Figure 25–46
The posterior labrum is attached to the glenoid with suture anchors, and the posterior capsule is sutured to the labrum.

After 3 weeks of isometric exercise, active and active assisted range of motion is begun. The emphasis is on elevation in the scapular plane of the body and on regaining rotation. For the first 4 to 6 weeks postoperatively, no motion is performed in the sagittal plane (i.e., forward flexion) to avoid placing increased stress on the newly repaired posterior capsule and soft tissues. At 6 weeks, forward flexion is allowed. At 12 weeks, resistance beyond 90 degrees of elevation can be added to increase strength and endurance. Attention should be focused on regaining synchrony of the scapula rotators, rotator cuff, and deltoid. When synchrony is firmly re-established, athletes may return to their sport, usually about 6 months postoperatively. Throwing athletes will generally require another 6 months to develop the endurance necessary to return to competitive throwing.

Posterior shoulder repair does not always allow athletes to return to their former throwing ability. Many athletes with posterior instability have little functional disability other than in their sport. The difficulty of returning to competitive throwing should not be underestimated; however, with careful surgical selection and meticulous rehabilitation, return is possible.

Posterior Lesions

Throwing athletes commonly have posterior glenoid spurs visible on radiographs. These spurs may or may not be symptomatic. Bennett described calcification in the posterior aspect of the shoulder.[10] He thought that these lesions were caused by a traction phenomenon at the insertion of the long head of the triceps in the posterior inferior glenoid. The symptom complex included pain referred to the posterior deltoid.

Occasionally, such lesions are noted in asymptomatic shoulders. Symptoms may develop gradually with increasing severity or, alternatively, may have a sudden onset. Bennett described an x-ray view to demonstrate the calcification of spurs: an anteroposterior view of the glenohumeral joint with the machine tilted 5 degrees cephalad and the arm positioned in both abduction and external rotation, as in the cocking position of throwing. The scapula is then rotated to a position that shows the exostosis on the inferior glenoid. A conventional axillary lateral view often shows the bone spur in this area as well.

In our experience, the calcification in a Bennett lesion is in the posterior inferior capsule and is due to repetitive stress to this area caused by the follow-through phase of pitching.[20] This lesion is a traction injury to the posterior inferior capsule. The lesion itself is often asymptomatic. However, in athletes with a fracture in the spur or a fibrous union at its base, the resultant symptoms will interfere with pitching. Furthermore, the calcification can cause a posterior inferior capsular contraction that can lead to symptomatic internal impingement. Generally, rest in these cases results in pain-free motion during normal activities and exercise. Return to pitching, however, causes severe pain after a few innings.

These athletes usually respond to conservative care, which includes not only rest but also anti-inflammatory medications and steroid injections. Physical therapy should concentrate on stretching out the posterior capsule. Athletes whose pain prevents them from throwing effectively have responded to an operative approach consisting of resection of the spur or calcification either arthroscopically or through the same deltoid-splitting approach described earlier. After exposing the capsule between the infraspinatus and the teres minor, the capsule is opened and the spur is identified and removed. The athlete can usually return to competitive throwing about 6 months after surgery. Lombardo and colleagues reported four athletes who successfully returned to competition after removal of a spur.[41] When the calcification, the spur, or both are removed arthroscopically, the posterior inferior capsule is opened. This part of the capsule should not be repaired after resection to avoid tightening the posterior capsule.

NEUROLOGIC PROBLEMS

Quadrilateral Space Syndrome

Cahill and Palmer described the quadrilateral space syndrome in 1983.[12] Axillary nerve function is compromised by fibrous bands in the quadrilateral space. The compromise occurs when the athlete abducts and externally rotates the arm as in the cocking maneuver in throwing. The patient experiences posterior shoulder pain, usually in the area of the teres minor muscle. The pain is exacerbated in the abducted and externally rotated position. Tenderness may or may not be noted directly in this area. The results of neurologic examination are generally normal, and electromyographic studies are not helpful. The diagnosis is usually confirmed by an arteriogram of the subclavian and axillary artery systems. With the shoulder in neutral position, the posterior humeral circumflex artery is visualized. With the arm in abduction and external rotation, arterial blood flow is compromised. It is also helpful to perform comparative studies on both arms to look for anatomic variations. Rest and cortisone injections may prove helpful in an athlete with this condition. If symptoms persist, however, operative decompression of the quadrilateral space is indicated. The standard approach is through a deltoid-splitting incision and release of the teres minor muscle. However, the authors of this chapter have found that the quadrilateral space can be approached through a vertical incision entering the quadrilateral space below the deltoid and not releasing the teres minor. The long head of the triceps is commonly partially released because it seems to be the offending structure rather than the teres minor.

Suprascapular Nerve Entrapment

In the general population, suprascapular nerve entrapment occurs most often in the suprascapular notch area. In an athlete, however, the nerve is often entrapped in the spinoglenoid notch or just distal to the notch.[14] This location spares the function of the supraspinatus muscle. The athlete may have what appears to be tendinitis. On closer examination, however, the surgeon notices atrophy of the infraspinatus muscle. This condition is seen most frequently in high-level pitchers and volleyball players. Most volleyball players, however, are asymptomatic and can be treated with an exercise program to strengthen the infraspinatus.[21] Surgical treatment of a symptomatic volleyball player or pitcher involves decompression of the suprascapular nerve at the spinoglenoid notch by releasing the spinoglenoid ligament. This ligament has recently been shown to be present in approximately 80% of shoulders.[15] In the authors' experience, surgical treatment of suprascapular nerve entrapment at the spinoglenoid notch has allowed recovery of some, but not all the muscle bulk. However, most of the athletes have been able to return to their sport. If the infraspinatus is not completely denervated, athletes have been able to return to throwing by maximizing the remaining infraspinatus function.

VASCULAR PROBLEMS

Axillary Artery

Occlusion of the axillary artery can typically occur when the arm is brought overhead. Most likely it is the secondary portion of the axillary artery that is occluded by pressure of the humeral head, as well as the overlying pectoralis minor muscle. Such occlusion can be observed in normal individuals and can be demonstrated by angiography.[57] Tullos and associates described occlusion of the axillary artery during pitching.[67] They thought that the transient occlusion in the axillary artery was due to the stretching under the pectoralis minor that occurred with each pitch. In rare cases, sufficient local trauma occurs over time to produce minimal damage and subsequent thrombosis. The clinical findings include various signs and symptoms that are often nonspecific. The diag-

nosis is difficult to make, and the athlete may complain of fatigue and muscle ache, lack of endurance, or intermittent paresthesia, as well as loss of control. If no objective findings are present, the symptoms may be dismissed as minor psychosomatic. An arteriogram is usually necessary to confirm the diagnosis. Vascular surgery relieves the blockage by either excision with reanastomosis or a bypass graft. In one well-known case, a professional baseball pitcher experienced progression of the thrombosis that resulted in a cerebral vascular accident and subsequent partial paralysis.

More recently, in a number of athletes, an aneurysm has developed in a branch of the axillary or subclavian artery.[52,59] In addition to the vascular occlusion symptoms mentioned earlier, these players sometimes have embolic phenomena in the hand distal to the aneurysm. Such embolism is thought to represent fragments of the thrombosis in the aneurysm.[22,33,43,56,63] Again, the diagnosis is confirmed by angiography, and treatment is surgery on the vasculature. Screening pitchers to identify those with an axillary artery compression aneurysm or thrombosis has not been shown to be effective.

Axillary Vein

Thrombosis of the axillary vein was originally described by Paget in 1875 and by van Schroether in 1884.[1] This condition has been called "effort thrombosis" because of the association with a forceful event that produces injury to the vein. It usually occurs in active athletic individuals and is preceded by strenuous effort or repetitive action. The athlete has pain and swelling in the arm. Objectively, venous distention involving the upper limb and secondary cyanosis may be present. A venogram will confirm the diagnosis. Treatment is usually conservative and involves rest and elevation. Anticoagulation is used in the initial phases to avoid progression of the thrombosis. After the initial episode, the athlete may continue to complain of external claudication. Vogel and Jensen reported on a college swimmer suffering from effort thrombosis of the subclavian vein.[71] They believed that the athlete had an unusual manifestation of thoracic outlet syndrome, although various provocative maneuvers did not induce any alternation in the radial pulse. A venogram revealed complete occlusion of the subclavian vein in the area of the first rib. Treatment consisted of therapy with intravenous streptokinase, heparin, and warfarin sodium (Coumadin). After 4 months, the first rib was removed and the patient became asymptomatic. Vogel and Jensen thought that the most likely site of compression at the subclavian vein was between the first rib and the clavicle in the costoclavicular area. A less likely mechanism of compression would be the tendon of the pectoralis minor, or the head of the humerus could also compress the axillary vein on its anterior aspect with shoulder abduction.

In a recent series presented by Arko and colleagues, 12 athletes were treated for subclavian vein thrombosis, initially with lytic therapy and anticoagulation.[4] However, eight patients later required thoracic outlet decompression and venolysis of the subclavian vein to relieve their symptoms. All the athletes in this series remained stable without further venous thrombosis and returned to their usual level of activity.

SUMMARY

Optimal performance tends to be the ultimate goal of an elite athlete; that of injury prevention and treatment tends to be somewhere behind. As health care practitioners, we want to assist athletes with their goals. If we can prevent injuries from occurring, we are helping to optimize performance. One of the ways that we can advocate prevention is to communicate an interest in and an understanding of their mechanics and potential pathomechanics. We can educate the athlete and the athletic staff on how to stay in the game longer at a higher level. We can share with them the subtle clinical and on-the-field mechanical signs of injury. By doing so, we can identify the potential injury earlier and get them back on the field more quickly. By increasing our understanding of these issues, we can better equip ourselves to select the appropriate intervention—be it rehabilitative or surgical.

REFERENCES AND BIBLIOGRAPHY

1. Adams JT and DeWeese JA: "Effort" thrombosis of the axillary and subclavian veins. J Trauma 11:923-929, 1971.
2. Allegrucci M, Whitney SL, and Irrgang JJ: Clinical implications of secondary impingement of the shoulder in freestyle swimmers. J Orthop Sports Phys Ther 20:307-318, 1994.
3. Andrews JR and Dugas JR: Diagnosis and treatment of shoulder injuries in the throwing athlete: The role of thermal-assisted capsular shrinkage. Instr Course Lect 50:17-21, 2001.
4. Arko FR, Harris EJ, Zarins CK, and Olcott C: Vascular complications in high-performance athletes. J Vasc Surg 77:935-942, 2001.
5. Arnoczky SP and Aksan A: Thermal modification of connective tissues: Basic science considerations and clinical implications. Instr Course Lect 50:3-11, 2001.
6. Babyar SR: Excessive scapular motion in individuals recovering from painful stiff shoulders: Causes and treatment strategies. Phys Ther 76:226-238, 1996.
7. Bain AM: Supraspinatus tendinitis. Physiotherapy 57:17-20, 1971.
8. Beall SM, Diefenbach G, and Allen A: Electromyographic biofeedback in the treatment of voluntary posterior instability of the shoulder. Am J Sports Med 15:175-178, 1987.
9. Belling Sorensen AK and Jorgensen U: Secondary impingement in the shoulder. An improved terminology in impingement. Scand J Med Sci Sports 10:266-278, 2000.
10. Bennett GE: Elbow and shoulder lesions of baseball players. Am J Surg 98:484-488, 1959.
11. Bigliani LU, Pollock RG, McIlveen SJ, et al: Shift of the posteroinferior aspect of the capsule for recurrent posterior glenohumeral instability. J Bone Joint Surg Am 77:1011-1020, 1995.
12. Cahill BR and Palmer RE: Quadrilateral space syndrome. J Hand Surg 8:65-69, 1983.
13. Cavallo RJ and Speer KP: Shoulder instability and impingement in throwing athletes. Med Sci Sports Exerc 30(4 suppl):S18-S25, 1998.
14. Cummins CA, Bowen M, Anderson K, and Messer T: Suprascapular nerve entrapment at the spinoglenoid notch in a professional baseball pitcher. Am J Sports Med 6:810-812, 1999.
15. Cummins CA, Messer TM, and Nuber GW: Suprascapular nerve entrapment. J Bone Joint Surg Am 82:415-424, 2000.
16. D'Alessandro DF, Bradley JP, Fleischli JE, and Connor PM: Prospective evaluation of thermal capsulorrhaphy for shoulder instability: Indications and results two to five year follow-up. Submitted to Am J Sports Med, April 2002.
17. DiGiovine NM, Jobe FW, Pink M, and Perry J: An electromyographic analysis of the upper extremity in pitching. J Shoulder Elbow Surg 1:15-25, 1992.
18. Ellenbecker TS and Mattalino AJ: Glenohumeral joint range of motion and rotator cuff strength following arthroscopic anterior stabilization with thermal capsulorrhaphy. J Orthop Sports Phys Ther 29:160-167, 1999.
19. Feltner M and Dapena J: Dynamics of the shoulder and elbow joints of the throwing arm during a baseball pitch. Int J Sports Biomech 2:235-259, 1986.
20. Ferrari JD, Ferrari DA, Coumas J, and Pappas AM: Posterior ossification of the shoulder: The Bennett lesion. Etiology, diagnosis, and treatment. Am J Sports Med 22:171-175, 1994.
21. Ferretti A, De Carli A, and Fontana M: Injury of the suprascapular nerve at the spinoglenoid notch. The natural history of infraspinatus atrophy in volleyball players. Am J Sports Med 26:759-763, 1998.
22. Fields W, Lemak N, and Ben-Menachem Y: Thoracic outlet syndrome: Review and reference to stroke in a major league pitcher. AJNR Am J Neuroradiol 7:73-78, 1986.
23. Fronek J, Warrer RF, and Bowen M: Posterior subluxation of the glenohumeral joint. J Bone Joint Surg Am 71:206-216, 1989.
24. Fu FH, Harner CD, and Klein AH: Shoulder impingement syndrome. A critical review. Clin Orthop 269:162-173, 1991.
25. Gainor BJ, Piotrowski F, Puhl J, et al: The throw: Biomechanics and acute injury. Am J Sports Med 8:114-118, 1980.
26. Goss TP and Costello G: Recurrent symptomatic posterior glenohumeral subluxation. Orthop Rev 17:1024-1032, 1988.
27. Hamner DL, Pink MM, and Jobe FW: A modification of the relocation test: Arthroscopic findings associated with a positive test. J Shoulder Elbow Surg 9:263-267, 2000.
28. Hawkins RJ, Koppert G, and Johnston G: Recurrent posterior instability (subluxation) of the shoulder. J Bone Joint Surg Am 66:169-174, 1984.
29. Herberts P and Kadefors R: A study of painful shoulder in welders. Acta Orthop Scand 47:381-387, 1976.
30. Hurley JA, Anderson TE, Dear W, et al: Posterior shoulder instability: Surgical vs non-surgical results. Orthop Trans 11:458, 1987.
31. Ianotti JP: Rotator Cuff Disorders: Evaluation and Treatment. American Academy of Orthopaedic Surgeons Monograph Series, 1991.
32. Inman VT, Saunders JB de CM, and Abbott LC: Observations on the functions of the shoulder joint. J Bone Joint Surg 26:1-30, 1944.
33. Itoh Y, Wakano K, Takeda T, and Murakami T: Circulatory disturbances in the throwing hand of baseball pitchers. Am J Sports Med 15:264-269, 1987.
34. Jobe CM: Posterior superior glenoid impingement: Expanded spectrum. Arthroscopy 11:530-536, 1995.
35. Jobe CM, Pink MM, Jobe FW, and Shaffer B: Anterior shoulder instability, impingement, and rotator cuff tear: Theories & concepts. In Jobe FW, Pink MM, Glousman RE, et al (eds): Operative Techniques in Upper Extremity Sports Injuries. St Louis: Mosby–Year Book, 1996, pp 164-176.
36. Jobe FW, Giangarra CE, Glousman RE, et al: Relationship of instability and impingement in throwing athletes: Review of the anterior capsulolabral reconstruction. Paper presented at a meeting of the American Shoulder and Elbow Surgeons, February 1989, Las Vegas, NV.
37. Jobe FW, Pink MM, Glousman RE, et al: Operative Techniques in Upper Extremity Sports Injuries. St Louis: Mosby–Year Book, 1996.
38. Johnston TB: The movements of the shoulder-joint: A plea for the use of the 'plane of the scapula' as the plane of reference for movements occurring at the humero-scapular joint. Br J Surg 25:252-260, 1937.
39. King W and Perry J: Personal communication, 1989.
40. Krishnan SG, Hawkins RJ, Karas SG, et al: Electrothermal arthroscopic shoulder capsulorrhaphy: A minimum two year follow-up. Paper presented at the Annual Meeting of AOSSM, June 30-July 3, 2002, Orlando, FL.
41. Lombardo SJ, Jobe FW, Kerlan RK, et al: Posterior shoulder lesions in throwing athletes. Am J Sports Med 5:106-110, 1977.
42. Mair SD, Zarzour RH, and Speer KP: Posterior labral injury in contract athletes. Am J Sports Med 24:753-758, 1998.
43. McCarthy W, Yao J, Schafer M, et al: Upper extremity arterial injury in athletes. J Vasc Surg 9:317-327, 1989.
44. McFarland EG, Campbell G, and McDowell J: Posterior shoulder laxity in asymptomatic athletes. Am J Sports Med 24:468-471, 1996.
45. Miniaci A, McBirnie J, and Miniaci SL: Thermal capsulorrhaphy of the treatment of multi-directional instability of the shoulder. Paper presented at a Specialty Day Meeting of the American Shoulder and Elbow Surgeons, March 2001, San Francisco.
46. Misamore GW and Facibene WA: Posterior capsulorrhaphy for the treatment of traumatic recurrent posterior subluxations of the shoulder in athletes. J Shoulder Elbow Surg 9:403-408, 2000.
47. Mishra DK and Fanton GS: Two-year outcome of arthroscopic Bankart repair and electrothermal-assisted capsulorrhaphy for recurrent traumatic anterior instability. Arthroscopy 17:844-849, 2001.
48. Monad H: Contractility of muscle during prolonged static and repetitive dynamic activity. Ergonomics 28:81-89, 1985.
49. Moseley JB, Jobe FW, Pink M, et al: EMG analysis of the scapular muscles during a shoulder rehabilitation program. Am J Sports Med 20:128-134, 1992.
50. Neer CS II: Anterior acromioplasty for the chronic impingement syndrome in the shoulder: A preliminary report. J Bone Joint Surg 54:41, 1972.
51. Neer CS II: Shoulder Reconstruction. Philadelphia: WB Saunders, 1990.
52. Nuber GW, McCarthy JW, Yao JS, et al: Arterial abnormalities of the shoulder in athletes. Am J Sports Med 18:514-519, 1990.
53. Paley KJ, Jobe FW, Pink MM, et al: Arthroscopic findings in the overhand throwing athlete: Evidence for posterior internal impingement of the rotator cuff. Arthroscopy 16:35-40, 2000.
54. Pappas AM, Zawacki RM, and Sullivan TJ: Biomechanics of baseball pitching: A preliminary report. Am J Sports Med 13:216-222, 1985.

55. Pink M, Perry J, Browne A, et al: The normal shoulder during freestyle swimming: An electromyographic and cinematographic analysis of twelve muscles. Am J Sports Med 19:569-576, 1991.

56. Reekers J, den Hartog B, Kromhout J, et al: Traumatic aneurysm of the posterior circumflex humeral artery: A volleyball player's disease? J Vasc Interv Radiol 4:405-408, 1993.

57. Rohrer MJ, Cardullo PA, Pappas AM, et al: Axillary artery compression and thrombosis in throwing athletes. J Vasc Surg 11:761-768, discussion 768-769, 1990.

58. Rowe C and Zarins B: Recurrent transient subluxation of the shoulder. J Bone Joint Surg Am 63:863-871, 1981.

59. Schneider K, Kasparyan NG, Altchek DW, et al: An aneurysm involving the axillary artery and its branch vessels in a major league baseball pitcher. A case report and review of the literature. Am J Sports Med 27:370-375, 1999.

60. Scovazzo ML, Browne A, Pink M, et al: The painful shoulder during freestyle swimming: An electromyographic and cinematographic analysis of twelve muscles. Am J Sports Med 19:577-582, 1991.

61. Shaffer BS, Conway JE, Jobe FW, et al: Infraspinatus splitting incision in posterior shoulder surgery. An anatomic and electromyographic study. Am J Sports Med 22:113-120, 1994.

62. Stocker D, Pink M, and Jobe FW: Comparison of shoulder injury in collegiate- and master's level swimmers. Clin J Sport Med 5:4-8, 1995.

63. Sugawara M, Ogino T, Minami A, and Ishii S: Digital ischemia in baseball players. Am J Sports Med 14:329-334, 1986.

64. Tibone JE and Bradley JP: The treatment of posterior subluxation in athletes. Clin Orthop 291:124-137, 1993.

65. Toth AP, Cordasco FA, Altchek DW, and O'Brien SJ: Thermal assisted capsular shrinkage for shoulder instability: Minimum two year follow-up. Paper presented at the Annual Meeting of the AOSSM, June 30-July 3, 2002, Orlando, FL.

66. Townsend H, Jobe FW, Pink M, and Perry J: Electromyographic analysis of the glenohumeral muscles during a baseball rehabilitation program. Am J Sports Med 19:264-272, 1991.

67. Tullos HS, Erwin WD, Woods WG, et al: Unusual lesions of the pitching arm. Clin Orthop 88:169, 1972.

68. Turkel SJ: Stabilizing mechanisms preventing anterior dislocation of the glenohumeral joint. J Bone Joint Surg Am 63:1208-1217, 1981.

69. Tyler TF, Calabrese GJ, Parker RD, and Nicholas SJ: Electrothermally-assisted capsulorrhaphy (ETAC): A new surgical method for glenohumeral instability and its rehabilitation considerations. J Orthop Sports Phys Ther 30:390-400, 2000.

70. Valadie AL, Jobe CM, Pink MM, et al: Anatomy of provocative tests for impingement syndrome of the shoulder. J Shoulder Elbow Surg 9:36-46, 2000.

71. Vogel CM and Jensen JE: 'Effort' thrombosis of the subclavian vein in a competitive swimmer. Am J Sports Med 13:269-272, 1985.

72. Walch G, Boileau P, Noel E, and Donel ST: Impingement of the deep surface of the supraspinatus tendon on the posterosuperior glenoid rim: An arthroscopic study. J Shoulder Elbow Surg 1:238-245, 1992.

73. Wall MS, Deng XH, Torzilli PA, et al: Thermal modification of collagen. J Shoulder Elbow Surg 8:339-344, 1999.

74. Wallace AL, Hollinshead RM, and Frank CB: Creep behavior of a rabbit model of ligament laxity after electrothermal shrinkage in vivo. Am J Sports Med 30:98-102, 2002.

75. Wong KL and Williams GR: Complications of thermal capsulorrhaphy of the shoulder. J Bone Joint Surg Am 83(suppl 2, part 2):151-155, 2001.

CHAPTER 26

FRACTURES, DISLOCATIONS, AND ACQUIRED PROBLEMS OF THE SHOULDER IN CHILDREN

James O. Sanders, M.D., and Mary Beth Cermak, M.D.

• • • •

FRACTURES OF THE PROXIMAL HUMERUS

Developmental Anatomy

The humerus and scapula form as a cartilaginous anlage at 5 weeks' gestation. During weeks 6 and 7, the glenohumeral joint forms by cavitation between the humerus and the scapula. By 12 weeks, the beginning of the fetal period, the region reaches its adult configuration and then progressively enlarges and matures. The proximal humeral ossification center becomes visible by ultrasound between 38 and 42 weeks' gestation,[83,106] but it does not generally appear on plain radiographs until 6 months of age.[83,111] The upper part of the humerus forms from three separate ossification centers: the head appears at 6 months, the lesser tuberosity in the fifth year, and the greater tuberosity in the second to third year. The tuberosities unite at 5 years of age, fuse with the head between 7 and 14 years of age, and then subsequently fuse to the shaft between 14 and 17 years in girls[35] and 16 and 19 years in boys.[35,11,136] Humeral head retroversion decreases with growth from about 65 degrees in infants to normal values by 6 to 12 years of age,[43] although throwing athletes may have persistent humeral retroversion.

Growth

The proximal humeral physis accounts for 80% of the growth of the humerus overall; however, this percentage varies with age. Before the age of 2, less than 75% of growth occurs at the proximal physis; it increases to 85% at age 8 and remains constant at 90% after age 11.[17,118,119] Stahl and Karpman[148] found very little growth of the proximal humeral physis beyond the skeletal age of 14, whereas Bortel and Pritchett found substantial growth remaining in boys until the skeletal age of 16 years.[17,118,119]

The proximal humeral physeal shape is unique. It has an inferior concavity, the apex of which is somewhat posteromedial. The epiphyseal contour remains essentially the same throughout growth, so injury does not cause significant deformity.[14] In contrast, in the proximal end of the femur, the relative size and shape of the bone change with skeletal maturation.

Surgical Anatomy

The articular surface covers both the epiphysis and a portion of the proximal medial metaphysis. Medially, the physis curves distally so that articular cartilage does not directly oppose metaphyseal bone but always lies over the epiphysis.[119] The joint capsule of the proximal end of the humerus extends to the metaphysis, thus making a portion of the metaphysis intra-articular.[38] Because the periosteum is strongest posteromedially, it the most common periosteal hinge.

The anterolateral ascending branch of the anterior circumflex artery supplies the humeral head[55]; it runs parallel to the lateral aspect of the biceps tendon and enters the humeral head where the proximal intertubercular groove meets the tuberosity. The posterior circumflex artery supplies only a small portion of the greater tuberosity and a small portion of the inferior head.[64]

Although proximal humeral physeal fractures typically propagate through the zone of hypertrophy adjacent to the zone of provisional calcification,[38,133] undulations do occur through other zones. Fractures rarely disturb physeal growth because these zones are distal to the proliferating cells. Remodeling potential is superb as a result of the large amount of growth from the proximal humeral physis.[7,35,107]

Because the physeal apex is somewhat posteromedial with strong posteromedial periosteum, most fractures displace anteriorly and laterally with the shaft protruding through the weaker anterolateral periosteum. The strong posteromedial periosteum remains attached and often avulses a metaphyseal fragment in older children. Occasionally, the periosteum or the biceps tendon becomes interposed and thus makes reduction difficult.[2,5,7,35,38,87,100,163]

Above the pectoralis major, displaced fractures have marked abduction of the proximal fragment from the rotator cuff with external rotation.[35,37] The deltoid pulls the distal fragment proximally, and the pectoralis major pulls it medially. Fractures between the pectoralis major and the deltoid insertions result in adduction of the proximal fragment from the pectoralis major and shortening by pull of the deltoid on the distal fragment. Diaphyseal fractures below the deltoid insertion result in abduction

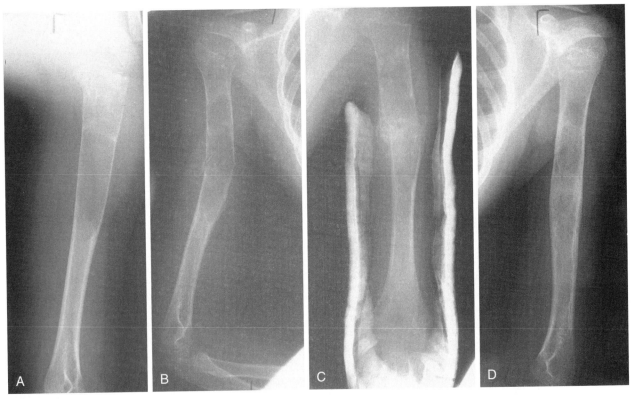

■ **Figure 26–1**
Asymptomatic simple bone cyst (**A**) noted on a chest radiograph and monitored until undergoing a spontaneous fracture with angulation (**B**). The fracture was treated with a "U" plaster (**C**) followed by two steroid injections, with good resolution of the cyst (**D**). *(From Rockwood CA, Wilkins KE, and Beaty J [eds]: Fractures in Children. Philadelphia: JB Lippincott, 1996.)*

of the long proximal fragment from the deltoid and shortening and medial displacement of the distal fragment from the biceps and triceps.[37] Recalling these anatomic factors can assist in fracture reduction.

Incidence

Proximal humeral fractures account for less than 5% of children's fractures,[4,35,62,64,69,84,89,160,173] with an incidence ranging from 1.2 to 4.4 per 10,000 per year.[10,173] They are the fourth most frequent epiphyseal fracture[126] and are most common in infants and adolescents, with the highest peak at 15 years of age, probably as a result of sports and other high-energy activities.[38,65,84,126] Proximal humeral physeal fractures represent 1.9% to 6.7% of physeal injuries and are some of the most common birth fractures.[70,87,116,117,121,144] Neonates and young children commonly have Salter-Harris type I injuries. By contrast, although children 5 to 11 years of age may sustain physeal fractures, metaphyseal fractures are more common, most likely because of the rapid growth phase occurring in the metaphyseal area in this age group, which leads to relative weakness.[38] In adolescents, 75% of these fractures are Salter-Harris type II, with type I fractures occurring in approximately 25%.[38]

Proximal humeral fractures can also occur through unicameral bone cysts, which are most often found in the proximal humeral metaphysis (Fig. 26–1). Thirty-eight

percent of simple bone cysts are localized to the proximal part of the humerus.[54] A pathologic fracture is likely if more than 85% of the transverse plane is involved on both anteroposterior and lateral radiographs.[1] Small cysts surrounded by cortical bone may heal without surgery if they are protected for an extended time.[6] The prognosis is best in patients who are older than 10 years and who have cysts farther from the physis.[6,109] The fallen leaf sign is pathognomonic but occurs in only 20% of cysts.[152] Growth arrest has been reported in both treated and untreated proximal humeral simple cysts.[63,105,109] Fractures through unicameral cysts are unlikely to speed the cyst's healing.[1,6,53,75] Steroid injections appear to be an effective treatment,* but the reason for their efficacy is unknown. It may be related to suppression of the high prostaglandin E_2 levels found in cysts.[143] Methylprednisolone also has a direct effect on synovial cells, possibly indicating an effect on the cyst's cellular component.[175] Repeated steroid injections result in healing in more than 90% of patients, with few complications. When injections fail, bone grafting usually succeeds. Cysts may also heal with osteotomy[150] and forceful injection of saline.[145] Recent reports have found injection of bone marrow aspirate or demineralized bone matrix efficacious.[13,30,127,129,170] A randomized trial comparing bone marrow aspirate with steroid injection is ongoing.

---

*See references 25, 26, 28, 33, 34, 46, 47, 123, 130, 135, 137-139.

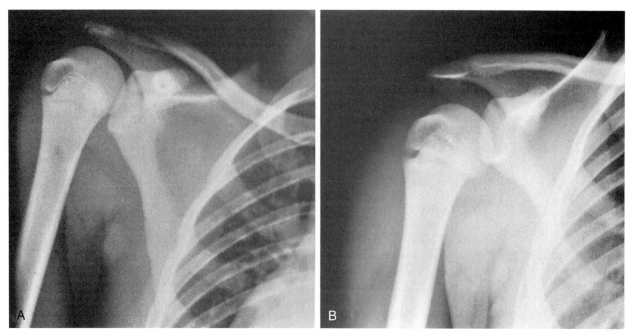

■ **Figure 26–2**
This 13-year-old Little League baseball pitcher complained of right shoulder pain for 2 weeks. **A,** This original anteroposterior radiograph shows a suggestion of widening at the lateral physis. **B,** The patient was allowed to continue pitching and suffered displacement of this proximal humeral stress fracture.

Mechanism of Injury

Birth Injuries

Although shoulder dystocia is strongly associated with macrosomia, it is difficult to predict prepartum.[27,52,72] Birth injuries may occur as the arm becomes hyperextended or rotated during delivery.[38,57,59,61,86,99,144] Dameron and Reibel[38] performed anatomic studies on stillborn infants, and all the injuries were Salter-Harris type I fractures. The metaphysis could not be displaced posteriorly by closed manipulation.[38] The physeal shape with its metaphyseal high point posterior and medial to the center and a stronger posterior periosteum attached to the periphery of the epiphysis caused anterior displacement of the metaphysis with respect to the epiphysis. These fractures reduced without interposition of the biceps tendon unless the tendon was manually forced into the site. With the humerus extended and adducted, the metaphysis could easily be displaced anteriorly. The top of the metaphysis penetrated the periosteum just lateral to the biceps tendon. Only after resecting the posterior periosteum could the metaphysis be displaced posteriorly.

Older Children

In older children, falls are the most common injury mechanism, followed by traffic accidents and sports.[79] Falls from horses account for a disproportionately large portion of proximal humeral fractures.[84] The older literature reports the most common mechanism to be a fall on an outstretched hand transmitting force through the arm and driving the metaphysis anteriorly and laterally.[2,18,68,72] Better studies indicate that a direct blow to the posterior aspect of the shoulder is the most common

mechanism.[38,107,146] Williams identified six potential mechanisms of injury as forced extension, flexion, lateral rotation, or medial rotation singly or in combination.[171]

Proximal humeral physeal slipping analogous to a slipped capital femoral epiphysis has been reported in gymnastics as a result of humeral weight bearing,[36] as a complication of radiotherapy,[42] and as a sequela of pituitary gigantism.[124] Repetitive pitching can cause physeal stress injuries (Fig. 26–2).[93,157,158] The fracture may result from child abuse.[51] Proximal humeral fractures are also reported with myelomeningocele,[94] perhaps related to upper extremity weight bearing or neuropathy from Arnold-Chiari malformations and syringomyelia.

Classification

Classification of proximal humeral fractures in children is simple and descriptive, although its reproducibility has not been tested. Fractures may be physeal or metaphyseal. *Physeal involvement* is classified by the Salter-Harris classification. In younger patients, fractures are predominantly Salter-Harris type I, whereas older patients typically have Salter-Harris type II fractures (Fig. 26–3). Taken together, most physeal fractures are Salter-Harris type II.[117] Type II fractures may have an additional anterolateral fragment.[22] Salter-Harris type III fractures are reported with[32,56] and without[154,172] associated shoulder dislocations. Type IV fractures have not been reported. Dameron and Reibel[38] classified fractures according to the Salter-Harris type and the age of the patient—0 to 5 years, 5 to 11 years, or 11 to 17 years. Metaphyseal fractures are classified by their displacement and by their relationship to the surrounding muscles as discussed earlier. After reduction, proximal humeral fractures may be stable or unstable.

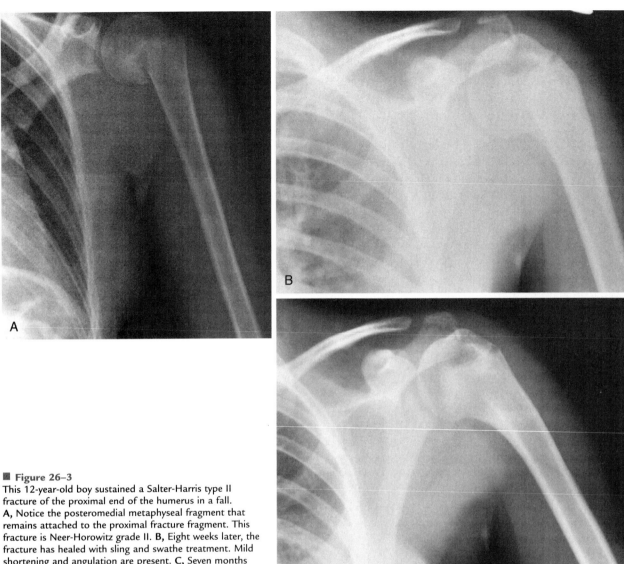

■ **Figure 26–3**
This 12-year-old boy sustained a Salter-Harris type II fracture of the proximal end of the humerus in a fall. **A,** Notice the posteromedial metaphyseal fragment that remains attached to the proximal fracture fragment. This fracture is Neer-Horowitz grade II. **B,** Eight weeks later, the fracture has healed with sling and swathe treatment. Mild shortening and angulation are present. **C,** Seven months after the fracture, significant remodeling has corrected most of the deformity.

DISPLACEMENT. Neer and Horowitz[107] classified proximal humeral physeal fractures according to the degree of displacement, with grade 1 representing up to 5 mm of displacement, grade 2 up to a third of the humeral shaft diameter, grade 3 up to two thirds of the humeral shaft diameter, and grade 4 greater than two thirds of the shaft diameter with total separation. Proximal humeral fractures may be in either varus angulation, which is the most common, or valgus angulation, which is quite rare.[59] The epiphysis slips into a varus position and usually responds well to nonoperative treatment.

STRESS INJURIES. Repetitive pitching can cause physeal stress injuries that respond to temporary cessation of pitching.[92,157,158]

OTHER FRACTURES. Other rare fractures include those of the greater tuberosity, which has been reported in association with luxatio erecta[49,80] or fracture through the lesser tuberosity.[74,128,167]

Fracture-dislocations may be anterior and associated with Salter-Harris type I, II, or III fractures,[32,51,56,110] or they may be posterior[161] or inferior.[49,80] Intrathoracic fracture-dislocations have been reported in adults[60] but not in children. Fractures may be segmental and involve the shaft and the neck[98,113] or the ipsilateral forearm or elbow.[70]

Signs and Symptoms

Evaluation of the Neonatal Shoulder

Infants who do not move their shoulder pose a diagnostic challenge. Certain aspects of the history are important for an accurate diagnosis. Was the delivery normal? When was the problem noticed? Does the child move any part of the extremity? Was there a history of maternal gestational diabetes or fetal macrosomia? Does the child nurse from each breast? A broad, useful differential diagnosis includes clavicular fracture, proximal humeral physeal fracture, humeral shaft fracture, shoulder dislocation, brachial plexus palsy, septic shoulder, osteomyelitis, hemiplegia, and child abuse.

The physical examination should include observation of the child for spontaneous motion of the upper extremity, including any hand or elbow motion, and evaluation of any areas of swelling, ecchymosis, or increased warmth and movement of the ipsilateral lower extremity. Each area of the upper extremity should be carefully palpated and compared with the opposite side for any change in soft tissue contour or tenderness, starting with the clavicle and continuing with the upper part of the arms and shoulders. Look for any tenderness in the supraclavicular fossa. Finally, examine the spine for tenderness or swelling.

After a proximal humeral fracture, the arm generally lies internally rotated with obvious deformity. Patients with a posterior fracture-dislocation have very limited, painful external rotation of the shoulder. Luxatio erecta with a greater tuberosity fracture is manifested as an abducted shoulder with the elbow flexed and the hand above the head with marked shoulder creases.[49] Lesser tuberosity fractures have tenderness anteriorly, limited internal rotation in adduction, and limited abduction in external rotation,[167] and impingement symptoms may occur with internal rotation.[74]

Radiographic Findings

Birth Injuries

Radiographs of the shoulder, clavicle, humerus, and cervical spine may be needed. Often, the shoulder, clavicle, and humerus can be seen on a single anteroposterior view of both the upper extremities and the chest. Birth injuries may be missed in children with an unossified humeral head. The only radiographic sign may be an alteration in the scapular-humeral relationship (Fig. 26–4). Scaglietti[136] and Kleinman and Akins[76] described the vanishing epiphysis sign in Salter-Harris type I fractures in which the posteriorly displaced epiphysis appears to vanish on an anteroposterior radiograph when compared with the opposite side. Although arthrograms can identify proximal humeral physeal separations,[40,168] ultrasound is

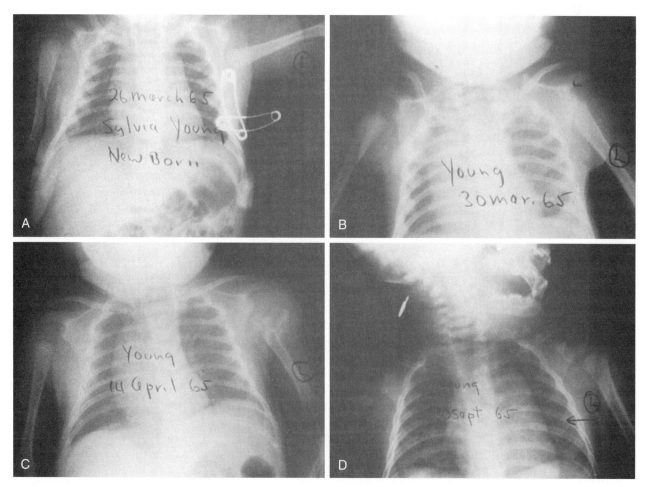

■ **Figure 26–4**

In a newborn, injury to the proximal part of the humerus is usually a completely displaced physeal injury, a so-called pseudodislocation. **A,** Radiographs at this age are sometimes misleading because of lack of ossification in the proximal epiphysis. **B,** Closed manipulation can be performed by applying longitudinal traction and gentle posterior pressure over the proximal end of the humerus. **C,** At 2½ weeks, abundant callus is present and the patient is clinically asymptomatic. **D,** A 6-month follow-up radiograph shows no asymmetry when compared with the opposite side.

noninvasive and diagnostic.[21,66,159] The ultrasound is obtained with a 7.5- or 10-MHz transducer, and the baby is positioned supine with the shoulder abducted. Birth fractures should have callus evident by day 10[96]; if not, child abuse should be suspected and high-detail shoulder radiographs obtained.[77] Posterior dislocations can be missed at birth and are best seen on a computed tomography (CT) scan.[156]

Older Children

Radiographs for any shoulder injury should include two perpendicular views to determine the glenohumeral relationship.[125,153] The true anteroposterior view, obtained with the beam parallel to the glenohumeral joint and shooting perpendicular to a line along the scapular spine, is very helpful. Although an axillary lateral is preferable, in an acutely injured shoulder, pain may necessitate a transthoracic or Y view. The apical oblique, a true anteroposterior view with a caudal tilt of 45 degrees, delineates the glenoid surface and the glenohumeral joint.[39] The apical oblique and the anteroposterior views together identify most injuries, and when these radiographs are combined with a transscapular lateral or axillary lateral view, almost all shoulder injuries can be demonstrated.[20] Lesser tuberosity fractures may require an axillary lateral radiograph.[67] Radionucleotide imaging is not very useful in the proximal end of the humerus because of physeal uptake. Occasionally in young children, an arthrogram or ultrasound may be necessary to establish the diagnosis of a proximal humeral Salter-Harris type I physeal fracture.[102,149] Magnetic resonance imaging (MRI) has been

reported to show fractures of the shoulder about the greater tuberosity and the glenoid rim and may be useful for occult fractures.[11,131,155] Posterior fracture-dislocations can be very difficult to determine without an axillary lateral or a transscapular view and are seen best on a CT scan.[66,156,164]

Occasionally, an upper humeral notch is visible on the medial aspect of the neck. This notch may be seen in pathologic conditions such as Gaucher's disease,[90] but it may also be a normal finding that probably represents the inferomedial capsular insertion.[114]

Treatment

The prognosis for birth and other injuries in infants is excellent (Fig. 26–5). Gentle manipulation usually reduces these fractures quite well without general anesthesia. Ultrasound can be used during the reduction maneuver to verify the reduction. Even if reduction is not achieved, the prognosis remains good. The arm is then immobilized to the chest with a soft dressing. The fracture usually heals by 2 to 3 weeks[38,59,72,87,144] and may be stable enough for the dressing to be removed after several days.[38]

Slipped Proximal Humeral Epiphysis Stress Fractures

A chronic *slipped proximal humeral epiphysis* is a rare disorder that can result from gymnastics,[36] radiotherapy,[42] and hyperpituitarism.[124] The proximal physis slips into varus and usually responds well to nonoperative treatment.

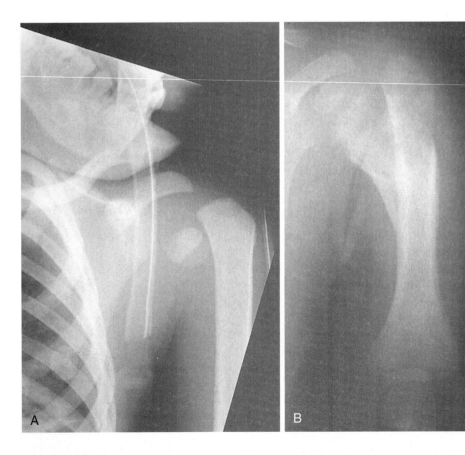

■ **Figure 26–5**
A and B, A proximal humeral physeal fracture from child abuse. Note the marked degree of early remodeling despite the severe displacement.

A

B

Stress injuries from repetitive pitching, termed "Little Leaguer's shoulder," are more common and usually heal well with temporary immobilization,[8,158] although growth arrest has been reported in untreated cases.[29]

Metaphyseal Fractures

Metaphyseal fractures are almost always amenable to closed treatment. Despite their displacement, they heal and remodel quite well (Figs. 26–6 and 26–7).

Nonoperative Treatment

Up to 5 years of age, proximal humeral physeal fractures are usually Salter-Harris type I, and accurate reduction of displaced fractures is not necessary. The arm is manipulated with traction, abduction, and flexion.[38] Older children with minimally displaced fractures can be managed with a sling and swathe.

REDUCTION. Potential barriers to reduction include the periosteum, the capsule,[48,85] the biceps tendon,[7,63] the

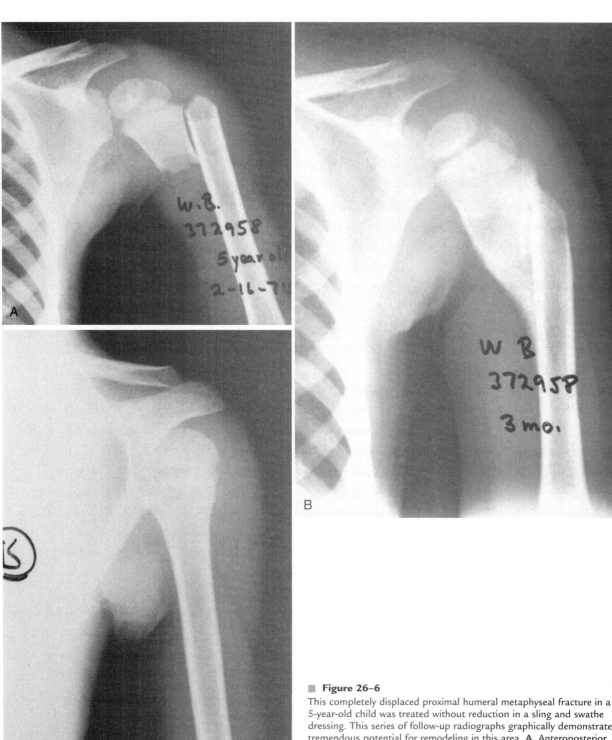

■ **Figure 26–6**

This completely displaced proximal humeral metaphyseal fracture in a 5-year-old child was treated without reduction in a sling and swathe dressing. This series of follow-up radiographs graphically demonstrates the tremendous potential for remodeling in this area. **A,** Anteroposterior radiograph of the injury. **B,** Three months after the injury, solid union has occurred without any clinical limitation. **C,** A 2-year follow-up film shows complete remodeling without shortening or angulation.

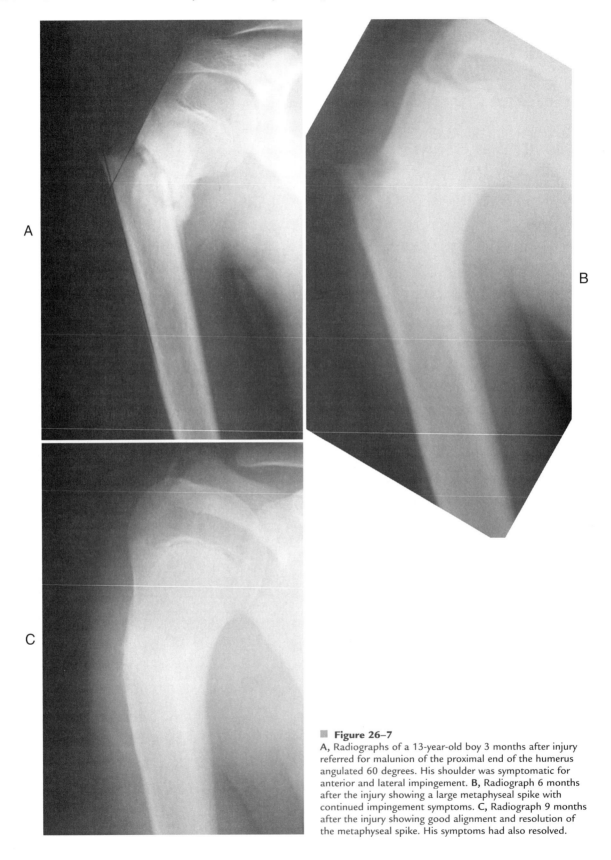

■ **Figure 26–7**

A, Radiographs of a 13-year-old boy 3 months after injury referred for malunion of the proximal end of the humerus angulated 60 degrees. His shoulder was symptomatic for anterior and lateral impingement. **B,** Radiograph 6 months after the injury showing a large metaphyseal spike with continued impingement symptoms. **C,** Radiograph 9 months after the injury showing good alignment and resolution of the metaphyseal spike. His symptoms had also resolved.

deltoid, and occasionally, a portion of the subscapularis.[146] Neer and Horowitz[107] recommend reduction by 90 degrees of forward flexion to correct the forward displacement of the shaft, moderate abduction to correct the shaft adduction, and slight external rotation. Alternatively, the fracture may be reduced by longitudinal traction with the shoulder in 135 degrees of abduction, 30 degrees of forward flexion, neutral rotation, and pushing posteriorly on the shaft.[18,72,169] Only partial bony apposition is required. Williams believes that by evaluating the mechanism of injury as a combination of forced flexion, extension, medial rotation, or lateral rotation on radiographs and by reversing the injury, stable closed reduction can be achieved.[171]

The difficult question for the physician becomes how aggressively to treat displaced fractures of the physis or metaphysis in older children. The displaced fracture may appear ominous on radiographs, but because of the tremendous remodeling potential, the result is often excellent if untreated. Smith notes:

The periosteum is extremely tough; for this reason it often tightens and closes under the extruded shaft end on attempts to reduce the fracture and thus renders closed reduction difficult or impossible. If reduction is not achieved, new bone is then formed within the periosteum in the triangular space formed by the displaced epiphysis, the shaft, and the periosteum itself. Bowing of the head and upper shaft thus result in the first few months of healing. However, with time, growth, and physical activity, this bowing becomes partially corrected and the originally displaced shaft becomes absorbed.[146]

Humeral fractures that *potentially* require closed or open reduction are most frequent after 11 years of age[107] because the results are extremely favorable in patients younger than 11 years, regardless of the method of treatment. Neer and Horowitz[107] recommend treating grade I and II fractures with a sling and swathe without reduction, reducing grade III fractures only if the angulation is severe, and reducing grade IV fractures and applying a spica cast in the "salute" position. Dameron and Reibel[38] based treatment on the patient's age and treated displaced Salter-Harris type I fractures in patients older than 11 years by reduction followed by a spica cast or thoracobrachial bandage for 3 weeks, whereas displaced Salter-Harris type II fractures were reduced and held in a thoracobrachial bandage or, if compliance is an issue, held in abduction, slight external rotation, and flexion in a cast in the salute position for 4 to 6 weeks. Larsen and associates[85] evaluated 64 unoperated patients with proximal humeral physeal fractures and found that although remodeling decreased with age, the results remained excellent and they recommended nonoperative treatment. The patients with greatest angulation at follow-up had Neer and Horowitz grade IV fractures and were 11 years or older.

Methods of nonoperative immobilization include a sling and swathe,[23] hanging arm cast,[23,85] shoulder spica, "Statue of Liberty" cast,[59] and traction. Because these fractures can generally be reduced by traction rather than by abduction, the shoulder spica and Statue of Liberty position are rarely necessary to maintain the position.[68]

Operative Treatment

Beringer and associates[12] reviewed Neer grade III and IV fractures. Only in those treated operatively did complications develop, whereas the results of nonoperative treatment, including a sling and swathe, were excellent.

Segmental fractures may be treated by open reduction and internal fixation or intramedullary pinning.[98] Alternatively, proximal humeral fractures may be treated nonoperatively, with standard treatment of the other injuries.[70,98]

INTRAMEDULLARY RODDING. Intramedullary rodding is possible with smooth flexible 2-mm-diameter nails inserted through the lateral epicondyle and placed intramedullary into the head (Fig. 26–8).[104] The rods can be used to manipulate the fracture into further reduction. The Hackethal technique may also be used.[120] Rush rods have been used in older adolescents.[166]

PERCUTANEOUS PINNING. Percutaneous pinning was described by Bohler,[15,16] and some minor modifications have been made.[73,78,103,112,115] The patient is placed supine, and an image intensifier is used to visualize the humeral head and neck. After closed reduction, the pins are placed either superiorly (Fig. 26–9) or inferiorly (Fig. 26–10) to avoid the axillary nerve. A Kirschner wire is placed over the shoulder anteriorly to determine the correct orientation of the pins. The pins are placed through the distal or proximal deltoid and advanced about 30 degrees to the humeral shaft. When the pins are inserted from an inferior direction, retroversion of the head relative to the shaft must be recognized. If the pins have a tendency to leave the shaft before entering the head, they may be tapped with a mallet to keep them in the medullary canal. In children, one pin is often satisfactory, although two pins or more are preferable. Although the pins may be placed through the acromion,[71] pin breakage may be increased. The pins are bent outside the skin with gauze placed between the pins and the skin to prevent excessive skin motion with resulting pain, skin irritation, and possibly infection. Open reduction and pinning are rarely needed for severely displaced proximal humeral fractures,[50,122] such as fracture-dislocations and Salter-Harris type III and IV fractures that cannot be adequately reduced by closed means.

OPEN REDUCTION. Open reduction is performed through the deltopectoral interval. To prevent hypertrophic scarring,[101] the approach should be made within Langer's lines and as inferiorly as possible toward the axilla.[58] The cephalic vein is reflected laterally with the deltoid after identifying the deltopectoral interval. The fracture or fracture-dislocation can usually be identified at this point. The axillary nerve on the inferior aspect of the subscapularis and the anterior circumflex vessels should be identified and protected. If the fracture cannot be adequately visualized, the subscapularis tendon and anterior capsule are opened in layers. After reducing and holding the fracture with provisional Kirschner wires, the final pins or screws are inserted (Fig. 26–11). The capsule and subscapularis tendons are repaired and the skin

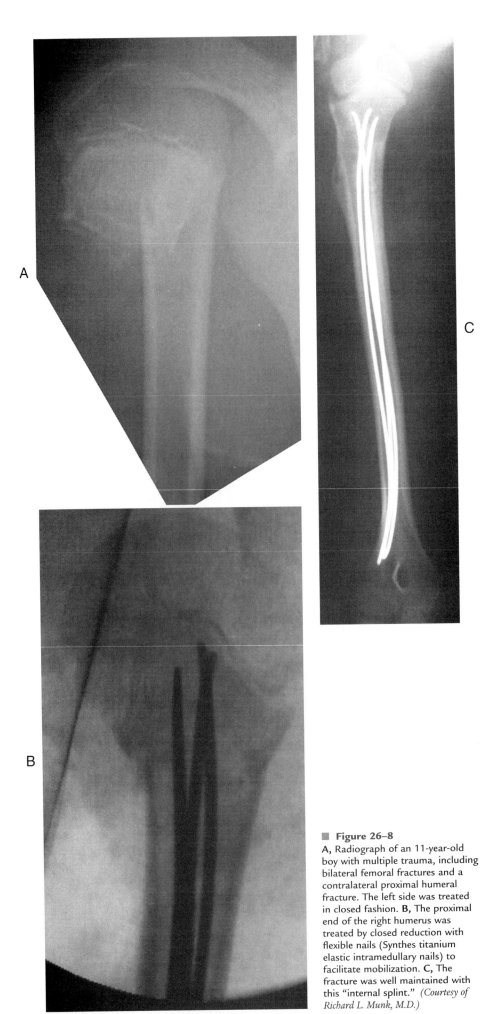

■ **Figure 26–8**
A, Radiograph of an 11-year-old boy with multiple trauma, including bilateral femoral fractures and a contralateral proximal humeral fracture. The left side was treated in closed fashion. **B,** The proximal end of the right humerus was treated by closed reduction with flexible nails (Synthes titanium elastic intramedullary nails) to facilitate mobilization. **C,** The fracture was well maintained with this "internal splint." *(Courtesy of Richard L. Munk, M.D.)*

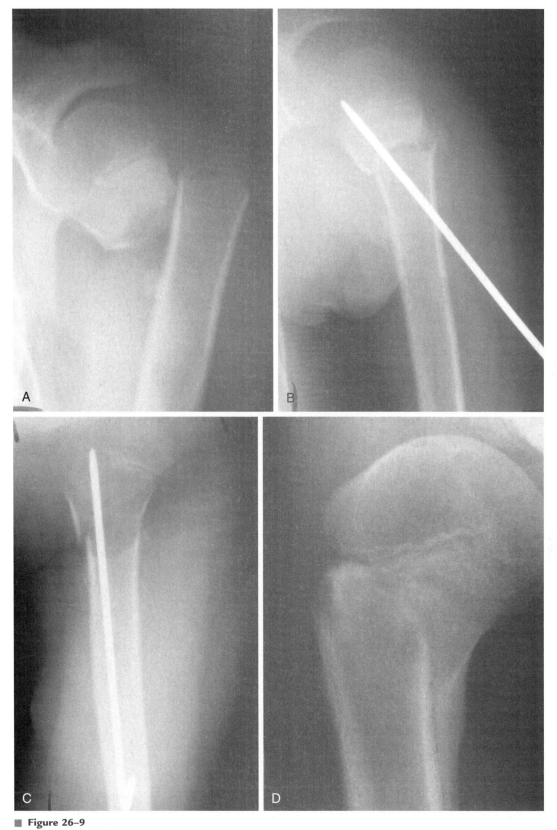

■ **Figure 26–9**

A-D, Technique of percutaneous pinning a proximal humeral metaphyseal fracture from a distal approach to avoid the axillary nerve. Although the ultimate outcome is good, its sole advantage in a younger patient is to speed up the remodeling process. *(From Rockwood CA, Wilkins KE, and Beaty J [eds]: Fractures in Children. Philadelphia: JB Lippincott, 1996.)*

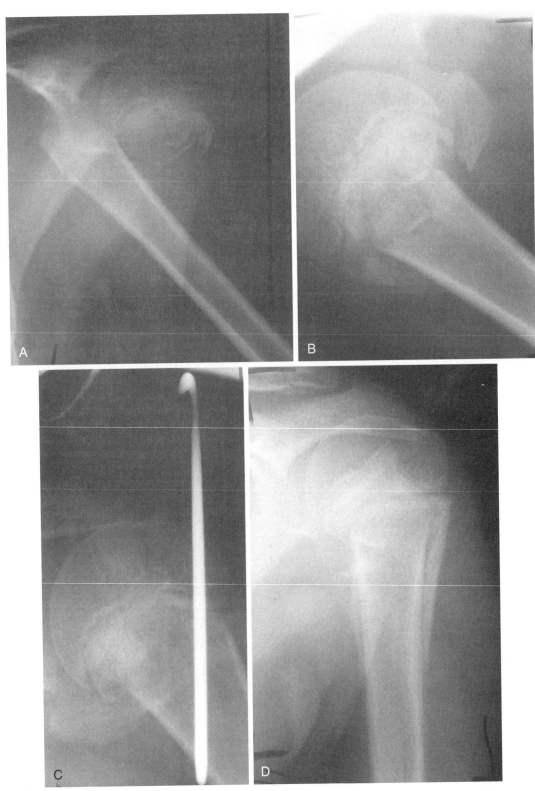

■ **Figure 26–10**

A-D, An unstable proximal humeral physeal fracture with an additional anterior lateral fragment treated by closed reduction (**B**) and pinned from a proximal direction (**C**). Valgus angulation is rare and probably results from a fall on the abducted arm. *(From Rockwood CA, Wilkins KE, and Beaty J [eds]: Fractures in Children. Philadelphia: JB Lippincott, 1996.)*

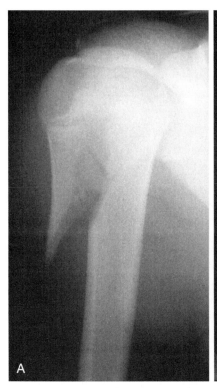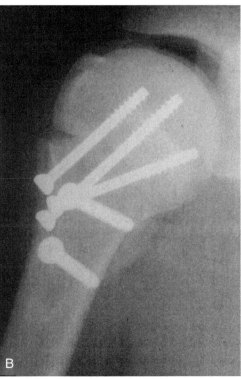

■ **Figure 26–11**

A and **B,** Proximal humeral fracture in a 14-year-old male multiple-trauma victim treated by open reduction and internal fixation to facilitate early mobilization. *(From Rockwood CA, Wilkins KE, and Beaty J [eds]: Fractures in Children. Philadelphia: JB Lippincott, 1996.)*

closed. The patient is placed in a soft thoracobrachial dressing or a commercial shoulder immobilizer.

EXTERNAL FIXATION. External fixation of proximal humeral fractures has been reported in adults but not in children, and it has very little utility except perhaps for extensively contaminated open fractures.[82]

FRACTURE-DISLOCATIONS. The most important issue in a Salter-Harris type I or II fracture-dislocation is the dislocation. The physeal fracture retains its ability to remodel.[110] Although Salter-Harris type III fractures may require open reduction,[56] they may also be treated successfully by closed reduction.[32] The mechanism of a Salter-Harris type III fracture appears to be anterior dislocation of the shoulder with the glenoid acting as a fulcrum, and the transepiphyseal fracture occurs as the shoulder retracts. The labrum may also be torn.[56] The dislocation must be reduced. The fracture is fixed with screws or pins if the reduction is unstable. Wang and coauthors reported a case in which devascularization of the head developed at 2 years but revascularization subsequently occurred.[165]

LESSER TUBEROSITY FRACTURES. In lesser tuberosity fractures, the subscapularis remains attached to the fracture fragment and is pulled medially. Old lesser tuberosity fractures may be treated nonoperatively.[128] If the fracture is seen acutely in an athlete, it may be repaired by open reduction and internal fixation. In athletes with symptomatic shoulder instability, the fragments should be excised and the anterior capsule and subscapularis reconstructed.[74,167]

GREATER TUBEROSITY FRACTURES. Aside from one case associated with an anterior dislocation treated by closed reduction (see Fig. 26–5),[35] all reported greater tuberosity fractures in children occurred with luxatio erecta and were treated nonoperatively. For older adolescents with greatly displaced greater tuberosity fractures,

the fracture should be treated like displaced greater tuberosity fractures in adults: open reduction, internal fixation, and repair of the rotator cuff.

Operative Indications

Because these fractures heal so well, surgery is rarely needed. The following quotation provides sage advice.[100]

The greatest concern in the treatment of the epiphyseal fracture of the proximal humerus is likely to be at the time of reduction when the surgeon reaches impasse in his ability to reduce the displacement of the fragments and maintain this position. Under parental pressure, expediency may supersede rationality in deciding on open reduction.

Because of the initial deformity, the surgeon often feels pressed to perform a reduction. However, because of the marked remodeling potential of the proximal part of the humerus, most fractures can be treated with a sling and swathe or a shoulder immobilizer, pain medications, and ice. Some authors state that open reduction–internal fixation is never indicated[2,12,38,146] and that nonoperative treatment is appropriate, even for markedly displaced fractures.[12,85] Other authors indicate that poorly reduced fractures in older children should be reduced and pinned or openly reduced and fixed.[70,141,151] Burgos-Flores and associates[22] recommended a more aggressive approach in patients older than 13 years because of persistent deformity and limitation of motion in older patients. Nevertheless, they noted that even these patients still function well without symptoms, despite some objective loss of motion. Older patients who are unlikely to have marked remodeling may be considered for either open reduction and internal fixation or closed reduction and pinning.

Unfortunately, no firm guidelines exist for determining which fractures will or will not remodel sufficiently. Clinically, remodeling ability is best determined by skeletal age and by looking at growth-remaining charts because those with little growth remaining are unlikely to remodel significantly.[17,118,119]

Multiple trauma is a potential indication for fixation to help mobilize the patient.[95]

Open fractures that require débridement may benefit from fixation to facilitate early rehabilitation of the soft tissue injury. Open treatment may be essential in rare cases when the periosteum is destroyed because much of the remodeling potential would be damaged.

■ AUTHORS' PREFERRED TREATMENT

NONOPERATIVE

We manage most proximal humeral physeal fractures nonoperatively, even if they are significantly displaced. We attempt closed reduction for very displaced fractures and then apply a thoracobrachial dressing or occasionally a hanging arm cast in older children. We prefer Bohler's "U" plaster with a soft wrap holding the arm to the patient's chest, although a sling and swathe or commercial shoulder immobilizer may be satisfactory (Fig. 26–12). Metaphyseal fractures are also usually treated by the closed method. Bayonet opposition with 1 to 2 cm of overlap is quite acceptable (Fig. 26–13).

OPERATIVE

The only advantage of reduction and pinning is more rapid remodeling of the proximal end of the humerus. This method does, however, provide a greater possibility

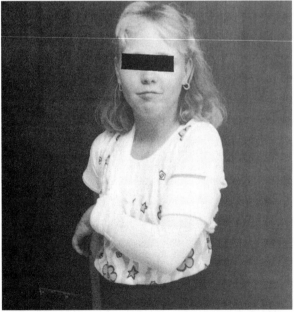

■ **Figure 26–12**
Clinical photograph of a 9-year-old girl wearing a homemade sling and swathe used in the treatment of proximal humeral fractures. A stockinette is padded at pressure points with cast padding and held in position with safety pins.

of complications.[12] The end result without complication will probably be equivalent to leaving the fracture unreduced.

Lesser tuberosity fractures that are diagnosed acutely in athletes should be repaired. The primary goal is to restore the subscapularis tendon and anterior capsule to prevent shoulder instability. Repair is accomplished by using either a lag screw for larger fragments or suture through drill holes for smaller fragments.

Greater tuberosity fractures associated with dislocations should be treated by closed reduction and simple immobilization. If the reduction is not satisfactory, the fracture should be openly reduced and the rotator cuff repaired.

Fracture-dislocations require reduction of the dislocation. If reduction cannot be obtained by closed means, open reduction must be performed. If closed reduction of the dislocation can be achieved in Salter-Harris type I or II fractures, the fracture portion can be treated nonoperatively. Attention is focused on the dislocation rather than the fracture. Salter-Harris type III fracture-dislocations should have an attempt at closed reduction. If successful, open reduction is not required. If the fracture or the dislocation cannot be reduced in closed fashion, open reduction is necessary.

Postfracture Care and Rehabilitation

Birth injuries do extremely well.[44] Although Scaglietti[136] reported several patients with late arm length inequality and limited external rotation, in retrospect, many of these patients probably had mild brachial plexus palsy rather than proximal humeral physeal fractures.

Proximal humeral metaphyseal fractures require a slightly longer period to heal than epiphyseal fractures do. Most epiphyseal fractures are stable by 2 to 3 weeks, but 3 to 4 weeks is needed for metaphyseal fractures. If the fracture pattern is stable, early pendulum exercises are started. However, if the fracture is unstable, exercise should be withheld 3 weeks before initiating motion. After the fracture is healing well, progressive passive forward flexion, external rotation, internal rotation, and extension are begun, followed by strengthening of the rotator cuff, trapezius, and deltoid. *In children,* epiphyseal and metaphyseal fractures display marked remodeling,[4,5,19,38,48,49,100,142] which may even occur in patients up to 17 years of age.[49] Patients with a marked angular deformity may have some limitation of motion, but this deformity is unlikely to be symptomatic.[108] Occasionally, patients report some aching with weather changes[22] or discomfort with heavy lifting.[108] Burgos-Flores[22] noted that only patients with a third anterolateral fragment in association with a Salter-Harris type II fracture experienced reduced mobility and the sensation of weakness. Significant limb length inequality is uncommon[9,35] and seldom sufficient to cause disability or poor cosmesis.

Complications

HUMERUS VARUS. *Humerus varus* is a very rare complication after neonatal or childhood trauma.[41,45,54,89,108]

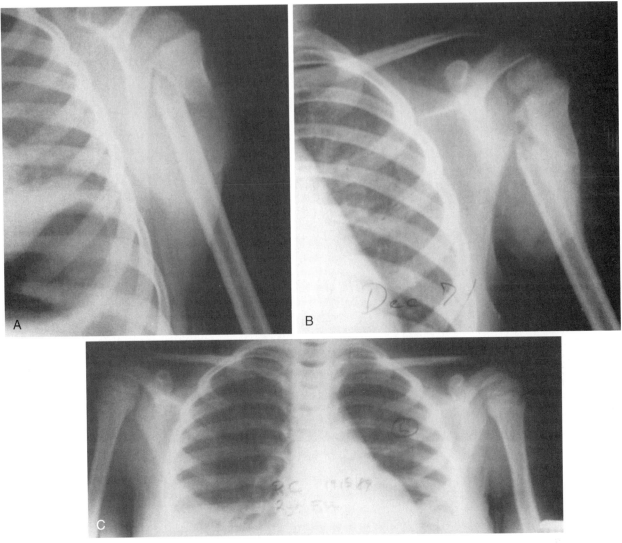

■ **Figure 26–13**
Metaphyseal fractures of the proximal part of the humerus are common in the 6- to 10-year-old age group, with healing and remodeling being the rule. **A,** This anteroposterior initial radiograph of the injury demonstrates a completely displaced metaphyseal facture of the proximal end of the humerus in an 8-year-old. **B,** Rapid healing has taken place with treatment in a sling and swathe in this 8-week follow-up radiograph. **C,** Complete remodeling is seen in this anteroposterior film taken at a 2-year follow-up.

According to Ellefsen and associates,[45] the injury usually occurs in the first year but may occur as late as 5 years of age. Two of their patients were victims of child abuse and suffered proximal humeral physeal fractures. The humeral neck-shaft angle may decrease to 90 degrees with marked shortening (Fig. 26–14). Trueta[156a] reported a similar clinical picture by experimentally damaging the proximal medial humeral physis. Functional impairment usually consists of mild to moderate limitation of glenohumeral abduction. Surgical realignment is unnecessary for most patients. Ellefsen and associates[45] recommend that if an osteotomy is performed, it be done to only 45 degrees rather than a complete 90 degrees. Solonen and Vastamaki[147] reported good results from osteotomy in five of seven cases operated on for limited active abduction and forward flexion.

LIMB LENGTH INEQUALITY. Limb length inequality is rarely significant from proximal humeral fractures. It is more common in patients treated surgically than in those treated nonoperatively.[9,38,132]

LOSS OF MOTION. Loss of motion is uncommon and reported primarily in patients treated surgically.[9,38,146] Loss of motion is more common in adolescents. We have seen one patient with a prominence causing limited forward flexion, but this problem appears to be improving (see Fig 26–7).

HYPERTROPHIC SCAR. Because hypertrophic scars from anterior reduction can be a problem with the anterior deltopectoral incision,[38,48] Fraser and associates stated that "open reduction should never be done in girls because any benefit will be more than offset by the result of the scar."[48] An axillary approach is more cosmetic than the anterior deltopectoral incision.[58,88]

INFERIOR SUBLUXATION. Inferior glenohumeral subluxation has been reported in two children with Salter-Harris type II fractures of the proximal end of the

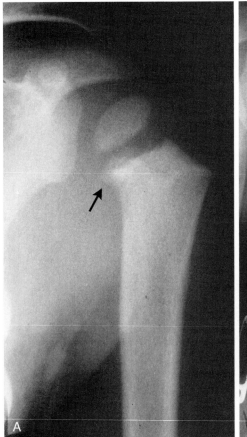
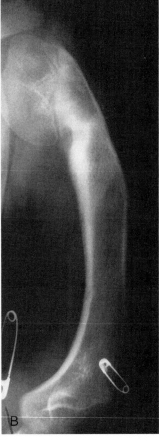

■ **Figure 26–14**
Proximal humeral varus resulting from an infection at
1½ years of age. **A,** Marked shortening. **B,** Varus.
*(From Rockwood CA, Wilkins KE, and Beaty J [eds]:
Fractures in Children. Philadelphia: JB Lippincott, 1996.)*

humerus.[174] This subluxation is probably secondary to a loss of deltoid and rotator cuff tone and is best treated by a sling to support the arm and early physical therapy. The outcome is generally good.

AVASCULAR NECROSIS. Osteonecrosis has been reported in only one child, and it occurred after a posterior fracture-dislocation that did not undergo reduction for 2 weeks.[161] During any shoulder surgery, the anterior humeral circumflex vessels and the lateral ascending branch should be avoided.

NERVE PALSY. Nerve injury may occur with fracture-dislocations[3,49,161] and has been reported in adolescents.[162] The axillary nerve usually recovers in 4 to 6 months. If an electromyogram does not demonstrate some recovery by this time, the nerve may be grafted. Recovery of the nerve is best after surgery performed within 1 year of the injury.[318] If the graft is successful, recovery usually occurs in 8 to 12 months.[3]

VASCULAR INJURY. Although vascular injury, including axillary artery disruption or thrombosis[92,140] and compartment syndrome after surgical neck fracture,[24] has been reported in adults, no reports have been made concerning children. A first-rib fracture potentially indicates rupture of the subclavian artery,[81] which is usually associated with signs of arterial insufficiency.

PIN MIGRATION. Pin migration is a life-threatening problem.[91,97] Pins should be bent outside the skin and removed after early healing. Any pins left underneath the skin must be monitored very closely with serial radiographs.

GROWTH ARREST. Growth arrest has been reported in a patient undergoing late open reduction of a displaced proximal humeral physeal fracture[38] and in patients with unicameral bone cysts.[72,105,109]

REFERENCES AND BIBLIOGRAPHY

1. Ahn JI and Park JS: Pathological fractures secondary to unicameral bone cysts. Int Orthop *18*:20-22, 1994.
2. Aitken AP: End results of fractures of the proximal humeral epiphysis. J Bone Joint Surg Am *18*:1036-1041, 1936.
3. Artico M, Salvati M, D'Andrea V, et al: Isolated lesion of the axillary nerve: Surgical treatment and outcome in 12 cases. Neurosurgery *29*:697-700, 1991.
4. Aufranc OE, Jones WN, and Bierbaum BE: Epiphyseal fracture of the proximal humerus. JAMA *207*:727-729, 1969.
5. Aufranc OE, Jones WN, and Butler JE: Epiphysial fracture of the proximal humerus. JAMA *213*:1476-1479, 1970.
6. Baker DM: Benign unicameral bone cyst. A study of forty-five cases with long-term follow up. Clin Orthop *71*:140-151, 1970.
7. Barlow IW and Newman RJ: Primary bone tumours of the shoulder: An audit of the Leeds Regional Bone Tumour Registry. J R Coll Surg Edinb *39*:51-54, 1994.
8. Barnett LS: Little League shoulder syndrome: Proximal humeral epiphyseolysis in adolescent baseball pitchers. A case report. J Bone Joint Surg Am *67*:495-496, 1985.
9. Baxter MP and Wiley JJ: Fractures of the proximal humeral epiphysis. Their influence on humeral growth. J Bone Joint Surg Br *68*:570-573, 1986.
10. Bengner U, Johnell O, and Redlund-Johnell I: Changes in the incidence of fracture of the upper end of the humerus during a 30-year period. A study of 2125 fractures. Clin Orthop *231*:179-182, 1988.
11. Berger PE, Ofstein RA, Jackson DW, et al: MRI demonstration of radiographically occult fractures: What have we been missing? Radiographics *9*:407-436, 1989.
12. Beringer DC, Weiner DS, Noble JS, and Bell RH: Severely displaced proximal humeral epiphyseal fractures: A follow-up study. J Pediatr Orthop *18*:31-37, 1998.
13. Biermann JS: Common benign lesions of bone in children and adolescents. J Pediatr Orthop *22*:268-273, 2002.

14. Blount WP: Osteoclasis of the upper extremity in children. Acta Orthop Scand 32:374-382, 1962.
15. Bohler L: The Treatment of Fractures. New York: Grune & Stratton, 1956.
16. Bohler L: The Treatment of Fractures—Supplement. New York: Grune & Stratton, 1966.
17. Bortel DT and Pritchett JW: Straight-line graphs for the predictions of growth of the upper extremities. J Bone Joint Surg Am 75:885-892, 1993.
18. Bourdillan JF: Fracture-separation of the proximal epiphysis of the humerus. J Bone Joint Surg Br 32:35-37, 1950.
19. Bovill EG Jr, Schneider FR, and Day L: Fracture of the proximal humerus with displacement in a child. JAMA 216:1188-1189, 1971.
20. Brems-Dalgaard E, Davidsen E, and Sloth C: Radiographic examination of the acute shoulder. Eur J Radiol 11:10-14, 1990.
21. Broker FHL and Burbach T: Ultrasonic diagnosis of separation of the proximal humeral epiphysis in the newborn. J Bone Joint Surg Am 72:187-191, 1990.
22. Burgos-Flores J, Gonzalez-Herranz P, Lopez-Mondejar JA, et al: Fractures of the proximal humeral epiphysis. Int Orthop 17:16-19, 1993.
23. Caldwell JA: Treatment of fractures in the Cincinnati General Hospital. Ann Surg 97:161, 1933.
24. Cameron SE: Acute compartment syndrome of the triceps. A case report. Acta Orthop Scand 64:107-108, 1993.
25. Campanacci M, De Sessa L, and Trentani C: Scaglietti's method for conservative treatment of simple bone cysts with local injections of methylprednisolone acetate. Ital J Orthop Traumatol 3:27-36, 1977.
26. Campos OP: Treatment of bone cysts by intracavity injection of methylprednisolone acetate: A message to orthopedic surgeons. Clin Orthop 165:43-48, 1982.
27. Camus M, Lefebvre G, Veron P, and Darbois Y: Obstetrical injuries of the newborn infant. Retrospective study apropos of 20,409 births [French]. J Gynecol Obstet Biol Reprod (Paris) 14:1033-1043, 1985.
28. Capanna R, Dal Monte A, Gitelis S, and Campanacci M: The natural history of unicameral bone cyst after steroid injection. Clin Orthop 166:204-211, 1982.
29. Carson WG Jr and Gasser SI: Little Leaguer's shoulder. A report of 23 cases. Am J Sports Med 26:575-580, 1998.
30. Chang CH, Stanton RP, and Glutting J: Unicameral bone cysts treated by injection of bone marrow or methylprednisolone. J Bone Joint Surg Br 84:407-412, 2002.
31. Coene LN and Narakas AO: Operative management of lesions of the axillary nerve, isolated or combined with other nerve lesions. Clin Neurol Neurosurg 94(suppl):6, 1992.
32. Cohn BT and Froimson AI: Salter 3 fracture dislocation of glenohumeral joint in a 10-year-old. Orthop Rev 15:403-404, 1986.
33. Connolly J and Secor M: Cortisone treatment of pathologic fracture through a bone cyst. Nebr Med J 67:286-287, 1982.
34. Croce F, Cuccurullo GD, Passaretti U, and Sadile F: Further experience in the therapy of juvenile osseous cyst using triamcinolone acetonide [Italian]. Arch Putti Chir Organi Mov 31:17-25, 1981.
35. Curtis RJJ, Dameron TB Jr, and Rockwood CA Jr: Fractures and dislocations of the shoulder in children. In Rockwood CA Jr, Wilkins KE, and King RE (eds): Fractures in Children, 3rd ed. Philadelphia: JB Lippincott, 1991, pp 829-919.
36. Dalldorf PG and Bryan WJ: Displaced Salter-Harris type I injury in a gymnast. A slipped capital humeral epiphysis? Orthop Rev 23:538-541, 1994.
37. Dameron TB Jr: Transverse fractures of distal humerus in children. Instr Course Lect 30:224-235, 1981.
38. Dameron TB Jr and Reibel DB: Fractures involving the proximal humeral epiphyseal plate. J Bone Joint Surg Am 51:289-297, 1969.
39. De Smet AA: Anterior oblique projection in radiography of the traumatized shoulder. AJR Am J Roentgenol 134:515-518, 1980.
40. DeSimone DP and Morwessel RM: Diagnostic arthrogram of a Salter I fracture of the proximal humerus in a newborn. Orthop Rev 17:782-785, 1988.
41. Di Filippo P, Mancini GB, and Gillio A: Humeral fractures with paralysis of the radial nerve [Italian]. Arch Putti Chir Organi Mov 38:405-409, 1990.
42. Edeiken BS, Libshitz HI, and Cohen MA: Slipped proximal humeral epiphysis: A complication of radiotherapy to the shoulder in children. Skeletal Radiol 9:123-125, 1982.
43. Edelson G: The development of humeral head retroversion. J Shoulder Elbow Surg 9:316-318, 2000.
44. Ekengren K, Bergdahl S, and Ekstrom G: Birth injuries to the epiphyseal cartilage. Acta Radiol 19:197-204, 1978.
45. Ellefsen BK, Frierson MA, Raney EM, and Ogden JA: Humerus varus: A complication of neonatal, infantile, and childhood injury and infection. J Pediatr Orthop 14:479-486, 1994.
46. Farber JM and Stanton RP: Treatment options in unicameral bone cysts. Orthopedics 13:25-32, 1990.
47. Fernbach SK, Blumenthal DH, Poznanski AK, et al: Radiographic changes in unicameral bone cysts following direct injection of steroids: A report on 14 cases. Radiology 140:689-695, 1981.
48. Fraser RL, Haliburton RA, and Barber JR: Displaced epiphyseal fractures of the proximal humerus. Can J Surg 10:427-430, 1967.
49. Freundlich BD: Luxatio erecta. J Trauma 23:434-436, 1983.
50. Frey C and Kloti J: Late results of sub-capital humerus fracture in children [German]. Z Kinderchir 44:280-282, 1989.
51. Friedlander HL: Separation of the proximal humeral epiphysis: A case report. Clin Orthop 35:163-170, 1964.
52. Gagnaire JC, Thoulon JM, Chappuis JP, et al: Injuries to the upper extremities in the newborn diagnosed at birth [French]. J Gynecol Obstet Biol Reprod (Paris) 4:245-254, 1975.
53. Galasko CS: The fate of simple bone cysts which fracture [letter]. Clin Orthop 101:302-304, 1974.
54. Gartland JJ and Cole FL: Modern concepts in the treatment of unicameral bone cysts of the proximal humerus. Orthop Clin North Am 6:487-498, 1975.
55. Gerber C, Schneeberger AC, and Vinh TS: The arterial vascularization of the humeral head. An anatomical study. J Bone Joint Surg Am 72:1486-1494, 1990.
56. Gregg-Smith SJ and White SH: Salter-Harris III fracture-dislocation of the proximal humeral epiphysis. Injury 23:199-200, 1992.
57. Gross SJ, Shime J, and Farine D: Shoulder dystocia: Predictors and outcome. Am J Obstet Gynecol 156:334-336, 1987.
58. Guibert L, Allouis M, Bourdelat D, et al: Fractures and slipped epiphyses of the proximal humerus in children. Place and methods of surgical treatment [French]. Chir Pediatr 24:197-200, 1983.
59. Haliburton RA, Barber JR, and Fraser RL: Pseudodislocation: An unusual birth injury. Can J Surg 10:455-462, 1967.
60. Hardcastle PH and Fisher TR: Intrathoracic displacement of the humeral head with fracture of the surgical neck. Injury 12:313-315, 1981.
61. Harris BA: Shoulder dystocia. Clin Obstet Gynecol 27:106-111, 1984.
62. Heim D, Herkert F, Hess P, and Regazzoni P: Surgical treatment of humeral shaft fractures—the Basel experience. J Trauma 35:226-232, 1993.
63. Herring JA and Peterson HA: Simple bone cyst with growth arrest. J Pediatr Orthop 7:231-235, 1987.
64. Hohl JC: Fractures of the humerus in children. Orthop Clin North Am 7:557-571, 1976.
65. Horak J and Nilsson BE: Epidemiology of fracture of the upper end of the humerus. Clin Orthop 112:250-253, 1975.
66. Howard CB, Shinwell E, Nyska M, and Meller I: Ultrasound diagnosis of neonatal fracture separation of the upper humeral epiphysis. J Bone Joint Surg Br 74:471-472, 1992.
67. Howard FM and Shafer SJ: Injuries to the clavicle with neurovascular complications. A study of fourteen cases. J Bone Joint Surg Am 47:1335-1346, 1965.
68. Howard NJ and Eloesser L: Treatment of fracture of the upper end of the humerus: An experimental and clinical study. J Bone Joint Surg Am 16:1-29, 1934.
69. Iqbal QM: Long bone fractures among children in Malaysia. Int Surg 59:410-415, 1974.
70. James P and Heinrich SD: Ipsilateral proximal metaphyseal and flexion supracondylar humerus fractures with an associated olecranon avulsion fracture. Orthopedics 14:713-716, 1991.
71. Jaschke W, Hopf G, Gerstner C, and Hiemer W: Proximal humerus fracture with dislocation in childhood, transacromial percutaneous osteosynthesis using Kirschner wires [German]. Zentralbl Chir 106:618-621, 1981.
72. Jeffrey CC: Fracture separation of the upper humeral epiphysis. Surg Gynecol Obstet 96:205-209, 1953.
73. Kapandji A: Osteosynthesis using the "palm-tree" nail technic in fractures of the surgical neck of the humerus [French]. Ann Chir Main 8:39-52, 1989.
74. Klasson SC, Vander Schilden JL, and Park JP: Late effect of isolated avulsion fractures of the lesser tubercle of the humerus in children. Report of two cases. J Bone Joint Surg Am 75:1691-1694, 1993.
75. Kleiger B: Unicameral bone cyst, 15 year follow-up. Bull Hosp Jt Dis 30:53-58, 1969.
76. Kleinman PK and Akins CM: The "vanishing" epiphysis: Sign of Salter type I fracture of the proximal humerus in infancy. Br J Radiol 55:865-867, 1982.
77. Kleinman PK and Marks SC Jr: A regional approach to the classic metaphyseal lesion in abused infants: The proximal humerus. AJR Am J Roentgenol 167:1399-1403, 1996.
78. Kocialkowski A and Wallace WA: Closed percutaneous K-wire stabilization for displaced fractures of the surgical neck of the humerus. Injury 21:209-212, 1990.
79. Kohler R and Trillaud JM: Fracture and fracture separation of the proximal humerus in children: Report of 136 cases. J Pediatr Orthop 3:326-332, 1983.
80. Kothari K, Bernstein RM, Griffiths HJ, et al: Luxatio erecta. Skeletal Radiol 11:47-49, 1984.
81. Kretz JG, Eisenmann B, El Badawy H, et al: Subclavian artery rupture during closed thoracobrachial injuries. Report on eleven cases [authors' transl] [French]. J Mal Vasc 6:107-109, 1981.
82. Kristiansen B and Kofoed H: External fixation of displaced fractures of the proximal humerus. Technique and preliminary results. J Bone Joint Surg Br 69:643-646, 1987.
83. Kuhns LR, Sherman MP, Poznanski AK, and Holt JF: Humeral head and coracoid ossification in the newborn. Radiology 107:145-149, 1973.
84. Landin LA: Fracture patterns in children: Analysis of 8682 fractures with special reference to incidence, etiology and secular changes in Swedish urban populations. Acta Orthop Scand Suppl 54:1-109, 1983.

85. Larsen CF, Kiaer T, and Lindequist S: Fractures of the proximal humerus in children. Nine-year followup of 64 unoperated on cases. Acta Orthop Scand 61:255-257, 1990.

86. Lemperg R and Liliequist B: Dislocation of the proximal epiphysis of the humerus in newborns. Acta Pediatr Scand 59:377-380, 1970.

87. Lentz W and Meuser P: The treatment of fractures of the proximal humerus. Arch Orthop Trauma Surg 96:283-285, 1980.

88. Leslie JT and Ryan TJ: The anterior axillary incision to approach the shoulder joint. J Bone Joint Surg Am 44:1193-1196, 1962.

89. Levitskii FA and Al'-Masri A: Characteristics of multiple fractures of the long bones of the upper limbs and their treatment [Russian]. Ortop Travmatol Protez April:42-45, 1989.

90. Li JK, Birch PD, and Davies AM: Proximal humeral defects in Gaucher's disease. Br J Radiol 61:579-583, 1988.

91. Liebling G and Bartel HG: Unusual migration of a Kirschner wire following drill wire fixation of a subcapital humerus fracture [German]. Beitr Orthop Traumatol 34:585-587, 1987.

92. Linson MA: Axillary artery thrombosis after fracture of the humerus. A case report. J Bone Joint Surg Am 62:1214-1215, 1980.

93. Lipscomb AB: Baseball pitching injuries in growing athletes. J Sports Med 3:25-34, 1975.

94. Lock TR and Aronson DD: Fractures in patients who have myelomeningocele. J Bone Joint Surg Am 71:1153-1157, 1989.

95. Loder RT: Pediatric polytrauma: Orthopaedic care and hospital course. J Orthop Trauma 1:48-54, 1987.

96. Lubrano di Diego JG, Chappuis JP, Montsegur P, et al: About 82 obstetrical astro-articular injuries of the new-born (excepting brachial plexus palsies). Limits of initial therapeutic aggression and follow-up of evolution, particularly concerning traumatic separation of upper femoral epiphysis [authors' transl] [French]. Chir Pediatr 19:219-226, 1978.

97. Lyons FA and Rockwood CA: Current concepts review. Migration of pins used in operations on the shoulder. J Bone Joint Surg Am 72:1262-1267, 1990.

98. Macfarlane I and Mushayt K: Double closed fractures of the humerus in a child. A case report. J Bone Joint Surg Am 72:443, 1990.

99. Madsen TE: Fractures of the extremities in the newborn. Acta Obstet Gynecol Scand 34:41, 1955.

100. McBride ED and Sisler J: Fractures of the proximal humeral epiphysis and the juxta-epiphysial humeral shaft. Clin Orthop 38:143-153, 1965.

101. McBride MT, Hennrikus WL, and Mologne TS: Newborn clavicle fractures. Orthopedics 21:317-319, 1998.

102. Merten DF, Kirks DR, and Ruderman RJ: Occult humeral epiphyseal fracture in battered infants. Pediatr Radiol 10:151-154, 1981.

103. Mestdagh H, Butruille Y, Tillie B, and Bocquet F: Results of the treatment of proximal humeral fractures by percutaneous nailing. Apropos of 142 cases [French]. Ann Chir 38:5-13, 1984.

104. Metaizeau JP and Ligier JN: Surgical treatment of fractures of the long bones in children. Interference between osteosynthesis and the physiological processes of consolidation. Therapeutic indications [French]. J Chir (Paris) 121:527-537, 1984.

105. Moed BR and LaMont RL: Unicameral bone cyst complicated by growth retardation. J Bone Joint Surg Am 64:1379-1381, 1982.

106. Nazario AC, Tanaka CI, and Novo NF: Proximal humeral ossification center of the fetus: Time of appearance and the sensitivity and specificity of this finding. J Ultrasound Med 12:513-515, 1993.

107. Neer CS and Horowitz BS: Fractures of the proximal humeral epiphysial plate. Clin Orthop 41:24-31, 1965.

108. Nilsson S and Svartholm F: Fracture of the upper end of the humerus in children. A follow-up of 44 cases. Acta Chir Scand 130:433-439, 1965.

109. Norman A and Schiffman M: Simple bone cysts: Factors of age dependency. Radiology 124:779-782, 1977.

110. Obremskey W and Routt ML Jr: Fracture-dislocation of the shoulder in a child: Case report. J Trauma 36:137-140, 1994.

111. Ogden JA, Conlogue GJ, and Jensen P: Radiology of postnatal skeletal development: The proximal humerus. Skeletal Radiol 2:153-160, 1978.

112. Olmeda A, Bonaga S, and Turra S: The treatment of fractures of the surgical neck of the humerus by osteosynthesis with Kirschner wires. Ital J Orthop Traumatol 15:353-360, 1989.

113. Olszewski W and Popinski M: Fractures of the neck and shaft of the humerus as a rare form of double fractures in children [Polish]. Chir Narzadow Ruchu Ortop Pol 39:121-123, 1974.

114. Ozonoff MB and Ziter FM Jr: The upper humeral notch. A normal variant in children. Radiology 113:699-701, 1974.

115. Peter RE, Hoffmeyer P, and Henley MB: Treatment of humeral diaphyseal fractures with Hackethal stacked nailing: A report of 33 cases. J Orthop Trauma 6:14-17, 1992.

116. Peterson CA and Peterson HA: Analysis of the incidence of injuries to the epiphyseal growth plate. J Trauma 12:275-281, 1972.

117. Peterson HA, Madhok R, Benson JT, et al: Physeal fractures: Part 1. Epidemiology in Olmsted County, Minnesota, 1979-1988. J Pediatr Orthop 14:423-430, 1994.

118. Pritchett JW: Growth and predictions of growth in the upper extremity. J Bone Joint Surg Am 70:520-525, 1988.

119. Pritchett JW: Growth plate activity in the upper extremity. Clin Orthop 268:235-242, 1991.

120. Putz P, Arias C, Bremen J, et al: Treatment of epiphyseal fractures of the proximal humerus using Hackethal's bundled wires. Apropos of 136 cases [French]. Acta Orthop Belg 53:80-87, 1987.

121. Rang M: Clavicle. In Children's Fractures, 2nd ed. Philadelphia: JB Lippincott, 1983, pp 139-142.

122. Reisig VJ and Grobler B: Proximal fractures of the humerus in children. Zentralbl Chir 105:25-31, 1980.

123. Robbins H: The treatment of unicameral or solitary bone cysts by the injection of corticosteroids. Bull Hosp Jt Dis Orthop Inst 42:1-16, 1982.

124. Robin GC and Kedar SS: Separation of the upper humeral epiphysis in pituitary gigantism. J Bone Joint Surg Am 44:189-192, 1962.

125. Rockwood CA Jr, Szalay EA, Curtis RJJ, et al: X-ray evaluation of shoulder problems. In Rockwood CA Jr and Matsen FA III (eds): The Shoulder, 1st ed. Philadelphia: WB Saunders, 1990, pp 178-207.

126. Rose SH, Melton LJ III, Morrey BF, et al: Epidemiologic features of humeral fractures. Clin Orthop 168:24-30, 1982.

127. Rosenthal RK, Folkman J, and Glowacki J: Demineralized bone implants for nonunion fractures, bone cysts, and fibrous lesions. Clin Orthop 364:61-69, 1999.

128. Ross GJ and Love MB: Isolated avulsion fracture of the lesser tuberosity of the humerus: Report of two cases. Radiology 172:833-834, 1989.

129. Rougraff BT and Kling TJ: Treatment of active unicameral bone cysts with percutaneous injection of demineralized bone matrix and autogenous bone marrow. J Bone Joint Surg Am 84:921-929, 2002.

130. Rud B, Pedersen NW, and Thomsen PB: Simple bone cysts in children treated with methylprednisolone acetate. Orthopedics 14:185-187, 1991.

131. Runkel M, Kreitner KF, Wenda K, et al: Nuclear magnetic tomography in shoulder dislocation [German]. Unfallchirurg 96:124-128, 1993.

132. Sakakida K: Clinical observations on the epiphysial separation of long bones. Clin Orthop 34:119-141, 1964.

133. Salter RB and Harris WR: Injuries involving epiphyseal plates. J Bone Joint Surg Am 45:587-622, 1963.

134. Samilson RL: Congenital and developmental anomalies of the shoulder girdle. Orthop Clin North Am 11:219-231, 1980.

135. Savastano AA: The treatment of bone cysts with intracyst injection of steroids. Injection of steroids will largely replace surgery in the treatment of benign bone cysts. R I Med J 62:93-95, 1979.

136. Scaglietti O: The obstetrical shoulder trauma. Surg Gynecol Obstet 66:868, 1938.

137. Scaglietti O, Marchetti PG, and Bartolozzi P: Rizulati a distanza dell'azione topica dell'acetato de methylprednisolone in microcristalli in alcune lesioni dello scheletro. Arch Putti 30:1, 1979.

138. Scaglietti O, Marchetti PG, and Bartolozzi P: The effects of methylprednisolone acetate in the treatment of bone cysts. Results of three years followup. J Bone Joint Surg Br 61:200-204, 1979.

139. Scaglietti O, Marchetti PG, and Bartolozzi P: Final results obtained in the treatment of bone cysts with methylprednisolone acetate (Depo Medrol) and a discussion of results achieved in other bone lesions. Clin Orthop 165:33-42, 1982.

140. Seitz J, Valdes F, and Kramer A: Acute ischemia of the upper extremity caused by axillary contused trauma. Report of 3 cases [Spanish]. Rev Med Chil 119:567-571, 1991.

141. Sessa S, Lascombes P, Prevot J, et al: Centromedullary nailing in fractures of the upper end of the humerus in children and adolescents [French]. Chir Pediatr 31:43-46, 1990.

142. Sherk HH and Probst C: Fractures of the proximal humeral epiphysis. Orthop Clin North Am 6:401-413, 1975.

143. Shindell R, Connolly JF, and Lippiello L: Prostaglandin levels in a unicameral bone cyst treated by corticosteroid injection. J Pediatr Orthop 7:210-212, 1987.

144. Shulman BH and Terhune CB: Epiphyseal injuries in breech delivery. Pediatrics 8:693-700, 1951.

145. Siegel IM: Brisement force with controlled collapse in treatment of solitary unicameral bone cyst. Arch Surg 92:109-114, 1966.

146. Smith FM: Fracture-separation of the proximal humeral epiphysis: A study of cases seen at the Presbyterian Hospital from 1929-1953. Am J Surg 91:627-635, 1956.

147. Solonen KA and Vastamaki M: Osteotomy of the neck of the humerus for traumatic varus deformity. Acta Orthop Scand 56:79-80, 1985.

148. Stahl EJ and Karpman R: Normal growth and growth predictions in the upper extremity. J Hand Surg [Am] 11:593-596, 1986.

149. Steiner GM and Sprigg A: The value of ultrasound in the assessment of bone. Br J Radiol 65:589-593, 1992.

150. Steinhauser J: "Dislocation osteotomy" in the treatment of large juvenile bone cysts [author's transl] [German]. Z Orthop Ihre Grenzgeb 119:331-335, 1981.

151. Stewart MJ and Hundley JM: Fractures of the humerus: A comparative study in methods of treatment. J Bone Joint Surg Am 37:681-692, 1955.

152. Struhl S, Edelson C, Pritzker H, et al: Solitary (unicameral) bone cyst. The fallen fragment sign revisited. Skeletal Radiol 18:261-265, 1989.

153. Szalay EA and Rockwood CA Jr: Injuries of the shoulder and arm. Emerg Med Clin North Am 2:279-294, 1984.

154. te Slaa RL and Nollen AJ: A Salter type 3 fracture of the proximal epiphysis of the humerus. Injury 18:429-431, 1987.

155. Tirman PF, Stauffer AE, Crues JV III, et al: Saline magnetic resonance arthrography in the evaluation of glenohumeral instability. Arthroscopy 9:550-559, 1993.
156. Troum S, Floyd WE III, and Waters PM: Posterior dislocation of the humeral head in infancy associated with obstetrical paralysis. A case report. J Bone Joint Surg Am 75:1370-1375, 1993.
156a. Trueta J: Studies of the Development and Decay of the Human Frame. Philadelphia, Saunders, 1968, pp 274-278.
157. Tullos HS, Erwin WD, Woods GW, et al: Unusual lesions of the pitching arm. Clin Orthop 88:169-182, 1972.
158. Tullos HS and Fain RH: Little League shoulder: Rotational stress fracture of proximal epiphysis. J Sports Med 2:152-153, 1974.
159. van den Broek JA and Vegter J: Echography in the diagnosis of epiphysiolysis of the proximal humerus in a newborn infant [Dutch]. Ned Tijdschr Geneeskd 132:1015-1017, 1988.
160. van Vugt AB, Severijnen RV, and Festen C: Neurovascular complications in supracondylar humeral fractures in children. Arch Orthop Trauma Surg 107:203-205, 1988.
161. Vastamaki M and Solonen KA: Posterior dislocation and fracture-dislocation of the shoulder. Acta Orthop Scand 51:479-484, 1980.
162. Visser CP, Coene LN, Brand R, and Tavy DL: Nerve lesions in proximal humeral fractures. J Shoulder Elbow Surg 10:421-427, 2001.
163. Visser JD and Rietberg M: Interposition of the tendon of the long head of biceps in fracture separation of the proximal humeral epiphysis. Neth J Surg 32:12-15, 1980.
164. Wadlington VR, Hendrix RW, and Rogers LF: Computed tomography of posterior fracture dislocations of the shoulder: Case reports. J Trauma 32:113-115, 1992.
165. Wang P Jr, Koval KJ, Lehman W, et al: Salter-Harris type III fracture-dislocation of the proximal humerus. J Pediatr Orthop B 6:219-222, 1997.
166. Weseley MS, Barenfeld PA, and Eisenstein AL: Rush pin intramedullary fixation for fractures of the proximal humerus. J Trauma 17:29-37, 1977.
167. White GM and Riley LHJ: Isolated avulsion of the subscapularis insertion in a child. A case report. J Bone Joint Surg Am 67:635-636, 1985.
168. White SJ, Blane CE, DiPietro MA, et al: Arthrography in evaluation of birth injuries of the shoulder. Can Assoc Radiol J 38:113-115, 1987.
169. Whitman RA: Treatment of epiphyseal displacement and fractures of the upper extremity of the humerus designed to assure deficit adjustment and fixation of the fragments. Ann Surg 47:706-708, 1908.
170. Wilkins RM: Unicameral bone cysts. J Am Acad Orthop Surg 8:217-224, 2000.
171. Williams DJ: The mechanisms producing fracture-separation of the proximal humeral epiphysis. J Bone Joint Surg Br 63:102-107, 1981.
172. Wong-Chung J and O'Brien T: Salter-Harris type III fracture of the proximal humeral physis. Injury 19:453-454, 1988.
173. Worlock P and Stower M: Fracture patterns in Nottingham children. J Pediatr Orthop 6:656-661, 1986.
174. Yosipovitch Z and Goldberg I: Inferior subluxation of the humeral head after injury to the shoulder. A brief note. J Bone Joint Surg Am 71:751-753, 1989.
175. Yu CL, D'Astous J, and Finnegan M: Simple bone cysts. The effects of methylprednisolone on synovial cells in culture. Clin Orthop 262:34-41, 1991.

FRACTURES OF THE CLAVICLE

The clavicle joins the thorax to the upper extremity through the sternoclavicular joint, the coracoclavicular ligaments, the acromioclavicular joint, and the muscular attachments of the deltoid, trapezius, and pectoralis major. It serves to anchor the scapula and provides a rigid base for muscular attachments that stabilize the shoulder for arm function. Without clavicular stability, the weight of the arm tends to protract the scapula and bring it forward, medial, and downward. The clavicle also provides bony protection for the subclavian and axillary vessels and the brachial plexus.[1] Although children with hypoplastic clavicles (i.e., complete congenital absence of the clavicles as a result of cleidocranial dysostosis) may function quite well,[1,5,84,85,92] such is not true of patients with trapezial or deltoid dysfunction from severe injury, in whom the results of clavicle excision are poor.[130]

Developmental Anatomy

EMBRYOLOGY AND DEVELOPMENT. The clavicle is one of the first two bones, along with the mandible, to ossify.

The clavicle initially forms as membranous bone, and growth cartilage secondarily develops at both ends.[44] By 7 to 8 weeks' gestation, the clavicle has already formed its adult characteristics with the typical S shape. Primary ossification starts from two separate centers, lateral and medial, either of which may have more advanced ossification.[44,118] The area in which these centers fuse corresponds to between a third and a quarter of the distance from the lateral end to the medial end at adulthood.[118] By 45 days in utero, these two ossification centers fuse to form one mass of clavicular shaft that predominates in growth to 5 years of age. Cartilaginous growth plates develop medially and laterally, and the medial physis provides approximately 80% of the longitudinal growth for the bone.[118,121] The medial epiphysis appears between ages 11 and 19 in girls and 14 and 19 in boys. It fuses to the shaft between 22 and 26 years of age in men and 22 and 25 years in women.[74,169] Medial clavicular epiphysiodesis is rare before 22 years of age (Fig. 26–15).[71] For this reason, many sternoclavicular dislocations are injuries through the medial physeal plate.[2,25] Laterally, the acromioclavicular ligaments attach densely into the periosteum of the lateral clavicular epiphysis and subsequently blend into the periosteum.[119] This fact is very important for understanding lateral clavicular injuries in children. Although a coracoclavicular joint is present in up to 10% of adults, it is not found in children.[82] Medially, the fossa for the rhomboid ligament's insertion on the inferior aspect of the clavicle is visible in only 0.59% of radiographs,[83] but it may be histologically present bilaterally in about half the population and unilaterally in approximately 20%.[83] The lateral or acromial epiphysis is not usually apparent on radiographs and has very little longitudinal growth. It rarely develops a secondary ossification center and fuses to the clavicle by 19 years of age.

The sternoclavicular joint is a diarthrodial joint made up of the large medial end of the clavicle, the sternum, and the first rib. It is incongruous with very little bony

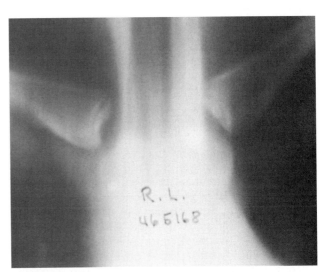

■ **Figure 26–15**

A tomogram of the medial aspect of the clavicle demonstrates open epiphyses. These epiphyses do not fuse to the clavicular shaft until 22 to 25 years of age. *(From Rockwood CA and Green DP [eds]: Fractures [3 vols], 2nd ed. Philadelphia: JB Lippincott, 1984.)*

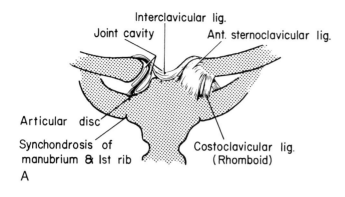

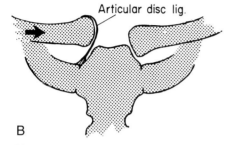

■ **Figure 26–16**

A, Schematic drawing of the anatomy of the sternoclavicular joint. Note the heavy ligamentous structure and articular disk. **B,** The articular disk ligament provides a checkrein for medial displacement of the clavicle. *(From Rockwood CA and Green DP [eds]: Fractures [3 vols], 2nd ed. Philadelphia: JB Lippincott, 1984.)*

stability in and of itself. A fibrocartilaginous disk or meniscus covers most of the articular surface. A strong series of ligaments bind the joint together. The intra-articular disk ligament is a dense fibrous structure that arises from the first rib and hemisects the joint, either completely or incompletely, and attaches anteriorly and posteriorly to the strong capsular ligaments. The anterior portion of the capsular ligament is heavier and stronger than the posterior portion. This anterior capsular ligament provides the primary support against upward and anterior displacement of the medial clavicle. The capsular ligaments attach predominantly to the epiphysis of the medial clavicle. The physis lies outside the joint capsule; therefore, in physeal injuries, the weak link is through the physis.[2,27,138] The joint is further protected by interclavicular and costoclavicular or rhomboid ligaments, which contribute to maintenance of the "poise of the shoulder" (Fig. 26–16).[109]

The sternoclavicular joint is positioned immediately anterior to many structures exiting the mediastinum, including the innominate artery and vein, the vagus and phrenic nerves, as well as the trachea and esophagus. Posteriorly displaced fractures of the medial part of the clavicle can impinge on these structures and cause an immediate and life-threatening emergency.[1,68,162] The sternoclavicular joint is movable and allows motion of 30 to 35 degrees of upward clavicular elevation, 35 degrees of motion in the anterior-to-posterior plane, and 45 to 50 degrees of rotation about the long axis of the clavicle. This joint provides the only true articulation between the upper extremity and the axial skeleton.[1]

Acromioclavicular Joint

The lateral third of the clavicle is surrounded by an extremely thick periosteal tube that remains intact circumferentially all the way to the acromioclavicular joint. The very strong coracoclavicular ligaments attach firmly to the inferior portion of this periosteal sleeve rather than to the bone itself. At the distal extent of the clavicle, a secondary ossification center is present, although it usually remains as an unossified epiphysis. When it does become ossified, the fusion process to the shaft occurs over a very short time sequence and is rarely seen on radiographs.[43,44] The acromioclavicular joint is a diarthrodial joint.[121] In adults, an intra-articular disk forms to cover the distal end of the clavicle. The joint is surrounded by a relatively weak capsule supported superiorly and inferiorly by acromioclavicular ligaments that in a child, blend with the thick periosteum of the distal part of the clavicle. The primary stabilizing ligaments are the strong conoid and trapezoid portions of the coracoclavicular ligaments, which arise from the coracoid and attach to the undersurface of the distal end of the clavicle and its periosteum. A fracture in this region is much more common than a dislocation. This thick periosteal tube usually remains intact inferiorly and distally along with the supporting ligamentous structures; therefore, even displaced fractures have tremendous potential for remodeling (Fig. 26–17).[9,27]

Clavicular Shaft

Incidence at Birth

Clavicle fractures are by far the most common skeletal injury during delivery, and reported rates range from 0.27% to 6.26%.* In children with a birth weight greater than 4000 g, the incidence increases to more than 13%.[96] The left-to-right ratio is slightly less than 2:1.[98] These fractures are occasionally bilateral.[8]

Incidence in Children

In older children, the clavicle is the fourth most commonly fractured bone,[87] and clavicular fractures represent between 8% and 15.5% of all children's fractures.[65,87,93,116] Nondisplaced fractures are most common in younger children, whereas displaced fractures are most common in adolescents. Almost 50% of all clavicular fractures occur in children who are 10 years or younger, and these fractures are more common in boys.[87,158] The incidence is 6.3 per 1000 per 6 months.[173] In all except one study, middle-third fractures were most common in children, and the incidence of lateral-third fractures increases with age.[65,116,156,158]

DISPLACEMENT. When the clavicle is fractured, the sternocleidomastoid pulls the medial portion proximally while the distal portion is pulled inferiorly by the pectoralis minor. The overall clavicle is shortened by the pectoralis and the subclavius.[27,120] Significant vascular injury is usually associated with direct blows.[175]

---

*See references 17, 22, 41, 49, 50, 60, 69, 76, 98, 123, 124, 140, 163, 167.

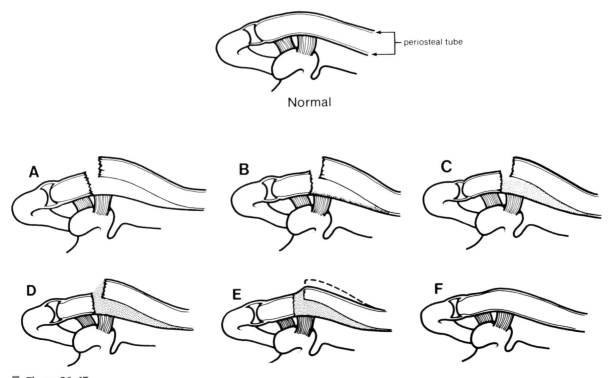

■ **Figure 26–17**
Phases of healing in fractures of the distal end of the clavicle in children. **A,** The clavicular shaft herniates through the periosteal tube with fracture. **B,** The coracoclavicular ligaments remain in continuity with the inferior portion of the periosteal tube. **C** and **D,** Periosteal callus is formed within the tube to stabilize the fracture. **E,** Remodeling occurs with resorption of the superior prominence of the shaft fragment. **F,** Final remodeling with good stability. *(From Rockwood CA and Green DP [eds]: Fractures [3 vols], 2nd ed. Philadelphia: JB Lippincott, 1984.)*

Mechanism of Injury

Birth

The upper part of the clavicle is the most frequently fractured bone during delivery,[41] probably because of the pressure of the symphysis pubis against the anterior aspect of the shoulder in the cephalic presentation, but this fracture is occasionally caused by the obstetrician pressing on the clavicle.[98] Fractures of the clavicle are strongly associated with shoulder dystocia and heavier birth weight.* However, most fractures of the clavicle occur in uneventful deliveries,[53,123,163,166,167] and a higher incidence of clavicular fractures is not necessarily an indication of poor obstetric care.[22,123,163] A cesarean section does not completely preclude fractures of the clavicle.[112] Five to 16 kg of force is required to produce a fracture of the clavicle in stillborn infants.[98] This force exceeds that in a routine delivery.[53,103] The incidence of concomitant brachial plexus palsy is very small,[91] although Oppenheim and associates[124] reported an incidence of 5%. Whether the clavicular fracture is protective of plexus injury or portends a worse outcome is uncertain.[68]

Older Children

In older children, falls are the most common cause of fractures of the clavicle.[87,116] Stanley and associates[157] analyzed

*See references 22, 41, 53, 67, 91, 98, 113, 123, 124, 163, 167.

the force required to fracture the clavicle and found that indirect mechanisms such as falling on an outstretched hand are highly unlikely to result in fracture of the clavicle. Most clavicle shaft fractures occur from a direct blow either to the clavicle or to the acromion.[141,157] Fractures of the clavicle frequently occur in sports.[87,116] Fractures from direct blows in sports may be preventable by adequate padding.[153] Stress fractures may also occur.[127] In addition, fractures of the clavicle may occur as a result of child abuse, but such fractures are not specific for abuse.[61,86]

Signs and Symptoms

Many fractures of the clavicle at birth are quite obvious. The most reliable clinical sign has been described as difficulty identifying the margins of the affected clavicle when compared with the normal clavicle.[78] The child generally has an asymmetric Moro reflex.[130] Uncommonly, it has been misdiagnosed as congenital muscular torticollis.[81] If the baby does not feed from one of the mother's breasts but will feed from the other breast, a fracture of the clavicle should be suspected.[168]

In older children, the diagnosis of a clavicle injury is usually quite evident (Fig. 26–18). Normally, ecchymosis and swelling are evident at the fracture site, which is usually quite tender. Plastic bowing, however, may not be accompanied by discrete tenderness (Fig. 26–19). The

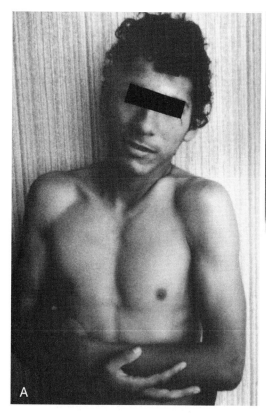

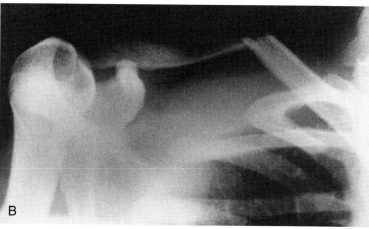

■ Figure 26–18

A, Clinical photograph of a young patient with a clavicle fracture. Note that the arm is supported by the good hand at the elbow and the head is tilted to the side of the fracture. **B,** The corresponding radiograph shows the clavicle fracture.

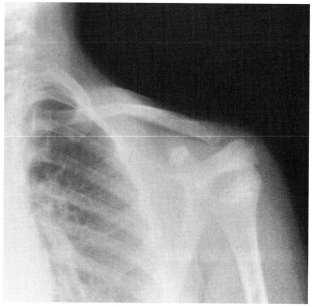

■ Figure 26–19

A greenstick fracture of the clavicle in an 8-year-old girl who had fallen on her outstretched arm. Note the soft tissue swelling superiorly at the fracture site. Such swelling is often a key to the diagnosis of a minimally displaced fracture.

most important part of the evaluation and treatment of an acute clavicular fracture is an examination to exclude injury to the underlying lungs, vascular structures, and brachial plexus.[27] Potential skin ischemia must also be evaluated.

Classification

The most common classification of fractures of the clavicle is that of Allman,[2] with type I representing the middle third, type II representing those distal to the coracoclavicular ligaments, and type III representing the medial third. The type I category is generally broadened to include all fractures lateral to the sternocleidomastoid and costoclavicular or rhomboid ligament and medial to the coracoclavicular ligaments. The clavicle may be plastically bowed rather than fully broken.[13] Fractures of the clavicle shaft in children may occur in association with anterior or posterior sternoclavicular injuries[59,61,90] or lateral clavicular injuries,[21] or they may be segmental.[90] They may rarely be associated with scapulothoracic dislocations or with scapular neck fractures.[91,123,150] The fractures are rarely bilateral and have also been reported to result from benign and malignant tumors.[139,144]

Radiographic Findings

Despite the S shape of the clavicle, a single anteroposterior view is usually sufficient to diagnose a fracture. However, to determine the displacement, a cephalically directed view is helpful. Two additional radiographic views have been described. The apical oblique projection is obtained with the injured side angled 45 degrees toward the tube and a 20-degree cephalic tilt of the beam. This view is primarily useful for detecting nondisplaced fractures of the middle third of the clavicle that are obscured by the clavicle's S shape.[166] An apical lordotic view has also been described to obtain a radiograph perpendicular to

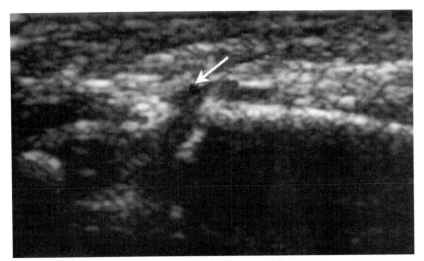

■ **Figure 26–20**
Ultrasound of a neonatal clavicular fracture demonstrating the fracture line. Such imaging is useful to determine the etiology of neonatal pseudoparalysis. *(From Rockwood CA, Wilkins KE, and Beaty J [eds]: Fractures in Children. Philadelphia: JB Lippincott, 1996.)*

the anteroposterior view; however, for this view, the shoulder must be placed in 135 degrees of abduction, which is not practical in acutely injured patients.[137] Nondisplaced fractures may show loss of soft tissue shadows when compared with the opposite side.[155] Ultrasound has proved useful in neonates (Fig. 26-20).[4,81] It has been used successfully in a 2-year-old as well,[55] although fractures at this age can usually be diagnosed by plain radiographs and clinical examination.

Differential Diagnosis

Birth fractures usually heal promptly. The absence of calcification in a neonate after 11 days of age should alert the physician to the possibility of child abuse.[25] Congenital pseudarthrosis is a rare and frequently asymptomatic disorder,[15,71,107,166] and the pseudarthritic ends often curve and are atrophic rather than hypertrophic (Fig. 26-21). It is generally right sided,[7,83,91,100,133] though occasionally bilateral.[16,60] Left-sided cases are quite rare and have not been well documented except with dextrocardia.[48] It is not associated with neurofibromatosis. The differential diagnosis includes a birth fracture and cleidocranial dysostosis.[39,133] Proposed etiologies of congenital pseudarthrosis include vascular pressure from the subclavian artery or failure of the two major ossification centers to unite.[7,23,79,100,133] However, the two ossification centers are always connected by areas of adjacent bone,[48] and the junction of the two ossification centers does not correspond with the site of the congenital pseudarthrosis.[118] Likewise, the clavicle is remote from the subclavian artery throughout its development.[118] These facts leave the etiology of congenital pseudarthrosis still unexplained.

CLAVICLE LESIONS. Clavicular abnormalities are numerous.[38,154] Many lesions can be confused with or cause fractures, including benign or malignant tumors[18,38,47,129,144,154,165] and erosions of the medial or lateral part of the clavicle that occur with hyperparathyroidism and renal osteodystrophy.[56,150,159] Clavicular stress reactions may be difficult to distinguish from neoplasia, and the use of ^{18}F-fluorodeoxyglucose has been described

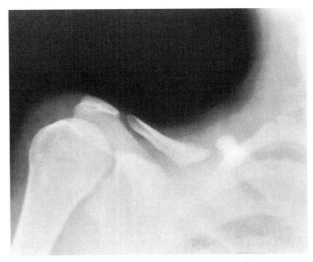

■ **Figure 26–21**
Congenital pseudarthrosis of the clavicle. This patient is asymptomatic but has an apparent clinical deformity.

for this purpose.[127] The rhomboid fossa appears as a radiolucent area,[73,161] and the coracoclavicular ligament may show some elevation of the bone surface simulating periostitis or callus formation.[161] These attachments may be confused with a tumor or fracture. The insertion of the sternocleidomastoid in infantile muscular torticollis can also create a medial lucency.[142] A lateral clavicular hook occurs with thrombocytopenia, radius aplasia syndrome, camptomelia, persistent brachial plexus palsy, and osteogenesis imperfecta[117,164]; it must be distinguished from plastic bowing, which may have a similar appearance.[13] Osteomyelitis,[46] including congenital syphilis[136] of the clavicle, is uncommon but can produce a periosteal reaction. The duration is usually longer than that of a fracture.[46,80,106,108] Idiopathic hyperostosis may be quite difficult to differentiate from a low-grade infection or from a fracture of the clavicle.[30,56,72,77,98,99] Some reported cases of idiopathic hyperostosis are very reminiscent of fractures occurring as a result of child abuse.[34] Clavicular periostitis is also attributed to prostaglandin infusion[172] and to subclavian catheter insertion.[40] A branch of the supraclavicular nerve frequently passes through the clavicle and is occasionally visible.[52,161] Gorham's disappearing bone disease[51] and Friedrich's juvenile chondrosis, which represents avascular necrosis of the medial part of the clavicle, may also occur.[35,97,149]

Treatment

Although more than 200 methods of treating clavicle fractures have been described, Nicoll[114] has stated:

> All that is really necessary is to support the elbow and brace the shoulders. The fractured clavicle cannot be immobilized (except perhaps by a shoulder spica incorporating the head). The usual compromise is that the patient attends daily to have his splint, strapping or bandage adjusted, thereby maintaining a reasonable degree of reduction for about a couple of hours a day, Sundays excepted.

Various splints, bandages, and dressings have been used to treat fractures of the clavicular shaft in children. Almost all clavicle shaft fractures in children can be treated nonoperatively.

PREVENTION. Obstetric care to prevent fractures of the clavicle can reduce the incidence by about half while maintaining the same fetal outcome.[146] Delivery of the posterior shoulder first and maneuvers are associated with a better outcome in shoulder dystocia.[58] It is generally difficult to prevent fractures of the clavicle in older children. Better pads for contact sports prevent some fractures of the clavicle by providing protection from direct blows.[153]

Birth Injuries

Birth injuries rarely require treatment. Parents are instructed to lift the child by the waist rather than by the arms and to gently care for the child for about 2 weeks.[130] Parents should be told that a bump will appear once the fracture is healed and will take several months to fully resolve. If the child is uncomfortable, pinning the shirt sleeve to the shirt with safety pins prevents motion sufficiently. The prognosis of *birth injuries* is excellent, and all children recover quite well.[22,49,95,112,163,167] Preferably, the physician rather than the parents makes the diagnosis.[122] A fracture of the clavicle is no reflection on the quality of the obstetric care, and a missed fracture of the clavicle causes no harm.

Plastic Bowing

Bowen[13] recommends treating plastically deformed fractures of the clavicle just like other clavicular fractures to prevent an overt fracture. Patients are evaluated and radiographs taken within 2 to 4 weeks.

Older Children

Nonoperative Indications

FIGURE-OF-EIGHT SPLINT. The figure-of-eight dressing is commonly used for fractures of the clavicle (Fig.

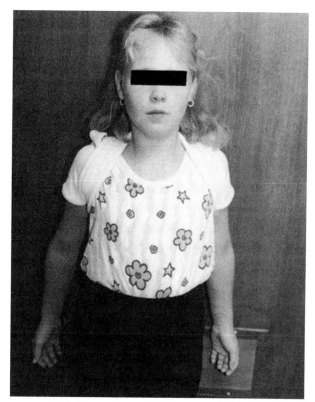

■ **Figure 26–22**
Figure-of-eight dressing applied to induce shoulder retraction. This position can be uncomfortable if it pushes directly on the fracture site or irritates the lower brachial plexus.

26–22). Usually, commercial soft splints are placed over the shoulders anteriorly and tied or buckled posteriorly to retract the shoulders. When used in children, the dressing can be made out of a stockinette with several sheets of cotton padding. The straps are tightened daily to remove any slackness. An additional anterior chest strap can prevent the tendency to slide laterally and exert a downward pull on the lateral aspect of the clavicle.[138] Older patients should powder their arms frequently to prevent chafing.

The figure-of-eight splint does not gradually reduce the fracture.[111,141] It can be quite uncomfortable, and if not used carefully, it can result in severe swelling, brachial plexus palsy, or compression of the neurovascular bundle.[36,88,111] The results are generally excellent. Ogden[120] indicates that no manipulation is needed in children younger than 6 years. In children older than 6 years, he recommends giving a local anesthetic, retracting the shoulders over a sandbag or a knee, and tying the figure-of-eight splint. This treatment is supplemented with plaster in older patients.[120] Figure-of-eight casts have been advocated for unstable fractures with vascular injury,[105] for noncompliant teenagers,[120,130] and for open fractures with less than optimal internal fixation.[67] Bohler[11] recommended the figure-of-eight splint for children younger than 10 years, not because of improved results, but to convince the parents that he was doing something.

SLING. Nondisplaced[130] and displaced fractures of the clavicle have good results when treated with a sling.[111,114] Comparative studies between slings and figure-of-eight bandages show the same ultimate outcome, but the sling provides more comfort.[3,70,157]

Operative Indications

SURGICAL. Fixation devices include suture, Kirschner wire fixation, modified Hagie pins, plate fixation, and external fixation. Intramedullary Kirschner wires result in a high incidence of pseudarthrosis with wires 2 mm in diameter or less and when they cause diastasis.[152] External fixation has the same indications as internal fixation but with the potential advantages of no periosteal stripping and no second operation for removal.[102,131,147,148,174] Plating, which is associated with complications such as superficial wound breakdown, refracture, malunion, nonunion, and difficulty obtaining fixation in a short bone segment, has been described with the 2.7-mm ASIF dynamic compression plate (DCP),[151] the 3.5-mm DCP,[128] and the low-contact DCP.[110]

Potential operative indications include irreducible fractures,[12,24,26,33,151,176] vascular injury,[128,176] severe skin damage in open fractures,[123] marked displacement with potential skin ulceration,[120] brachial plexus palsy from clavicle compression, impingement of the clavicle on the great vessels,[110,176] and established symptomatic pseudarthrosis.[35,153,273] Severe shortening of the clavicle in adults may be associated with subjective abduction weakness,[32,121] but it is unlikely to be a functional problem. Ogden described skin ulceration from an unreduced clavicular fracture requiring subsequent débridement.[120] An irreducible clavicle has been described in a 13-year-old girl who had a fracture of the clavicle and a dislocation of the sternoclavicular joint with the medial part of the clavicle caught between the trapezius and the platysma. The girl was treated with an osseous suture and a plaster body jacket.[67] Vascular injury is not an absolute indication for internal fixation, and good results have been reported with both bed rest and open reduction with periosteal repair.[105,162] A displaced scapular neck fracture in conjunction with a clavicular fracture may require internal fixation because of potential loss of shoulder support.[62,90] A recent study, however, casts doubt on this indication.[54] Symptomatic pathologic fractures may also require fixation.[125]

Union without permanent deformity is inevitable in children 10 years and younger. To our knowledge, only one nonunion has been reported in a child.[20] In a series of children up to 17 years of age with head injuries and unable to have any treatment for fractures of the clavicle, all patients had excellent results with remodeling of up to 90 degrees of angulation and up to 4 cm of overlap.[170] Two patients with lateral clavicular injuries formed a double clavicle. One had complete reabsorption of the extra clavicle, whereas the other required excision later. In older teenagers and adults, shortening may be associated with some pain and subjective weakness of abduction.[32] However, this effect may be secondary to the surrounding soft tissue damage rather than the injury to the clavicle itself.

■ AUTHORS' PREFERRED TREATMENT

Treatment of birth injuries is based on the symptoms. If the child is uncomfortable, we ask the parent to safety-pin the sleeve to the shirt for a few weeks to keep the arm from moving into uncomfortable positions. If the child is comfortable, we inform the parents that a bump will develop over the fracture site. It remodels over a period of several months and does not result in long-term disability.

A number of older children are initially seen with figure-of-eight splints applied in emergency departments and are quite uncomfortable. We usually remove the splint and replace it with a sling, sometimes to the parent's chagrin, but to the patient's delight. We inform the parents that a bump will form over the area of the fracture, that the bone takes several months to remodel, and that it is extremely uncommon to have any subsequent difficulties. We prohibit contact sports until adequate healing is apparent clinically or radiographically.

Very few indications exist for *operative treatment* of fractures of the clavicle in children. Such indications include severe displacement with potential skin ulceration and direct impingement of the clavicle on the subclavian vessels and brachial plexus. Even these patients can sometimes be treated by closed manipulation of the fracture and by the application of a figure-of-eight dressing or a plaster cast. This situation is one of the few times that we prefer a figure-of-eight dressing over a sling. However, the figure-of-eight splint must be applied carefully to keep the shoulders retracted without causing lower brachial plexus irritation. Because the periosteum in children is stout, the clavicle can, if necessary, simply be placed back into the periosteal sleeve, the clavicle sutured through drill holes, and the periosteal sleeve repaired. This repair does not require a second operation for removal of hardware, and there is no chance of pin migration.

Complications

MALUNION. *Malunion* of displaced fractures in children is inevitable.[11,135,158] However, as mentioned previously, children remodel quite well and generally have no long-term problems (Fig. 26–23). Other potential complications include early or late *brachial plexus palsy*,[5,28,29,95] which may be caused by a figure-of-eight harness.[89,111] If the plexus is explored, it has been suggested that the clavicular deformity be corrected, the first rib possibly be resected, and any vascular lesions be corrected at the same time.[29] The *supraclavicular nerve* may be stretched[45]; however, irritation from fracture entrapment has not been reported. Reflex sympathetic dystrophy has been described in a 15-year-old boy who was hit by a football helmet.[66] *Pneumothorax* may occur in severe trauma and has been reported with birth trauma.[94] A *pseudocyst* of the clavicle has been described after a fracture; however, it is unclear what the pseudocyst represents.[63]

VASCULAR INJURIES. Vascular injuries include subclavian artery disruption, subclavian artery or vein compression, and arteriovenous fistulas.[5,51,64,75,162] Subclavian artery compression in a child can be treated with a figure-of-eight bandage and bed rest, but open reduction of the

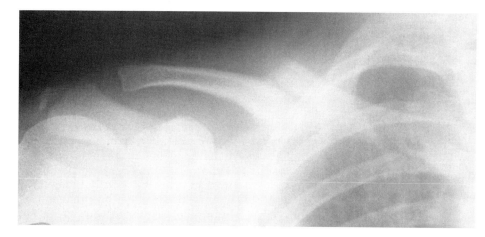

■ **Figure 26–23**
Even displaced malunited clavicular fractures in children cause few, if any problems. This 15-year-old was initially evaluated 6 weeks after a clavicular fracture, and marked shortening was noted. He has full, painless motion and a small palpable mass. The patient was allowed to return to contact sports and has had no further difficulties. *(From Rockwood CA, Wilkins KE, and Beaty J [eds]: Fractures in Children. Philadelphia: JB Lippincott, 1996.)*

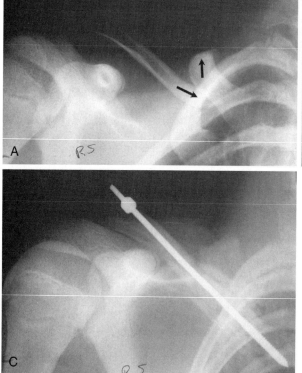

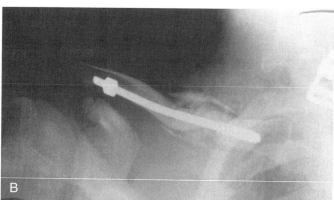

■ **Figure 26–24**
A-C, Radiographs showing the technique of repairing congenital pseudarthrosis of the clavicle with a modified Hagie pin. Refer to the text for details. *(From Rockwood CA, Wilkins KE, and Beaty J [eds]: Fractures in Children. Philadelphia: JB Lippincott, 1996.)*

clavicle may be required.[64,162] Subclavian vein compression has been reported in a 13-year-old boy with a greenstick, posteroinferiorly angulated, midshaft clavicular fracture who was treated by fracture reduction with towel clips and held with a shoulder spica.[105] It is important to check the patient's pulses. Always look for evidence of vascular insufficiency, and obtain an angiogram if necessary.[14] Pay attention to a first-rib fracture and mediastinal widening in severe trauma. Generally, vascular surgeons can perform the repair through a supraclavicular approach[143]; however, a portion of the clavicle can be resected for exposure.[104]

INTERNAL FIXATION. Internal fixation is associated with many problems, including pin migration,[37,42,96,142] nonunion,[38,151,152] refracture after plate removal,[151] infec-

tion, and cosmetically unacceptable scars from both internal and external fixation.[147,152]

PSEUDARTHROSIS. Pseudarthrosis may result from a pathologic fracture,[125] or it may be traumatic or congenital. Traumatic pseudarthrosis has been reported in children[11,101,115,132] and is often, but not necessarily[171] more symptomatic than congenital pseudarthrosis.[166] Techniques for treating traumatic pseudarthrosis were developed in adults and involve surgical intervention with compression of the site and bone grafting.[10,19,79,101,134,171] The compression can be applied with either a DCP or a threaded screw such as a modified Hagie pin. Complications of pseudarthrosis repair include pneumothorax, subclavian vein damage, air embolism, and brachial plexus palsy.[33]

Congenital pseudarthrosis may be completely asymptomatic.[15] Surgery is indicated for pain or cosmesis.[16] Congenital pseudarthrosis may heal without an iliac crest bone graft.[57,145] Because of the short fragments, it may be difficult to get good fixation with a DCP,[31] and the repair can be complicated by brachial plexus palsy.[160] An arcuate incision over the second rib avoids the supraclavicular nerves and hides any keloid.[126]

For traumatic nonunion or pseudarthrosis, we prefer the technique of Rockwood that was reported by Boehme and associates (Fig. 26–24).[10] In this technique, the entire extremity is draped from the base of the neck to the hand. These authors described making the incision directly over the clavicle in the lines of Langer; however, making the incision slightly inferior to the clavicle provides better cosmesis. The pseudarthrosis is exposed and débrided until bleeding bone is identified. The intramedullary canal is drilled with sequential curets and a hand drill. A modified Hagie pin* of proper diameter is selected. One end of the pin has fine threads with a nut on it, and the other end has coarse built-up threads and a trocar point. The end of the pin with the fine threads is drilled through the lateral fragment into the posterior cortex of the clavicle posterior and medial to the acromioclavicular joint. It is then drilled out to the skin through a small incision. The hand drill is then attached to the lateral end of the pin. With the pseudarthrosis held reduced, the trocar point is fed into the medullary canal and the coarse threaded end of the pin is drilled into the medial fragment. The nonthreaded portion of the pin is at the pseudarthrosis site. The nut is tightened on the pin until compression is achieved. A bone graft is placed. The pin or plate is removed once healing is complete.

REFERENCES AND BIBLIOGRAPHY

1. Abbott L and Lucas D: Function of the clavicle: Its surgical significance. Ann Surg 140:583-599, 1954.
2. Allman FL: Fractures and ligamentous injuries of the clavicle and its articulations. J Bone Joint Surg Am 49:774, 1967.
3. Andersen K, Jensen PO, and Lauritzen J: Treatment of clavicular fractures. Figure-of-eight bandage versus a simple sling. Acta Orthop Scand 58:71-74, 1987.
4. Bartoli E, Saporetti N, and Marchetti S: The role of echography in the diagnosis of neonatal clavicular fractures [Italian]. Radiol Med (Torino) 77:466-469, 1989.
5. Bateman JE: Neurovascular syndromes related to the clavicle. Clin Orthop 58:75-82, 1968.
6. Beall MH and Ross MG: Clavicle fracture in labor: Risk factors and associated morbidities. J Perinatol 21:513-515, 2001.
7. Behringer BR and Wilson FC: Congenital pseudarthrosis of the clavicle. Am J Dis Child 123:511-517, 1972.
8. Bianchi G and Bertoni GP: Bilateral fracture of the clavicle in the newborn [Italian]. Minerva Pediatr 19:2226-2229, 1967.
9. Blount WP: Osteoclasis of the upper extremity in children. Acta Orthop Scand 32:374-382, 1962.
10. Boehme D, Curtis RJ, DeHaan JT, et al: Nonunion of fractures of the midshaft of the clavicle. Treatment with a modified Hagie intramedullary pin and autogenous bone grafting. J Bone Joint Surg Am 73:1219-1226, 1991.
11. Bohler L: The Treatment of Fractures—Supplement. New York: Grune & Stratton, 1966.
12. Bonnet J: Fracture of the clavicle. Arch Chir Neerl 27:143-151, 1975.
13. Bowen A: Plastic bowing of the clavicle in children. A report of two cases. J Bone Joint Surg Am 65:403-405, 1983.
14. Bowers VD and Watkins GM: Blunt trauma to the thoracic outlet and angiography. Am Surg 49:655-659, 1983.
15. Brooks S: Bilateral congenital pseudarthrosis of the clavicles—case report and review of the literature. Br J Clin Pract 38:432-433, 1984.
16. Brunner C and Morger R: Congenital non-union of the clavicle [authors' transl] [German]. Padiatr Padol 16:137-141, 1981.
17. Camus M, Lefebvre G, Veron P, and Darbois Y: Obstetrical injuries of the newborn infant. Retrospective study apropos of 20,409 births [French]. J Gynecol Obstet Biol Reprod (Paris) 14:1033-1043, 1985.
18. Capanna R, Sudanese A, Ruggieri P, and Biagini R: Aneurysmal cyst of the clavicle [Italian]. Chir Organi Mov 70:157-161, 1985.
19. Capicotto PN, Heiple KG, and Wilbur JH: Midshaft clavicle nonunions treated with intramedullary Steinmann pin fixation and onlay bone graft. J Orthop Trauma 8:88-93, 1994.
20. Caterini R, Farsetti P, and Barletta V: Posttraumatic nonunion of the clavicle in a 7-year-old girl. Arch Orthop Trauma Surg 117:475-476, 1998.
21. Celenza M, Bertini G, De Tullio V, et al: A case of a fracture of the clavicle associated with an acromio-clavicular luxation [Italian]. Minerva Med 81:127-129, 1990.
22. Chez RA, Carlan S, Greenberg SL, and Spellacy WN: Fractured clavicle is an unavoidable event. Am J Obstet Gynecol 171:797-798, 1994.
23. Colavita N, La Vecchia G, Book E, and Vincenzoni M: Congenital pseudarthrosis of the clavicle: Roentgenographic appearance and discussion of the aetiological and pathogenetical theories [authors' transl] [Italian]. Radiol Med (Torino) 66:923-926, 1980.
24. Cooper SB: Fractures of the clavicle in infants and young children. ONA J 4:187-188, 1977.
25. Cumming WA: Neonatal skeletal fractures. Birth trauma or child abuse? J Can Assoc Radiol 30:30-33, 1979.
26. Curtis RJJ: Operative management of children's fractures of the shoulder region. Orthop Clin North Am 21:315-324, 1990.
27. Curtis RJJ, Dameron TB Jr, and Rockwood CA Jr: Fractures and dislocations of the shoulder in children. In Rockwood CA Jr, Wilkins KE, and King RE (eds): Fractures in Children, 3rd ed. Philadelphia: JB Lippincott, 1991, pp 829-919.
28. Della Santa DR and Narakas AO: Fractures of the clavicle and secondary lesions of the brachial plexus [French]. Z Unfallchir Versicherungsmed 85:58-65, 1992.
29. Della Santa D, Narakas A, and Bonnard C: Late lesions of the brachial plexus after fracture of the clavicle. Ann Chir Main Memb Super 10:531-540, 1991.
30. Eftekhari F, Jaffe N, Schwegel D, and Ayala A: Inflammatory metachronous hyperostosis of the clavicle and femur in children. Report of two cases, one with long-term follow-up. Skeletal Radiol 18:9-14, 1989.
31. Engert J, Klumpp H, and Simon G: Clavicular pseudarthroses in childhood [German]. Chirurg 50:631-635, 1979.
32. Eskola A, Vaininonpaa S, Myllynen P, et al: Outcome of clavicular fracture in 89 patients. Arch Orthop Trauma Surg 105:337-338, 1986.
33. Eskola A, Vaininonpaa S, Myllynen P, et al: Surgery for ununited clavicular fracture. Acta Orthop Scand 57:366-367, 1986.
34. Finsterbush A and Husseini N: Infantile cortical hyperostosis with unusual clinical manifestations. Clin Orthop 144:276-279, 1979.
35. Fischel RE and Bernstein D: Friedrich's disease. Br J Radiol 48:318-319, 1975.
36. Fowler AW: Treatment of fractured clavicle [letter]. Lancet 1:46-47, 1968.
37. Fowler AW: Migration of a wire from the sternoclavicular joint to the pericardial cavity [letter]. Injury 13:261-262, 1981.
38. Franklin JL, Parker JC, and King HA: Nontraumatic clavicle lesions in children. J Pediatr Orthop 7:575-578, 1987.
39. Freedman M, Gamble J, and Lewis C: Intrauterine fracture simulating a unilateral clavicular pseudarthrosis. J Can Assoc Radiol 33:37-38, 1982.
40. Friedman AP, Velcek FT, Haller JO, and Nagar H: Clavicular periostitis: An unusual complication of percutaneous subclavian venous catheterization. Radiology 148:692, 1983.
41. Friedrich I, Junge WD, and Fischer B: Causes of clavicular fracture in newborns [authors' transl] [German]. Zentralbl Gynakol 101:1528-1531, 1979.
42. Fueter-Tondury M: Migration of the wire after osteosynthesis [German]. Schweiz Med Wochenschr 106:1890-1896, 1976.
43. Gardner E: Prenatal development of the human shoulder joint. Surg Clin North Am 92:219-276, 1953.
44. Gardner E: The embryology of the clavicle. Clin Orthop 58:9-16, 1968.
45. Gelberman RH, Verdeck WN, and Brodhead WT: Supraclavicular nerve-entrapment syndrome. J Bone Joint Surg Am 57:119, 1975.
46. Gerscovich EO and Greenspan A: Osteomyelitis of the clavicle: Clinical, radiologic, and bacteriologic findings in ten patients. Skeletal Radiol 23:205-210, 1994.
47. Gerscovich EO, Greenspan A, and Szabo RM: Benign clavicular lesions that may mimic malignancy. Skeletal Radiol 20:173-180, 1991.
48. Gibson DA and Carroll N: Congenital pseudarthrosis of the clavicle. J Bone Joint Surg Br 52:629-643, 1970.
49. Gilbert WM and Tchabo JG: Fractured clavicle in newborns. Int Surg 73:123-125, 1988.
50. Gitsch G and Schatten C: Incidence and potential factors in the genesis of birth injury–induced clavicular fractures [German]. Zentralbl Gynakol 109:909-912, 1987.
51. Glass-Royal M and Stull MA: Musculoskeletal case of the day. Gorham syndrome of the right clavicle and scapula. AJR Am J Roentgenol 154:1335-1336, 1990.

*A full set of clavicle pins and drills is produced by De Puy Orthopedic Co., Warsaw, Indiana.

52. Goldenberg DB and Brogdon BG: Congenital anomalies of the pectoral girdle demonstrated by chest radiography. J Can Assoc Radiol 18:472-477, 1967.
53. Gonik B, Hollyer VL, and Allen R: Shoulder dystocia recognition: Differences in neonatal risks for injury. Am J Perinatol 8:31-34, 1991.
54. Goodnight JM, Rockwood CA Jr, and Wirth MA: Ipsilateral fractures of the clavicle and scapula [abstract]. Submitted for publication, 1996.
55. Graif M, Stahl-Kent V, Ben Ami T, et al: Sonographic detection of occult bone fractures. Pediatr Radiol 18:383-385, 1988.
56. Griffiths HJ and Ozer H: Changes in the medial half of the clavicle—new sign in renal osteodystrophy. J Can Assoc Radiol 24:334-336, 1973.
57. Grogan DP, Love SM, Guidera KJ, and Ogden JA: Operative treatment of congenital pseudarthrosis of the clavicle. J Pediatr Orthop 11:176-180, 1991.
58. Gross SJ, Shime J, and Farine D: Shoulder dystocia: Predictors and outcome. Am J Obstet Gynecol 156:334-336, 1987.
59. Hardy JR: Complex clavicular injury in childhood. J Bone Joint Surg Br 74:154, 1992.
60. Herman S: Congenital bilateral pseudarthrosis of the clavicles. Clin Orthop 91:162-163, 1973.
61. Herndon WA: Child abuse in a military population. J Pediatr Orthop 3:73-76, 1983.
62. Herscovici D Jr, Fiennes AG, Allgower M, and Ruedi TP: The floating shoulder: Ipsilateral clavicle and scapular neck fractures [see comments]. J Bone Joint Surg Br 74:362-364, 1992.
63. Houston HE: An unusual complication of clavicular fracture. J Ky Med Assoc 75:170-171, 1977.
64. Howard FM and Shafer SJ: Injuries to the clavicle with neurovascular complications. A study of fourteen cases. J Bone Joint Surg Am 47:1335-1346, 1965.
65. Iqbal QM: Long bone fractures among children in Malaysia. Int Surg 59:410-415, 1974.
66. Ivey M, Britt M, and Johnston RV Jr: Reflex sympathetic dystrophy after clavicle fracture: Case report. J Trauma 31:276-279, 1991.
67. Jablon M, Sutker A, and Post M: Irreducible fracture of the middle third of the clavicle. Report of a case. J Bone Joint Surg Am 61:296-298, 1979.
68. Jackson ST, Hoffer MM, and Parrish N: Brachial-plexus palsy in the newborn. J Bone Joint Surg Am 70:1217-1220, 1988.
69. Jelic A, Marin L, Pracny M, and Jelic N: Fractures of the clavicle in neonates [Serbo Croatian (Roman)]. Lijec Vjesn 114:32-35, 1992.
70. Jensen PO, Andersen K, and Lauritzen J: Treatment of mid-clavicular fractures. A prospective randomized trial comparing treatment with a figure-eight dressing and a simple arm sling [Danish]. Ugeskr Laeger 147:1986-1988, 1985.
71. Jinkins WJ Jr: Congenital pseudarthrosis of the clavicle. Clin Orthop 62:183-186, 1969.
72. Jirik FR, Stein HB, and Chalmers A: Clavicular hyperostosis with enthesopathy, hypergammaglobulinemia, and thoracic outlet syndrome. Ann Intern Med 97:48-50, 1982.
73. Jit I and Kaur H: Rhomboid fossa in the clavicles of North Indians. Am J Phys Anthropol 70:97-103, 1986.
74. Jit I and Kulkarni M: Times of appearance and fusion of epiphysis at the medial end of the clavicle. Indian J Med Res 64:773-782, 1976.
75. Jojart G and Nagy G: Ultrasonographic screening of neonatal adrenal apoplexy. Int Urol Nephrol 24:591-596, 1992.
76. Jojart G, Zubek L, and Toth G: Clavicle fracture in the newborn [Hungarian]. Orv Hetil 132:2655-2657, 1991.
77. Jones ET, Hensinger RN, and Holt JF: Idiopathic cortical hyperostosis. Clin Orthop 163:210-213, 1982.
78. Joseph PR and Rosenfeld W: Clavicular fractures in neonates [see comments]. Am J Dis Child 144:165-167, 1990.
79. Jupiter JB and Leffert RD: Non-union of the clavicle. Associated complications and surgical management. J Bone Joint Surg Am 69:753-760, 1987.
80. Jurik AG and Moller BN: Inflammatory hyperostosis and sclerosis of the clavicle. Skeletal Radiol 15:284-290, 1986.
81. Katz R, Landman J, Dulitzky F, and Bar-Ziv J: Fracture of the clavicle in the newborn. An ultrasound diagnosis. J Ultrasound Med 7:21-23, 1988.
82. Kaur H and Jit I: Brief communication: Coracoclavicular joint in Northwest Indians. Am J Phys Anthropol 85:457-460, 1991.
83. Kite JH: Congenital pseudarthrosis of the clavicle. South Med J 61:703-710, 1968.
84. Kochhar VL and Srivastava KK: Unusual lesions of the clavicle. Int Surg 61:51-53, 1976.
85. Kochhar VL and Srivastava KK: Anatomical and functional considerations in total claviclectomy. Clin Orthop 118:199-201, 1976.
86. Kogutt MS, Swischuk LE, and Fagan CJ: Patterns of injury and significance of uncommon fractures in the battered child syndrome. AJR Am J Roentgenol 121:143-149, 1974.
87. Landin LA: Fracture patterns in children: Analysis of 8682 fractures with special reference to incidence, etiology and secular changes in Swedish urban populations. Acta Orthop Scand Suppl 54:1-109, 1983.
88. Leffert RD: Brachial-plexus injuries. N Engl J Med 291:1059-1067, 1974.
89. Lemire L and Rosman M: Sternoclavicular epiphyseal separation with adjacent clavicular fracture. J Pediatr Orthop 4:118-120, 1984.
90. Leung KS and Lam TP: Open reduction and internal fixation of ipsilateral fractures of the scapular neck and clavicle. J Bone Joint Surg Am 75:1015-1018, 1993.

91. Levine MG, Holroyde J, Woods JR Jr, et al: Birth trauma: Incidence and predisposing factors. Obstet Gynecol 63:792-795, 1984.
92. Lewis MM, Ballet FL, Kroll PG, and Bloom N: En bloc clavicular resection: Operative procedure and postoperative testing of function. Case reports. Clin Orthop 193:214-220, 1985.
93. Lichtenberg RP: A study of 2,532 fractures in children. Am J Surg 87:330-338, 1954.
94. Longo R and Ruggiero L: Left pneumothorax with subcutaneous emphysema secondary to left clavicular fracture and homolateral obstetrical paralysis of the arm [Italian]. Minerva Pediatr 34:273-276, 1982.
95. Lubrano di Diego JG, Chappuis JP, Montsegur P, et al: About 82 obstetrical astro-articular injuries of the new-born (excepting brachial plexus palsies). Limits of initial therapeutic aggression and follow-up of evolution, particularly concerning traumatic separation of upper femoral epiphysis [authors' transl] [French]. Chir Pediatr 19:219-226, 1978.
96. Lyons FA and Rockwood CA: Current concepts review. Migration of pins used in operations on the shoulder. J Bone Joint Surg Am 72:1262-1267, 1990.
97. Macule F, Ferreres A, Palliso F, et al: Aseptic necrosis of the sternal end of the clavicle: Friedrich's disease. Acta Orthop Belg 56:613-615, 1990.
98. Madsen TE: Fractures of the extremities in the newborn. Acta Obstet Gynecol Scand 34:41, 1955.
99. Magnus L and Sauerbrei HU: Two cases of infantile cortical hyperostosis (monostotic form) [authors' transl] [German]. Rofo Fortschr Geb Rontgenstr Nuklearmed 128:530-533, 1978.
100. Manashil G and Laufer S: Congenital pseudarthrosis of the clavicle: Report of three cases. AJR Am J Roentgenol 132:678-679, 1979.
101. Manske DJ and Szabo RM: The operative treatment of mid-shaft clavicular non-unions. J Bone Joint Surg Am 67:1367-1371, 1985.
102. Maurin X: External fixation of fractures of the clavicle [French]. Chirurgie 101:367-375, 1975.
103. Meghdari A, Davoodi R, and Mesbah F: Engineering analysis of shoulder dystocia in the human birth process by the finite element method. Proc Inst Mech Eng [H] 206:243-250, 1992.
104. Meyer JP, Goldfaden D, Barrett J, et al: Subclavian and innominate artery trauma: A recent experience with nine patients. J Cardiovasc Surg (Torino) 29:283-289, 1988.
105. Mital MA and Aufranc OE: Venous occlusion following greenstick fracture of clavicle. JAMA 206:1301-1302, 1968.
106. Mollan RA, Craig BF, and Biggart JD: Chronic sclerosing osteomyelitis. An unusual case. J Bone Joint Surg Br 66:583-585, 1984.
107. Morin LR, Fossey FP, Besselievre A, et al: Congenital pseudarthrosis of the clavicle. Acta Obstet Gynecol Scand 72:120-121, 1993.
108. Mortensson W, Edeburn G, Fries M, and Nilsson R: Chronic recurrent multifocal osteomyelitis in children. A roentgenologic and scintigraphic investigation. Acta Radiol 29:565-570, 1988.
109. Mulimba JA: Fractures of the humerus. East Afr Med J 60:843-847, 1983.
110. Mullaji AB and Jupiter JB: Low-contact dynamic compression plating of the clavicle. Injury 25:41-45, 1994.
111. Mullick S: Treatment of mid-clavicular fractures [letter]. Lancet 1:499, 1967.
112. Nadas S, Gudinchet F, Capasso P, and Reinberg O: Predisposing factors in obstetrical fractures. Skeletal Radiol 22:195-198, 1993.
113. Nadas S and Reinberg O: Obstetric fractures. Eur J Pediatr Surg 2:165-168, 1992.
114. Nicoll EA: Annotation. Miners and mannequins. J Bone Joint Surg Br 36:171-172, 1954.
115. Nogi J, Heckman JD, Hakala M, and Sweet DE: Non-union of the clavicle in a child. A case report. Clin Orthop 110:19-21, 1975.
116. Nordqvist A and Petersson C: The incidence of fractures of the clavicle. Clin Orthop 300:127-132, 1994.
117. Oestreich AE: The lateral clavicle hook—an acquired as well as a congenital anomaly. Pediatr Radiol 11:147-150, 1981.
118. Ogata S and Uhthoff HK: The early development and ossification of the human clavicle—an embryologic study. Acta Orthop Scand 61:330-334, 1990.
119. Ogden JA: Distal clavicular physeal injury. Clin Orthop 188:68-73, 1984.
120. Ogden JA: Skeletal Injury in the Child, 2nd ed. Philadelphia: WB Saunders, 1990, pp 323-423.
121. Ogden JA, Conlogue GJ, and Bronson ML: Radiology of postnatal skeletal development. III. The clavicle. Skeletal Radiol 4:196-203, 1979.
122. O'Halloran MJ: Clavicular fractures in neonates: Frequency vs significance [letter; comment]. Am J Dis Child 145:251, 1991.
123. Ohel G, Haddad S, Fischer O, and Levit A: Clavicular fracture of the neonate: Can it be predicted before birth? Am J Perinatol 10:441-443, 1993.
124. Oppenheim WL, Davis A, Growdon WA, et al: Clavicle fractures in the newborn. Clin Orthop 250:176-180, 1990.
125. O'Rourke IC and Middleton RWD: The place and efficacy of operative management of fractured clavicle. Injury 6:236-240, 1975.
126. Owen R: Congenital pseudarthrosis of the clavicle. J Bone Joint Surg Br 52:644-652, 1970.
127. Paul R, Ahonen A, Virtama P, et al: F-18 fluorodeoxyglucose: Its potential in differentiating between stress fracture and neoplasia. Clin Nucl Med 14:906-908, 1989.
128. Poigenfurst J, Rappold G, and Fischer W: Plating of fresh clavicular fractures: Results of 122 operations. Injury 23:237-241, 1992.

129. Pointu J, Kehr P, Sejourne P, et al: Aneurysmal cyst of the clavicle: An uncommon lesion and a difficult diagnosis [authors' transl] [French]. Sem Hop 58:1141-1143, 1982.

130. Post M: Current concepts in the treatment of fractures of the clavicle. Clin Orthop 245:89-101, 1989.

131. Putnam MD and Walsh TM: External fixation for open fractures of the upper extremity. Hand Clin 9:613-623, 1993.

132. Pyper JB: Non-union of fractures of the clavicle. Injury 9:268-270, 1978.

133. Quinlan WR, Brady PG, and Regan BF: Congenital pseudarthrosis of the clavicle. Acta Orthop Scand 51:489-492, 1980.

134. Rabenseifner L: Etiology and therapy of clavicular-pseudarthrosis [author's transl] [German]. Aktuelle Traumatol 11:130-132, 1981.

135. Rang M: Clavicle. In Children's Fractures, 2nd ed. Philadelphia: JB Lippincott, 1983, pp 139-142.

136. Rasool MN and Govender S: Infections of the clavicle in children. Clin Orthop 265:178-182, 1991.

137. Riemer BL, Butterfield SL, Daffner RH, and O'Keeffe RMJ: The abduction lordotic view of the clavicle: A new technique for radiographic visualization. J Orthop Trauma 5:392-394, 1991.

138. Rowe CR: An atlas of anatomy and treatment of midclavicular fractures. Clin Orthop 58:29-42, 1968.

139. Salam A, Eyres K, and Cleary J: Malignant Langerhans' cell histiocytosis of the clavicle: A rare pathological fracture. Br J Clin Pract 44:652-654, 1990.

140. Salonen IS and Uusitalo R: Birth injuries: Incidence and predisposing factors. Z Kinderchir 45:133-135, 1990.

141. Sankarankutty M and Turner BW: Fractures of the clavicle. Injury 7:101-106, 1975.

142. Sartoris DJ, Mochizuki RM, and Parker BR: Lytic clavicular lesions in fibromatosis colli. Skeletal Radiol 10:34-36, 1983.

143. Schaff HV and Brawley RK: Operative management of penetrating vascular injuries of the thoracic outlet. Surgery 82:182-191, 1977.

144. Schmelzeisen H: Eosinophilic granuloma. Risk of fracture and rare site [German]. Aktuelle Traumatol 18(suppl 1):67-75, 1988.

145. Schoenecker PL, Johnson GE, Howard B, and Capelli AM: Congenital pseudarthrosis. Orthop Rev 21:855-862, 1992.

146. Schrocksnadel H, Heim K, and Dapunt O: The clavicular fracture—a questionable achievement in modern obstetrics [German]. Geburtshilfe Frauenheilkd 49:481-484, 1989.

147. Schuind F, Pay-Pay E, Andrianne Y, et al: External fixation of the clavicle for fracture or non-union in adults. J Bone Joint Surg Am 70:692-695, 1988.

148. Schuind F, Pay-Pay E, Andrianne Y, et al: Osteosynthesis of the clavicle using an external fixator [French]. Acta Orthop Belg 55:191-196, 1989.

149. Schumacher R, Muller U, and Schuster W: Rare localisation of osteochondrosis juvenilis [authors' transl] [German]. Radiologe 21:165-174, 1981.

150. Schwartz EE, Lantieri R, and Teplick JG: Erosion of the inferior aspect of the clavicle in secondary hyperparathyroidism. AJR Am J Roentgenol 129:291-295, 1977.

151. Schwarz N and Hocker K: Osteosynthesis of irreducible fractures of the clavicle with 2.7- mm ASIF plates. J Trauma 33:179-183, 1992.

152. Schwarz N and Leixnering M: Failures of clavicular intramedullary wire fixation and their causes [German]. Aktuelle Traumatol 14:159-163, 1984.

153. Silloway KA, McLaughlin RE, Edlich RC, and Edlich RF: Clavicular fractures and acromioclavicular joint dislocations in lacrosse: Preventable injuries. J Emerg Med 3:117-121, 1985.

154. Smith J, Yuppa F, and Watson RC: Primary tumors and tumor-like lesions of the clavicle. Skeletal Radiol 17:235-246, 1988.

155. Snyder LA: Loss of the accompanying soft tissue shadow of the clavicle with occult fracture [letter]. South Med J 72:243, 1979.

156. Stanley D and Norris SH: Recovery following fractures of the clavicle treated conservatively. Injury 19:162-164, 1988.

157. Stanley D, Trowbridge EA, and Norris SH: The mechanism of clavicular fractures. A clinical and biomechanical analysis. J Bone Joint Surg Br 70:461-464, 1988.

158. Taylor AR: Some observations on fractures of the clavicle. Proc R Soc Med 62:1037-1038, 1969.

159. Teplick JG, Eftekhari F, and Haskin ME: Erosion of the sternal ends of the clavicles. A new sign of primary and secondary hyperparathyroidism. Radiology 113:323-326, 1974.

160. Toledo LC and MacEwen GD: Severe complication of surgical treatment of congenital pseudarthrosis of the clavicle. Clin Orthop 139:64-67, 1979.

161. Treble NJ: Normal variations in radiographs of the clavicle: Brief report. J Bone Joint Surg Br 70:490, 1988.

162. Tse DH, Slabaugh PB, and Carlson PA: Injury to the axillary artery by a closed fracture of the clavicle. A case report. J Bone Joint Surg Am 62:1372-1374, 1980.

163. Turnpenny PD and Nimmo A: Fractured clavicle of the newborn in a population with a high prevalence of grand-multiparity: Analysis of 78 consecutive cases [see comments]. Br J Obstet Gynaecol 100:338-341, 1993.

164. Van Goethem H and Van Goethem C: Bilateral aplasia of the radius with abnormal hooking of the claviculae and sucrose-maltose intolerance. Helv Paediatr Acta 36:271-280, 1981.

165. Waldman RS and Powell T: Eosinophilic granuloma of the clavicle simulating primary bone neoplasm. Clin Orthop 64:150-152, 1969.

166. Wall JJ: Congenital pseudarthrosis of the clavicle. J Bone Joint Surg Am 52:1003-1009, 1970.

167. Walle T and Hartikainen-Sorri AL: Obstetric shoulder injury. Associated risk factors, prediction and prognosis. Acta Obstet Gynecol Scand 72:450-454, 1993.

168. Waninger KN and Chung MK: A new clue to clavicular fracture in newborn infants [letter]? Pediatrics 88:657, 1991.

169. Webb PA and Suchey JM: Epiphyseal union of the anterior iliac crest and medial clavicle in a modern multiracial sample of American males and females. Am J Phys Anthropol 68:457-466, 1985.

170. Wilkes JA and Hoffer MM: Clavicle fractures in head-injured children. J Orthop Trauma 1:55-58, 1987.

171. Wilkins RM and Johnston RM: Ununited fractures of the clavicle. J Bone Joint Surg Am 65:773-778, 1983.

172. Woo K, Emery J, and Peabody J: Cortical hyperostosis: A complication of prolonged prostaglandin infusion in infants awaiting cardiac transplantation. Pediatrics 93:417-420, 1994.

173. Worlock P and Stower M: Fracture patterns in Nottingham children. J Pediatr Orthop 6:656-661, 1986.

174. Xiao XY: Treatment of clavicular fracture patient with a percutaneous bone-embracing external clavicular microfixer [Chinese]. Chung Hua Wai Ko Tsa Chih 31:657-659, 1993.

175. Yates DW: Complications of fractures of the clavicle. Injury 7:189-193, 1976.

176. Zenni EJ Jr, Krieg JK, and Rosen MJ: Open reduction and internal fixation of clavicular fractures. J Bone Joint Surg Am 63:147-151, 1981.

MEDIAL CLAVICLE AND STERNOCLAVICULAR INJURIES

Anatomic Considerations

The epiphysis at the medial end of the clavicle is the last epiphysis of the long bones to appear, and it fuses to the shaft of the clavicle at the start of the third decade (see Fig. 26–15).[14,18,32,42] The anatomy of the clavicle was discussed previously. Posterior to the joint are the great vessels and mediastinal structures. The joint allows movement in three axes. It can elevate 45 degrees, depress 5 degrees, protract and retract 15 degrees, and rotate 45 to 50 degrees.[2,8,11,28]

Incidence

The true incidence of injuries to the medial end of the clavicle in children is unknown. Knowledge of these injuries is limited to case reports and small series with a variety of treatments and short-term follow-up.* Rowe reports that fractures and dislocations of the medial part of the clavicle constitute less than 6% of all injuries of the clavicle for all age groups.[36] Medial clavicular injuries account for only 1% to 3% of all clavicle injuries in children.[30,34]

Mechanism of Injury

Injuries to the medial part of the clavicle may be secondary to direct or indirect trauma.[6,17,19,20,30,33,40] Biomechanical analysis and clinical experience suggest that most medial clavicular injuries are a result of indirect trauma, such as a fall onto the shoulder leading to compressive loading on the clavicle. The direction of the load determines the subsequent displacement.[5]

---

*See references 1, 4, 6, 10, 17, 20, 22, 39, 41, 43, 44.

Classification

Extraphyseal fractures of the medial part of the clavicle have been described in children,[15,16] but the majority of reported injuries to this region in children are Salter-Harris type I and type II injuries (Fig. 26–25).[1,4,10,20,22,43,44] The displacement can be anterior or posterior. Anterior displacement of sternoclavicular joint injuries occurs twice as often as posterior displacement[35,37] in large series, but most case reports in the literature involve retrosternal displacement because of the morbidity associated with these injuries. True dislocation of the sternoclavicular joint in children is rare. Most reported cases of younger patients are part of a larger series of adults and do not exclude Salter-Harris injuries as a possibility.[17,27,38,39] Painful chronic instability has been reported in a 12-year-old patient.[25]

Signs and Symptoms

Minimally displaced injuries may have few symptoms or clinical findings, and the diagnosis is often delayed. The child or parent may only notice a mass secondary to callus formation. Children with displaced injuries to the medial part of the clavicle have swelling and pain. They will often tilt their head toward the side of the injury.[38] Initial assessment of the deformity may be difficult because of the swelling, but the contour of the chest will generally be altered (Figs. 26–26 and 26–27). Anterior dislocations are obvious on examination. Posterior dislocations can be more difficult to diagnose and may be associated with injury to the retrosternal structures. Venous congestion, choking, difficulty swallowing, diminished pulses, difficulty breathing, and neurologic complaints related to the brachial plexus have been all reported in association with these injuries and must be taken seriously.[35] These signs and symptoms may suggest underlying pneumothorax, brachial plexus injury, laceration of the superior vena cava, rupture of the esophagus, occlusion of the subclavian artery, or rupture of the trachea requiring urgent attention.

Radiographic Findings

Several specialized radiographic techniques can aid in the imaging of fractures and dislocations of the medial part of the clavicle and sternoclavicular joint. A 40-degree cephalic tilt view (serendipity view) allows the sternoclavicular joints and medial clavicle to be seen apart from other overlapping structures (Fig. 26–28).[35] The use of

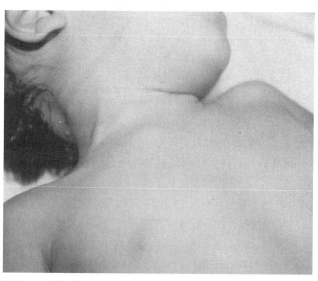

■ **Figure 26–26**
Clinical photograph of a young boy with a right anteriorly displaced medial clavicular injury.

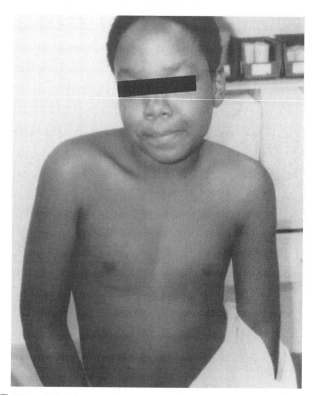

■ **Figure 26–27**
Posterior displacement of a medial clavicular injury. Notice the loss of contour of the left clavicle in comparison to the normal right side.

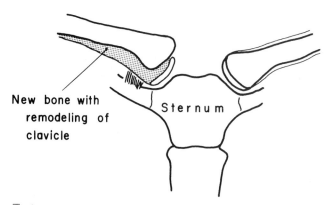

■ **Figure 26–25**
Diagram depicting a Salter-Harris type I injury to the medial clavicular physis. Healing is by periosteal new bone formation with significant potential for remodeling.

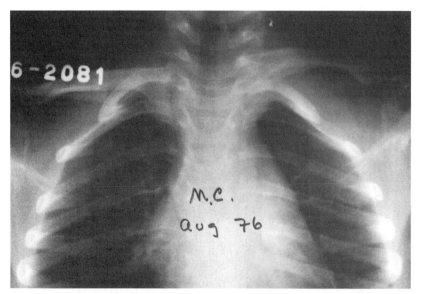

■ **Figure 26–28**
Serendipity view of the medial aspect of the clavicles. This 40-degree tangential radiograph demonstrates an anterior dislocation of the left sternoclavicular joint. *(From Rockwood CA and Green DP [eds]: Fractures [3 vols], 2nd ed. Philadelphia: JB Lippincott, 1984.)*

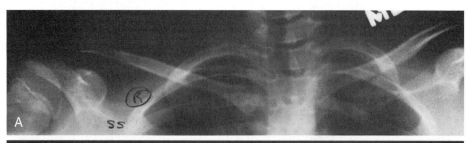

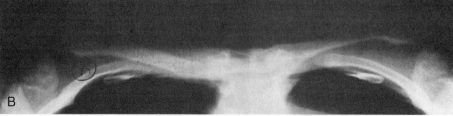

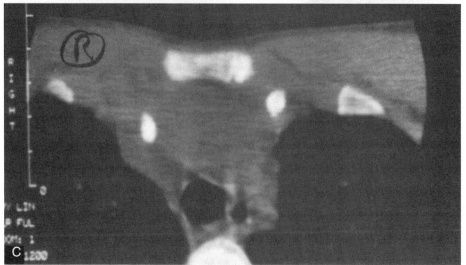

■ **Figure 26–29**
Posterior sternoclavicular dislocation of the medial aspect of the right clavicle. **A,** A plain anteroposterior radiograph shows asymmetry but is difficult to interpret. **B,** A tangential view demonstrates posterior displacement. **C,** A computed tomographic scan clearly demonstrates the injury, as well as the relationship of the displaced medial clavicle to the mediastinal structures.

plain tomography and CT scans has greatly improved the diagnosis and assessment of injuries and displacement in this anatomic region (Fig. 26–29).[11,12,21,24] Ultrasound has also been useful in diagnosing and managing the reduction of retrosternal dislocations.[3]

Treatment

A child with a minimally displaced medial clavicular fracture has few symptoms or clinical findings. Only symptomatic treatment is necessary. A sling can be used for comfort with early range of motion. No reduction is necessary. The tremendous growth potential of the medial clavicular physis allows for a great deal of remodeling of malunions. Anteriorly dislocated fractures and physeal injuries that mimic anterior dislocations of the sternoclavicular joint may have a bony prominence. In a growing child, this prominence will remodel,[35] and routine reduction of these injuries is probably not warranted. Symptomatic treatment with a sling or figure-of-eight harness for comfort yields good results.[9,35] If reduction is attempted, local or general anesthesia may be used. The patient is placed supine with a bolster between the shoulders. The arm is abducted 90 degrees, and longitudinal traction is applied. Posterior pressure is then gently applied over the fracture. The shoulders are held with limited immobilization (e.g., a padded figure-of-eight dressing or cast) for 3 to 4 weeks until stable.[9,35,37] Despite immobilization, many fractures remain unstable, and the surgeon is tempted to use internal fixation.[4,10,15] Many problems are reported with internal fixation in this area. Pin migration, which can be seen as early as 5 days after implantation,[13] can lead to pneumothorax, pericardial tamponade, and sudden death.[7,23,26,29]

Physeal fractures with posterior displacement may require emergency reduction because of compromise of surrounding vital structures.[4,6,10,15,16,20,22,44] Closed reduction is best attempted with a general anesthetic. The patient is placed supine with a bolster under the shoulders. Lateral traction is applied to the arm with pressure over the lateral aspect of the shoulder. The medial part of the clavicle may be grabbed with a towel clip after sterilely preparing the area and pulling anteriorly. A palpable pop often occurs. An alternative method is to adduct the arm to the trunk with caudal traction on the arm or hand while forcing both shoulders posteriorly by direct pressure. The reduction is generally stable,[27,35,44] and internal fixation is not necessary. If open reduction is needed, suture fixation or repair of the periosteal tube[20,38,39] can hold the reduction. Limited immobilization is used for 3 to 4 weeks. Rapid healing and remodeling of the injury generally occur.[35,44]

True sternoclavicular joint dislocation can be managed with closed reduction as described earlier. Anterior dislocations are more common than posterior dislocations.[35] As with physeal fractures in this region, a posterior dislocation associated with symptoms of retrosternal visceral injury should be treated by urgent reduction. A delay in performing closed reduction for more than 48 hours has been associated with a higher likelihood of needing to perform an open reduction.[17,27] Clavicular osteotomy may be helpful in assisting with open reduction.[31,38] Few problems occur with chronic anterior dislocations, but persistent pain can occur and necessitate late reconstruction.[25] Symptomatic, chronic dislocation of the sternoclavicular joint has been reported in a child[25] with successful late reconstruction.

■ AUTHORS' PREFERRED METHOD OF TREATMENT

We prefer nonoperative treatment of all true fractures and dislocations in this region. The remodeling potential is

great. Markedly displaced injuries in an older adolescent may merit an attempt at closed reduction under a local block. If redisplacement occurs, we do not favor operative intervention with internal fixation because of the high incidence of complications reported. Brief immobilization of these injuries for 2 to 4 weeks should provide enough healing and stability to allow for rehabilitation. Posterior dislocations or physeal fractures with compromise of the mediastinal structures warrant urgent reduction under a general anesthetic. The method of reduction was previously described. Internal fixation other than suture is not necessary for stabilization.

REFERENCES AND BIBLIOGRAPHY

1. Asher MA: Dislocations of the upper extremity in children. Orthop Clin North Am 7:583-591, 1976.
2. Bearn JG: Direct observations on the function of the capsule of the sternoclavicular support. J Anat 101:159-170, 1967.
3. Benson LS, Donaldson JS, and Carroll NC: Use of ultrasound in management of posterior sternoclavicular dislocation. J Ultrasound Med 10:115-118, 1991.
4. Brooks AL and Hennison GD: Injury to the proximal clavicular epiphysis. J Bone Joint Surg Am 54:1347, 1972.
5. Browne JE, Stanley RF, and Tullos HS: Acromioclavicular joint dislocations. Comparative results following operative treatment with and without primary distal clavisectomy. Am J Sports Med 5:258-263, 1977.
6. Buckerfield CT and Castle ME: Acute traumatic retrosternal dislocation of the clavicle. J Bone Joint Surg Am 66:379-385, 1984.
7. Clark RL, Milgram JW, and Yawn DH: Fatal aortic perforation and cardiac tamponade due to a Kirschner wire migrating from the right sternoclavicular joint. South Med J 67:316-318, 1974.
8. Corrigan GE: The neonatal clavicle. Biol Neonat 2:79-92, 1959.
9. Curtis RJJ: Operative management of children's fractures of the shoulder region. Orthop Clin North Am 21:315-324, 1990.
10. Denham RH and Dingley AF: Epiphyseal separation of the medial end of the clavicle. J Bone Joint Surg Am 49:1179-1183, 1967.
11. DePalma AF: The role of the disks of the sternoclavicular and the acromioclavicular joints. Clin Orthop 13:222-232, 1959.
12. Destouet JM, Gilula LA, Murphy WA, and Sagel SS: Computed tomography in the diagnosis of dislocations of the sternoclavicular joint. Radiology 138:123-128, 1981.
13. Engel W: Results of stable osteosynthesis in clavicular fractures [German]. Chirurg 41:234-235, 1970.
14. Gardner E and Gray DJ: Prenatal development of the human shoulder and acromioclavicular joints. Am J Anat 92:219-276, 1953.
15. Gaudernak T and Poigenfurst J: Simultaneous dislocation-fracture of both ends of the clavicle [German]. Unfallchirurgie 17:362-364, 1991.
16. Hardy JR: Complex clavicular injury in childhood. J Bone Joint Surg Br 74:154, 1992.
17. Heinig CF: Retrosternal dislocation of the clavicle: Early recognition, x-ray diagnosis, and management. J Bone Joint Surg Am 50:830, 1968.
18. Jit I and Kulkarni M: Times of appearance and fusion of epiphysis at the medial end of the clavicle. Indian J Med Res 64:773-782, 1976.
19. Landin LA: Fracture patterns in children: Analysis of 8682 fractures with special reference to incidence, etiology and secular changes in Swedish urban populations. Acta Orthop Scand Suppl 54:1-109, 1983.
20. Lemire L and Rosman M: Sternoclavicular epiphyseal separation with adjacent clavicular fracture. J Pediatr Orthop 4:118-120, 1984.
21. Levisohn EM, Bunnell WP, and Yuan HA: Computed tomography in the diagnosis of dislocations of the sternoclavicular joint. Clin Orthop 140:12-16, 1979.
22. Lewonowski K and Bassett GS: Complete posterior sternoclavicular epiphyseal separation. A case report and review of the literature. Clin Orthop 281:84-88, 1992.
23. Longo R and Ruggiero L: Left pneumothorax with subcutaneous emphysema secondary to left clavicular fracture and homolateral obstetrical paralysis of the arm [Italian]. Minerva Pediatr 34:273-276, 1982.
24. Lourie AA: Tomography in the diagnosis of posterior dislocation of the sternoclavicular joint. Acta Orthop Scand 51:579-580, 1980.
25. Lunseth PA, Chapman KW, and Frankel VH: Surgical treatment of chronic dislocation of the sterno-clavicular joint. J Bone Joint Surg Br 57:193-196, 1975.
26. Lyons FA and Rockwood CA: Current concepts review. Migration of pins used in operations on the shoulder. J Bone Joint Surg Am 72:1262-1267, 1990.
27. McKenzie JMM: Retrosternal dislocation of the clavicle. J Bone Joint Surg Br 45:138-141, 1963.
28. Moseley HF: The clavicle: Its anatomy and function. Clin Orthop 58:17-27, 1968.

29. Norback I and Markkula H: Migration of Kirschner pin from clavicle into ascending aorta. Acta Chir Scand 151:177-179, 1985.

30. Nordqvist A and Petersson C: The incidence of fractures of the clavicle. Clin Orthop 300:127-132, 1994.

31. Omer GE Jr: Osteotomy of the clavicle in surgical reduction of anterior sternoclavicular dislocation. J Trauma 7:584-590, 1967.

32. Owings-Webb PA: Epiphyseal union of the anterior iliac crest and medial clavicle in a modern multiracial sample of American males and females. Am J Phys Anthropol 68:457-466, 1985.

33. Paterson DC: Retrosternal dislocation of the clavicle. J Bone Joint Surg Br 43:90-94, 1961.

34. Rang M: Clavicle. In Children's Fractures, 2nd ed. Philadelphia: JB Lippincott, 1983, pp 139-142.

35. Rockwood CA: Dislocation of the sternoclavicular joint. Instr Course Lect 24:144-159, 1975.

36. Rowe CR: An atlas of anatomy and treatment of midclavicular fractures. Clin Orthop 58:29-42, 1968.

37. Salvatore JE: Sternoclavicular joint dislocation. Clin Orthop 58:51-55, 1968.

38. Selesnick FH, Jablon M, Frank C, and Post M: Retrosternal dislocation of the clavicle. Report of four cases. J Bone Joint Surg Am 66:287-291, 1984.

39. Simurda MA: Retrosternal dislocation of the clavicle: A report of four cases and a method of repair. Can J Surg 11:487-490, 1968.

40. Stanley D, Trowbridge EA, and Norris SH: The mechanism of clavicular fractures. A clinical and biomechanical analysis. J Bone Joint Surg Br 70:461-464, 1988.

41. Thomas CB and Friedman RJ: Ipsilateral sternoclavicular dislocation and clavicle fracture. J Orthop Trauma 139:68-69, 1989.

42. Todd TW and D'Errico J: The clavicular epiphyses. Am J Anat 25-50, 1928.

43. Wheeler ME, Laaveg SJ, and Sprague BL: S-C joint disruption in an infant. Clin Orthop 139:68, 1979.

44. Winter J, Sterner S, Maurer D, et al: Retrosternal epiphyseal disruption of medial clavicle: Case and review in children. J Emerg Med 7:9-13, 1989.

LATERAL CLAVICLE INJURIES

Anatomic Considerations

The anatomy of the clavicle was discussed previously.

Incidence

Rowe[22] reported 52 lateral clavicular injuries out of 690 clavicle fractures seen in a mixed population, for an incidence of 7.5%. Nordqvist and Petersson[17] found that Allman type II injuries constitute 21% of clavicular fractures in all age groups. These injuries are four to five times as common as sternoclavicular injuries,[20,22] but the true incidence of lateral clavicular injuries in children is unknown.

Mechanism of Injury

Most injuries to the distal end of the clavicle are due to direct shoulder trauma from falls or sports.[1,5,8] As the scapula is driven inferiorly, a fracture of the clavicle occurs through the lateral epiphyseal growth plate. The periosteum surrounding the distal end of the clavicle splits, and the bone displaces with the coracoclavicular ligaments still attached to the inferior periosteum (Fig. 26–30).[5,21]

Classification

Though rare, true dislocation of the acromioclavicular joint can occur in older children.[5,8,21] These injuries are classified as in adults.[1] Most lateral clavicle injuries in children younger than 13 years will be Salter-Harris type I or II fractures with displacement of the medial fragment

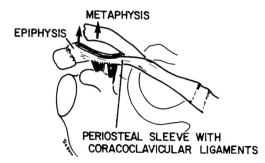

■ **Figure 26–30**

Schematic drawing of the injury pattern of the distal end of the clavicle showing how the clavicular metaphysis is displaced superiorly *(arrows)* through a tear in the periosteum while the acromioclavicular joint remains intact. Similarly, the coracoclavicular ligaments, which are attaching directly into the periosteum during much of development, remain intact, so the distance between the periosteal sleeve and coracoid process remains normal. *(From Ogden JA: Distal clavicular physical injury. Clin Orthop 188:7, 1984.)*

from the periosteal tube.[5,7-9,19,21,25] This fracture can be difficult to demonstrate radiographically because the distal clavicular epiphysis is often not ossified.[10,11] Rockwood has classified injuries to the distal end of the clavicle and acromioclavicular joint in children as follows[21] (Fig. 26–31):

Type I—Mild injury to the acromioclavicular ligaments without disruption of the periosteal tube. The distal end of the clavicle is stable, and radiographs are normal.

Type II—Partial disruption of the periosteal tube with mild instability of the distal end of the clavicle. Slight widening of the acromioclavicular joint is noted on radiographs, and the coracoclavicular interval is normal.

Type III—A large disruption of the periosteal tube with elevation of the distal portion of the clavicle and gross instability. The coracoclavicular interval is increased 25% to 100% more than in the normal shoulder.

Type IV—Similar to a type III injury, but with posterior displacement and buttonholing of the distal end of the clavicle through the trapezius muscle. Little superior migration is apparent on anteroposterior radiographs, but the axillary view will show posterior displacement of the clavicle relative to the acromion.[14]

Type V—Complete disruption of the periosteal tube with marked superior displacement of the clavicle into subcutaneous tissue. The deltoid and trapezius muscle attachments to the clavicle may be disrupted. The coracoclavicular distance is increased 100% more than in the opposite side.

Type VI—Complete disruption of the periosteal tube with inferior dislocation of the distal end of the clavicle to a position below the coracoid process.[13]

Because the periosteal tube remains contiguous, it will form a new clavicle while the bone displaced from the periosteal tube is being resorbed. During this interval, the patient will have a double clavicle.

An injury that can mimic a physeal fracture of the distal end of the clavicle is separation of the physis at the base of the coracoid with an acromioclavicular joint injury. The

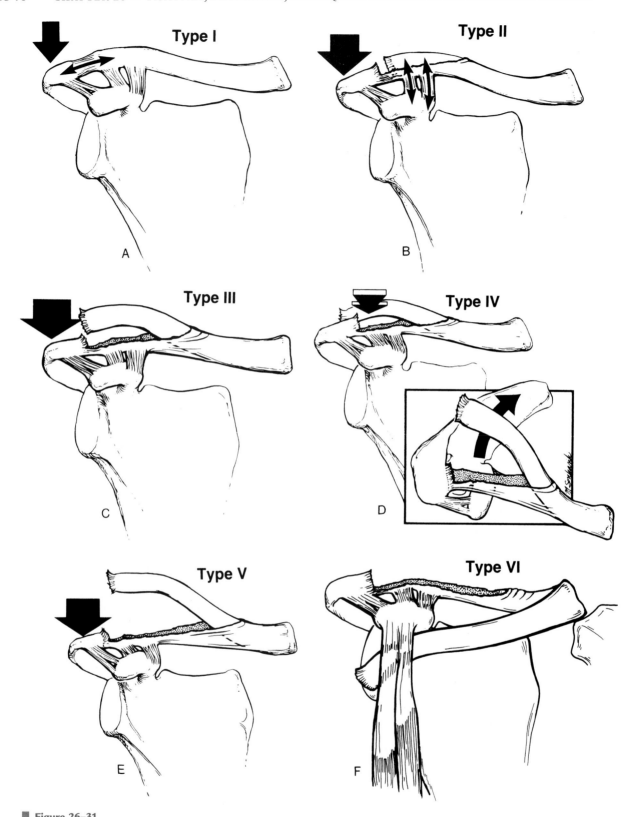

■ Figure 26–31
A-F, Rockwood's classification of clavicular-acromioclavicular joint injuries in children. (See text for description.) *(From Rockwood CA and Green DP [eds]: Fractures [3 vols], 2nd ed. Philadelphia: JB Lippincott, 1984.)*

periosteal tube of the distal part of the clavicle generally remains intact. This intact tube causes superior migration of the distal end of the clavicle and is a true injury of the acromioclavicular joint. These injuries have not been reported in children younger than 12 years.[3,16,23]

Signs and Symptoms

Type I and II fractures do not have significant displacement of the lateral aspect of the clavicle. Mild swelling and tenderness with some restriction of motion because of pain will be noted. With the progressive displacement seen in type III through type V injuries, there is obvious deformity with prominence of the clavicle. When these injuries heal as a double clavicle, the old superior clavicle can become quite prominent and may occasionally be symptomatic. Swelling and pain are present along with instability and tenderness of the distal end of the clavicle.[6,21] Type IV injuries can be easily missed because of posterior displacement of the clavicle.[19] Little deformity is evident once the swelling subsides, and radiographs look very similar to those of a type II injury. Type VI injuries are easily identified clinically but are rare. Swelling, pain, and restricted motion are present. The acromion is prominent, and the distal end of the clavicle is not palpable. Injury to the brachial plexus and axillary vessels can occur.[13]

Radiographic Findings

Anteroposterior radiographs of this area should center on the acromioclavicular joint and are best when a soft tissue technique is used. The axillary lateral view and a 20-degree cephalic tilt view help assess the degree and direction of displacement. Stress radiographs may be helpful when injury is suspected but is not seen on routine views. Both acromioclavicular joints should be viewed simultaneously on the same x-ray plate, first without and then with a light weight to provide distal traction on the extremities. The coracoclavicular distance increases on the injured side if the injury is sufficient. The Stryker notch view can be very helpful to look for a fracture of the common physis of the superior glenoid and the base of the coracoid (Fig. 26–32). This radiograph is taken as an anteroposterior view of the shoulder with the patient's hand resting on top of the head.

Treatment

Because most distal clavicular injuries in children are physeal injuries without true acromioclavicular separation, they have great potential for healing and remodeling (Fig. 26–33). Concern about the prominence of the distal clavicular fragment with permanent deformity has been suggested as a reason for closed reduction and pin fixation in a small series of patients without long-term follow-up.[9,15,19] Larger reviews, however, have found that nonoperative treatment leads to predictably excellent results without any functional sequelae.[5,8,15] If the distal clavicular prominence leads to difficulty in the future, the

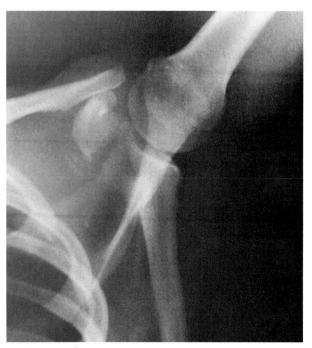

■ **Figure 26–32**
The Stryker notch view is best for demonstrating a fracture at the base of the coracoid.

prominence of the double clavicle can be excised at that time with predictably good results. For true acromioclavicular separations in older children, a series of adult patients has demonstrated that conservative treatment of complete dislocations will result in good functional and clinical outcomes.[2,4,18,24] All these data suggest that surgery for distal clavicular injuries in children is mainly for cosmetic reasons.

For the rare situation with marked displacement of the distal end of the clavicle and tenting of the skin or an open fracture, open reduction and internal fixation may be necessary. In some situations, the periosteal tube can be repaired after replacing the clavicle back into its periosteal bed. Temporary internal fixation for 4 to 6 weeks with a coracoclavicular lag screw or a transacromial Kirschner wire may be used.[7,9,12,19] Displaced fractures of the coracoid or glenoid physis are usually associated with an acromioclavicular joint dislocation. Open reduction plus internal fixation of the coracoid fracture is recommended for these injuries. Nondisplaced fractures can be treated nonoperatively with a sling.[3,16]

■ AUTHORS' PREFERRED METHOD OF TREATMENT

We prefer to treat most distal clavicular injuries in children nonoperatively. Initially, patients are placed in a sling with mild analgesics given to control early pain. Early range-of-motion and return-to-play activities are begun as soon as pain allows. Clinical healing is usually complete by 6 weeks, and resumption of full activities is allowed. For widely displaced (types IV to VI) fractures or open fractures, we recommend open reduction and temporary

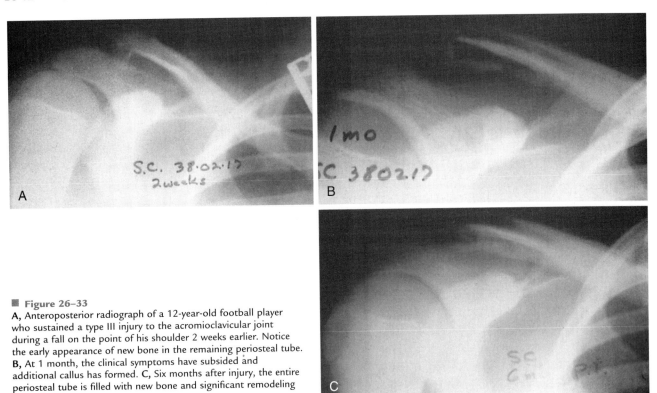

■ **Figure 26–33**

A, Anteroposterior radiograph of a 12-year-old football player who sustained a type III injury to the acromioclavicular joint during a fall on the point of his shoulder 2 weeks earlier. Notice the early appearance of new bone in the remaining periosteal tube. **B,** At 1 month, the clinical symptoms have subsided and additional callus has formed. **C,** Six months after injury, the entire periosteal tube is filled with new bone and significant remodeling is under way.

internal fixation by either repairing the periosteal tube or placing a coracoclavicular lag screw or Kirschner wires across the acromioclavicular joint.

Children older than 13 years can have true acromioclavicular dislocations. Most of these injuries have an excellent functional outcome if treated conservatively. The reader is referred to Chapter 11 on adult clavicle injuries for further references on treatment and outcome.

REFERENCES AND BIBLIOGRAPHY

1. Allman FL: Fractures and ligamentous injuries of the clavicle and its articulations. J Bone Joint Surg Am 49:774, 1967.
2. Bakalim G and Wilppula E: Surgical or conservative treatments of total dislocation of the acromioclavicular joint. Acta Chir Scand 141:43-47, 1975.
3. Bernard TN, Brunet ME, and Haddad RJ: Fractured coracoid process in acromioclavicular dislocations. Report of four cases and review of the literature. Clin Orthop 175:227-232, 1983.
4. Bjerneld H, Hovelius L, and Thorling J: Acromio-clavicular separations treated conservatively. A 5-year follow-up study. Acta Orthop Scand 54:743-745, 1983.
5. Black GB, McPherson JA, and Reed MH: Traumatic pseudodislocation of the acromioclavicular joint in children. A fifteen year review. Am J Sports Med 19:644-646, 1991.
6. Curtis RJJ: Operative management of children's fractures of the shoulder region. Orthop Clin North Am 21:315-324, 1990.
7. Edwards DJ, Kavanagh TG, and Flannery MC: Fractures of the distal clavicle: A case for fixation. Injury 23:44-46, 1992.
8. Eidman DK, Siff SJ, and Tullos HS: Acromioclavicular lesions in children. Am J Sports Med 9:150-154, 1981.
9. Falstie-Jensen S and Mikkelsen P: Pseudodislocation of the acromioclavicular joint. J Bone Joint Surg Br 64:368-369, 1982.
10. Gardner E and Gray DJ: Prenatal development of the human shoulder and acromioclavicular joints. Am J Anat 92:219-276, 1953.
11. Garn SM, Rohmann CG, and Silverman FN: Radiographic standards for postnatal ossification and tooth calcification. Med Radiogr Photogr 43:45-66, 1967.
12. Gaudernak T and Poigenfurst J: Simultaneous dislocation-fracture of both ends of the clavicle [German]. Unfallchirurgie 17:362-364, 1991.
13. Gerber C and Rockwood CA Jr: Subcoracoid dislocation of the lateral end of the clavicle. A report of three cases. J Bone Joint Surg Am 69:924-927, 1987.
14. Gunther WA: Posterior dislocation of the clavicle. J Bone Joint Surg Am 31:878, 1949.
15. Havrŷnek P: Injuries of distal clavicular physis in children. J Pediatr Orthop 9:213-215, 1989.
16. Montgomery SP and Loyd RD: Avulsion fracture of the coracoid epiphysis with acromioclavicular separation. Report of two cases in adolescents and review of the literature. J Bone Joint Surg Am 59:963-965, 1977.
17. Nordqvist A and Petersson C: The incidence of fractures of the clavicle. Clin Orthop 300:127-132, 1994.
18. Nordqvist A, Petersson C, and Redlund-Johnell I: The natural course of lateral clavicle fracture. 15 (11-21) year follow-up of 110 cases. Acta Orthop Scand 64:87-91, 1993.
19. Ogden JA: Distal clavicular physeal injury. Clin Orthop 188:68-73, 1984.
20. Rockwood CA: Dislocation of the sternoclavicular joint. Instr Course Lect 24:144-159, 1975.
21. Rockwood CA Jr: The shoulder: Facts, confusions and myths. Int Orthop 15:401-405, 1991.
22. Rowe CR: An atlas of anatomy and treatment of midclavicular fractures. Clin Orthop 58:29-42, 1968.
23. Taga I, Yoneda M, and Ono K: Epiphyseal separation of the coracoid process associated with acromioclavicular sprain. A case report and review of the literature. Clin Orthop 207:138-141, 1986.
24. Walsh WM, Peterson DA, Shelton G, and Neumann RD: Shoulder strength following acromioclavicular injury. Am J Sports Med 13:153-158, 1985.
25. Wilkes JA and Hoffer MM: Clavicle fractures in head-injured children. J Orthop Trauma 1:55-58, 1987.

BIPOLAR CLAVICLE INJURIES

Fractures or fracture-dislocations of both ends of the clavicle are rare injuries that are described in small series and case reports.[1-3] In adults, the injury is typically an anterior sternoclavicular dislocation and a posterior or type IV acromioclavicular dislocation. Sanders and associates recommend open reduction of the acromioclavicular dislocation in active individuals and symptomatic treatment of the coracoclavicular dislocation.[3] Beckman reported a child with a bipolar injury who was treated successfully by replacing the clavicle back into its periosteal tube without further fixation.[1]

REFERENCES AND BIBLIOGRAPHY

1. Beckman T: A case of simultaneous luxation of both ends of the clavicle. Acta Chirurg Scand 56:156-163, 1924.
2. Gaudernak T and Poigenfurst J: Simultaneous dislocation-fracture of both ends of the clavicle [German]. Unfallchirurgie 17:362-364, 1991.
3. Sanders JO, Lyons FA, and Rockwood CA: Management of dislocations of both ends of the clavicle. J Bone Joint Surg Am 72:399-402, 1990.

FRACTURES AND DISLOCATIONS OF THE SCAPULA

Developmental Anatomy

The scapula first appears as a cartilaginous anlage at the C4 to C5 level in the fifth gestational week. During the sixth and seventh gestational weeks, it enlarges to extend from C4 to C7. During the seventh week, the shoulder joint forms, and the scapula descends from the cervical area to its position overlying the first through fifth ribs. Failure of the scapula to descend results in Sprengel's deformity.[60]

Most of the scapula is formed by membranous ossification. The multiple ossification centers about the scapula can be confused with fractures (Fig. 26-34). The body's ossification center is present at birth.[57] The coracoid process ossifies from two separate centers. The first is distal, and ossification closely follows the proximal humeral epiphysis but is more erratic.[39] The base of the coracoid process begins ossifying in the 10th year, forms

a portion of the glenoid, and unites with the body at about 15 years of age. Initially, the coracoid process is larger than the acromion,[45] but it gradually assumes the adult form. The acromion forms from two to five ossification centers that appear at puberty; they may fail to unite and result in a bipartite or tripartite acromion.[13] The most anterior portion is the pre-acromion, the middle portion is the meso-acromion, and the portion at the angle between the scapular spine and the acromion is the meta-acromion, which is separate from the base of the acromion. Persistence of these centers may be confused with an acromion fracture.[42,45,49] The most common os acromiale type is failure of the meso-acromion to join the meta-acromion. The junction of an os acromiale with the spine may have a distinct joint cavity and is differentiated from a fracture by round, uniform cleavage lines, in contrast to a fracture's sharp, ragged edges. An os acromiale (Fig. 26-35) is rarely visible except on the axillary lateral view and is more commonly bilateral than unilateral.[45] It normally fuses to the remaining scapula at approximately 22 years of age.[57] The glenoid forms from the ossification center at the base of the coracoid and a second horseshoe-shaped center. Centers for the vertebral border and the inferior scapula angle appear at puberty and unite with the body at about 21 years of age. Developmental anomalies of the scapula include a bipartite coracoid, coracoid duplication, absent acromion,[34] glenoid hypoplasia,[8] scapular hypoplasia, and Sprengel's anomaly.[2,12,13,45,57] Because of these numerous ossification centers, comparison radiographs and a careful clinical examination are important.

Surgical Anatomy

The scapula is a flat triangular bone, and its 17 muscular attachments control scapulothoracic motion. The scapula

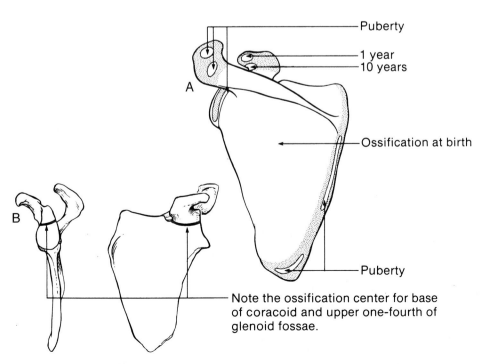

Puberty

1 year
10 years

Ossification at birth

Puberty

Note the ossification center for base of coracoid and upper one-fourth of glenoid fossae.

■ **Figure 26–34**
A and **B,** Multiple ossification centers of the scapula.

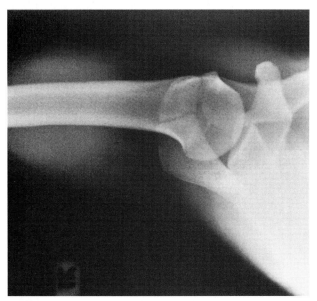

■ Figure 26–35
An unfused os acromiale seen on the axillary lateral view. This process can be mistaken for an acute fracture of the acromion, which is a rare injury in a child.

is highly mobile and provides approximately 60 degrees of shoulder elevation. The scapular spine divides the dorsal surface into fossae that accommodate the supraspinatus and infraspinatus muscles.

The scapula is encased in muscle and is relatively protected from trauma. Fractures and dislocations of the scapula constitute only 1% of all fractures and 5% of shoulder fractures[25,27] and are even more uncommon in children. Fractures of the scapula are often associated with other life-threatening, severe injuries that are more important than the fracture of the scapula itself.[20,46,60,63]

Classification

Several classification schemes have been devised for fracture of the scapula, but none are specific for children. A summary of various types of fractures is included in the following outline. The proportion of fracture types is 12% for acromion, 11% for spine, 7% for coracoid, 27% for neck, 10% for glenoid, and 35% for body fractures.[1]

A few scapular fractures have potential pitfalls. Scapular neck fractures associated with clavicular fractures or sternoclavicular or acromioclavicular dislocations (the so-called floating shoulder) are potentially unstable and allow the scapular neck to displace and change the normal muscle configuration about the shoulder. Fractures through the coracoid with lateral clavicular fractures are a childhood equivalent of acromioclavicular joint dislocations (Fig. 26–36).[48] Acromial fractures with narrowing result in subacromial impingement.[38]

Scapulothoracic dissociations are classified as intrathoracic and are described as the "locked scapula"[52] or as being laterally displaced.[3,40] Open lateral dislocations are essentially incomplete forequarter amputations. The patient's neurovascular status is at great risk. To sustain this injury, the attachment with the thorax must be broken at either the sternoclavicular joint or the acromioclavicular joint, or a clavicular fracture must occur. Ebraheim and associates distinguish scapulothoracic dissociation from scapulothoracic dislocation, which is traumatic dislocation of the inferior scapulothoracic articulation with less devastating vascular and neurologic damage.[16] We find it difficult to distinguish dissociation from dislocation of an articulation.

Ideberg classified glenoid fractures as types I to V based on their location in the glenoid and the course of the fracture through the rest of the scapula.[30,31] Type I, or anterior avulsion fracture, results from dislocations, subluxations, or direct injury and may be associated with glenohumeral instability. Large fragments with instability should be distinguished from the more common rim fractures resulting from dislocations.[5] Type II is a transverse or oblique fracture occurring through the glenoid with an inferior free glenoid fragment that results in inferior glenohumeral subluxation. Type III fractures involve the upper third of the glenoid, including the coracoid, and are often associated with an acromial fracture, a clavicle fracture, or an acromioclavicular dislocation. A type III fracture has been reported in an adolescent.[6] A type IV fracture is a horizontal glenoid fracture extending through the body all the way to the vertebral border. Type V is a combination of type IV with a transverse fracture through the scapular neck or its inferior half with the inferior fragment floating free. Goss expanded type V to include combinations of types II, III, and IV, and Goss added a type VI that consists of a severely comminuted glenoid cavity.[23]

Goss groups scapular injuries by stability. He defined the superior shoulder suspensory complex as a bony and soft tissue ring on the end of a superior and inferior bony strut.[23-25] The ring consists of the glenoid process, coracoid process, coracoclavicular ligaments, distal part of the clavicle, acromioclavicular ligaments, and acromial process. The superior strut is the middle part of the clavicle, and the inferior strut is the lateral scapular body and spine. A double disruption of this complex can result in severe displacement with potential implications for treatment.

Classification

Body
    Nondisplaced
    Displaced
Neck[43]
    Isolated
    Clavicular axis disrupted
Coracoid[48]
    Isolated
    Acromioclavicular joint disruption
Acromion[38]
    I—Nondisplaced; A, avulsion; B, direct trauma
    II—Displaced with no subacromial narrowing
    III—Displaced with subacromial narrowing
Glenoid fractures[30,31]
    I—Anterior avulsion fracture
    II—Transverse with an inferior free fragment
    III—Upper third, including the coracoid

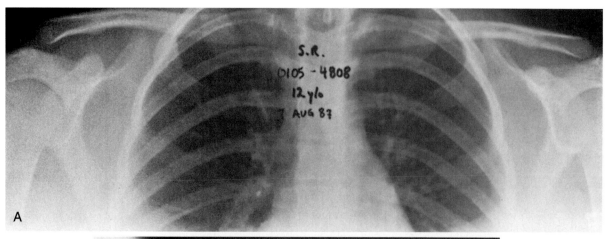

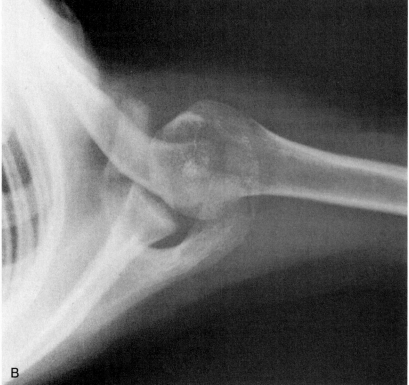

■ **Figure 26–36**
From the clinical examination, this 12-year-old boy was thought to have a distal clavicular–acromioclavicular joint injury after falling on his right shoulder. **A,** Comparison anteroposterior views of both shoulders reveal slight depression of the right scapula but no difference in comparative coracoclavicular distance. **B,** An axillary lateral view demonstrates the condition to be a fracture of the base of the coracoid.

IV—Horizontal fracture extending through the body
V—Combination of II and III
VI—Extensively comminuted
Scapulothoracic dissociation[54]
 Open or closed
 Complete or incomplete amputation (traumatic fore-
  quarter amputation)
 Neurovascular status:
  a. Intact
  b. Partially disrupted
  c. Completely disrupted
   I. Intrathoracic
   II. Lateral

A. Acromioclavicular joint injury
B. Sternoclavicular joint injury
C. Clavicle fracture

Mechanisms of Injury

Avulsion fractures associated with glenohumeral joint injuries are the most commonly encountered fractures of the scapula. Other fractures of the scapula generally occur with great violence.[20,46,60,63] They are uncommon in infants and children but quite specific for child abuse unless a clear mechanism exists.[36] Coracoid fractures generally occur with injury to the acromioclavicular joint through the weak bone rather than the stronger ligaments.[48] Stress fractures of the acromion,[14,26,59,62] coracoid,[9,58] and glenoid[7] and at the teres minor insertion[10] are reported in adults, but the only stress fractures reported in children are a scapular body stress fracture in a gymnast[50] and a coracoid process fracture in an archer.[51]

Signs and Symptoms

Seventy-five percent or more of patients with scapula fractures have associated injuries[1,56] that may be life-threatening.[1,32,56,60] The most frequent injuries are to the head, chest, kidneys, and especially the ipsilateral lung, chest wall, and ipsilateral shoulder girdle, including the neurovascular structures.[60] Mortality in one series was 14.3%.[60] Victims of severe trauma should be assessed and managed by the ABCs (airway, breathing, and circulation). Clinically, scapular fractures are characterized by swelling, pain, and tenderness about the scapular area if the patient is responsive. Scapular neck fractures additionally exhibit flattening of the overall shoulder contour. A careful neurovascular and chest examination is essential in all injuries to the scapula.

Imaging Studies and Differential Diagnosis

An anteroposterior view and a scapulolateral view define most scapular fractures (Fig. 26–37). Several scapular abnormalities can mimic fractures, especially os acromiale. Although acromial fractures are a strong indicator of child abuse, ossification adjacent to the tip of the

acromion can be a normal finding.[35] This center is generally on the inferior portion and is anterior on the axillary view. A bone scan may be necessary to distinguish it from a fracture.[35] Andrews and associates describe a 20-degree caudal tilt lateral view with the shoulder adducted to show the lateral aspect of the acromion, which may help profile an os acromiale.[4] Defects in glenoid ossification, including an ununited epiphysis, a pseudoforamen of the scapula, and a scapular notch, must be distinguished from a fracture.[21] Coracoid fractures are best seen on a Stryker notch view (Fig. 26–38), although a CT scan may be necessary.[29] Glenoid fractures may be difficult to visualize and are best seen on the axillary lateral view.[56] A true anteroposterior view, a West Point view, and an apical oblique view are often necessary. A CT scan is best for intra-articular fractures (Fig. 26–39), and computerized reconstructions may be needed. Scapulothoracic dislocations are best identified on a nonrotated anteroposterior chest radiograph with the medial border of the scapula displaced laterally relative to the uninjured side.[16,33] This injury must be considered in patients with massive trauma to the upper extremity and nerve or vascular deficits and whose radiographs demonstrate lateral displacement of the scapula, complete acromioclavicular joint separation, or fracture of the clavicle.[55]

Treatment

The scapula is very flexible in children. As rare as scapular fractures are in adults, they are extremely uncommon in children, and treatments must be based on those that are

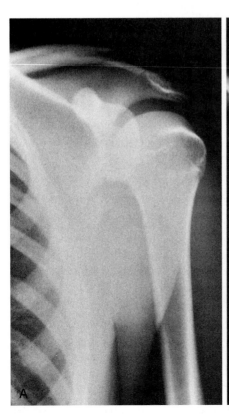
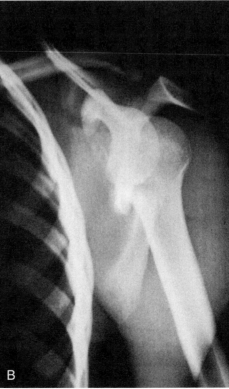

■ **Figure 26–37**
Fractures of the body of the scapula are usually associated with high-energy injuries. **A,** An anteroposterior radiograph shows a displaced body fracture. **B,** True scapular lateral view.

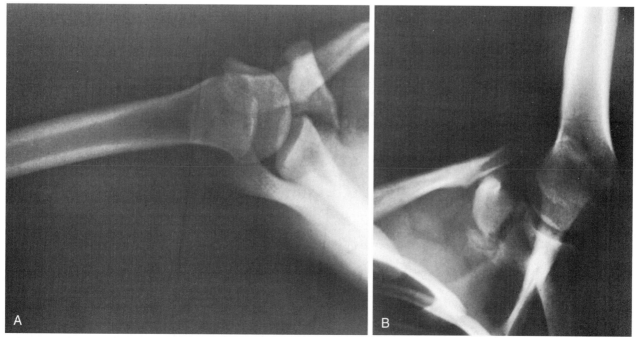

■ **Figure 26–38**

Fractures of the base of the coracoid are best seen on the Stryker notch view. **A,** Axillary lateral view of the injury. **B,** Healing callus shown on the Stryker notch view.

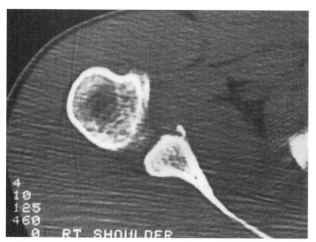

■ **Figure 26–39**

Displaced fractures of the anterior glenoid are associated with dislocations of the glenohumeral joint. A computed tomographic scan is very good for assessing this lesion.

found most useful in adults. It is crucial to consider child abuse except in major vehicular trauma.

BODY. Most scapular body fractures respond to conservative treatment.[18,32,56,63] The muscles around the scapula tend to keep the fragments in reasonable proximity with good healing potential. In the few fractures that fail to unite, partial body fragments can be excised. Treatment of scapula body fractures is usually defined by the associated injuries.[19]

SCAPULA NECK. Nondisplaced fractures of the scapular neck that are not associated with fractures of the clav-

icle can be treated expectantly. If they are displaced significantly, closed reduction and application of a thoracobrachial cast may be sufficient. If the clavicle or its joints are disrupted, Herscovici and associates recommend open reduction of the clavicle to preserve the suspensory function of the coracoclavicular ligaments, but they leave the scapula alone.[28] Leung and Lam recommend fixing both the scapular neck fracture and the clavicle fracture.[43] Skeletal traction is an acceptable alternative.[15] Several more recent reviews cast doubt on the need to fix these fractures.[17,22,61] In children with their stout periosteum and remodeling potential, it is doubtful that this injury would require fixation.

CORACOID FRACTURES. Coracoid fractures that are nondisplaced can be simply treated with a sling. Displaced fractures are usually associated with an acromioclavicular joint or lateral clavicular injury. These fractures should be treated by open reduction and internal fixation.[48,56]

ACROMIAL FRACTURES. Nondisplaced acromial fractures are treated with a sling. Only nondisplaced acromial fractures have been reported in children.[38] Displaced acromial fractures with subacromial impingement should be reduced and stabilized with pins, screws, or a small plate.[27,38] Nonunion is reported in adults but not in children.[47]

GLENOID FRACTURES. The majority of glenoid fractures, except those associated with shoulder instability, are rarely symptomatic when they heal, and these fractures can be treated in closed fashion.[64] Large fractures involving a large portion of the glenoid fossa associated with glenohumeral instability should be fixed.[37] For glenoid fractures that do not involve the anterior rim or the superior half of the glenoid, a posterior approach is easier.[44,53,56] Ideberg[30,31] suggests open reduction for persistent subluxation or an unstable reduction. Although he reports patients as young as 6 years,[31] the youngest patient treated surgically was 30 years of age.[31] Type II fractures associated with glenohumeral instability or inferior subluxation may require open reduction,[41] although the approach and fixation may be quite difficult. This finding has been reported in a 16-year-old who appeared to have an open proximal humeral physis that was successfully treated by open reduction and internal fixation through a deltopectoral approach.[6] If no subluxation is present, it can be treated by shoulder rehabilitation. Type III fractures occur through the junction between the ossification centers of the glenoid and are often accompanied by a fractured acromion or clavicle or acromioclavicular separation. Early motion tends to improve the position.[11,30,31] Type IV, V, and VI fractures are not reported in children and can be extremely difficult to treat by open reduction because the scapula has very little bone for good fixation.[23,30,31] In children who can tolerate prolonged immobilization, skeletal traction followed by protected motion may be satisfactory treatment.

SCAPULOTHORACIC DISLOCATIONS AND DISSOCIATION. Intrathoracic dislocation is rare. The medial border is caught between either the third and fourth ribs or the fourth and fifth ribs. It can usually be reduced by closed means. DePalma[15] described reduction by hyperabduction and manual manipulation of the axillary border to rotate the scapula forward while at the same time pushing it back into location. The reduction is usually stable. The patient may be more comfortable with some immobilization such as strapping or a collar and cuff. Nettrour and associates[52] reported open reduction of this injury in an 11-year-old boy. The rhomboid muscle is typically torn. Late reduction may require soft tissue reattachment to maintain stability.

Lateral scapulothoracic dissociation is potentially life-threatening.[3] Initially, the patient should be stabilized by using the ABCs of trauma care. It is important to perform a detailed neurovascular examination. Generally, massive injury to the entire extremity has occurred. Arteriography can help plan the vascular reconstruction if time allows. In a massive injury with brachial plexus avulsion, amputation should be considered.[55] If any of the plexus remains intact, it is best to salvage the limb.[55] Salvage may require shoulder arthrodesis and above-elbow amputation. A successful muscular repair has been reported in a child and should be considered in patients with an intact brachial plexus after the artery has been repaired.

REFERENCES AND BIBLIOGRAPHY

1. Ada JR and Miller ME: Scapular fractures: Analysis of 113 cases. Clin Orthop 269:174-180, 1991.
2. Ahn JI and Park JS: Pathological fractures secondary to unicameral bone cysts. Int Orthop 18:20-22, 1994.
3. An HS, Vonderbrink JP, Ebraheim NA, et al: Open scapulothoracic dissociation with intact neurovascular status in a child. J Orthop Trauma 2:36-38, 1988.
4. Andrews JR, Byrd JW, Kupferman SP, and Angelo RL: The profile view of the acromion. Clin Orthop 263:142-146, 1991.
5. Aston JW and Gregory CF: Dislocation of the shoulder with significant fracture of the glenoid. J Bone Joint Surg Am 55:1531-1533, 1973.
6. Aulicino PL, Reinert C, Kornberg M, and Williamson S: Displaced intra-articular glenoid fractures treated by open reduction and internal fixation. J Trauma 26:1137-1141, 1986.
7. Bennett GE: Shoulder and elbow lesions of the professional baseball pitcher. JAMA 117:510-514, 1941.
8. Borenstein ZC, Mink J, Oppenheim W, et al: Case report 655: Congenital glenoid dysplasia (congenital hypoplasia of the glenoid neck and fossa of the scapula, with accompanied deformity of humeral head, coracoid process, and acromion). Skeletal Radiol 20:134-136, 1991.
9. Boyer DW Jr: Trapshooter's shoulder: Stress fracture of the coracoid process. Case report. J Bone Joint Surg Am 57:862, 1975.
10. Brower AC, Neff JR, and Tellema DA: An unusual scapular stress fracture. AJR Am J Roentgenol 129:519-520, 1977.
11. Butters KP: Fractures and dislocations of the scapula. In Rockwood CA Jr, Green DP, and Bucholz RW (eds): Fractures in Adults, 3rd ed. Philadelphia: JB Lippincott, 1991, pp 990-1019.
12. Chung SM and Farahvar H: Surgery of the clavicle in Sprengel's deformity. Clin Orthop 116:138-141, 1976.
13. Chung SMK and Nissenbaum MM: Congenital and developmental defects of the shoulder. Orthop Clin North Am 6:381-392, 1975.
14. Dennis DA, Ferlic DC, and Clayton ML: Acromial stress fractures associated with cuff-tear arthropathy. A report of three cases. J Bone Joint Surg Am 68:937-940, 1986.
15. DePalma AF: Surgery of the Shoulder, 3rd ed. Philadelphia: JB Lippincott, 1983, pp 362-372.
16. Ebraheim NA, An HS, Jackson WT, et al: Scapulothoracic dissociation. J Bone Joint Surg Am 70:428-432, 1988.
17. Egol KA, Connor PM, Karunakar MA, et al: The floating shoulder: Clinical and functional results. J Bone Joint Surg Am 83:1188-1194, 2001.
18. Eskola A, Vainionpaa S, Korkala O, and Rokkanen P: Acute complete acromioclavicular dislocation. A prospective randomized trial of fixation with smooth or threaded Kirschner wires or cortical screw. Ann Chir Gynaecol 76:323-326, 1987.
19. Findlay RT: Fractures of the scapula. Ann Surg 93:1001-1008, 1931.
20. Gelberman RH, Verdeck WN, and Brodhead WT: Supraclavicular nerve-entrapment syndrome. J Bone Joint Surg Am 57:119, 1975.
21. Goldenberg DB and Brogdon BG: Congenital anomalies of the pectoral girdle demonstrated by chest radiography. J Can Assoc Radiol 18:472-477, 1967.
22. Goodnight JM, Rockwood CA Jr, and Wirth MA: Ipsilateral fractures of the clavicle and scapula [abstract]. Submitted for publication, 1996.
23. Goss TP: Current concepts review: Fractures of the glenoid cavity. J Bone Joint Surg Am 72:299-305, 1992.
24. Goss TP: Double disruptions of the superior shoulder suspensory complex. J Orthop Trauma 7:99-106, 1993.
25. Goss TP: Scapular fractures and dislocations: Diagnosis and treatment. J Am Acad Orthop Surg 3:22-33, 1995.
26. Hall RJ and Calvert PT: Stress fracture of the acromion: An unusual mechanism and review of the literature. J Bone Joint Surg Br 77:153-154, 1995.
27. Hardegger FH, Simpson LA, and Weber BG: The operative treatment of scapular fractures. J Bone Joint Surg Br 66:725-731, 1984.
28. Herscovici D Jr, Fiennes AG, Allgower M, and Ruedi TP: The floating shoulder: Ipsilateral clavicle and scapular neck fractures [see comments]. J Bone Joint Surg Br 74:362-364, 1992.
29. Holst AK and Christiansen JV: Epiphyseal separation of the coracoid process without acromioclavicular dislocation. Skeletal Radiol 27:461-462, 1998.
30. Ideberg R: Fractures of the scapula involving the glenoid fossa. In Bateman JE, Walsh RD (eds): Surgery of the Shoulder. Toronto: BC Decker, 1984, pp 63-66.
31. Ideberg R: Unusual glenoid fractures. Acta Orthop Scand 58:191-192, 1987.
32. Imatani RJ: Fractures of the scapulae: A review of 53 fractures. J Trauma 15:473-478, 1975.
33. Kelbel JM, Jardon OM, and Huurman WW: Scapulothoracic dislocation. Clin Orthop 209:210-214, 1986.
34. Kim SJ and Min BH: Congenital bilateral absence of the acromion. A case report. Clin Orthop 300:117-119, 1994.
35. Kleinman PK and Spevak MR: Variations in acromial ossification simulating infant abuse in victims of sudden infant death syndrome. Radiology 180:185-187, 1991.
36. Kogutt MS, Swischuk LE, and Fagan CJ: Patterns of injury and significance of uncommon fractures in the battered child syndrome. AJR Am J Roentgenol 121:143-149, 1974.
37. Kreitner KF, Runkel M, Grebe P, et al: MR tomography versus CT arthrography in glenohumeral instabilities [German]. Rofo Fortschr Geb Rontgenstr Neuen Bildgeb Verfahr 157:37-42, 1992.
38. Kuhn JE, Blasier RB, and Carpenter JE: Fractures of the acromion process: A proposed classification system [see comments]. J Orthop Trauma 8:6-13, 1994.
39. Kuhns LR, Sherman MP, Poznanski AK, and Holt JF: Humeral head and coracoid ossification in the newborn. Radiology 107:145-149, 1973.
40. Lange RH and Noel SH: Traumatic lateral scapular displacement: An expanded spectrum of associated neurovascular injury. J Orthop Trauma 7:361-366, 1993.
41. Lee SJ, Meinhard BP, Schultz E, and Toledano B: Open reduction and internal fixation of a glenoid fossa fracture in a child: A case report and review of the literature. J Orthop Trauma 11:452-454, 1997.
42. Leslie JT and Ryan TJ: The anterior axillary incision to approach the shoulder joint. J Bone Joint Surg Am 44:1193-1196, 1962.
43. Leung KS and Lam TP: Open reduction and internal fixation of ipsilateral fractures of the scapular neck and clavicle. J Bone Joint Surg Am 75:1015-1018, 1993.

44. Leung KS, Lam TP, and Poon KM: Operative treatment of displaced intra-articular glenoid fractures. Injury 24:324-328, 1993.

45. McClure JG and Raney RB: Anomalies of the scapula. Clin Orthop 110:22-31, 1975.

46. McGahan JP, Rab GT, and Dublin A: Fractures of the scapula. J Trauma 20:880-883, 1980.

47. Mick CA and Weiland AJ: Pseudoarthrosis of a fracture of the acromion. J Trauma 23:248-249, 1983.

48. Montgomery SP and Loyd RD: Avulsion fracture of the coracoid epiphysis with acromioclavicular separation. Report of two cases in adolescents and review of the literature. J Bone Joint Surg Am 59:963-965, 1977.

49. Mudge MK, Wood VE, and Frykman GK: Rotator cuff tears associated with os acromiale. J Bone Joint Surg Am 66:427-429, 1984.

50. Nagle CE and Freitas JE: Radionuclide imaging of musculoskeletal injuries in athletes with negative radiographs. Physician Sports Med 15:147-155, 1987.

51. Naraen A, Giannikas KA, and Livesley PJ: Overuse epiphyseal injury of the coracoid process as a result of archery. Int J Sports Med 20:53-55, 1999.

52. Nettrour LF, Krufky EL, Mueller RE, and Raycroft JF: Locked scapula: Intrathoracic dislocation of the inferior angle. J Bone Joint Surg Am 54:413-416, 1972.

53. Norwood LA, Matiko JA, and Terry GC: Posterior shoulder approach. Clin Orthop 201:167-172, 1985.

54. Oni OO, Hoskinson J, and McPherson S: Closed traumatic scapulothoracic dissociation. Injury 23:138-139, 1992.

55. Oreck SL, Burgess A, and Levine AM: Traumatic lateral displacement of the scapula: A radiographic sign of neurovascular disease. J Bone Joint Surg Am 66:758-763, 1984.

56. Rowe CR: Fractures of the scapula. Surg Clin North Am 43:1565-1571, 1963.

57. Samilson RL: Congenital and developmental anomalies of the shoulder girdle. Orthop Clin North Am 11:219-231, 1980.

58. Sandrock AR: Another sports fatigue fracture. Radiology 117:274, 1975.

59. Schils JP, Freed HA, Richmond BJ, et al: Stress fracture of the acromion [letter]. AJR Am J Roentgenol 155:1140-1141, 1990.

60. Thompson DA, Flynn TC, Miller PW, and Fischer RP: The significance of scapular fractures. J Trauma 25:974-977, 1985.

61. van Noort A, te Slaa RL, Marti RK, and van der Werken C: The floating shoulder. A multicentre study. J Bone Joint Surg Br 83:795-798, 2001.

62. Ward WG, Bergfeld JA, and Carson WG Jr: Stress fracture of the base of the acromial process. Am J Sports Med 22:146-147, 1994.

63. Wilber MC and Evans EB: Fractures of the scapula. J Bone Joint Surg Am 59:358-362, 1977.

64. Zdravkovic D and Damholt VV: Comminuted and severely displaced fractures of the scapula. Acta Orthop Scand 45:60-65, 1974.

GLENOHUMERAL SUBLUXATION AND DISLOCATION IN CHILDREN

The diagnosis and management of glenohumeral dislocation in adults and adolescents is covered extensively in Chapter 14. This section focuses on special considerations for shoulder dislocations in younger children and infants.

Anatomic Considerations

In children, the humeral attachment of the glenohumeral joint capsule is along the anatomic neck, so the capsular attachment is epiphyseal except for the medial portion, which is metaphyseal. The proximal humeral epiphysis develops from three ossification centers. Union of these centers occurs at approximately 7 years of age, with union of the humeral head to the humeral shaft at 14 to 17 years in girls and 16 to 18 years in boys.[12] The strong capsular attachments to the epiphysis make failure of the physis a more common injury than dislocations in children with open growth plates. When dislocations occur, a Bankart lesion is found in 80% of cases.[51] Hill-Sachs lesions occur in over half the patients.[27,28,36]

Incidence

Shoulder dislocations in children younger than 12 years are uncommon. The incidence is reported to be 2.5% to 4.7% of all shoulder dislocations.[54,65] Atraumatic dislocation appears to be more common in younger patients, and the incidence of traumatic dislocation rises with age. Several authors have reported on traumatic and atraumatic dislocations in adolescents with open physes, but the ages of the patients are not generally reported.[1,26,27,40,54,56,64]

Classification

Classification schemes should enable a clinician to identify the etiology of the injury, give a prognosis for the natural history of the problem, and define the treatment. The rarity of dislocations in younger children makes this difficult, and no universally accepted classification scheme exists. Curtis and associates devised a classification scheme based on the etiology of dislocation that has been useful in children.[12] This classification can be further subdivided into the direction of dislocation.

Traumatic
    Anterior
    Posterior
    Inferior (luxatio erecta)
Atraumatic
    Congenital
    Developmental
        Infection, neurologic
    Joint laxity problems
        Ehlers-Danlos syndrome
    Emotional and psychiatric problems

Mechanism of Injury

Traumatic dislocations in children, as in adults, are most commonly anterior dislocations associated with significant trauma from contact sports, falls, and motor vehicle accidents.[1,2,23,40,54,65] Typically, a longitudinal force applied to an outstretched arm forces the arm into an abducted, externally rotated position and levers the humeral head out of the glenoid anteriorly. These injuries may be associated with physeal fractures of the proximal end of the humerus[10,20,46,47] and must be differentiated from true physeal fractures, which can mimic dislocations in infants and neonates.[12,13,22,37] Posterior traumatic dislocation has also been reported in children secondary to trauma and severe spasticity but is very uncommon.[17,19,43] Inferior dislocation with luxatio erecta of the shoulder is likewise rare but has been reported in association with forced manipulation of an infant with a brachial plexus injury.[35]

Atraumatic dislocations occur without a history of significant trauma. Frequently, patients have bilateral involvement with multidirectional or posterior instability and an associated generalized ligamentous laxity.[4,41,44] The dislocations may be voluntary or involuntary.[43,56] In voluntary dislocations, suppression of supraspinatus and infraspinatus muscle activity with firing of the pectoralis major and deltoid while positioning the arm in a vulnerable position produces a dislocation. Congenital dysplasia of the glenoid, excessive retroversion of the glenoid, and developmental abnormalities of the proximal end of the humerus have also been associated with recurrent dislocations.[9,49,66] In addition, dislocation and subluxation of the glenohumeral joint in children have been reported to be secondary to brachial plexus injuries, septic arthritis, Apert's syndrome, and arthrogryposis.[3,9,11,15,30,39,52,61] Three cases of congenital dislocation of the shoulder have also been reported along with reference to several other cases with no history of birth trauma.[24,33,48] Progressive subluxation can occur in fibrodysplasia ossificans progressiva from continued growth in the presence of a humeral-chest wall synostosis.[57]

Signs and Symptoms

A child with a traumatic anterior dislocation has initial signs and symptoms identical to those seen in adults.[40] Pain and swelling develop with an obvious loss of normal shoulder contours as a result of displacement of the humeral head. As in adults, neurologic injury can occur but may be difficult to document in a younger child. In infants and neonates, physeal fractures of the proximal part of the humerus may be clinically indistinguishable from true dislocation of the glenohumeral joint at initial evaluation. The arm will be held abducted and externally rotated.[3,13,22,37,58] Making the diagnosis can be very difficult in children with developmental delay.[31]

Traumatic posterior dislocations of the glenohumeral joint are as rare in children as they are in adults. Marked limitation of shoulder external rotation can be noted, as well as loss of the normal contour of the humeral head anteriorly.[17,43]

Atraumatic dislocations do not have much pain associated with the dislocation. Frequently, clinical findings of generalized joint laxity and multidirectional instability are present.[7,44,53,56] Dislocations associated with congenital anomalies or with brachial plexus injuries are also generally not painful in childhood.[3,9,11,15,61]

Radiographic Findings

The x-ray findings of traumatic dislocations in children are similar to those seen in adults. An anteroposterior film with an axillary lateral and West Point lateral view may demonstrate an associated Hill-Sachs lesion (Fig. 26–40), fracture of the glenoid rim, and congenital abnormalities of the glenoid or proximal end of the humerus.[12] The West Point view is also useful for identifying anteroinferior bony abnormalities.[14] CT-arthrography scans can be useful in defining the anatomy. Recently, MRI has proved helpful in evaluating the pathology associated with shoulder dislocations.[8,45,63] Retroversion of the glenoid can be demonstrated in recurrent posterior dislocators by CT scans.[66] Radiographs for atraumatic dislocations are often normal,[6,6,44,56] but stress views may demonstrate inferior instability (Fig. 26–41).

Treatment

All acute traumatic shoulder dislocations should be reduced.[2,12] Many closed methods have been described in the section on adult shoulder dislocations. The use of intra-articular lidocaine has been popular because it avoids the need for sedation and has been shown to be effective.[42] Closed reduction of a shoulder dislocation associated with a proximal humeral fracture is best attempted under a general anesthetic; however, the result is often unsuccessful and open reduction is required.[10,20,46,47] Immobilization for comfort is achieved with a sling or a sling and swathe. The period of immobilization has not been shown to affect the rate of recurrent dislocations in younger patients.[25,26,40]

The rate of recurrence of shoulder dislocations in adolescents and young adults has been reported to be 25% to 100% within 2 years of the initial dislocation, and most authors have reported a very high rate of redislocation.[1,7,16,25-27,40,53,55,64,65] The presence of an associated tuberosity fracture is associated with a lower rate of redislocation.[26,27] The lowest rates of recurrence have been found in series emphasizing an early and aggressive rotator cuff strengthening program, although the series involved older teenagers.[1,7] However, a recent review found a lower than expected incidence of redislocation,[36] and it will be discussed further.

The rarity of acute traumatic shoulder dislocations in children and adolescents, along with the uncertainty of the natural history of recurrence, leaves surgical indications for this disorder poorly defined. A wide variety of surgical techniques have been used successfully for repair of recurrent dislocations in adults. These techniques are described in Chapter 14 on glenohumeral instability in adults. Most series report young adults and adolescents within their patients but do not separate the results of their younger patients from the overall series. The use of a coracoid bone block technique and an arthroscopically assisted labral repair in adolescents has been reported.[5,18] Lawton and colleagues[36] recently reviewed a large series from the Mayo Clinic. They found recurrent instability in 24% of patients in short-tem and in 9% in medium-term follow-up. Surgical treatment was associated with higher success rates and more stability, particularly for those with a traumatic onset, anterior instability, multidirectional instability, and subluxation. Conversely, surgery did not affect the outcome of patients with posterior instability, voluntary instability, and atraumatic onset.

The initial management of an atraumatic dislocation is a careful history and physical examination, followed by reduction of the dislocation. It is important to be certain that the dislocation was truly atraumatic and to search for anatomic, neurologic, behavioral, or connective tissue abnormalities that may have contributed to the dislocation.[2,7,9,11,46,50,56,66] Reduction of the dislocation is generally easily accomplished. Rapid institution of a vigorous rehabilitation program is usually recommended and has been successful in improving shoulder stability when psychiatric problems are not present.[7,43,44,56] Management of atraumatic recurrent dislocations can be difficult. Habitual dislocators have not been found to have degenerative joint disease or pain over time unless they have undergone shoulder surgery.[29,43,56] In patients with involuntary dislocations, pain may develop with recurrent dislocations. The instability can be unidirectional or multidirectional. Takwale and coauthors[59] reported good results with

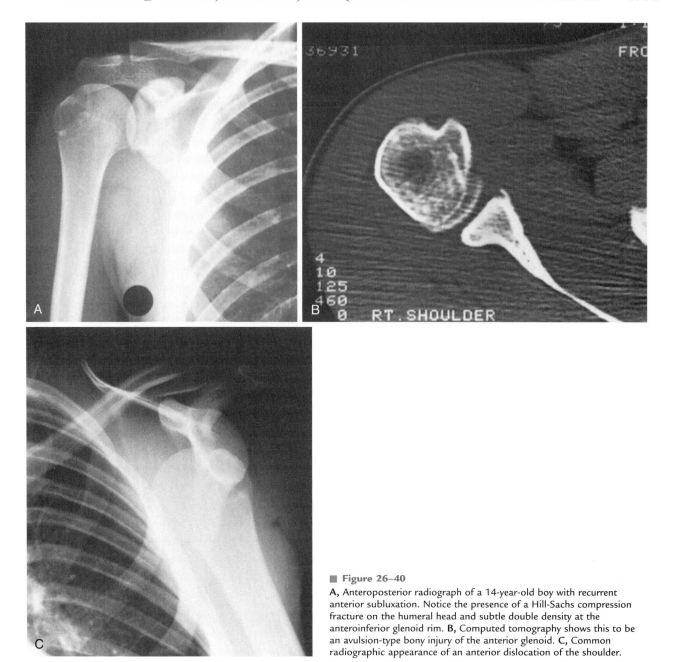

■ **Figure 26–40**

A, Anteroposterior radiograph of a 14-year-old boy with recurrent anterior subluxation. Notice the presence of a Hill-Sachs compression fracture on the humeral head and subtle double density at the anteroinferior glenoid rim. **B,** Computed tomography shows this to be an avulsion-type bony injury of the anterior glenoid. **C,** Common radiographic appearance of an anterior dislocation of the shoulder.

retraining of muscle patterns in these patients. Successful results have also been recorded with the inferior capsular shift as described by Neer and Foster and detailed in the section on glenohumeral instability in Chapter 14.[6,44] Recurrent posterior dislocation may benefit from the combination of a posterior soft tissue and bony procedure.[32,38]

Reduction of chronic shoulder dislocations associated with brachial plexus injuries or obstetric trauma is unlikely to be achieved by closed methods. Open reduction via an anterior approach has been used successfully with capsulorrhaphy and release of the deltoid insertion.[3,15,19,34,35] The subscapularis may be very adherent to the capsule and make dissection difficult.[60] A combined anterior/posterior approach has also been

described.[62] To our knowledge, the natural history of untreated dislocations in these patients has not been documented.

The natural history of shoulder instability associated with congenital or other musculoskeletal abnormalities such as Apert's syndrome is unknown.[11,21,30] Correction of bony abnormalities is recommended if surgical reconstruction is undertaken, but the long-term outcomes of these procedures have not been reported.[9,66] The management of a few cases of true congenital dislocation of the shoulder in small newborns delivered by cesarean section with no radiographic evidence of fracture has been reported.[24,33,48] Treatment consisting of adduction and internal rotation resulted in a stable and normally functioning shoulder and arm by 6 weeks.

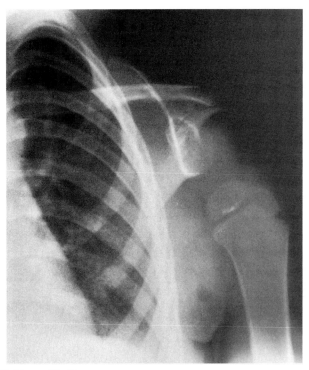

■ **Figure 26–41**
Dramatic demonstration of inferior subluxation of the glenohumeral joint in a patient with multidirectional instability. The clinical correlate is the "sulcus sign."

■ AUTHORS' PREFERRED METHOD OF TREATMENT

For young children or adolescents with a traumatic shoulder dislocation, gentle closed reduction should be performed after a careful physical examination and history. Intra-articular lidocaine with chloral hydrate or intravenous midazolam (Versed) provide excellent analgesia for a closed reduction in children. Alternatively, a more conventional traction/countertraction method under intravenous sedation can be performed. If the child has an associated proximal humeral shaft fracture, the reduction maneuver is done under a general anesthetic because the likelihood of needing an open reduction is high. Immobilization is used for 3 to 4 weeks until the child is comfortable, and a rehabilitation program emphasizing rotator cuff and deltoid strengthening is then instituted. If recurrent anterior dislocations occur, surgical intervention is indicated. We prefer an anterior approach with repair of a Bankart lesion if encountered and capsular advancement to reduce any redundancy found at the time of repair. The techniques for this treatment are described in Chapter 14 on glenohumeral instability in adults. Immobilization in a sling is maintained for 6 weeks, with early pendulum shoulder motion and elbow range of motion instituted in the first month. Resisted external rotation exercises are avoided until 3 months. Progressive strengthening exercises are begun at 3 months and continued until 6 months after surgery. Stiffness and contractures about the shoulder are not generally encountered.

Children with atraumatic dislocations need reduction after an acute dislocation, which is generally easily accomplished. Habitual dislocation should be discouraged. We prefer to manage these children with a rehabilitation program that emphasizs rotator cuff strengthening and behavior modification to discourage voluntary dislocations. If involuntary dislocations persist after 6 to 12 months of supervised rehabilitation in patients with multidirectional instability, we proceed with the capsular procedure described by Neer.[44] Habitual dislocators are treated with rehabilitation and skillful neglect.

We prefer to reduce chronic shoulder dislocations associated with brachial plexus injury or birth trauma by way of an anterior approach and capsulorrhaphy. The supraspinatus and deltoid muscles are generally contracted and may need release or lengthening distally to achieve reduction. In very young children, immobilization of the arm at the side for 6 weeks can stretch these muscles sufficiently so that winging of the scapula does not persist.

Children with congenital anomalies or with shoulder subluxation associated with other musculoskeletal deformities should be carefully assessed for their overall function before embarking on reconstructive surgical procedures to reduce the shoulder. Clearly defined functional goals should guide the surgical efforts. No reported surgical series are available to guide reconstructive efforts.

REFERENCES AND BIBLIOGRAPHY

1. Aronen JG and Regan K: Decreasing the incidence of recurrence of first time anterior shoulder dislocations with rehabilitation. Am J Sports Med *12*:382-391, 1984.
2. Asher MA: Dislocations of the upper extremity in children. Orthop Clin North Am *7*:583-591, 1976.
3. Babbitt DP and Cassidy RH: Obstetrical paralysis and dislocation of the shoulder in infancy. J Bone Joint Surg Am *50*:1447-1452, 1968.
4. Banas MP, Dalldorf PG, Sebastianelli WJ, and DeHaven KE: Long-term followup of the modified Bristow procedure [see comments]. Am J Sports Med *21*:666-671, 1993.
5. Barry TP, Lombardo SJ, Kerlan RD, et al: The coracoid transfer for recurrent anterior instability of the shoulder in adolescents. J Bone Joint Surg Am *67*:383-387, 1985.
6. Bigliani LU, Pollock RG, McIlveen SJ, et al: Shift of the posteroinferior aspect of the capsule for recurrent posterior glenohumeral instability. J Bone Joint Surg Am *77*:1011-1120, 1995.
7. Burkhead WZ Jr and Rockwood CA Jr: Treatment of instability of the shoulder with an exercise program [see comments]. J Bone Joint Surg Am *74*:890-896, 1992.
8. Chandnani VP, Yeager TD, Deberardino T, et al: Glenoid labral tears: Prospective evaluation with MR imaging, MR arthrography, and CT arthrography. Am J Radiol *161*:1229-1235, 1993.
9. Chung SMK and Nissenbaum MM: Congenital and developmental defects of the shoulder. Orthop Clin North Am *6*:381-392, 1975.
10. Cohn BT and Froimson AI: Salter 3 fracture dislocation of glenohumeral joint in a 10-year-old. Orthop Rev *15*:403-404, 1986.
11. Cozen L: Congenital dislocation of the shoulder and other anomalies. Arch Surg *35*:956-966, 1937.
12. Curtis RJJ, Dameron TB Jr, and Rockwood CA Jr: Fractures and dislocations of the shoulder in children. *In* Rockwood CA Jr, Wilkins KE, and King RE (eds): Fractures in Children, 3rd ed. Philadelphia: JB Lippincott, 1991, pp 829-919.
13. Dameron TB Jr and Reibel DB: Fractures involving the proximal humeral epiphyseal plate. J Bone Joint Surg Am *51*:289-297, 1969.
14. De Smet AA: Anterior oblique projection in radiography of the traumatized shoulder. AJR Am J Roentgenol *134*:515-518, 1980.
15. Dunkerton MC: Posterior dislocation of the shoulder associated with obstetric brachial plexus palsy. J Bone Joint Surg Br *71*:764-766, 1989.
16. Elbaum R, Parent H, Zeller R, and Seringe R: Traumatic scapulo-humeral dislocation in children and adolescents. Apropos of 9 patients [French]. Acta Orthop Belg *60*:204-209, 1994.
17. Foster WS, Ford TB, and Drez D Jr: Isolated posterior shoulder dislocation in a child. A case report. Am J Sports Med *13*:198-200, 1985.

18. Goldberg BJ, Nerschl RP, McConnell JP, and Pettrone FA: Arthroscopic trans-glenoid suture capsulolabral repairs: Preliminary results. Am J Sports Med 21:656-665, 1993.
19. Green NE and Wheelhouse WW: Anterior subglenoid dislocation of the shoulder in an infant following pneumococcal meningitis. Clin Orthop :125-127, 1978.
20. Gregg-Smith SJ and White SH: Salter-Harris III fracture-dislocation of the proximal humeral epiphysis. Injury 23:199-200, 1992.
21. Grieg DM: True congenital dislocation of the shoulder. Edinb Med J 30:157-175, 1923.
22. Haliburton RA, Barber JR, and Fraser RL: Pseudodislocation: An unusual birth injury. Can J Surg 10:455-462, 1967.
23. Heck CC: Anterior dislocation of the glenohumeral joint in a child. J Trauma 21:174-175, 1981.
24. Heilbronner DM: True congenital dislocation of the shoulder. J Pediatr Orthop 10:408-410, 1990.
25. Henry JH and Genung JA: Natural history of glenohumeral dislocation—revisited. Am J Sports Med 10:135-137, 1982.
26. Heolen MA, Burgers AM, and Rozing PM: Prognosis of primary anterior shoulder dislocation in young adults. Arch Orthop Trauma Surg 110:51-54, 1990.
27. Hovelius L: Anterior dislocation of the shoulder in teen-agers and young adults. Five-year prognosis. J Bone Joint Surg Am 69:393-399, 1987.
28. Hovelius L: The natural history of primary anterior dislocation of the shoulder in the young. J Orthop Sci 4:307-317, 1999.
29. Huber H and Gerber C: Voluntary subluxation of the shoulder in children. A long-term follow-up study of 36 shoulders. J Bone Joint Surg Br 76:118-122, 1994.
30. Kasser J and Upton J: The shoulder, elbow, and forearm in Apert syndrome. Clin Plast Surg 18:381-389, 1991.
31. Kawaguchi AT, Jackson DL, and Otsuka NY: Delayed diagnosis of a glenohumeral joint dislocation in a child with developmental delay. Am J Orthop 27:137-140, 1998.
32. Kawam M, Sinclair J, and Letts M: Recurrent posterior shoulder dislocation in children: The results of surgical management. J Pediatr Orthop 17:533-538, 1997.
33. Kelly SW: In Surgical Diseases of Children. St Louis: CV Mosby, 1924.
34. Kuhn D and Rosman M: Traumatic, nonparalytic dislocation of the shoulder in a newborn infant. J Pediatr Orthop 4:121-122, 1984.
35. Laskin RS and Sedlin ED: Luxatio erecta in infancy. Clin Orthop 80:126-129, 1971.
36. Lawton RL, Choudhury S, Mansat P, et al: Pediatric shoulder instability: Presentation, findings, treatment, and outcomes. J Pediatr Orthop 22:52-61, 2002.
37. Lemperg R and Liliequist B: Dislocation of the proximal epiphysis of the humerus in newborns. Acta Pediatr Scand 59:377-380, 1970.
38. Letts M: Posterior habitual dislocation of the shoulder [abstract]. Paper presented at a meeting of the Pediatric Orthopaedic Society of North America, 1996, Phoenix, AZ.
39. Lev-Toaff AS, Karasick D, and Rao VM: "Drooping shoulder"—nontraumatic causes of glenohumeral subluxation. Skeletal Radiol 12:34-36, 1984.
40. Marans HJ, Angel KR, Schemitsch EH, and Wedge JH: The fate of traumatic anterior dislocation of the shoulder in children. J Bone Joint Surg Am 74:1242-1244, 1992.
41. Matsen FA, Thomas SC, and Rockwood CA: Glenohumeral instability. In Rockwood CA Jr and Matsen FA (eds): The Shoulder, 1st ed. Philadelphia: WB Saunders, 1990, pp 526-622.
42. Matthews DE and Roberts T: Intraarticular lidocaine versus intravenous analgesic for reduction of acute anterior shoulder dislocations. A prospective randomized study. Am J Sports Med 10:135-137, 1995.
43. May VR Jr: Posterior dislocation of the shoulder: Habitual, traumatic, and obstetrical. Orthop Clin North Am 11:271-285, 1980.
44. Neer CS and Foster CR: Inferior capsular shift for involuntary inferior and multidirectional instability of the shoulder. A preliminary report. J Bone Joint Surg Am 62:897-908, 1980.
45. Neumann CH, Petersen SA, Jahnke AH Jr, et al: MRI in the evaluation of patients with suspected instability of the shoulder joint including a comparison with CT-arthrography. Rofo Fortschr Geb Rontgenstr Neuen Bildgeb Verfahr 154:593-600, 1991.
46. Nicastro JF and Adair DM: Fracture-dislocation of the shoulder in a 32-month-old child. J Pediatr Orthop 2:427-429, 1982.
47. Obremskey W and Routt ML Jr: Fracture-dislocation of the shoulder in a child: Case report. J Trauma 36:137-140, 1994.
48. Peckham FE: Two cases of congenital dislocation of the shoulder. Arch Pediatr 21:509-511, 1904.
49. Petersson CJ and Redlund-Johnell I: Radiographic joint space in normal acromioclavicular joints. Acta Orthop Scand 54:431-433, 1983.
50. Pettersson H: Bilateral dysplasia of the neck of the scapula and associated anomalies. Acta Radiol 22:81-84, 1981.
51. Postacchini F, Gumina S, and Cinotti G: Anterior shoulder dislocation in adolescents. J Shoulder Elbow Surg 9:470-474, 2000.
52. Resnik CS: Septic arthritis: A rare cause of drooping shoulder. Skeletal Radiol 21:307-309, 1992.
53. Rockwood CA Jr: The shoulder: Facts, confusions and myths. Int Orthop 15:401-405, 1991.
54. Rowe CR: Prognosis in dislocations of the shoulder. J Bone Joint Surg Am 38:957-977, 1956.
55. Rowe CR: Anterior dislocations of the shoulder. Prognosis and treatment. Surg Clin North Am 43:1609-1614, 1963.
56. Rowe CR, Pierce DS, and Clark JG: Voluntary dislocation of the shoulder. A preliminary report on a clinical, electromyographic, and psychiatric study of twenty-six patients. J Bone Joint Surg Am 55:445-460, 1973.
57. Sawyer JR, Klimkiewicz JJ, Iannotti JP, and Rocke DM: Mechanism for superior subluxation of the glenohumeral joint in fibrodysplasia ossificans progressiva. Clin Orthop 130-133, 1998.
58. Scaglietti O: The obstetrical shoulder trauma. Surg Gynecol Obstet 66:868, 1938.
59. Takwale VJ, Calvert P, and Rattue H: Involuntary positional instability of the shoulder in adolescents and young adults. Is there any benefit from treatment? J Bone Joint Surg Br 82:719-723, 2000.
60. Torode I and Donnan L: Posterior dislocation of the humeral head in association with obstetric paralysis. J Pediatr Orthop 18:611-615, 1998.
61. Travlos J, Goldberg I, and Boome RS: Brachial plexus lesions associated with dislocated shoulders. J Bone Joint Surg Br 72:68-71, 1990.
62. Troum S, Floyd WE III, and Waters PM: Posterior dislocation of the humeral head in infancy associated with obstetrical paralysis. A case report. J Bone Joint Surg Am 75:1370-1375, 1993.
63. Uri DS, Kneeland B, and Dalinka MK: Update in shoulder magnetic resonance imaging. Magn Reson Q 11:21-44, 1995.
64. Vermeiren J, Handelberg F, Casteleyn PP, and Opdecam P: The rate of recurrence of traumatic anterior dislocation of the shoulder. A study of 154 cases and a review of the literature. Int Orthop 17:337-341, 1993.
65. Wagner KT Jr and Lyne ED: Adolescent traumatic dislocations of the shoulder with open epiphyses. J Pediatr Orthop 3:61-62, 1983.
66. Wirth MA, Lyons FR, and Rockwood CA Jr: Hypoplasia of the glenoid. A review of sixteen patients. J Bone Joint Surg Am 75:1175-1184, 1993.

BRACHIAL PLEXUS PALSY IN CHILDREN

Brachial plexus palsy occurs in 0.1% to 0.4% of all births.[71] Occasionally, it can result from trauma, congenital masses, and viral or Parsonage-Turner syndrome.* Although early examiners saw a number of late cases and had difficulty discerning subsequent deformity from the initial etiology,[55] both experimental[11,43,57] and clinical[7,11] evidence strongly implicates a traction injury. (Fig. 26–42) The incidence is higher in children over 4000 g, particularly in those with shoulder dystocia.[35,66,68] The more difficult the delivery, the greater the likelihood of a plexus injury (Fig. 26–43).[7,30,43] Occasionally, however, the problem may occur without noticeable delivery problems.[31]

Smellie[60] initially described upper root injuries in 1764, whereas Duchenne,[15] in 1861, described the entity in detail. Using electrical studies, Erb[18] showed in 1874 that paralysis at the junction of the fifth and sixth roots, or Erb's point, produces the typical palsy. Flaubert[19] described the characteristic lower plexus palsy in 1827, but Klumpke's later description associated her name with this palsy.[33] Newborn plexus palsies are almost always supraclavicular. The upper plexus is more susceptible to traction within the roots and trunk, whereas the lower plexus is less susceptible to traction injuries but more susceptible to avulsion.

An accurate description of a brachial plexus injury requires anatomic localization and a description of the degree and type of disruption (Figs. 26–44 to 26–47). Typical proximal C5 and C6 injuries produce weak shoulder external rotation, abduction, and elbow flexion (Fig. 26–48). Loss of the extensor carpi radialis brevis and longus causes weak wrist dorsiflexion and radial deviation. The triceps pulls the elbow out into full extension. Upper plexus palsies may also have diaphragmatic

---

*See references 2, 12, 29, 35, 43, 45, 46, 57, 68, 72.

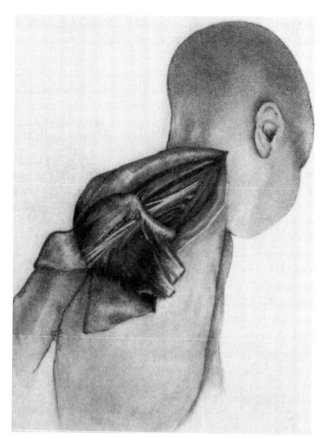

■ **Figure 26–42**

When the head and neck are separated, considerable tension is applied to the junction of the fifth and sixth cervical roots. *(From Sever JW: Obstetric paralysis. Am J Dis Child 12:541-578, 1916.)*

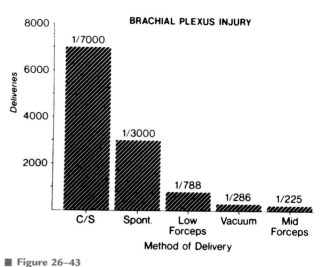

■ **Figure 26–43**

Incidence of Erb's palsy by method of delivery. *(Reprinted with permission from the American College of Obstetricians and Gynecologists. McFarland LV, Raskin M, Daling JR, and Benedetti TJ: Erb/Duchenne's palsy: A consequence of fetal macrosomia and method of delivery. Obstet Gynecol 68:784-788, 1986.)*

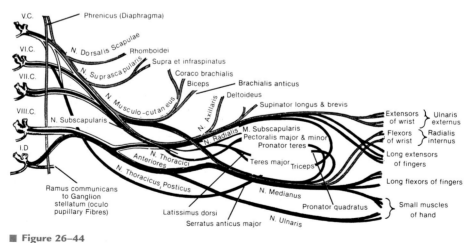

■ **Figure 26–44**

Semidiagrammatic scheme of the brachial plexus demonstrating the nerve supply to the muscles of the upper extremities. *(From Taylor AS: Conclusions derived from further experience in the surgical treatment of brachial birth palsy. Am J Med Sci 146:836-856, 1913.)*

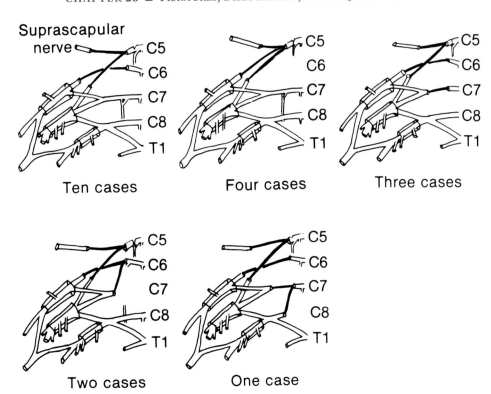

Ten cases   Four cases   Three cases

Two cases   One case

■ **Figure 26–45**
Patterns of placement of sural nerve grafts in 20 patients. Absence of the nerve roots indicates those that were avulsed. *(From Boome RS and Kaye JC: Obstetrical traction injuries of the brachial plexus. J Bone Joint Surg Br 70:571-576, 1988.)*

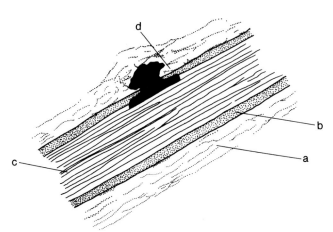

■ **Figure 26–46**
Schematic representation of the pathology in incomplete lesions. Initial rupture of the perineural sheath produces a hematoma (d) involving the epineurium (a), perineurium (b), and nerve bundles (c). *(From Clark LP, Taylor AS, and Prout TP: A study of brachial birth palsy. Am J Med Sci 130:670-707, 1905.)*

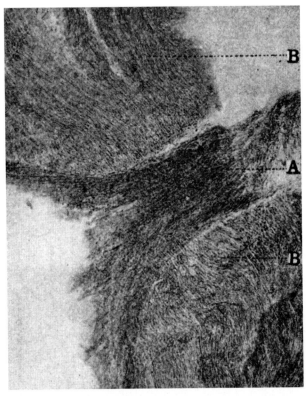

■ **Figure 26–47**
Photomicrograph demonstrating the constricting fibrous tissue (A) across the torn nerve fibers (B). *(From Clark LP, Taylor AS, and Prout TP: A study of brachial birth palsy. Am J Med Sci 130:670-707, 1905.)*

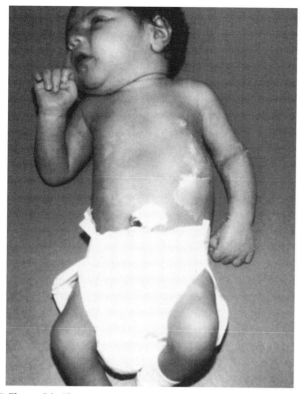

■ **Figure 26–48**
The typical posture of the upper extremity in a newborn with an upper root injury.

involvement via the C4 phrenic roots. If C7 is additionally involved, the triceps will be weak, and the elbow positions in slight flexion. A weak triceps also implies a weak latissimus dorsi, thus making later transfers less predictable. Further weakness of wrist dorsiflexion and radial deviation occurs. Lower plexus palsies (C8, T1) are characterized by weakness of the wrist flexors, particularly the flexor carpi ulnaris, weak forearm pronation, and weakness of finger flexion and extension and weakness of the intrinsic musculature. The forearm is held in supination and the fingers are partially flexed (Fig. 26–49). Total plexus palsies create a flail arm. Zancolli and Zancolli[74] usefully group palsies into proximal, distal, posterior cord,[2] and flaccid. Pure lower plexus or Klumpke's palsies are quite rare.[4]

Although the severity of a nerve injury may be classified according to Seddon and associates' classification of neurapraxia, neurotmesis, or axonotmesis[56] or according to the more detailed Sunderland classification of grades 1 to 5,[62] determination of the grade of injury clinically, especially in a newborn, can be quite difficult. Gilbert and associates recommend a repeat examination after 48 hours, when the examination is easier.[22,23,25] The examination focuses on an asymmetric Moro reflex, an asymmetric tonic neck reflex, the resting posture of the extremity, and any evidence of a cord injury (e.g., no leg function). Other causes of an asymmetric Moro reflex should also be sought, such as a fracture of the clavicle or humerus. Once the infant is a little older, play is useful to examine for active motor function. Particular functions to watch for are active elbow flexion, shoulder abduction, hand opening, and grasp. The typical contracture of an upper plexus palsy is shoulder internal rotation and adduction

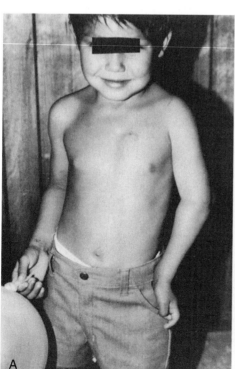

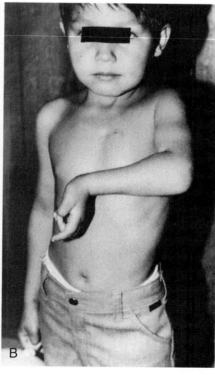

■ **Figure 26–49**
The usual posture of an arm with a lower root lesion: the elbow is extended (**A**) and flexed (**B**).

A   B

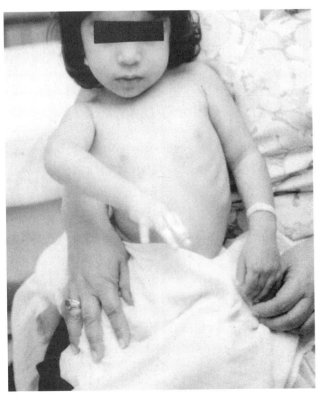

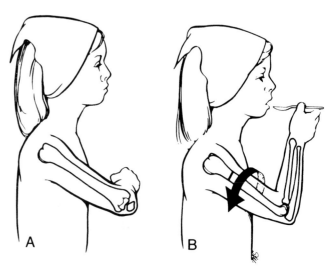

■ **Figure 26–52**

A, With limited abduction and forward flexion, the internal rotation contracture prevents the forearm and hand from reaching the face. **B,** Derotating the humerus approximately 90 degrees enables the hand to be brought to the head and face. *(From Blount WP: Osteoclasis of the upper extremity in children. Acta Orthop Scand 32:374-382, 1962.)*

■ **Figure 26–50**

Even though this patient has shoulder abduction to 75 degrees, she is unable to put her hand to her mouth because of a 45-degree internal rotation contracture.

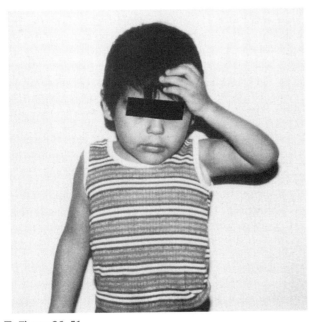

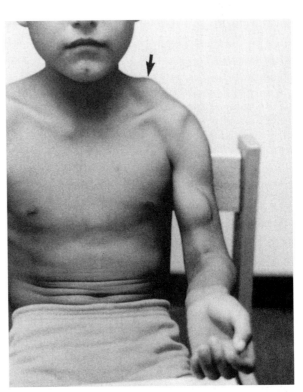

■ **Figure 26–53**

Clinical picture demonstrating elevation of the superior border of the scapula *(arrow)* with external rotation of the humerus and abduction of the arm—the "scapular sign of Putti."

■ **Figure 26–51**

The goal in recovery is to enable the patient to reach the hand to the head or mouth.

and forearm pronation (Fig. 26–50). A severe internal rotation contracture can be a functional problem (Figs. 26–51 and 26–52). Rarely, the shoulder is contracted in abduction or external rotation, but this position is usually secondary to excessively vigorous splinting. A shoulder

contracture can be visualized by Putti's sign (Fig. 26–53)[73]—a contracted glenohumeral joint causes the scapula to wing away from the thorax when the arm is manipulated. In lower plexus palsies, the forearm may be stuck in supination. Once the child is about 3 years of age, a more detailed motor and sensory examination is possible. The involved limb is shorter than the normal side and may have contractures. Once contractures develop, it is difficult to examine a muscle's strength.

In general, recovery of a nerve to a bulky muscle such as the deltoid is better than recovery of nerves to finer muscles such as the rotator cuff. Motor nerves such as musculocutaneous nerves recover better than mixed nerves such as the ulnar nerve. Upper root stretch injuries have a better prognosis than lower root stretch injuries do, and infraclavicular injuries have a better prognosis than supraclavicular injuries do. Factors that indicate a worse prognosis are lower or total plexus palsy, a slow recovery indicative of a more severe disruption, and evidence of root avulsion such as scapular winging (the long thoracic nerve has a very high takeoff), Horner's syndrome (primarily the T1 root), and lower extremity spasticity or a phrenic nerve palsy. A lot of shoulder bruising or physeal separation portends a poor prognosis because of the degree of trauma. The prognostic value of a fracture of the clavicle is less certain.[4] It may decompress the plexus and lead to a better prognosis, or the degree of trauma may portend a worse prognosis. Myelograms, CT-myelograms, or MRI can show traumatic meningoceles in root avulsions but can be misleading.[28,41,44,46] State-of-the-art MRI has been shown to be as effective in diagnosing cervical root avulsion as CT-myelography.[14] Electromyograms may lead to an overly optimistic prognosis in that only minimal nerve regrowth is necessary for reinnervation potentials.[59]

Treatment is made more difficult because of a lack of consensus regarding the prognosis for injuries. Some authors report a very low incidence of recovery, whereas others report full recovery in more than 95% of patients.[8,12,26,29,35,45,73] Early observation should identify the level of the lesion and the rapidity of recovery while treatment should concentrate on range of motion to prevent contractures. Splinting, which was attempted vigorously in the past, can result in debilitating shoulder abduction contractures, luxatio erecta, and radial head dislocations and is rarely used now except on a limited basis for elbow flexion contractures and perioperatively. Bracing has a very limited role, except for rare, specific functions. Children find the braces cumbersome. The braces provide little benefit, and children usually discard them. After a while, even range-of-motion exercises tend to be abandoned.

Early complications that can be overlooked are posterior shoulder dislocation[6,16,36,37,42,65,70,72] and infection.[21,69] To be certain that no shoulder dislocation is present, children with a brachial plexus palsy and limited shoulder external rotation should have an axillary lateral radiograph taken. Findings on clinical examination are similar to those for a dislocated hip—apparent shortening, skin fold asymmetry, deep axilla, posterior shoulder fullness, and occasionally a palpable click. The most important is loss of external rotation. In a paper out of the Texas Scottish Rite, their incidence is 9%.[47] This problem can be treated by open reduction through an anterior or a combined anterior and posterior approach, along with tendon transfer. A neonatal septic shoulder can also be manifested as a brachial plexus palsy.[21,69] Typically, the shoulder and elbow move after birth and stop moving a few

days later. This part of the history is extremely important because infants may not have a fever and early radiographs are usually normal. Any discomfort of the shoulder should bring this diagnosis to mind. Although some of the literature advocates aspiration and intravenous antibiotics,[37] we strongly recommend open drainage through a posterior approach and intravenous antibiotics. In our experience, it still takes several weeks for the "brachial plexus palsy" to resolve.

The last decade has emphasized early exploration and nerve grafting, and Gilbert and associates have advocated the most aggressive approach.[22,23,25] Mallet[40] graded end results on the degree of active motion possible at the shoulder and elbow (Fig. 26-54). Using this scale, Gilbert and Tassin's review[25] indicated that all patients without return of deltoid and biceps function by 3 months of age had poor results; therefore, if biceps function is not present (it is easier to see than deltoid function) by 3 months of age, the patient is scheduled for surgery. Part of the reason for the aggressive scheduling is the worry that some function will return during the next month and parents will refuse the operation. A supraclavicular incision explores the upper plexus, and a continued transclavicular incision explores the lower plexus if needed. With both complete sural nerves harvested, any questionable areas of the plexus are excised, grafted, and held with fibrin glue. Gilbert reports that the surgery improves the natural history by one Mallet grade. Full recovery cannot be ascertained before 4 years.[58]

Only recently have good comparative studies been presented from other centers. Waters[71] reviewed patients with brachial plexus palsies at Boston Children's Hospital. He found that children who recovered biceps function by 1 month of age had essentially normal function. Those who had recovery of biceps function by 3 months of age did better than did those grafted by 6 months of age. However, children observed beyond 6 months did worse than those grafted at the same time. It appears from Waters' study that if no biceps recovery is made by 6 months, nerve exploration is justified. Waters published an algorithm for the treatment of infants with incomplete recovery (Fig. 26-55).[71] However it is still uncertain whether exploration between 3 and 6 months of age would improve the results.

Smith and associates[60a] followed 170 patients. Only 29 did not recover biceps function by 3 months. Among those, patients regaining biceps function before 6 months had better function than those with later return. Likewise, more extensive injuries had poorer results.

Some surgeons try to restore elbow flexion by grafting into the musculocutaneous nerve.[49,74] Neurotization can be performed with the intercostals, the spinal accessory, the phrenic, or any other cervical motor nerve.[27,32,34,46,53,54] Neurotization of nerves to bulk muscles such as the deltoid or biceps is more successful than neurotization of nerves to smaller muscles.[10,61] It has been used successfully to restore shoulder abduction by grafting into the suprascapular and axillary nerves.[10]

In older children, contracture release may allow better muscle function from moderately functional muscles that are unable to overpower the contracture. The mainstay of shoulder contracture release has been the subscapularis release of Sever.[57] This release has been modified by others

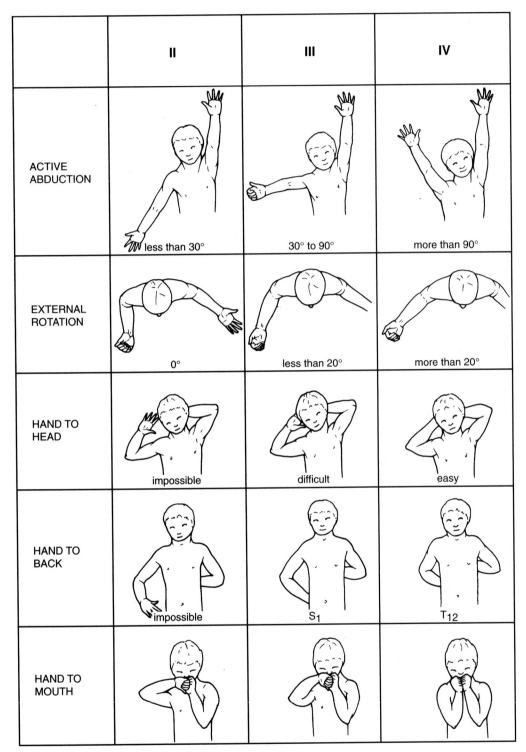

	II	III	IV
ACTIVE ABDUCTION	less than 30°	30° to 90°	more than 90°
EXTERNAL ROTATION	0°	less than 20°	more than 20°
HAND TO HEAD	impossible	difficult	easy
HAND TO BACK	impossible	S_1	T_{12}
HAND TO MOUTH			

■ **Figure 26–54**
Mallet classification of end results from brachial plexus palsy in newborns. *(Adapted from Mallet J: Paralysie obstétricale du plexus brachial. Traitement des séquelles. Primauté du traitement de l'épaule. Méthode d'expression des résultats. Rev Chir Orthop 58[suppl 1]:115, 1972.)*

to prevent anterior subluxation of the humerus. Zancolli and Zancolli lengthen the posterior cuff to allow the subluxation to reduce.[74] An increasingly popular operation is release of the subscapularis origin at an early age as described by Carlioz and Brahimi.[9] We have performed this procedure in patients younger than 2 years and found it quite useful. The approach is made in a virtually blood-

less plane between the latissimus dorsi and the teres minor posteriorly. The small latissimus insertion on the interior angle of the scapula is released to provide direct access to the anterior of the scapula. The scapula is then held with a towel clip or a strong suture on the interior angle to allow manipulation. The subscapularis origin is released, and the muscle is elevated extraperiosteally until

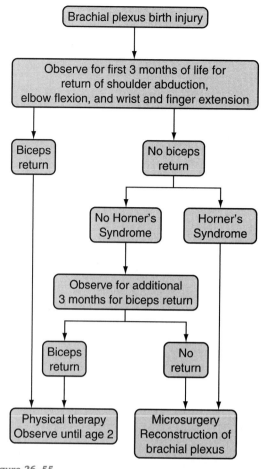

■ **Figure 26–55**

Algorithm for the treatment of brachial plexus birth injury. *(From Waters PM: Obstetrical brachial plexus injuries: Evaluation and management. J Am Acad Surg 5:205-214, 1997.)*

the contracture is freed. The patient is then maintained in a shoulder spica for 4 weeks with the shoulder in external rotation, followed by physical therapy. This procedure must be done while the glenohumeral joint remains congruous. Transfer of the latissimus can be accomplished at the same time or later. Incidentally, we learned this approach from Mary Beth Ezaki and have made it our utilitarian approach to the anterior scapula area for surgeries such as removing benign tumors like osteochondromas.

Numerous tendon transfers to restore motion have been described.[13,17,24,50,52] L'Episcopo[38] released the shoulder contracture and transferred the latissimus dorsi and teres major to the posterior of the humerus to restore active external rotation (Figs. 26–56 and 26–57). Numerous variations of this operation are described. Weakness of internal rotation after this procedure prompted Tachdjian to lengthen the pectoralis major rather than resect it.[63] Zancolli and Zancolli[74] lengthen the latissimus dorsi and circle part of it around the posterior of the humerus, suture it back on itself, and transfer the pectoralis major to the distal subscapularis to restore internal rotation (Fig. 26–58). Phipps and Hoffer transfer the latissimus to the posterior superior rotator cuff to restore active abduction as well as external rotation.[51] Some authors, such as

Gilbert and associates,[24] have modified the Mayer operation by using the trapezius to restore abduction but have not found it to be a very satisfactory operation.

Once deformity is fully established, the humeral head becomes flattened and retroverted and may subluxate or dislocate posteriorly. The entire extremity, including the clavicle and scapula, are smaller with a dysplastic, flattened glenoid. The coracoid process becomes lengthened. In the presence of a deformed humeral head, transfers alone are contraindicated. A humeral osteotomy to relieve the internal rotation contracture can be quite helpful for these patients. It has also been described with some additional flexion to assist in forward elevation,[5] although we have no experience with this modification. We make a deltopectoral approach and expose the proximal end of the humerus. The pectoralis major tendon is step-cut for lengthening. A four-hole plate is used, and the proximal screws are placed. The plate is removed, and the osteotomy is completed. The arm is externally rotated until the hand can be placed at the hip and on top of the head and then slightly externally rotated beyond this point to account for some recurrence. The patient is then placed in a shoulder spica cast. Although this operation does not change the patient's range of motion, it can place the shoulder in a much more functional position.

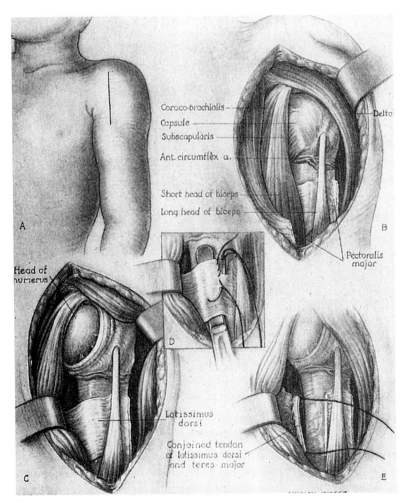

Coraco-brachialis
Capsule
Subscapularis
Ant. circumflex a.
Short head of biceps
Long head of biceps
Delto
Pectoralis major
Head of humerus
Latissimus dorsi
Conjoined tendon of latissimus dorsi and teres major

■ Figure 26-56
The anterior approach for the L'Episcopo procedure. **A,** The incision. **B,** The deep anterior structures after the pectoralis major has been cut. **C,** In the original description both the anterior capsule and subscapularis were cut to expose the head of the humerus. **D,** Presuturing the conjoined tendon of the latissimus dorsi and teres major. **E,** Release of the conjoined tendon. *(Reprinted by permission from the New York State Journal of Medicine, copyright by the Medical Society of the State of New York. From L'Episcopo JB: Restoration of muscle balance in the treatment of obstetrical paralysis. N Y State J Med 39:357-363, 1939.)*

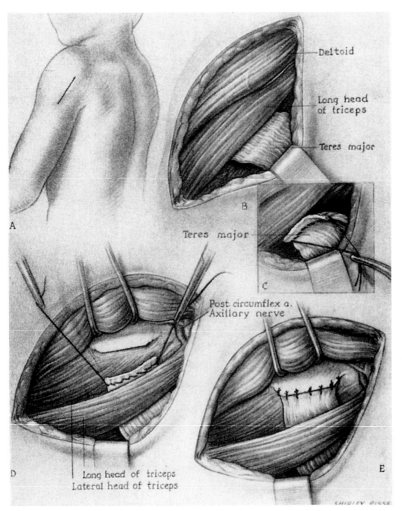

■ **Figure 26–57**

The posterior approach for the L'Episcopo procedure. **A,** Posterior incision parallel to the posterior deltoid. **B,** Exposure of the relaxed teres major posterior to the long head of the triceps. **C,** The conjoined tendons of the teres major and latissimus dorsi are pulled out of the posterior incision of the sutures. **D,** The conjoined tendons are passed under the long head of the triceps. **E,** The tendons are sutured to an anterior periosteal flap. *(Reprinted by permission from the New York State Journal of Medicine, copyright by the Medical Society of the State of New York. From L'Episcopo JB: Restoration of muscle balance in the treatment of obstetrical paralysis. N Y State J Med 39:357-363, 1939.)*

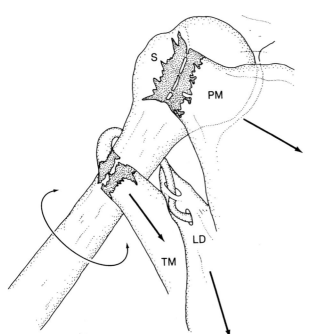

■ **Figure 26–58**

Zancolli's modification of the L'Episcopo procedure. The teres major (TM) is left intact. The distal portion of the Z-plasty of the latissimus dorsi (LD) has been passed posteriorly around the shaft of the humerus and sutured to the proximal portion. The pectoralis major (PM) is sutured to the insertion of the subscapularis (S). *(From Zancolli EA: Classification and management of the shoulder in birth palsy. Orthop Clin North Am 12:433-457, 1981.)*

REFERENCES AND BIBLIOGRAPHY

1. Adler JB and Patterson RL: Erb's palsy. J Bone Joint Surg Am 49:1052-1064, 1967.
2. al-Qattan MM and Clarke HM: A new type of brachial plexus lesion to be added to the classical types [letter]. J Hand Surg [Br] 19:673, 1994.
3. al-Qattan MM, Clark HM, and Curtis CG: The prognostic value of concurrent clavicular fractures in newborns with obstetric brachial plexus palsy. J Hand Surg [Br] 19:729-730, 1994.
4. al-Qattan MM, Clarke HM, and Curtis CG: Klumpke's birth palsy. Does it really exist? J Hand Surg [Br] 20:19-23, 1995.
5. al Zahrani S: Modified rotational osteotomy of the humerus for Erb's palsy. Int Orthop 17:202-204, 1993.
6. Babbit DP and Cassidy RH: Obstetrical paralysis and dislocation of the shoulder in infancy. J Bone Joint Surg Am 50:1447-1452, 1968.
7. Baskett TF and Allen AC: Perinatal implications of shoulder dystocia. Obstet Gynecol 86:14-17, 1995.
8. Bodensteiner JB, Rich KM, and Landau WM: Early infantile surgery for birth-related brachial plexus injuries: Justification requires a prospective controlled study [editorial; comment]. J Child Neurol 9:109-110, 1994.
9. Carlioz H and Brahimi L: La place de la désinsertion interne du sous-scapulaire dans le traitement de la paralysie obstétricale du membre supérieur chez l'enfant. Ann Chirurg Infantile Paris 12:159-168, 1971.
10. Chuang DC, Lee GW, Hashem F, and Wei FC: Restoration of shoulder abduction by nerve transfer in avulsed brachial plexus injury: Evaluation of 99 patients with various nerve transfers. Plast Reconstr Surg 96:122-128, 1995.
11. Clark LP, Taylor AS, and Prout TP: A study of brachial plexus palsy. Am J Med Sci 130:670-674, 1905.
12. Clarke HM and Curtis CG: An approach to obstetrical brachial plexus injuries. Hand Clin 11:563-580, 1995.
13. Comlei JJ, Herzburg C, and Nassan AI: Biomechanical basis of transfers for shoulder paralysis. Hand Clin 5:10, 1989.
14. Doi K, Otsuka K, Okamoto Y, et al: Cervical root avulsion in brachial plexus injuries: Magnetic resonance imaging classification and comparison with myelography and computerized tomography myelography. J Neurosurg 96(suppl):277-284, 2002.
15. Duchenne C: De l'Eléctrisation Localisée et de Son Application á la Pathologic et á la Thérupeutique. Paris: JB Balliére, 1861.
16. Dunkerton MC: Posterior dislocation of the shoulder associated with obstetric brachial plexus palsy. J Bone Joint Surg Br 71:764-766, 1989.
17. Egloff DF, Raffoul W, Bonnard C, and Stadler J: Palliative surgical procedures to restore shoulder function in obstetric brachial palsy: Critical analysis of Narakas' series. Hand Clin 11:597-606, 1995.
18. Erb W: Uber eine eigenthumliche Localisation von Lahmungen im Plexus Brachialis. Verh Naturhistorische Midizin Heidelberg 2:130-136, 1874.
19. Flaubert: 1827. Referenced in Clark LP, Taylor AS, and Prout TP: A study of brachial plexus palsy. Am J Med Sci 130:670-674, 1905.
20. Francel PC, Koby M, Parks TS, et al: Fast spin-echo magnetic resonance imaging for radiologic assessment of neonatal brachial plexus injury. J Neurosurg 83:461-466, 1995.
21. Gabriel SR, Thometz JG, and Jaradeh S: Septic arthritis associated with brachial plexus neuropathy: A case report. J Bone Joint Surg Am 78:103-105, 1996.
22. Gilbert A: Long-term evaluation of brachial plexus surgery in obstetric palsy. Hand Clin 11:583-594, 1995.
23. Gilbert A, Razaboni R, and Amar-Khodja S: Indication and results of brachial plexus surgery in obstetric palsy. Orthop Clin North Am 19:91-105, 1988.
24. Gilbert A, Romana C, and Ayatti R: Tendon transfers for shoulder paralysis in children. Hand Clin 4:633-642, 1988.
25. Gilbert A and Tassin JL: Surgical repair of the brachial plexus in obstetric paralysis [French]. Chirurgie 110:70-75, 1984.
26. Greenwald AG, Shure PC, and Shiveley JL: Brachial plexus birth palsy: A 10-year report on the incidence and prognosis. J Pediatr Orthop 4:689-692, 1984.
27. Gu YD, Zhang GM, Chen DS, et al: Seventh-cervical nerve root transfer from the contralateral healthy side for treatment of brachial plexus root avulsion [see comments]. J Hand Surg [Br] 17:518-521, 1992.
28. Gudinchel F, Maeder P, Oberson JC, and Schnyder P: Magnetic resonance imaging of the shoulder in children with brachial plexus birth palsy. Pediatr Radiol 25(suppl 1):S125-S128, 1995.
29. Hardy AE: Birth injuries of the brachial plexus: Incidence and prognosis. J Bone Joint Surg Br 63:98-101, 1981.
30. Iffy L, Varadi V, and Jakobovits A: Common intrapartum denominators of shoulder dystocia related birth injuries. Zentralbl Gynakol 116:33-37, 1994.
31. Jennett RJ, Tarby TJ, and Kreinick CJ: Brachial plexus palsy: An old problem revisited. Am J Obstet Gynecol 166:1673-1676, 1992.
32. Kawabata H, Kawai H, Masatomi T, and Yasui N: Accessory nerve neurotization in infants with brachial plexus birth palsy. Microsurgery 15:768-772, 1994.
33. Klumpke A: Contribution a lénide des paralysie radiculaires du plexus brachial. Rev Med (Paris) 5:591-593, 1885.
34. Laurent JP, Lee R, Shenaq S, et al: Neurosurgical correction of upper brachial plexus birth injuries. J Neurosurg 79:197-203, 1993.
35. Laurent JP and Lee RT: Birth-related upper brachial plexus injuries in infants: Operative and nonoperative approaches. J Child Neurol 9:111-117, 1994.
36. Leibolt FL and Furey JC: Obstetric paralysis with dislocation of the shoulder—a case report. J Bone Joint Surg Am 35:227-230, 1953.
37. Lejman T, Strong M, Michuo P, and Hayman M: Septic arthritis of the shoulder during the first 18 months of life. J Pediatr Orthop 15:172-175, 1995.
38. L'Episcopo JB: Tendon transplantation in obstetrical paralysis. Am J Surg 25:122-125, 1934.
39. Lichtblau PD: Shoulder dislocation in the infant: Case report and discussion. J Fla Med Assoc 61:313-320, 1977.
40. Mallet J: Parakysie obstetricale du plexus brachial. Traitement des séquelles. Priznaute' du traitement de Lépanle-Méthode d'expression des resultats. Rev Chir Orthop 58(suppl 1): 115, 1972.
41. Mancias P, Slopis JM, Yeakley JW, and Vriesendorp FJ: Combined brachial plexus injury and root avulsion after complicated delivery. Muscle Nerve 17:1237-1238, 1994.
42. May VR Jr: Posterior dislocation of the shoulder: Habitual, traumatic and obstetrical. Orthop Clin North Am 11:271-285, 1980.
43. Meghdari A, Davoodi I, and Meshbah F: Engineering analysis of shoulder dystocia in the human birth process by the finite element method. Proc Inst Mech Eng [H] 4:213-250, 1994.
44. Mehta VS, Hanerji AK, and Tripathi RP: Surgical treatment of brachial plexus injuries. Br J Neurosurg 7:491-500, 1993.
45. Michelow BJ, Clarke HM, Curtis CG, et al: The natural history of obstetrical brachial plexus palsy. Plast Reconstr Surg 93:675-680, 1994.
46. Miller SF, Flasier CM, Griebel ML, and Boop FA: Brachial plexopathy in infants after traumatic delivery: Evaluation with MR imaging. Radiology 189:481-484, 1993.
47. Moukoko D, Wilkes D, Ezaki MB, and Carter PR: Posterior shoulder dislocation in infants with Erb's palsy. Texas Scottish Rite handout. Dallas: American Society of Surgery of the Hand, 2002.
48. Nagano A, Yamamolo S, and Mikami Y: Intercostal nerve transfer to restore upper extremity functions after brachial plexus injury. Ann Acad Med Singapore 24(suppl):42-45, 1995.
49. Narakas A: Surgical treatment of traction injuries of the brachial plexus. Clin Orthop 133:71-90, 1978.
50. Nakaras AO: Paralytic disorders of the shoulder girdle. Hand Clin 4:619-632, 1988.
51. Phipps GJ and Hoffer MM: Latissimus dorsi and teres major transfer to rotator cuff for Erb's palsy. J Shoulder Elbow Surg 4:124-129, 1995.
52. Price AE and Grossmaj JA: A management approach for secondary shoulder and forearm deformities following obstetrical brachial plexus injury. Hand Clin 11:607-617, 1995.
53. Rutowski R: Neurotizations by means of the cervical plexus in over 100 patients with from one to five root avulsions of the brachial plexus. Microsurgery 14:285-288, 1993.
54. Samardzie M, Grujicic D, and Antunovie V: Nerve transfers in brachial plexus traction injuries. J Neurosurg 76:191-197, 1992.
55. Scagliotti O: The obstetrical shoulder trauma. Surg Gynecol Obstet 66:868, 1938.
56. Seddon HJ, Medawar PB, and Smith H: Rate of regeneration of peripheral nerves in man. J Physiol (Paris) 102:191-215, 1943.
57. Sever JW: Obstetric paralysis: Its etiology, pathology, clinical aspects and treatment, with a report of four hundred and seventy cases. Am J Dis Child 12:541-578, 1916.
58. Slooff AC: Obstetric brachial plexus lesions and their neurosurgical treatment. Clin Neurol Neurosurg 95(suppl):S73-S77, 1993.
59. Slooff AC: Obstetric brachial plexus lesions and their neurosurgical treatment. Microsurgery 16:30-34, 1995.
60. Smellie W: A Collection of Cases Preternatural and Observations in Midwifery. London: Wilson & Durham, 1764.
60a. Smith NC, Rowan P, Ezaki M, Carter PR: Neonatal brachial plexus palsy: Long-term follow-up of patients with absent biceps function at three months. J Bone Joint Surg Am. Accepted and pending publication.
61. Songcharoen P: Brachial plexus injury in Thailand: A report of 520 cases. Microsurgery 16:35-39, 1995.
62. Sunderland S: Rate of regeneration in human peripheral nerves. Arch Neurol Psychiatry 58:251-295, 1947.
63. Tachdjian MO: Pediatric Orthopedics. Philadelphia: WB Saunders, 1990, pp 2009-2082.
64. Travlos J, Goldberg I, and Boome RS: Brachial plexus lesions associated with dislocated shoulders. J Bone Joint Surg Br 72:68-71, 1990.
65. Troum S, Floyd WE 3d, and Waters PM: Posterior dislocation of the humeral head in infancy associated with obstetrical paralysis: A case report. J Bone Joint Surg Am 75:1370-1375, 1993.
66. Ubachs JM, Slooff AC, and Peeters LL: Obstetric antecedents of surgically treated obstetric brachial plexus injuries. Br J Obstet Gynaecol 102:813-817, 1995.
67. Vassalos E, Prevedorakis C, and Paraschopoulou P: Brachial plexus palsy on the newborn. Am J Obstet Gynecol 11:554-556, 1968.
68. Walle T and Hartikainen-Sorri AL: Obstetric shoulder injury: Associated risk factors, prediction and prognosis. Acta Obstet Gynecol Scand 72:450-454, 1993.
69. Wang YC, Lin FK, Hung KI, and Wu DY: Brachial plexus neuropathy secondary to septic arthritis and osteomyelitis: Report of two cases. Acta Paediatr Sin 35:449-454, 1994.

70. Waters PM: Is biceps recovery a reliable prognosticator for brachial plexus birth palsy [abstract]? Paper presented at a meeting of the Pediatric Orthopaedic Society of North America, 1996, Phoenix, AZ.
71. Waters PM: Obstetrical brachial plexus injuries: Evaluation and management. J Am Acad Surg 5:205-214, 1997.
72. Wickstrom J: Birth injuries of the brachial plexus: Treatment of defects of the shoulder. Clin Orthop 23:196, 1962.
73. Wilkins KE: Special problems with the child's shoulder. In Rockwood CA Jr and Matsen FA III (eds): The Shoulder. Philadelphia: WB Saunders, 1990, pp 1033-1087.
74. Zancolli EA and Zancolli ER Jr: Palliative surgical procedures in sequelae of obstetrical palsy. Hand Clin 4:643-669, 1988.

ARTHROGRYPOSIS

Arthrogryposis multiplex congenita is a poorly understood condition that is nonprogressive and characterized by multiple joint contractions and muscle wasting.[9,12] More than 150 different disorders with multiple joint contractures have been classified as a type of arthrogryposis.[11] The syndrome is classically grouped into two major types: a neurogenic form and a myopathic form. A high percentage of infants who die of arthrogryposis in the perinatal period will be found to have neurogenic forms.[3] The more classic myopathic form is often called "amyoplasia" and is the type typically seen in orthopaedic clinics. It accounts for up to 40% of patients with arthrogryposis in clinical surveys.[2]

The etiology of this disorder is as yet unknown. Many authors believe that the myopathic form represents a type of congenital muscular dystrophy.[5,8,14] Abnormalities or an absence of anterior horn cells has been found in autopsy specimens.[7] Distal arthrogryposis (type 1) appears to have an autosomal dominant pattern of inheritance and has been mapped to the pericentromeric region of chromosome 9.[1,6] However, many believe that arthrogryposis is a nongenetic disease of early pregnancy associated with multiple intrauterine problems.[16] Viral infections have also been shown to have a connection with arthrogryposis.[14]

The pattern of involvement varies greatly. Forty-six percent of patients have four-extremity involvement, 11% have only upper extremity involvement, and 43% have only lower extremity involvement.[13] Generally, the involvement is bilateral and symmetrical. Patients with upper extremity involvement typically have internal rotation of the shoulders, extension contractures of the elbows, and flexion contractures of the wrists and fingers (Fig. 26-59). The diagnosis of arthrogryposis should meet the following criteria: (1) joint contractures at birth in two different areas of the body (not bilateral clubfeet), (2) no progression, and (3) muscle wasting with fusiform joint configuration.[4]

Treatment

Management of upper extremity deformities in arthrogryposis depends on the motor function of the upper extremity, the degree of contracture present, and the functional needs of the patient.[3,5,11,15] Functionally, the upper extremities should be able to assist in feeding and toileting and should be able to oppose each other.[3,5] Most early surgical interventions should consist of soft tissue surgery, but not before the age of 3 or 4. Individuals with arthrogryposis demonstrate remarkable compensatory

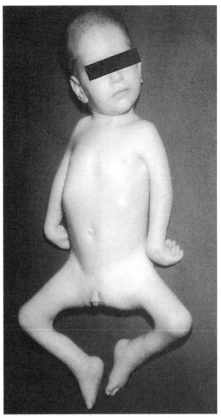

■ Figure 26-59
A photograph of a young child with arthrogryposis involving all four extremities. The upper extremities demonstrate the typical internal rotation of the shoulders, extension of the elbows, and flexion of the wrists and fingers.

strategies. The goal of treatment should be to enhance function and not just create a different appearance. Apparently severe contractures may not limit the individual, and repositioning the extremity may worsen its function. Careful assessment by an experienced occupational therapist is important before intervention is considered.[3,5,11,14,15] The deformities become more fixed as the child grows, even though the disease is nonprogressive. Fusions should not be performed until skeletal maturity.

Nonoperative Treatment

Early stretching and splinting should be considered for infants.[10] Patients often use compensatory strategies involving the trunk and back to make up for absent actions.[3,15] Special adaptive equipment for activities of daily living and clothing can help a great deal to facilitate independence. Most patients with arthrogryposis function well in adult life, but a high percentage remain partially dependent on others. The degree of dependence has been linked more to nonphysical factors than to physical deformity, thus underscoring the need for providing coping skills for these individuals.[4]

Operative Treatment

The shoulder is involved in the majority of individuals with arthrogryposis, but surgical intervention is rarely

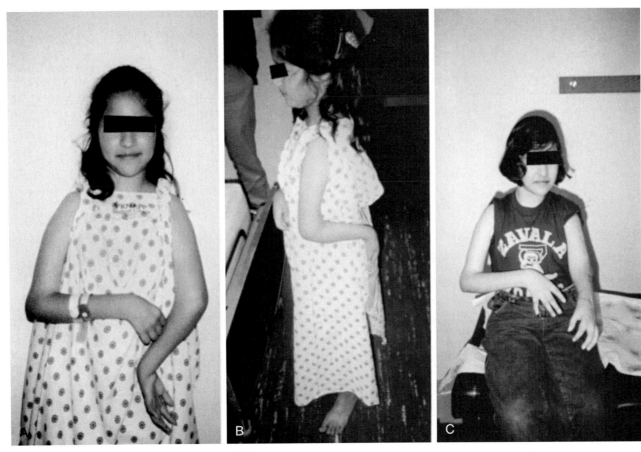

■ **Figure 26–60**
A, Preoperative view of a young teenager who has arthrogryposis primarily involving the upper extremities. The severe internal rotation of the shoulder limits the ability of the hand to reach the face. **B,** Photograph demonstrating the extreme internal rotation of the left upper extremity. **C,** Postoperative view after humeral derotation osteotomy and wrist fusion. The hand can now be brought to a much more functional position.

required. Adduction contractures have not been found to be a major problem for most patients. Occasionally, internal rotation contracture of the shoulder limits access to the face and mouth. Furthermore, if the hands cannot be brought together, manipulation of objects can be difficult, particularly if the hands are severely involved. Tenotomy of the pectoralis major and subscapularis advancement have not been found to be helpful in the management of this problem.[5] Derotational osteotomy of the humerus may be indicated in some situations to allow enough external rotation so that the hand can reach the face and mouth or enough internal rotation so that it may oppose the opposite hand (Fig. 26–60).[3,8,11] Postoperative immobilization should be with a cast or custom orthosis in the optimal position for function.

■ AUTHORS' PREFERRED METHOD OF TREATMENT

Shoulder surgery is rarely needed. Wrist, finger, and elbow function is much more important and should be addressed first. If severe internal or external rotation is present, a derotational osteotomy may be indicated. A proximal osteotomy with pin or plate fixation and post-

operative immobilization in a shoulder spica cast or custom orthosis in the position of optimal function are recommended.

REFERENCES AND BIBLIOGRAPHY

1. Bamshad M, Watkins WS, Zeager RK, et al: A gene for distal arthrogryposis type I maps to the percentromeric region of the chromosome 9. Am J Hum Genet 55:1153-1158, 1994.
2. Banker BQ: Neuropathologic aspects of arthrogryposis multiplex congenita. Clin Orthop 194:30-43, 1985.
3. Bennett JB, Hansen PE, Granberry WM, and Cain TE: Surgical management of arthrogryposis in the upper extremity. J Pediatr Orthop 5:281-286, 1995.
4. Carlson WO, Spec GJ, Vicaro V, and Wagner DR: Arthrogryposis multiplex congenital: A long-term follow-up study. Clin Orthop 194:115-128, 1985.
5. Drummond DS, Siller TN, and Cruess RL: Management of arthrogryposis multiplex congenita. Instr Course Lect 23:79-95, 1974.
6. Kasai T, Oki T, Osuga T, and Nogami H: Familial arthrogryposis with distal involvement of the limbs. Clin Orthop 166:182-184, 1982.
7. Krugliak L, Gadoth N, and Behar AJ: Neuropathic form of arthrogryposis multiplex congenita: Report of 3 cases with complete necropsy, including the first reported case of agenesis of muscle spindles. Neurol Sci 37:179-185, 1978.
8. Lloyd-Roberts GC and Lettin AWF: Arthrogryposis multiplex congenita. J Bone Joint Surg Br 52:494-508, 1970.
9. O'Brien PS, Grapper PT, Tredwell SJ, and Hill JG: Orthopaedic aspects of the Trinsic pseudocamptodactyly syndrome. J Pediatr Orthop 4:469-471, 1984.
10. Palmer PM, MacEwin GD, Bowen JR, and Mithius PA: Passive motion therapy for infants with arthrogryposis. Clin Orthop 194:54-59, 1985.

11. Shapiro F and Specht L: Current concepts review: The diagnosis and orthopaedic treatment of childhood spinal muscular atrophy, peripheral neuropathy, Friedreich ataxia, and arthrogryposis. J Bone Joint Surg Am 75:1699-1715, 1993.

12. Sheldon W, Thursfield W, and Miller R: Amyoplasia congenita. Arch Dis Child 7:119-136, 1932.

13. Swinyard CA and Mayer V: Multiple congenital contractures. JAMA 183:23, 1963.

14. Williams P: The management of arthrogryposis. Orthop Clin North Am 9:67-88, 1978.

15. Williams PF: Management of upper limb problems in arthrogryposis. Clin Orthop 194:60-67, 1985.

16. Wynne-Davies R, Williams PF, and O'Conner JCT: The 1960s epidemic of arthrogryposis multiple congenita: A survey from the United Kingdom, Australia, and the United States of America. J Bone Joint Surg Br 63:76-82, 1981.

CHAPTER 27

OCCUPATIONAL SHOULDER DISORDERS

Manny Halpern, Ph.D.,   Arash Araghi, D.O.,   and Joseph D. Zuckerman, M.D.

• • • •

Musculoskeletal disorders can be characterized as "work-related diseases." The World Health Organization[142] (WHO) defines these diseases as multifactorial, with work contributing significantly, though not exclusively, to causation of the disease. The term "disorder" is more appropriate when some of the outcomes are of uncertain pathogenesis and may consist of symptoms without obvious clinical signs.[135] The term "work-related musculoskeletal disorders" (WMSDs) has come to replace repetitive strain injuries or cumulative trauma disorders. The National Safety Council Standards Committee, accredited by the American National Standards Institute (ANSI), combined these notions and defined musculoskeletal disorders (MSDs) as a disturbance in the regular or normal function of muscle, tendon, tendon sheath, nerve, bursa, blood vessel, bone, joint, or ligament that results in altered structure or impaired motor or sensory function. Accordingly, WMSDs are MSDs that may be caused, aggravated, or precipitated by intense, repeated, or sustained work activities with insufficient recovery; they generally develop over a period of weeks, months, and years.[100] It follows that MSDs can be partially caused by adverse work conditions, can be exacerbated by workplace exposure, and can impair work capacity. The National Research Council adopted a similar definition but emphasized that none of the common MSDs are uniquely caused by work exposure and that physical and social aspects of life outside work need to be considered.[99] In this respect, MSDs would be more accurately defined as activity-related conditions rather than work-related ones. Nevertheless, this chapter will focus on the impact of occupational factors.

The umbrella term MSD comprises a variety of conditions that affect the trunk and the upper extremities. WMSDs of the upper extremities are diffuse neuromuscular illnesses with significant proximal upper body findings that affect distal function.[106] The boundaries of the shoulder region are not clearly defined because the neck, shoulders, and upper part of the arms operate as a functional unit. The boundaries are further complicated in that most of the musculoskeletal problems of this region are nonspecific without well-defined diagnoses. Aside from variable location, the current definitions of MSDs lack criteria for the intensity, frequency, and duration of the symptoms that will be indicative of a "case." Case status is currently based on symptoms that have occurred within a specific time frame (such as a week), at a specific frequency (such as three episodes in the past year), for a given duration (such as a single episode lasting more than 5 days), or with a combination of frequency and severity.[16]

This chapter defines occupational shoulder disorders (OSDs) as work- or activity-related MSDs of the shoulder region. The diagnoses consist of trapezial and parascapular myalgia, rotator cuff and bicipital tendinitis, impingement syndrome, and subacromial/subdeltoid bursitis. Tension neck and cervical syndrome may be viewed as other terms for trapezial myalgia. This chapter will cover primarily myalgias; the other entities are covered elsewhere in this textbook.

The chapter also excludes several other clinical diagnoses. Primary frozen shoulder is idiopathic, and secondary frozen shoulder is usually due to progression of one of the aforementioned conditions or is a consequence of systemic disease. Therefore, it does not conform to the definition of MSD. Thoracic outlet syndrome (TOS) has been defined as an essentially vascular phenomenon that can be objectively documented. Neurogenic TOS, however, is a controversial diagnosis that may rely on physical findings when laboratory tests are often negative. Pascarelli and Hsu[106] encountered neurogenic TOS in 70% of shoulder and upper extremity patients, mostly computer operators and musicians, and postulated that the condition is related to postural derangement. We cannot comment on the etiologic relationship or its work-relatedness and do not consider this condition under OSDs at this point.

The chapter reviews the epidemiology, etiology, and suggested treatment of OSDs. The relationship of acromioclavicular and glenohumeral arthritis with occupational factors is also explored. The chapter further provides general information on primary and secondary prevention of MSDs in occupational settings. The workers' compensation system has been implicated as a contributing factor in the reporting of MSDs. Therefore, the influence of workers' compensation on the outcome of treatment is examined. Finally, the chapter reviews the current disability compensation systems.

OCCUPATIONAL SHOULDER DISORDERS

This chapter uses the descriptive term *occupational shoulder disorder* to denote WMSDs of the shoulder.[9,88] The previous edition of this chapter referred to WMSDs of the neck and shoulder as *occupational cervicobrachial disorders.* This term, which was mainly used in the Japanese, Australian, and Scandinavian literature in the 1970s and 1980s, has not been adopted in the United States. The term *work-related upper extremity musculoskeletal disorders* has also been used, but it includes the elbow, forearm, wrist, and hand.[92]

An OSD refers to a symptom complex that is characterized by vague pain about the shoulder girdle, including the paracervical, parascapular, and glenohumeral musculature.[9,45,57,90,134] It may also be associated with pain that radiates into the region of the upper part of the arm.[7] OSDs are thought to be the result of cumulative trauma associated with the performance of certain activities and tasks.[15,136,138]

Epidemiology

The variable definitions of the disorders make it difficult to estimate the burden of OSDs in the general population. The National Health Interview Survey for 1995 showed a 1.74% prevalence of impairment from upper extremity or shoulder MSDs. However, estimates of incidence in the *general* population, as opposed to the *working* population, are unreliable because more than 80% of the adult population in the United States is in the workforce.[99]

The annual survey of occupational injuries and illnesses conducted by the Bureau of Labor Statistics (BLS) is the most frequently referenced source of information on WMSDs in the United States. The number of occupational injuries and illnesses involving days away from work has been declining since the mid-1990s. Cases attributed to repetitive trauma peaked at 332,000 in 1994 (out of 2.25 million lost workday cases in the private industry); they were down to 247,000 in 1999 (out of 2.75 million). These cases are not all MSDs because under repeated trauma the BLS also includes conditions such as hearing loss. Musculoskeletal illnesses and injuries in the private industry amounted to 582,340 that year, with 56,834 shoulder MSDs and 11,945 neck cases.[25] Connective tissue diseases and disorders, rheumatism, and tendinitis were the most frequent conditions affecting the shoulder. Courtney and Webster[34] cross-tabulated the BLS data and found that the most frequent shoulder injuries were sprains, strains, and tears caused by overexertion; they ranked second to overexertion back injuries. In half the cases, these injuries resulted in 6 days' absence from work. The most severe shoulder injuries, however, were "general symptoms" resulting from bodily reaction and overexertion, with a median of 128 days away from work.

The Safety & Health Assessment and Research for Prevention (SHARP) program of the Department of Labor and Industries in Washington State used Washington State fund–accepted claims data to estimate the burden of workers' compensation claims for rotator cuff syndrome (International Classification of Diseases [ICD] codes 7261, 72611, and 8404; Current Procedural Terminology [CPT] codes 23410, 23412, 23415, and 23420) and shoulder WMSDs.[115] Men accounted for about two thirds of the claims, and the median age of the claimants was the mid-30s. Of all WMSDs of the upper extremity, rotator cuff syndrome incurred the highest median cost per compensable claim: the cost increased from $3570 in 1987 to $9410 in 1992 and then decreased to $6462 in 1995. The median cost of shoulder WMSDs in that period was $350. In both cases, the average burden is much higher than the median because of skewed distribution. Thus, the average cost was $15,790 per case of rotator cuff syndrome and $7980 per shoulder WMSD. The average time lost per claim was 263 days (median, 97) for the first and 213 (median, 41) for the latter. The data for Washington State are probably representative of other states: the data for WMSDs of the upper extremity collected by Liberty Mutual across the United States (10% of the private workers' compensation market) were similarly skewed.[59]

Most of what we know about the etiology of MSDs comes from epidemiologic studies,[99] which show that MSDs are not unique to any occupational group. Occupations reportedly range from meat processors, to apparel workers or assemblers in the manufacturing industries, to data entry operators in offices.

The data published in various studies of the prevalence and incidence of neck and shoulder WMSDs should be viewed critically. In the absence of agreement on case definitions in epidemiologic studies, it has been difficult to estimate the burden associated with these disorders. Contrasting between two extreme definitions, differences were found in prevalence (55% versus 20%), overall disability (14.6% versus 23.2%), difficulty at work (8% versus 15.5%), and the proportion reporting pain interfering with work (27.3% versus 16.2%). Studies using different case definitions therefore lack comparability.[16]

The common trait of the occupational groups reporting high OSD rates is intense exposure to specific work attributes. The attributes associated with an increased probability of MSDs are considered risk factors. It is plausible that individuals who engage in light static occupations would be more likely to suffer from trapezius myalgia, whereas those involved in heavy labor would be more susceptible to rotator cuff disease. However, this hypothesis needs to be verified by epidemiologic surveys.

In 1997, the National Institute of Occupational Safety and Health (NIOSH) studied the epidemiologic evidence for the work-relatedness of neck, shoulder, and upper extremity disorders.[19] The focus of this review was to assess evidence for a relationship between shoulder tendinitis and workplace exposure to the following: (1) repetitive exertion, (2) awkward posture, (3) forceful exertion, and (4) hand-arm vibration. Included were studies relevant to shoulder disorders. These disorders were defined by a combination of symptoms and physical examination findings or by symptoms alone, but not specifically defined as tendinitis. NIOSH also included studies for which the health outcome combined neck and shoulder disorders (tension neck, cervical syndrome, TOS, frozen shoulder, tendinitis, acromioclavicular syndrome), but in which the exposure was likely to have been specific to the shoulder. Diagnoses of shoulder disorders (e.g., tendinitis, acromioclavicular syndrome, frozen shoulder) were based on symptoms determined by interview and physical examination. Shoulder tendinitis included supraspinatus, infraspinatus, and bicipital tendinitis.

The review used five criteria for assessing the evidence: strength of association, temporal relationship, consistency of association, coherence of evidence, and exposure-response relationship. These studies generally compared workers in jobs that involved higher levels of exposure with workers who had lower levels of exposure, with the degree of exposure determined by observation or measurement of job characteristics. The epidemiologic evidence for upper extremity MSDs is summarized in Table 27-1. In the following we focus on risk factors that could be associated with shoulder MSDs. Over 20 epidemiologic studies have provided evidence regarding the relationship between these disorders and the four physical workplace factors.

The review found *evidence* of a positive association between highly repetitive work (factor 1) and OSDs. Of the seven studies that met at least one of the criteria, five reported significant associations (odds ratios varying from 1.6 to 5.0). The evidence has important limitations. Only three studies specifically address the health outcome of shoulder tendinitis, and these studies involve combined exposure to repetition with awkward shoulder postures or static shoulder loads. The other six studies with significant positive associations dealt primarily with symptoms.

The NIOSH review also found *evidence* of a relationship between repeated or sustained shoulder postures (factor 2) with greater than 60 degrees of flexion or abduction and OSDs. Of 13 studies examined, 7 reported significant risk estimates (odds ratios, 2.3 to 10.6). Evidence of both shoulder tendinitis and nonspecific shoulder pain was found. The evidence for specific shoulder postures was strongest in those with combined exposure to several physical factors, such as holding a tool while working overhead. The association was positive and consistent in the six studies that used diagnosed cases of shoulder tendinitis or a constellation of symptoms and physical findings compatible with tendinitis as the health outcome. Only 1 of the 13 studies failed to find a positive association between exposure and symptoms or a specific shoulder disorder. This result was consistent with evidence in the biomechanical, physiologic, and psychosocial literature.

Based on the available epidemiologic studies, the NIOSH 1997 report found *insufficient evidence* for a positive association between shoulder MSDs and force (factor 3) or exposure to segmental vibration (factor 4).

Hildebrandt and coworkers[64] reviewed 27 studies that related climatic factors to MSDs, although none of these studies specifically addressed the subject. In a questionnaire distributed to 2030 workers in 24 different occupations, they found that a third of the workers related symptoms at the lower back and neck-shoulder region to climatic conditions. They perceived that these conditions aggravate their symptoms. Sick leave as a result of neck-shoulder symptoms was associated with climatic factors, particularly draughts. The authors concluded that researchers, workers, and patients consider such a relationship plausible but that the epidemiologic evidence is still very weak.

The NIOSH review of the epidemiologic evidence for WMSDs of the lower part of the back found the strongest associations with combined risk factors. Few studies attempted to investigate combined effects on OSDs. Nevertheless, NIOSH needed to combine risk factors to estimate some risk indicators, for example, force exertion and exposure to hand-arm vibration while operating powered hand tools. The combined effect of the latter risk factors for the upper extremities was demonstrated empirically by Armstrong and colleagues.[11]

OSDs are multifactorial in origin and may be associated with both occupational and nonoccupational factors. The relative contributions of these covariates may be specific to particular disorders. For example, the confounders for nonspecific shoulder pain may differ from those for shoulder tendinitis. Two of the most important confounders or effect modifiers for shoulder tendinitis are age and sport activities. Subjects who have been extremely active in sports seem to have an increased risk for shoulder tendinitis and acromioclavicular osteoarthrosis, and those who have been extremely active in sports and also report high exposure to load lifting during work are at even higher risk.[120] In other words, sports activities add to the workload on the shoulder and increase the risk for OSDs.

TABLE 27–1. Evidence for Causal Relationship between Physical Work Factors and Musculoskeletal Disorders of the Upper Extremities

MSD Location or Diagnosis	Risk Factors					
	Number of Studies	Force	Static or Extreme Postures	Repetition	Vibration (Segmental)	Combination
Neck and neck/shoulder	>40	++	+++	++	+/0	(−)
Shoulder	>20	+/0	++	++	+/0	(−)
Elbow	>20	++	+/0	+/0	(−)	+++
Carpal tunnel	>30	++	+/0	++	++	+++
Hand/wrist tendinitis	8	++	++	++	(−)	+++
Hand-arm vibration	20	(−)	(−)	(−)	+++	(−)

Note: +++, strong evidence; ++, evidence; +/0, insufficient evidence; (−), evidence of no effect.
Based on Bernard BP (ed): Musculoskeletal Disorders and Workplace Factors: A Critical Review of Epidemiologic Evidence for Work-Related Musculoskeletal Disorders of the Neck, Upper Extremity and Low Back. Washington, DC: DHHS (NIOSH), Publication No. 97-141, 1997.

Most of the shoulder studies considered the effects of age in their analysis. However, the NIOSH review concluded that it is unlikely that the majority of the positive associations between physical exposure and OSDs are due to the effects of non–work-related confounders.[19] In view of the NIOSH review estimate of an average risk ratio for OSDs of 4.76 (median, 3.3), it is possible to calculate that on average, 79% of the OSD cases may be attributable to exposure to risk factors at work (the median attributable fraction is close to 70%).

Etiology

Two theories have been proposed to explain the etiology of OSDs: the *organic* or *physiologic* theory and the *psychosocial* theory.[90]

The *organic* or *physiologic* theory is based on the premise that shoulder pain is secondary to overuse caused by static overload. For example, a high prevalence of OSDs has been reported among dental care workers; some were 5.4 times more likely to experience symptoms than a control group of pharmacists.[91] This increased risk is considered to be secondary to maintaining an unsupported awkward working posture with cervical flexion of 45 to 90 degrees and shoulder flexion and abduction of more than 30 degrees for extended periods (Fig. 27–1). Some of the significant associations reported in the epidemiologic studies may have been related to exposure to repetitive work with the distal

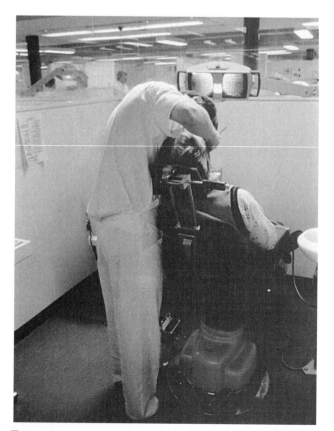

■ **Figure 27–1**
The exceptionally high rate of occupational cervicobrachial disorder among dentists is thought to result from maintenance of an awkward posture for extended periods.

part of the upper extremity while the shoulder and upper part of the arm were maintained in a static posture. However, it is not possible to use the arm/hand without stabilizing the rotator cuff girdle and the glenohumeral joint. Therefore, the dynamic load resulting from repetitive arm, hand, or finger movements is superimposed on top of a static load component at the shoulder.

Much research has been conducted to provide objective evidence in support of the organic or physiologic theory of myalgia. Such studies have involved the use of electromyography (EMG), muscle biopsy, and serum enzyme analysis.

The level of activity at which a static, isometric contraction of shoulder muscles can be sustained without injury is not known.[130] Several researchers have attempted to identify the endurance limit, defined as the highest force possible to maintain for an "unlimited" period. Jonsson and associates suggested that the static load level should always be below 5% of the maximal voluntary contraction (MVC).[76-78] In further support of this suggestion, Sjogaard and coworkers have shown that muscle fatigue occurs at 5% of MVC after 1 hour of sustained contraction.[116]

Various EMG studies suggest that myalgia is manifested as muscle tension. Myalgia has the following characteristics: (1) symptomatic patients exhibit higher muscle tension as evident by EMG records,[41,114] (2) muscle tension is higher at the painful site,[41] (3) pain is reported even when static muscle contraction is as low as 2% to 5% of MVC,[32] (4) the painful side fatigues faster,[53] and (5) patients with neck and shoulder disorders have shorter muscle endurance.[75]

The EMG findings may be explained by evidence of skeletal muscle damage. Decrements in generation of muscle force in the face of repetitive use without nerve damage are evidence of either fatigue of motor units or skeletal fiber damage. The difference is important because loss of force as a result of fatigue is recovered within minutes to hours of rest, whereas fiber damage is repaired more slowly and may be irreversible. Muscle contraction involves metabolic changes in the working tissue, changes in blood flow and consequently intramuscular pressure, and changes in motor unit recruitment. These changes signify fatigue but under some conditions may result in a persistent reduction in generation of force. One of the mechanisms of reduced force generation is damage to contractile structures, such as molecular damage to myosin heads or cross-bridges; methods for testing this hypothesis in intact muscle have not been developed yet.[99] Even though any sustained contraction involves reduced blood flow, interstitial myofibrosis can cause a persistent reduction in blood flow, which in turn may lead to muscle ischemia and fatigue.[12] Muscle biopsy studies have demonstrated degenerated mitochondria and increased glycogen deposits.[42] Fiber structural damage is also accompanied by products of cell inflammation and necrosis, edema, and leaking of intrafiber proteins and enzymes.[99] Thus, Larsson and associates performed bilateral open biopsies of the trapezius muscle in 17 patients with chronic myalgia related to static loads during repetitive assembly work.[83-85] Pathologic muscle fibers were identified and found to be related to the presence of myalgia. Such changes were thought to be secondary to mitochondrial dysfunction as a consequence of reduced local blood flow.

Muscle contraction results in an increase in intramuscular pressure. Ischemic conditions occur when intramuscular pressure exceeds capillary closing pressure at about 30 mm Hg. The increased metabolic demands of the working muscle and the relative ischemia caused by increased intramuscular pressure may contribute to derangements in intracellular pH/lactic acid, calcium, and potassium balance. However, this mechanism probably relates mainly to the onset of muscle fatigue rather than fiber damage.[99]

Disuse and overprotection of the symptomatic extremity have also been suggested to account for the easy fatigability found in the EMG studies.[36] This explanation suggests that muscle injury may be mediated by mechanisms related to muscle recruitment. As muscles fatigue, alternative muscles may be recruited as replacements, even though they may be less suitable for the task. Localized fatigue can occur in very low level contractions, such as those needed to hold the arms in an elevated posture. Slow-twitch fibers are characteristic of the small motor units recruited for low-force, repetitive endurance work. The smaller fibers are also recruited first and remain in action throughout the low-level contractions. Because they carry a disproportionate burden, they are referred to as "Cinderella" fibers.[99] The small, slow-twitch motor units of larger muscles such as the trapezius are therefore vulnerable to fatigue and damage.

The trapezius muscle has been found to be affected by jobs that place high static loads on the muscle.* Excessive scapular elevation as a result of mental stress or workstation design may also contribute to the increased trapezius load.[55,103] In a study of 20 assembly line workers with neck and shoulder pain, Bjelle and colleagues found significantly high levels of muscle enzymes, including creatinine phosphokinase and aldolase, in eight workers, without any underlying pathology.[20,21] The elevated muscle enzyme levels were found to diminish after 2 to 8 weeks of sick leave. Elevated serum creatinine kinase levels have been found in welders, cash register operators, and assembly line workers.[54] Such high levels have not been observed in the control groups (controllers and forklift drivers). The sustained high load necessary for light, static work has been theorized to cause severe adenosine triphosphate depletion, increased permeability, and resultant release of muscle enzymes.[56]

Edwards has proposed that muscle fatigue results from an imbalance between recruitment and relaxation.[38] An alteration in central motor control apparently leads to an imbalance in the use of muscles for static activity as opposed to their use in dynamic work. This theory may serve to explain how mental stress could play a role in causing these disorders.

The *psychosocial* theory[17,18,68,69,125,137] maintains that emotional stress is an etiologic factor in the development of OSDs. The proponents of this theory contend that OSDs occur in jobs that do not involve excessive muscle strain

and, consequently, they are not related to overuse but are more a result of psychosocial factors.[44,89,129] In a study of 607 metal industry workers, depression and distress symptoms were found to be predictors of low back pain, neck-shoulder pain, and other musculoskeletal complaints.[88] Workers may also fear that if they ignore their symptoms, the symptoms may progress and become permanently disabling. Finally, the workers' compensation system can contribute to this problem by awarding benefits based on the recognition that cumulative trauma can cause significant disability. In a study of 201 patients with chronic pain, Tait and associates found that patients with litigation claims reported having pain of significantly longer duration and had significantly more disability than nonlitigating patients did.[124] Bongers and colleagues found that monotonous work, high perceived workload, and time pressure were causally related to musculoskeletal symptoms.[23]

In an effort to address the complex, multifactorial nature of OSDs, Armstrong and coworkers proposed a model that incorporates both the organic and psychosocial theories.[10] In this model, *exposure* refers to external factors such as work requirements that produce an internal *dose*, which in turn disturbs the internal state of the individual. Such disturbances may be mechanical, physiologic, or psychological, and these disturbances in turn evoke a certain *response* that includes the mechanical and metabolic changes that occur at the tissue level of the individual. Finally, *capacity*, which can be either physical or psychological, refers to the ability of the individual to resist destabilization after various doses of exposure. This model provides a framework to explain the relationship between work exposure factors and the different responses that occur, both psychological and physiologic. A similar model was adopted by the panel of the National Research Council.[99]

Management

Evaluation of a patient with a suspected OSD involves a thorough history and physical examination. The hallmark of OSDs is musculoskeletal pain or discomfort that occurs on the job. It typically includes a vague pain associated with burning or numbness and tingling, which may radiate proximally to the neck or distally down the upper part of the arm. Other symptoms may include fatigue and loss of strength. The quality of the pain along with radiation, intensity, rapidity of onset, and aggravating/alleviating factors should be determined. Usually, the diagnosis will fall in one of the categories of myalgia, tendinitis, or bursitis.

Once the diagnosis has been made, successful treatment requires not only an understanding of the basic pathophysiology of the condition but also knowledge of the specific workplace, ergonomics, and any psychosocial and economic aspects that would have an impact on patient management. Feuerstein and Hickey suggested the use of a multidisciplinary approach with a focus on the physical, ergonomic, and psychological factors that may contribute to prolonged disability.[43] In their study they noted that patients treated with a multidisciplinary

---

*See references 22, 32, 49, 52, 58, 72, 77, 78, 139, 140.

approach had a significantly higher rate of return to work than did those treated with usual care. Before making a diagnosis, it is important to consider and rule out other predisposing organic conditions. Sikorski and associates, in a prospective study of 204 workers with occupationally related upper limb or neck pain, found that in the majority (58%) of cases a discrete MSD existed.[114] Neurologic and vascular conditions such as cervical radiculopathy, TOS, and Raynaud's phenomenon could all be associated with OSDs. Congenital or developmental deformities of the shoulder or cervical spine can also predispose a worker to OSDs. Musculoskeletal neoplasms, both benign (e.g., osteochondroma) and malignant, can be found about the shoulder girdle and should be considered. Referred sources of pain from other organ systems, including the cardiac, pulmonary, and gastrointestinal systems, should also be ruled out.

Several classifications of OSDs have been proposed, and such systems have been used for the development of treatment protocols. A five-grade classification system was developed by the OCD committee of the Japanese Association of Industrial Health (Table 27-2). This system includes tendinitis as well as several neurologic and vascular symptoms that often accompany occupational shoulder pain.

A simplified three-stage system was developed by the Occupational Repetition Strain Advisory Committee in Australia. This system is based on persistence of symptom and interference with work (Table 27-3).

Luck and Andersson[90] proposed a pathophysiologic grading system that is a modification of the Australian classification (Table 27-4). This system focuses on myogenic pain.

The pathophysiologic basis for pain in grade I is metabolic changes that occur in response to a sustained static load. Progression to grade II involves pain that does not resolve overnight and is secondary to muscle inflammation and early interstitial fibrosis. Grade III is characterized by progression to severe myopathy with interstitial fibrosis. The more advanced the grade, the longer and more aggressive treatment must be in terms of having time off work and using a multidisciplinary approach.

A large portion of patients in whom an OSD is diagnosed will have signs and symptoms consistent with trapezial myalgia. Patients will complain of pain, tenderness, stiffness, and burning of the upper part of the back and shoulder. On examination, they may demonstrate muscle tightness, increased tone, and multiple "trigger points." Occasionally, subtle decreases in range of motion will be seen. Risk factors for myalgia are unvarying stationary positioning of the shoulder and neck, along with prolonged static loading. Management consists of modalities such as the application of ice and heat. Range-of-motion exercises together with strengthening exercises should also be instituted. Anti-inflammatory agents may be used in moderate cases, supplemented with low doses of tricyclic antidepressants in more refractory cases.

TABLE 27-2.   Japanese Grading System

Grade I
Subjective complaints without clinical findings

Grade II
Subjective complaints with induration and tenderness of the neck, shoulder, and arm muscles

Grade III
Includes grade II and any of the following:
1. Increased tenderness or enlargement of affected muscles
2. Positive neurologic tests
3. Paresthesia
4. Decrease in muscle strength
5. Tenderness of spinous processes of the vertebrae
6. Tenderness of the paravertebral muscles
7. Tenderness of the nerve plexus
8. Tremor of the hand or eyelid
9. Cinesalgia of the neck, shoulder, and upper extremity
10. Functional disturbance of the peripheral circulation
11. Severe pain or subjective complaints of the neck, shoulder, or upper extremity

Grade IV
Type 1
Severe type of grade III

Type 2
Direct development from grade II without passing through grade III, but having specific findings as follows:
1. Orthopaedic diagnosis of the neck-shoulder-arm syndrome
2. Organic disturbances such as tendinitis or tenosynovitis
3. Autonomic nervous disturbances such as Raynaud's phenomenon, passive hyperemia, or disequilibrium
4. Mental disturbance such as anxiety, sleeplessness, thinking dysfunction, hysteria, or depression

Grade V
Disturbances not only at work but also in daily life

TABLE 27-3.   Australian Staging System

Stage I
Aching and tiredness of the affected limb that occurs during the work shift but subsides overnight and during days off work. There is no significant reduction in work performance, and there are no physical signs. This condition can persist for months and is reversible.

Stage II
Symptoms fail to settle overnight, cause a sleep disturbance, and are associated with a reduced capacity for repetitive work. Physical signs may be present. The condition usually persists for months.

Stage III
Symptoms persist at rest. Sleep is disturbed, and pain occurs with nonrepetitive movement. The person is unable to perform light duties and has difficulty with nonoccupational tasks. Physical signs are present. The condition may persist for months to years.

TABLE 27-4.   Pathophysiologic Grading System

Grade I (Mild)
Shoulder girdle muscle pain that occurs during work or similar activities and resolves a few hours later; no findings on physical examination

Grade II (Moderate)
Shoulder girdle muscle pain that persists for several days after work; muscle belly and insertional tenderness on examination

Grade III (Severe)
Shoulder girdle muscle pain that is constant for weeks or longer; multiple tender areas; palpable induration indicative of muscle fibrosis; muscle belly contracture; reduced range of motion of myogenic origin

Introducing more frequent rest breaks along with altering the posture and exertion of force at work can help in alleviating this condition.

Patients can also have signs and symptoms consistent with rotator cuff or bicipital tendinitis and bursitis. The diagnosis and management of these disorders have already been covered elsewhere in this textbook; however, these disorders have specific predisposing risk factors when they are occupational in origin. For rotator cuff tendinitis, repetitive motion, particularly abduction, flexion, and rotation, places the worker at risk, along with heavy lifting and static posturing.[62] Repetitive motion, especially in the overhead position, is a risk factor for the development of tendinitis and bursitis.[119] Bicipital tendinitis, though less common, can occur with repetitive motion in flexion and abduction.[119]

Stress in the workplace can be external, internal, and physiologic. All these factors can contribute to the development of OSDs. External stress resulting from personal issues outside the workplace has been found to increase baseline shoulder girdle muscle tension and reduce the ability to relax these muscles, particularly during high-repetition, static load positions.

Emotional stress results from exposure to environmental and organizational risk factors in the workplace. Such factors include poor lighting, high background noise, cramped working conditions, inadequate work breaks, job dissatisfaction, and excess productivity demands.

Physiologic stress will result from the muscle pain itself. Such muscles are difficult to relax, and consequently, a vicious cycle is established in which sustained static load levels and their duration are increased. This increased stress, in turn, may interfere with a worker's concentration, performance, and productivity. Persistent pain may eventually interrupt the worker's sleep, which further increases the stress level.

Himmelstein and associates suggested that in addition to medical management, more aggressive approaches to obtain control, avoidance of unnecessary surgery, assistance to patients in managing residual pain and stress, and attention to employer-employee conflicts are all-important in preventing prolonged work disability secondary to upper extremity disorders.[65]

DEGENERATIVE JOINT DISEASE

Although the relationship between cumulative trauma and injury to soft tissues about the shoulder girdle has been delineated, the association of glenohumeral arthritis with occupational factors is less clear.[8,30,87,125,128,144] Unlike the hip and knee, the shoulder is not a weight-bearing joint. As such, symptomatic degenerative arthritis of the glenohumeral joint is less common.

A few studies have investigated the association of glenohumeral arthritis with various occupations. Although some of these studies have reported a relationship between certain occupations and osteoarthritis of the shoulder, a direct association has not been found. Kellgren and Lawrence[80] and later Lawrence[86] found that the prevalence of glenohumeral arthritis in men was influenced by occupation. Waldron and Cox studied the skeletons of 367 workers buried in London between 1729 and 1869 and found no significant relationship between occupation and osteoarthritis of the shoulder.[133] Similarly, in a study that included 151 shoulder dissections, Petersson did not find any convincing evidence to support the notion that occupation is a factor in the development of osteoarthritis of the glenohumeral joint.[107]

As with OSDs, sustained load may be associated with the development of glenohumeral arthritis. Dentists seem to be susceptible as a result of sustained static loads while maintaining the shoulder in a position of flexion and abduction with elevation of the scapula. In a Finnish study that included 40 dentists, Katevuo and coworkers found that 46% had radiographic evidence of osteoarthritis and 44% had bilateral disease.[79] In contrast, only 13% in the control group—82 farmers presumably unexposed to static load—had findings consistent with osteoarthritis.

It has been speculated that pneumatic drilling may predispose workers to degenerative arthritis. To examine the effect of vibration exposure on the shoulder, Bovenzi and colleagues compared 67 foundry workers who used vibratory tools with 46 heavy manual laborers.[24] They found no significant difference between the two groups in the prevalence of radiographic changes in the shoulder. In general, it has been difficult to differentiate degenerative changes caused by vibration from those that can simply be attributed to heavy manual work.

Degeneration of the acromioclavicular joint is more common than glenohumeral arthritis. As with glenohumeral arthritis, there is little evidence for a relationship with specific occupations. The NIOSH review cites one study as evidence for an association between acromioclavicular osteoarthritis and occupational force exertion, as well as a dose-response relationship. In a radiographic study of bricklayers and blasters, Stenlund and associates[121] found that the odds ratios increased with the level of lifetime weight handled on the job. When adjusted for age, construction workers had more than a two times greater risk for osteoarthritis of the acromioclavicular joint than their supervisors did. The authors found that construction workers who also engaged in sports activity were more susceptible to acromioclavicular osteoarthritis. Unlike tendinitis, the risk for those with high workloads did not show job-specific trends: although the left side seems to have been mostly loaded at work, the risk for the left shoulder was not higher than that for the right side.[120] It is possible, though, that the odds ratios for the left side in these studies may have been underestimated.[19]

Other studies report contrary findings. In a cadaver study, De Palma found degenerative changes in almost all subjects older than 50 years.[37] Petersson often identified degeneration in 30- to 50-year-old people and regularly in individuals older than 60 years.[108] Because degeneration occurred with equal frequency in men and women and was of the same severity in the right and left shoulders, the occupation may not have been a contributing factor. In a retrospective study that included 83 patients who underwent distal clavicular resection for arthritis, Worcester and Green found no relationship to occupation.[141]

Although a few studies have suggested that the risk factors for OSDs may apply to arthritis, the insidious onset of degenerative disorders makes them more difficult to attribute to work. In summary, there is little evidence that glenohumeral and acromioclavicular osteoarthritis is work related.

PREVENTION

"Ergonomics" is the study of work—the tasks, the technology, and the environment—in relation to human capabilities. In practice, ergonomics is a process of problem solving. The process requires answers to several questions:

- Where is the problem?—the jobs or positions targeted for intervention.
- What is the problem?—the specific risk factors for MSD present on the job, their magnitude, and the body parts at risk.
- Why is there a problem?—the possible ergonomic root causes of the risk factors, specifically, design hazards that may exacerbate MSDs, such as the design of the workstation, tools, and products that need to be handled, as well as the way that work is organized or the techniques that are used by the individual.
- What to do?—prioritizing hazard control measures.

The first two steps require a surveillance of job hazards. Prevention of WMSDs requires methods that focus on assessment of risk factors. Such assessment characterizes the stresses that act on the worker. It establishes the circumstances under which people are affected and the severity of the problems. The physical stresses associated with OSDs rely on the findings of epidemiologic studies. Although the strength of their association with OSDs varies, the epidemiologic evidence suggests that several physical stressors play a role in the etiology, either separately or jointly. Therefore, the following occupational data should be collected:

- Excessive or sustained exertion of force
- Awkward postures, mainly shoulder flexion/extension or abduction
- Repetitive motions of the shoulder and neck*
- Contact with vibrating power tools
- Ambient temperature

Knowledge of the dimensions of the exposure—magnitude, duration, repetitiveness (frequency)—is necessary to assess the risk. The choice of a method is a tradeoff between time, resources, and the level of detail desired. The most cursory task analysis involves a description of the sequence of functions or actions with the use of terms such as transportation, operation, inspection, or storage. The activities of the upper extremities often require a more detailed analysis. The methods range from indirect measures such as self-reports in interviews or questionnaires, through observations, to direct instrumented measures such as electrogoniometry, heart rate monitors, or EMG.

In summary, the multifactorial nature of WMSDs implies that several categories of ergonomic hazard induce a variety of stressors. It therefore follows that several solutions are often possible. By modifying the design of the workstation or the tools, redesigning the work objects, reorganizing the sequence of tasks, or implementing any combination of these solutions, exposure to physical stressors is reduced. The preferable solution would effectively control all or most of the stressors identified on the job. To deal with multiple risk factors, numerous root causes, and a variety of possible solutions, professional and administrative strategies need to be developed.

The strategies adopted to prevent WMSDs can be classified as *primary* and *secondary*. Primary prevention addresses the clinical manifestation of a disease before it occurs. Secondary prevention measures attempt to arrest the development of a disease while it is still in the early symptomatic stage.[109] The first aims at groups of workers, whereas the second focuses on the individual.

By following established practices for controlling exposure to hazardous materials, NIOSH[98] lists four areas of strategy to control and prevent musculoskeletal injuries:

1. Engineering controls to redesign tools, tasks, and workstations
2. Administrative controls, including
   ○ Work practices (job rotation or enrichment, limited overtime, rest breaks)
   ○ Safe work practice training, including body mechanics
   ○ Worker placement evaluation (employee selection)
3. Personal protective equipment such as gloves, padding, and wrist rests and armrests; NIOSH and the Occupational Safety and Health Administration (OSHA) consider braces medical devices rather than personal protective equipment
4. Medical management to minimize the impact of the health problems

The goal of NIOSH's intervention strategy is to eliminate, reduce, or control the presence of ergonomic hazards. These interventions can be used in both primary and secondary prevention and will be discussed in more detail under secondary prevention.

Primary Prevention

For primary prevention, NIOSH recommends a tiered hierarchy of controls in which engineering changes are viewed as the first preference, administrative changes are a second preference, and personal protective equipment is the last choice.

The increase in reported cases of MSD and the increase in workers' compensation costs in the United States prompted some regulatory efforts. Until 1991, attempts to standardize or control exposure to MSD risk factors were limited to specific tasks or situations. American and international standards on exposure to vibration have

---

*Studies usually define repetitive work for the shoulder as activities that involved cyclic flexion, extension, abduction, or rotation of the shoulder joint. The studies operationalize repetitiveness in four different ways: (1) the observed frequency of movements past predefined angles of shoulder flexion or abduction, (2) the number of pieces handled per time unit, (3) short cycle time/repeated tasks within the cycle, and (4) a descriptive characterization of repetitive work or repetitive arm movements.

been available. The Human Factors Society (HFS) together with ANSI issued ergonomic guidelines for video display terminals (VDTs) of computer workstations. These guidelines were not specifically aimed at addressing WMSDs, although they contained technical standards for workstation design, chairs, keyboards, and monitors (ANSI/HFS 100-1988). These standards have been updated in 2002. The International Standards Organization has also established a technical committee for ergonomics (ISO TC 159), with a subcommittee for standardizing the terminology, methodology, and data on anthropometry and biomechanics. Another subcommittee standardizes the dimensions of control stations to prevent awkward postures. The subcommittee for human systems interaction issued standards for VDT workplaces (ISO 9241). These standards will supersede existing directives and guidelines in place in the European Union regarding furniture, hardware, software, and environments for VDT stations.[117]

After high-profile citations under the General Duty Clause, as well as improper reporting of injuries, OSHA issued guidelines in 1993 for managing ergonomics programs.[104] These guidelines were limited to the meatpacking industry. This industry was targeted because of a high incidence and severity of MSDs of the upper extremities. OSHA further emphasized that these guidelines were not a standard or regulation. OSHA's approach focused on ergonomics as a process. The guidelines consisted of a discussion of the importance of management commitment and employee involvement, recommended program elements, and detailed guidance and examples for the program elements. The ANSI-accredited committee for controlling MSDs adopted a similar approach and added medical management to the program elements.[100] The working draft was limited to disorders of the upper extremities.

Unlike the *program* standards, the American Conference of Governmental Industrial Hygienists (ACGIH) chose to develop a *performance* standard for the upper extremities by using an expert consensus process (Physical and Biological Hazards of the Workplace). ACGIH has been involved in several lawsuits in 2001 (see http://www.ACGIH.org). The lawsuits targeted the threshold limit values for chemical exposure only, but they might be applied to physical threshold limit values as well. Thus, it appears that OSHA's reliance on consensus standards such as those of ACGIH and ANSI could face legal challenges in the future.

In the absence of federal regulations regarding the prevention of WMSDs, some local initiatives attempted to fill the gap, with varying degrees of success. Thus, the states of California and Washington introduced ergonomic regulations on their own; those of Washington have been withdrawn in 2003.

Secondary Prevention

The hierarchy of controls in secondary prevention is somewhat different from that of primary prevention because the focus here is on individual patients. Ergonomic accommodations for employees with MSDs fall under the category of secondary prevention. Accommodations are interventions intended to reduce exposure to factors that limit the activities of an impaired individual. More detailed knowledge is required about the residual abilities and limitations of the individual.

Three principal means of accommodating impaired or disabled employees may be implemented: client matching, job restructuring, and job modifications.

A form of employee selection—*client matching*—is the simplest and most effective way to return a person with a disability to work. It involves ensuring that the job requirements are consistent with the present abilities of the employee. If an employee cannot return to the previous job, an alternative job is found that can be performed without risk of reinjury. This strategy does not attempt to fit the job to the worker because it requires hardly any modifications to the job.

Job restructuring is an administrative control to reduce exposure to a risk factor. Two techniques have been proposed for reducing static load on the shoulder: the introduction of rest breaks and job rotation.

Many studies have attempted to find the optimal rest break frequency, duration, and content to prevent shoulder disorders caused by static, repetitive work. Many of the studies have focused on VDT work. NIOSH has recommended a 15-minute rest break after 1 to 2 hours of VDT work.[123] Similarly, the Swedish National Board of Occupational Safety and Health has recommended an upper limit of 1 to 2 hours of continuous video terminal work.[123]

The optimal frequency and length of breaks will depend mainly on the type of work that is being performed, the length of time that it can be sustained, and the posture or load that is held. Breaks can be active, with static load being relieved by dynamic muscle work. Short exercise and stretch periods constitute such breaks, and they seem to be more effective than those that involve complete rest.

By rotating from one job to another, static loading of the shoulders can be avoided. This technique requires careful assessment of task demands to ensure that the shoulders will be relieved occasionally. Although this technique is more easily accomplished in manufacturing industries, it is difficult to introduce in office work, which involves fewer tasks with sufficient variability. Workers may, however, arrange their tasks so that the tasks will periodically take them away from their workstation, for example, interrupting typing activities with photocopying, filing, or other errands. This technique can be viewed as a form of active break rather than formal job rotation.

In secondary prevention, job restructuring entails assigning the impaired employee to restricted duties. For example, restructuring the job by assigning heavy lifting tasks to another person would enable a worker with an OSD or low back pain to work while recovering from the injury.

Job modifications and redesign usually involve the use of assistive technology to enable individuals to perform the required tasks. Other employees may also benefit from similar devices. Occasionally, some tasks can be eliminated in the process of introducing new technology.

The Office of Disability Employment Policy annually examines about 80,000 cases handled by the Job Accommodation Network, a service offered by the Department of Labor to employers and rehabilitation and medical professionals.[102] In 20% of cases, employers were able to accommodate impaired workers at "no cost," probably by rearranging the layout of a workplace, among other factors. Engineering accommodations that require purchasing do not need to be expensive. A survey indicated that between 1992 and 1999, 51% of the accommodations might be called "quick fixes" because they cost between $1 and $500 and only 4% cost more than $5000. Companies reported an average return of $34.58 in benefits for every dollar invested in making an accommodation.[73]

Case Examples

The following are examples of three cases of secondary prevention of OSDs. The first outlines the medical management of a clerical worker with an OSD. The second case focuses on risk factors and their root causes. The third example demonstrates application of the ergonomic solving process in secondary prevention.

Case 1

A 41-year-old, right-hand-dominant secretary at a large investment banking corporation has a chief complaint of right shoulder pain. She described a gradual onset of pain that began approximately 1 year before evaluation. She reports diffuse, poorly localized pain about the right side of her neck and right shoulder region. Her pain is intermittent and varies in terms of severity. In general, however, her pain worsens with work and is alleviated with rest. Specific work activities that exacerbate her symptoms include typing on a keyboard and writing. She spends approximately 9 hours a day in front of a VDT. Initially, her pain occurred solely during work and seemed to resolve at night.

Over the past few months, however, her pain has lingered into the evening and occasionally persists into the first part of the weekend. She has been evaluated previously by several physicians.

She underwent a rheumatologic workup for inflammatory disease, and the result was negative. She has undergone electrophysiologic studies, and the results were also negative. Her physical examination was negative other than the finding of diffuse tenderness of the right trapezius muscle belly. The results of radiographs of the cervical spine and shoulder were negative.

An OSD was diagnosed, and she started on a course of physical therapy that included shoulder and neck range-of-motion and stretching exercises. She was instructed in muscle relaxation techniques and counseled with regard to limiting the number of hours spent at the computer keyboard, as well as the value of rest breaks during her workday.

Her workstation was evaluated by an ergonomist, and several modifications were implemented. These modifications included the procurement of a chair with height adjustment, a wider computer keyboard, and an adjustable stand for holding hard copy that is being transcribed.

After 6 months her symptoms were much improved, and by 1 year she had only minor discomfort that occurred exclusively during her workday and responded to basic stretching maneuvers.

Case 2

Figure 27–2 shows the posture adopted by a standing worker while assembling a fixture at a workbench with a manual screwdriver. The risk factor immediately obvious is the awkward posture of the shoulder—right arm abduction; the task also entails the exertion of force applied to the screwdriver. What are then the ergonomic root causes for these risk factors?

The fixture requires the use of screws, so a screwdriver is needed. The design of the fixture could be modified to simplify the assembly.

The length of the handle of the screwdriver may be one of the reasons that the operating arm needs to be raised. A tool with a shorter handle may enable working in a different posture. Because a manual screwdriver requires repetitive forearm and wrist motion, a powered tool could speed up the assembly and reduce the amount of time working with the arm abducted.

The overall design of the workplace can have a significant influence with regard to the stress placed on the worker's shoulder.[43,66,67,81,82] The specific dimensions and space requirements of the workplace can dictate the amount of load that is placed on the shoulder. Shoulder loads are influenced by arm position,[29,101] the external load that is being handled, and the specific movements of the arm. Chaffin calculated the average time that the arm could be held in various positions of flexion, abduction, and forward-reach.[28] He found that the larger the flexion

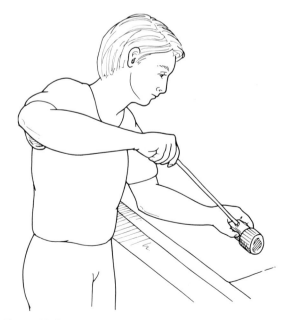

■ **Figure 27–2**
The repeated arm abduction and force exertion involved in assembling a fixture with a screwdriver makes this an example of a high-risk job for musculoskeletal disorders of the upper extremities.

or abduction angle or forward-reach position, the higher the load moment and, consequently, the earlier that fatigue will develop.

Any external load held in the worker's hand or a force applied by the hand will increase the moment acting on the shoulder proportional to the weight of the object, the force applied by the hand, and the distance that the object is held from the shoulder joint. Arm and forearm positions are affected by the orientation of the hand. A supinated hand requires the arm to be adducted and close to the trunk, whereas with a pronated hand, the arm will be more abducted and elevated.

The degree of shoulder abduction is often determined by the vertical height of the work surface. Shoulder abduction can, in turn, lead to rotator cuff disease. Adjustable tables can help limit the degree of shoulder abduction. In a study by Tichauer, it was found that metabolic expenditure increased when the arm abduction angle exceeded 20 degrees.[126,127]

Arm movements influence shoulder load because muscle contractions are needed to accomplish them. In general, the larger the arc of motion, the faster the movement, and the farther that the center of mass of the arm is away from the shoulder, the greater the biomechanical torque acting around the shoulder. In either case, muscle tension increases.

Several methods have been proposed to reduce the load placed on the shoulder. These methods can be divided into two groups: those that reduce the moment arm and those that reduce the external load. To reduce the moment arm, several things can be done, including bringing the workstation closer, standing or sitting close to the workstation, sloping the work surface, adjusting the table height, and adjusting the chair height. The external load can be reduced by dividing it into several individual loads, choosing lighter tools, and providing arm support by using armrests and balance slings. It is also important to

recognize that there is an area of joint reach limits. The workstation may be designed so that the reach target is below the shoulder height of a small woman and the waist level of a large man. In this way, most cases of severe shoulder flexion and abduction can be avoided, as well as trunk flexion.

Case 3

A 43-year-old woman complained of pain in her right shoulder, elbow, and index finger. She was living in a suburban area, divorced without children. She had been experiencing the symptoms for about 6 months, a few weeks after starting working on the assembly line of a plant producing electric engines for adjusting car seats. At first, the symptoms appeared at the second part of her shift work and usually disappeared on the weekend. When a new engine was introduced, production quotas increased. The symptoms became more severe and frequent, and she sought medical care. OSD and lateral epicondylitis were diagnosed. She was on leave for a week but was being paid by the piece, and she preferred returning to work part-time. She encountered difficulty shopping, dressing, and washing. OSHA had cited the plant for various violations, including underreporting of WMSDs. A review of the recordable cases revealed that the incidence rate at the department of the patient was 13 times higher than the national rate for the manufacturing sector.

As part of medical management of the case, an ergonomic assessment of the workstations on the assembly line was conducted. The patient was observed at her position inserting an element into the assembled fixture with a magnetic clip inserter. The results of the assessment are summarized in Table 27–5. Detailed analysis revealed that the task required six operations with the right hand, one of which entailed an awkward posture, exertion of force, and repetitive motion. While using the

TABLE 27–5. Summary of Ergonomic Assessment of a Patient with an Occupational Shoulder Disorder

Job Title: Magnetic clip inserter
Number of Task Elements: Right hand 6/left hand 5

Total Cycle Time: 7 sec
Date:

Where Is the Problem?	What Is the Problem?	Why Is There a Problem?	What to Do?
Task element #5 for right hand: Use magnetic clip inserter	*Posture:* —Shoulder asymmetry —Right arm abduction >45° —Right forearm pronation *Repetitiveness:* —Wrist radial deviation and dorsal flexion *Force:* —Right elbow —Right wrist —Right hand palm contact pressure —Right hand finger 3 and 4 for guiding hand tool	*Tool Design:* T-handle of magnetic clip inserter *Product Design:* Location of insertion on the fixture	*Priority 1:* —Change handle of inserter to a power grip —Looser glove with palm padding *Priority 2:* —Anti-fatigue mats —Foot railing *Priority 3:* —Change location of clip insertion on the fixture —Tilt the conveyor belt toward the operator

Conclusion: High-risk job for right shoulder and right elbow clip inserter, the right shoulder had to be elevated; the arm was abducted more than 45 degrees and stabilized to enable the transmission of force to the hand tool through the forearm and wrist. The hand tool could not be grasped in a power grip and needed to be steered with the index finger. The operation also required leaning forward while flexing the neck to see the insertion.

Job rotation was not deemed an advisable accommodation because other positions on the assembly line had similar risk factors. Various engineering solutions were proposed, with a focus on a new hand tool and better gloves as first priority.

OUTCOMES OF TREATMENT

Few studies have examined nonoperative treatment outcomes for upper extremity MSDs, and fewer still have focused on OSDs. The outcome measure in occupational health for assessing success in the management of work-related injuries has been return to work. However, besides medical intervention, other factors such as age, gender, wages, education, and job characteristics contribute to this outcome.[65] Cheng and coworkers [31] investigated the relationship among employer, provider, and patient outcome measures and how they relate to occupational and clinical factors in a New England workplace physical therapy clinic. They found that 42 OSD patients demonstrated significant improvement in self-assessed physical functioning and body pain scores after an average of about seven visits during a 30-day period of physical therapy. Employer and provider outcomes were moderately correlated: full-time workers were more likely to remain on or return to their jobs, and so did patients who achieved the physical therapist's goals. Although 77% of the patients remained on or returned to their premorbid jobs, pain scores on discharge were still higher than the standard, thus suggesting that the treatment outcome may not be considered successful from the patient's perspective.

Medicolegal factors play an important role in returning to work after an illness or injury. Although conflicting results and opinions have been reported in the literature, most studies find that patients with workers' compensation do not respond to surgery with the same success as other patients do.[14,46,60,61,110,111] The potential for secondary gain is in many cases believed to complicate the recovery of these patients.[50,51] On behalf of compensation patients, one study has been reported by Frieman and Fenlin in which the effect of litigation and workers' compensation claims on the outcome of anterior acromioplasty was examined in patients with chronic inflammation of the supraspinatus tendon caused by impingement syndrome.[46] A comparison of three groups consisting of workers' compensation patients, litigation patients, and those with no apparent financial gain revealed a significantly longer time to return to work (an average of 14.2 weeks versus 4.7 weeks versus 2.5 weeks, respectively), although the patients in the compensation group were involved in heavy labor demanding a more complete return of shoulder endurance. Overall, satisfactory pain relief plus return to preinjury work activities was achieved, with 91% of employed patients returning to full employment despite the potential for secondary gain.

Much more prevalent in the literature is a less optimistic outlook on the postoperative outcome of compensation patients. Misamore and associates reported a comparison of results in two populations of patients undergoing primary repair of the rotator cuff.[96] Twenty-four patients were receiving workers' compensation and 79 were not. The two groups were comparable with regard to age, sex, size of the tear, and preoperative strength, pain, and active range of motion. At a mean follow-up of 45 months, only 54% of the compensation group was rated as good or excellent versus 92% of the noncompensation patients. Similarly, 42% of the compensation group returned to full activity as opposed to 94% of their counterparts in the study. No significant differences were noted between the two groups with regard to the amount of time required to return to work, although fewer of the compensation patients returned to full activity. The average return to work in this study was 6 months, which concurs with a previous report.[14] These authors also noted that most of the unsatisfactory results were due to subjective criteria such as pain, function, and strength. Although both groups had similar active range of motion, fewer than half the patients who were receiving compensation returned to full work activity. After repair of the rotator cuff, those who did return to work were able to do so just as quickly as patients who were not receiving compensation.

Hawkins and coauthors reported similar unsuccessful results in the compensation population after anterior acromioplasty for chronic impingement syndrome with an intact rotator cuff.[60] Of 108 patients, 87% were graded as satisfactory at an average follow-up of 5.2 years. Several factors influenced the results of a 13% failure rate. Most significant was the comparison of patients claiming workers' compensation with those who did not. No differences were found in preoperative profiles or operative findings; however, 22.9% of the compensation group had unsatisfactory results versus 9.2% of the noncompensation group.

EVALUATION OF UPPER EXTREMITY DISABILITY AND IMPAIRMENT

The BLS, the National Center for Health Statistics, and Workers' Compensation Awards are primary sources of estimates for occupational illness and injury data. Statistics on disabilities are collected by National Center for Health Statistics through the National Health Interview Survey; the U.S. Census Bureau collects data as part of the Current Population Survey (CPS) and the Survey of Income and Program Participation (SIPP). Each agency and instrument for data collection uses a different definition of disability. At the present time, the United States does not have any comprehensive national system to keep track of work-related illness, injury, impairment, or disability. In recent years, participation by working-age people in Social Security disability programs has grown from less than 4 million people in 1985 to 6.6 million in 1995. The inflation-adjusted cost of cash benefits rose 66%

from $23 billion in 1985 to $53 billion in 1994. In addition, the cost of providing Medicare and Medicaid to these beneficiaries was about $48 billion. Thus, the cost of cash and health care benefits for disabled beneficiaries in 1994 was $101 billion. The burden of disabilities is naturally larger than the population served by the Social Security programs. The SIPP reports that 32.1 million working-age people (or 18.7% of the population 15 to 64 years of age) have a *disability;* 10% of the people with disabilities have a nonsevere disability. The CPS reports that 17.2 million people, or 9.9% of the 1998 working-age U.S. population (16 to 64 years old), had a disability that prevents or limits work. About a third have a nonsevere work disability. According to the National Health Interview Survey, 16.2 million working-age people have a work limitation (10.5% of the population 18 to 64 years of age).[70]

Disability versus Impairment

In 2000, the WHO introduced a new framework of reference for classifying the consequences of disease or dysfunction that complemented the ICD. The *International Classification of Functioning, Disability, and Health* (ICF) is a classification of health and health-related domains that describe body functions and structures, activities, and participation.[143] The domains are classified with regard to body, individual, and societal perspectives. Because an individual's functioning and disability occur in a context, the ICF also includes a list of environmental factors that describe the context in which individuals live. Having a problem may mean an impairment, limitation, restriction, or barrier, depending on the construct. The WHO moved away from a classification of *"impairments"* to a classification of problems with body structure and function. Similarly, *"disability"* is now viewed as limitations in activities, and *"handicap"* is defined as restrictions in participation.

The classification can be applied to document the impact of a shoulder impairment. For example, symptoms of pain in the shoulder would be classified under sensory and pain body functions; changes in range of motion or stability of the joint would be coded under neuromusculoskeletal and movement-related body functions. The location of the disorder may be coded under shoulder structures related to movement (bones, joints, muscles, etc.). Activities related to mobility may be affected, such as lifting or carrying objects or self-care tasks such as dressing. A disability may ensue if the individual is limited in the performance of these activities. If these limitations cannot be accommodated through assistive technology or social and medical support, participation at work may be restricted, and the person becomes handicapped.

The extent of the problems encountered by an individual may be further expressed as scales called "qualifiers." For example, the extent of impairment may be rated (qualified) on a scale of 0 for "no impairment" to 4 for "complete impairment." Impairments in body structure use qualifiers of the nature of the change and location ranging from 0 for "no change in structure" to 7 for "qualitative changes in structure, including accumulation of fluid." Although the system itself does not provide a link between scores of clinical assessment tools and these qualifiers,

Cieza and coworkers[33] found a high level of agreement between health care professionals regarding the ICF constructs and eight common health status measurements (e.g., Short Form-36, Pain Disability Index and Sickness Impact Profile).

The clinical utility of ICF as well as its usefulness for policy making and planning health services is currently under investigation throughout the world. Thus, the International Paris Task Force on Back Pain adopted the ICF as a framework for its recommendations.[1] In 2001, the National Committee on Vital and Health Statistics of the Centers for Disease Control and Prevention recommended that the U.S. Department of Health adopt the ICF in national studies.[97]

For rehabilitation physicians, the ICF has two notable limitations regarding its practicality. One limitation is that it does not yet relate consequences to specific diagnoses, thus limiting its use in clinical practice and in planning services. In 2002 the WHO began to select core sets of constructs that may be useful for addressing specific disorders or groups of disorders, such as low back pain.[122] Future efforts may address shoulder disorders. A second limitation lies in the scope of the ICF. The system covers consequences in areas such as sexual activity, recreation, home management, self-care, family membership, and social integration, which are not the domain of government regulation in the United States. Compensation systems such as the Social Security Administration (SSA) and workers' compensation are limited to participation in work and employment. For establishing work disability, only a limited set of the ICF taxonomy may be useful.

In 1994, the SSA acknowledged that its disability determination process lacks a conceptually coherent framework.[118] The agency considered the precursor of the ICF as a model,[94] but it has not formally adopted one yet. The SSA and other agencies involved in determination of disability maintain the medical model that focuses on impairment, although they do allow considerations regarding limitation of activities, age, work experience, and others in the process. The process that these agencies implement is described next.

Disability Determination

Determination of disability is an administrative process in which the orthopaedist plays a key role in the evaluation of impairment.[26] When a disability-determining agency requests that a form be filled out or that an examination be performed, usually an assessment of impairment is being sought. Determination of the impact of an individual's impairment on functioning of that individual in society or, more specifically, on employment is usually performed by the determining agency. The complicated infrastructure of disability determination is based not only on medical impairment but also on the interplay of educational level, work experience, available job opportunities, psychological factors, age, and socioeconomic background. Judgments that are based on such a wide range of factors are open to some degree of variation and subjectivity.[2,35,105,112,132] A major source of difficulty in the determination of disability is that medical evaluations are relied on to make decisions regarding work capacity. Such evaluations may very well be performed in the absence of an actual assessment of work-related functional capacity.

Medical impairment encompasses both physical and mental entities, of which the orthopaedic surgeon evaluates anatomic or physiologic defects that interfere with an individual's ability to perform certain functions in a standard fashion. Upper extremity impairments are usually expressed in terms of physical signs such as joint range of motion or decrement in generation of force.[2] Several agencies request that impairment be expressed as a percentage in relation to the whole body. Compensation agencies frequently ask the orthopaedist to determine work restrictions based on the medical evaluation so they can match abilities and disabilities to specific jobs.

The orthopaedist is frequently called on to provide an objective medical evaluation of the impairment in the process of determination of disability. This specialist may be asked to play different roles as an advisor, objective third-party examiner, patient advocate, or adjudicator, depending on different agencies' needs within the various disability programs. In addition, the orthopaedist may be asked to determine and document medical restrictions based on a worker's illness or injury. It is therefore essential that there be a clear understanding of exactly what information the requesting agency wants to know. It should be recognized that in a "gatekeeper" role, the doctor-patient relationship might be directly affected.

The orthopaedist should be knowledgeable and have current information regarding federal and state regulations, as well as employers' work rules. Knowledge of the workplace is an essential component when evaluating a person's disability and return to work. The orthopaedist should have a clear understanding of the factors leading to work-related injuries and disorders. A review of work tasks is essential when determining work-relatedness, as well as contributing factors from previous work experience. A comprehensive assessment should include information about non–work-related activities as well, such as spare-time and sports activities.

One of the most challenging tasks is to ascertain whether the illness or injury is work related. This undertaking can be somewhat complex because not only can there be variations in diagnostic criteria and definitions, but the same disorder may also be considered work related in one case and not in another. The orthopaedist usually has little formal training specific to the workplace. At the request of the Quebec Research Institute on Occupational Health and Safety, an international expert group has created by consensus a database that can be referred to on WMSDs, including those of the upper extremity.

Guidelines for Degree of Impairment

The following sources are helpful references that the orthopaedist can use to evaluate impairment.

The American Academy of Orthopaedic Surgeons' publication *The Clinical Measurement of Joint Motion*[4] provides a standardized, reproducible, and efficient method for assessment of joint motion. Considerable emphasis is placed on range of motion when evaluating shoulder

impairment. Thus, when the various agencies request an assessment of impairment, the orthopaedist can accurately base the assessment of shoulder impairment on range of joint motion on the unaffected side or can refer to the normal comparative data provided in this publication. Normal joint kinesiology, the range of normal joint motion, and the change in joint motion with age are also discussed.

The American Academy of Orthopaedic Surgeons also has a *Manual for Orthopaedic Surgeons in Evaluating Permanent Physical Impairment.*[3] This publication was an attempt to address the problem of inconsistencies that the orthopaedist might face when formulating an opinion on impairment in relation to workers' compensation and personal injury litigation. A scoring system is proposed for the shoulder that can be used as a guide in calculating the percentage of permanent impairment and loss of function in relation to the whole arm.

The American Medical Association has updated their *Guides to the Evaluation of Permanent Impairment*; it is currently in its fifth edition. The *Guides* represents a consensus of experts concerning the best practice for evaluation. A format is specified in which data are acquired to analyze, record, and report information about the impairment. The medical evaluation is based on three components. First, the nature of the impairment and its consequences are documented. Second, protocols are provided to evaluate specific organ systems. The musculoskeletal section contains a protocol that can be used to systematically evaluate upper extremity impairment. Third, tables are provided that relate to the evaluation protocols. For the upper extremity, the range of active motion is rounded to the nearest 10 degrees, and a table is provided to calculate the relationship of impairment of the upper extremity to impairment of the whole person. It should be noted that the validity of these measures for determination of disability has not been adequately studied. The degree to which the procedures predict work disability as a result of soft tissue musculoskeletal impairment has been questioned.[93]

The Minnesota Medical Association has developed a *Revised Temporary Disability Duration Guide*[95] to evaluate a disability that lasts for less than 52 weeks. Impairment is based primarily on the diagnosis and is supported by the medical history, physical findings, and diagnostics.

CURRENT DISABILITY COMPENSATION SYSTEMS

The Americans with Disabilities Act

On July 26, 1990, Congress enacted Public Law 336, the Americans with Disabilities Act (ADA) (http://www.usdoj.gov/crt/ada/adahom1.htm). The act prohibits discrimination and ensures equal opportunity for persons with disabilities in employment, state and local government services, public accommodations, commercial facilities, and transportation. Employment issues are covered by Title I, and the Equal Employment Opportunity Commission (EEOC) is the federal agency that interprets employment discrimination laws and enforces Title I of the ADA. People already in the workforce who incur an MSD have tried to use coverage of the ADA to seek solution to grievances. These cases have been handled by the EEOC. An idea of the impact of the ADA on OSDs may be obtained from the Job Accommodation Network. In the first quarter of 2002, 12% of the cases handled involved the upper extremities and 13% were related to the back. The total caseload since 1984 has exceeded 305,000. This number is much lower than the burden expected from population surveys. Assuming that only a third of the upper extremity cases were related to the shoulder, the ADA may have affected about 12,000 people with shoulder disabilities.[74]

The ADA intends to protect qualified individuals with disabilities from employment discrimination. To understand who is protected by the ADA, it is necessary to understand the definition of an "individual with a disability" and then determine whether the individual meets the definition of a "qualified individual with a disability." An individual is protected by the ADA only if both definitions are met.

The ADA defines an *individual with disability* as a person who meets one of the following criteria:

- Has a physical or mental impairment that *substantially limits* one or more major life activities
- Has a *record of* a statutory disability
- Is *regarded as* being disabled

Neck and shoulder MSDs are a "physical impairment" in the ADA sense because they are a "physiologic disorder" and not a physical trait or characteristic. To qualify as an individual with disability, the impairment has to limit major life activities such as sitting, standing, lifting, and reaching.* A limitation has to be described by its *severity*, *duration* (how long it is expected to last), and *impact* (permanent or long term). The diagnosis does not determine disability, only the impact of the impairment. Individuals with shoulder MSD have encountered the same treatment by the courts as those with low back impairments. The courts have given various interpretations regarding limitations on lifting or reaching as qualifying for disability. To qualify as "substantial," the limitation is expected to affect activities outside work as well as work activities. Limitations on housework, gardening, or child care may not be sufficient.† Limitations on performing manual material handling tasks have been rejected on the ground that the limitation has to affect performance in a class of jobs or a broad range of jobs.‡ Even a "30% service-connected" limitation as a result of shoulder impairment

may not be sufficient if it is not shown that a major life activity is affected.§

A *qualified individual with disability* is an individual ". . . who meets the skill, experience, education, and other job-related requirements of a position held or desired and who, with or without reasonable accommodation, can perform the essential functions of a job."

It is sometimes necessary to identify the *essential functions* of a job to know whether an individual with a disability is qualified to do the job. Written job descriptions provide one form of evidence when determining whether a function is essential. Job or task analyses that focus on the results or outcomes of a function are considered more helpful than those focused on the way that it is performed.[39] These analyses are particularly important when the function can be performed in only a limited way. As industry attempts to increase efficiency through developing a more flexible system of labor specification, each employee may be asked to perform a wide variety of tasks and functions. The lack of detail in these new forms of job descriptions may make it easier to qualify for a job, but it may also make it more difficult to define the essential functions.

Practices covered by the ADA include, among others, testing, evaluation, medical examination, compensation, and leave. The ADA does not eliminate preplacement medical examination as a selection tool. It mandates that medical screening criteria be job related and consistent with business necessity. The latter may require that the individual pose no direct threat to the health and safety of others. The EEOC[40] interprets "direct threat" to include threat to the health and safety of the applicant, but the EEOC interpretation was rejected by a federal district court in Illinois.¶ For a physician examiner to make the required assessment, the specific requirements of the job must be determined, including which duties are essential and which are not. The decision making can be greatly facilitated if job descriptions address the physical requirements of the job and the environmental hazards associated with the work.[27] The ADA limits assessment of an individual's physical capacity if it is unknown what functional abilities are required or what environmental hazards are present.

The EEOC[40] has attempted to clarify some of the issues related to medical examination and testing. In general, tests that measure an applicant's physiologic response, such as heart rate or maximal oxygen uptake, to a physical task, such as running, renders the test a medical examination. As a rule, these tests are interpreted by a health professional. They can be administered after a conditional offer of employment, provided that all candidates are subjected to the same examination regardless of disability (42 U.S.C. §12112(d)(3)). Strength tests depend on the context in which the test is given. If it is used to determine the capability of performing a specific task (lifting a 30-lb box and carrying it for 20 ft), the test is not "medical" and could be administered pre-offer. The test measures the weight of the object handled and the distance carried, not

---

*Currently, the SIPP is the main survey that collects information consistent with the ADA definition. The 1998 survey reported that only 27% of those unable to lift or carry 10 lb were employed.[70]

†Toyota Motor Manufacturing, Kentucky, Inc., v. Williams, Supreme Court No 00-1089. http://www.usdoj.gov:80/osg/briefs/2000/3mer/1ami/2000-1089.mer.ami.pdf

‡See Burgard v. Super Value Holdings, Inc., or 1997 U.S. App. Lexis 12228 (10th Cir. 1997) regarding the lower part of the back and Sherrod v. American Airlines, Case No. 97-10011 (5th Cir, January 28, 1998), or McKay v. Toyota Motor Manufacturing, 110 F.3d 369 (1997), regarding neck impairments.

§Bailey v. Runyon, Postmaster General, U.S. Postal Service.

¶Kohnke v. Delta Airlines, Inc., 8 NDLR§221 (N.D. Ill. 1966) (No. 93 C 7096).

the person's physiologic response. The distinction is subtle but legally significant.

Workers' Compensation

Workers' compensation is a no-fault insurance system for work-related accidental injury and occupational disease for federal and state workers. Federal government employees receive benefits under the Federal Employees' Compensation Act, and state employees are provided for by separate legislation in state workers' compensation laws enacted by each state. Worker compensation laws share many characteristics but also have important differences in the federal and state systems. To further complicate the issue of what is compensable under workers' compensation, compensable conditions can vary from one state to the next, as well as benefit amounts, processing of claims, and settlement of disputes.[63] It is important that the orthopaedist understand the requirements of the state workers' compensation system. Under workers' compensation, employers must provide medical treatment and compensation benefits to employees for work-related illness or injury. Employers must demonstrate their ability to pay for workers' compensation costs by obtaining insurance coverage through a state fund or private carrier or by self-insurance. Four categories of compensable disabilities may be provided for under state workers' compensation: temporary total disability, temporary partial disability, permanent total disability, and permanent partial disability. The largest number of workers' compensation cases is for temporary disability, which accounts for about three fourths of compensable claims. In addition to paying medical expenses and compensating workers for lost wages, state workers' compensation provides for survivors' benefits and vocational rehabilitation. In a study conducted by the Minnesota Blue Cross, workers' compensation costs were found to be almost twice the cost for similar conditions when compared with general liability claims.

To qualify for an award, a worker has to demonstrate that the injury occurred as a result of and in the course of employment. Satisfying criteria for a compensation claim is not an issue in the case of injuries induced by overt external force; however, in the absence of trauma, assertions of work-relatedness may be more difficult to establish. Most states require that injured employees be unable to perform their level of work or obtain employment that is suitable to their qualifications and training.

The American Medical Association's *Guides to the Evaluation of Permanent Impairment* provides a standard framework and method of analysis through which physicians can evaluate, report on, and communicate information about shoulder impairment.[5,48] It is either recommended or mandated by law in workers' compensation cases in 38 states and two territories in the United States. The most current edition should be used.

Under workers' compensation, impairment is a medical issue and is defined as an alteration in an individual's health status that interferes with activities of daily living. When using the American Medical Association's guidelines, the orthopaedist can represent to what degree

an individual's capacity to carry out daily activities has been diminished. Permanent impairment is defined as one that has become static or stabilized during a period sufficient to allow optimal tissue repair and one that is unlikely to change despite further medical or surgical therapy.

Under workers' compensation, the evaluation or rating of a disability is a nonmedical assessment. Disability is defined as a decrease or loss or absence of the capacity of an individual to meet personal, social, or occupational demands or to meet statutory or regulatory requirements because of an impairment. A disability refers to a task that an individual cannot do; it arises out of the interaction between impairment and external requirements, with an emphasis on the person's occupation. It logically follows that "impaired" individuals are not necessarily "disabled" with regard to their occupation. Impaired individual are considered handicapped if they have obstacles to accomplish basic activities that can be overcome by compensating in some way for the effects of the impairment. The most common cause of a dispute over compensation claims is determination of the extent of the disability. A physician's expert opinion is then requested, and a hearing is held before the workers' compensation agency.

Railroad and Maritime Workers' Compensation

The Federal Employer's Liability Act (FELA) supersedes state compensation laws and provides for a comprehensive injury compensation system for railroad workers. Unlike state compensation laws, there are no limits on awards, and consequently the system is expensive. Although the physician determines the magnitude of impairment, under FELA a jury decides the degree of the injured worker's disability. The Jones Act provides compensation for maritime workers and provides the same rights and remedies as FELA.

Social Security

Two disability compensation programs are administered by the SSA. Workers with a recent work history in Social Security–covered employment are eligible for the Social Security Disability Insurance program. Individuals who have no recent work history but who meet a financial needs test receive benefits under the disability portion of the Supplemental Security Income Program. Both programs use the same definition of disability and the same regulations for determining disability. Disability under the Social Security Program is defined in economic terms and in terms of the person's ability to work.[71] Individuals are considered disabled if the impairment is of such severity that they are unable to do the work previously performed and are not able to be engaged in any other kind of substantial gainful work as a result of the person's age, education, and occupational experience. To be considered for benefits, a worker must be unable to work for at least 6 months. This definition of disability is more restrictive than that of other agencies in that the medically determined physical or mental impairment is expected to result in death or to last for at least 12 months. The impairment must have demonstrable anatomic, physiologic, or psychological abnormalities demonstrated by medically accepted clinical and laboratory diagnostic techniques. The Social Security Program has established medical criteria referred to as the "listing of impairments" that define disorders and the level of severity that supposedly prevents a person from working. Unlike workers' compensation, recipients of Social Security are subject to periodic review to determine continued eligibility.

Approximately two thirds of the initial disability claims are denied by Social Security. A claimant's eligibility is determined by a team of examiners based on a review of the records. If a person is denied benefits, there is an appeal process whereby the case is reconsidered by another team of examiners. If benefits are still denied, the claimant is seen in person by a decision maker and the claim may go to the Appeals Council of the SSA and ultimately to the federal courts.

The orthopaedist is required to furnish sufficient medical evidence to Social Security, including the medical history, clinical findings, laboratory findings, diagnosis based on signs and symptoms, prescribed treatment and prognosis, and a medical source statement describing what the patient can do despite the impairment (i.e., work-related activities such as sitting, walking, lifting, or carrying).

Private Insurance Companies

Individual disability income policies pay a fixed monetary amount of coverage and may be integrated with other public disability programs. They are provided on both an individual and a group basis. In general, benefits may be provided either for a stated period or until the attainment of a specific age. Most policies require that the beneficiary be re-examined by a physician designated by the insurance company to ensure continuation of benefits. Disability is defined in various ways, and the requirements of coverage are determined by each company individually.

Private agencies may request that the orthopaedic surgeon determine either short-term or permanent ability to work. The calculation of time off work is often determined by the orthopaedist's experience with a similar diagnosis. Good communication and candor between the orthopaedist, the patient, and the insurance company are necessary to achieve the desired goal of return to work.

CONCLUSION

Occupational shoulder disorders refer to a symptom complex that is characterized by vague pain about the shoulder girdle, including the paracervical, parascapular, and glenohumeral musculature; this chapter did not address tendinitis and nerve impingement syndromes, which are also included under OSDs. Though not clearly defined, epidemiologic evidence has shown a relationship between mechanical stress, such as static or awkward posture and repetitive motions, and health outcomes classified as OSDs.

Several hypotheses have been postulated to explain the injury mechanism triggered by exposure to the mechanical stressors. Decrements in generation of muscle force have been demonstrated in EMG studies, as well as by physical and laboratory findings. Damage to contractile structure and reduced blood flow secondary to increased intramuscular pressure have been reported. In addition, there is evidence for a muscle recruitment mechanism whereby the slow-twitch fibers characteristic of small motor units are recruited first for force and for repetitive, endurance work and remain in action throughout low-level contractions. These motor units of larger muscles such as the trapezius are therefore vulnerable to fatigue and damage manifested as myalgia.

Several classifications of OSDs have been proposed, and such systems have been used for the development of treatment protocols. Management consists of modalities such as the application of ice and heat. Range-of-motion exercises along with strengthening exercises should also be used. Anti-inflammatory agents may likewise be helpful. Ergonomic modifications can serve to reduce the exposure to mechanical stress. These modifications are used in primary and secondary prevention of OSDs. The intervention starts with an assessment of the risk factors present in occupational and recreational activities. Engineering modifications are the preferred strategy because they remove the risk at the source, although administrative measures that reduce the exposure are often the first line of action.

Nonoperative treatment can achieve satisfactory outcomes such as reduction of pain and return to the preinjury activity level. Litigation and workers' compensation claims complicate the recovery, particularly in cases treated surgically.

The WHO approved an international classification of functioning that can serve to distinguish between disability and impairment. Accordingly, OSDs are structural and functional body impairments. A disability occurs when various activities are limited. Many estimates of impairment from OSDs and disability have been made in the United States, and they depend on the case definition and the method used to collect the data. About 3 million people with disability have a nonsevere condition, whereas about 16 million people of working age have some work limitation. However, determination of disability is largely an administrative process in which the orthopaedist plays a key role in evaluation of the impairment. The American Academy of Orthopaedic Surgeons and the American Medical Association issued the most commonly used guidelines to grade the impairment. The most challenging task is to ascertain whether the illness or injury is work related.

The decision regarding public assistance in the case of disability caused by OSDs is framed by the current compensation systems. The most common venue for covering medical costs is private insurance. Workers' compensation is a more common venue for indemnity, as well as the treatment costs involved in managing OSDs. However, in the absence of trauma, assertions of work-relatedness may be difficult to establish. The ADA provides a mechanism for accommodations, but it is questionable whether the impact of OSDs will qualify individuals for it. The

Railroad and Maritime Workers' Compensation and Social Security are probably the less common systems for OSD compensation.

REFERENCES AND BIBLIOGRAPHY

1. Abenheim L, Rossignol M, Valat JP, et al: The role of activity in the therapeutic management of back pain: Report of the International Paris Task Force on Back Pain. Spine 25(suppl):1S-33S, 2000.
2. Abreu BC (ed): Physical Disability Manual. New York: Raven Press, 1981.
3. American Academy of Orthopaedic Surgeons: Manual for Orthopaedic Surgeons in Evaluating Permanent Physical Impairment. Chicago: AAOS, 1975.
4. American Academy of Orthopaedic Surgeons: The Clinical Measurement of Joint Motion. Chicago: AAOS, 1994.
5. American Medical Association: Guides to the Evaluation of Permanent Impairment, 4th ed. Chicago: AMA, 1993.
6. American National Standards Institute: Accredited Standards Committee Z-365: Control of Work-Related Musculoskeletal Disorders (working draft). Itasca, IL: National Safety Council, August 2002.
7. Anderson JAD: Shoulder pain and tension neck and their relation to work. Scand J Work Environ Health 10:435-442, 1984.
8. Anderson JAD: Industrial rheumatology and the shoulder. Br J Rheumatol 26:326-328, 1987.
9. Andersson GBJ: Epidemiology of occupational neck and shoulder disorders. In Repetitive Motion Disorders of the Upper Extremity. Chicago: American Academy of Orthopaedic Surgeons, 1995.
10. Armstrong T, Buckle P, Fine L, et al: A conceptual model for work-related neck and upper limb musculoskeletal disorders. Scand J Work Environ Health 19:73-84, 1993.
11. Armstrong TJ, Marshall MM, Martin BJ, et al: Exposure to forceful exertions and vibration in a foundry. Int J Ind Ergon 30:163-179, 2002.
12. Awad EA: Interstitial myofibrosis: Hypothesis of mechanism. Arch Phys Med Rehabil 54:449-453, 1973.
13. Backman AL: Health survey of professional drivers. Scand J Work Environ Health 9:30-35, 1983.
14. Bakalim G and Pasila M: Surgical treatment of rupture of the rotator cuff tendon. Acta Orthop Scand 46:751-757, 1975.
15. Barton NJ, Hooper G, Noble J, and Steel WM: Occupational causes of disorders in the upper limb. BMJ 304:309-311, 1992.
16. Beaton DE, Cole DC, Manno M, et al: Describing the burden of upper-extremity musculoskeletal disorders in newspaper workers: What difference do case definitions make? J Occup Rehabil 10:39-53, 2000.
17. Bergenudd H and Johnell O: Somatic versus nonsomatic shoulder and back pain experience in middle age in relation to body build, physical fitness, bone mineral content, gamma-glutamyltransferase, occupational workload, and psychosocial factors. Spine 16:1051-1055, 1991.
18. Bergenudd H, Lindgarde F, Nilsson B, and Petersson CJ: Shoulder pain in middle age: A study of prevalence and relation to occupational work load and psychosocial factors. Clin Orthop 231:234-238, 1988.
19. Bernard BP (ed): Musculoskeletal Disorders and Workplace Factors: A Critical Review of Epidemiologic Evidence for Work-Related Musculoskeletal Disorders of the Neck, Upper Extremity and Low Back. Washington, DC: DHHS (NIOSH), Publication No. 97-141, 1997.
20. Bjelle A, Hagberg M, and Michaelson G: Occupational and individual factors in acute shoulder-neck disorders among industrial workers. Br J Ind Med 38:356-363, 1981.
21. Bjelle A, Hagberg M, and Michaelson G: Work-related shoulder-neck complaints in industry: A pilot study. Br J Rheumatol 26:365-369, 1987.
22. Bjorksten M, Itani T, Jonsson B, and Hoshizawa M: Evaluation of muscular load in shoulder and forearm muscles among medical secretaries during occupational typing and some non-occupational activities. In Jonsson B (ed): Biomechanics, vol X. Baltimore: University Park Press, 1987.
23. Bongers P, deWinter C, Kompier M, and Hildebrandt V: Psychosocial factors at work and musculoskeletal disease. Scand J Work Environ Health 19:297-312, 1993.
24. Bovenzi M, Fiorito A, and Volpe C: Bone and joint disorders in the upper extremities of chipping and grinding operators. Int Arch Occup Environ Health 59:189-198, 1987.
25. Bureau of Labor Statistics (BLS): Number of nonfatal occupational injuries and illnesses involving days away from work involving musculoskeletal disorders by selected worker and case characteristics, 1999 [http://stats.bls.gov/iif/oshwc/osh/case/ostb0911.pdf - 3/28/01].
26. Carey TS and Hadler NM: The role of the primary physician in disability determination for social security insurance and workers' compensation. Ann Intern Med 104:706-710, 1986.
27. Carmean G: Tie medical screening to the job. HR Magazine 37(7):85-87, 1992.
28. Chaffin DB: Localized muscle fatigue—definitions and measurement. J Occup Med 15:346-354, 1973.
29. Chaffin DB and Andersson GBJ: Occupational Biomechanics. New York: John Wiley, 1984.
30. Chakravarty K and Webley M: Shoulder joint movement and its relationship to disability in the elderly. J Rheumatol 20:1359-1361, 1993.
31. Cheng MSS, Amick BC, Watkins MP, and Rhea CD: Employer, physical therapist, and employee outcomes in the management of work-related upper extremity disorders. J Occup Rehabil 12:257-267, 2002.
32. Christensen H: Muscle activity and fatigue in the shoulder muscles of assembly-plant employees. Scand J Work Environ Health 12:582-587, 1986.
33. Cieza A, Borckow T, Ewert T, et al: Linking health status measurements to the International Classification of Functioning, Disability and Health. J Rehabil Med 34:1-6, 2002.
34. Courtney TK and Webster BW: Antecedent factors and disabling occupational morbidity—insights from the new BLS data. Am Ind Hyg Assoc J 62:622-632, 2001.
35. Croft P, Pope D, Zonca M, et al: Measurement of shoulder related disability: Results of a validation study. Ann Rheum Dis 53:525-528, 1994.
36. Danneskiold-Samsoe B, Christiansen E, Lund B, and Andersen R: Regional muscle tension and pain ("fibrosis"). Scand J Rehabil Med 15:17-20, 1983.
37. De Palma AF: Degenerative Changes in the Sternoclavicular and Acromioclavicular Joints in Various Decades. Springfield, IL: Charles C Thomas, 1957.
38. Edwards RHT: Hypothesis of peripheral and central mechanisms underlying occupational muscle pain and injury. Eur J Appl Physiol 57:275-281, 1988.
39. Equal Employment Opportunity Commission (EEOC): Technical Assistance Manual on the Employment Provisions (Title 1) of the Americans with Disabilities Act. EEOC-M-1A January 1992. EEOC, 1992.
40. Equal Employment Opportunity Commission (EEOC): ADA Enforcement Guidance: Preemployment Disability-Related Questions and Medical Examinations, October 1995.
41. Erdelyi A, Sihvonen T, Helin P, and Hanninen O: Shoulder strain in keyboard workers and its alleviation by arm supports. Int Arch Occup Environ Health 60:119-124, 1988.
42. Fassbender H and Wegner K: Morphologic and Pathogenese des Weichteirheumatimus. Z Rheumaforsch 32:355-374, 1973.
43. Feuerstein M and Hickey PF: Ergonomic approaches in the clinical assessment of occupational musculoskeletal disorders. In Turk DC and Melzack R (eds): Handbook of Pain Assessment. New York: Gilford Press, 1992, pp 71-99.
44. Flodmark BT and Aase G: Musculoskeletal symptoms and type A behaviour in blue collar workers. Br J Ind Med 49:683-687, 1992.
45. Friedenberg ZB and Miller WT: Degenerative disc disease of the cervical spine. J Bone Joint Surg Am 45:1171-1178, 1963.
46. Frieman BG and Fenlin JM: Anterior acromioplasty: Effect of litigation and worker's compensation. J Shoulder Elbow Surg 4:175-181, 1995.
47. Gartsman GM: Arthroscopic acromioplasty for lesions of the rotator cuff. J Bone Joint Surg Am 72:169-197, 1990.
48. Gloss DS and Wardle MG: Reliability and validity of American Medical Association's guide to ratings of permanent impairment. JAMA 248:2292-2296, 1982.
49. Granstrom B, Kvarnstrom S, and Tiefenbacher F: Electromyography as an aid in the prevention of excessive muscle strain. Appl Ergon 16:49-54, 1985.
50. Hadler NM: Occupational illness: The issue of causality. J Occup Med 26:587-593, 1984.
51. Hadler NM: Occupational Musculoskeletal Disorders. New York: Raven Press, 1993.
52. Hagberg M, Jonsson B, Brundin L, et al: Musculoskeletal pain in butchers: An epidemiologic, ergonomic and electromyographic study [in Swedish]. Work Health 12:6-52, 1983.
53. Hagberg M and Kvarnstrom S: Muscular endurance and electromyographic fatigue in myofascial shoulder pain. Arch Phys Med Rehabil 65:522-525, 1984.
54. Hagberg M, Michaelson G, and Ortelius A: Serum creatinine kinase as an indicator of local muscular strain in experimental and occupational work. Int Arch Occup Environ Health 50:377-386, 1982.
55. Hagberg M and Sundelin G: Discomfort and load on the upper trapezius muscle when operating a word processor. Ergonomics 29:1637-1645, 1986.
56. Hagberg M and Wegman DH: Prevalence rates and odds ratios of shoulder-neck diseases in different occupational groups. Br J Ind Med 44:602-610, 1987.
57. Hagg GM and Suurkula J: Zero crossing rate of electromyograms during occupational work and endurance tests as predictors for work related myalgia in the shoulder/neck region. Eur J Appl Physiol 62:436-444, 1991.
58. Hagner IM, Hagberg M, Hammerstrom U, et al: Physical load when cleaning floors using different techniques [in Swedish]. Work Health 29:7-27, 1986.
59. Hashemi L, Webbster BS, Clancy EA, and Courtney TK: Length of disability and cost of work-related musculoskeletal disorders of the upper extremity. J Occup Environ Med 40:261-269, 1998.
60. Hawkins RJ, Brock RM, Abrams JS, and Hobeika P: Acromioplasty for impingement with an intact rotator cuff. J Bone Joint Surg Br 70:795-797, 1988.
61. Hawkins RJ, Misamore GW, and Hobeika PE: Surgery for full thickness rotator cuff tears. J Bone Joint Surg Am 67:1349-1355, 1985.
62. Herbert R, Dropkin J, Levin S, et al: Diagnosis and medical management of work-related neck and upper extremity musculoskeletal disorders in dental care workers. In Murphy DC (ed): Ergonomics and the Dental Care Worker. Washington, DC: American Public Health Association, 1998, pp 375-417.
63. Herington TN and Morse LH: Occupational Injuries: Evaluation, Management, and Prevention. St Louis: CV Mosby, 1995.

64. Hildebrandt VH, Bongers PM, van Duk FJH, et al: The influence of climatic factors on non-specific back and neck-shoulder disease. Ergonomics 45:32-48, 2002.

65. Himmelstein JS, Feuerstein M, Stanek EJ, et al: Work-related upper extremity disorders and work disability: Clinical and psychosocial presentation. J Occup Environ Med 37:1278-1286, 1995.

66. Hinnen U, Laubli T, Guggenbuhl U, and Krueger M: Design of check-out systems including laser scanners for sitting work posture. Scand J Work Environ Health 18:86-94, 1992.

67. Ho SF and Lee HS: An investigation into complaints of wrist pain and swelling among workers at a factory manufacturing motors for refrigerators. Singapore Med J 35:274-276, 1994.

68. Holstrom EB, Lindell J, and Moritz U: Low back and neck/shoulder pain in construction workers: Occupational workload and psychosocial risk factors. Part 1. Relationship to low back pain. Spine 17:663-671, 1992.

69. Holmstrom EB, Lindell J, and Moritz U: Low back and neck/shoulder pain in construction workers: Occupational workload and psychosocial risk factors. Part 2. Relationship to neck and shoulder pain. Spine 17:672-677, 1992.

70. InfoUse: Chartbook on Disability in the United States, 1998. Washington, DC: National Institute on Disability and Rehabilitation Research [http://www.infouse.com/disabilitydata/addresources.html].

71. International Labour Organization: ILO Encyclopaedia of Occupational Health and Safety. Geneva: International Labour Organization, 1983.

72. Itani T, Yoshizawa M, and Jonsson B: Electromyographic evaluation and subjective estimation of the muscular load in shoulder and forearm muscles during some leisure activities. In Johnson B (ed): Biomechanics X-A. Champaign, IL: Human Kinetics Publishers, 1987, pp 241-247.

73. Job Accommodation Network (JAN): Accommodation Cost/Benefit Data—July 1999. Washington, DC: Office of Disability Employment Policy, Department of Labor [http://www.jan.wvu.edu/media/Stats/BenCosts0799.html].

74. Job Accommodation Network (JAN): U.S. Quarterly Report January—March 2002. Washington, DC: Office of Disability Employment Policy, Department of Labor [http://www.jan.wvu.edu].

75. Johansson JA and Rubenowitz S: Risk indicators in the psychosocial and physical work environment for work-related neck, shoulder and low back symptoms: A study among blue- and white-collar workers in eight companies. Scand J Rehabil Med 26:131-142, 1994.

76. Jonsson B: The static load component in muscle work. Eur J Appl Physiol 57:305-310, 1988.

77. Jonsson B, Brundin L, Hagner IM, et al: Operating a forwarder: An electromyographic study. In Winter DA, Nouman RW, Wells RP, et al (eds): Biomechanics IX-B. Champaign, IL: Human Kinetics Publishers, 1985, pp 21-26.

78. Jonsson B, Hagberg M, and Sima S: Vocational electromyography in shoulder muscles in an electronics plant. In Morecki A, Fidelus K, Kedzior K, and Wit A (eds): Biomechanics VII-B. Baltimore: University Park Press, 1981, pp 10-15.

79. Katevuo K, Aitasalo K, Lehtinen R, and Pietila J: Skeletal changes in dentists and farmers in Finland. Commun Dent Oral Epidemiol 13:23-25, 1985.

80. Kellgren JH and Lawrence JS: Rheumatism in miners. Part II. X-ray study. Br J Ind Med 9:197-207, 1952.

81. Keyserling WM, Punnett L, and Fine LJ: Postural stress of the trunk and shoulders: Identification and control of occupational risk factors. In Ergonomic Interventions to Prevent Musculoskeletal Injuries in Industry. Chelsea, MI: Lewis Publishers, 1987, pp 11-26.

82. Kluth K, Bohlemann J, and Strasser H: Rapid communication: A system for a strain-oriented analysis of the layout of assembly workplaces. Ergonomics 37:1441-1448, 1994.

83. Larsson B, Libelius R, and Ohlsson K: Trapezius muscle changes unrelated to static work load: Chemical and morphologic controlled studies of 22 women with and without neck pain. Acta Orthop Scand 63:203-206, 1992.

84. Larsson SE, Bengtsson A, Bodegard L, et al: Muscle changes in work-related chronic myalgia. Acta Orthop Scand 59:552-556, 1988.

85. Larsson SE, Bodegard L, Henriksson KG, and Oberg PA: Chronic trapezius myalgia: Morphology and blood flow studied in seventeen patients. Acta Orthop Scand 61:394-398, 1990.

86. Lawrence JS: Rheumatism in cotton operatives. Br J Ind Med 18:270-276, 1961.

87. Lawrence JS, Bremner JM, and Bier F: Osteoarthrosis: Prevalence in the population and relationship between symptoms and x-ray changes. Ann Rheum Dis 25:1-24, 1966.

88. Leino P and Magni G: Depressive and distress symptoms as predictors of low back pain, neck-shoulder pain, and other musculoskeletal morbidity: A 10-year follow-up study of metal industry employees. Pain 53:89-94, 1993.

89. Linton SJ and Kamwendo K: Risk factors in the psychosocial work environment for neck and shoulder pain in secretaries. J Occup Med 31:609-613, 1989.

90. Luck JV and Andersson GBJ: Occupational shoulder disorders. In Rockwood CA Jr and Matsen FA III (eds): The Shoulder. Philadelphia: WB Saunders, 1990, pp 1088-1108.

91. Mangharam J and McGlothan JD: Ergonomics and dentistry: A literature review. In Murphy DC (ed): Ergonomics and the Dental Care Worker. Washington, DC: American Public Health Association, 1998, pp 25-82.

92. Mani L and Gerr F: Work-related upper extremity musculoskeletal disorders. Prim Care 27:845-864, 2000.

93. Matheson L, Guadino E, Mael F, and Hesse B: Improving the validity of the impairment evaluation process: A proposed theoretical framework. J Occup Rehabil 10:311-320, 2000.

94. Matheson LN, Kane M, and Rudbard D: Development of new methods to determine work disability in the United States. J Occup Rehabil 11:143-154, 2001.

95. Minnesota Medical Association: Worker's Compensation Permanent Partial Disability Schedule. Minneapolis: Minnesota Medical Association, 1984.

96. Misamore GW, Ziegler DW, and Rushton JC: Repair of the rotator cuff: A comparison of results of two populations of patients. J Bone Joint Surg Am 77:1335-1339, 1995.

97. National Committee on Vital and Health Statistics (NCVHS): Classifying and Reporting Functional Status. Washington, DC: Department of Health and Human Services, 2001 [http://www.ncvhs.hhs.gov/010716rp.html].

98. National Institute for Occupational Safety and Health (NIOSH): A National Strategy for Occupational Musculoskeletal Injuries: Implementation Issues and Research Needs—1991 Conference Summary. DHHS (NIOSH) Publication No. 93-101, 1992.

99. National Research Council: Musculoskeletal Disorders and the Workplace: Low Back and Upper Extremities. Washington, DC: National Academy Press, 2001 [http://www.nap.edu/books/0309072840/html].

100. National Safety Council: ANSI-Accredited Standards Committee Z-365: Control of Work-Related Musculoskeletal Disorders (working draft). Itasca, IL: NSC, August 2002.

101. Nayha S, Anttonen H, and Hassi J: Snowmobile driving and symptoms of the locomotive organs. Arctic Med Res Suppl 3:41-44, 1994.

102. Office of Disability Employment Policy (ODEP): Costs and Benefits of Accommodation. July 1996 [http://www.dol.gov/odep/archives/ek96/benefits.html].

103. Onishi N, Sakai K, and Kogi K: Arm and shoulder muscle load in various keyboard operating jobs of women. J Hum Ergol (Tokyo) 11:89-97, 1982.

104. OSHA: Ergonomics Program Management Guidelines for Meatpacking Plants. DOL/OSHA 3123, 1993.

105. Osterweis M, Kleinman A, and Mechanic D (eds): Pain and Disability, Behavioral and Public Policy Perspectives. Washington, DC: National Academy Press, 1982.

106. Pascarelli EF and Hsu YP: Understanding work-related upper extremity disorders: Clinical findings in 485 computer users, musicians, and others. J Occup Rehabil 11:1-21, 2001.

107. Petersson CJ: Degeneration of the glenohumeral joint: An anatomical study. Acta Orthop Scand 54:277-283, 1983.

108. Petersson CJ: Degeneration of the acromioclavicular joint: A morphological study. Acta Orthop Scand 54:434-438, 1983.

109. Pope MH and Andersson GBJ: Prevention. In Nordin M, Andersson GBJ, and Pope MH (eds): Musculoskeletal Disorders in the Workplace. New York: Mosby, 1997, pp 244-249.

110. Post M and Cohen J: Impingement syndrome: A review of late stage II and early stage III lesions. Clin Orthop 207:126-132, 1986.

111. Saddemi S, Hawkins R, Morr J, and Hawkins A: Arthroscopic subacromial decompression: Two- to four-year follow-up study. Paper presented at the Ninth Open Meeting of the American Shoulder and Elbow Surgeons, February 1993, San Francisco.

112. Salen BA, Spangfort EV, Lygren AL, and Nordenar R: The disability rating index: An instrument for the assessment of disability in clinical settings. J Clin Epidemiol 47:1423-1434, 1994.

113. Shugars HA, Miller D, Williams D, et al: Musculoskeletal pain among general dentists. Gen Dent 35:272-276, 1987.

114. Sikorski J, Molan R, and Askin G: Orthopaedic basis for occupationally related arm and neck pain. Aust N Z J Surg 59:471-478, 1989.

115. Silverstein B, Welp E, Nelson N, Kalat J: Claims incidence of work-related disorders of the upper extremities: Washington state, 1987 through 1995. Am J Public Health 88:1827-1833, 1998.

116. Sjogaard G, Kiens B, Jorgensen K, and Saltin B: Intramuscular pressure: EMG and blood flow during low-level prolonged static contraction in man. Acta Physiol Scand 128:475-484, 1996.

117. Smith WJ: ISO and ANSI: Ergonomic Standards for Computer Products. Upper Saddle River, NJ: Prentice Hall, 1996.

118. Social Security Administration (SSA): Plan for a New Disability Claim Process. Washington, DC: SSA, September 1994.

119. Sommerich CM, McGlothlin JD, and Marras WS: Occupational risk factors associated with soft tissue disorders of the shoulder: A review of recent investigations in the literature. Ergonomics 36:697-717, 1993.

120. Stenlund B: Shoulder tendinitis and osteoarthritis of the acromioclavicular joint and their relation to sports. Br J Sports Med 27:125-130, 1993.

121. Stenlund B, Goldie I, Hagberg M, et al: Radiographic osteoarthrosis in the acromioclavicular joint resulting from manual work or exposure to vibration. Br J Ind Med 49:588-593, 1992.

122. Stucki G, Ewert T, and Cieza A: Value and application of the ICF in rehabilitation medicine. Disabil Rehabil 25(11-12):628-634, 2003.

123. Swedish National Board of Occupational Safety and Health: Ordinance. In ASF 12: Concerning Work with Visual Display Units (VDUS). Stockholm, 1985.

124. Tait R, Chibnall J, and Richardson W: Litigation and employment status: Effects on patients with chronic pain. Pain 43:37-46, 1990.

125. Takala J, Sievers K, and Klaukka T: Rheumatic symptoms in the middle-aged population in southwestern Finland. Scand J Rheumatol Suppl 47:15-29, 1982.
126. Tichauer ER: Potential of biomechanics for solving specific hazard problems. In Proceedings of ASSE 1968 Conference. Park Ridge, IL: American Society of Safety Engineers, 1968, pp 149-187.
127. Tichauer ER: The Biomechanical Basis of Ergonomics: Anatomy Applied to the Design of Work Situations. New York: Wiley, 1978.
128. Tiddia F, Cherchi GB, Pacifico L, and Chiesa C: Yersinia enterocolitica causing suppurative arthritis of the shoulder. J Clin Pathol 47:760-761, 1994.
129. Tola S, Riihimaki H, Videman T, et al: Neck and shoulder symptoms among men in machine operating, dynamic physical work and sedentary work. Scand J Work Environ Health 14:299-305, 1988.
130. Vasseljen O and Westgaard RH: A case-control study of trapezius muscle activity in office and manual workers with shoulder and neck pain and symptom-free controls. Int Arch Occup Environ Health 67:11-18, 1995.
131. Vasseljen O, Westgaard RH, and Larsen S: A case-control study of psychological and psychosocial risk factors for shoulder and neck pain at the workplace. Int Arch Occup Environ Health 66:375-382, 1995.
132. Vasudevan SV: Impairment, disability, and functional capacity assessment. In Turk DC and Melzack R (eds): Handbook of Pain Assessment. New York: Gilford Press, 1992.
133. Waldron HA and Cox M: Occupational arthropathy: Evidence from the past. Br J Ind Med 46:420-422, 1989.
134. Waris P: Occupational cervicobrachial syndromes: A review. Scand J Work Environ Health 6 (suppl 3):3-14, 1980.
135. Wells R: Task analysis. In Ranney D (ed): Chronic Musculoskeletal Injuries in the Workplace. Philadelphia: WB Saunders, 1997, pp 41-63.
136. Westgaard RH and Jansen T: Individual and work-related factors associated with symptoms of musculoskeletal complaints. II. Different risk factors among sewing machine operators. Br J Ind Med 49:154-162, 1992.
137. Westgaard RH, Jensen C, and Hansen K: Individual and work-related factors associated with symptoms of musculoskeletal complaints. Int Arch Occup Environ Health 64:405-413, 1993.
138. Westgaard RH, Jensen C, and Nilsen K: Muscle coordination and choice-reaction time tests as indicators of occupational muscle load and shoulder-neck complaints. Eur J Appl Physiol 67:106-114, 1993.
139. Winkel J, Ekblom B, Hagberg M, and Jonsson B: The working environment of cleaners: Evaluation of physical strain in mopping and swabbing as a basis for job redesign. In Ergonomics of Work-station Design. London: Butterworths, 1983, pp 35-44.
140. Winkel J, Ekblom B, and Tillberg B: Ergonomics and medical factors in shoulder/arm pain among cabin attendants as a basis for job redesign. In Malsvi H and Kobayashi K (eds): Biomechanics VIII-A. Champaign, IL: Human Kinetics Publishers, 1983, pp 563-567.
141. Worcester JN and Green DP: Osteoarthritis of the acromioclavicular joint. Clin Orthop 58:69-73, 1968.
142. World Health Organization (WHO): Identification and Control of Work-Related Diseases, Technical Report 174. Geneva: WHO, 1985, pp 7-11.
143. World Health Organization (WHO): International Classification of Functioning, Disability and Health (ICF). Geneva: WHO [http://www3.who.int/icf/icftemplate.cfm].
144. Zenz C: Occupational Medicine: Principles and Practical Applications: Chicago: Year Book, 1988.

CHAPTER 28

EFFECTIVENESS EVALUATION AND THE SHOULDER

Frederick A. Matsen III, M.D., Kevin L. Smith, M.D., and Moby Parsons, M.D.

• • • •

. . . which was merely the common-sense notion that every hospital should follow every patient it treats, long enough to determine whether or not the treatment has been successful, and then to inquire "if not, why not?" with a view to preventing similar failures in future.

- E. A. Codman 1934

Outcomes research has seen an explosion of interest in recent years across all fields of medicine.[29,41,58] This growth has been driven by a number of factors that include increasing health care costs, inadequacies of research methodology, and regional variations in practice without apparent reason.[134] It has piqued the interest of groups, including epidemiologists, physicians, third-party payers, health care systems, and patients. It is now apparent that individual practicing physicians can document their results with specific treatment programs. Because treatment interventions in orthopaedic surgery are aimed at preserving and improving quality of life, assessing the benefit of a treatment program is best done in terms of variables that are directly relevant to the self-assessed quality of life of the patient.[4]

The trend is now to emphasize patient self-assessment as the standard method for understanding the natural history of shoulder conditions and the effectiveness of their treatment.*

HISTORY

In the past, clinical studies in orthopaedics were mainly investigations of small groups of patients reviewed retrospectively with the use of objective parameters assessed by health care professionals. We might call these variables "medical metrics," including examples such as fracture union, deformity, recurrence, strength, and range of motion. Occasionally, when patients' subjective perceptions were reported, such as pain relief and overall satisfaction, they would recommend similar treatment to others, and they would agree to the same procedure if necessary in the future. Reported perceptions would often include whether patients were better, the same, or worse. Results were often divided into categories of relative success, such as poor, fair, good, and excellent.

Many studies lacked statistical rigor, strict inclusion or exclusion criteria, standardization of treatment methods, and consistent measures of comfort and function before and after treatment. Scores were proposed that arbitrarily attached a relative weight to various elements of the examination.[90] Most clinical studies have been reported by specialists in the procedure of interest rather than by individuals in the general practice of orthopaedics, where the preponderance of care is rendered. Thus, the degree to which the reported results are relevant to the bulk of practicing physicians in the United States is uncertain.

The concept of systematically documenting the results of treatment was formalized when Codman proposed his "end result" idea in Boston just after the turn of the century.[24] He advocated critical evaluation of the results of each patient's treatment over time in order to identify and understand treatment failures. It is obvious from the quotation at the beginning of this chapter that Codman was an advocate of quality control for all treatment rendered rather than only considering the results of specialists. In the current age, the rising cost of health care mandates quality control through the practice of evidence-based medicine. With the goal of finding reliable and cost-effective disease-specific treatments, outcomes data are essential for determining the effectiveness of treatment interventions.

Donabedian was the first to use the term "outcome" in expressing Codman's end result idea.[36] In addition, he defined two other major dimensions of quality of care, namely, structure and process. Structural factors include the number of hospital beds in an institution and the quality control practices of its laboratory. These factors are easy to quantify and measure and were an early focus of the Joint Commission. Process indicators monitor the steps and actions involved in patient care and include variables such as who gives medications, how specimens are handled, and conformity with set protocols of care. Proximate outcomes relate specifically to the steps in the overall process of care. For example, the radiology department may consider the final, accurate report as its outcome. Finally, ultimate outcome measures what

*See references 17, 37, 43, 51-53, 59-61, 96, 111, 113, 124, 125, 128, 142, 156.

exactly happens to the patient as a result of the entire course of action, including patient satisfaction, morbidity, and mortality. This concept is closely linked to the process of care and is the current focus of outcome studies.

Karnofsky and Burchenal introduced the use of surveys for evaluating the success of cancer treatment in the 1940s.[69] A patient-oriented approach to evaluation of results was advocated by Lembcke.[86] Katz and colleagues used activities of daily living (ADLs) scales to measure outcomes in elderly patients[72]; Bradburn looked at psychological well-being and its effect on patients[18]; Breslow introduced methods of measuring physical, mental, and social well-being[19]; and Bush and associates developed the Health Status Index and the Quality of Well-Being (QWB) Scale.[22] These milestones set the stage for the current understanding and methodology of outcome measurement via self-assessment questionnaires.

In the 1970s, Wennberg and Gittelsohn's epidemiologic study documented that health care utilization varied widely from one region to another.[151] This compelling finding was the catalyst that sparked much of the current interest in outcomes research. The methodology used, termed small-area analysis, demonstrated large variations in the rate of tonsillectomy, hysterectomy, prostatectomy, and other procedures between regions despite controlling for variations in population demographics.[152] A patient living in New Haven, for instance, was found to be twice as likely to undergo spine surgery for degenerative disk disease than one living in Boston, yet the latter was twice as likely to undergo total hip replacement than the former.[150] Whatever the explanation for this phenomenon, it posed the key question regarding what information is needed to justify a specified treatment.

Starting with the shoulder surgeon Codman, orthopaedics has been a leader in outcomes research.[76,78] The American Academy of Orthopaedic Surgeons has promoted this kind of investigation to provide specific outcome measurement instruments.[1,2] Keller has advocated the use of certain terminology for different aspects of outcomes research.[77] *Efficacy* indicates whether a procedure or technology works in the hands of select individuals in a specific setting. *Effectiveness* indicates that an efficacious procedure works when used throughout the general medical community. An *efficacious* procedure may indeed prove to be *ineffective* when used by general practitioners. Finally, *appropriateness* indicates that a treatment is indicated in the patients receiving it. An improperly used procedure may lead to better or worse results than expected, thus clouding the understanding of its value.

Some studies have applied the emerging methodologies to measure the effectiveness of various orthopaedic treatments.* When considering these studies, it becomes apparent that measuring the effectiveness of management methods for musculoskeletal conditions is more complex than measuring the effectiveness of an antihypertensive medication for lowering blood pressure. In the treatment of hypertension, the inclusion criteria can be simply

defined, the evaluation tool is straightforward, and the person administering the treatment and the technique used are relatively unimportant. The nature of the treatment can be blinded from the patient and the evaluator, thus permitting double-blind, side-by-side comparisons of the effectiveness of treatment. None of these statements are true when we try to compare the effectiveness of surgical management of rotator cuff disease with nonoperative treatment, for example.

The literature on acromioplasty illustrates the challenges and difficulties with outcome measurement in orthopaedics.[90] In each study, different inclusion criteria were applied. Distinct evaluation tools were used, many based principally on medical metrics (i.e., change in acromial shape on radiographs). The evaluation methods often were not used before and after treatment so that the success or failure of treatment could be quantified. Different definitions of "success" were used. As a result, it is difficult to compare and contrast the results and to define the indications for this most commonly performed shoulder procedure.[3,38,42,62,108,109,118]

Some research has been based on large databases, such as Medicare claims data.[152] Although these databases have the advantage of being applicable to the broad range of practice in the United States, results from these sources do not reflect change in comfort, function, or health status. Other studies involve a meta-analysis of all related literature for a given area to look for rigorous evidence to support the use of a particular treatment.[31,84,93] Although much research has been retrospective, an increasing number are using prospectively designed protocols.[9,14,15,21] Some authors promote the use of treatment algorithms and practice guidelines to facilitate the analysis of results and to minimize the practice variability noted through small-area analysis.[13]

Another important concept is that of *cost-effectiveness*.[22,39,50,54,65,85,114,132] The current medical cost climate dictates that health care not only be effective and appropriate but also be worthy of the expenditures related to it.

Although effectiveness, appropriateness, and cost-effectiveness are straightforward in concept, they are challenging to measure in a clinical context:

How is effectiveness measured and by whom?
What does the "general medical community" mean?
How can an "indication" be rigorously defined?
How can the full "cost" of a treatment be determined?

EVALUATION OF INSTRUMENTS

As recognition of the importance of outcome measurement has increased, so too has the understanding of what constitutes accurate and effective measurement. The requirements for obtaining accurate data from an outcome measurement instrument include *validity, reproducibility, internal consistency,* and *responsiveness to change*.[144] The term *validity* is used to describe whether a given instrument actually measures what it is purported to measure. *Reproducibility* refers to the ability of a tool to yield the same result when administered on separate occasions. This attribute is commonly referred to as test-

---

*See references 8, 16, 23, 31, 57, 66, 67, 73, 82, 87, 95, 107, 116, 126.

retest reliability. The *internal consistency* of a tool implies that it is able to adequately measure a single concept irrespective of extraneous effectors. Thus, an internally consistent assessment of shoulder function should not be affected by problems with the elbow, wrist, or hand. Finally, to be of value, a tool must show *responsiveness to change*. If purported to measure knee function, a tool should be able to demonstrate a difference before and after knee arthroplasty, for example. For clinical studies on the effectiveness of a treatment intervention, validated measurement instruments must be able to track not only differences in an individual patient over time but also differences between patients with the same condition.[133]

Precision analysis is another parameter for assessing the accuracy of a measurement tool. Precision refers to the equality with which a tool measures different initial levels of the same trait.[34] For example, does it equally measure patients with mild, moderate, and severe pain. Many measurement instruments make the general assumption that function is measured with equal precision at all levels. This assumption may affect the accuracy of tracking individual status over time.[27] Because most questionnaire items target the midrange of function, with few items targeting the extremes, the measurement error in determining function that falls outside the midrange increases as these ranges of function are not precisely measured. This point highlights the conflict of designing clinically useful scoring systems. There must be enough items to be precise across a range of functions, but not so many that it compromises their ease of administration, wide acceptance, and low cost.

The effectiveness of outcome measurement instruments and the ability to compare different outcomes between related groups of patients depend on the definition of the condition to which the instrument is applied, as well as the reliability and timing of methods used to gather data. Strict criteria outlining the necessary information for making a diagnosis have not been established for the majority of musculoskeletal conditions as they have for conditions such as hypertension. Without uniform definitions, valid and reliable disease-specific outcome measures cannot be developed.[56] Because different scoring systems may rely on different outcome criteria, assign different weights to each criterion, and accord different ranges of values to each categorical ranking, comparison of outcomes between different scoring systems is difficult.[139] This comparison is further complicated by the lack of standardization for estimating clinically relevant and significant changes in patient outcomes for individual shoulder disorders. Determination of the degree to which a pretreatment and post-treatment change is clinically significant depends on the existence of normative values for determining whether a treated individual can be distinguished from normal individuals serving as a reference group. Such normative values have not been categorically established for general or joint-specific musculoskeletal function.[64] Currently, the definition of clinically significant depends largely on the judgment of individual physicians and patients.[140] For observer-based scoring systems that rely on objective measurement of function, variability in measurement methods and the absence of standardized measurement protocols complicate the comparison of results between different clinical studies.[63]

TYPES OF OUTCOME MEASUREMENTS

Patient Self-assessment versus Observer-Based Measurement Instruments

Medical metrics uses factors observed by health care professionals, including physical examination findings (e.g., range of motion, strength), radiographic analysis (e.g., union, loosening), and the incidence of complications such as deep venous thrombosis and infection.[47,57] By contrast, *patient assessments* include documentation of parameters evident to the individual, such as mental health, social well-being, role function (as worker, parent, spouse), physical function, and ability to carry out activities of daily living (ADLs).[67,68,75,76,78] These patient assessments are most practically obtained by self-assessment questionnaires because they are *inexpensive* to use when compared with measurements of strength or range, *convenient* (they can be completed without the patient having to return to the physician's office), and *free from variability* because of differences among medical observers.

Increasing recognition of the biases introduced by objective measurement of shoulder function has led to greater reliance on patient self-assessment of outcome as the best means of determining whether a given treatment intervention has effected a clinically significant change. Differences between subjective and objective perception of outcome depend on differences in the objectives of physicians and patients.[154] Subjective perception may also be modulated by the stage of the condition, and this perception may differ from functional assessment. For example, in the postoperative period, patients are focused on recovery, but 6 months later, they may be focused on performance. Although their functional score may be the same at these intervals, their perception is markedly different. For disorders in which the clinical examination can be unreliable and may not correlate with patients' subjective perception of their function, objective outcome measures may be inaccurate.[81]

Tingart and colleagues correlated the subjective and objective results of the Constant and Neer scores and found that the overall correlation was only fair.[137] More patients subjectively rated their outcome as excellent or good than were classified accordingly by the objective scoring system. Differences between subjective and objective outcomes also depended on the age of the patient. This study suggests that treatment recommendations from clinical studies that rely solely on objective measurement may not be accurate for certain groups of patients. Dawson and associates studied the benefits of using patient-based methods of assessment by correlating the Oxford Shoulder Score, Constant Score, and the Short Form-36 (SF-36) in 93 patients undergoing shoulder surgery for conditions of the rotator cuff. All scores improved significantly at 6 months, but the Constant score was reduced at 4 years. This decline in objective measurement did not correlate with the patient's subjective judgment of the change in symptoms or the success of the operation.[34] Hoving and coworkers studied the reliability of a standardized protocol of measurement of shoulder movement and found that intra- and inter-rater reliability varied widely. This study demonstrates that objective assessment of shoulder function suffers from differences in interpretation of measurements between providers.[63]

Taken together, the results of these studies support the use of patient self-assessment measurement tools as opposed to those that rely on objective determination of shoulder function. Thus, to the extent that patient self-assessment instruments remove observer judgment from the measurement equation, they probably provide the most clinically relevant estimate of outcome. For determining the effectiveness of treatment, self-assessment tools provide a better measure of success that is patient based rather than process based.

Categorization of Measurement Tools

Measurement instruments for evaluation of the musculoskeletal system can be categorized as generalized, joint specific, or diagnosis specific. Generalized measurement instruments focus on measuring the impact of musculoskeletal disease on the overall health status of the patient. Although these types of assessment tools are important for determining the effect of the condition on lifestyle and emotional function, they may be poor at detecting small, but clinically significant changes in quality of life.[81] Joint-specific measurement tools are the most commonly used in outcomes assessment and must be widely applicable and valid across a range of disorders. However, items in these measurement tools are often less disease specific and may therefore be less sensitive in detecting change for different diagnoses.[91] Diagnosis-specific instruments are the most sensitive for detecting differences in self-assessed outcome between patients with the same diagnosis and at different times for the diagnosis of interest.[91] To the extent that measurement of disease-specific quality of life is required to accurately determine the benefit of an orthopaedic intervention, diagnosis-specific quality-of-life measurement tools may be the most valid, responsive, and reproducible. However, the cost-efficiency and acceptance of diagnosis-specific instruments may be prohibitive to their administration in a community-based setting where the bulk of orthopaedic care takes place and where evidence-based treatments may be the most important in terms of assessing the cost-effectiveness of individual treatment interventions.[133,154]

Despite the complexities of accurately determining treatment effectiveness, the principles of evaluating patient outcomes in terms of quality of life remain simple and unchanged by methodologic and statistical rigor. The ideal approach enables every practitioner to comply with Codman's admonition to follow every patient treated, long enough to determine whether or not the treatment has been successful, and then to inquire if not, why not? A plan can then be devised to prevent similar failures in the future. From this admonition we can derive the characteristics of the desired results assessment tool:

Every practitioner requires that the tool be inexpensive and easy to administer and record such that all can use it.

Follow every patient necessitates that the tool be applicable to as many different conditions as possible, simple to complete, and achievable without requiring the patient's return to the office (e.g., otherwise, patients who are poor or who live a long distance away may be systematically excluded).

Long enough implies that the tool enable follow-up for many years after the treatment.

Determine whether or not the treatment has been successful proposes that the tool measure factors that are important to the patient (e.g., comfort and function) and that the same tool be applied before and after treatment so that success or failure can be meaningfully defined rigorously and quantitatively in terms of a change in the results.

"If not, why not?" makes it imperative that differences between the pretreatment and post-treatment measurements reliably reveal every patient who has improved and those who have worsened after implementing the treatment.

Preventing similar failures in the future means that the results need to be available to the specific provider such that appropriate changes can be made because failures are often due to the individual provider's patient selection, technique, or postoperative management rather than solely to the type of operation or implant used.

It is evident that existing methods involving hospital discharge data, meta-analysis, or studies confined to largely specialized practices do not provide the individualized quality control advocated by Codman.

SHOULDER ASSESSMENT INSTRUMENTS

The different shoulder assessment tools currently available can be evaluated against Codman's criteria. The following includes a sampling of the various types used, from general to specific. Multiple studies have been performed to compare different outcome measurement instruments in terms of validity, reliability, and responsiveness.* Beaton and Richards prospectively compared the validity of five self-assessment questionnaires that measure shoulder function.[6] All performed similarly in describing patients' shoulder function and in discriminating relative severity. Beaton and Richards also compared the test-retest reliability and responsiveness of five different shoulder questionnaires in 99 patients with shoulder pain. All questionnaires had acceptable reliability except the Subject Shoulder Rating Scale. All questionnaires were more sensitive in detecting change in function than general health status instruments were.[7] In light of these similarities, they proposed that one might choose a questionnaire for practical reasons, such as ease of administration or scoring.

---

*See references 5, 7, 27, 28, 122, 127, 129, 137, 140, 141.

TABLE 28-1. Simple Shoulder Test*

1.	Is your shoulder comfortable with your arm at rest by your side?	Yes	No
2.	Does your shoulder allow you to sleep comfortably?	Yes	No
3.	Can you reach the small of your back to tuck in your shirt with your hand?	Yes	No
4.	Can you place your hand behind your head with the elbow straight out to the side?	Yes	No
5.	Can you place a coin on a shelf at the level of your shoulder without bending your elbow?	Yes	No
6.	Can you lift 1 lb (a full pint container) to the level of your shoulder without bending your elbow?	Yes	No
7.	Can you lift 8 lb (a full gallon container) to the level of the top of your head without bending your elbow?	Yes	No
8.	Can you carry 20 lb (a bag of potatoes) at your side with the affected extremity?	Yes	No
9.	Do you think you can toss a softball underhand 10 yards with the affected extremity?	Yes	No
10.	Do you think you can throw a softball overhand 20 yards with the affected extremity?	Yes	No
11.	Can you wash the back of your opposite shoulder with the affected extremity?	Yes	No
12.	Would your shoulder allow you to work full-time at your regular job?	Yes	No

*The Simple Shoulder Test (SST) is used for patient self-assessment of general shoulder function.
From Lippitt SB, Harryman DT II, and Matsen FA III: A practical tool for evaluation function: The simple shoulder test. *In* Matsen FA III, Fu FH, and Hawkins RJ (eds): The Shoulder: A Balance of Mobility and Stability. Rosemont, IL: American Academy of Orthopaedic Surgeons, 1993, pp 501-518.

Simple Shoulder Test

The Simple Shoulder Test (SST) is a short and simple shoulder-specific self-assessment tool that has proved to be practical within the context of busy practices.* The SST consists of a set of 12 "yes" or "no" questions derived from the common complaints of patients evaluated at the University of Washington Shoulder Service. These 12 questions are listed in Table 28-1. The SST has been shown to (1) be reproducible in test-retest situations,[89,102] (2) be practical in a busy practice setting,[89,102] (3) be sensitive to a wide variety of shoulder disorders,[6,89,102] and (4) be able to quantitate the change in shoulder function as a result of treatment and permit identification of treatment failures.[100]

Normal subjects have been shown to be able to perform essentially all the SST functions. Conversely, the SST is sensitive to the shoulder disabilities perceived by patients undergoing evaluation and management of a wide range of shoulder disorders.[6,7,89,102,122]

The SST can be viewed as a minimal data set of functional information that can be collected on all patients at the time of initial evaluation. If additional functional data are needed to make the questionnaire more sensitive, questions can be added to the original 12 while keeping

the minimal data set intact. For example, when studying high-performance athletes, one could add such questions as "Does your shoulder allow you to pitch (or serve) with your usual speed and control?" "Does your shoulder allow you to swim your normal workout?" or "Does your shoulder allow you to compete at the varsity level in your sport?"

The simplicity of this test allows characterization of the shoulder function of an individual patient or a group of patients meeting specified inclusion criteria. The effectiveness of a management program can easily be characterized in terms of change in the patient's assessment and ability to perform the different functions before and after the treatment.

Rowe's Rating Sheet for Bankart Repair

One of the earliest attempts at standardizing the evaluation of shoulder function was Rowe's rating of the results of Bankart repair (Table 28-2).[123] It includes a maximal potential score of 100 points, which are subdivided into stability (50 points), motion (20 points), and function (30 points). This disease-specific instrument provides a measure of the relative success of instability surgery. The rating scale is heavily weighted to the recurrence of instability (50 points) but does not include the evaluation of ADLs, ability to sleep, and pain. It includes medical metrics, and thus it requires that the patient return to the office for serial examination.

UCLA Shoulder Scoring System

The UCLA scale has been widely used since Ellman introduced it in 1986 (Table 28-3).[38] It has a total score of 35 points, with pain and function each allotted 1 to 10 points and active forward flexion, strength of forward flexion, and patient satisfaction each totaling 1 to 5 points. The overall score is then classified as excellent (34 to 35 points), good (29 to 33 points), or poor (<29 points). The weighting of the questions has interesting consequences; for example, if a patient is unable to internally rotate to T8 (e.g., fasten a brassiere), she loses 4 points and can have only a good result at best. This score includes medical metrics, so the patient must return to the office for serial examination.

Hospital for Special Surgery Shoulder-Rating Score Sheet

Altchek and associates proposed a scoring system based on a maximal possible score of 100 points for a normal shoulder (Table 28-4).[3] Pain accounts for 30 points, functional assessment for 28 points, tenderness for 5 points, impingement maneuvers for 32 points, and range of motion for 5 points. Pain was given the most weight because it is the primary symptom of concern to these authors. They developed an overall results rating scale defining excellent results as those scoring 90 to 100 points, good scoring 70 to 89 points, fair scoring 50 to 69 points, and poor with less than 50 points. The Hospital

*See references 17, 37, 43, 51-53, 60, 61, 89, 100-104, 111, 113, 124, 128, 142.

TABLE 28-2. Rowe Scoring System*

Scoring System	Units	Excellent (100-90)	Good (89-75)	Fair (74-51)	Poor (50 or Less)
Stability, no recurrence, subluxation, or apprehension	50	No recurrences	No recurrences	No recurrences	Recurrence of dislocation
Apprehension when placing arm in certain positions	30	No apprehension when placing arm in complete elevation and external rotation	Mild apprehension when placing arm in elevation and external rotation	Moderate apprehension during elevation and external rotation	Marked apprehension during elevation and extension
Subluxation (not requiring reduction)	10	No subluxation	No subluxation	No subluxation	
Motion 100% of normal external rotation, internal rotation, and elevation	20	100% of normal external rotation, internal rotation, and complete elevation	75% of normal external rotation, internal rotation, and complete elevation	50% of normal external rotation; 75% of internal rotation and elevation	No external rotation; 50% of elevation (can get hand only to face) and 50% of internal rotation
75% of normal external rotation; normal elevation and internal rotation	15				
50% of normal external rotation; 75% of internal rotation and elevation	5				
50% of normal external and internal rotation; no elevation	0				
Function: No limitation in work or sports; little or no discomfort	30	Performs all work and sports; no limitation in overhead activities; shoulder strong in lifting, swimming, tennis, throwing; no discomfort	Mild limitation in work and sports; shoulder strong; minimal discomfort	Moderate limitation doing overhead work and heavy lifting; unable to throw, serve hard in tennis, or swim; moderate disabling pain	Marked limitation; unable to perform overhead work and lifting; cannot throw, play tennis, or swim; chronic discomfort
Mild limitation in work or sports; little or no discomfort	25				
Moderate limitation and discomfort	10				
Marked limitation and pain	0				
Total units possible	100				

*The Rowe scoring system is used for evaluating the results of Bankart repairs.
From Rowe CR, Patel D, and Southmayd WW: The Bankart procedure: A long-term end-result study. J Bone Joint Surg Am *60*:1-16, 1978.

TABLE 28-3. UCLA Scoring System*,†

Function/Reaction Measured	Points
Pain	
Present all of the time and unbearable; strong medication used frequently	1
Present all of the time but bearable; strong medication used occasionally	2
None or little at rest, present during light activities; salicylates used frequently	4
Present during heavy or particular activities only; salicylates used occasionally	6
Occasional and slight	8
None	10
Function	
Unable to use limb	1
Only light activities possible	2
Able to do light housework or most activities of daily living	4
Most housework, shopping, and driving possible; able to fix hair and dress and undress, including fastening brassiere	6
Slight restriction only; able to work above shoulder level	8
Normal activities	10
Active Forward Flexion	
150 degrees or more	5
120 to 150 degrees	4
90 to 120 degrees	3
45 to 90 degrees	2
30 to 45 degrees	1
Less than 30 degrees	0
Strength of Forward Flexion (Manual Muscle Testing)	
Grade 5 (normal)	5
Grade 4 (good)	4
Grade 3 (fair)	3
Grade 2 (poor)	2
Grade 1 (muscle contraction)	1
Grade 0 (nothing)	0
Satisfaction of the Patient	
Satisfied and better	5
Not satisfied and worse	0

*The University of California–Los Angeles (UCLA) scoring system is used for evaluating shoulder function and patient satisfaction.
†Maximal score of 35 points.
From Ellman H, Hanker G, and Bayer M: Repair of the rotator cuff: End-result study of factors influencing reconstruction. J Bone Joint Surg Am 68:1136-1144, 1986.

TABLE 28-4. Hospital for Special Surgery Scoring System*

	No. of Points
Pain (30 points)	
None = 6 points, mild = 3, moderate = 2, severe = 0 during	
1. Sports	___
2. Non–sports-related overhead reaching	___
3. Activities of daily living	___
4. Sitting at rest	___
5. Sleeping	___
Total	___
Functional limitation (28 points)	
None = 7 points, mild = 4, moderate = 2, severe = 0 during:	
1. Sports with hand overhead	___
2. Sports not involving use of the shoulder	___
3. Reaching overhead	___
4. Nonspecific activities of daily living	___
Total	___
Tenderness (5 points)	
None = 5 points, at one or two sites = 3, at more than two sites = 0	
Total	___
Impingement maneuvers (32 points)	
Indicated numbers of points are assigned for each maneuver in an all-or-none fashion, 0 points being assigned if the maneuver is	
1. Impingement sign (15)	___
2. Abduction sign (12)	___
3. Adduction sign (5)	___
Total	___
Range of motion (5 points)	
One point is assigned for each 20-degree loss of motion in any plane, to a maximum of 5 points	
Total	___

*The Hospital for Special Surgery (HSS) scoring system is used for evaluating the results of acromioplasty.
From Altchek DW, Warren RF, Wickiewicz TL, et al: Arthroscopic acromioplasty: Technique and results. J Bone Joint Surg Am 72:1198-1207, 1990.

for Special Surgery Shoulder-Rating Scale relies heavily on medical metrics and thus requires that the patient return to the office for serial examination.

Constant Scoring System

In 1987, Constant and Murley presented their approach for measuring shoulder function (Table 28–5).[26] It involves a numeric estimation of the patient's function and evaluates the patient's pain. Point allocation includes 15 points for pain, 20 points for ADLs, 40 points for range of motion, and 35 points for strength. With the Constant score, 75% of the points are based on medical metrics; it therefore requires the patient to return to the office for serial examination.

American Shoulder and Elbow Surgeons' Form

This form includes both a patient self-evaluation section and medical metrics.[120] The patient self-evaluation section takes approximately 3 minutes to complete, requires no assistance, and includes an ADL section measured on a 4-point ordinal scale and visual analog scales to measure pain and instability. A shoulder score can be derived from the pain scales (50%) and a cumulative (ADL) score (50%). The medical metrics section includes demographic data and assessments of range of motion, physical signs, strength, and stability.

A modified version of this form is now available that reflects dysfunction of the entire upper extremity, including the hand, wrist, elbow, and shoulder (Table 28–6). It is based on the premise that the arm is a kinematic chain that acts in concert because all the elements are important in positioning the hand for grasp and manipulation of the environment.

TABLE 28–5. Constant Scoring System*

Pain	Points
None	15
Mild	10
Moderate	5
Severe	0

Activities of Daily Living

Acitivity Level	Points	Positioning	Points
Full work	4	Up to waist	2
Full recreation/sport	4	Up to xiphoid	4
Unaffected sleep	2	Up to neck	6
		Up to top of head	8
		Above head	10

Total for activities of daily living: 20

Points for Forward and Lateral Elevation

Elevation (Degrees)	Points
0–30	0
31–60	2
61–90	4
91–120	6
121–150	8
151–180	10

External Rotation Scoring

Position	Points
Hand behind head with elbow held forward	2
Hand behind head with elbow held back	2
Hand on top of head with elbow held forward	2
Hand on top of head with elbow held back	2
Full elevation from on top of head	2
Total: 10	

Internal Rotation Scoring

Position	Points
Dorsum of hand to lateral-thigh area	0
Dorsum of hand to buttock	2
Dorsum of hand to lumbosacral junction	4
Dorsum of hand to waist (3rd lumbar vertebra)	6
Dorsum of hand to 12th dorsal vertebra	8
Dorsum of hand to interscapular region (DV 7)	10

*The Constant scoring system is used for evaluating general shoulder function both objectively and subjectively.
From Constant CR and Murley AHG: A clinical method of functional assessment of the shoulder. Clin Orthop *214*:160-164, 1987.

TABLE 28–6. ASES Scoring System*

ASES Patient Self-evaluation: Instability Questionnaire

Does your shoulder feel unstable (as though it is going to dislocate)?	YES	NO

How unstable is your shoulder (mark line)?

0 |____|____|____|____|____|____|____|____|____|____| 10
Very Stable   Very Unstable

ASES Patient Self-evaluation: Activity of Daily Living Questionnaire

Circle the number in the box that indicates your ability to do the following activities:
0 = unable to do; 1 = very difficult to do; 2 = somewhat difficult; 3 = not difficult

Activity	Right Arm				Left Arm			
1. Put on a coat	0	1	2	3	0	1	2	3
2. Sleep on your painful or affected side	0	1	2	3	0	1	2	3
3. Wash back or do up bra in back	0	1	2	3	0	1	2	3
4. Manage toileting	0	1	2	3	0	1	2	3
5. Comb hair	0	1	2	3	0	1	2	3
6. Reach a high shelf	0	1	2	3	0	1	2	3
7. Lift 10 lb above shoulder	0	1	2	3	0	1	2	3
8. Throw a ball overhand	0	1	2	3	0	1	2	3
9. Do usual work—list:	0	1	2	3	0	1	2	3
10. Do usual sport—list:	0	1	2	3	0	1	2	3

ASES Physician Assessment: Range of Motion

Range of Motion	Right		Left	
Total shoulder motion; goniometer preferred	Active	Passive	Active	Passive
Forward elevation (maximal arm-trunk angle)				
External rotation (arm comfortably at side)				
External rotation (arm at 90 degrees of abduction)				
Internal rotation (highest posterior anatomy reached with the thumb)				
Cross-body adduction (antecubital fossa to the opposite acromion)				

ASES Physician Assessment: Signs

0 = none; 1 = mild; 2 = moderate; 3 = severe

Sign	Right				Left			
Supraspinatus/greater tuberosity tenderness	0	1	2	3	0	1	2	3
Acromioclavicular joint tenderness	0	1	2	3	0	1	2	3
Biceps tendon tenderness (or rupture)	0	1	2	3	0	1	2	3
Other tenderness—list:	0	1	2	3	0	1	2	3
Impingement I (passive forward elevation in slight internal rotation)	Y	N			Y	N		
Impingement II (passive internal rotation with 90 degrees of flexion)	Y	N			Y	N		
Impingement III (90 degrees of active abduction—classic painful arc)	Y	N			Y	N		
Subacromial crepitus	Y	N			Y	N		
Scars—location:	Y	N			Y	N		
Atrophy—location:	Y	N			Y	N		
Deformity—describe:	Y	N			Y	N		

*The American Shoulder and Elbow Surgeons (ASES) scoring system is used for evaluating general shoulder function both objectively and subjectively.
MRC, Medical Research Council.
From Richards RR, An K-N, Bigliani LU, et al: A standardized method for assessment of shoulder function. J Shoulder Elbow Surg 3:347–352, 1994.

Continued

TABLE 28–6. ASES Scoring System—cont'd

ASES Physician Assessment: Strength (Record MRC grade)
0 = no contraction; 1 = flicker; 2 = movement with gravity eliminated;
3 = movement against gravity; 4 = movement against some resistance; 5 = normal power

	Right						Left					
Testing affected by pain?	Y		N				Y		N			
Forward elevation	0	1	2	3	4	5	0	1	2	3	4	5
Abduction	0	1	2	3	4	5	0	1	2	3	4	5
External rotation (arm comfortably at side)	0	1	2	3	4	5	0	1	2	3	4	5
Internal rotation (arm comfortably at side)	0	1	2	3	4	5	0	1	2	3	4	5

ASES Physician Assessment: Instability
0 = none; 1 = mild (0- to 1-cm translation)
2 = moderate (1- to 2-cm translation or translates to glenoid rim)
3 = severe (>2-cm translation or over rim of glenoid)

Anterior translation	0	1	2	3	0	1	2	3
Posterior translation	0	1	2	3	0	1	2	3
Interior translation (sulcus sign)	0	1	2	3	0	1	2	3
Anterior apprehension	0	1	2	3	0	1	2	3
Reproduces symptoms?	Y	N			Y	N		
Voluntary instability?	Y	N			Y	N		
Relocation test positive?	Y	N			Y	N		
Generalized ligamentous laxity?			Y	N				

Other physical findings:

Examiner's name: Date

Shoulder Severity Index

Conceived by Patte, this tool seeks to assess chronically painful shoulder disabilities (Table 28–7).[115] It takes approximately 7 minutes to complete and evaluates pain in different situations of daily life, functional activities, strength, and daily handicap. It includes 7 questions concerning pain, 20 for function, and 1 each for strength, handicap, and satisfaction.[6]

Other Tools

Many groups have altered the aforementioned scoring systems to suit various specific clinical conditions. Kay and Amstutz revised the UCLA score to apply specifically to hemiarthroplasty results.[74] This modified, treatment-specific version is shown in Table 28–8.

Other assessment tools are very disease specific. One example is the form proposed by Poigenfurst and colleagues to specifically evaluate the results of acromioclavicular separation and its management (Table 28–9).[117] Dawson and associates devised a self-assessment questionnaire specifically for evaluation of shoulder instabil-

ity. This instrument correlated well with the Rowe score in terms of validity and reliability.[33]

Specific patient groups are the focus of other questionnaires. Tibone and Bradley proposed a scoring system whose goal was the assessment of athletic shoulder problems and results.[136] This form is shown in Table 28–10.

Dawson and colleagues published their questionnaire for evaluating patients' perceptions before and after shoulder surgery.[32] This 12-item questionnaire was specifically created to measure the outcome of operations on the shoulder, excluding stabilization procedures (Table 28–11).

Others have used batteries of questions aimed at documenting the patient's history and functional status, as well as postoperative results. For example, the Hughston Clinic and the Steadman-Hawkins Clinic use the inventories shown in Tables 28–12 and 28–13.

The Academy of Orthopaedic Surgeons has developed a questionnaire to evaluate upper extremity function, including the hand, wrist, elbow, and shoulder. This questionnaire is part of their thrust toward a specialty-wide outcomes evaluation system for essentially all

Text continued on p. 1403

TABLE 28-7.   Shoulder Severity Scoring System*

Algofunctional Index of Patte for Shoulders

Family name: First name: Date:

_____   _____   _____

Shoulder: *Right/Left*
File Number: Documented:

_____   _____

Diagnosis:

_____

Pain (P)

Choose the figure that most appropriately describes your pain:
  0: No pain
  1: Mild pain
  2: Moderate pain
  3: Severe pain
  4: Unbearable pain
Place this figure in each column and then multiply by the coefficient:
  When resting with the arm hanging or bent   _____ X   2   = _____
  As soon as you try to raise your arm   _____ X   1.5 = _____
  Only when you repeat the movement   _____ X   1   = _____
  During a sudden movement   _____ X   0.5 = _____
If you can't sleep on the affected shoulder, add 1 point: +1   = _____
If you have the feeling that something "blocks" when you raise the arm:
  Forward, add 2 points   +2   = _____
  Sideways, add 1 point   +1   = _____
If you take painkillers
  All the time: add 4 points   +4   = _____
  From time to time: add 2 points   +2   = _____

                                                   Points = [   ] /30*

Functional Index (I)
Movements must be performed with the affected shoulder, even if these are unusual movements, and **without the help of the other hand** and without "cheating" by using the head or the trunk.

Please reply to each question using the following point system:
  0: Without difficulty
  1: With difficulty/0.5/1.5
  2: Impossible

Can you:
1. Hygiene
     Wash your forehead or apply makeup yourself   = _____
     Wash your hair completely (even behind)   = _____
     Wash under the armpit on the opposite side   = _____
     Wash your opposite scapula (from in front)   = _____
     Wipe yourself (after going to the toilet)   = _____
                                                  ..../10

2. Dressing
     Put tight trousers on and buckle the belt   = _____
     Put a pullover on or off by passing it over your head = _____
     Put a jacket on, finishing with the affected shoulder = _____
     Put your shirt into skirt or trousers (including behind) = _____
                                                  ..../8

3. Eating: sitting at a table
     Eat your soup with a spoon (elbow not on the table) = _____
     Lift a full bottle (1 L) with your arm outstretched = _____
     Pour yourself a drink from this bottle   = _____
                                                  ..../6

*The Shoulder Severity scoring system was developed by Patte for patient self-assessment of painful or chronically disabled shoulders.
From Patte D: Directions for the use of the index severity for painful and/or chronically disabled shoulders [abstract]. Paper presented at the first Open Congress of the European Society of Surgery of the Shoulder and Elbow [SECEC], Paris, 1987, pp 36–41.   *Continued*

TABLE 28-7.   Shoulder Severity Scoring System—cont'd

4. Daily gestures (try to do them even if they are not usual)
    Knitting, ironing, planing   = _____
    Military salute   = _____
    Open and close a window (or shelve light things):
      At eye level   = _____
      Above your head   = _____
    Change an electric light bulb on the ceiling   = _____
    Clean the window panes above the level of your head   = _____
    Push open a door with your arm stretched sideways   = _____
    Change gears in a car (put into reverse gear)   = _____
                           ..../16

                       I = [   ] /40

Total Functional Index

Muscle Strength (MS)
How much lifting strength do you think you have lost when lifting an object (2 kg) with the arm stretched out horizontally?
    Normal strength   =   0
    Less than normal strength with fatigability   = 3 to 5
    Half of usual strength   = 6 to 10
    No lifting strength   =   15

                       MS = [   ] /15

Daily Handicap (H)
Rate your handicap between 0% and 100%

0% |___|___|___|___|___|___|___|___|___|___|___|___| 100%
(No handicap)   (Unbearable handicap)

(The figure to be noted is that marked in centimeters by the patient.)   H = [   ] /15
Total = (P + 1 + MS + H)

The algofunctional index (AF)[†] for functional value of the shoulder examined is:
100—total   AF + = %

Evaluation of the Result

	Favorable			Unfavorable		
	TB 1	B 2	M + 3	M − 4	E 5	1
Algofunctional index (postoperative)	>90%	>75%	>66%	>50%	<50%	2 3
Comparison of preoperative and postoperative algofunctional index			>25%	<25%		4 5

Adjustments   Painful chronic shoulder: pain must be <5 for favorable result
                   Active patient: muscular strength must be multiplied by 2   MS × 2

                   Elderly patient with limited activity or prosthetic replacement:
                   Muscular strength must be divided by 2   MS / 2

Subjective result   Very pleased [   ]   Pleased [   ]   Dissatisfied [   ]

[†]This algofunctional index can be used only if the pain (P) is less than 15. Otherwise, the index must be calculated again once the painful episode is over.

TABLE 28–8. UCLA Scoring System–Modification for Hemiarthroplasty*

	Score	Findings
Pain		
	1	Constant, unbearable; strong medication used frequently
	2	Constant, but bearable; strong medication used occasionally
	4	None or little at rest; occurs with light activity; salicylates used frequently
	5	With heavy or particular activities only; salicylates used occasionally
	8	Occasional and slight
	10	No pain
Function		
	1	Unable to use arm
	2	Very light activity only
	4	Light housework or most daily living activities
	5	Most housework, washing hair, putting on brassiere, shopping, driving
	8	Slight restrictions only; able to work above shoulder level
	10	Normal activities
Muscle Power and Motion		
	1	Ankylosis with deformity
	2	Ankylosis with good functional position
	4	Muscle power poor to fair; elevation less than 60 degrees; internal rotation less than 45 degrees
	5	Muscle power fair to good; elevation of 90 degrees; internal rotation of 90 degrees
	8	Muscle power good or normal; elevation of 140 degrees; external rotation of 20 degrees
	10	Normal muscle power; motion near normal

*A modification of the UCLA scoring system is used for evaluating the results of shoulder hemiarthroplasty.
From Kay SP and Amstutz HC: Shoulder hemiarthroplasty at UCLA. Clin Orthop 228:42-44, 1988.

TABLE 28–9. Acromioclavicular Separation Scoring System*

Rating Criteria According to Poigenfurst et al (1987)

Excellent
Maximal limitation of mobility of no more than 10 degrees when compared with the contralateral side
No complaints (except sensitivity to changes in weather)
Full athletic fitness (no paresthesia)
Radiographic findings: no dislocation or subluxation

Good
Limitation of mobility ranging between 1 and 20 degrees when compared with the contralateral side
Minor complaints during load
Full athletic fitness (minor paresthesia lateral from the scar)
Radiographic findings: no dislocation; subluxation as much as half of the clavicular diameter

Poor
Limitation of mobility of more than 20 degrees when compared with the contralateral side
Complaints during normal activities or even at rest
Obvious reduction in athletic fitness (paresthesia lateral from the scar)
Radiographic findings: dislocation

*The scoring system was developed by Poigenfurst and associates specifically for evaluating results after acromioclavicular separation.
From Poigenfurst J, Orthner E, and Hoffman J: Technik und ergebnisse der koraklavikularen verschraubung bei frischen Akromioklavikularzerreissungen. Acta Chir Austriaca 1:11-16, 1987.

TABLE 28-10. Athletic Shoulder Outcome Scoring System*

Name _____ Age _____ Sex _____

Dominant Hand _____(R)_____(L)_____ (Ambidextrous) _____

Type of Sport _____

Position Played _____

Years Played _____

Prior Injury _____

Activity Level
1. Professional (Major League)
2. Professional (Minor League)
3. College
4. High school
5. Recreational (full-time)
6. Recreational (part-time)

Diagnosis
1. Anterior instability
2. Posterior instability
3. Multidirectional instability
4. Recurrent dislocations
5. Impingement syndrome
6. Acromioclavicular syndrome
7. Acromioclavicular arthrosis
8. Rotator cuff repair (partial)
9. Rotator cuff repair (complete)
10. Biceps tendon rupture
11. Calcific tendinitis
12. Fracture

Subjective (90 Points)

I. Pain	Points
No pain with competition	10
Pain after competing only	8
Pain while competing	6
Pain preventing competing	4
Pain with ADLs	2
Pain at rest	0

II. Strength/Endurance |
--- | ---
No weakness; normal competition fatigue | 10
Weakness after competition; early competition fatigue | 8
Weakness during competition; abnormal competition fatigue | 6
Weakness or fatigue preventing competition | 4
Weakness or fatigue with ADLs | 2
Weakness or fatigue preventing ADLs | 0

III. Stability |
--- | ---
No looseness during competition | 10
Recurrent subluxations while competing | 8
Dead arm syndrome while competing | 6
Recurrent subluxations prevent competition | 4
Recurrent subluxations during ADLs | 2
Dislocations | 0

IV. Intensity |
--- | ---
Preinjury versus postinjury hours of competition (100%) | 10
Preinjury versus postinjury hours of competition (<75%) | 8
Preinjury versus postinjury hours of competition (<50%) | 6
Preinjury versus postinjury hours of competition (<25%) | 4
Preinjury versus postinjury hours of ADLs (100%) | 2
Preinjury versus postinjury hours of ADLs (<50%) | 0

V. Performance |
--- | ---
At the same level, same proficiency | 50
At the same level, decreased proficiency | 40
At the same level, decreased proficiency, not acceptable to an athlete | 30
Decreased level with acceptable proficiency at that level | 20
Decreased level, unacceptable proficiency | 10
Cannot compete, had to switch sport | 0

Objective (10 Points)

Range of Motion |
--- | ---
Normal external rotation at 90-degree to 90-degree position; normal elevation | 10
Less than 5-degree loss of external rotation; normal elevation | 8
Less than 10-degree loss of external rotation; normal elevation | 6
Less than 15-degree loss of external rotation; normal elevation | 4
Less than 20-degree loss of external rotation; normal elevation | 2
Greater than 20-degree loss of external rotation or any loss of elevation | 0

Overall Results

Excellent	90–100	Points
Good	70–89	Points
Fair	50–69	Points
Poor	<50	Points

*The Athletic Shoulder Outcome scoring system is used for evaluating general shoulder function specifically in athletes.

ADLs, activities of daily living.

From Tibone JE and Bradley J: Evaluation of treatment outcomes for the athlete's shoulder. *In* Matsen FA III, Fu FH, and Hawkins RJ (eds): The Shoulder: A Balance of Mobility and Stability. Rosemont, IL: American Academy of Orthopaedic Surgeons, 1993, pp 526–527.

9553

ity.

TABLE 28-11.   Shoulder Surgery Scoring System*

Item	Scoring Categories
During the Past 4 Weeks	
1. How would you describe the worst pain you had from your shoulder?	1 None 2 Mild 3 Moderate 4 Severe 5 Unbearable
2. Have you had any trouble dressing yourself because of your shoulder?	1 No trouble at all 2 Little trouble 3 Moderate trouble 4 Extreme difficulty 5 Impossible to do
3. Have you had any trouble getting in and out of a car or using public transportation because of your shoulder (whichever you tend to use)?	1 No trouble at all 2 Little trouble 3 Moderate trouble 4 Extreme difficulty 5 Impossible to do
4. Have you been able to use a knife and fork at the same time?	1 Yes, easily 2 With little difficulty 3 With moderate difficulty 4 With extreme difficulty 5 No, impossible
5. Could you do the household shopping on your own?	1 Yes, easily 2 With little difficulty 3 With moderate difficulty 4 With extreme difficulty 5 No, impossible
6. Could you carry a tray containing a plate of food across a room?	1 Yes, easily 2 With little difficulty 3 With moderate difficulty 4 With extreme difficulty 5 No, impossible
7. Could you brush or comb your hair with the affected arm?	1 Yes, easily 2 With little difficulty 3 With moderate difficulty 4 With extreme difficulty 5 No, impossible
8. How would you describe the pain that you usually had from your shoulder?	1 None 2 Mild 3 Moderate 4 Severe 5 Unbearable
9. Could you hang your clothes up in a wardrobe with the affected arm?	1 Yes, easily 2 With little difficulty 3 With moderate difficulty 4 With extreme difficulty 5 No, impossible
10. Have you been able to wash and dry yourself under both arms?	1 Yes, easily 2 With little difficulty 3 With moderate difficulty 4 With extreme difficulty 5 No, impossible
11. How much has pain from your shoulder interfered with your usual work (including housework)?	1 Not at all 2 A little bit 3 Moderately 4 Greatly 5 Totally
12. Have you been troubled by pain from your shoulder in bed at night?	1 No nights 2 Only 1 or 2 nights 3 Some nights 4 Most nights 5 Every night

*The shoulder surgery scoring system was developed by Dawson and associates for patient self-assessment of general shoulder function after surgery.
From Dawson J, Fitzpatrick R, and Carr A: Questionnaire on the perceptions of patients about shoulder surgery. J Bone Joint Surg Br 78:593–600, 1996.

TABLE 28–12. Hughston Sports Medicine Foundation Follow-up Shoulder History*

1. How often does your shoulder hurt?	0 1 2 3 4 5 6 7 8 9 10 None · · · · · · · · · · All the time
2. How severe is the pain at its worst	0 1 2 3 4 5 6 7 8 9 10 None · · · · · · · · Excruciating, requiring pain pills
3. Does your shoulder hurt at night?	0 1 2 3 4 5 6 7 8 9 10 No · · · · · · · · Severe, doesn't allow me to sleep
4. Does the pain in your shoulder radiate to your neck or down your arm?	0 1 2 3 4 5 6 7 8 9 10 Never · · · · · · · · · · All the time
5. Do you feel popping when your shoulder moves?	0 1 2 3 4 5 6 7 8 9 10 None · · · · · · · · Severe, all the time
6. Does your shoulder catch when you move it?	0 1 2 3 4 5 6 7 8 9 10 None · · · · · · · · Severe, all the time
7. Does your shoulder slip when you move it?	0 1 2 3 4 5 6 7 8 9 10 No · · · · · · · · Severe, all the time
8. Is your shoulder stiff?	0 1 2 3 4 5 6 7 8 9 10 No · · · · · · · · Cannot move my shoulder
9. Do you have the feeling of your arm "going dead" with certain activities?	0 1 2 3 4 5 6 7 8 9 10 No · · · · · · · Every time I perform that activity
10. How would you grade the strength of your shoulder in comparison to your normal shoulder?	0 1 2 3 4 5 6 7 8 9 10 Same · · · · · · · · · · No strength
11. Are you able to push objects?	0 1 2 3 4 5 6 7 8 9 10 No problem · · · · · · · · · · Unable
12. Are you able to pull objects?	0 1 2 3 4 5 6 7 8 9 10 No problem · · · · · · · · · · Unable
13. Are you able to throw objects?	0 1 2 3 4 5 6 7 8 9 10 No problem · · · · · · · · · · Unable
14. Are you able to lift objects (up to 10 to 15 lb)?	0 1 2 3 4 5 6 7 8 9 10 No problem · · · · · · · · · · Unable
15. Are you able to carry objects (10 to 15 lb) with your arms at your side?	0 1 2 3 4 5 6 7 8 9 10 No problem · · · · · · · · · · Unable
16. Are you able to comb your hair?	0 1 2 3 4 5 6 7 8 9 10 No problem · · · · · · · · · · Unable
17. Are you able to eat with utensils?	0 1 2 3 4 5 6 7 8 9 10 No problem · · · · · · · · · · Unable
18. Are you able to sleep on the involved side?	0 1 2 3 4 5 6 7 8 9 10 No problem · · · · · · · · · · Unable
19. Are you able to wash the opposite underarm?	0 1 2 3 4 5 6 7 8 9 10 No problem · · · · · · · · · · Unable
20. Are you able to use the involved hand for toilet care?	0 1 2 3 4 5 6 7 8 9 10 No problem · · · · · · · · · · Unable
21. Are you able to reach your back pocket or fasten your bra?	0 1 2 3 4 5 6 7 8 9 10 No problem · · · · · · · · · · Unable
22. Are you able to dress?	0 1 2 3 4 5 6 7 8 9 10 No problem · · · · · · · · · · Unable
23. Are you able to use your involved hand at shoulder level?	0 1 2 3 4 5 6 7 8 9 10 No problem · · · · · · · · · · Unable
24. Are you able to use your involved hand over your head?	0 1 2 3 4 5 6 7 8 9 10 No problem · · · · · · · · · · Unable
25. Are you able to perform your usual work?	0 1 2 3 4 5 6 7 8 9 10 No problem · · · · · · · · · · Unable
26. Are you able to perform your usual sport?	0 1 2 3 4 5 6 7 8 9 10 No problem · · · · · · · · · · Unable
27. Has your lifestyle changed because of your shoulder?	0 1 2 3 4 5 6 7 8 9 10 Not at all · · · · · · · · · · Dramatically
28. Are you satisfied with your shoulder function since surgery?	0 1 2 3 4 5 6 7 8 9 10 Yes · · · · · · · · · · No

COMMENTS:

*The Hughston Sports Medicine Foundation follow-up shoulder history form is used for patient self-assessment of general shoulder function and satisfaction.
From J. C. Hughston, Hughston Sports Medicine Clinic, Columbus, GA.

TABLE 28–13.   Hawkins Shoulder Evaluation Form*

Pain Assessment Postoperatively

1. Is your overcall pain better than it was before surgery?   Y
                                                               N

2. How bad is your pain today? (Mark line)

| | | | | | | | | | | | |

No pain at all   Pain as bad as it can be

3. Is your pain . . . (Circle one):
        Improving   Staying the same   Getting worse
4. Do you require pain medications?   Y   N
5. Do you require narcotic analgesics?   Y   N
6. If yes, how many per day? (Average)   # ___ Pills

Function

Circle the number that indicates your ability to do the following activities:
0 = Unable; 1 = very difficult; 2 = somewhat difficult; 3 = not difficult

Activity	Right Arm				Left Arm			
Put on a coat	0	1	2	3	0	1	2	3
Sleep on your side	0	1	2	3	0	1	2	3
Wash back/hook brassiere	0	1	2	3	0	1	2	3
Manage toileting	0	1	2	3	0	1	2	3
Comb hair	0	1	2	3	0	1	2	3
Reach a high shelf	0	1	2	3	0	1	2	3
Lift 10 lb above shoulder	0	1	2	3	0	1	2	3
Throw a ball overhead	0	1	2	3	0	1	2	3
Do usual work (List):	0	1	2	3	0	1	2	3
Do modified work (List):	0	1	2	3	0	1	2	3
Do usual sport (List):	0	1	2	3	0	1	2	3
Do modified sport (List):	0	1	2	3	0	1	2	3

At what level can you participate in sports? (Check one)

_____   1. Significantly below my preinjury level

_____   2. Slightly below my preinjury level

_____   3. Equal to my preinjury

_____   4. Above my preinjury level

Overall Satisfaction

| | | | | | | | | | | |

Very satisfied   Unsatisfied

*The Hawkins shoulder evaluation form is used for patient self-assessment of general shoulder function and satisfaction.
From R. J. Hawkins, Steadman Hawkins Clinic, Vail, CO.

---

musculoskeletal systems.[2] These questionnaires also include an overall health status portion. The upper extremity–specific portion is shown in Table 28–14. Normative values have also been established. These data are important for determining whether treated individuals can be distinguished from normal individuals serving as a reference group and for ascertaining the degree to which pretreatment and post-treatment change is clinically significant.[64]

In 1991, a group of rheumatologists presented their approach to shoulder evaluation, the Shoulder Pain and Disability Index.[121] It includes five visual analog scales that test pain and eight scales that test function. The index requires 3 to 5 minutes for patients to complete and is moderately easy to score. This index also aims at overall shoulder function and pain.

The Subjective Shoulder Rating Scale, presented in 1992, uses multiple-choice questions that are weighted by response.[63] It takes less than 3 minutes to fill out and

is easy to score. This form is oriented to a determination of impairment and deals more with overall shoulder function.[6]

The Shoulder Disability Questionnaire is a 16-item self-assessment instrument designed to evaluate functional status limitation and may be useful for assessing functional disability in longitudinal studies.[140,141]

The Disability of the Arm, Shoulder and Hand questionnaire is a region-specific measurement tool that was developed to evaluate disability and symptoms in a single or multiple disorders of the upper extremity at a single or multiple points in time. It may be applied to conditions involving only a single joint.[5,129]

The Single Assessment Numeric Evaluation (SANE) is determined by a subject's written response to the question "How would you rate your shoulder today as a percentage of normal (0% to 100% scale)?" The SANE score has been shown to correlate well with other outcome measures, thus suggesting that it may be a good adjunct

TABLE 28-14. AAOS Upper Extremity Scoring System*

	No Difficulty	Mild Difficulty	Moderate Difficulty	Severe Difficulty	Unable
Open a tight or new jar	1	2	3	4	5
Write	1	2	3	4	5
Turn a key	1	2	3	4	5
Prepare a meal	1	2	3	4	5
Push open a heavy door	1	2	3	4	5
Place an object on a shelf above your head	1	2	3	4	5
Do heavy household chores (e.g., wash walls, wash floors)	1	2	3	4	5
Garden or do yardwork	1	2	3	4	5
Make a bed	1	2	3	4	5
Carry a shopping bag or briefcase	1	2	3	4	5
Carry a heavy object (over 10 lb)	1	2	3	4	5
Change a lightbulb overhead	1	2	3	4	5
Wash or blow-dry your hair	1	2	3	4	5
Wash your back	1	2	3	4	5
Put on a pullover sweater	1	2	3	4	5
Use a knife to cut food	1	2	3	4	5
Recreational activities that require little effort (e.g., card playing, knitting, etc.)	1	2	3	4	5
Recreational activities in which you take some force or impact through your arm, shoulder, or hand (e.g., golf, hammering, tennis)	1	2	3	4	5
Recreational activities in which you move your arm freely (e.g., playing frisbee, badminton)	1	2	3	4	5
Manage transportation needs (getting from one place to another)					
Sexual activities	1	2	3	4	5

	Not at All	Slightly	Moderately	Quite a bit	Extremely
During the **past week, to what extent** has your arm, shoulder, or hand problem interfered with your normal social activities with family, friends, neighbors, or groups? (Circle number.)	1	2	3	4	5

	Not Limited at All	Slightly Limited	Moderately Limited	Very Limited	Unable
During the **past week** were you limited in your work or other regular daily activities as a result of your arm, shoulder, or hand problem? (Circle number.)	1	2	3	4	5

Please rate the severity of the following symptoms in the **last week**. (Circle number.)

	None	Mild	Moderate	Severe	Extreme
Arm, shoulder, or hand pain	1	2	3	4	5
Arm, shoulder, or hand pain when you performed any specific activity	1	2	3	4	5
Tingling (pins and needles) in your arm, shoulder, or hand	1	2	3	4	5
Weakness in your arm, shoulder, or hand	1	2	3	4	5
Stiffness in your arm, shoulder, or hand					

*The American Academy of Orthopaedic Surgeons (AAOS) upper extremity portion of their scoring system is used for patient self-assessment of general upper extremity function.
From the American Academy of Orthopaedic Surgeons/Council of Musculoskeletal Specialty Societies/Institute for Work and Health Outcomes Data Collection Package. Version 2.0. May 1997.

Continued

TABLE 28-14.   AAOS Upper Extremity Scoring System—cont'd

	No Difficulty	Mild Difficulty	Moderate Difficulty	Severe Difficulty	So Much Difficulty That I Can't Sleep
During the **past week**, how much difficulty have you had sleeping because of the pain in your arm, shoulder, or hand? (Circle number.)	1	2	3	4	5

	Strongly Disagree	Disagree	Neither Agree nor Disagree	Agree	Strongly Agree
I feel less capable, less confident, or less useful because of my arm, shoulder, or hand problem. (Circle number)	1	2	3	4	5

The following questions relate to the impact of your arm, shoulder, or hand problem on **playing your musical instrument or sport or both**. If you play more than one sport or instrument (or play both), please answer with respect to the activity that is most important to you. Please indicate the sport or instrument that is most important to you:

Please circle the number that best describes your physical ability in the past week. Did you have any difficulty:

	No Difficulty	Mild Difficulty	Moderate Difficulty	Severe Difficulty	Unable
Using your usual technique for playing your instrument or sport?	1	2	3	4	5
Playing your musical instrument or sport because of arm, shoulder, or hand pain?	1	2	3	4	5
Playing your musical instrument or sport as well as you would like?	1	2	3	4	5
Spending your usual amount of time practicing or playing your instrument or sport?	1	2	3	4	5

The following questions relate to the impact of your arm, shoulder, or hand problem on **your work**.

Please circle the number that best describes your physical ability in the *past week*. Did you have any difficulty:

	No Difficulty	Mild Difficulty	Moderate Difficulty	Severe Difficulty	Unable
Using your usual technique for your work?	1	2	3	4	5
Doing your usual work because of arm, shoulder, or hand pain?	1	2	3	4	5
Doing your work as well as you would like?	1	2	3	4	5
Spending your usual amount of time doing your work?	1	2	3	4	5

for assessing outcomes with little demand in time or resources.[154]

Investigators in Canada have sought to develop disease-specific quality-of-life instruments for instability, rotator cuff disease, and osteoarthritis. These instruments include the Western Ontario Shoulder Instability Index (WOSI), the Western Ontario Rotator Cuff Index (WORC), and the Western Ontario Osteoarthritis of the Shoulder Index (WOOS).[79-81,91]

HEALTH STATUS INSTRUMENTS

Shoulder disorders do not exist in isolation, but rather in the context of the overall health of the individual. Health status self-assessment tests have been developed to document patients' perception of their overall health and function. Because shoulder-specific instruments perform differently than health status instruments do (e.g., SF-36), both disease-specific and overall health status measures are needed for the complete evaluation of patients with shoulder problems.[6] Although joint-specific instruments are more sensitive in detecting change in patient status over time, they do not reliably measure the effect of a condition or treatment intervention on the overall health status of the patient. Because patient quality of life depends on the overall health condition, understanding patient perception in terms of general health status is important for estimating the relative contribution of musculoskeletal disease.

History

Health status assessments and psychological indicators have been used extensively throughout medicine, including evaluation of low back pain.[14,20,35,46,138,143,155] Similarly, problems of the shoulder are not without influences other than joint-specific issues. The importance of overall health status in disorders of the shoulder is not a new idea. Even Codman noted the impact of various psychological and medical issues on patients with shoulder complaints.[25] Lorenz and Musser[92] and Coventry[30] noted the effect of health variables on conditions of the shoulder in the 1950s. Several subsequent studies evaluated the characteristics of patients with frozen shoulders, once again looking at factors other than those related to the shoulder itself.[21,45,112] Green and associates presented data examining the effect of psychological and psychiatric factors on failed shoulder surgery.[55] Using the SF-36 form, Gartsman and colleagues sought to determine whether perception of health status had an effect on assessment of shoulder function for five common shoulder disorders, including anterior instability, rotator cuff tear, adhesive capsulitis, osteoarthritis, and impingement syndrome. Data were compared with published norms and indicated that these shoulder conditions rank in severity with five major medical conditions, including hypertension, congestive heart failure, acute myocardial infarction, diabetes mellitus, and clinical depression.[48]

Variability in both the manifestation of specific shoulder conditions and the degree of improvement after shoulder surgery is not well understood and probably relates to the contribution of physical and psychological comorbidity. Matsen and coworkers studied preoperative health status and shoulder function in patients undergoing total shoulder arthroplasty for degenerative joint disease. Preoperative physical and social function correlated highest with postoperative comfort and function. This study highlights the importance of general health assessment in predicting patients who are likely to benefit most from a treatment intervention.[101]

The four most widely used and evaluated scales that are appropriate for use in musculoskeletal disease/injury are the SF-36, the QWB that forms the backbone of the quality-adjusted life years (QALYs) methodology, the Nottingham Health Profile, and the Sickness Impact Profile (SIP). These scales share the common goal of assessing many characteristics of human activity, including physical, psychological, social, and role functioning. Additionally, they share the characteristic of assessing the patient as a whole (from the patient's perspective) and not as an organ system, disease, or limb. They are internally consistent and reproducible and can discriminate between clinical conditions of different severity. The scales are also sensitive to change in health status over time. Additional benefits are derived from the fact that they are not administered by a physician, which increases their reliability.

Self-assessments of health status have been in wide clinical use; some include evaluation of anxiety and depression, pain scales, and symptom inventories.[44,110,116]

Brief descriptions of these instruments follow.

Short Form-36

The SF-36 is a widely used general health status questionnaire that has been used to demonstrate the health status of control populations and populations with defined medical and psychological conditions, including the effectiveness of orthopaedic management.[4,16,67,70,71,130,131,135,144-148] This form is shown in Table 28-15.

By means of a standard algorithm, the responses to the questions are used to calculate eight SF-36 parameters. The maximal score for each parameter is 100.[148] The variables evaluated include "physical role function," "comfort (pain)," "physical function," "emotional role function," "social function," "vitality (energy/fatigue)," "mental health," and "general health."

Radosevich and associates used this instrument to collect reference data from large populations.[119] Control data for the SF-36 were derived from three separate population-based health status surveys. These reference data cohorts did not exclude individuals with chronic back pain, arthritis, and other chronic conditions; thus, these control data represent a population cross-section and not the health status of "normal" individuals. As shown in Figures 28-1 to 28-8, the results from population-based controls decrease with age. Accordingly, if patients from different age groups are to be compared, it is useful to normalize patients' scores with the average of control patients of similar age.[119]

The SF-36 demonstrates face validity; for instance, among 1200 randomly selected subjects completing the questionnaire, patients with arthritis had the second worst body pain score and the second most limited physical role function score. They also had the second best emotional role function score and the best mental health score out of all the chronic conditions investigated. For social function, vitality, and general health perceptions, individuals with arthritis scored in the middle of the group.[94]

The SF-36 has been validated to be reliable by self-administration (by the patient), by interviewer, by telephone, and by mail, and the form takes only 5 to 7 minutes to complete. These features make its use appealing; it is the most practical for use in a busy office or clinic setting. This instrument, however, may well have a "floor effect" for musculoskeletal conditions, which means that patients with musculoskeletal problems may "bottom out" on the scale so that it does not differentiate different degrees of impairment. Our experience in administering the SF-36 shows that some patients with musculoskeletal disease or injury misinterpret the questions on general health as being exclusive of their musculoskeletal disease. The SF-36 also emphasizes lower extremity rather than upper extremity function.[40,99] Various groups have begun to develop an algorithm yielding a composite score for mental and physical overall function.

The SF-36 is helpful in responding to Codman's admonition. The form documents health status from the standpoint of the patient, it is practical and easy to complete, and it has been shown to be sensitive to musculoskeletal disease and orthopaedic treatment.

Quality of Well-Being Scale

Quality-of-life data are becoming increasingly important for evaluating the cost utility or cost-effectiveness of various health care programs. The QWB forms the basis

TABLE 28–15. Health Status Questionnaire (SF-36)*

This survey asks for your views about your health. Please answer every question by circling the appropriate number: 1, 2, 3, etc. If you are unsure about how to answer a question, please give it the best answer you can and make a comment in the left margin or on the back. Thank You.

1. **In general, would you say your health is (circle one number):**

Excellent	1
Very good	2
Good	3
Fair	4
Poor	5

2. **Compared to 1 year ago**, how would you rate your health in general now? (Circle one number.)

Much better now than 1 year ago	1
Somewhat better now than 1 year ago	2
About the same	3
Somewhat worse now than 1 year ago	4
Much worse now than 1 year ago	5

3. **The following questions are about activities you might do during a typical day.**
   Does your health limit you in these activities? If so, how much? (Circle 1, 2, or 3 on each line.)

	Yes, Limited a Lot	*Yes, Limited a Little*	*No, Not Limited at All*
a. Vigorous activities such as running, lifting heavy objects, participating in strenuous sports	1	2	3
b. Moderate activities such as moving a table, pushing a vacuum cleaner, bowling, or playing golf	1	2	3
c. Lifting or carrying groceries	1	2	3
d. Climbing several flights of stairs	1	2	3
e. Climbing one flight of stairs	1	2	3
f. Bending, kneeling, or stooping	1	2	3
g. Walking more than 1 mile	1	2	3
h. Walking several blocks	1	2	3
i. Walking one block	1	2	3
j. Bathing and dressing yourself	1	2	3

4. **During the past 4 weeks**, have you had any of the following problems with your work or other regular daily activities **as a result of your physical health?**
   (Please answer YES or NO for each question by circling 1 or 2 on each line.)

	Yes	*No*
a. Cut down on the amount of time you spent on work or other activities	1	2
b. Accomplished less than you would like	1	2
c. Were limited in the kind of work or other activities	1	2
d. Had difficulty performing the work or other activities (e.g., it took extra effort)	1	2

5. **During the past 4 weeks**, have you had any of the following problems with your work or other regular daily activities as a result of any emotional problems (e.g., feeling depressed or anxious)?
   (Please answer YES or NO for each question by circling 1 or 2 on each line.)

	Yes	*No*
a. Cut down on the amount of time you spent on work or other activities	1	2
b. Accomplished less than you would like	1	2
c. Didn't do work or other activities as carefully as usual	1	2

6. **During the past 4 weeks**, to what extent has your physical health or emotional problems interfered with your normal social activities with family, friends, neighbors, or groups? (Circle one number.)

Not at all	1
Slightly	2
Moderately	3
Quite a bit	4
Extremely	5

7. **How much body pain have you had during the past 4 weeks?** (Circle one number.)

None	1
Very mild	2
Mild	3
Moderate	4
Severe	5
Very severe	6

*The Health Status Questionnaire (SF-36) form is used for patient self-assessment of overall health status.
From Ware JE and Sherbourne CD: The MOS 36 item short-form health survey (SF-36). I. Conceptual framework and item selection. Med Care *30*:473–481, 1992.

Continued

TABLE 28-15.   Health Status Questionnaire (SF-36)—cont'd

8. During the <u>past 4 weeks</u>, how much did pain interfere with your normal work (including work both outside the home and housework)? (Circle one number.)

Not at all	1
A little	2
Moderately	3
Quite a bit	4
Extremely	5

9. These questions are about how you feel and how things have been with you <u>during the past month</u>. For each question, please indicate the one answer that comes closest to the way you have been feeling.
   How much of the time during <u>the past month</u>

	All of the Time	Most of the Time	A Good Bit of the Time	Some of the Time	A Little of the Time	None of the Time
a. Did you feel full of pep?	1	2	3	4	5	6
b. Have you been a very nervous person?	1	2	3	4	5	6
c. Have you felt so down in the dumps nothing could cheer you up?	1	2	3	4	5	6
d. Have you felt calm and peaceful?	1	2	3	4	5	6
e. Did you have a lot of energy?	1	2	3	4	5	6
f. Have you felt downhearted and blue?	1	2	3	4	5	6
g. Did you feel worn out?	1	2	3	4	5	6
h. Have you been a happy person?	1	2	3	4	5	6
i. Did you feel tired?	1	2	3	4	5	6
j. Has your health limited your social activities (like visiting your friends or close relatives)?	1	2	3	4	5	6

10. Please choose the answer that best describes how true or false each of the following statements is for you. (Circle one number on each line.)

	Definitely True	Mostly True	Not Sure	Mostly False	Definitely False
a. I seem to get sick a little easier than other people	1	2	3	4	5
b. I am as healthy as anybody I know	1	2	3	4	5
c. I expect my health to get worse	1	2	3	4	5
d. My health is excellent	1	2	3	4	5

11. Please answer YES or NO for each question by circling 1 or 2 on each line.

	Yes	No
a. In the past year, have you had 2 weeks or more during which you felt sad, blue, or depressed or when you lost all interest or pleasure in things you usually care about or enjoyed?	1	2
b. Have you had 2 years or more in your life when you felt depressed or sad most days, even if you felt okay sometimes?	1	2
c. Have you felt depressed or sad much of the time in the past year?		

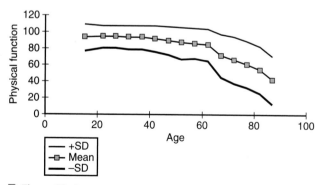

■ Figure 28–1
Population-based control data demonstrating change in the SF-36 physical function score with age.

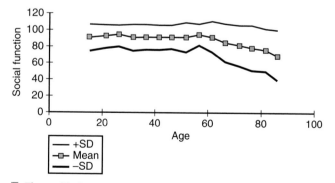

■ Figure 28–2
Population-based control data demonstrating change in the SF-36 social function score with age.

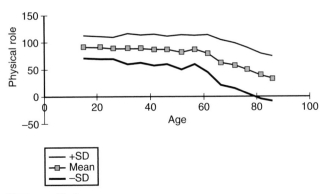

■ **Figure 28–3**
Population-based control data demonstrating change in the SF-36 physical role score with age.

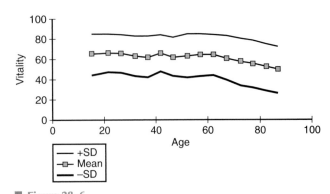

■ **Figure 28–6**
Population-based control data demonstrating change in the SF-36 vitality score with age.

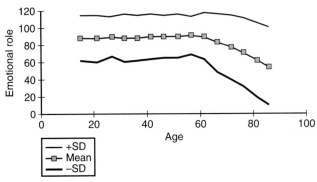

■ **Figure 28–4**
Population-based control data demonstrating change in the SF-36 emotional role score with age.

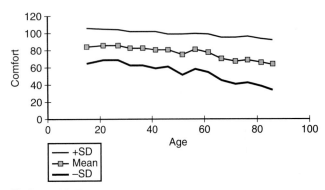

■ **Figure 28–7**
Population-based control data demonstrating change in the SF-36 comfort score with age.

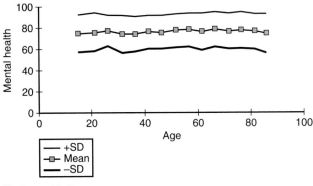

■ **Figure 28–5**
Population-based control data demonstrating change in the SF-36 mental health score with age.

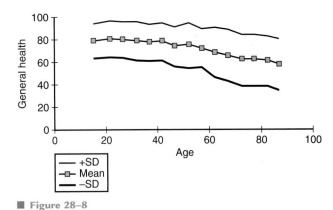

■ **Figure 28–8**
Population-based control data demonstrating change in the SF-36 general health score with age.

for QALYs[149] and was designed to be used as an effectiveness measure for policy analysis and resource allocation. Patients respond to questions from an interviewer regarding their level of physical activity (three levels), mobility (three levels), social activity (five levels), and the one symptom or problem that bothers them the most on the day when the questionnaire is administered (choice of 22 symptom complexes). Almost 80% of the population reports at least one symptom during any given 6-day period. The QWB is then calculated by factoring in preference weights, which were derived from responses to a

household survey that queried respondents concerning their preferences for various health states on a scale of 1 to 10 ranging from death to perfect health. QWB scores are calculated separately for each of the 6 days preceding the interview, and the final score is the average of these six scores. Scores range from zero, implying death, to 1, denoting perfect health. By using data from large populations multiplied by years of life expectancy and cost per intervention, the QALY is obtained, or cost per year of well-life expectancy. QALYs provide a method for making decisions regarding resource allocation. When orthopaedic interventions such as hip arthroplasty and hip fracture fixation have been studied with this methodology, they have fared well.[114,153] The QWB physical function scale probably suffers from the floor effect in which degrees of musculoskeletal function cannot be differentiated.

Sickness Impact Profile

The SIP includes 136 endorsable statements developed by Bergner and associates at the University of Washington. It is best administered by trained interviewers and takes 25 to 35 minutes to complete.[10-12] Its 12 domains are addressed by simple "yes" or "no" questions. These 12 areas are scored independently and combined into a physical and a psychosocial subscale, as well as one aggregate score. Its scoring scale is 0 to 100 points, with high scores denoting severe disability and low scores implying minimal deficit. Scores in excess of the mid-30s bring serious quality-of-life issues into question. It has been used in multiple health conditions and facilitates a comparison of the impact of various diseases on health. It has been used in musculoskeletal trauma with good success.[97,98] Because of the difficulty and time taken to administer the test, it may be most useful for well-funded outcome studies or controlled trials. It is likely that it also suffers from the floor effect.

Nottingham Health Profile

The Nottingham Health Profile is administered via an interview and has been used to assess functional outcomes of limb salvage versus early amputation.[49,105,106] It has been shown to be valid in other studies in Great Britain and Sweden. Part I of the profile measures subjective health status with 38 weighted questions that assess impairments in sleep, emotional reaction, mobility, energy level, pain, and social isolation. For each variable a score of 100 points represents maximal disability, whereas 0 points indicates no limitations. Part II includes seven "yes" or "no" statements that measure the influence of health problems on job, home, family life, sexual function, recreation, and enjoyment of holidays. Responses to both portions of the profile can be compared with average scores for the general population by taking into consideration such demographic factors as age and sex distribution.

The aforementioned examples are general health status instruments that have broad acceptance and enable comparison of the functional impact of various diseases. Disease- or condition-specific instruments offer increased sensitivity and maximal limitation of floor and ceiling effects.[87]

RESULTS

Self-assessment tools reflect differences among diagnoses. The application of self-assessment tools to conditions of the shoulder is relatively recent. The authors now have a 4-year experience in applying a combination of the SF-36 and the SST to shoulder self-assessment.[103] Two

previous investigations combined with the results presented here indicate that the patient's self-assessment can document and call attention to important aspects of the patient's condition that might not otherwise be detected.[100,104]

The authors used the SF-36 to evaluate the compromise in general health status of 777 patients with nine well-characterized conditions of the shoulder by comparing them with age-matched population controls.[88] These patients met the necessary and sufficient criteria for one of nine shoulder diagnoses (number of patients/average age of patients): traumatic instability (TUBS, 90/30), frozen shoulder (FS, 74/56), degenerative joint disease (DJD, 160/63), partial-thickness cuff lesion (PTCL, 102/46), atraumatic instability (AMBRII, 65/27), full-thickness rotator cuff tear (RCT, 132/60), secondary DJD (second-degree DJD, 42/54), post-traumatic stiff shoulder (PTSS, 76/45), and rheumatoid arthritis (RA, 36/56). For each patient, each of the SF-36 scores (physical role [PR], comfort [C], physical function [PF], social function [SF], emotional role [ER], vitality [V], general health [GH], and mental health [MH]) was expressed as a percentage of the average for the age-matched control population.[119] The data are summarized here (Fig. 28–9) as the means of these percentages.

The SF-36 data from this large series of shoulder patients indicate that the physical role and comfort scores were less than 60% of those of age-matched controls for all nine diagnoses. Although the mental health for all groups was high, the physical function, vitality, and general health scores were particularly low for patients with rheumatoid arthritis. Self-assessment data enable orthopaedic surgeons to document the compromise in health status associated with musculoskeletal conditions and the rationale for treating them. In that a goal of treatment is to restore these parameters to 100% of the population-based values, these data also provide a benchmark against which treatment effectiveness can be determined.[103] Within this highly selected population, standardized self-assessment indicated substantial, yet variable compromise in shoulder function and overall health status. Patients with rheumatoid arthritis showed major and significantly worse health status deficits than did those with osteoarthritis. These differences may be important considerations when selecting approaches for the management of patients with shoulder arthritis. For example, patients with severely limited vitality or social function scores may warrant different treatment than individuals with high scores for these parameters. Other examples of how similar data can be displayed in an understandable manner are shown in Figures 28–10 and 28–11.

Finally, the application of this methodology before and after treatment is extremely compelling. The authors have used it to evaluate the results of total shoulder arthroplasty for degenerative arthritis of the shoulder.[100] The SF-36 and SST data of a group of 54 patients before and after joint replacement are presented in Figures 28–12 and 28–13. We have been able to document a significant improvement in many of the variables examined, thus exemplifying its effectiveness as a management scheme for shoulder arthritis in some patients.

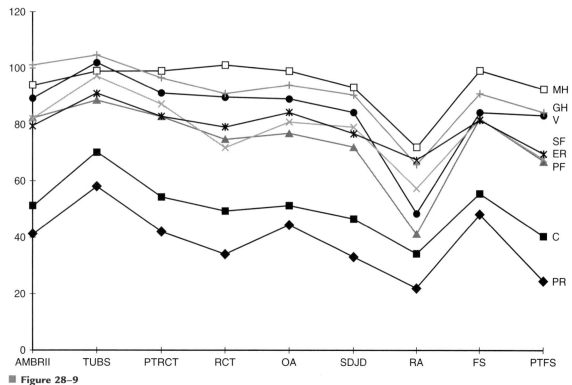

■ Figure 28–9
Relative compromise in general health status for patients with various shoulder conditions demonstrated by SF-36 scores as
a percentage of the average for the age-matched control population. See text for definitions of abbreviations.

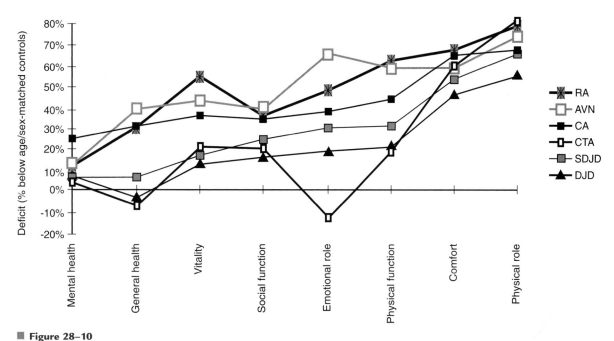

■ Figure 28–10
Relative compromise in general health status for patients with various shoulder conditions demonstrated by SF-36 scores as a
percent deficit versus the age-matched control population. AVN, avascular necrosis; CA, cancer; DJD, degenerative joint disease;
RA, rheumatoid arthritis.

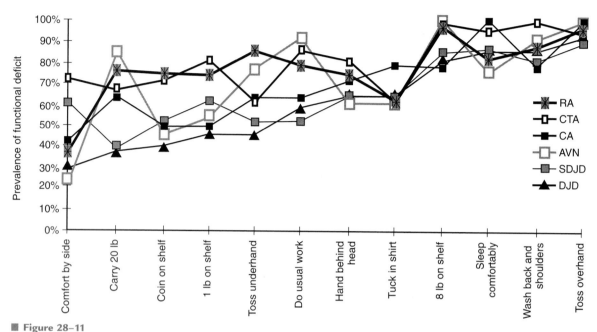

■ Figure 28–11

Relative compromise in shoulder function for patients with various shoulder conditions demonstrated by percentages of patients perceiving deficits on the Simple Shoulder Test. See Figure 28–10 for definitions.

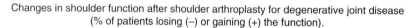

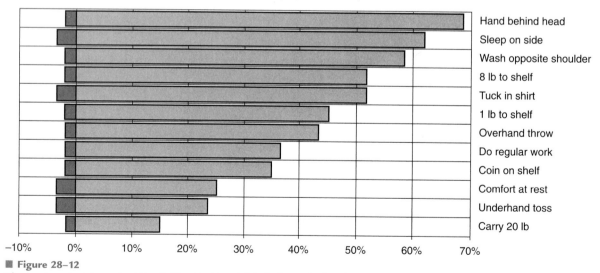

■ Figure 28–12

Changes in patients' perceived Simple Shoulder Test deficits before and after shoulder arthroplasty.

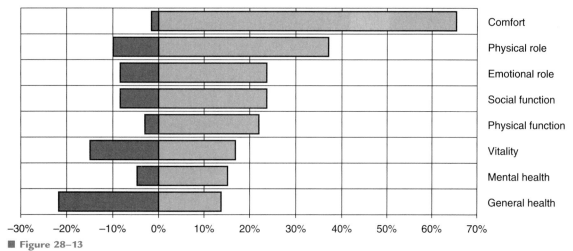

Changes in health status after shoulder arthroplasty for degenerative joint disease (% of patients worsened (−) or improved (+) by more than standard deviation)

■ **Figure 28–13**

Changes in patients' perceived Health Status Questionnaire (SF-36) deficits before and after shoulder arthroplasty.

SELF-ASSESSMENT TOOLS IN THE MEASUREMENT OF COST-EFFECTIVENESS

Measuring cost-effectiveness is challenging. The cost of various treatment methods varies substantially. Compare, for example, the cost of nonoperative and operative management of rotator cuff tears. To initiate a method by which the cost-effectiveness of different treatment methods might be compared, the authors conducted a preliminary study of 67 unmatched patients who were being evaluated for treatment of documented, symptomatic full-thickness tears. Based on our clinical assessment and the desires of the patient, one of three treatment methods was selected for each patient: nonoperative management, subacromial smoothing without repair, and surgical repair. The number of patients, average age, gender, and length of follow-up for the patients in each of the three groups are shown in Table 28–16.

All patients completed SSTs measuring shoulder function and SF-36 health status questionnaires preoperatively and at follow-up. The effectiveness of treatment was measured in terms of the postoperative-preoperative change in the number of "yes" responses on the SST and the postoperative-preoperative change in the SF-36 comfort score. This analysis indicated that the

greatest improvement was found in the group that underwent surgical repair. The changes in SST and SF-36 comfort score results for each patient were then divided by the total charges for the treatment to yield the average change per $1000 charge. In this analysis, nonoperative treatment was associated with the greatest change per unit charge (Figs. 28–14 and 28–15).

Although no conclusions can be drawn from these preliminary results, it is hoped that further studies of this type will help determine the value of different treatment methods.

CONCLUSION

The examples presented earlier indicate that patient self-assessment of health status and shoulder function allows each physician to fulfill Codman's admonition. Such

TABLE 28–16. Patient Characteristics for Three Groups of Rotator Cuff Tear Treatment

	No. of Patients	Average Age	Percent Female	Average Follow-up (yr)
Nonoperative	36	62.4	36	1.7
Subacromial smoothing	11	67.8	45	1.7
Cuff repair	20	60.3	10	2.0

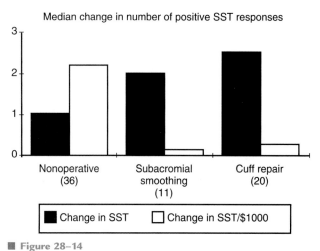

Median change in number of positive SST responses

■ **Figure 28–14**

Change in the number of positive Simple Shoulder Test (SST) responses regarding shoulder function relative to the cost of three rotator cuff tear treatments.

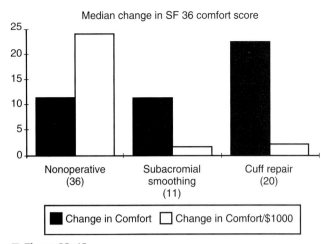

■ Figure 28–15
Change in the Health Status Questionnaire (SF-36) comfort score relative to the cost of three rotator cuff tear treatments.

assessments provide practical, standardized, and meaningful characterization of the status of the patient at the time of initial evaluation, which we refer to as the "ingo," as well as the patient's status after treatment, which is the outcome. The difference between the outcome and the ingo is the effectiveness of the treatment for the patient. Patients for whom the difference between outcome and ingo is not positive call up Codman's question—if not, why not? What is it about the disease, the patient, the treatment, or the doctor that has given rise to the failure? What are the predictors of success and failure? Dividing the effectiveness by the cost of the treatment yields a tangible measure of cost-effectiveness.

The use of standardized tools across practices will permit the combination of data in a statistically valid way so that we can better understand factors contributing to the success and value of treatment. By using patient self-assessment as the cornerstone of these analyses, we keep our focus on the persons submitting themselves to the risks, benefits, and costs of treatment rather than exclusively on medical metrics. In the end, the results of the analyses are easy for the individual physician to communicate to those who need to know how they are likely to benefit if this treatment is performed.

We would like to conclude with a synopsis of a letter published in the *American Academy of Orthopaedic Surgeons Bulletin* (vol 45, No. 4, October 1997):

OUTCOMES DATA HELPS PATIENTS, PRACTITIONERS

by Frederick A. Matsen III, MD

Frederick A. Matsen III, MD, is Professor and Chairman, Department of Orthopaedics, University of Washington School of Medicine, Seattle, Washington.

Orthopaedic surgeons make a difference! It is virtually axiomatic that orthopaedic surgery improves the well-being of millions of individuals each year. Each of us can recount case after case in which our care restored someone's functional independence, ability to work or to resume his or her favorite recreational activities.

Wouldn't it be wonderful if each of us could measure the amount of good we do for the conditions we treat? This information would be of great value to share with our patients and their families: "85 percent of my patients who couldn't walk a block before hip arthroplasty can do so within three months of my surgery." How nice it would be to have our own data on our own efficacy, rather than having to quote the results presented by some other Medical Center.

On the other hand, occasionally our best efforts produce no change in the patient's well-being and, rarely, we may make them worse. We're not talking about complications here, but rather those patients who just didn't get any improvement in function from our treatment. How often does this happen in my practice? If I could easily identify the patients who didn't improve, I could learn whether I have a problem in patient selection, surgical technique, implant selection, aftercare or patient compliance. I might find that my operation works less well for individuals hurt on the job, or those over a certain age or those who want to resume weight lifting.

By identifying these factors in my own practice, I could have an even more reasonable preoperative discussion with my patients. I could say, "While I know you've got a bad problem there, my success in getting folks injured longshoring back to work after disk surgery has been less than 10 percent."

While many other reasons can be advanced for measuring the efficacy of our treatment, one of the best reasons is that it provides the most personal continuing medical education. If the individual practitioner keeps track of the differences in patients' function and well-being resulting from his/her treatment, and if this information is used to optimize patient selection and treatment, everyone involved benefits.

In order to know if a specific treatment made a difference, it is essential that the status of the patient before treatment (the "ingo") and after treatment (the "outcome") are quantitated using the same tool. In this way the difference is obtained by simple subtraction. If only the outcome of treatment is known, the efficacy of the treatment cannot be known. Thus, the routine measurement of "ingo" becomes a matter of great importance: unless these data are collected before treatment, it is virtually impossible to collect them in a reliable way later.

Because we are all getting increasingly busy, "ingo" and outcome data are ideally collected in a way that is minimally intrusive to our practice. Since a major reason for measuring the difference we make is to communicate this information to our patients, the data need to be expressible in terms patients can readily understand, rather than in terms of medical metrics (such as range of motion, foot-pounds of torque or scores on a grading system). In this regard, patients are most likely to be interested in information regarding changes in function, comfort and well-being. Fortunately, the most direct way to obtain this information also is the most efficient in the context of a busy office practice: patient self-assessment. Because patient self-assessment questionnaires can be completed at home, they have the additional advantage of not requiring the patient to return to the office every time outcome data are needed.

Short, simple lists of "yes" or "no" questions regarding the patient's ability to perform different functions are often sufficient to measure the difference resulting from treatment. These simple tests can be designed to reflect deficits common to the problem being treated: "Does your knee allow you to get in and out of a car easily?" "Does your shoulder allow you to sleep comfortably on that side?" Such lists of questions, structured so that a positive response indicates the ability to perform the function, are easily answered and recorded. Ingos and outcomes are easily compared for individual patients and groups of patients (e.g., those men under age 50 having total knee arthroplasty). The data can be easily communicated to patients considering a procedure: "Only 20 percent of my patients answered 'yes' to this question before surgery, whereas 85 percent answered 'yes' one year after the procedure." These data also identify the 15 percent who are still unable and motivate the question, "Why not?" Using this simple test paradigm, both our patients and we become more informed.

The right reason for measuring our individual efficacy as physicians and surgeons is because it shows us where we've made a difference to our patients and when we have not. It helps us inform them of reasonable expectations of treatment in our hands. It helps us inform ourselves on where we have room for improvement. In short, measuring the difference we make helps make good orthopaedics better.

REFERENCES AND BIBLIOGRAPHY

1. Academy plans data collection system. AAOS Bull 43:24, 1995.
2. Academy proceeds on outcomes database. AAOS Bull 44:29-30, 1996.
3. Altchek DW, Warren RF, Wickiewicz TL, et al: Arthroscopic acromioplasty: Technique and results. J Bone Joint Surg Am 72:1198-1207, 1990.
4. Bayley KB, London MR, Grunkemeier GL, et al: Measuring the success of treatment in patient terms. Med Care 33(suppl 4):AS226-AS235, 1995.
5. Beaton DE, Katz JN, Fossel AH, et al: Measuring the whole or the parts? Validity, reliability, and responsiveness of the Disabilities of the Arm, Shoulder and Hand outcome measure in different regions of the upper extremity. J Hand Ther 14:128-146, 2001.
6. Beaton DE and Richards RR: Measuring function of the shoulder. J Bone Joint Surg Am 78:882-890, 1996.
7. Beaton D, and Richards RR: Assessing the reliability and responsiveness of 5 shoulder questionnaires. J Shoulder Elbow Surg 7:565-572, 1998.
8. Bellamy N, Buchanan WW, Goldsmith CH, et al: Validation study of WOMAC: A health status instrument for measuring clinically important patient relevant outcomes following total hip or knee arthroplasty in osteoarthritis. J Orthop Rheumatol 1:95-108, 1988.
9. Benirschke SK, Melder I, Henley MB, et al: Closed interlocking nailing of femoral shaft fractures: Assessment of technical complications and functional outcomes by comparison of a prospective database with retrospective review. J Orthop Trauma 7:118-122, 1993.
10. Bergner M, Bobbitt RA, Carter WB, et al: The sickness impact profile: Development and final revision of a health status measure. Med Care 19:787-805, 1981.
11. Bergner M, Bobbitt RA, Kressel S, et al: The sickness impact profile: Conceptual formulation and methodological development of a health status index. Int J Health Services 6:393-415, 1976.
12. Bergner M, Bobbitt RA, Pollaro WE, et al: The sickness impact profile: Validation of a health status measure. Med Care 14:57-67, 1976.
13. Bigos SJ: The practitioner's guide to the industrial back problem. Part II. Helping the patient with the return to work predicament. Semin Spine Surg 4:55-63, 1992.
14. Bigos SJ, Battie MC, Fisher LD, et al: A longitudinal, prospective study of industrial back injury reporting. Clin Orthop 279:21-34, 1992.
15. Binder AI, Bulgen DY, Hazleman BL, et al: Frozen shoulder: A long-term prospective study. Ann Rheum Dis 43:361-364, 1984.
16. Bombardier C, Melfi CA, Paul J, et al: Comparison of a generic and a disease-specific measure of pain and physical function after knee replacement surgery. Med Care 33(suppl 4):AS131-AS144, 1995.
17. Boorman R, Kopjar B, Fehringer E, et al: The effect of total shoulder arthroplasty on self-assessed health status is comparable to that of total hip arthroplasty and coronary artery bypass grafting. J Shoulder Elbow Surg 12:158-163, 2003.
18. Bradburn NM: The Structure of Psychological Well-Being. Chicago: Aldine Publishing, 1969.
19. Breslow L: A quantitative approach to the World Health Organization definition of health; physical, mental and social well-being. Int J Epidemiol 1:347-355, 1972.
20. Brown T, Nemiah JC, Barr JS, et al: Psychologic factors in low-back pain. N Engl J Med 251:123-128, 1954.
21. Bruckner FE and Nye CJS: A prospective study of adhesive capsulitis of the shoulder (frozen shoulder) in a high risk population. Q J Med 198:191-204, 1981.
22. Bush JW, Chen MM, and Patrick DL: Health status index in cost-effectiveness and analysis of PKU program. In Berg RL (ed): Health Status Indexes. Chicago: Hospital Research and Educational Trust, 1973, pp 172-208.
23. Cleary PD, Reilly DT, Greenfield S, et al: Using patient reports to assess health-related quality of life after total hip replacement. Q Life Res 2:3-11, 1993.
24. Codman EA: The product of a hospital. Surg Gynecol Obstet 18:491-496, 1914.
25. Codman EA: Hysteria, neurasthenia, neurosis, traumatic neuritis, malingering. In The Shoulder. Malaber, FL: Krieger Publishing, 1934, pp 400-410.
26. Constant CR and Murley AHG: A clinical method of functional assessment of the shoulder. Clin Orthop 214:160-164, 1987.
27. Cook KF, Gartsman GM, Roddey TS, and Olson SL: The measurement level and trait-specific reliability of 4 scales of shoulder functioning: An empiric investigation. Arch Phys Med Rehabil 82:1558-1565, 2001.
28. Cook KF, Roddey TS, Olson SL, et al: Reliability by surgical status of self-reported outcomes in patients who have shoulder pathologies. J Orthop Sports Phys Ther 32:336-346, 2002.
29. Cotton P: Orthopedics research now asks, "does it work?" rather than just, "how is the procedure performed?" JAMA 265:2164-2165, 1991.
30. Coventry MB: Problem of painful shoulder. JAMA 151:177-185, 1953.
31. Crandell D, Richmond J, Lau J, et al: A meta-analysis of the treatment of injuries of the anterior cruciate ligament. Paper presented at the Annual Meeting of the American Orthopaedic Society for Sports Medicine, 1994, Palm Springs, FL.
32. Dawson J, Fitzpatrick R, and Carr A: Questionnaire on the perceptions of patients about shoulder surgery. J Bone Joint Surg Br 78:593-600, 1996.
33. Dawson J, Fitzpatrick R, and Carr A: The assessment of shoulder instability. The development and validation of a questionnaire. J Bone Joint Surg Br 81:420-426, 1999.
34. Dawson J, Hill G, Fitzpatrick R, and Carr A: The benefits of using patient-based methods of assessment. Medium-term results of an observational study of shoulder surgery. J Bone Joint Surg Br 83:877-882, 2001.
35. Deyo RA, Andersson G, Bombardier C, et al: Outcome measures for studying patients with low back pain. Spine 19 (suppl):2032S-2036S, 1994.
36. Donabedian A: Evaluating the product of medical care. Milbank Q 44:166-203, 1966.
37. Duckworth DG, Smith KL, Campbell B, and Matsen FA 3rd: Self-assessment questionnaires document substantial variability in the clinical expression of rotator cuff tears. J Shoulder Elbow Surg 8:330-333, 1999.
38. Ellman H, Hanker G, and Bayer M: Repair of the rotator cuff: End-result study of factors influencing reconstruction. J Bone Joint Surg Am 68:1136-1144, 1986.
39. Emery DD and Schneiderman LJ: Cost-effectiveness analysis in health care. Hastings Cent Rep 19:8-13, 1989.
40. Engelberg R, Martin DP, Agel J, et al: The musculoskeletal functional assessment instrument: Criterion and construct validity. J Orthop Res 14:182-192, 1996.
41. Epstein A: The outcomes movement—will it get us where we want to go. N Engl J Med 373:266-270, 1990.
42. Esch J, Ozerkis L, Helgager J, et al: Arthroscopic subacromial decompression: Results according to the degree of rotator cuff tear. Arthroscopy 4:241-249, 1988.
43. Fehringer EV, Kopjar B, Boorman RS, et al: Characterizing the functional improvement after total shoulder arthroplasty for osteoarthritis. J Bone Joint Surg Am 84:1349-1353, 2002.
44. Fitzpatrick R, Ziebland S, Jenkinson C, et al: The social dimension of health status measures in rheumatoid arthritis. Int Dis Stud 13:34-37, 1991.
45. Fleming A, Dodman S, Beer TC, et al: Personality in frozen shoulder. Ann Rheum Dis 35:456-457, 1976.
46. Frymoyer JW, Rosen JC, Clements J, et al: Psychologic factors in low-back pain disability. Clin Orthop 195:178-184, 1985.
47. Gartland JJ: Orthopaedic clinical research: Deficiencies in experimental design and determination of outcome. J Bone Joint Surg Am 70A:1357-1364, 1988.
48. Gartsman GM, Brinker MR, Khan M, and Karahan M: Self-assessment of general health status in patients with five common shoulder conditions. J Shoulder Elbow Surg 7:228-237, 1998.

49. Georgiadis GM, Behrens FF, Joyce MJ, et al: Open tibial fractures with severe soft tissue loss—limb salvage compared with below knee amputation. J Bone Joint Surg Am 75:1431-1441, 1993.

50. Gillespie WJ and Daellenbach HG: Assessing cost-effectiveness in orthopaedic outcome studies. Orthopaedics 15:1275-1277, 1992.

51. Goldberg BA, Lippitt SB, and Matsen FA III: Improvement in comfort and function after cuff repair without acromioplasty. Clin Orthop 390:142-150, 2001.

52. Goldberg BA, Nowinski RJ, and Matsen FA III: Outcome of nonoperative management of full-thickness rotator cuff tears. Clin Orthop 382:99-107, 2001.

53. Goldberg BA, Smith KL, Jackins SE, et al: The magnitude and durability of functional improvement after total shoulder arthroplasty for degenerative joint disease. J Shoulder Elbow Surg 10:464-469, 2001.

54. Gordon TA, Burleyson GP, Tielsch JM, et al: The effects of regionalization on cost and outcome for one general high-risk surgical procedure. Ann Surg 221:43-49, 1995.

55. Green A, Norris TR, Becker GE, et al: Failed shoulder surgery: Psychological and psychiatric considerations. Paper presented at Specialty Day, American Shoulder and Elbow Surgeons, 1996, Atlanta,.

56. Green S, Buchbinder R, Glazier R, and Forbes A: Systematic review of randomized controlled trials of interventions for painful shoulder: selection criteria, outcome assessment and efficacy. BMJ 316:354-360, 1998.

57. Gross M: A critique of the methodologies used in clinical studies of hip joint arthroplasty published in the English literature. J Bone Joint Surg Am 70:1364-1371, 1988.

58. Guadagnoli E and McNeil BJ: Outcomes research: Hope for the future or the latest rage? Inquiry 31:14-24, 1994.

59. Hanscom B, Lurie JD, Homa K, and Weinstein JN: Computerized questionnaires and the quality of survey data. Spine 27:1797-1801, 2002.

60. Harryman DT II, Hettrich C, Smith KL, et al: A prospective multipractice investigation of patients with full thickness rotator cuff tears: The importance of comorbidities, practice, and other covariables on self-assessed shoulder function and health status. J Bone Joint Surg Am 85:690-696, 2003.

61. Hasan SS, Leith JM, Campbell B, et al: Characteristics of unsatisfactory shoulder arthroplasties. J Shoulder Elbow Surg 11:431-441, 2002.

62. Hawkins RJ, Brock R, Abrams J, et al: Acromioplasty for impingement with an intact rotator cuff. J Bone Joint Surg Br 70:795-797, 1988.

63. Hoving JL, Buchbinder R, Green S, et al: How reliably do rheumatologists measure shoulder movement? Ann Rheum Dis 61:612-616, 2002.

64. Hunsaker FG, Cioffi DA, Amadio PC, et al: The American Academy of Orthopaedic Surgeons outcomes instruments: Normative values from the general population. J Bone Joint Surg Am 84:208-215, 2002.

65. Jensen I, Nygren A, Gamberale F, et al: The role of the psychologist in multidisciplinary treatments for chronic neck and shoulder pain: A controlled cost-effectiveness study. Scand J Rehabil Med 27:19-26, 1995.

66. Johanson NA, Charlson ME, Szatrowski TP, et al: A self administered hip-rating questionnaire for the assessment of outcome after total hip replacement. J Bone Joint Surg Am 74:587-597, 1992.

67. Kantz ME, Harris WJ, Levitsky K, et al: Methods for assessing condition-specific and generic functional status outcomes after total knee replacement. Med Care 30(suppl):MS240-MS252, 1990.

68. Kaplan RM and Bush JW: Health-related quality of life measurement for evaluation research and policy analysis. Health Psychol 1:61-80, 1982.

69. Karnofsky DA and Burchenal JH: The clinical evaluation of chemotherapeutic drugs. In MacLeod CM (ed): Evaluation of Chemotherapeutic Agents. New York: Columbia University Press, 1949, pp 191-194.

70. Katz JN, Harris TM, Larson MG, et al: Predictors of functional outcomes after arthroscopic partial meniscectomy. J Rheumatol 19:1938-1942, 1992.

71. Katz JN, Larson MG, Phillips CB, et al: Comparative measurement sensitivity of short and longer health status instruments. Med Care 30:917-925, 1992.

72. Katz S, Ford AB, Moskowitz RW, et al: Studies of illness in the aged. JAMA 185:914-919, 1963.

73. Kay A, Davison B, Badley E, et al: Hip arthroplasty: Patient satisfaction. Br J Rheumatol 22:243-249, 1983.

74. Kay SP and Amstutz HC: Shoulder hemiarthroplasty at UCLA. Clin Orthop 228:42-44, 1988.

75. Keller R, Soule DN, Wennberg JE, et al: Dealing with geographic variations in the use of hospitals: The experience of the Maine Medical Assessment Foundation orthopaedic study group. J Bone Joint Surg Am 72:1286-1293, 1990.

76. Keller RB: Outcomes research in orthopaedics. J Am Acad Orthop Surg 1:122-129, 1993.

77. Keller RB: How outcomes research should be done. In Matsen FA III, Fu FH, and Hawkins RJ (eds): The Shoulder: A Balance of Mobility and Stability. Rosemont, IL: American Academy of Orthopaedic Surgeons, 1993, pp 487-499.

78. Keller RB, Rudicel SA, and Liang MH: Outcomes research in orthopaedics. J Bone Joint Surg Am 75:1562-1574, 1993.

79. Kirkley A: Western Ontario Rotator Cuff (WORC) Index. 1996.

80. Kirkley A: Western Ontario Shoulder Instability (WOSI) Index. 1996.

81. Kirkley A, Griffin S, McLintock H, and Ng L: The development and evaluation of a disease-specific quality of life measurement tool for shoulder instability. The Western Ontario Shoulder Instability Index (WOSI). Am J Sports Med 26:764-772, 1998.

82. Kirwan JR, Currey HL, Freeman MA, et al: Overall long-term impact of total hip and knee joint replacement surgery on patients with osteoarthritis and rheumatoid arthritis. Br J Rheumatol 33:357-360, 1990.

83. Kohn D, Geyer M, and Wulker N: The Subjective Shoulder Rating Scale (SSRS): An examiner-independent scoring system. Paper presented at the International Congress on Surgery of the Shoulder, 1992, Paris.

84. L'Abbe KA, Detsky AS, and O'Rourke K: Meta-analysis in clinical research. Ann Intern Med 107:224-233, 1987.

85. Lavernia CJ, Guzman JF, Gachupin-Garcia A, et al: Cost effectiveness and quality of life in knee arthroplasty. Clin Orthop 345:134-139, 1997.

86. Lembcke PA: Measuring the quality of medical care through vital statistics based on hospital service areas: A comparative study of appendectomy rates. Am J Health 42:276-286, 1952.

87. Levine DW, Simmons BP, Koris MJ, et al: A self-administered questionnaire for the assessment of severity of symptoms and functional status in carpal tunnel syndrome. J Bone Joint Surg Am 75:1585-1592, 1993.

88. Levinsohn DG and Matsen FA III: Evaluation of nine common mechanical shoulder disorders with the SF-36 Health Status Instrument. Paper presented at the 64th Annual Meeting of the American Academy of Orthopaedic Surgeons, 1997, San Francisco.

89. Lippitt SB, Harryman DT II, and Matsen FA III: A practical tool for evaluating function: The Simple Shoulder Test. In Matsen FA III, Fu FH, and Hawkins RJ (eds): The Shoulder: A Balance of Mobility and Stability. Rosemont, IL: American Academy of Orthopaedic Surgeons, 1993, pp 501-518.

90. Lirette R, Morin F, and Kinnard P: The difficulties in assessment of results of anterior acromioplasty. Clin Orthop 278:14-16, 1992.

91. Lo IK, Griffin S, and Kirkley A: The development of a disease-specific quality of life measurement tool for osteoarthritis of the shoulder: The Western Ontario Osteoarthritis of the Shoulder (WOOS) index. Osteoarthritis Cartilage 9:771-778, 2001.

92. Lorenz TH and Musser MJ: Life stress, emotions and painful stiff shoulder. Ann Intern Med 37:1232-1244, 1952.

93. Lu-Yao GL, Keller RB, Littenberg B, et al: A meta-analysis of 106 published reports. J Bone Joint Surg Am 76:15-25, 1994.

94. Lyons RA, Lo SV, and Littlepage BNC: Comparative health status of patients with 11 common illnesses in Wales. J Epidemiol Community Health 48:388-390, 1994.

95. Lysholm J and Gillquist J: Evaluation of knee ligament surgery results with special emphasis on use of a scoring scale. Am J Sports Med 10:150-154, 1982.

96. MacDermid JC, Richards RS, Donner A, et al: Responsiveness of the Short Form-36, disability of the arm, shoulder, and hand questionnaire, patient-rated wrist evaluation, and physical impairment measurements in evaluating recovery after a distal radius fracture. J Hand Surg [Am] 25:330-340, 2000.

97. MacKenzie EJ, Burgess AR, McAndrew MP, et al: Patient-oriented functional outcome after unilateral lower extremity fracture. J Orthop Trauma 7:393-401, 1993.

98. MacKenzie EJ, Cushing BM, Jurkovich GJ, et al: Physical impairment and functional outcomes six months after severe lower extremity fractures. J Trauma 34:528-539, 1993.

99. Martin D, Engelberg R, Agel J, et al: Development of the musculoskeletal functional assessment instrument. J Orthop Res 14:173-181, 1996.

100. Matsen FA III: Early effectiveness of shoulder arthroplasty for patients who have primary glenohumeral degenerative joint disease. J Bone Joint Surg Am 78:260-264, 1996.

101. Matsen FA III, Antoniou J, Rozencwaig R, et al: Correlates with comfort and function after total shoulder arthroplasty for degenerative joint disease. J Shoulder Elbow Surg 9:465-469, 2000.

102. Matsen FA III, Lippitt SB, Sidles JA, and Harryman DT II: Practical Evaluation and Management of the Shoulder. Philadelphia: WB Saunders, 1994.

103. Matsen FA III, Smith KL, DeBartolo SE, et al: A comparison of patients with late-stage rheumatoid arthritis and osteoarthritis of the shoulder using self-assessed shoulder function and health status. Arthritis Care Res 10:43-47, 1997.

104. Matsen FA III, Ziegler DW, and DeBartolo SE: Patient self-assessment of health status in glenohumeral degenerative joint disease. J Shoulder Elbow Surg 4:345-351, 1995.

105. McDowell I and Newell C: Measuring Health: A Guide to Rating Scales and Questionnaires. New York: Oxford University Press, 1987, pp 125-133.

106. McEwen J: The Nottingham Health Profile: A measure of perceived health. In Teeling-Smith G (ed): Measuring the Social Benefits of Medicine. London: Office of Health Economics, 1983, pp 75-84.

107. Mohtadi GH and Nicholas GH: Quality of life assessment as an outcome in anterior cruciate ligament reconstruction surgery. In Jackson DW, et al (eds): The Anterior Cruciate Ligament: Current and Future Concepts. New York: Raven Press, 1993.

108. Neer CS II: Anterior acromioplasty for the chronic impingement syndrome in the shoulder: A preliminary report. J Bone Joint Surg Am 54:41-50, 1972.

109. Neer CS II: Impingement lesions. Clin Orthop 173:70-77, 1983.

110. Nerenz DR, Repasky DP, Whitehouse FW, et al: Ongoing assessment of health status in patients with diabetes mellitus. Med Care 30:MS112-MS124, 1992.

111. Norquist BM, Goldberg BA, and Matsen FA III: Challenges in evaluating patients lost to follow-up in clinical studies of rotator cuff tears. J Bone Joint Surg Am 82:838-842, 2000.

112. Oesterreicher W and Van Dam G: Social psychological researches into brachialgia and periarthritis. Arthritis Rheum 7:670-683, 1964.

113. O'Kane JW, Jackins S, Sidles JA, et al: Simple home program for frozen shoulder to improve patients' assessment of shoulder function and health status. J Am Board Fam Pract 12:270-277, 1999.

114. Parker MJ, Myles JW, Anand JK, et al: Cost-benefit analysis of hip fracture treatment. J Bone Joint Surg Br 74:261-264, 1992.

115. Patte D: Directions for the Use of the Index Severity for Painful and/or Chronically Disabled Shoulders. Paris: 1987.

116. Pitson D, Bhaskaran V, Bond H, et al: Effectiveness of knee replacement surgery in arthritis. Int J Nurs Stud 31:49-56, 1994.

117. Poigenfurst J, Orthner E, and Hoffman J: Technik und Ergebnisse der koraklavikularen Verschraubung bei frischen Akromioklavikularzerreissungen. Acta Chir Austriaca 1:11-16, 1987.

118. Post M and Cohen J: Impingement syndrome: A review of late stage II and early stage III lesions. Clin Orthop 207:126-132, 1986.

119. Radosevich DM, Wetzler H, and Wilson SM: Health Status Questionnaire (HSQ) 2.0: Scoring Comparisons and Reference Data. Bloomington, MN: Health Outcomes Institute, 1994.

120. Richards R-N, An K-N, Bigliani LU, et al: A standardized method for assessment of shoulder function. J Shoulder Elbow Surg 3:347-352, 1994.

121. Roach KE, Budiman-Mak E, Songsiridej N, et al: Development of a shoulder pain and disability index. Arthritis Care Res 4:143-149, 1991.

122. Roddey TS, Olson SL, Cook KF, et al: Comparison of the University of California–Los Angeles Shoulder Scale and the Simple Shoulder Test with the shoulder pain and disability index: Single-administration reliability and validity. Phys Ther 80:759-768, 2000.

123. Rowe CR, Patel D, and Southmayd WW: The Bankart procedure: A long-term end-result study. J Bone Joint Surg Am 60:1-16, 1978.

124. Rozencwaig R, van Noort A, Moskal MJ, et al: The correlation of comorbidity with function of the shoulder and health status of patients who have glenohumeral degenerative joint disease. J Bone Joint Surg Am 80:1146-1153, 1998.

125. Sen SS, Gupchup GV, and Thomas J III: Selecting among health-related quality-of-life instruments. Am J Health Syst Pharm 56:1965-1970, quiz 1971, 1999.

126. Shapiro ET, Rockett SE, Richmond JC, et al: Use of a patient-based health assessment for evaluation of ACL patients. Paper presented at the Annual Meeting of the American Orthopaedic Society for Sports Medicine, 1994, Palm Springs, FL.

127. Skutek M, Fremerey RW, Zeichen J, and Bosch U: Outcome analysis following open rotator cuff repair. Early effectiveness validated using four different shoulder assessment scales. Arch Orthop Trauma Surg 120:432-436, 2000.

128. Smith KL, Harryman DT II, Antoniou J, et al: A prospective, multipractice study of shoulder function and health status in patients with documented rotator cuff tears. J Shoulder Elbow Surg 9:395-402, 2000.

129. SooHoo NF, McDonald AP, Seiler JG III, and McGillivary GR: Evaluation of the construct validity of the DASH questionnaire by correlation to the SF-36. J Hand Surg [Am] 27:537-541, 2002.

130. Stewart AL, Hays RD, and Ware JE: The MOS short form general health survey; reliability and validity in a patient population. Med Care 26:724-735, 1988.

131. Stewart AL, Ware JE, Brook RH, et al: Conceptualization and Measurement of Health for Adults in the Health Insurance Study. Vol II. Physical Health in Terms of Functioning. Santa Monica, CA: Rand Corp, 1978.

132. Swiontkowski MF and Chapman JR: Cost and effectiveness issues in care of injured patients. Clin Orthop 318:17-24, 1995.

133. Swiontkowski MF, Engelberg R, Martin DP, and Agel J: Short musculoskeletal function assessment questionnaire: Validity, reliability, and responsiveness. J Bone Joint Surg Am 81:1245-1260, 1999.

134. Tarlov AR: Multiple influences propel outcomes field. Med Outcomes Trust Bull 3:5, 1995.

135. Tarlov AR, Ware JE, Greenfield S, et al: The medical outcomes study: An application of methods for monitoring the results of medical care. JAMA 262:925-930, 1989.

136. Tibone JE and Bradley JP: Evaluation of treatment outcomes for the athlete's shoulder. In Matsen FA III, Fu FH, and Hawkins RJ (eds): The Shoulder: A Balance of Mobility and Stability. Rosemont, IL: American Academy of Orthopaedic Surgeons, 1993, pp 519-529.

137. Tingart M, Bathis H, Lefering R, et al: Constant Score and Neer Score. A comparison of score results and subjective patient satisfaction. Unfallchirurg 104:1048-1054, 2001.

138. Troup JDG, Foreman TK, Baxter CE, et al: The perception of back pain and the role of psychophysical tests of lifting capacity. 1987 Volvo Award in Clinical Sciences. Spine 12:645-657, 1987.

139. Turchin DC, Beaton DE, and Richards RR: Validity of observer-based aggregate scoring systems as descriptors of elbow pain, function, and disability. J Bone Joint Surg Am 80:154-162, 1998.

140. van der Heijden GJ, Leffers P, and Bouter LM: Shoulder disability questionnaire design and responsiveness of a functional status measure. J Clin Epidemiol 53:29-38, 2000.

141. van der Windt DA, van der Heijden GJ, de Winter AF, et al: The responsiveness of the Shoulder Disability Questionnaire. Ann Rheum Dis 57(2):82-87, 1998.

142. Viola RW, Boatright KC, Smith KL, et al: Do shoulder patients insured by workers' compensation present with worse self-assessed function and health status? J Shoulder Elbow Surg 9:368-372, 2000.

143. Waddell G, McCulloch JA, Kummel E, et al: Non-organic physical signs in low back pain. Spine 5:117-125, 1980.

144. Ware JE: Methodological considerations in the selection of health status assessment procedures. In Wenger NK, et al (eds): Assessment of Quality of Life in Clinical Trials of Cardiovascular Therapies. New York: Le Jac, 1984, pp 87-111.

145. Ware JE, Johnston SA, Davies-Avery A, et al: Conceptualization and measurement of health for adults in the Health Insurance Study. Vol III. Mental Health. Santa Monica, CA: Rand Corp, 1979.

146. Ware JE and Sherbourne CD: The MOS 36 item short-form health survey (SF-36). I. Conceptual framework and item selection. Med Care 30:473-481, 1992.

147. Ware JE, Sherbourne CD, and Davies AR: Developing and testing the MOS 20-item short-form health survey: A general population application. In Stewart AL and Ware JE (eds): Measuring Function and Well-Being: The Medical Outcomes Study Approach. Durham, NC: Duke University Press, 1992, pp 277-290.

148. Ware JE Jr, Snow KK, Kosinski M, et al: SF-36 Health Survey, Manual and Interpretation Guide. Boston: The Health Institute, New England Medical Center, 1993.

149. Weinstein MC and Stason WB: Hypertension: A Policy Perspective. Cambridge, MA: Harvard University Press, 1976.

150. Wennberg JE, Freeman JL, and Culp WJ: Are hospital services rationed in New Haven or over-utilised in Boston? Lancet 1:1185-1188, 1987.

151. Wennberg J and Gittelsohn A: Small area variations in health care delivery. Science 182:1102-1108, 1973.

152. Wennberg JE and Gittelsohn A: Variations in medical care among small areas. Sci Am 246:120-134, 1987.

153. Williams A: Setting priorities in health care: An economist's view. J Bone Joint Surg Br 73:365-367, 1991.

154. Williams GN, Gangel TJ, Arciero RA, et al: Comparison of the Single Assessment Numeric Evaluation method and two shoulder rating scales. Outcomes measures after shoulder surgery. Am J Sports Med 27:214-221, 1999.

155. Wiltsie LL and Rocchio PD: Preoperative psychological tests as predictors of success of chemonucleolysis in the treatment of the low back syndrome. J Bone Joint Surg Am 57:478-484, 1975.

156. Wolf JM and Green A: Influence of comorbidity on self-assessment instrument scores of patients with idiopathic adhesive capsulitis. J Bone Joint Surg Am 84:1167-1173, 2002.

INDEX

Note: Page numbers followed by f indicate figures; those followed by t indicate tables.

Scapulothoracic bursitis, 442-443, 443f, 444f
  arthroscopic management of, 315
  crepitus in, 442
  treatment of, 451
  vs. rotator cuff tear, 833
Scapulothoracic bursoscopy, arthroscopic,
  346-347
Scapulothoracic crepitus, 180-181, 442-443,
  443f, 444f
  treatment of, 451
Scapulothoracic dislocation, in children, 1344,
  1346, 1348
Scapulothoracic dissociation, 440-441, 441f
  in children, 1344, 1348
  treatment of, 450-451
  with acromioclavicular injury, 578, 579f
Scapulothoracic fusion, for long thoracic
  nerve injury, 1016
Scapulothoracic joint
  arthroscopic examination of, 289, 289f
  contribution of to shoulder motion, 157-
    158, 158f, 232-234, 233f, 234f
  glenohumeral motion and, 157-158, 158f,
    232-234, 233f, 234f
  motion of, 38, 237, 237f
    after arthrodesis, 237
  with frozen shoulder, 237
Scapulothoracic motion interface (STMI),
  1124, 1126, 1129-1130, 1130f
Scarecrow test, 884f, 956
Scars, hypertrophic, 1321
Scholasticism, 34, 37-38
Scoliosis
  in amputees, 1276
  Sprengel's deformity and, 118-120, 119t
Screw displacement axis (SDA), 229-230, 231f,
  235, 236f
Screw fixation. *See also specific fractures and
  techniques.*
  complications of, in anterior shoulder
    repair, 736f, 737f, 741-742, 741f
Seat belt fractures, 468, 469f
  nonunion of, 481
Sedation, preoperative, 276
Seizures
  humeral fractures in, 358, 363
  posterior glenohumeral dislocation in,
    688, 689f
  scapular fractures in, 438
Self-assessment instruments. *See also
  Outcomes research.*
  in arthritis, 895, 897-899, 899t
  in arthroplasty outcomes measurement,
    981, 982t, 983f
Semi-sitting position, 276-277, 277f
Semitendinous graft, in sternoclavicular
  reconstruction, 624, 624f
Sensory testing, 167
Sepsis. *See* Infection; Osteomyelitis; Septic
  arthritis.
Septic arthritis, 912, 1233-1253. *See also
  Infection.*
  acromioclavicular, 586, 1239, 1242
  after arthroplasty, 1234f, 1243, 1249-1251,
    1250f-1252f
  anatomic aspects of, 82, 1234-1237, 1235f,
    1236f
  bacterial attachment in, 1240-1241, 1240f,
    1241f
  bacterial pathogens in, 1238-1239, 1238f,
    1241-1242
  bursal infection and, 1235
  cell biology and, 1234-1237, 1235f, 1236f
  classification of, 1237, 1237t

Septic arthritis (*Continued*)
  complications of, 1246
  differential diagnosis of, 1243
  etiology of, 1237
  fungal, 1241
  gonococcal, 1242, 1247
  hematogenous spread of, 1237
  historical perspective on, 1233-1234, 1233-
    1254
  imaging in, 1242, 1244-1245, 1244f-1246f
  in neonatal brachial plexus injury, 1358
  in rheumatoid arthritis, 1243
  incidence of, 1239, 1239t
  involved joints in, 1239t
  laboratory evaluation in, 1243-1245
  microbial adhesion in, 1240-1241, 1240f,
    1241f
  natural history of, 1238, 1238f
  outcome of, 1247
  pathogenesis of, 1238-1239
  resectional arthroplasty in, 919
  routes of infection in, 1234-1235, 1235f
  signs and symptoms of, 1242-1243
  spontaneous, 1239
  sternoclavicular, 608-609, 609f, 610f, 627,
    1239, 1242
    treatment of, 627, 643
  synovial fluid analysis in, 1243-1244, 1244t
  treatment of, 1246-1249, 1249t
    antibiotics for, 1246-1249, 1249t, 1253
    arthroscopic, 313, 314, 1246, 1251-1253
    author's method of, 1251-1253
    surgical, 1246-1249, 1251-1253, 1251f
  tubercular, 1242, 1245f
    shoulder stiffness in, 1135
    vs. tumor, 1213
  viral, 1243
  vs. tumor, 1212-1213
  Serendipity view, 208, 208f, 209f
    of sternoclavicular joint, 613-614, 614f
Serratus anterior muscle
  action of, 54
  anatomy of, 54-55, 55f, 1015
  dysfunction of, 54
    in long thoracic nerve injury, 1015-
      1017, 1016
    scapular winging in, 153, 154f
  evaluation of, 167t
  evolutionary development of, 5
  exercise for, 1287, 1287f
  function of, 258-259, 1287
    in arm elevation, 258-259
    in shoulder stability, 258-259, 1287
    in swimmers, 1282, 1284f
    in throwing athletes, 1279, 1280f, 1287
  innervation of, 54-55, 1015
  relative to scapula, 43f, 45, 49, 49f
Serratus anterior space, arthroscopic
  examination of, 289, 289f
Sever release, for brachial plexus palsy, 1359
Shock, electrical
  humeral fractures due to, 358, 363
  posterior glenohumeral dislocation due to,
    688, 689f
  scapular fractures due to, 438
Short form 36 (SF-36), 825, 826f, 1406, 1407t-
  1408t, 1408f-1409f, 1410, 1411f, 1413f
  after full-thickness rotator cuff tear repair,
    864, 864f
  before and after arthroplasty, 981, 982t
  in arthritis, 895, 897, 899, 899t
  in cost-effectiveness evaluation, 1413,
    1414f
  in shoulder stiffness, 1147

Short thoracic nerve, 55
Shoulder. *See also constituent parts.*
  anatomy of, 666f
    comparative, 1-5, 2f-4f, 1068-1069,
      1069f
    gross, 33-91
    historical perspective on, 33-38, 35f-
      37f
    variational, 97-115
  development of
    evolutionary, 1-5, 2f-4f
    postnatal, 11-12, 12f, 13f
    prenatal
      in embryologic period, 5-9, 6f-9f
      in fetal period, 9-11, 10f, 11f
  dislocation of. *See* Glenohumeral
    dislocation; Glenohumeral
    instability.
  division of motion in, 38. *See also
    Shoulder motion.*
  elevation of. *See* Arm elevation.
  embryology of, 5-11, 6f-10f
  flail, as treatment option, 1221
  floating, 434, 435f, 473
  Little League, 1309, 1309f, 1313
  motion of. *See* Shoulder motion.
  ossification of
    postnatal, 11-12
    prenatal, 6, 7, 9, 11
  poise of, maintenance of, 599, 600f, 1326,
    1326f
  stiffness in. *See* Stiffness.
Shoulder arthrodesis. *See* Arthrodesis.
Shoulder arthroplasty. *See* Arthroplasty.
Shoulder assessment instruments, 1390-1405.
  See also Outcomes research.
Shoulder capsule
  anatomy of, 15-16, 22, 22f
  histology of, 22, 22f
Shoulder compartments, 82-83, 1190-1192,
  1191f
  compression syndromes and, 82. *See also
    Compression syndromes.*
  infection in, 82
  regional anesthesia, 82-83
  tumor, 82, 1190
Shoulder contracture release, for brachial
  plexus palsy, 1358-1360
Shoulder disarticulation, 1257, 1260-1262,
  1261f. *See also* Amputation(s).
Shoulder dystocia. *See* Birth trauma.
Shoulder function tests, in rotator cuff tear,
  825, 826f
Shoulder fusion. *See* Arthrodesis.
Shoulder hiking, in throwing athletes, 1287
Shoulder instability. *See* Glenohumeral
  dislocation; Glenohumeral instability;
  Glenohumeral subluxation.
Shoulder motion, 38
  acromioclavicular joint in, 223-227, 225f,
    226f
  adipose tissue in, 83f-87f, 84-85
  articular distribution of, 38, 157-158,
    158f
  articular surface and orientation in, 232,
    232f
  bursae in, 86-87, 87f
  center of rotation in, 235
  clavicle in, 225-226, 226f, 459f, 460
  clinical relevance of, 235-238, 262-263
  Codman's paradox and, 227-228, 228f, 230
  constraints on, 238-254. *See also* Shoulder
    stability.
  description of, 229-230